The Art and Science of
Assisted Reproductive Technology

The Art and Science of
Assisted Reproductive Technology

Editor

Sunita R Tandulwadkar
MD FICS FICOG
Chief
Ruby Hall IVF and Endoscopy Center
Head
Department of Obstetrics and Gynecology
Ruby Hall Clinic
Pune, Maharashtra, India

Forewords

Bomi Bhote
Togas Tulandi
Prakash Trivedi

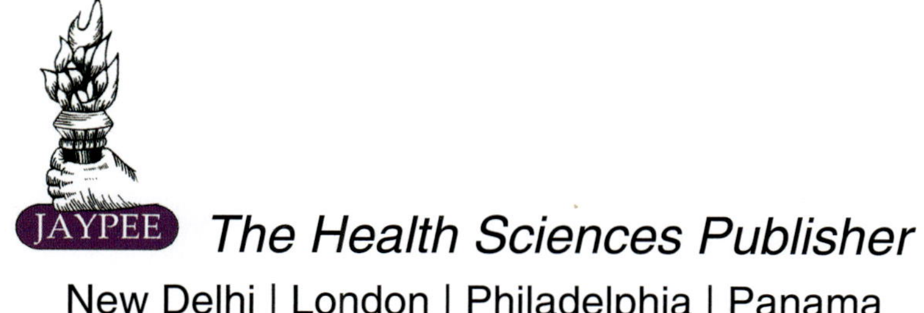

The Health Sciences Publisher

New Delhi | London | Philadelphia | Panama

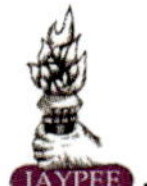 **Jaypee Brothers Medical Publishers (P) Ltd.**

Headquarters
Jaypee Brothers Medical Publishers (P) Ltd.
4838/24, Ansari Road, Daryaganj
New Delhi 110 002, India
Phone: +91-11-43574357
Fax: +91-11-43574314
E-mail: jaypee@jaypeebrothers.com

Overseas Offices

J.P. Medical Ltd.
83, Victoria Street, London
SW1H 0HW (UK)
Phone: +44-20 3170 8910
Fax: +44 (0)20 3008 6180
E-mail: info@jpmedpub.com

Jaypee-Highlights Medical Publishers Inc.
City of Knowledge, Bld. 237, Clayton
Panama City, Panama
Phone: +1 507-301-0496
Fax: +1 507-301-0499
E-mail: cservice@jphmedical.com

Jaypee Medical Inc.
The Bourse
111, South Independence Mall East
Suite 835, Philadelphia, PA 19106, USA
Phone: +1 267-519-9789
E-mail: jpmed.us@gmail.com

Jaypee Brothers Medical Publishers (P) Ltd.
17/1-B, Babar Road, Block-B
Shaymali, Mohammadpur
Dhaka-1207, Bangladesh
Mobile: +08801912003485
E-mail: jaypeedhaka@gmail.com

Jaypee Brothers Medical Publishers (P) Ltd.
Bhotahity, Kathmandu, Nepal
Phone: +977-9741283608
E-mail: kathmandu@jaypeebrothers.com

Website: www.jaypeebrothers.com
Website: www.jaypeedigital.com

The Art and Science of Assisted Reproductive Technology

First Edition: **2015**

ISBN: 978-93-5152-475-5

Printed at Ajanta Offset & Packagings Ltd., New Delhi

Dedicated to

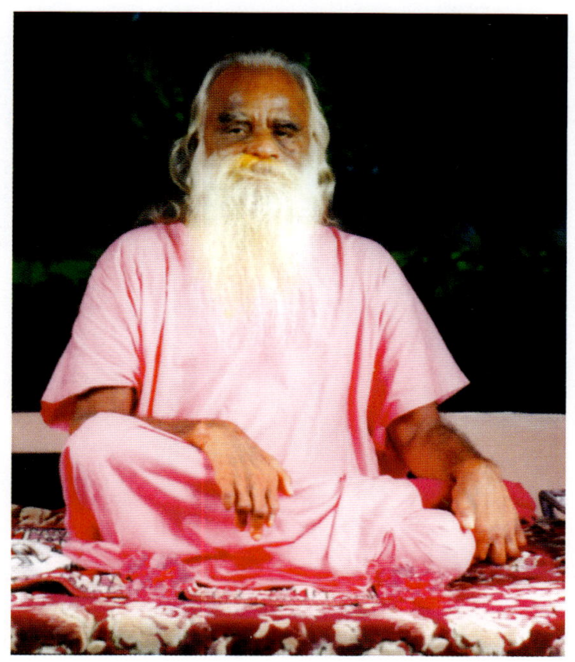

My Guru
Param Pujya Swami Shree Gagangiri Maharaj

गुरूः ब्रह्मः गुरुः विष्णुः गुरुः देवमहेश्वरः ।
गुरुः साक्षात् परं ब्रह्मः तस्मै श्रीगुरुवे नमः ॥

Guru Brahma Guru Vishnu Guru Devo Maheshwaraha |
Guru Saakshat Para Brahma Tasmai Sree Gurave Namaha ||

Contributors

Abha Majumdar
Director
Centre of IVF and Human Reproduction
Department of Obstetrics and Gynecology
Sir Ganga Ram Hospital
New Delhi, India

Alain Chanson
Center of Reproductive Medicine
Lausanne, Switzerland

Alfred Senn
Center of Reproductive Medicine
Lausanne, Switzerland

Anupama Singh
Fellow in Reproductive Medicine
Ruby Hall IVF and Endoscopy Center
Ruby Hall Clinic
Pune, Maharashtra, India

Arveen Vohra
Cosultant
Reproductive Medicine
Bengaluru, Karnataka, India

Ashok Agarwal
Director
Andrology Center and
Center for Reproductive Medicine
Cleveland Clinic
Ohio, USA

Ashwini S
Fellow in Reproductive Medicine
Gunasheela Fertility Center
Bengaluru, Karnataka, India

Bhavana Mittal
Infertility and IVF Specialist
Pushpanjali Institute of IVF and Infertility
Shivam Surgical and Maternity Center
New Delhi, India

Bina Vasan
Manipal Hospital
Bengaluru, Karnataka, India

Bindu Chimote
Vaunshdhara Clinic
Nagpur, Maharashtra, India

Capalbo A
Center for Reproductive Medicine
Clinica Valle Giulia
Rome, Italy

Chaitanya Nagori
Director
Dr Nagori's Institute for infertility and IVF
Ahmedabad, Gujarat, India

Chaithra SK
Fellow in Reproductive Medicine
Ruby Hall IVF and Endoscopy Centre
Ruby Hall Clinic
Pune, Maharashtra, India

Chauhan Kumudini
Associate Consultant Infertility Unit
Department of Obstetrics and Gynecology
Sir Ganga Ram Kolmet Hospital
New Delhi, India

Christophe Blockeel
Center for Reproductive Medicine
Universitair Ziekenhuis Brussel
Vrije Universiteit Brussel (VUB)
Laarbeeklaan, Brussels, Belgium

Cimadomo D
GENERA Center for Reproductive Medicine
Clinica Valle Giulia
Rome, Italy

Daniel R Franken
Department of Obstetrics and Gynecology
Faculty of Health Science
University of Stellenbosch and Tyberberg Hospital
Cape Town, South Africa

Devika Chopra
Fellow in Reproductive Medicine
Ruby Hall IVF and Endoscopy Centre
Ruby Hall Clinic
Pune, Maharashtra, India

Devika Gunasheela
Managing Director
Gunasheela Fertility Center
Bengaluru, Karnataka, India

Dominic Stoop
Center for Reproductive Medicine
Dutch Speaking Free University of Brussels
Brussels, Belgium

Engie Al Salman
Department of Obstetrics and Gynecology
Faculty of Medicine
University of Alexandria
Egypt

Fabien Murisier
Center of Reproductive Medicine
Lausanne, Switzerland

Fessy Louis T
CIMAR Fertility center
Cochin, Kerala, India

Françoise Urner
Center of Reproductive Medicine
Lausanne, Switzerland

Giulia Brigante
Department of Biomedical
Metabolic and Neural Sciences
University of Modena and
Reggio Emilia and Azienda USL of Modena
Via Giardini, Modena, Italy

Hrishikesh Pai
Consultant
Gynaecologist and IVF Specialist
Bloom IVF Center
Lilavati Hospital
Mumbai, Maharashtra, India

Ian Cooke
Academic Unit of Reproductive and
Developmental Medicine
Sheffield, UK

Israel Ortega
IVI-Madrid
Rey Juan Carlos University
Madrid, Spain

Jaideep Malhotra
Director
Rainbow Hospitals
Agra, Uttar Pradesh, India

Jana AlShalati
Department of Obstetrics and Gynecology
McGill University
Montreal, Quebec, Canada

Juan A García-Velasco
IVI-Madrid
Rey Juan Carlos University
Madrid, Spain

Jure Knez
Department of Reproductive Medicine
University Medical Centre
Maribor, Slovenia

Jyothi Patil
Fellow in Reproductive Medicine
Gunasheela Fertility Centre
Bengaluru, Karnataka, India

Kamala Selvaraj
GG Hospital
Chennai, Tamil Nadu, India

Kamini A Rao
Chief Consultant
Department of Reproductive Medicine
Bengaluru, Karnataka, India

Madhuri Patil
Dr Patil's Endoscopy and Fertility Center
Bengaluru, Karnataka, India

Manuela Simoni
Department of Biomedical, Metabolic and Neural Sciences
University of Modena and Reggio Emilia and
Azienda USL of Modena
Via Giardini 1355-Modena, Italy

Marc Germond
Center of Reproductive Medicine
Lausanne, Switzerland

Meenakshi Dua
Southend Fertility and
IVF Centres
Delhi NCR, India

Nalini Mahajan
Clinical Director
NOVA IVI Fertility
New Delhi, India

Nandan Roongta
Consultant
Gynaecologist and IVF Specialist
Bloom IVF Center
Lilavati Hospital
Mumbai, Maharashtra, India

Nandita Palshetkar
Consultant
Gynaecologist and IVF Specialist
Bloom IVF Center
Lilavati Hospital
Mumbai, Maharashtra, India

Narendra Malhotra
Director
Rainbow Hospitals
Agra, Uttar Pradesh, India

Natachandra Chimote
Director
Vaunshdhara Clinic
Nagpur, Maharashtra, India

Nayana Patel
Akanksha IVF Clinic
Anand, Gujarat, India

Neena Malhotra
Professor
ART Center
Department of Obstetrics and Gynecology
All India Institute of Medical Sciences
New Delhi, India

Nirzari Mangeshikar
DNB OBGY Student (Final Year)
Ruby Hall IVF and Endoscopy Center
Ruby Hall Clinic
Pune, Maharashtra, India

Nishad Chimote
Vaunshdhara Clinic
Nagpur, Maharashtra, India

Padma Rekha Jirge
IVF Specialist
Shreyas Hospital
Kolhapur, Maharashtra, India

Pankaj Kaingade
Akanksha IVF Clinic
Anand, Gujarat, India

Parinaaz Parhar
Fellow in Reproductive Medicine
Ruby Hall IVF and Endoscopy Centre
Ruby Hall Clinic
Pune, Maharashtra, India

Partha Guha Roy
Senior Clinical Consultant
Fertility Clinic and IVF Center
Mumbai, Maharashtra, India

Parul Arora
Rainbow Hospitals
Agra, Uttar Pradesh, India

Pooja Lodha
Lead Consultant
Department of Fetal Medicine
Ruby Hall Clinic
Pune, Maharashtra, India

Pratap Kumar
Department of Obstetrics and Gynecology
Kasturba Medical College
Manipal University
Manipal, Karnataka, India

Prathiba G
Department of Obstetrics and Gynecology
Gunasheela Fertility Center
Bengaluru, Karnataka, India

Priya Bhave Chittawar
Reproductive Endocrinologist
Fertility Specialist
Gynecological Endoscopic Surgeon
Bhopal, Madhya Pradesh, India

Rajvi H Mehta
Director
Trivector Embryology Support Academy
Bengaluru, Karnataka, India

Ranjana Mangoli
Fertility Clinic and IVF Center
Mumbai, Maharashtra, India

Rienzi L
Genera Center for Reproductive Medicine
Clinica Valle Giulia
Rome, Italy

Rishma Pai
Consultant
Gynaecologist and IVF Expert
Lilavati and Jaslok Hospitals
Mumbai, Maharashtra, India

Sadhana K Desai
Founder Director
Fertility Clinic and IVF Center
Mumbai, Maharashtra, India

Sanjay Patel
Gynec-Endoscopic Surgeon
Infertility and IVF Specialist
Director,
Mayflower Women's Hospital
Ahmedabad, Gujarat, India

Sejal Naik
Rahul Hospital and Well Woman Clinic
Surat, Gujarat, India

Sejal Doshi
MD Candidate (2015)
Northeast Ohio Medical University
Ohio, USA

Sesh Kamal Sunkara
King's College, London
Division of Women's Health
United Kingdom

Sonal Panchal
Dr Nagori's Institute for Infertility and IVF
Ahmedabad, Gujarat, India

Sonal Vaidya
Chief Embryologist
Ruby Hall IVF and Endoscopy Center
Ruby Hall Clinic
Pune, Maharashtra, India

Sonia Malik
Southend Fertility and IVF Centers
Delhi NCR, India

Sunita R Tandulwadkar
Chief
Ruby Hall IVF and Endoscopy Center
Head
Department of Obstetrics and Gynecology
Ruby Hall Clinic
Pune, Maharashtra, India

Susmitha Dulipalla
Fellow in Reproductive Medicine
Ruby Hall IVF and Endoscopy Center
Ruby Hall Clinic
Pune, Maharashtra, India

Togas Tulandi
Professor
Department of Obstetrics and Gynecology, and
Milton Leong Chair in Reproductive Medicine
McGill University, Montreal, QC, Canada

Ubaldi F
Clinical Director
Genera Centre for Reproductive Medicine
Clinica Valle Giulia
Rome, Italy

Vandana Bhatia
Southend Fertility and IVF Centers
Delhi NCR, India

Vijay Mangoli
Fertility Clinic and IVF Center
Mumbai, Maharashtra, India

Yasser Orief
Department of Obstetrics and Gynecology
Faculty of Medicine
University of Alexandria, Egypt

Foreword

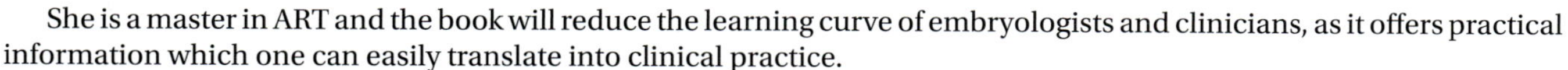

The past few decades have witnessed momentous advances in the field of assisted human reproduction and assisted reproductive technology, which has given hope to millions of women who cannot conceive after undergoing basic treatment. Thus, ART process has given hope to millions of childless couples and is an added new dimension to gynecology and obstetrics.

Assisting in creation is not only an art but also a science, because there are many procedures to be followed meticulously to achieve success. Procedures such as IVF, ICSI, IMSI, freezing of eggs and embryos and surrogacy are all a part of ART.

Dr Sunita Tandulwadkar is a successful gynecologist, and I have known her for the last twenty years. Her rapport and bond with the patients is something which I have always appreciated over the years. Her other quality of always striving for excellence is what has brought her to the pinnacle in her field.

She is a master in ART and the book will reduce the learning curve of embryologists and clinicians, as it offers practical information which one can easily translate into clinical practice.

I am very pleased to write the foreword for *The Art and Science of Assisted Reproductive Technology* which aims to highlight the ongoing future of ART.

Her knowledge and expertise along with contributions from other experts makes this a beacon and a reference book for all the people in this field.

Bomi Bhote
Chief Executive Officer
Ruby Hall Clinic
Pune, Maharashtra
India

Foreword

The most beautiful thing we can experience is the mysterious.
It is the source of all true art and science.
—Albert Einstein
(1879-1955)

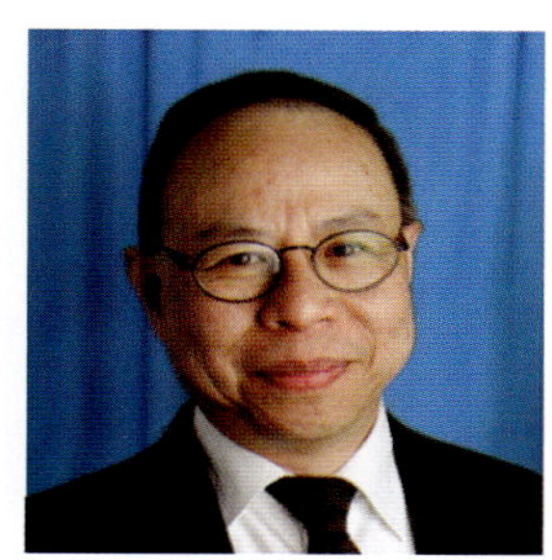

Creating life in the test tube is not a mystery anymore, it has become a reality. Indeed, advances in assisted reproductive technology have revolutionized the science and the treatment of infertility. It has increased our understanding about oocyte development, fertilization, gamete development and gamete cryopreservation. The contents of *The Art and Science of Assisted Reproductive Technology* are comprehensive. As the title indicates, Dr Sunita Tandulwadkar has combined art and science in producing the book. It covers different aspects of reproduction including laboratory aspect of infertility, medical and surgical treatments, gamete manipulation, the use of gamete donation and the obstetrical outcome. This is a complete text for infertility and reproduction that serves the clinicians, scientists and the trainees. It is a good addition to the medical literature.

Togas Tulandi MD MHCM
Professor
Department of Obstetrics and Gynecology, and
Milton Leong Chair in Reproductive Medicine
McGill University
Montreal, QC, Canada

Foreword

During the last 2-3 decades, the field of assisted reproductive technologies have surged with many peaks. Many pioneers and successful ART consultants reached a point of saturation; their growth though high came to a plateau.

Being in the field of endoscopy and ART for more than two decades, I have seen a few specialists to have maintained enthusiasm, passion to learn and excel.

Their spirits have never died in spite of scientific and professional success. One such person is Dr Sunita Tandulwadkar, a woman with a broad and long-term vision. It is my privilege to write the foreword of such an exceptional talent from India, having this aptly titled book *The Art and Science of Assisted Reproductive Technology*.

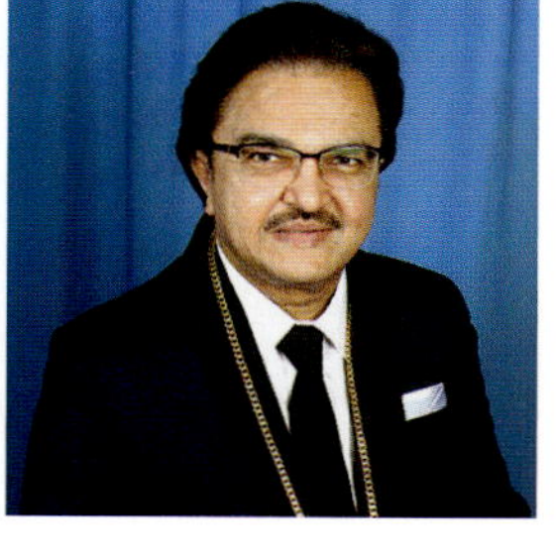

The book with national and international experts covers all aspects; whether from the laboratory, research clinical and technologies of the future.

I, as both President of the Federation of Obstetric and Gynaecological Societies of India (FOGSI) and Indian Association of Gynaecological Endoscopists (IAGE) and actively involved with ART-ISAR, appreciate her great work. The contributing experts are handpicked.

The book is a wealth for both experts and amateurs in the field of ART.

Long live the fire, passion, interest and expertise of Sunita to learn and share.

Prakash Trivedi
President FOGSI 2015
President IAGE 2013-2015

Preface

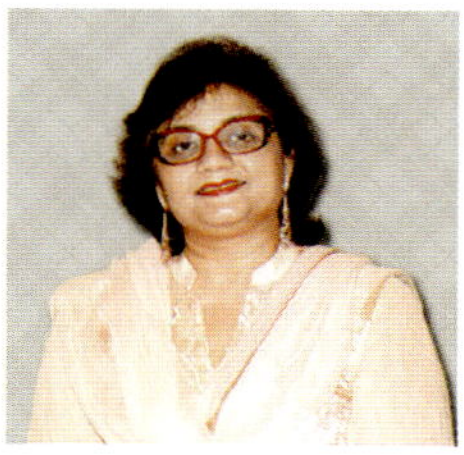

It is remarkable to see how ART as a specialty has matured and established itself over the years since the birth of the world's first IVF baby Louise Brown in the UK in 1978.

Infertility affects 10 to 15% of couples in the current scenario owing to various causes. Whatever be the reason, it is clear that more and more couples are seeking help about their fertility issues. With this backdrop, there is an increased needs for all of us to be more thorough with our knowledge of infertility and come up with sound economical and effective solutions.

This book has been motivated by the desire, we had to further the evolution of understanding of human reproduction and ART. The book presents research-based best practices related to ART aiming to specifically provide a sound basis for evaluation and treatment of infertile couples. It has brought together experts from the field of ART across the globe to provide their valuable inputs on the subject.

I have made sincere efforts to focus on issues starting from basics in infertility to the emerging issues, such as third party reproduction, especially in the Indian scenario, outcomes of children conceived through the ART as well as laboratory aspects of ART.

I am dedicating the book to the readers and hoping that they find it immensely useful and imparts extra confidence in handling the many demands in the field. We also look forward to feedbacks and inputs from all which will help us improve further.

Sincerely thanking to all my team members and the esteemed contributors without whose efforts the book would have not been the same. My special thanks to Dr Nirzari Mangeshikar who has worked with me tirelessly for more than 12 months to complete the book. I really appreciate her efforts. Thanks to Dr Pooja Lodha, Dr Parinaaz Parhar, Dr Anupama Singh and Dr Chaithra SK who have helped for proofreading apart from contributing to chapters. My heartfelt thanks to my husband Dr Rajesh Tandulwadkar and my son Rishi for their constant, unwavering support and encouragement as well as criticism which as given the book its current shape.

I am heartily thankful to Shri Jitendar P Vij (Group Chairman), Mr Ankit Vij (Group President), Mr Tarun Duneja (Director-Publishing), Mr KK Raman (Production Manager), Mr Sunil Kumar Dogra (Production Executive), Mr Neelambar Pant (Production Coordinator), Mr Sabarish Menon (Commissioning Editor—Mumbai Branch), Mr Quaisher Hossain (Medical Editor), Mr Girish Pandey (Typesetter), Mr Rohan (Graphic Designer), and Mr Himanshu Sharma (Proofreader) of M/s Jaypee Brothers Medical Publishers (P) Ltd, New Delhi, India, and their highly professional publishing team to work in such a professional manner. Thanks to their editorial efforts to improve the book overall.

Furthermore, the outlook for the future looks stunning including novel technologies that may facilitate quantum advances in the clinic and laboratory and we hope to be a part of this movement.

Sunita R Tandulwadkar

Contents

Section 4 Endocrinology and Stimulation Protocols

Section 8 Culture of Embryos and Transfer

Section 9 Implantation

Section 10   Cryopreservation

Section 14   Pregnancy and ART

Section 15   Complications in ART

Setting-up an ART Laboratory

1 — How to Set-up an ART Laboratory?

Sunita R Tandulwadkar, Devika Chopra

INTRODUCTION

The journey of a successful in vitro fertilization (IVF) program starts from the clinician's office, goes through the assisted reproductive technology (ART) laboratory and ends in a successful delivery at the hospital. What most people fail to recognize is that the heart of a successful IVF or intracytoplasmic sperm injection (ICSI) cycle lies in the laboratory. The laboratory is the place where the semen is analyzed, oocytes are assessed after retrieval and finally, where embryos are formed and cryopreserved. A well-equipped and organized laboratory is what separates an excellent IVF fertility center from an average one.

Many aspects need to be looked into before setting-up an ART laboratory. The location, construction, the equipment and ventilation are a few important parameters that need to be kept in mind while implementing a successful ART program. This chapter has highlighted the important steps that need to be taken whilst starting an ART laboratory.

LOCATION OF THE ART LABORATORY

The location of the ART laboratory with respect to the ART unit as well as the local area in which the ART unit is placed may play an important role in the success rates of that particular ART unit. The locality of the ART unit should be in a low-traffic, secure area, which is easily accessible.[1] It should be reviewed whether the building site or nearby area is scheduled to undergo construction or renovation. This is of particular importance as activity related to any type of demolition; construction or renovation will adversely affect laboratory results. Air in urban areas may contain high levels of pollutants such as carbon monoxide, nitrous oxide, sulfur dioxide and heavy metals. This may affect the ambient atmosphere within the laboratory. The importance of air handling units is discussed elsewhere in this chapter.

The laboratory should be physically isolated. It should be in proximity to the procedure room where oocyte retrieval, embryo transfer and microsurgical epididymal sperm aspiration (TESA)/percutaneous epididymal sperm aspiration (PESA) is performed. The IVF unit should be a no-smoking zone. The use of cosmetics and strong fragrances by laboratory staff should be monitored and controlled.

CONSTRUCTION MATERIALS

Construction materials including internal finishes, doors, air vents, floor and ceiling elements should be selected based on their durability and maintenance requirements. All surfaces should be made of smooth, impervious and non-shedding materials that offer no surface roughness or porosity which might allow retention of particulate matter or the development of microbiological contamination.

Paints, adhesives, glues and sealants may be implicated for releasing VOCs like alkanes, aromatics, alcohol, aldehyde and ketones, etc. Therefore, wall surfaces are covered with low-VOC water-based paint with acrylic, vinyl acrylic or acrylic latex polymers. Interior paint should not contain formaldehyde, acetaldehyde, isocyanates, reactive amines and phenols. Emission testing of paints should be done.[2] Stainless steel and anodized aluminum can be used in doors as well as in workstations. Water-based low-VOC adhesives can be used when needed.

Indoors; construction materials such as MDF, PVC flooring, paints and adhesives constitute the major source of Volatile Organic Compounds (VOCs) leading to the phenomenon called "sick building syndrome". Other sources of indoor chemical hazards are cleaning fluids, floor waxes, cosmetics and cigarette smoke.

CONSTRUCTION DESIGN

The embryology laboratory should have adequate space for:

- Aseptic and optimal handling of gametes and embryos.
- Storage areas and equipment such as incubators, centrifuges and cryo equipment—logical planning for efficiency and safety within each working area.
- Record keeping, data entry, and related administrative functions. Computer equipment should be available for data collection compliance.
- A general wet area in which washing of equipment, sterilization, etc. is performed should be separate from the embryology laboratory. Moreover, if fixatives are applied, a fume-hood will be required for handling of gametes and embryos.[3]

When designing a laboratory, recent developments in equipment and facilities should be considered. Work-benches should have a height which permits to work comfortably. Ducts and equipment must be laid out in such a way that repair work when needed can be performed outside the laboratory, without disturbing its functionality. Incubators, laminar flow units and micromanipulation work station should be placed in such a way that an embryologist should be able to finish one complete procedure without moving more than 3 meters in any direction. Air inlets and outlets should be carefully spaced for prevention of changes in local temperature. Micromanipulation work stations and laminar flow hoods should not be placed too close to air supply fixtures that it impacts on sterility or temperature.[4]

Burning In

At the end of the construction, there should be a 3-month waiting period before first occupation of the new facilities. During this period, the temperature is increased by 10–20°C and the air-handling ventilation unit should be set up to continuously bring in fresh air. After this period, testing should be carried out for particulate matter and microbes.

CONFIGURATION OF THE AIR-HANDLING VENTILATION AND FILTRATION SYSTEM

It has been suggested that control of VOC levels within the ambient air is critical for successful conception in vitro.[5] Outside air, which is relatively VOC free, may in fact be a cleaner source than inside air, since each of the fixed and transient laboratory components used may produce gaseous emissions. Air handling systems should probably be designed with these findings in mind **(Fig. 1)**.[6]

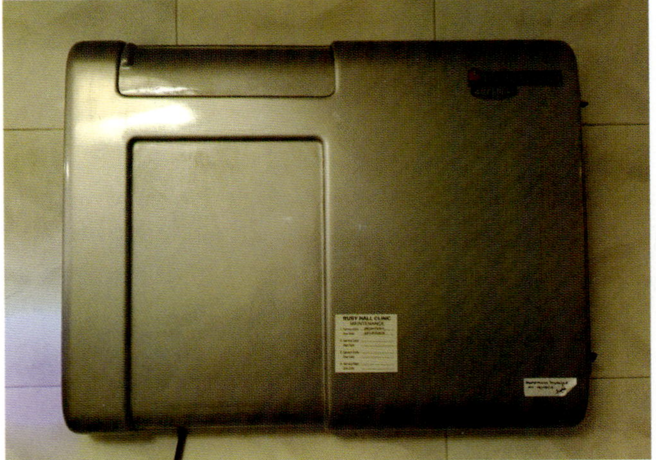

Fig. 1 Air-handling system

There is an association between the presence of air contaminants in the IVF laboratory and impairment of embryonic development.[7] Controlling air quality in an ART laboratory has shown beneficial effects regarding fertilization and embryo development.[8] Therefore IVF laboratories are equipped with various filters. The outside air brought into the unit is first filtered with activated carbon, which removes various hydrocarbons, and then high-efficiency particulate absorption (HEPA) removes the particulate materials (0.3 microns).[6] The purified air should be supplied to positively pressured room (0.10–0.20 inches of water) that uses around 7–15 fresh air changes per hour (FACH). A room with positive pressure has higher air volume entering than exiting the room. As a result, it is difficult for unpurified air to enter the room from the surrounding areas. However air entry cannot be prevented when doors are opened and closed.[9] The system must be capable of supplying air with temperature of 30–35% at least 40% relative humidity.

USE OF ULTRAVIOLET LAMPS IN IN VITRO FERTILIZATION LABORATORY

Ultraviolet radiation acts as an antibacterial agent but system's effectiveness depends on air quality. Sterilized environment can only be achieved if the room in question is hermetically sealed and completely subjected to 254 nm ultraviolet radiation. The object is to reduce the number of microorganisms to a minimum. The lamps are installed between the activated carbon filter and HEPA filters.[10]

Sequential ultraviolet illumination is highly effective in eliminating or reducing fungal and bacterial contaminants. During the construction of laboratory installation of a sequential ultraviolet illuminator with the intention of decreasing circulating biological contaminants is advisable.[11]

■ LAMINAR AIR FLOW HOODS

There are two types of laminar air flow (LAF) hoods **(Fig. 2)**, vertical and horizontal flow. The main goal of the LAF hood is to protect the gametes and embryos. Laminar flow cabinets create particle-free working environments by projecting air through a filtration system and removing it across a work surface in a laminar or unidirectional air stream. They provide an excellent clean air environment for a number of laboratory requirements. Laminar flow cabinets work by the use of in-flow laminar air drawn through one or more HEPA filters, designed to create a particle-free working environment and provide product protection. Commonly, the filtration system comprises of a pre-filter and a HEPA filter. The laminar flow cabinet is enclosed on the sides and constant positive air pressure is maintained to prevent the intrusion of contaminated room air.[12,13]

■ INCUBATORS

CO_2 incubator: CO_2 incubators mimic the environmental conditions that sperm, oocytes, blastocysts and developing embryos encounter in vivo **(Figs 3A and B)**.

A minimum of two CO_2 incubators are essential in any program as a backup in case of unexpected malfunction. One is exclusively for media equilibration and another one for fertilization/embryo culture.

Triple gas incubator: Incubators with an atmosphere comprising CO_2, O_2, and N_2 provide a more natural environment than a plain CO_2 incubator, giving better embryo quality and higher success rate. Gas cylinders should be placed outside or in a separate room with an automatic backup system.

Benchtop incubator: This system places a heated surface directly above and below the culture dish **(Fig. 3C)**. The small volume of the chambers within this incubator allows rapid recovery from exposure to room air (lid opening). Temperature, humidity, and CO_2 inside of the chamber return to pre-opening levels rapidly.

■ MICROSCOPES

Oocyte pick-up, embryo handling and micromanipulation require various types of microscopes. Most of the available models of stereo zoom microscopes, transmitted light sources and inverted microscopes can be integrated into

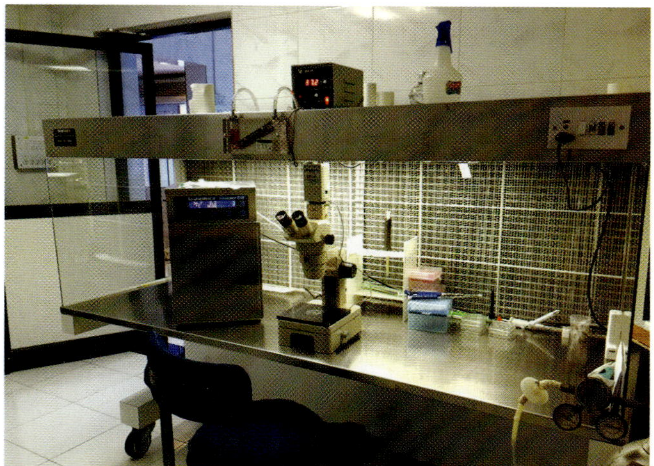

Fig. 2 Laminar air flow hood

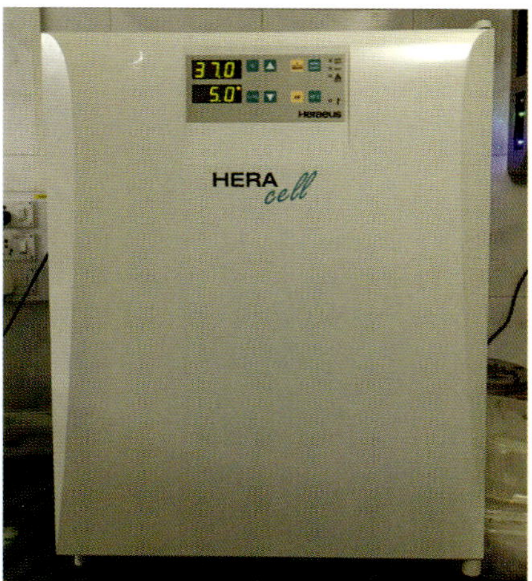

Fig. 3A CO_2 incubator

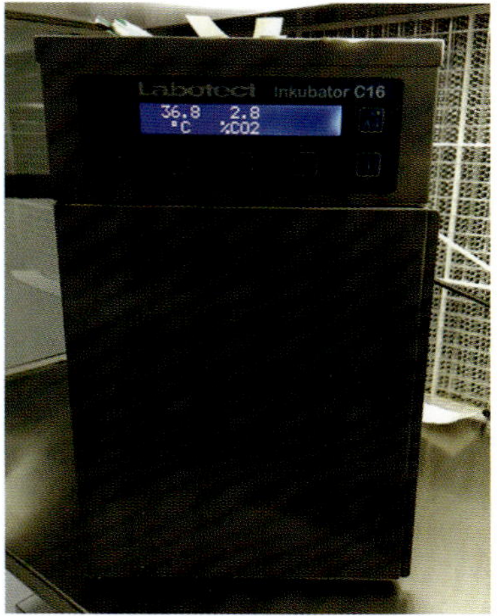

Fig. 3B CO_2 working incubator

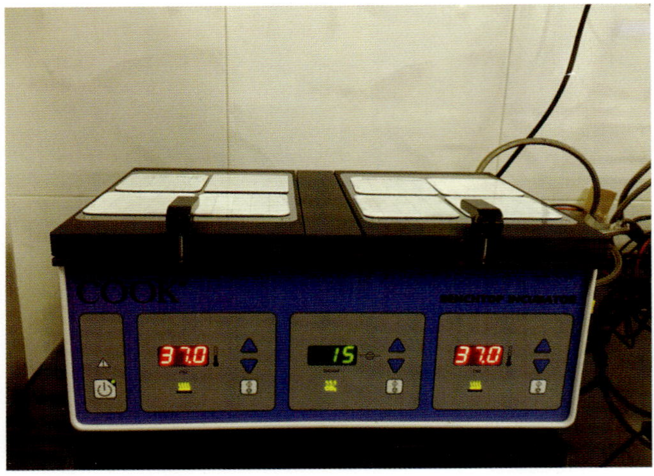

Fig. 3C CO_2 benchtop incubator

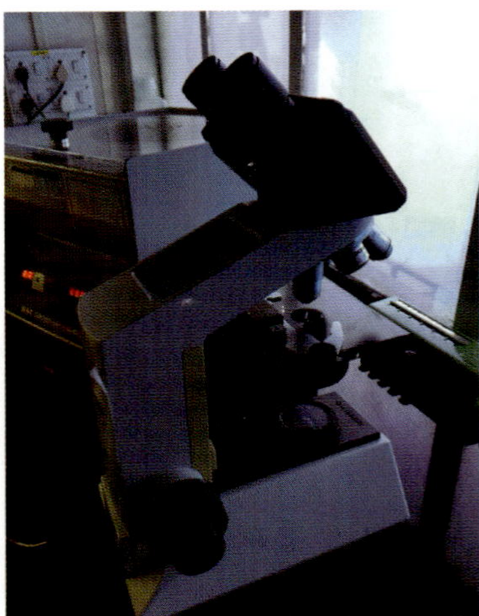

Fig. 4A Upright microscope

IVF workstations. Different types of microscopes used for various IVF applications:

- *Upright microscope* used for sperm vitality tests and oocyte collections **(Fig. 4A)**.
- *Inverted microscope* used with micromanipulator for processes such as ICSI, intracytoplasmic morphologically-selected sperm injection (IMSI) **(Fig. 4B)**. Inverted microscopes are available from Nikon, Olympus, Leica, Carl Zeiss, etc. The micromanipulators those are available in the market are Narishige, Eppendorf, Research Instruments, Cell Robotics, etc., to mention a few.
- *Stereo zoom microscopes:* Stereo zoom microscope is used in IVF laboratory for egg harvesting during ovum pick up, for insemination, embryo changes from media to media, embryo loading to embryo transfer catheter, etc. Stereo zoom microscope is usually integrated into the heated laminar flow table **(Fig. 4C)**.

CENTRIFUGES

Centrifuge machine with swing-out rotor is ideal for the sperm preparation in IVF **(Fig. 5)**. Centrifugation or vigorous mixing of open containers has a high potential for creating aerosols or droplets. Centrifuges may be placed in exhaust hoods during use or non-aerosol centrifuges may be used. Capped tubes must be used for centrifugation.[1]

LIQUID NITROGEN CANS

Liquid nitrogen dewars are essential for storage of sperm and embryos **(Fig. 6)**. Nitrogen tanks should be cleaned and sanitized at least every year. Sufficient number of

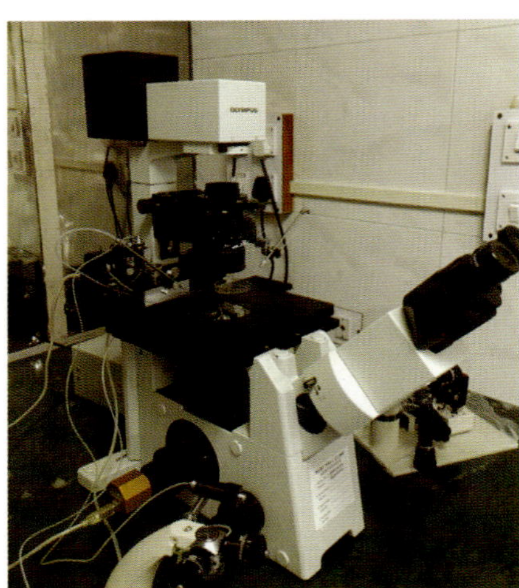

Fig. 4B Inverted microscope

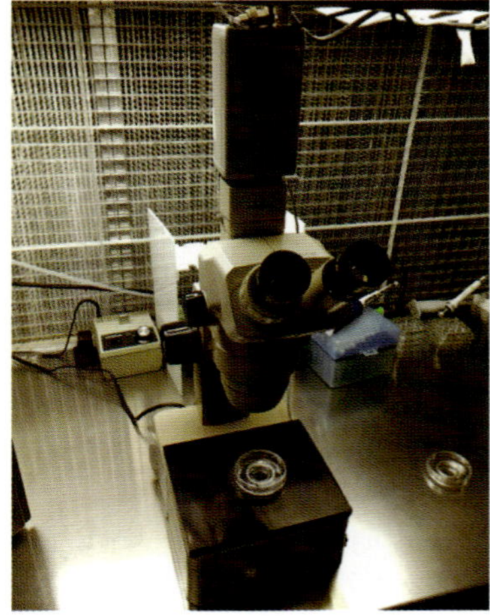

Fig. 4C Stereo zoom microscope

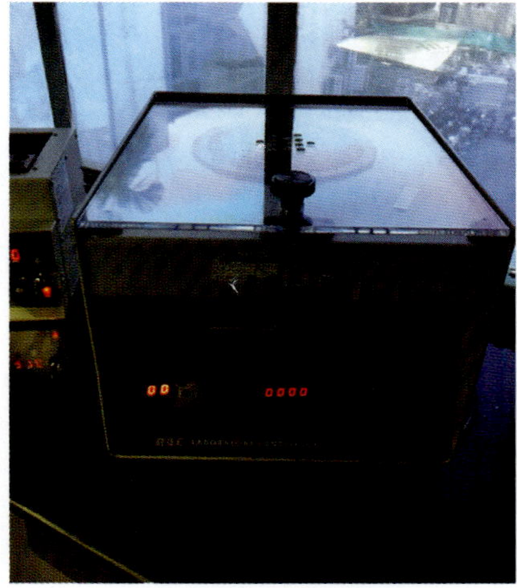

Fig. 5 Centrifuge

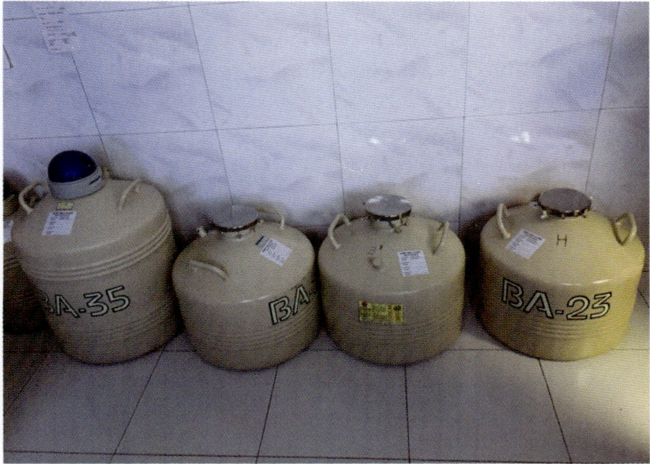

Fig. 6 Liquid nitrogen cans

dewars should be available depending on case load. The samples must be labeled clearly before placing them into the liquid nitrogen tanks. Records must be kept so that samples are easier to find. Liquid nitrogen tanks come attached with alarms that go off when the temperature in the tank reaches a critical level that is deleterious to the stored embryos and/or gametes.

■ CONCLUSION

Many factors need to be kept in mind before setting up an ART unit and laboratory. The success of any ART program depends upon the laboratory, its equipment and its upkeep. In conclusion, IVF success rates can be correlated with a well-functioning and state-of-the-art laboratory.

■ REFERENCES

1. The Practice Committee of the American Society for Reproductive Medicine and the Practice Committee of the Society for Assisted Reproductive Technology. Revised guidelines for human embryology and andrology laboratories. Fertil Steril. 2008;90(Suppl 3):S45-59.
2. Giligan A. Guidelines for material use in USA during construction of tissue culture laboratory. New Jersey: Alpha Environmental; 2006.
3. Gianaroli L, Plachot M, van Kooij R, Al-Hasani S, et al. ESHRE guidelines for good practice in IVF laboratories. Committee of the Special Interest Group on Embryology of the European Society of Human Reproduction and Embryology. Hum Reprod. 2000;15:2241-6.
4. Cohen J, Alikani M, Gilligan A, et al. Setting up an ART laboratory. In: Gardner DK, Weissman A, Howles CM, Shoham Z (Eds). Textbook of Assisted Reproductive Techniques, 4th edition. United Kingdom: Informa; 2011.
5. Mahran AM, Sharma RK, Abdel-Maguid E, et al. Evaluation of sperm chromatin damage with two routine sperm processing procedures used for assisted reproduction. Fertil Steril. 2008;76(Suppl 3):S16.
6. Cohen J, Gilligan A, Schimmel E, et al. Ambient air and its potential effects on conception in vitro. Hum Reprod. 1997;12(Suppl 8):1742-9.
7. Esteves SC, Verza Junior S, Gomes AP. Comparison between ISO type 5 and type 6 cleanrooms combined with VOC's filtration system for micromanipulation and embryo culture in severe male factor infertility. Fertil Steril. 2006;86:2.
8. Boone W, Johnson J, Locke A, et al. Control of air quality in an assisted reproductive technology laboratory. Fertil Steril. 1997;71(Suppl 1):150-4.
9. Angtrakool P. International Standard (ISO 14644). Cleanrooms and associated controlled environments. USA: Food and Drug Administration; 2001.
10. Mukherjee T, Duke M, Alan C, et al. Value of sequential ultraviolet illumination in reducing ambient fungi, bacteria, and nonviable fungal structures (NVFS) in an IVF laboratory. Fertil Steril. 2003;80(Suppl 3):289-90.
11. Khoudja YF. Better IVF outcomes following improvements in laboratory air quality. J Assist Reprod Genet. 2013;30:69-76.
12. Lee M, Grazi R, Seifer D. Incorporation of the Cook K-Minc incubator and media system into the IVF lab: the future of IVF. J Clin Embryol. 2010;13(3):21-32.
13. Esteves SC, Bento FC. Implementation of air quality control in reproductive laboratories in full compliance with the Brazilian Cells and Germinative Tissue Directive. Reproduct Bio Medicine Online. 2013;26:9-21.

2 Quality Control in an ART Laboratory

Vijay Mangoli, Ranjana Mangoli

Every time an embryologist sees an in vitro fertilization (IVF) baby, he recollects its journey from gamete collection to embryo transfer. He truly experiences what Aristotle had said, *"those who see things grow from the beginning will have the finest view of them"*. An embryologist does not just observe them grow, but create them under optimum culture conditions.

Creating a human being in laboratory is indeed a responsible task that requires technical skill and adequate knowledge about the subject. IVF laboratory is a cluster of many sections, each with a specific purpose affecting final outcome. Hence, it also demands strict quality control not only for establishment, but also on a continuous basis till the program is running. It becomes responsibility of the embryologist to establish and maintain optimum standards at all time with motto of "Zero Tolerance" for mistakes and negligence. Mistakes in IVF have the potential for very serious consequences. Therefore, we should have a holistic approach of prophylactic management for prevention of errors.

Although there is a steady rise in pregnancy rate over last two decades, still there is lot of uncertainty in IVF outcome. Many times, the embryologists are surprised not because they are not getting expected pregnancy rate but because they are confused—why all of a sudden so many patients are getting pregnant. On the other hand, sometimes they wonder, in spite of everything looking perfect, why there is a sudden drop in pregnancy rate! Though there is no magic formula available as yet which can give us consistent high pregnancy rate, there are some quality control Dos and Don'ts that can prevent pregnancy rate from falling below unacceptable level. Another important aspect to keep in mind is, there can be vast differences between two assisted reproductive technology (ART) laboratories—structure wise, material wise and technique wise. Therefore, quality indices criteria should be based on basic principles of ART.

There are two main aspects of quality management: (1) quality control and (2) quality assurance. Quality control is the standardization of all techniques, tests and procedures so that the outcome becomes reproducible and not person specific, e.g. if a laboratory director has standardized a technique of semen freezing to get more than 70% post thaw survival, the protocol should be mentioned in standard operative procedure (SOP) in such a way that anybody in the laboratory doing semen freezing should get same results.

Whereas quality assurance is more expansive term that encompasses not only quality control but involves monitoring and control of the ultimate outcome of the test or technique. In the above example, quality assurance not only confirms 70% survival, but ensures that the sample is collected, processed, stored, recorded and utilized properly.

It is practically not possible to do quality control checking of all stages on a daily basis. Therefore, such monitoring is divided in durations as daily, weekly, monthly and yearly basis. These are some practical quality control points that help us getting reproducible results.

LABORATORY PERSONNEL

To maintain a good quality control program, center should have fully trained keen interested and committed staff. Apart from sound knowledge in their respected field, they should have basic knowledge about the instruments maintenance and troubleshooting. Second very important requirement is willingness to admit and rectify the mistakes. It is not a crime to make mistake, but it is a crime to hide and try to cover them. Experience, skill and ability to handle difficult situations by laboratory staff, contribute to the success of an ART center. As there is no government-recognized training centers in India at present, the person is trained "on job". It is responsibility of the project director to have adequate staff depending upon number of cases. Overburden can cause fatigue and more seriously, irreversible mistakes like specimen misidentification. It was speculated before the era of intracytoplasmic sperm injection (ICSI) that a center performing 100 IVF cases per year should have one embryologist and two technicians. However, in today's scenario of ICSI, intracytoplasmic morphologically selected sperm injection (IMSI) and detailed data entry, the same center needs two fully trained embryologists and three technicians. Quality control in this aspect includes upgradation of knowledge to latest developments in the field and experimentation, within permissive limits, by laboratory director. All protocols and procedures of every step involved should be in written form of SOP that can be accessed easily by each laboratory person. Any change should be immediately mentioned in SOP with date of rectification so that its effect can be analyzed. Every new person joining the team should be given adequate time to get accustomed to working conditions and protocols. Considering significance of the job, the proficiency of staff to demonstrate competency can be evaluated periodically.

■ PROCEDURES

Consistent results are obtained when there is uniformity in procedures irrespective of person performing. Each procedure should be available in written form near the site of performance. All protocols should be written in simple language and stepwise manner giving details of materials, equipment, solutions and disposable required. Formulae of calculation, if any, should be mentioned simply, preferably citing examples. The laboratory director should supervise performance of juniors till it is done in the same manner that gives reproducible results. It is also his responsibility to review SOPs at least annually and upgrade if required.

Air

Ambient air is an important but often ignored part in the laboratory. Air pollution often goes unnoticed because it is invisible. **Table 1** illustrates some of the sources that can

Table 1 Common pollutants and their sources in an IVF laboratory

Pollutants	Sources
Enflurane, halothane	Anesthetic gases
Toluene, butane	Pesticides, aerosoles
Aldehydes	Paints, vinyl flooring
Freones, chloroethanes	Refrigerators, air conditioners
Ethylene oxide	Disposables
Isopropyl alcohol	Disinfectant

contribute to air pollution. Almost all these pollutants have strong affinity for water molecule and hence can easily get dissolved in culture media, changing its composition to toxic level. In an IVF laboratory, scents, perfumes or any such volatile material are strictly prohibited.

Culture room should have air purification class 10,000 maintained continuously with about 40 air changes/hour. It is necessary to maintain continuous positive pressure in one direction—from culture room to operating theater and outwards. Prefilters and high-efficiency particulate air filters should be changed regularly. Its frequency depends upon location of the center. Alcohols, acids or batteries of uninterruptible power supply (UPS) system should not be stored near culture room. Establishments like adjacent petrol pump or chemical godown will increase criteria air contaminants including volatile organic compounds in the culture room to very high level.

Instruments and Equipment

These are the backbones of an ART center. We depend a lot on them to achieve the goal of creating and maintaining viable embryos. In fact quality control of instruments itself is a separate topic if discussed in detail. The best way to deal with them is to give annual maintenance contract to respected companies and maintain a fix schedule for their servicing. But equal important is to counter check the readings displayed on the panel with standardized calibrating instruments on a daily basis—particularly temperature, CO_2 level, humidity of incubators and optics maintenance of microscopes. Generally major instruments like incubators, freezing machine, micro-manipulators are taken care of, but temperature of dry air oven, stage warmer of microscope, refrigerator, proper steam pressure of autoclave, revolutions per minute of centrifuge are generally ignored. If instruments are in perfect working conditions, then half the job is done!

Medium

The importance of media is next to the experience of the embryologist. Embryos are cultured in micro-environments and any deviation from optimum requirements immediately reflects in their growth pattern. One should understand science and logic behind its composition. If medium is made in house, it should be checked for these three parameters—physicochemical, biological and functional. Physicochemical includes pH and osmolarity. Biological control includes proper sterilization, and testing endotoxin level. Functional tests are carried out mainly to check potential of medium through sperm survival test, mouse embryo assay, and cell culture growth such as the culture of the mouse hybridoma cell line. The centers using ready-made media should confirm proper handling and temperature control during transport.

Electricity

In vitro fertilization center should have a continuous power supply. There are many delicate and sensitive instruments which are calibrated with great care. Sudden fluctuations in the electric current can change the internal settings of electronic circuit completely. They may display set values, but the actual values may vary. Installation of proper stabilizer, and spike suppressor along with a good UPS system should be part of equipment.

Disposables

It is advisable to use disposables from a reputed company. They are to be rinsed before use whenever possible, e.g. before equilibrating media, oocyte pickup (OPU), sperm preparation and transfer catheters. Minimum 10 days of proper ventilation is required for ethylene oxide treated disposables because these products are known for their property called "Off-Gassing" for few days after sterilization.

■ CULTURE ROOM

Temperature of culture room is to be balanced between ambient air and that of incubators or ICSI platform. Proper ventilation will minimize the discomfort to embryologists. In many countries, another major problem is to get consistent medical grade CO_2. One should not use industrial grade CO_2. Purity certification should be demanded form supplier. It is advantageous to keep separate cylinders for each incubator rather than giving same connection. The gas tubing and filters should be changed regularly. User manuals of all instruments should be kept in an easily accessible manner.

■ INFECTION/CONTAMINATION CONTROL

As we try to create ideal conditions for the growth of embryos in the culture room, it invites unwanted growth as well. Warm, humid atmosphere inside the incubator is good for many pathogens and even normal flora like *Escherichia coli*. Source of contamination can be materials like pens, markers, spectacles, cell phones, papers, cartons, etc. Minimum material should be stored in the culture room. At the same time, care has to be taken of main storage room, which is generally overlooked, thus carrying yeast and fungal spores directly into the culture room. Source of infections can be biological fluids like semen, follicular fluid and blood, or it can be through staff. It is responsibility of clinicians to inform laboratory staff clearly about any such known infection of husband or wife. Because generally laboratory staff does not interact with patient till they come for OPU. Maintaining sterility of incubators, good awareness and personal hygiene habits of the staff can prevent both infection and contamination from spreading to the culture room.

■ INSTRUCTIONS TO PATIENTS

This is an extremely important aspect of quality assurance which is often underestimated. It is important to tell patient not only what to do, but equally important to instruct what not to do, e.g. husband is asked to keep abstinence from sex of 3 days but not instructed to includes masturbation and night falls as well. Similarly, patient is asked to collect sample in sterile container but not instructed that if sample is spilled on the floor, not to pick it up and put it in the collection jar. Giving proper instructions is collective responsibility of clinicians, nurses, laboratory people and even administration persons.

■ RECORD KEEPING

Another mandatory requirement in the quality control procedure is to maintain proper records in detail of all methodologies adopted, materials used, and account of each egg and embryo obtained through IVF. As aim of quality control is primarily to assess performance, it becomes absolutely essential to keep records of all variables, personnel, techniques and material both in favorable and adverse situations. Analysis of such data helps us to find out cause of poor results and also factors that improves pregnancy rates. For years, data has been recorded as hard copies in registers. However, for quick access and immediate analysis, data should be backed up in electronic form. This also minimizes space required to store large data for longer duration, as may be required by local authorities. The importance of paperwork is much more than we anticipate academically, research wise, for retrospective analysis and in legal issues.

■ OTHER ASPECT OF QUALITY CONTROL

Till now we discussed one side of quality control, which can be applied to maintain and enhance pregnancy rate. Quality control in IVF has one more perspective, which is more important than getting pregnancies. And which should be considered with highest priority that is to avoid accidents while handling human genetic material. Many types of error may occur, for example, miscommunication (putting embryos into the wrong patient), technique (carryover of sperm between patients), forgetfulness (leaving dishes out of the incubator, not filling nitrogen vessels), accident (dropping dishes), forced errors (due to excessive workload, interruption, inexperience), poor checking (misprogramed machines), and so on. All of these mistakes can happen, probably more than once, but most are avoidable. One role of quality assurance is to reduce the likelihood of mistakes. Nevertheless, where human being is involved, errors and mistakes are bound to occur. Moreover, there is the, thankfully rare, additional possibility of malicious or criminal activity, which is particularly difficult to guard against.

One incident in the Netherlands in March 1993 shook the whole world when a twin of different races was born to a couple undergoing IVF treatment. Similar incidents were reported in the United Kingdom in 2009 and in the United States of America in 2011. Of course, these may be some of the incidents that came into light out of numerous that we are not aware of. In any other establishment, if a mistake is found, then the product can be withdrawn from the market, or if it is a general laboratory then the reports can be canceled and tests can be repeated. But the same rule does not apply to an IVF laboratory. Once the baby is born, or even the pregnancy is established, the issue becomes much complicated ethically, emotionally and legally. Therefore, each step in all the procedures should be performed keeping this potential risk in mind. Extreme care has to be taken while processing many semen samples, distributing many patient's eggs and embryos for insemination and growth medium, preparing ICSI plates, adding sperm to the PVP droplet, during insemination and while freezing more than one patient's embryos. Each step has to be done with full concentration.

In near future, there will be more uniformity throughout global ART centers in techniques and procedures for infertility treatments to give high pregnancy rate in terms of take-home babies. This will further narrow quality control indices that can be monitored by single internationally accredited body. Till then each center should set and follow rigorous quality control program to achieve best possible results.

■ BIBLIOGRAPHY

1. American Society for Reproductive Medicine. Revised minimum standards for in vitro fertilization, gamete intra fallopian transfer, and related procedure. Fertil Steril. 1998;53: 225-6.
2. Hall J, Gilligan A, Schimmel T, et al. The origin, effect and control of air pollution in laboratories used for human embryo culture. Hum Reprod. 1998;13(Suppl 4):146-55.
3. Jhonson MT, Gardner DK. Embryo culture in the twenty-first century. In: Gardner DK, Rizk BRMB, Falcone T, (Eds). Human Assisted Reproductive Technology: Future trends in Laboratory and Clinical Practice. Cambridge: Cambridge University Press. 2011.
4. Lane M, Mitchell M, Cashman KS, et al. To QC or not to QC: the key to a consistent laboratory. Reprod Fertil Dev. 2008;20: 23-32.
5. McCulloh DH. Quality control and quality assurance: record keeping and impact on ART performance and outcome. Infertil Reprod Med Clin North Am. 1998;9:285-309.
6. Nijs M, Franssen K, Cox A, et al. Reprotoxicity of intra uterine insemination and in vitro fertilization–embryo transfer disposables and products: a retrospective analysis of 4 year study. Fertile Steril. 2009;92:527-35.
7. Svalander P, Anderson E, Hyllner J, et al. Quality assurance methods for production of culture media and equipment essential for high success rate. In: Maximizing the Potential of Every Embryo to Minimize Multiple Embryo Transfer. Textbook for Postgraduate Course at the Meeting of American Society for Reproductive Medicine. American society for Reproductive Medicine. San Francisco, October; 1998.pp.1-15.

3 Quality Care Management in ART Clinic

Madhuri Patil

INTRODUCTION

In vitro fertilization (IVF) laboratories and fertility clinics are under constant pressure to improve quality of their services and increase the percentage of successful treatment cycle. Today newer techniques, modifications of existing ones, and new approaches characterize this specialization and all these need to pass through quality control (QC).[1]

The aim of QC is to establish standard working methods, which ensures that the established levels of quality is reached and maintained. The results must be visible and measureable in order to prove that standards are being adhered to and met. Documentation should be established, effectively implemented, reviewed, controlled and revised depending on the latest evidence.

OBJECTIVES OF QUALITY CONTROL AND ASSURANCE

Today despite improvement in the quality of medication and protocols used and the various laboratory variables, there has not been much increase in the live birth rates following infertility treatment. This makes it mandatory for all service providers in this field to adhere to internal QC programs and external quality assurance (QA) schemes to provide good service to patients to improve the success rates. Every contemporary assisted reproductive technology (ART) laboratory should implement a quality management system (QMS) to establish and maintain strict QC and QA programs. QC includes operational techniques and activities, which are carried out in order to meet the quality requirements. QC is the main goal to establishing a quality standard or specifications for each aspect of the testing procedures and determination of how close to the quality standard the testing procedure is, evaluate effectiveness of policies and procedures, identify and correct problems, assume the accuracy and precision of procedures and monitor the competency and performance of the laboratory staff and clinician.

On the other hand, QA is the total sum of all planned and systematic activities required in order to establish sufficient trust that a product or service meets the quality requirements as determined.

Total quality improvement (TQI) is comprehensive monitoring process designed not only to detect and eliminate problems, but also to enhance performance of the ART clinic by exploring innovation and developing flexibility and effectiveness in all processes and involves proactive strategy of ongoing evaluation and monitoring. Indicators used in a TQI plan should be objective, relevant to the laboratory and clinician, and measure a broad range of specific events or aspects of treatment that reflect the quality of care (equipment, personnel, consumables and drugs used). TQI has three key elements viz., understanding the situation, analyzing data and improving performance **(Fig. 1)**.

Documentation forms an very important part of the QC, as it defines approach and responsibility, and also outlines the structure of documentation, which consists of quality manual, detailed written standard procedures (SOPs), working instructions and laboratory forms or records (log books).

Quality assessments require internal and external audit, management review and interprofessional assessment.

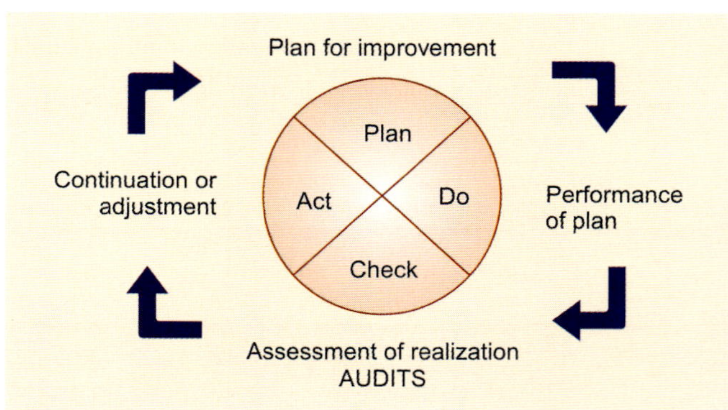

Fig. 1 Quality management in ART clinics

Internal audit requires a quality manager and/or qualified personnel with defined and documented standard procedure protocols. Internal audit should be performed periodically and systematically evaluated. Nonconformities (deficiencies or deviations) should be noted and preventive and corrective measures taken. It should have internal and external QA programs.

An independent external body with national or international standard does external audit, periodically and systematically. Nonconformities (deficiencies or deviations) should be noted and preventive and corrective measures taken. Internal and external QA programs are important. Formal recognition with certification and accreditation is of great value. Accreditation of ART clinic is an efficient and effective tool to achieve and demonstrate technical competence. It can guarantee a constant improvement of the work. It has a major advantage of being able to unify all the different national and international standards and guidelines. It also may provide a new impulse for ART clinics to achieve and maintain the highest level of patient care and the highest success rates.

Management review should be done annually to know the suitability and effectiveness QMS. It involves assessment of outcome of internal or external audits. Preventive and corrective measures against nonconformities and complaints are checked and verified. It evaluates the performance measures by studying the quality indicators and patient satisfaction.

Interprofessional assessment is done periodically by independent (external) colleagues and is based on defined and documented regulation. It assesses the professional competence of an ART clinic.

Problem management involves correction and prevention of accident, complaint, defect, deficiency, deviation, error, failure, infection, mistake and nonconformity. Thus, risk analysis along with corrective and preventive activities is very important.

All aspects of our work in laboratories and clinics involved in the diagnosis and treatment of human infertility can benefit from such programs and schemes, moving the work from being a subjective art form to an objective science. Equally, many clinical procedures are amenable to such scrutiny. Acceptance and introduction of such schemes and programs will rely initially on the self-motivation of the laboratories themselves and personnel involved for the same along with the accrediting authorities. This will help in maintaining the highest level of patient care.

A committee for monitoring infertility treatment and ART is essential and should actively pursue several different strategies to achieve comprehensiveness and quality in all ART clinics. It is in this context that the National Guidelines for Accreditation, Supervision and Regulation of ART clinics in India was formulated by the Indian Council of Medical Research (ICMR) and the National Academy of Medical Sciences, India, in 2005, and over time it has been modified according to the recent evidence.[1] Guidelines are required to implement a quality system for all clinicians, embryologists and IVF laboratory staff.

In the ART clinic, the ART laboratory plays a basic and crucial role in the treatment of infertile individuals. Management of an infertile couple requires a multidisciplinary approach involving the physicians, embryologists, scientists, nurses, counselors and clerical staff. All of them have to cooperate closely to provide optimal service to the patients. Deficiencies or poor performance in one of the disciplines involved undermine efforts to achieve the highest level of patient care and the highest success rates.

Quality management is thus needed to ensure consistency and reproducibility of all methods, and this is particularly necessary in light of the possible risks of ART. Quality in the ART unit depends on the history and organization of the clinic, its objectives and standard, its logistics and cost-benefits and the end point of treatment, which includes the success rate and patient satisfaction.

■ MINIMAL PHYSICAL REQUIREMENTS OF AN ART CLINIC

Non-sterile Area

Reception and Waiting Room

Reception and waiting room should be large enough to accommodate the patients and their relatives. It should also be well ventilated and have clean and hygienic toilets.

Consulting or Doctor's Room

A separate examination room with privacy for interviewing and examining male and female partners independently is essential. It is essential to maintain strict privacy while taking the detailed history, which is very important to direct our investigations and treatment. In case a male doctor examines a female patient, there must always be a female attendant present. The room must be equipped with an examination table and gynecological instruments for examining the female per vaginum, and an appropriate ultrasound machine. Examination of an infertile woman is not complete without a transvaginal ultrasound examination, which is going to direct us for the further management.

Imaging services are provided as per the scope of services of the organizations.[2] The organization should be aware of the legal and other requirements of imaging services and the same are documented for informational and compliance by all concerned in the organization. The organization maintains and updates its compliance status of legal and other requirements in the regular manner.

Apart from a consulting room for doctors, there should be a dedicated room for counseling, which forms a very important part of infertility management.

General Purpose Clinical Laboratory

General purpose clinical laboratory will make it convenient for the patient to undergo investigations? This is essential as hormonal test and tests for infection form an important part of evaluation of an infertile couple. At times microbiology and histopathology examination may also be required. If not available in the premises it can also be outsourced.

Store Room

Store room facilities must be available for storing sterile (media, needles, catheters, petri dishes and such-like items) and non-sterile material under refrigerated and non-refrigerated conditions as appropriate.

Record Room

Records may be maintained as a hardcopy or soft copy, so that the entire data can be accessed, when required. The data must include essential details of the patient's records, which contains history, records of clinical examination and investigations done earlier and carried out recently and the treatment options advised. It also should contain the details of the treatment carried out and the outcome of treatment, and follow-up if any. Any other point such as possible adverse reaction to drugs must be recorded. Today it is best to maintain all the records computerized and the software must have archival, retrieval and multivariate statistical analysis capabilities.

Sterilization Area

A separate facility must be available for sterilizing and autoclaving all surgical items as well as some of those to be used in the ART laboratory.

Vermin Proofing

Adequate steps should be taken for vermin proofing, which should be taken prior to starting clinical work in the clinic because no pesticide can be used in a fully functional IVF clinic, as it could be toxic to the gametes and embryos.

Semen Collection Room

There must be a stand-alone room with privacy and an appropriate environment, which is located in a secluded area close to the laboratory for semen collection. It is important that the patient collects the sample in the premises of the ART clinic, rather than bringing it to the laboratory for analysis and processing after collecting it outside the clinic. If the sample is collected outside the ART clinic, the semen quality and identity is likely to be compromised.

The procedures for collection of semen must be as described in the WHO semen analysis manual. The container used must be sterile, maintained at body temperature and nontoxic. This room must have a wash basin with availability of soap and clean towels. The room must also have a toilet and must not be used for any other purpose.

Room for Intrauterine Insemination

There must be a separate clean room with an appropriate table for intrauterine insemination (IUI).

Changing Room

Changing rooms and hand washing facilities should be located near to the laboratory.

Sterilization Room

Sterilization room should have an autoclave and hot air oven. Autoclave is required for sterilization of instruments required for surgical procedures, IUI, oocyte pickup and embryo transfer. Ultrasonic cleaner along with the hot air oven is required for sterilization of glassware.

Sterile Area

The sterile area houses the operation theater, a room for oocyte retrieval and embryo transfer which should be present adjoining the embryology laboratory, semen processing laboratory and embryology laboratory. An anteroom for changing footwear, an area for changing into sterile garments and a scrub area must strictly control entry to the sterile area. The sterile area must be air conditioned where fresh air filtered through an approved and appropriate filter system is circulated at ambient temperature. Proper training of all the laboratory staff accordingly to these procedures is mandatory.

The instruction manual for every instrument should be available in the laboratory.

Operation Theater

Operation theater must be well equipped with facilities for carrying out surgical endoscopy. The operation theater must be equipped for emergency resuscitative procedures.

Operation Theater or Room for Transvaginal Ovum Pickup and Embryo Transfer

Operation theater room or room for transvaginal ovum pickup and embryo transfer must be in the sterile area and have an examination table on which the patient can be placed for carrying out the procedure and then rest undisturbed for a period of time. If the oocyte retrieval is done under anesthesia or analgesia it should have all facilities and equipped for emergency resuscitation.

Embryology Laboratory Complex

Laboratory design should provide adequate space to permit good laboratory practice and must be as close as possible to operating room. Construction should permit aseptic and optimal handling of gametes, zygotes or embryos throughout treatment; high-efficiency particulate air (HEPA) and volatile organic compound (VOC) filtration of air as well as positive air pressure with an appropriate number of air exchanges per hour to maintain a clean air environment. Access to the laboratory should be permitted only to authorized personnel.

Walls and floors must be composed of materials that can be easily washed and disinfected; use of carpeting must be strictly avoided. The laboratory equipment must be adequate for laboratory work and easy to clean and to disinfect. All critical equipment, including incubators and frozen gamete, zygote and embryo storage facilities, should be appropriately alarmed and monitored. An automatic emergency uninterrupted power source (UPS) or generator backup in the event of power failure is very important.

Location of storage areas and equipment should be planned for efficiency and safety within the working area. Separate office space should be provided for administrative work, so that the embryology laboratory is not used for the same.

The embryology laboratory must have the following equipments:

CO_2 or triple gas incubators: A minimum number of two incubators is a must. Gas cylinders should be placed outside or in a separate room with an automatic backup system. Incubators should be frequently cleaned and sterilized. The incubator should be monitored daily for appropriate temperature and gas content before first opening when used for patient procedures. Incubators should be monitored using calibrated thermometers and independent methods of gas analysis and pH meters and not by digital display alone. Record of these measurements, as well as those shown by the digital displays of each device, must be retained. The CO_2 and triple gas cylinders should also be monitored for calibration and validation especially the triple gas mixture.

Documented procedures in an ART clinic govern procurement, handling, storage, distribution, usage and replenishment of medical gases.[3] The organization shall adhere to statutory requirements under the provisions of the Indian explosives act, Gas Cylinder Rules, and Static and Mobile Pressure Vessel (Unfired) Rules.[4] Medical gases should be handled, stored, distributed and used in a safe manner.

A laminar flow bench with a thermostatically controlled heating plate houses the stereo microscope.

Stereo microscope: Microscopes suitable for oocyte identification in the follicular fluid for its maturity and quality, determination of fertilization and zygote and embryo grading, loading of embryo transfer catheter, oocyte or embryo or sperm cryopreservation, storage and thawing should be used.

Inverted microscope with micromanipulator: A high-resolution inverted microscope with phase contrast or Hoffman optics, preferably with facilities for video recording should be available. It should have a microma-nipulator with or without laser for micromanipulation of oocytes or embryos. Procedures requiring microma-nipulation of human oocytes and/or embryos include intracytoplasmic sperm injection (ICSI), assisted hatching (AH), polar body or embryo biopsy for preim-plantation genetic diagnosis (PGD) removal of fragments from highly fragmented embryos.

Devices to maintain the temperature and pH of media, oocytes, and embryos during various phases of the procedure of IVF should be available (slide warmers, incubators, water baths, heating block, test tube heaters, etc.). Regular checks of functional parameters for these devices used to maintain temperature of media, gametes, zygotes and embryos during each phase of the procedure, when they are out of the incubators, should be in place.

Disposable materials and culture media: Disposable article like petri dishes, test tubes and pipettes should be of tissue culture grade plastic for steps that involve exposure to tissue and body fluids. A pH meter and osmometer for regular monitoring of media is essential. All laboratory chemicals and reagents must be labeled to indicate date received, date opened, and shelf life, where applicable.

Each batch of culture media should be tested before use for osmolarity and pH testing should be performed following equilibration with CO_2 at concentrations used for ART procedures.

Equipment for freezing embryos: Freezing can be done either by slow freezing or vitrification.

Liquid N_2 cans: Liquid nitrogen cans with canisters and straw holders are required for cryopreservation of gametes, embryos and ovarian or testicular tissue.

Refrigerator: For storing culture media and oil, PVP and hyaluronidase.

It is the responsibility of laboratory personnel to ensure that any material that comes into contact with sperm, eggs or embryos is not toxic, and tested for toxicity by appropriate bioassay or animal model system. This includes, aspiration needles, transfer catheters, plastic ware, glassware, culture media, and protein source.

Identification of Patients and their Gametes, Zygotes and Embryos

Before commencing any procedure related to a treatment cycle, the embryologist should check that the patient has signed the corresponding consent form. The clinical and serological exams undergone by the patients before undergoing any treatment for infertility should be checked in order to detect any possible positivity to viral infections. For correct handling and identification of gametes, zygotes and embryo samples there should be rules established by a system of checks and, where needed, double checks by a second person. All material from the operation room, culture dishes and falcon tubes used for sperm preparation (including lids), must bear the name of the patient. In the incubator, identified oocytes and sperm should be kept together on the same tray and double-checked. All pipettes should be immediately discarded after use. Appropriate steps need to be taken for the correct identification of gametes and embryos to avoid mix-ups.

Incubators should be organized in order to facilitate identification of embryos, zygotes, oocytes and sperm. Verification of patient's identity should be performed at all critical steps, which include—before ovum pickup, at semen recovery, at insemination or ICSI, at cryopreservation and at embryo transfer procedures. Documentation of all critical steps for each patient is essential and one copy of the documented data should be given to the patient and one has to be retained by the

ART clinic. The identity of the laboratory person handling the samples at each point of the process, from receipt through final disposition, date and time, should be clearly indicated. This permits tracking of the sample throughout its period in the laboratory and also at later dates.

The embryology laboratory must have daily log book in which all the day's activities are recorded, including the performance of the equipment. Records of ordinary and extraordinary maintenance on all the equipment must be maintained.

Written instructions should be available to all members of the staff describing in detail the various phases of IVF techniques, including all the laboratory operative procedures, in which the protocols, the equipment and the material list should be specified along with actions that need to be taken in the case of equipment failure. The laboratory director should review and update all procedures on at least an annual basis. Any changes must be approved, signed and dated by the laboratory director.

Protective Measures

All body fluids (follicular fluid, semen, etc.) should be treated as potentially contaminated. The purpose of the protective measures is both to protect laboratory staff and to ensure aseptic conditions for gametes, zygotes and embryos. There should be strict observation of staff hygiene by using of laboratory clothing with cap and mask, use of non-toxic (non-powdered) gloves, use of eye and face protection, and of cryogloves if cryogenic materials are handled. All the laboratory work should be performed in a laminar flow benches, it is best to use mechanical pipetting devices. Contaminated laboratory equipment and/or work surfaces should be disinfected and sterilized using 70% alcohol. All disposable material; after usage should be discarded immediately in the proper waste containers. Potential infectious materials must be disposed of in a manner that protects laboratory workers and maintenance, service, and housekeeping staff from exposure to infectious materials in the course of their work. Needles and other sharp objects like holding and injection pipette, strippers and micropipettes should be handled with extreme caution and discarded in special containers. Glassware in the laboratory including pasteur pipettes and broken glassware should be discarded in special containers. Food, drinks, cigarettes and cigars are strictly forbidden. The use of make up and strong perfumes should be avoided. Cross-contamination with infectious material could happen when straws with semen, oocytes, zygotes or embryos are filled by dipping the straw in semen or in patient medium with gametes, zygotes or embryos, sealing it and passing it into liquid nitrogen without external disinfection.[5] It is advisable to keep the material stored in the cryopreservation tanks in a way that avoids contact of the liquid nitrogen phase with the biological substances. Specimens known to be contaminated should be stored in high-security straws and preferably, in dedicated tanks. Also samples containing body fluids, such as seminal plasma, should be cryopreserved in high-security straws. Another way to avoid contact with liquid nitrogen is to store samples in the gaseous phase of liquid nitrogen.[6]

This makes it mandatory to have an established laboratory safety programme:[7]

- A well-documented laboratory safety manual should be available in the laboratory. This takes care of the safety of the workforce as well as the equipment in the laboratory. It shall be in consonance with the risks and hazards identified.
- This program is aligned with the ART clinics safety program.
- Written procedures guide the handling and disposal of infectious and hazardous materials.
- Laboratory personnel are appropriately trained in safe practices.
- Laboratory personnel are provided with appropriate safety equipment or devices, e.g. fire extinguisher, disinfectants, etc. All laboratory staff shall be appropriately immunized especially against hepatitis B.

Semen Processing Room

Semen processing room must be a separate room with a laminar air flow and centrifuge for semen processing, preferably close to the semen collection room. This laboratory must also have facilities for microscopic examination of semen and postcoital test smears, which includes a light microscope, Makler's chamber or hemocytometer, slides with coverslip, disposable and sterile Finnpipettes, pipettes, round bottom and conical test tubes, embryo toxicity tested syringes. Care must be taken for the safe disposal of biological waste and other materials (syringes, glass slides, etc.).

■ DOCUMENTATION

Information Management System[8]

Information is an important resource for effective and efficient delivery of health care. Provision of health care and its continued improvement is dependent to a large extent on the information generated, stored and utilized appropriately by the organization. All clinical and laboratory aspects of the ART cycles for each patient should be maintained. All investigations and treatment records along with the steps throughout the ART procedure must be traceable. The oocytes must be accounted for from retrieval to embryo transfer or cryopreservation or disposal. Though not revealed to the patient information on the sperm and oocyte donors should be maintained, if required in the future.

Like all QMSs documentation is an essential component. It is suggested that the organization prepare an apex manual (quality manual) incorporating the various standards and objective elements and providing appropriate linkages. Documented policies and procedures should exist for maintaining confidentiality, security integrity of records, data and information. The organization shall control the accessibility to the medical records department (MRD) and to its hospital information system. These documented policies and procedures are in consonances with the applicable laws and the procedures for the same incorporate safeguarding of data or record against loss, destruction and tampering. In case of physical records and data, there should be adequate pest and rodent control measures. There must also be fire safe cabinets or there must be adequate fire fighting equipment.

The organization uses developments in appropriate technology for improving confidentiality, integrity and security. Privileged health information is used for the purposes identified or as required by law and not disclosed without the patient's authorization. Documented policies and procedures exist for retention time of record, data and information and regularly carry out review of medical record to analyze it on regular basis and the information gathered should be used to identify and resolve problems.

A documented procedure exists on how to respond to patients or physicians and other agencies requests for access to information in the medical record in accordance with the local and national law.

Composition and Qualifications of the Members of the ART Team

An ART clinic requires a well-orchestrated teamwork between the reproductive endocrinologist, gynecologist, andrologist and clinical embryologist, which is supported by a counselor and a program coordinator or director.

Reproductive Endocrinologist or Gynecologist

Reproductive endocrinologist or gynecologist must be a licensed physician with training and experience in reproductive endocrinology, particularly in the use of ovulation—inducing agents and hormonal control of the menstrual cycle and having knowledge of diagnostic methods for determining the cause of infertility.

The clinician should also have a specialized training and experience in gynecologic ultrasonography for monitoring of follicular development and ultrasound-guided oocyte retrieval. Experience in laparoscopic and hysteroscopic surgery, both diagnostic and therapeutic is essential.

Andrologist

An individual experienced in male reproduction (andrology) with special competence in semenology and with expertise in reproductive surgery should be available.

Clinical Embryologist

Clinical embryologist should be appropriately qualified and experienced responsible person with qualifications of diploma and expertise in the field of embryology and biological or medical sciences according to national rules. Should have personal experience in maintenance of a clinical embryology laboratory and in tissue culture techniques. There should also be an individual with specialized training and experience in gamete and embryo cryopreservation techniques, when gamete and/or embryo cryopreservation is offered.

Counselor

Counselor is an individual with a minimum degree in psychology or social sciences with expertise in reproductive issues.

Nurse

The nurse should provide appropriate nursing support. The registered nurse in the ART setting provides education, counseling, support, and nursing care to patients seeking assistance for conception and for those who attain pregnancy with treatment. The nurse should have orientation to the clinical setting and demonstrated competence in the specialty field of infertility with the knowledge of investigations, treatment and medicines used in this field.

Genetic Counselor

Genetic counselor is who has specialized expertise in genetics or genetic counseling.

Program Coordinator or Director

Program coordinator or director is a senior person with experience in all aspects of ART. Is responsible for coordinating all activities in the ART clinic and taking care of staff administration, stock keeping, finance and maintenance of patient records. The program coordinator should have good public relation skills to satisfy the patient's needs and complaints.

■ QUALITY CONTROL AND QUALITY ASSURANCE

The clinical and embryology team should regularly audit the internal indicators of success and analyze the problems and take a corrective action. The indicators include fertilization and cleavage rate, blastocyst formation rate and number of top quality embryos, biochemical and ongoing clinical pregnancy rate after fresh and frozen thawed transfers. It is also important to make a note of the number of patients who have had failed fertilization. All these parameters will tell us about the implantation rate and also survival of zygotes or embryos after thawing. Compliance with a QMS is mandatory.

Elements of Quality Control

Maintenance of the Laboratories

Laminar flow hoods, laboratory tables, incubators and other areas where sterility is required must be periodically checked for microbial contamination using standard techniques, and a record of such checks must be kept.

A log book must be maintained which records the temperature, carbon dioxide content and humidity of the incubators and the manometer readings of the laminar air flow.

All equipment should be maintained and calibrated on a daily, monthly, and annual basis as appropriate to the type of equipment. One must maintain a record of instrument calibration, functional checks of equipment when possible, and evidence of an active review of records. Documentation or corrective action when instruments and/or procedures malfunction should be kept. QC testing is recommended when commercial media is purchased and used within its labeled expiration period. Laboratories should also establish quality assessment for acceptable receiving conditions for transported commercial media. The ART clinic should plan for engineering support services.

System function checks should be made and documented for power off, high temperature and low CO_2. After hours, alarms should be transmitted in case of problem to a person who can respond to these emergencies immediately.

Quality of Consumables Used in the Laboratory

All disposable plastic ware must be procured from reliable sources after ensuring that they are not toxic to the embryo. Culture media used for processing gametes or growing embryos in vitro should be preferably procured from reliable manufacturers. Each batch of culture medium needs to have been tested for sterility, endotoxins, osmolality and pH. The embryologist should know the composition of the media that are being used. Most media are supplemented with serum; they should, therefore, be tested for antibodies to HIV 1 and 2, hepatitis B and C, syphilis and HTLV-I and -II. Use sterile techniques, appropriate disease screens, and safe laboratory procedures will come a long way in maintain the quality and results in an ART clinic.

The treatment of patients positive for HIV or hepatitis B or C (diagnosed as infectious after PCR control for the presence of the viral genome) should be only performed in laboratories having dedicated areas, in which the adequate safety measures are followed. Alternatively, patients with positivity for HIV or hepatitis B or C could be allocated to specific series or time slots during the working day, which are followed by an accurate cleaning and disinfection of the laboratory. A class II laminar flow cabinet that protects both the operator and the specimen should be used when contaminated samples are handled.

A systematic monitoring of the testing process can be performed under QA, aimed at improving the entire process by identifying problems, errors or improvements that may have occurred. For this internal QA, results should be evaluated on a regular basis, indicators should be objective and relevant, and adequate thresholds set up. In order to prevent bias due to patient variation, a representative number of procedures in relation of the total number of procedures performed should be selected to establish the corresponding thresholds. Critical levels of laboratory performance for each indicator should be defined and numbers or rates of errors and adverse events noted. Protocols should be available for fire and electrical safety and internal and external disaster, including provisions for equipment backup in the event of equipment failure.

To complement the internal quality assessments, participation in external QAs programs, either commercial, or in collaboration with other laboratories, is recommended.

Problem management: Problem management includes notification procedure for non-conformities, identification of critical steps for the same and corrective and preventive measures. Internal and external audits and management reviews along with performance indicators will provide an insight into the problem and also help in rectifying it.

Prerequisites for a good ART outcome require the following:
- Knowledge and scientific background
- Competence and practical skills
- Awareness of problems and risk management
- A good and mutual cooperation between the clinician and laboratory personnel.

Apart from this the ART clinic should also look into parameters like user satisfaction, patient safety and monitor and evaluate quality of care given to them. A multitude of factors, often appearing in combination, can affect providers' ability to deliver quality reproductive health services. Common factors include changes in the health care system, strengths or deficiencies within systems or individual facilities, availability of supplies and equipment, regulatory constraints, and providers' level of competence.[9]

Before attempting to improve the quality of care, it is important to determine what factors contribute to lower quality care. Quantitative approaches and self assessment tools, such as continuous quality improvement (CQI), client-oriented, provider-efficient services (COPE), and performance improvement (PI), can help organizations determine strengths and weaknesses in service delivery and help identify solutions.

Experts recommend that program managers incorporate service delivery guidelines that reflect internationally accepted norms, such as sterilizing clinical equipment, in order to protect clients' health.

Quality Assurance

Quality assurance is a comprehensive program designed to look at the laboratory as a whole and to identify problems or errors that exist in an attempt to improve the entire process. Indicators used in a QA program should be objective, relevant to the laboratory, and measure a broad range of specific events or aspects of treatment that reflect the quality of care. For an IVF laboratory, some common components of a QA program would include: QC activities, a comprehensive written procedure manual, continuing educational activities, a program for employee evaluation, a safety program for the protection of both laboratory staff and patients, and the use of an external proficiency program. QA programs are designed to identify problems or errors that exist in the laboratory and correct these defects. For each indicator incorporated into the laboratory's QA program, an appropriate threshold needs to be established. The threshold sets the critical level of quality laboratory performance for each indicator. Since clinical protocols are not uniform among

Table 1 Impact of setting threshold

Threshold values	Result
Threshold values set too low	Failure to detect laboratory errors and correct poor performance
Threshold value set too high	Standards are impossible to achieve; improvement efforts are misdirected
Threshold values appropriately se	The laboratory has true view of its performance and can effectively direct its effort towards improvements

ART laboratories, the threshold values must be specific for each individual clinical laboratory.

Threshold values for each of the indicators need to be based on how the specific protocols used in the laboratory impact the outcomes and the nature of indicator's effect on quality of care. As illustrated in **Table 1**, thresholds that are set too high will erroneously indicate a problem with the laboratory performance. Conversely, a threshold set too low may fail to detect a laboratory deficiency or a poor level of performance.[10]

There is an established laboratory QA program, which is documented. The program addresses verification and/or validation of test methods. These could either be modified official methods or methods developed in-house or methods extended to a component, analysis or matrix not previously tested or included in validation. A note needs to be made of changes involving new technology or automation.

Verification usually includes accuracy, precision and linearity. Validation in addition includes sensitivity and specificity. The program addresses surveillance of test results and includes periodic calibration and maintenance of all equipment (traceability certificate of all calibration done shall also be documented and maintained).

Mechanisms to detect clerical, transcriptional, clinical or analytical mistakes should be in place. When problems and/or adverse trends are identified, corrective measures should be implemented to resolve the issue to ensure quality patient care. There should be documentation whether corrective measures instituted were able to effectively resolve the problem. QA also includes the review of reports and consistency of service as well as statistical analysis of outcomes data.

■ DISCUSSION

Clinical services are available to meet patient needs and all such services meet applicable local and national standards, laws and regulations. The organization has a system for providing services, required by its patient population, clinical services offered and health care practitioner needs. The laboratory services are organized and provided in a manner that meets the emergency requirements by the organization itself or by outsourcing or both. Patients should be informed when an outside source of laboratory services is used.[11]

The ethical guidelines should go beyond technicalities and build effective safeguards so that the unequal power relationship between the providers and users of new technology is minimized. The guidelines should also keep in mind the unequal gender balance and ensure that the rights of the users of these technologies are not compromised in any manner and full information should be given to the users. In this context, particular care needs to be taken to protect the rights of the subjects of research as well as the consumers of these techniques. Infertile couple, given the social pressure to reproduce as well as their own intense desire to conceive, is particularly vulnerable to commercial interests and experimentation in the medical field, since desperation might lead them to consent to hazardous techniques in the hope of conceiving.[12]

The existing evidences clearly show that setting standards, QC and certification has multiple beneficial effect; improving in efficiency and safety increases in overall quality and credibility of the center, as well as promotion of a new way of thinking and acting.

It is also vital to understand what can motivate medical staff to provide high-quality care. There is little data about why providers persevere under difficult conditions or about what would motivate them to make additional efforts to improve the quality of their care, although providers' main motivation seems to be their desire to do something good for others or to give back to the community.[13,14] Understanding provider's needs and motivations can help those interested in designing ways to improve quality of care. Experts have developed several interventions, largely under the control of managers of reproductive health facilities and programs that could lead to better provision of reproductive health services. But despite widespread application, the options have not yet been rigorously tested through controlled experiments. Most programs use multiple interventions, so it is difficult to determine the effectiveness of any single intervention. In general, the most effective interventions seem to be those that combine multiple approaches.

Quality assessment studies usually measure one of three types of outcomes: medical outcomes, costs, and client satisfaction.

Unlike most medical laboratories that play a diagnostic role, laboratories for ART, are involved in the treatment of infertile couples. Handling human gametes and producing human embryos in order to achieve much-sought pregnancies form the key tasks of an ART laboratory. The impact of the activities and the possible risks makes it necessary to ensure the safety and reproducibility of all methods. To achieve and maintain the highest level of patient care and the highest success rates, a QMS should be implemented. Several guidelines, compiled by professional associations of ART experts, official international standards and quality management models have been developed and issued and can be applied. Irrespective of the choice, establishing a QMS in an ART laboratory leads to a huge amount of additional work and requires a lot of investment in all kind of areas. However, due to the increased standardization and efficiency of all procedures as well as the improved transparency and traceability of all actions performed, the quality of service provided by the laboratory will improve substantially and the effort will be worthwhile.

Laboratories staffed with properly trained personnel, operating with a close attention to issues of quality with equally efficient clinical personnel are crucial in maintaining high pregnancy rates following assisted reproduction. The use of internal QC procedures and external QA programs are useful tools in monitoring the performance of the laboratory and has positive repercussions on pregnancy rates.

Thus each ART clinic is challenged for achieving and maintaining not only the highest level of patient care but also the highest success rates. To achieve and maintain the highest level of patient care and the highest success rates, a QMS should be implemented. Several guidelines, compiled by professional associations of ART experts, official international standards and quality management models have been developed and issued and can be applied. This allows for increased standardization and efficiency of all procedures as well as the improved transparency and traceability of all actions performed, the quality of service provided by the laboratory will improve substantially and the effort will be worthwhile.

■ CONCLUSION

Ensuring optimal conditions in an ART clinic involves a detailed written standard procedure for both clinical and laboratory work, which also specifies safety policies. Appropriately educated and trained personnel in the field of reproductive endocrinology and andrology should do the evaluation and treatment of the infertile couple. Laboratory director should be qualified, experienced and responsible for correct operation and calibration of instruments, maintenance of a correct system for patient sample collection and management, for consistent and proper execution of appropriate technique and methods, documentation and record keeping and maintain a system for the appraisal of performance and correction of deficiencies.

Surveillance of optimal conditions by ongoing methods of assessing staff competency in terms of their clinical and clerical skills is a must. It is important to monitor and evaluate the number and type of accidents, mistakes and deviations that have occurred and implement corrective measures. It is also desirable to have a system in place for the implementation of advances and improvements both on the clinical and laboratory aspect of the ART clinic. One should also have a system in place for documenting and addressing the complaints of the patients, who are under great stress. It is the experience of physicians, embryologists, and staff members along with the consistency of approach, attention to detail, and good communication as being vital to excellent outcomes thereby ensuring a holistic approach to patient care.

Quality is never an accident; it is always the result of high intention, sincere effort, intelligent direction and skillful execution; it represents the wise choice of many alternatives.

APPENDIX
Key Practices in an ART Clinic

Patient Evaluation

- Ovarian reserve screening of all patients [cycle day 3 follicle-stimulating hormone (FSH), anti-Müllerian hormone and antral follicle counts]
- Evaluation of uterine cavity and tubes (3D USG, saline infusion sonography, hysterosalpingography, hysteroscopy and laparoscopy)
- Evaluation for hydrosalpinges
- Trial embryo transfer (ET) before IVF stimulation cycle
- Referral of male factor cases to a urologist with training in andrology.

Ovarian Stimulation

- Use of a step-down approach to gonadotropin dosing
- Preferential use of a mixed protocol of FSH and luteinizing hormone
- Correct choice in using gonadotropin-releasing hormone (GnRH) analogs—agonist or antagonist
- Recommend cycle cancellation for less than three mature follicles
- Human chorionic gonadotropins (hCG) or GnRH agonist trigger when at least three dominant follicles of more than 18 mm mean diameter.

Oocyte Retrieval and ET

- Preferential use of a single-lumen needle for USG guided transvaginal retrieval
- Use of ultrasound guidance for ET
- Use of progesterone supplementation after retrieval and continued at least until fetal cardiac activity documented after pregnancy.

Laboratory Practices

- Selective use of correct procedure—IUI, IVF or ICSI
- Use of single or group culture of embryos in microdrops of media
- Adjustment of incubator—percentage of CO_2 based on media pH 5–6
- Selective use of AH and preimplantation genetic screening
- Choosing between cleavage stage and blastocyst ET.

Laboratory Environment

- Positive air pressure in the laboratory
- HEPA filtration of laboratory air
- Filtration of laboratory air for volatile and chemically active compounds
- Use of laminar flow hoods
- Use of heated microscope stages.

■ REFERENCES

1. Indian Council of Medical Research, National Academy of Medical Sciences (India). National guidelines for accreditation, supervision and regulation of ART clinics in India. New Delhi: Ministry of Health and Family Welfare, Government of India; 2005.
2. Access assessment and continuity care (AAC.9). In: National Accreditation Board for Hospitals and Healthcare Providers (NABH). Accreditation Standards for Hospitals, 3rd edition. New Delhi: NABH; 2011. pp. 18-9.
3. Facility management system (FMS.3). In: National Accreditation Board for Hospitals and Healthcare Providers (NABH). Accreditation Standards for Hospitals, 3rd edition. New Delhi: NABH; 2011. pp. 154-56.
4. National Fire Protection Association (NFPA). Medical Gas and Vacuum Systems Installation Handbook: NFPA's new NFPA 99C solution. Massachusetts: NFPA; 2012.
5. Tedder RS, Zuckerman MA, Goldstone AH, et al. Hepatitis B transmission from contaminated cryopreservation tank. Lancet. 1995;346:137-40.
6. Bielanski A. Non-transmission of bacterial and viral microbes to embryos and semen stored in the vapour phase of liquid nitrogen in dry shippers. Cryobiology. 2005;50:206-10.
7. Access Assessment and continuity care (AAC.8). In: National Accreditation Board for Hospitals and Healthcare Providers (NABH). Accreditation Standards for Hospitals, 3rd edition. New Delhi: NABH; 2011. pp. 16-7.
8. Information Management System (IMS). In: National Accreditation Board for Hospitals and Healthcare Providers (NABH). Accreditation Standards for Hospitals, 3rd edition. New Delhi: NABH; 2011. pp. 183-96.
9. Lantis K, Green CP, Joyce S. Providers and Quality of Care. In: New Perspectives on Quality of Care, No. 3. Washington, DC: Population Council and Population Reference Bureau; 2002.
10. Mayer JF, Jones EL, Dowling-Lacey D, et al. Total quality improvement in the IVF laboratory: choosing indicators of quality. Reprod Biomed Online. 2003;7(6):695-9.
11. Laboratory services: Assessment of patients (AOP.5). In: Joint Commission International (JCI). Joint Commission International Accreditation Standards for Hospitals, 4th edition. Illinois: JCI; 2010.
12. Murthy L, Subramanian V. ICMR guidelines on assisted reproductive technology: lacking in vision, wrapped in red tape. 2007;4(3):123-4.
13. Tavrow P, Namate D, Mpemba N. Quality of care: an assessment of family planning providers' attitudes and client-provider interactions in Malawi. Centre for Social Research, University of Malawi, Blantyre; 1995.
14. Huezo C. Improving the quality of care by improving the motivation of service providers: a study based in Uganda and Bangladesh. Paper presented at MAQ Mini-University, Washington, DC, April 20, 2001.

How to Investigate an Infertile Couple?

4

Evaluation of the Male Partner

Madhuri Patil

■ INTRODUCTION

There are several recognized causes of infertility along with numerous undetectable defects in the oocyte and sperm quality that might prevent conception among infertile couples. The unrecognized causes may result in persistent failure to conceive after multiple attempts with the conventional treatments such as ovarian stimulation or intrauterine insemination (IUI) and even in vitro fertilization (IVF). At times, the conventional diagnostic test done in the male partner may not be able to identify and pinpoint the exact cause of infertility. In this group of patients, IVF itself may be able to throw some light on the problems of sperm, fertilization and embryo quality. Approximately, 8–15% of the couples are unable to conceive after 1 year of unprotected intercourse.[1] A male factor is solely responsible for subfertility in approximately 20% of infertile couples and contributes in another 20–25% of couples along with the female factor.[2] A male infertility factor is often defined by abnormal semen parameters but may be present even when the semen analysis is normal. A history of previous fertility does not exclude the possibility of a newly acquired, secondary, male infertility factor and involves a workup similar to primary male factor.

Role of spermatozoa during fertilization is contribution of haploid set of chromosomes with paternal pattern of gene imprinting, triggering oocyte activation with cortical granule exocytosis, meiosis resumption and completion with spindle formation and subsequent initiation of metabolic events required to support embryonic development, epigenetic and structural inheritance (centrosome).

The natural process of fertility involves fusion of spermatozoon with the oocyte requires both gametes to be structurally normal, viable and functionally competent. Sperm characteristic important for fertilization:
- Normal morphology
- Normal intact acrosome
- Straight line velocity (VSL) and linearity (LIN)
- Ability to bind to zona pellucida
- Ability to penetrate the zona pellucida
- Ability to fuse with the oolemma
- Activate the oocyte
- Ability to form an pronucleus.

Spermatogenesis is a tightly regulated process that starts in the seminiferous tubules and ends in functional terms in the female reproductive tract **(Table 1)**. It is under somatic control and is influenced by environmental and genetic factors and its output is extremely variable even in fertile population and certain subtle conditions in the male cannot be identified and treated.

Abnormal semen parameters and rarely, patients with normal semen quality may have sperm that are either incapable of oocyte fertilization or harbor genetic abnormalities that prevent normal fetal development. Two systems that police abnormal sperm production are

Table 1 The acquisition of full functional sperm competence in vivo occurs in female reproductive tract

Seminiferous tubules	From spermatogenesis to immature sperm
Epididymis	1. Acquisition of progressive motility
	2. Membrane changes
	3. Cross linking of protamine's
Female reproductive tract	**Capacitation**
	1. Ion-mediated modification ensuring a more fluid cell membrane
	2. Hyper-activation of sperm movement by massive calcium entry
Cumulus-oocyte complex	Acrosome exocytosis by calcium influx

apoptosis and DNA repair and remodeling. Apoptosis limit germ cell population to the numbers that can be supported by Sertoli cells with selective depletion of abnormal sperm cells enabling production of normal mature spermatozoa. DNA repair and remodeling results in base excision repair protein (BER) excise and replace damaged DNA base, mainly those arising from endogenous oxidative and hydrolytic decay of DNA. At times altered gene expression also results in production of abnormal sperms.

The cause for male subfertility remains frequently obscure in about 30% of the cases (idiopathic infertility). In another 25% chromosomal abnormalities and mutations [Klinefelter syndrome (47,XXY), chromosomal aberrations, cystic fibrosis (CF), congenital bilateral absence of vas deferens or Y-chromosomal azoospermia factor (AZF) deletions] are responsible.[3] In the remaining fertility impairment may be due to maldescended testis, infections, varicocele, idiopathic testicular tumors, lymphomas, leukemia, sarcoma, secondary hypogonadism, obstructions and vasectomy. Causes of male infertility are given in **Table 2**.

■ EVALUATION OF MALE PARTNER

All male partners need to undergo evaluation primarily in the form of semen analysis when a couple presents to us with failure to achieve a successful pregnancy after 12 months or more of regular unprotected intercourse. At times earlier evaluation may be justified, based on medical history and physical findings and is warranted after 6 months for couples in which the female partner is over the age of 35 years.[4]

Evaluation of the infertile male aims at identifying any abnormality in the semen and underlying medical conditions that may present as infertility. This is important because we need to identify and treat the correctable conditions, so that couple is given a chance to achieve conception naturally or with assistance. It is important that semen be collected in an ideal container which is 60–100 mL wide mouth plastic jar made of polypropylene with a screw cap that fits tightly to prevent any loss of semen when it is transported.

If the initial evaluation of the semen is abnormal, then a repeat semen analysis is done one month apart **(Fig. 1)**. Depending on the semen analysis further investigations are done, which includes complete evaluation of the male partner, hormonal assay, ultrasound examination of the scrotum, karyotyping and molecular genetics, examination of postejaculatory urine sample **(Flow charts 1 to 3)**, sperm function test and testicular biopsy.

Table 2 Causes of male infertility

Etiology	Frequency

1. Primary testicular disorders
  • Klinefelter's syndrome and variants
  • Cryptorchidism
  • Orchitis
  • Irradiation
  • Cytotoxic therapy
  • Partial androgen resistance
	10–13%

2. Hypothalamic-pituitary disease idiopathic, tumors, hyperprolactinemia	1%
3. Genital tract obstruction • Congenital or acquired obstruction of vas deferens or epididymis	8–10%
4. Previous vasectomy	
5. Sperm autoimmunity	4–6%
6. Drugs, toxins, stress, illness	?
7. Life style—smoking, occupation, dress habits • Less consumption of omega–3 fatty acids, time spent in commuting	?
8. Coital problems	1%
9. Idiopathic	70–75%
10. Poor sperm motility, teratozoospermia, varicocele, chronic prostatitis	?

There is no known treatment for partial androgen resistance syndrome **(Flow chart 4)** where the man has azoospermia with normal follicle-stimulating hormone (FSH) levels but elevated luteinizing hormone (LH) and testosterone levels.

The diagnostic andrological evaluation will give the clinician direction to further management. It will help the clinician identify a treatable or a non-treatable fertility factor.

Now we would discuss the detailed evaluation of the male partner.

Semen Analysis

Semen analysis (SA) is the cornerstone of the laboratory evaluation of the infertile male and helps to define the severity of the male factor. All patients should be provided

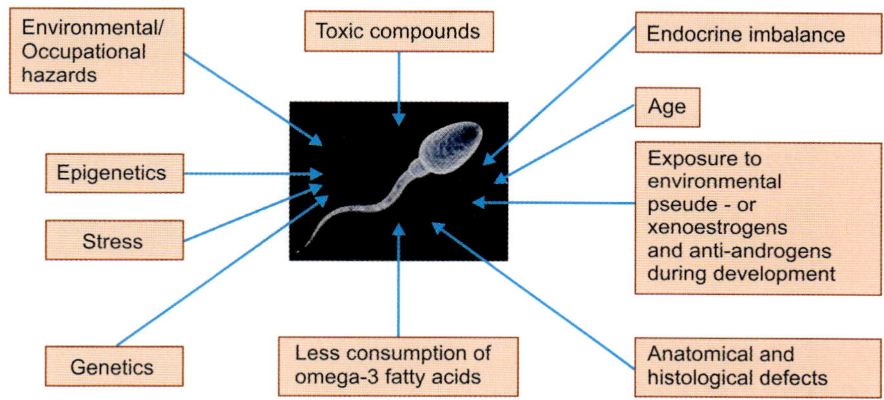

Fig. 1 Disruptors of spermatogenesis

Flow chart 1 Diagnostic-therapeutic algorithm in azoospermia and severe oligozoospermia

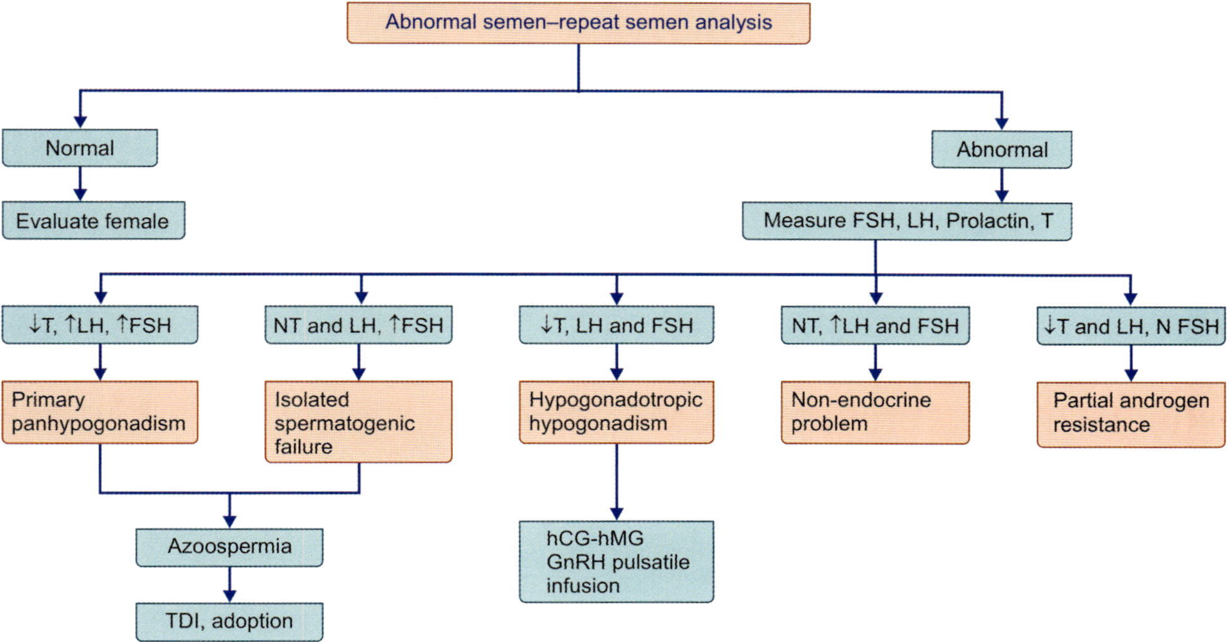

with standardized instructions for semen collection, including a defined pre-test abstinence interval of 2–5 days. Although a standard duration of abstinence is important for evaluation of semen parameters, some men with severe oligospermia can have equal or better sperm concentration with a short (hours) period of abstinence, supporting the potential use of multiple semen analyses during assisted reproductive technology (ART) treatment cycles.[5-7]

If the first semen sample is abnormal, a second sample should be evaluated. It is important that the second sample examined is separated by at least 1 month.

Semen can be collected by masturbation into a specimen collection bottle made of polypropylene or by intercourse using special semen collection condoms that do not contain spermicidal substances toxic to sperm. Ideally, the specimen should be collected in the premises

Flow chart 2 Evaluation of azoospermia with normal FSH, LH and testosterone values

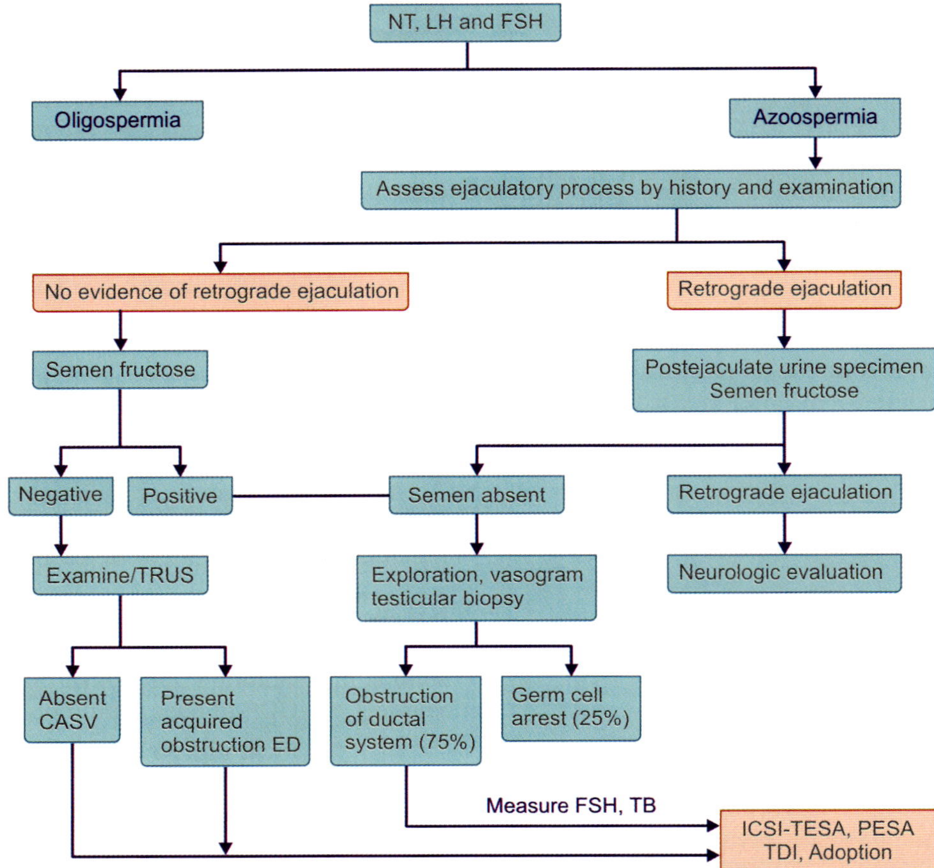

of the laboratory in specially designated semen collection rooms and not the toilet. If the semen sample is collected at home, the specimen should be kept at room or body temperature during transport and examined in the laboratory within 30 minutes to 1 hour of collection. To ensure accurate results, the laboratory should have a good quality control program for semen analysis that conforms to the standards outlined in the standard operating procedures based on recent evidence.

The semen analysis provides information on semen volume, pH, liquefaction, viscosity, sperm concentration, motility, viability, morphology and agglutination, semen cytology and biochemistry and when required sperm function test.

Clinical reference ranges have been established for sperm concentration, motility, and morphology to help classify men as fertile or subfertile **(Table 3)**.[8]
The detailed semen analysis should be done as follows:

Color

Normally, the color of the semen is opaque and grayish. It is yellowish when the number of days of abstinence is more or in the presence of infection or inflammation. Usually, the sperm concentration is low when the semen is transparent and has watery consistency.

Odor

A semen sample has a strong distinctive odor derived from prostatic secretion. One should make a note only when there is absence of odor or in the presence of uncharacteristic odor.

Liquefaction

In normal sample, liquefaction occurs within 10–20 minutes. Liquefaction is caused by proteolytic enzymes

Flow chart 3 Evaluation of oligoasthenospermia with normal FSH, LH and testosterone levels

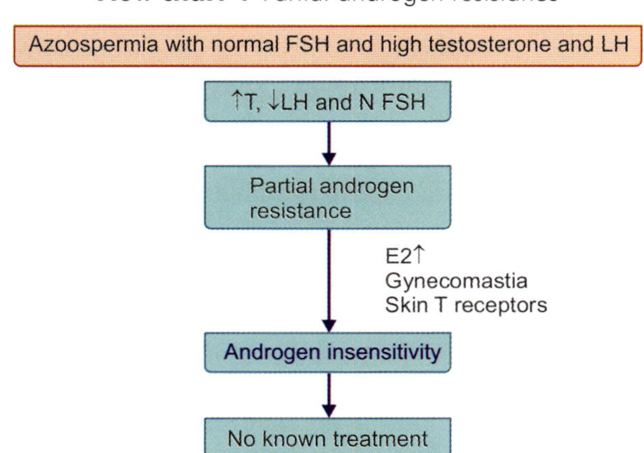

Flow chart 4 Partial androgen resistance

fibrinolysin, secreted by prostate and fibrinogenase and aminopeptidase. Liquefaction serves as an indicator of normal prostate function.

If liquefaction delayed for more than 20 minutes or does not occur at all, it indicates prostatic dysfunction or previous prostatitis.

When the post-liquefaction thread is less than 2 cm it is said to be normal. Increased viscosity apart from abnormal prostatic function may be due to an infection in the genital tract, prostate or seminal vesicle, artifact as a result of the use of an unsuitable type of plastic container or frequent ejaculation.

Volume

Normal volume should be anywhere between 1.4 mL and 1.7 mL. Low volume is seen in obstruction due to a previous infection of the genital tract, congenital absence of the seminal vesicles and vas deferens (associated with absence of fructose) and retrograde ejaculation especially in those patients who have a history of previous surgery of the prostate or the bladder neck (**Flow chart 5**).

pH

Normal pH should be more than or equal to 7.2. pH may be more than 8.0 in acute prostatitis, vesiculitis and bilateral epididymitis. It may be less than 7.2 in chronic infection and may be less than 7.0 in obstruction of the ejaculatory duct or cases where only prostatic fluids are secreted.

Table 3 Lower limit of accepted reference values according to WHO 2010 manual

Parameter	Lower reference limit
Semen volume (mL)	1.5 (1.4–1.7)
Total sperm number (10^6 per ejaculate)	39 (33–46)
Sperm concentration (10^6 per mL)	15 (12–16)
Total motility (PR + NP in %)	40 (38–42)
Progressive motility (PR in %)	32 (31–34)
Vitality (Live sperms %)	58 (55–63)
Sperm morphology (Normal forms %)	4 (3.0–4.0)
Other consensus threshold values	
pH	≥7.2
Peroxidase positive leukocytes (10^6 per mL)	<1
MAR test (motile spermatozoa with bound particles %)	<50
Immunobead test (motile spermatozoa with bound particles %)	<50
Seminal zinc (μmol/ejaculate)	≥2.4
Seminal fructose (μmol/ejaculate)	≥13
Seminal neutral glucosidase (mU/ejaculate)	≥20

Abbreviations: MAR, mixed antiglobulin reaction; NP, nonprogressive motility; PR, progressive motility

Flow chart 5 Abnormalities in the semen volume

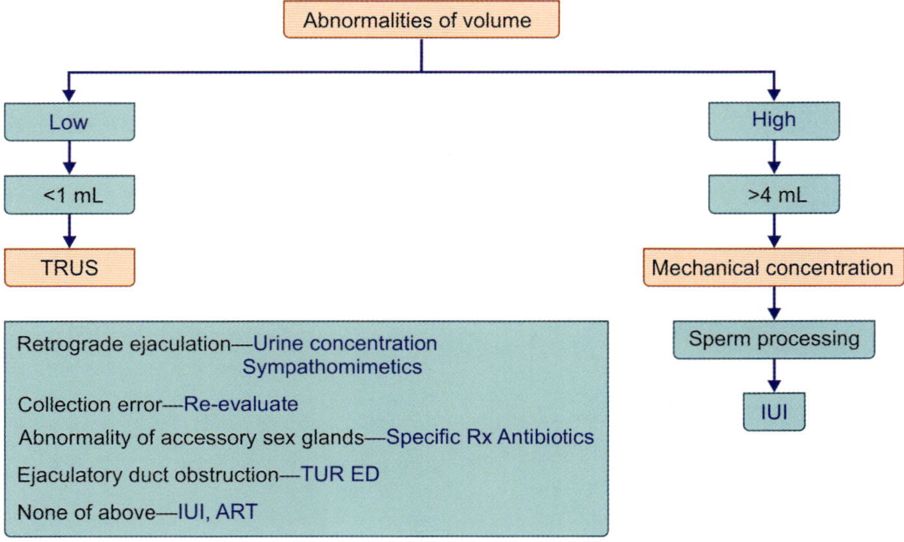

Sperm Concentration

According to the WHO manual, the sperm concentration should be 15 million/mL and the total number of sperms per ejaculate should be between 33 and 46 million. The diagnosis of azoospermia should be established only after the specimen is centrifuged (preferably at 3000 g) for 15 minutes and the pellet is examined meticulously under high power for presence of sperms.

The sperm concentration can be counted either using the hemocytometer **(Fig. 2)** or the Makler's chamber **(Fig. 3)**.

The advantage of the Makler's chamber is that, there is no need to dilute the semen sample as in a hemocytometer. Counting the total number of sperms in ten squares gives the total count **(Fig. 4)**.

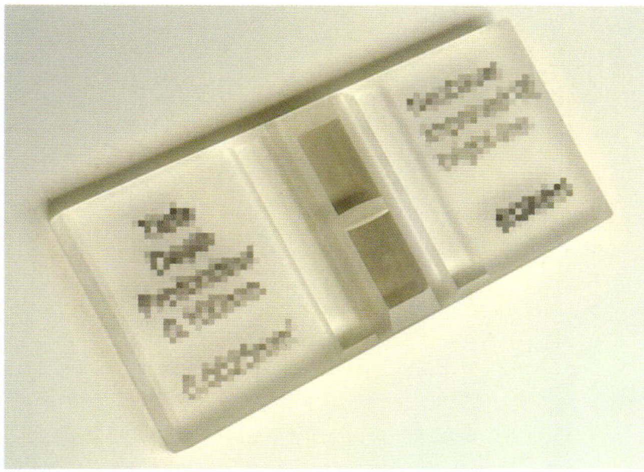

Fig. 2 Hemocytometer

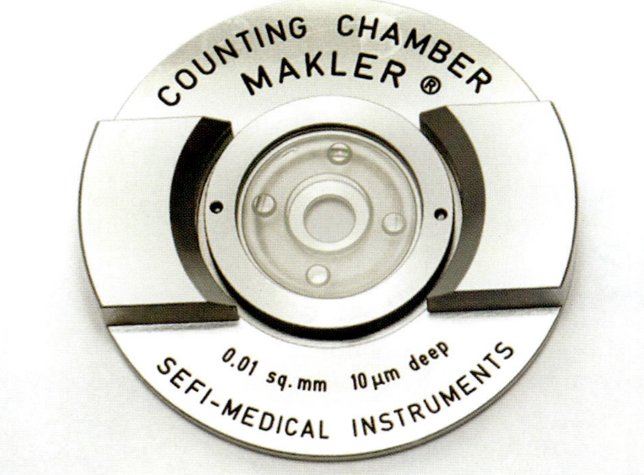

Fig. 3 Makler's chamber

Motility and Forward Progression

When we talk about motility one should consider kind and aggressiveness of movement (speed of forward progression), percentage of inactive and active spermatozoa (% motile) and duration of motility (in vitro) for at least for 24 hours.

The total motility, which includes progressive and nonprogressive motile sperms should be 40% and progressive motility, which included the rapid and slow linear should be 32%.

Progressive motility and total motile sperm count are important characteristics that determine the mode of therapy. Post-wash total motile count (TMC) represents the total number of motile sperm that are present after preparation and is one of the best parameters to choose treatment in patients with borderline count and motility. Total motile sperm count of 5 million/mL is a useful threshold value for decisions about treating a couple with IUI or IVF or intracytoplasmic sperm injection (ICSI). It was noted that no pregnancies occurred with IUI in cases with a total motile sperm count of less than 1 million/mL. Thus, IUI is effective therapy for male factor infertility when the:

- Total count is 10 million/mL,
- Initial sperm motility of greater than or equal to 30%, and
- Total motile sperm count is greater than or equal to 1 million.

Morphological Evaluation of Spermatozoa

According to the WHO 2010 criteria the normal forms should be 4%, but according to the strict Tygerberg Kruger criteria the normal forms should be 14%.

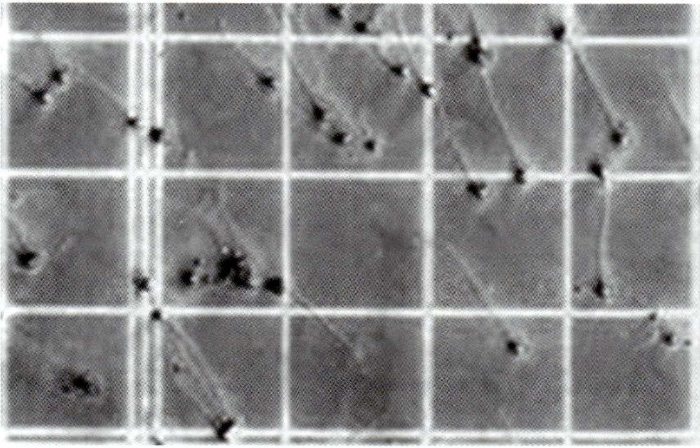

Fig. 4 Counting the total number of sperms in ten squares gives the total count

According to strict Tygerberg criteria, a normal spermatozoon should be:

- Oval form with a smooth contour
- An acrosome comprising between 40% and 70% of the distal part of the sperm head
- Without any abnormalities of the neck, mid-piece or tail
- No cytoplasmic droplets of more than half of the sperm head.

The teratozoospermia index (TZI) is a good predictor of fertilization and pregnancy rate. It is a multiple anomalies index, where a total of 100–200 sperms are counted and the record of normal and abnormal sperms kept. The abnormal sperms can have a maximal of four abnormalities and all these are noted down. Total number of all separate abnormalities is then divided by total number of abnormal spermatozoa counted and this gives the TZI. The normal TZI is less than 1.6 and a TZI of more than 1.85 requires ICSI irrespective of the count and motility.

Strict sperm morphology has been used to identify couples at risk for poor or failed fertilization using standard in vitro fertilization (IVF) techniques[9] and thus to identify those who may be candidates for ICSI.[10]

Sperm Viability Tests

Sperm viability can be assessed by mixing fresh semen with a supravital dye such as eosin Y or trypan blue, or by the use of the hypo-osmotic swelling (HOS) test.[8] Viability tests identify viable non-motile sperms. HOS identifies sperms that have intact cell membranes. When stained viable sperm actively exclude the dye and remain colorless **(Fig. 5A)**, while nonviable sperm **(Fig. 5B)** readily take up the stain. However, sperm judged viable by dye tests cannot be used for IVF. On the other hand with HOS test, viable non-motile sperm, which swell when incubated in a hypo-osmotic solution, can be used successfully for ICSI.[11] Viable non-motile sperm can also be identified by incubation in pentoxifylline. Viable sperm will develop motility after exposure to pentoxifylline.[12]

Semen Cytology

We need to looks for debris, white blood cells, polymorphs, epithelium cells, histiocytes and ghost cells (cytoplasm without a nucleus) **(Fig. 6A)** and premature germ cells **(Figs 6B and C)**. The white blood cells should be less than 1 million/mL and the premature germ cells should be less than 5 million/mL.

Increased numbers of white blood cells in semen have been associated with deficiencies in sperm function and motility. Under wet mount microscopy, leukocytes

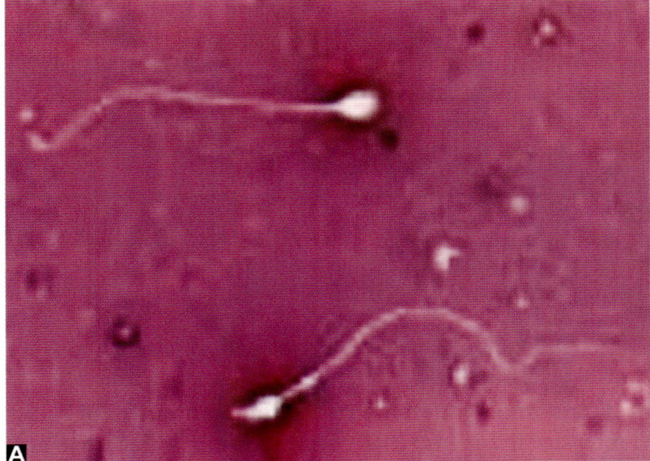
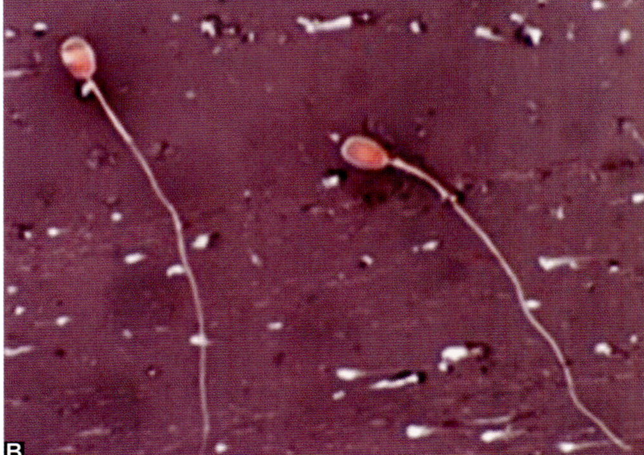

Figs 5A and B (A) Viable; and (B) Nonviable

and immature germ cells appear quite similar and are properly called 'round cells.' All andrology laboratories must ensure that the two types of cells are differentiated. The leukocytes can be differentiated from immature germ cells by traditional cytological staining and immunohistochemical techniques **(Figs 7A and B)**.[13] Men with true pyospermia (greater than 1 million leukocytes per mL) should be specifically evaluated to exclude genital tract infection or inflammation. They should also undergo semen culture with antibiotic sensitivity testing.

Semen Biochemistry

Specific analyses of semen biochemistry are relevant to accessory sex gland functions.

These include:

- Fructose from seminal vesicles
- Zinc and acid phosphatase from prostate gland
- Alpha-glycosidase and carnitine from epididymis.

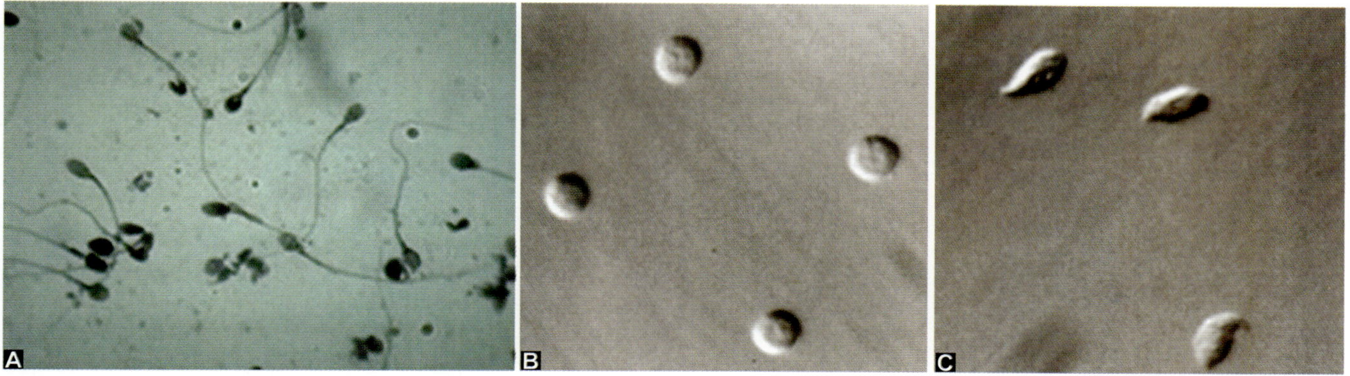

Figs 6A to C (A) Debris and WBCs; (B) Round spermatid; and (C) Elongated spermatid

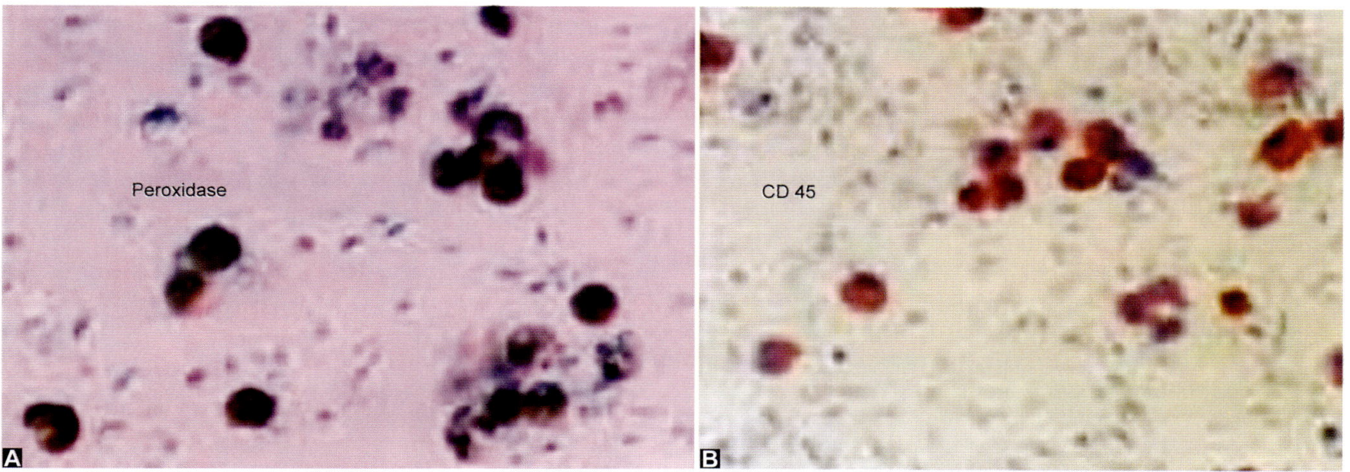

Figs 7A and B Differentiated from immature germ cells

The seminal fluid fructose has to be more than 13 mmol per ejaculate and the zinc levels should be more than 2.4 mmol per ejaculate. If epididymal dysfunction is suspected one could do seminal fluid alpha glucosidase levels, which should be more than 20 mU per ejaculate. Routine evaluation of glucosidase and carnitine levels is not required.

Agglutination

Sperm agglutination **(Figs 8A and B)** in the presence of normal count, motility and morphology can impair fertility in the male.

There are two types of agglutinations:

1. *Non-specific agglutination* where sperm adhere to cells present in the seminal plasma.
2. *Specific agglutination* **(Fig. 9)** which is caused by antisperm antibodies which can be detected by

immunobead test and mixed antiglobulin reaction (MAR test). Normally both these test have less than 50% sperm bound to the particles. Sperm-bound antibodies are thought to be clinically important because they can decrease motility, block penetration of the cervical mucus and prevent fertilization and thereby decrease the likelihood for conception.[14]

Sperm agglutination indirectly indicates the presence of sperm antibodies and is associated with infection (orchitis), testicular trauma, torsion and biopsy and history of vasectomy. Antisperm antibodies (ASA) **(Flow chart 6)** are a rare cause of male subfertility that do not require routine testing and are typically treated with ICSI though IUI may be tried but with a low success rate. ASAs can be found in the serum, seminal plasma, or bound directly to sperm. ASAs can form when there is a breach in the blood-testis barrier and the immune system is exposed to large quantities of sperm antigens. Men with

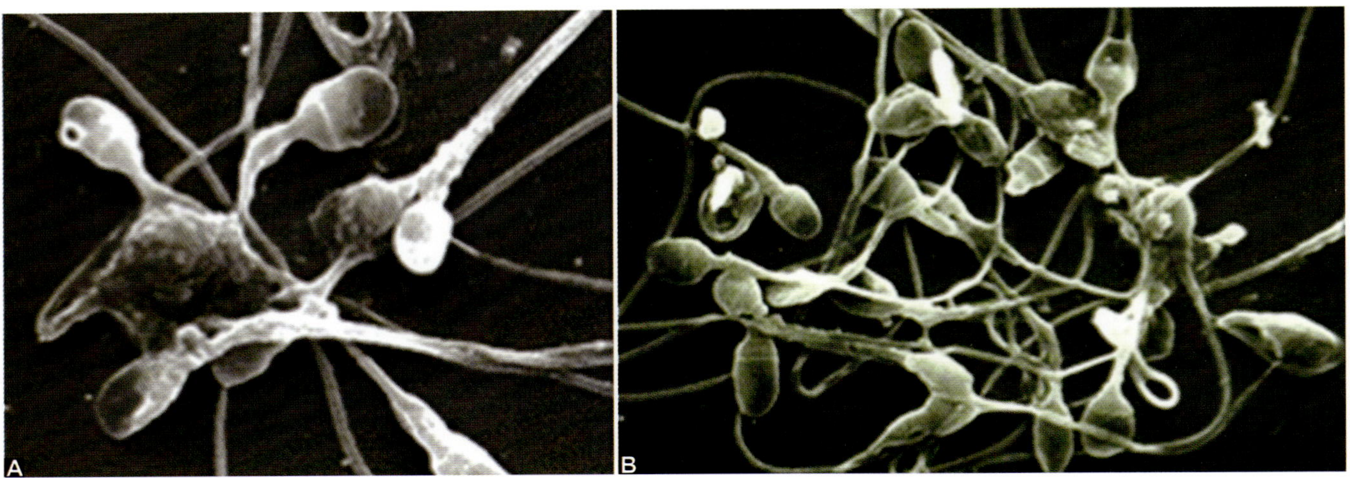

Figs 8A and B Sperm agglutination

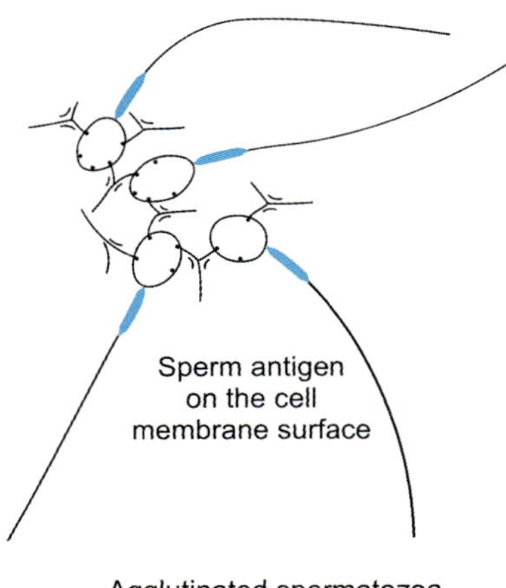

Fig. 9 Specific agglutination

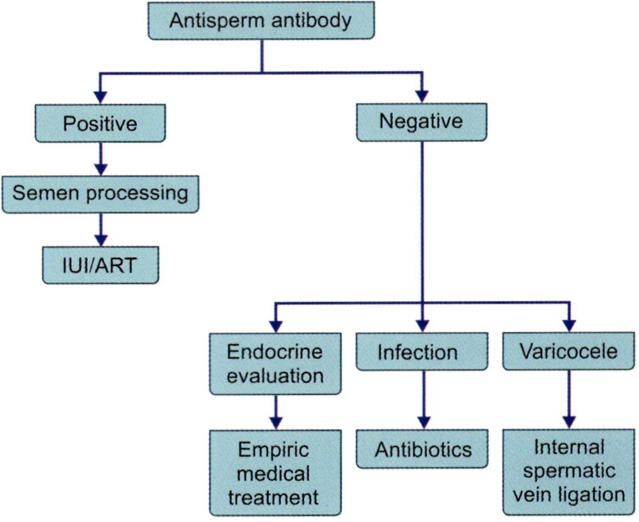

Flow chart 6 Evaluation of men with agglutination, pus cells and compromised motility

azoospermia and ASA are likely to have reproductive tract obstruction.[15]

Sperm Functional Assessment

Apart from count, progressive motility and morphology several other test like postcoital test (PCT), HOS, trial wash and sperm survival which determine quantitative and qualitative yields, computer-aided sperm analysis (CASA), mucus penetration test which can identify capable sperm population in semen, sperm DNA fragmentation (DFI) and reactive oxygen species (ROS) activity in the semen. Oxidative stress **(Fig. 10)** can result in lipid peroxidation, protein damage, biomembrane damage and sperm head DNA damage. This in turn can affect fertility, motility and gamete binding.

Sperm function test can diagnose some subtle changes in function by a particular test/assay, which helps clinically to direct therapy: which treatment is most appropriate and what are the chances of failure?

Postcoital Test

This test is based on the principle that penetration of sperm into cervical mucus can indicate defective cells.[16]

This test does not have a positive or negative predictive value for pregnancy and similar cumulative pregnancy

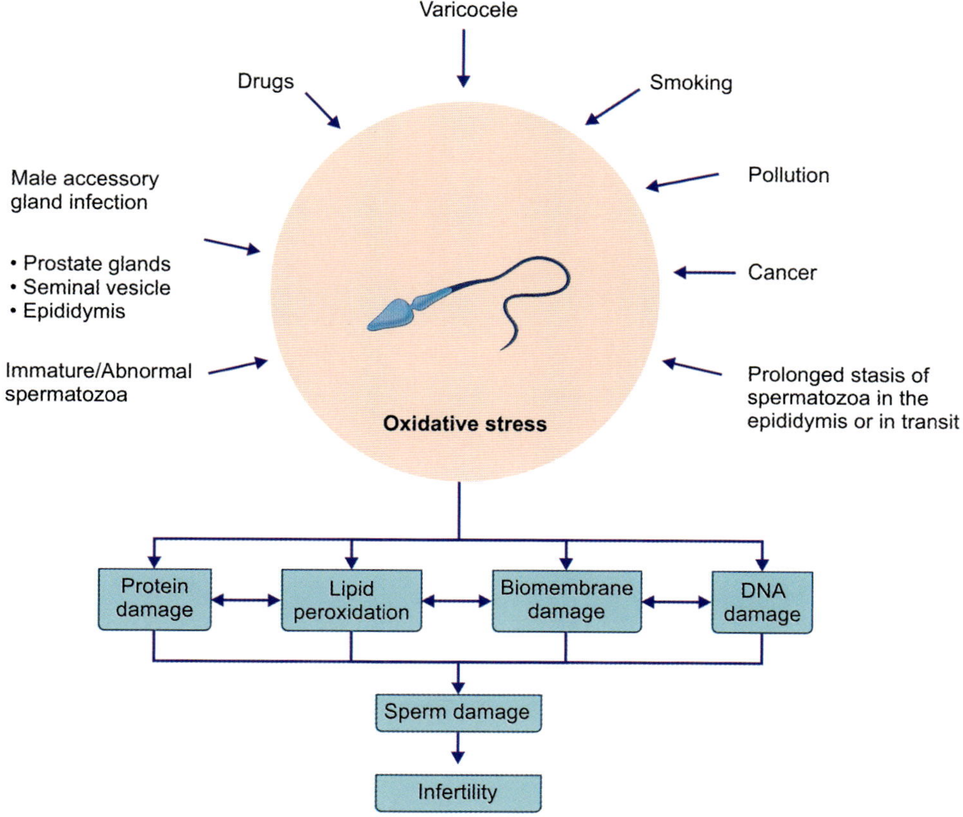

Fig. 10 Oxidative stress and male subfertility

rates were observed at 24 months when impact of infertility investigations with and without PCT were compared.[17]

It may be of value in the following conditions diagnosis of sexual dysfunction and ejaculatory problems. But results of PCT may have little effect on treatment strategy in the light of the widespread use of IUI for fertility problems in today's practice. Moreover, the lack of effective treatment for ASA may render PCT unnecessary.

Sperm Penetration Assays and Sperm Zona Binding Tests

Detect defects in sperm-fertilizing capacity and can identify patients who will benefit from ICSI. Oligozoospermic and severely teratospermic men have a higher number of defective sperm–zona pellucida interactions, which may account for their low fertility potential in both spontaneous and IVF pregnancies. However, today ICSI is routinely used during IVF for male-factor infertility couples, and in those who have failed to conceive with previous IUI or IVF cycles and so probably today this test is not done routinely. It is a significant problem in 35% of subfertile men with normal semen parameters.

Hypo-osmotic Swelling Test

It gives information on membrane integrity of sperm and is aimed at determining spermatozoa with intact plasma membrane. It has good correlation between spermatozoa showing positive HOS reaction and fertilization rate at in vitro fertilization (IVF). It has also been observed that surface toxin factor, which immobilizes the sperm are present in HOS negative sperms. Patients with good count and motility but less than 50% HOS positive sperms result in fertilization and cleavage with IVF, but the surface toxin factor is transferred to zona pellucida, which prevents implantation and so ICSI is preferred. Normally more than 60% of the sperms should show curling of the tail **(Fig. 11)** when subjected to HOS. This group can benefit with IUI or timed intercourse. Those with HOS between 50–60% are in the gray zone and may be subjected to IVF if the post-wash count is at least 10 million/mL. Those men

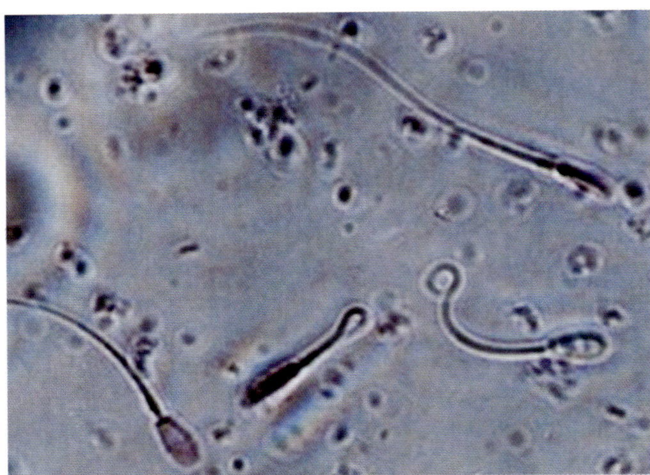

Fig. 11 Hypo-osmotic swelling

who have a HOS of less than 50% benefit with ICSI and should not undergo either IUI or IVF despite a good count and motility.

Trial Wash and Sperm Survival

Threshold value for decisions to treat with IUI or IVF or ICSI is a total motile sperm count of 5 million/mL. No pregnancies occurred with IUI in cases with a total motile sperm count of less than 1 million/mL.

Postwash Sperm Survival

Postprocessing sperm survival is a good determinant of the fertilizing potential of the sperms. A 24-hour survival should be more or equal to 70% for a couple to achieve pregnancy with IUI. If the survival is less, the couples would require some form of ART (IVF or ICSI).[18]

Acrosome Reaction

The acrosome reaction of human sperm can be detected using specialized staining techniques. Rates of spontaneous acrosome reactions and acrosome reactions induced by agents such as calcium ionophore and progesterone have been measured. Sperm from infertile men tend to demonstrate higher acrosome levels spontaneously, but lower levels in the presence of inducers.[19] It is labor-intensive and expensive and so may be recommended in cases of profound abnormalities of head morphology or in unexplained infertility and repeated IVF failures. The other inconsistencies when performing acrosome reaction are sperm capacitation conditions, methods used to induce acrosomal exocytosis, methods used to evaluate acrosome reaction. There were also differences in definition of thresholds for acrosome reaction and IVF rates. Acrosome reaction has a positive predictive value (PPV) of greater than or equal to 75% but the negative predictive value (NPV) tended to be more variable. It has a sensitivity of 80% with little more than 20% false positive rate.[20]

Acrosin Activity Test

Acrosin is serine protease-like enzyme that exhibits a lectin like carbohydrate binding activity to the zona pellucida glycoproteins. Low acrosin activity has been associated with low sperm density, motility and poor normal morphology.

Computer-assisted Sperm Analysis (CASA)

It is a semi-automated technique with high precision and gives the quantitative assessment of sperm kinetics. It also provides data on sperm density, motility, straight line and curvilinear velocity, linearity, and average path velocity, amplitude of lateral head displacement, flagellar beat frequency and hyperactivation. Predictive statistics demonstrated low specificity and sensitivity and a high rate of false positives.

But according to evidence based medicine, CASA is not superior to conventional semen analysis (Grade A). The disadvantages of CASA are following:

- Sperm concentration, sample preparation and frame rate can affect accuracy of CASA
- Stains used also affect the accuracy of determining morphology
- Does not add any advantages in clinical practice
- Requires expensive equipment and still requires the active participation of a technician.

Sperm DNA Fragmentation Tests

DNA integrity is important for normal embryo development. Sperm DNA integrity is maintained in part by the effect of disulfide cross-links between protamines that allow for the compaction of chromatin in the nucleus. Sperm DNA damage can occur as a result of necrosis, apoptosis, oxidative stress and alteration in sperm chromatin packaging **(Fig. 12)**.

Sperm DNA damage can occur as a result of intrinsic factors, such as protamine deficiency and mutations affecting DNA compaction, or from extrinsic factors such as heat, radiation, and gonadotoxins **(Flow chart 7)**.

A number of clinical tests have been developed to measure sperm DNA fragmentation rates **(Fig. 13)**. Direct methods, such as the single-cell gel electrophoresis assay (Comet assay) and terminal deoxynucleotidyl transferase

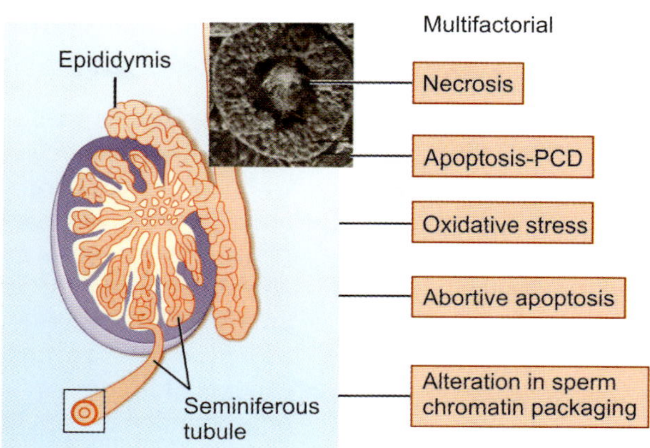

Fig. 12 Etiology of sperm DNA damage

Flow chart 7 Causes of sperm DNA fragmentation

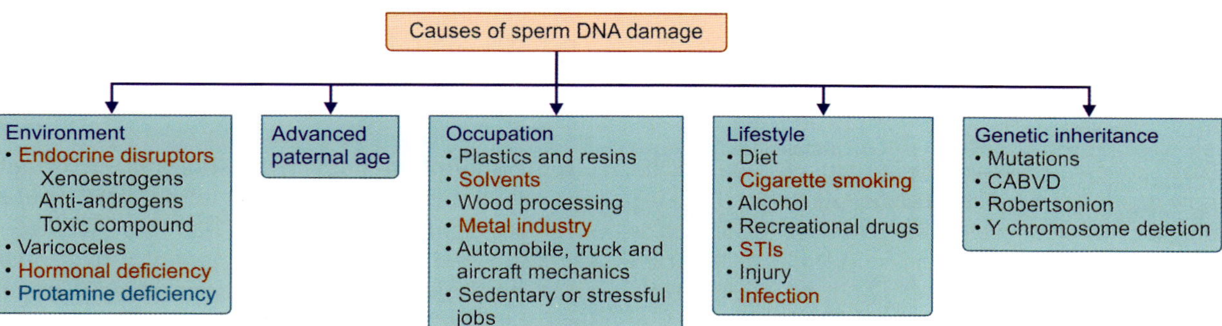

Detection of sperm DNA damage

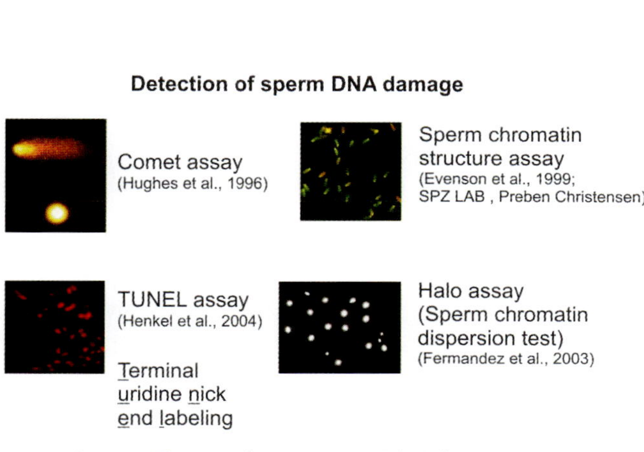

Fig. 13 Tests to detect sperm DNA fragmentation

dUTP nick end labeling (TUNEL) assays, specifically analyze the number of breaks in the DNA. Indirect tests like the sperm chromatin structure assay (SCSA) define abnormal chromatin structure as an increased susceptibility of sperm DNA to acid-induced denaturation in situ.[21]

Threshold values used to define an abnormal test are greater than or equal to 25–27% for the SCSA[22] and greater than or equal to 36% for TUNEL assays[23] and greater than 30% for Comet assay.

Infertile men, especially those with abnormal semen parameters have increased DNA damage. It was also observed that 8% of infertile men have abnormal DNA integrity despite normal semen parameters (concentration, motility, and morphology). There is evidence linking sperm DNA fragmentation to poor reproductive outcome with impact on embryo/blastocyst development, progress of pregnancy and pregnancy loss. It has been observed that nuclear DNA anomalies lead to failure of fertilization in IVF, failure to implant in ICSI cycles and increased time to conception. It is important to remember that all spermatozoa are not equally exposed to the risk of DNA damage.

The existing data relating to the relationship between abnormal DNA integrity and reproductive outcomes are too limited to routinely recommend any of these tests for males in an infertile couple, but the effect of abnormal sperm DNA fragmentation on the value of IUI or IVF and ICSI results may be clinically informative.[24]

Indications for DFI Testing: The test should be offered before IVF/ICSI to male partners of couples with a history of:
- Unexplained or persistent infertility
- Failure to conceive after 5–6 IUI cycles despite good count and motility
- Low fertilization rates or poor embryo quality in IVF cycles
- Implantation failure after IVF
- Recurrent miscarriage
- Prolonged stay in an environment that exposes to reproductive toxins
- Abnormal semen analysis
- Advancing male age (>45 years).

High levels of sperm DNA damage have some correlation with oligozoospermia,[25-34] poor motility and morphology oligoasthenoteratozoospermia (OAT) cytoplasmic retention and mitochondrial DNA damage.

Relationship between sperm DNA damage and pregnancy:
- In IUI: strong negative effect (OR = 9.9)
- In IVF : mild negative effect (OR = 1.7)
- In ICSI: no effect (OR = 1.2).

Thus, increasing intervention from IUI to IVF to ICSI, the less impact sperm DNA damage has on early fertility check points. But in both in IVF and ICSI pregnancy loss, DNA damage has a moderate positive effect (OR = 2.5).[35] Sperm retrieved from the testis tend to have better sperm DNA quality in men with abnormal ejaculated sperm DNA integrity. Because the prognostic clinical value of DNA integrity testing may not affect treatment of couples, the routine use of DNA integrity tests in the clinical evaluation of male factor infertility is controversial.[36]

Estimation of Sperm Creatine Kinase and Reactive Oxygen Species (ROS)[34]

Reactive oxygen species (ROS) appear to be generated by both seminal leukocytes and sperm cells and can interfere with sperm function by peroxidation of sperm lipid membranes and creation of toxic fatty acid peroxides.[37] Leukocytes or WBCs are the main source of ROS, though abnormal spermatozoa are minor source of ROS, and they are caused by retention of cytoplasmic droplets during defective spermiogenesis. Smoking, alcohol abuse and exposure to radiation and toxic chemicals can also result in production of high ROS.

Increased levels are seen in subfertile males. The assays include a gelatinolysis technique and spectrophotometric assay. Its activity has been correlated inversely with low fertility rates in IVF and is good predictor of IVF success, independent of sperm morphology.

High ROS levels causes sperm damage by lipid peroxidation of the plasma membrane, germ cell apoptosis, and DNA strand breakage resulting in the passage of defective paternal DNA to conceptus. It can also result in damage to sperm membrane, decreasing sperm motility and its ability to fuse with the oocyte.

Estimation of sperm creatine kinase has similar prediction value as ROS.

Research Setting

Other tests and procedures have been used to select sperm for ICSI and may identify gametes with better quality, including hyaluronic acid binding, membrane maturity testing, apoptotic evaluation, and magnified sperm examination.[38] However, these tests have a very limited role in the evaluation of male infertility because they have limited clinical utility and typically do not affect treatment.

Sperm function test should not be routine investigations as they are complex, expensive, not rigorously tested, do not always provide clinically useful information and typically do not affect treatment.[39]

Extended Screening in Male Subfertility

When the initial screening evaluation reveals an abnormal male reproductive history or demonstrates abnormal semen parameters, a thorough evaluation by an andrologist is indicated. More detailed evaluation of the male partner is also important in couples with unexplained infertility and those who remain infertile after successful treatment of identified female infertility factors.

The more thorough evaluation for male infertility should include a complete medical history and physical examination performed by an andrologist and based on the clinical findings, additional tests and procedures may be recommended. These tests may include serial semen analyses, endocrine evaluation [FSH, LH, total and free testosterone, prolactin, thyroid stimulating hormone (TSH), SHBG, inhibin B and anti-Müllerian hormone (AMH)], postejaculatory urinalysis, ultrasonography (scrotal and transrectal), specialized tests on semen and sperm, genetic screening [karyotyping, "Y" chromosome microdeletion and congenital bilateral aplasia of the vasa deferens (CBAVD) and CF gene mutations] and testicular biopsy.

Reproductive and Sexual History

The reproductive history should include coital frequency and timing, duration of infertility and prior fertility, childhood illnesses and developmental history, systemic medical illnesses (such as diabetes mellitus and upper respiratory diseases), previous surgery, medications and allergies, history of sexually transmitted infections, exposure to gonadal toxins (including environmental and chemical toxins and heat) and past or current use of anabolic steroids, recreational drugs, tobacco, and alcohol.

Physical Examination and Ultrasound

Physical examination and ultrasound (scrotal and transrectal ultrasound) is recommended in cases of abnormal male history, abnormal semen analysis, unexplained infertility and treated female factor with persistent infertility. At the onset, it is important to look for secondary sexual characteristics (body habitus, hair distribution, and breast development) followed by detailed examination of the penis (length, defects and location of external urethral meatus) and testis (size and consistency), examination for the presence and consistency of vas and epididymis, evaluation of the pampiniformis plexus and a transrectal examination for accessory glands, seminal vesicles and prostate. Today for diagnosis of CBAVD, physical examination is enough and scrotal exploration is unnecessary.

Ultrasonography

Ultrasonography is a useful tool for detecting abnormalities of the male genital tract that may adversely affect fertility but is usually indicated only in a small fraction of cases.

Transrectal ultrasonography (TRUS) helps in detecting abnormalities of the seminal vesicle, prostate and ejaculatory duct. TRUS may be recommended in all oligospermic men having low volume ejaculates, palpable vasa, and normal testicular size with normal serum testosterone. One could diagnose complete or partial ejaculatory duct obstruction in the presence of dilated seminal vesicles or ejaculatory ducts and/or midline cystic prostatic structures.[40,41]

Men with ejaculatory duct obstruction usually produce a low volume, acidic ejaculate containing no sperm or fructose. Men with CBAVD may exhibit similar findings because they often have absent or atrophic seminal vesicles. Men with partial ejaculatory duct obstruction exhibit low semen volume, oligoasthenospermia, and poor progressive motility.

Scrotal Ultrasonography

Normally a careful physical examination by the clinician can identify most scrotal pathology, including varicoceles, spermatoceles, absent vasa, epididymal induration, and testicular masses. Scrotal ultrasonography can identify occult varicoceles that are not palpable, but evidence has showed that such lesions have no clinical significance.[36] Scrotal ultrasonography can be helpful for better defining vague or ambiguous physical examination findings or abnormalities (including apparent masses) and can be performed in men having testes located in the upper scrotum, a small scrotal sac, or other anatomy that hinders physical examination. Testicular ultrasonography is useful for men presenting with infertility and risk factors for testicular cancer, such as cryptorchidism or a previous testicular neoplasm.

Endocrine Evaluation

Endocrine evaluation identifies abnormalities of the hypothalamic-pituitary-testicular axis. It is indicated for men having abnormal semen parameters, particularly when the sperm concentration is below 10 million/mL, impaired sexual function and in the presence of other clinical findings that suggest a specific endocrinopathy.

The minimum initial hormonal evaluation should include measurement of serum FSH and total testosterone concentrations. When the total testosterone level is low (< 300 ng/mL), a more extensive evaluation is indicated and should include a second measurement of total testosterone and measurements of serum free testosterone, LH, prolactin, SHBG and TSH. Most men with abnormal spermatogenesis have a normal serum FSH level, a markedly elevated serum FSH concentration clearly indicates an abnormality in spermatogenesis.

Recently, the serum inhibin B and AMH concentration has emerged as a marker for spermatogenesis. Inhibin B levels are significantly lower in infertile men than in fertile men and correlate better with sperm parameters than FSH levels.[42,43] Levels correlate with testicular cytology but are not superior to FSH as predictors of the presence of sperm in testicular sperm extraction (TESE)/fine-needle aspiration (FNA) in men with azoospermia. It was also observed that stimulated levels of serum inhibin B and AMH levels do not add clinically relevant information in subfertile men compared to basal levels of these hormones.

Postejaculatory Urinalysis

A low volume or absent antegrade ejaculate suggests incomplete semen collection, retrograde ejaculation, lack of emission, ejaculatory duct obstruction, hypogonadism, or CBAVD. To exclude retrograde ejaculation, a post-ejaculatory urinalysis should be performed in men having an ejaculate volume less than 1.0 mL, except in those diagnosed with hypogonadism or CBAVD. Before advising examination of postejaculate urine it is important to determine whether there was an improper or incomplete collection or a very short abstinence interval (less than 1 day) might be the cause.

The postejaculatory urinalysis is performed by centrifuging the urine specimen for 10 minutes at 300 g, followed by microscopic examination of the pellet at 400 magnification. In men with azoospermia or aspermia, the presence of any sperm in the postejaculatory urinalysis suggests retrograde ejaculation. In men with low ejaculate volume and oligospermia, 'significant numbers' of sperm must be observed to support the diagnosis of retrograde ejaculation; there is no consensus of expert opinion on the minimum number required.

Genetic Screening

Normal sperm morphology is not always indicative of euploidy. Genetic abnormalities can cause infertility by affecting sperm production or sperm transport. Men with nonobstructive azoospermia (NOA) and severe oligospermia (<5 million/mL) are more likely to have.

The prevalence of chromosomal abnormalities is 10–15% in azoospermic men (approximately 5% in men with severe oligospermia (< 5 million/mL), and less than 1% in men with normal sperm concentrations.[44]

Genetic screening includes karyotyping to rule out numerical chromosomal abnormalities like Klinefelters syndrome XXY **(Fig. 14)** and its variants, which accounts for about two-third of all chromosomal abnormalities observed in infertile men.[45]

The prevalence of structural autosomal abnormalities, such as inversions and balanced translocations is also higher in infertile men than in the general population.[46]

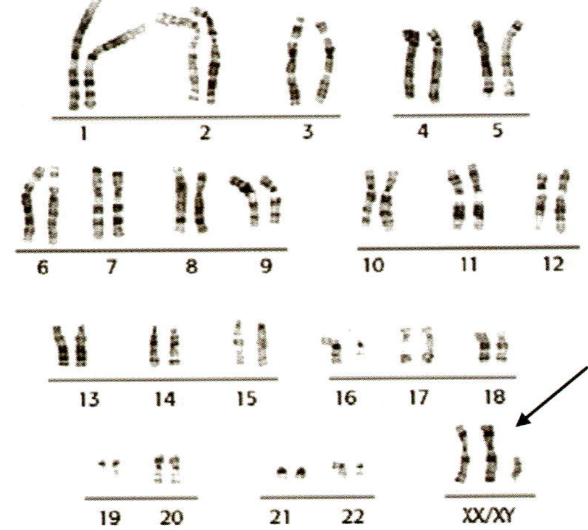

Fig. 14 Karyotype of a male with Klinefelter's syndrome

Moreover, those couples where the male partner has gross karyotypic abnormality are at increased risk for miscarriages and having children with chromosomal and congenital defects. Therefore, all men with non-obstructive azoospermia or severe oligospermia should be evaluated with a karyotype before using their sperm to perform ICSI.

Molecular genetics (polymerase chain reaction techniques to analyze sequence tagged sites) is required to identify Y chromosome micro-deletions that are associated with isolated defects in spermatogenesis and abnormality of the cystic fibrosis trans-membrane conductance regulator (CFTR) gene in men with CBAVD. These tests are important to identify genetic causes for infertility and have a major impact on the choice and outcome of treatment.

Y chromosome micro-deletions have been found in 7% of infertile men with severely impaired spermatogenesis and 16% with azoospermia as compared with 2% of normal men.[47] Therefore, it must be offered to those men who have NOA or severe oligospermia before performing ICSI with their sperm.

Most deletions causing azoospermia or oligospermia occur in regions of the long arm of the Y chromosome (Yq11) known as the AZF regions, designated as AZFa (proximal), AZFb (central), and AZFc (distal). AZFa, AZFb and AZFc were established as the Y chromosome regions regulating spermatogenesis. Subsequent DNA sequencing approaches demonstrated that these regions harbor a total of 12 different genes/gene families necessary for spermatogenesis.[48-50]

For example, the DAZ (deleted in azoospermia) gene, which encodes a transcription factor usually present in men with normal fertility, is located in the AZFc region.

The specific location of the deletion along the Y chromosome will influences the prognosis and help in deciding the further line of treatment. The deletions involving the entire AZFa and AZFb region appear to predict a very poor prognosis for sperm retrieval.[51,52]

Men with microdeletion in the AZFc region of the Y chromosome have severe oligospermia or azoospermic but still may produce sufficient numbers of sperm to allow TESE.[53]

When ICSI is done with testicular sperm in men with AZFc microdeletion of Y chromosome, it is important to counsel the couple that the male progeny could inherit the abnormality and thus be infertile.[54]

Absence of Y chromosome micro;deletion does not rule out genetic abnormality, because there may be other, currently unknown, gene sequences on the Y or other chromosomes that also might be required for normal spermatogenesis.

There is a strong association between CBAVD and mutations of the cystic fibrosis gene mutations (CFTR) gene, which is located on chromosome 7.[55]

Almost all men with clinical cystic fibrosis exhibit CBAVD and 80% of men with CBAVD have documented mutations of the CFTR gene. Failure to detect a CFTR abnormality in men with CBAVD does not exclude the presence of a mutation that cannot be identified with currently available methods. Therefore, men with CBAVD should be assumed to have a CFTR gene mutation. The risk of conceiving a child affected with CF is higher if the female partner is also a carrier.

The prevalence of CFTR mutations also is increased among men with azoospermia related to congenital bilateral obstruction of the epididymides and those with unilateral vasa agenesis. Consequently, genetic evaluation should be considered for those having either abnormality. Some men are presented with either unilateral or bilateral vasal agenesis, and unilateral renal agenesis have the mesonephric duct abnormalities associated with hereditary renal adysplasia (HRA) which has an autosomal dominant form of inheritance with incomplete penetrance and variable expression. These patients do not have CFTR mutations and require genetic counseling prior to IVF.[56,57]

Sperm Chromosome Aneuploidy

Sperm DNA aneuploidy can be assessed by fluorescent in situ hybridization (FISH) technology.[58] Men with karyotypic abnormalities, severely abnormal sperm morphology, and NOA have highest risk of sperm aneuploidy.[58] Men presenting with infertility and a normal karyotype had an increased frequency of meiotic alterations detectable in their sperm and one study reported an incidence of 6%.[59] Patients with recurrent pregnancy loss and recurrent IVF failure may also benefit from sperm aneuploidy testing.[60,61] But the cost, inability to screen the actual sperm used in ICSI, and difficulty in assigning a meaningful risk assessment to couples based on the test results has limited its use in routine evaluation of the male partner.[62]

Testicular Biopsy

When sperm retrieval for ICSI is considered in azoospermic men a testicular biopsy should be performed for prognostic purposes to determine whether spermatozoa are likely to be retrieved via testicular aspiration or extraction. Presence or absence of sperm in a biopsy specimen does not predict absolutely whether sperm are present elsewhere within that testicle. Today there is no consensus on which group of patients will benefit with testicular biopsy. The FSH and inhibin B values do not serve as a marker, which will prognosticate the outcome of testicular biopsy. A diagnostic testicular biopsy may be indicated in men having a normal serum FSH concentration an average or just smaller than normal size testis. This is because it has been observed that the incidence of obtaining sperms from the biopsy specimen is very low in the presence of high FSH and low inhibin B levels and when the testicular size is very small and the consistency is very soft. A unilateral or bilateral testicular biopsy can be done; though currently no clear consensus of opinion on the issue. If a unilateral biopsy is performed, it should be on the larger testis.

Moreover it is important that the testicular biopsy should be done only where facilities are available for cryopreservation of the testicular sample in case sperms are obtained. These frozen sperms can then be used for ICSI without repeating the biopsy. Testicular biopsy also helps in differentiating obstructive from NOA. Thus testicular biopsy serves as a diagnostic as well as therapeutic procedure in this group of patients.

A normal testicular biopsy implies obstruction at some level in the reproductive system, and the location must then be determined. Most men with obstructive azoospermia that cannot be attributed to iatrogenic vasal injury have bilateral epididymal obstruction, which can be confirmed by surgical exploration. Vasography may help to identify obstruction in the vas deferens or ejaculatory ducts. Due to the risk for vasal scarring and obstruction, vasography should not be performed at the time of diagnostic testicular biopsy unless reconstructive surgery is performed at the same time.

Testicular biopsy can be performed using a standard open incision technique called as TESE or by percutaneous testicular sperm aspiration (TESA) **(Figs 15A to C)**. Open testicular biopsy performed under local anesthesia and can be from a single site **(Fig. 15B)** or multiple sites **(Fig. 15C)**. It was introduced by Silber in 1995.[63,64] The single site has an advantage that it avoids multiple testicular incisions and thus prevents injury to testicular arteries which are end-arteries. Injury at biopsy may result in partial testicular infarction if multiple incisions are taken.[65]

Testicular fine-needle aspiration or TESA was introduced in 1995 by Bourne. In obstructive azoospermia (OA), it usually allows sperm retrieval sufficient for ICSI, but not for cryopreservation but in NOA there may be no recovery of sperms. One of the complications of TESA is intratesticular hematoma which has been reported in 7% of cases.[66]

Sperm recovery rate (SRR) in NOA is 51.3% with TESE and 21.1% with TESA. TESA is not indicated in NOA because of its low sperm retrieval rate and it works only in cases of hypospermatogenesis.[67]

The overall SRR was 54% by mTESE and 10% by FNA, whereas total complication rate following mTESE was 10% in the early phase and none in the long-term follow-up compared to 24% of FNA.[68] Thus, mTESE is superior to FNA as regards SRR and lower incidence of complications in NOA patients.

At histology in a TESE samples from NOA more than 50% men with germinal failure have minute foci of spermatogenesis, which are insufficient to produce spermatozoa in the ejaculate. It is also observed that incomplete testicular failure may involve a sparse multifocal distribution of spermatogenesis throughout the entire testicle.[63,64]

Predictor for Sperm Recovery

- Histology of testicular biopsy gives information on pattern of spermatogenesis and is predictive of the likelihood of finding sperm in TESE procedure in 85% of patients (HR 12:2422)
- AZF 'Y' deletion site (AZFc SRR good)
- FSH not predictive (but may be helpful)
- Inhibin B? – some recent data doubted its value.

■ DISCUSSION

An initial screening evaluation of the male partner should be done if pregnancy has not occurred within one year of unprotected intercourse. An earlier evaluation may be warranted if a known male or female infertility risk factor exists or if a male wants to know about his fertility potential. The initial evaluation should include a detailed semen analysis and if abnormal repeated after one month. If abnormality persist a comprehensive history taking, complete physical examination and further evaluations by ultrasound (scrotal, transrectal), hormonal test (FSH and serum testosterone), sperm function test (sperm DNA fragmentation testing, acrosome reaction, ROS) and testicular biopsy is warranted. Scrotal ultrasonography is indicated for men whose physical examination is difficult or inadequate and when a testicular mass is suspected. TRUS is indicated for men with oligospermia, low volume ejaculates, palpable vasa, ejaculatory duct obstruction, azoospermia, low ejaculate volumes and normal testicular size. A postejaculatory urinalysis is indicated for men having an ejaculate volume less than 1.0 mL, except in those diagnosed with hypogonadism or CBAVD. Sperm function test are useful investigative tools but are not recommended for the routine evaluation of infertile men. There is a higher

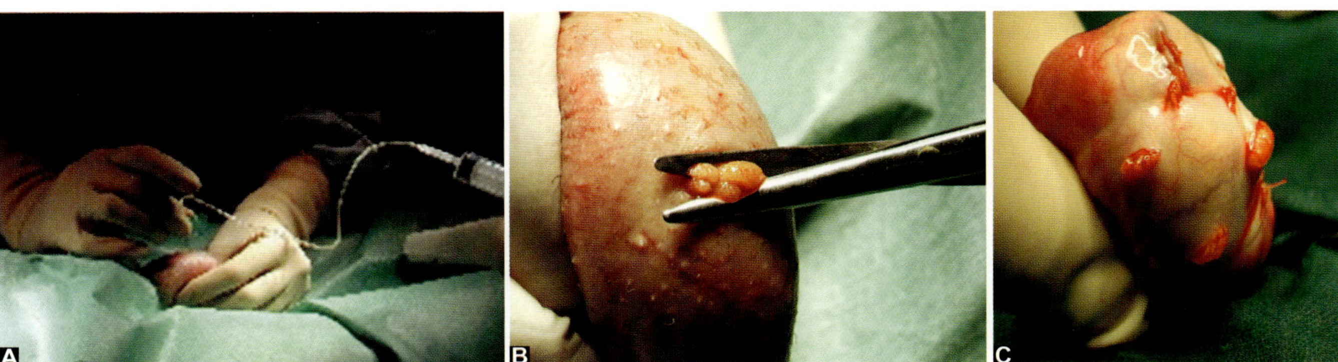

Figs 15A to C (A) Testicular sperm aspiration; (B and C) Testicular sperm extraction

incidence of genetic abnormality in men with NOA or severe oligospermia (<5 million/mL) and therefore should be offered karyotype and Y chromosome analysis before performing ICSI using their sperm. Genetic testing for CFTR mutations is done in men with CBAVD. This test should also be offered to the female partner of men with CBAVD before proceeding with treatments that use sperm from the affected man. Genetic counseling is offered to all couples where the male or female partner has a suspected genetic abnormality. Diagnostic testicular biopsy may be indicated for men having normal sized testicles with azoospermia, and a normal serum FSH concentration.

Although each sperm parameter could predict fertility and subfertility, none was a powerful discriminator. It is important to remember that normal reference values for semen parameters projected in the WHO 2010 manual do not reflect normal sperm concentration in the general population, nor do they equate with the minimum values required for conception. This is because men with semen variables outside the reference ranges may be fertile and, conversely, men having values within the reference range still may be infertile.

Problems of WHO 2010 Reference Limits

- Lowered reference limits calculated from results on semen provided by recent fathers and men in a general population who are not subfertile.[69]
- Data was collected during a long period of time, and external quality control not been implemented in all contributing laboratories thus the validity of the suggested reference limits can be questioned.[70]
- Data came from studies on semen samples obtained after 2–7 days of abstinence and so reference values were not standardized.
- Ejaculate volume, and sperm concentration in particular, increase considerably with each day of increasing abstinence.[71,72]

■ CONCLUSION

Etiology of azoospermia and severe oligospermia in most cases is idiopathic and can affect the clinical outcome. One must remember that spermatogenesis cannot be readily altered for therapeutic benefit. Further investigations for specific spermatozoal factors will contribute to the development of novel and more personalized approaches to test and treat male factor infertility. Thus the main problem to be solved in future is effective treatment of defective sperm production or function. Till then we need to identify as far as possible the underlying etiology and in cases of azoospermia predicting the chances of finding

spermatozoa from the testis. Predictions of results are often unreliable and a final answer can frequently only be achieved only after the couple undergoes treatment. This makes it essential for us to counsel patients desiring paternity.

The end-point of the infertile male evaluation is to find, if possible, pathology for the problem and to see if any specific treatment is available. Our goal should be to achieve spontaneous pregnancy and reduce the need for ART, downgrade the level of ART needed and increase the pregnancy rates when ART is unavoidable.

■ REFERENCES

1. Stephen EH, Chandra A. Declining estimates of infertility in the United States: 1982-2002. Fertil Steril. 2006;86:516-23.
2. Thonneau P, Marchand S, Tallec A, et al. Incidence and main causes of infertility in a resident population (1,850,000) of three French regions (1988-1989). Hum Reprod. 1991;6:811-6.
3. Vogt PH. Molecular genetics of human male infertility: from genes to new therapeutic perspectives. Curr Pharm Des. 2004; 10:471-500.
4. Practice Committee of American Society for Reproductive M. Definitions of infertility and recurrent pregnancy loss. Fertil Steril. 2008;90:S60.
5. Marshburn PB, Alanis M, Matthews ML, et al. A short period of ejaculatory abstinence before intrauterine insemination is associated with higher pregnancy rates. Fertil Steril. 2010;93:286-8.
6. Jurema MW, Vieira AD, Bankowski B, et al. Effect of ejaculatory abstinence period on the pregnancy rate after intrauterine insemination. Fertil Steril. 2005;84:678-81.
7. Raziel A, Friedler S, Schachter M, et al. Influence of a short or long abstinence period on semen parameters in the ejaculate of patients with nonobstructive azoospermia. Fertil Steril. 2001;76:485-90.
8. World Health Organization. WHO laboratory manual for the examination and processing of human semen, 2010. Available at: http://www.who.int /reproductivehealth/publications/ infertility/9789241547789/en/index.html. [Accessed on May 2012].
9. Kruger TF, Acosta AA, Simmons KF, et al. Predictive value of abnormal sperm morphology in in vitro fertilization. Fertil Steril. 1988;49:112-7.
10. Pisarska MD, Casson PR, Cisneros PL, et al. Fertilization after standard in vitro fertilization versus intracytoplasmic sperm injection in subfertile males using sibling oocytes. Fertil Steril. 1999;71:627-32.
11. Liu J, Tsai YL, Katz E, et al. High fertilization rate obtained after intracytoplasmic sperm injection with 100% nonmotile spermatozoa selected by using a simple modified hypo-osmotic swelling test. Fertil Steril. 1997;68:373-5.
12. de Mendoza MV, Gonzalez-Utor AL, Cruz N, et al. In situ use of pentoxifylline to assess sperm vitality in intracytoplasmic sperm injection for treatment of patients with total lack of sperm movement. Fertil Steril. 2000;74:176-7.

13. Wolff H, Anderson DJ. Immunohistologic characterization and quantitation of leukocyte subpopulations in human semen. Fertil Steril. 1988;49:497-504.

14. Ayvaliotis B, Bronson R, Rosenfeld D, et al. Conception rates in couples where autoimmunity to sperm is detected. Fertil Steril. 1985;43:739-42.

15. Lee R, Goldstein M, Ullery BW, et al. Value of serum antisperm antibodies in diagnosing obstructive azoospermia. J Urol. 2009;181:264-9.

16. Barratt CLR, Osborn JC, Harrison PE, et al. The hypo-osmotic swelling test and the sperm mucus penetration test in determining fertilization of the human oocyte. Hum Reprod. 1989;4:430-4

17. Oei SG, Helmerhorst FM, Keirse MJ. When is the post-coital test normal? A critical appraisal. Hum Reprod. 1995;10:1711-4.

18. Branigan EF, Estes MA, Muller CH. Advanced semen analysis: a simple screening test to predict intrauterine insemination success. Fertil Steril. 1999;71(3):547-51.

19. Fenichel P, Donzeau M, Farahifar D, et al. Dynamics of human sperm acrosome reaction: relation with in vitro fertilization. Fertil Steril. 1991;55:994-9.

20. Sergio Oehninger, Daniel R Franken, Ellen Sayed, et al. Sperm function assays and their predictive value for fertilization outcome in IVF therapy: a meta-analysis. Hum Reprod Update. 2000;6(2):160-8.

21. Evenson DP, Jost LK, Marshall D, et al. Utility of the sperm chromatin structure assay as a diagnostic and prognostic tool in the human fertility clinic. Hum Reprod. 1999;14:1039-49.

22. Larson-Cook KL, Brannian JD, Hansen KA, et al. Relationship between the outcomes of assisted reproductive techniques and sperm DNA fragmentation as measured by the sperm chromatin structure assay. Fertil Steril. 2003;80:895-902.

23. Henkel R, Hajimohammad M, Stalf T, et al. Influence of deoxyribonucleic acid damage on fertilization and pregnancy. Fertil Steril. 2004;81:965-72.

24. Collins JA, Barnhart KT, Schlegel PN. Do sperm DNA integrity tests predict pregnancy with in vitro fertilization? Fertil Steril. 2008;89:823-31.

25. Irvine DS, Twigg JP, Gordon EL, et al. DNA integrity in human sperm: relationships with semen quality. J Androl. 2000;21:33-44.

26. Menezo YJ, El Mouatassim S, Chavrier M, et al. Human oocytes and preimplantation embryos express mRNA for growth hormone receptor. Zygote. 2003;11:293-7.

27. Schmid TE, Kamischke A, Bollwein H, et al. Genetic damage in oligozoospermic patients detected by fluorescence in situ hybridization, inverse restriction site mutation assay, sperm chromatin structure assay and the Comet assay. Hum Reprod. 2003;18:1474-80.

28. O'Connell MJ. Never say never. The NIMA-related protein kinases in mitotic control. Trends Cell Biol. 2003;13(5):221-8

29. Saleh RA, Agarwal A, Nada EA, et al. Negative effects of increased sperm DNA damage in relation to seminal oxidative stress in men with idiopathic and male factor infertility. Fertil Steril. 2003a;79(Suppl 3):1597-605.

30. Gandini L, Lombardo F, Paoli D, et al. Study of apoptotic DNA fragmentation in human spermatozoa. Hum Reprod. 2000;15:830-9.

31. Siddighi S, Patton WC, Jacobson JD, et al. Correlation of sperm parameters with apoptosis assessed by dual fluorescence DNA integrity assay. Arch Androl. 2004;50:311-4.

32. Trisini AT, Singh NP, Duty SM, et al. Relationship between human semen parameters and deoxyribonucleic acid damage assessed by the neutral comet assay. Fertil Steril. 2004;82:1623-32.

33. Appasamy M, Muttukrishna AR, Pizzey O, et al. Relationship between male reproductive hormones, sperm DNA damage and markers of oxidative stress in infertility. Reprod Biomed Online. 2007;14:159-65.

34. Huszar G, Vigue L, Morshedi M. Sperm creatine phosphokinase M-isoform ratios and fertilizing potential of men: a blinded study of 84 couples treated with in vitro fertilization. Fertil Steril. 1992;57:882-8.

35. Zini A, Boman JM, Belzile E, et al. Sperm DNA damage is associated with an increased risk of pregnancy loss after IVF and ICSI: systematic review and meta-analysis. Hum Reprod. 2008;23:2663-8.

36. Practice Committee of American Society for Reproductive M. The clinical utility of sperm DNA integrity testing. Fertil Steril. 2008;90:S178-80.

37. Kim JG, Parthasarathy S. Oxidation and the spermatozoa. Semin Reprod Endocrinol. 1998;16:235-9.

38. Foresta C, Garolla A, Bartoloni L, et al. Genetic abnormalities among severely oligospermic men who are candidates for intracytoplasmic sperm injection. J Clin Endocrinol Metab. 2005;90:152-6.

39. Oehninger S. Clinical and laboratory management of male infertility: an opinion on its current status. J Androl. 2000;21:814-21.

40. Carter SS, Shinohara K, Lipshultz LI. Transrectal ultra-sonography in disorders of the seminal vesicles and ejaculatory ducts. Urol Clin North Am. 1989;16:773-90.

41. Jarow JP. Transrectal ultrasonography of infertile men. Fertil Steril. 1993;60:1035-9.

42. Kumanov P, Nandipati K, Tomova A, et al. Inhibin B is a better marker of spermatogenesis than other hormones in the evaluation of male factor infertility. Fertil Steril. 2006;86:332-8.

43. Van Assche E, Bonduelle M, Tournaye H, et al. Cytogenetics of infertile men. Hum Reprod. 1996;11(Suppl 4):1-25.

44. Ravel C, Berthaut I, Bresson JL, et al. Genetics Commission of the French Federation of C. Prevalence of chromosomal abnormalities in phenotypically normal and fertile adult males: large-scale survey of over 10,000 sperm do- nor karyotypes. Hum Reprod. 2006;21:1484-9.

45. De Braekeleer M, Dao TN. Cytogenetic studies in male infertility: a review. Hum Reprod. 1991;6:245-50.

46. Debiec-Rychter M, Jakubowski L, Truszczak B, et al. Two familial 9;17 translocations with variable effect on male carriers fertility. Fertil Steril. 1992;57:933-5.

47. Pryor JL, Kent-First M, Muallem A, et al. Microdeletions in the Y chromosome of infertile men. N Engl J Med. 1997;336:534-9.

48. Kuroda-Kawaguchi T, Skaletsky H, Brown LG, et al. The AZFc region of the Y chromosome features massive palindromes and uniform recurrent deletions in infertile men. Nat Genet. 2001;29:279-86.

49. Skaletsky H, Kuroda-Kawaguchi T, Minx PJ, et al. The male-specific region of the human Y chromosome is a mosaic of discrete sequence classes. Nature. 2003;423:825-37.

50. Tilford CA, Kuroda-Kawaguchi T, Skaletsky H, et al. A physical map of the human Y chromosome. Nature. 2001;409:943-5.

51. Brandell RA, Mielnik A, Liotta D, et al. AZFb deletions predict the absence of spermatozoa with testicular sperm extraction: preliminary report of a prognostic genetic test. Hum Reprod. 1998;13:2812-5.

52. Krausz C, Quintana-Murci L, McElreavey K. Prognostic value of Y deletion analysis: what is the clinical prognostic value of Y chromosome microdeletion analysis? Hum Reprod. 2000;15:1431-4.

53. Oates RD, Silber S, Brown LG, et al. Clinical characterization of 42 oligo-spermic or azoospermic men with microdeletion of the AZFc region of the Y chromosome, and of 18 children conceived via ICSI. Hum Reprod. 2002;17:2813-24.

54. Kent-First MG, Kol S, Muallem A, et al. The incidence and possible relevance of Y-linked microdeletions in babies born after intracytoplasmic sperm injection and their infertile fathers. Mol Hum Reprod. 1996;2:943-50.

55. Anguiano A, Oates RD, Amos JA, et al. Congenital bilateral absence of the vas deferens. A primarily genital form of cystic fibrosis. JAMA. 1992;267:1794-7.

56. McCallum T, Milunsky J, Munarriz R, et al. Unilateral renal agenesis associated with congenital bilateral absence of the vas deferens: phenotypic findings and genetic considerations. Hum Reprod. 2001;16:282-8.

57. McPherson E, Carey J, Kramer A, et al. Dominantly inherited renal adysplasia. Am J Med Genet. 1987;26:863-72.

58. Carrell DT. The clinical implementation of sperm chromosome aneuploidy testing: pitfalls and promises. J Androl. 2008;29:124-33.

59. Egozcue S, Blanco J, Vendrell JM, et al. Human male infertility: chromosome anomalies, meiotic disorders, abnormal spermatozoa and recurrent abortion. Hum Reprod Update. 2000;6:93-105.

60. Carrell DT, Wilcox AL, Lowy L, et al. Elevated sperm chromosome aneuploidy and apoptosis in patients with unexplained recurrent pregnancy loss. Obstet Gynecol. 2003;101:1229-35.

61. Petit FM, Frydman N, Benkhalifa M, et al. Could sperm aneuploidy rate determination be used as a predictive test before intracytoplasmic sperm injection? J Androl. 2005;26:235-41.

62. Tempest HG, Martin RH. Cytogenetic risks in chromosomally normal infertile men. Curr Opin Obstet Gynecol. 2009;21:223-7.

63. Silber SJ, Van Steirteghem AC, Liu J, et al. High fertilization and pregnancy rate after intracytoplasmic sperm injection with sperm obtained from testicle biopsy. Hum Reprod. 1995;10:148-52.

64. Silber SJ, Nagy Z, Liu J, et al. The use of epididymal and testicular spermatozoa for intracytoplasmic sperm injection the genetic implication for male infertility. Hum Reprod. 1995;10:2031-43.

65. Schlegel PN, Palermo GD, Goldstein M, et al. Testicular sperm extraction with intracytoplasmic sperm injection for non-obstructive azoospermia. Urology. 1997;49:435-40.

66. Lewin A, Reubinoff B, Porat-Katz A, et al. Testicular fine needle aspiration: the alternative method for sperm retrieval in non-obstructive azoospermia. Hum Reprod. 1999;14:1785-90.

67. Dohle GR, Colpi GM, Hargreave TB, et al. The EAU Working Group on Male Infertility. EAU Guidelines on male infertility. Eur Urol. 2005;48:703-11.

68. El-Haggar S, Mostafa T, Abdel Nasser T, et al. Fine needle aspiration vs. mTESE in non-obstructive azoospermia. Int J Androl. 2007;27:32-6.

69. Björndahl L. What is normal semen quality? On the use and abuse of reference limits for the interpretation of semen analysis results. Hum Fertil (Camb). 2011;14(3):179-86.

70. Cooper TG, Noonan E, von Eckardstein S, et al. World Health Organization reference values for human semen characteristics. Hum Reprod Update. 2010;16:231-45.

71. Menkveld R. The basic semen analysis. In: Oehninger S, Kruger TF (Eds). Male Infertility. Diagnosis and Treatment. Oxford: Informa Healthcare; 2007. pp. 141-70.

72. Bjorndahl L, Mortimer D, Barratt CLR, et al. A Practical Guide to Basic Laboratory Andrology. Cambridge: Cambridge University Press; 2010.

5

Investigation of Infertile Female

Sonia Malik, Meenakshi Dua, Vandana Bhatia

One in every four couples in developing countries has been found to be affected by infertility.[1] According to the World Health Organization, 1.9% of women in the reproductive age group (20–44 years) suffer from primary infertility. Out of these women who had had at least one live birth and were exposed to the risk of pregnancy, 10.5% find it difficult to have another child (secondary infertility). Females account for 33%, males in 20%, both male and female in 39% and in 8% no cause for infertility is found. Infertile couples are usually advised to start their investigations after 12 months of trying to conceive or after 6 months if the female partner is more than 35 years old or immediately if there is an obvious cause for their infertility or subfertility.

For a woman to conceive, she should produce a healthy egg, which is picked up by a healthy tube, fertilizes with healthy sperm at ampullary region of tube, blastocyst transported to uterine cavity, implants and grows into a fetus. Any factor affecting this process will lead to infertility. Hence, a conscious effort should be made.

INDIVIDUALIZED PRETREATMENT ASSESSMENT

Most common cause of female infertility is ovulation disorders (32%), followed by tubal factor (26%). Other causes like uterine cavity abnormality, endometrial factor and immunological factors accounts for 18%.[2] Grossly while assessing a female for causes of infertility, her ovaries, tubes and uterus should be healthy and function properly. Investigation of an infertile female starts from detailed history taking. It helps the clinician to prioritize investigation. History taking is an integral part in evaluation of female infertility.

GENERAL ASSESSMENT

While taking detailed history related to infertility, her general health should not be ignored. History of chronic illness (diabetes, hypertension, thyroid disorders and childhood tuberculosis), current and past medications, previous surgeries, chronic infections, genetic disorders and personal history regarding smoking and alcohol intake should be taken carefully. Detailed sexual history should include frequency and timing of intercourse and any sexual dysfunction. Both couple should be tested for human immunodeficiency virus, hepatitis B, hepatitis C and syphilis serology. Diabetes screening should be offered to all polycystic ovary syndrome patients and women more than 35 years age presenting with infertility. The goal of evaluation is to identify the cause for infertility, which may be medically or surgically correctable.

HISTORY AND PHYSICAL EXAMINATION

At first consultation, sufficient time should be taken to obtain a detailed medical, reproductive and family history.[3]

Relevant history includes the following:
- Age of patient
- Type and duration of infertility
- Duration of cohabitation
- Detailed menstrual history (including age at menarche, cyclicity, presence or severity of dysmenorrhea and amount of estimated blood loss)
- Obstetric history (number of conceptions, live children, any pregnancy complications, last child birth)
- Comorbid illness (thyroid dysfunction, galactorrhea, diabetes and hypertension)
- Past treatment records (investigation results, treatment taken, response to treatment, operative findings in case any surgery done)
- Any occupational hazard (shift or touring jobs, stress at work)
- Current medications and allergies.

Physical examination should include:

- General examination (weight, body mass index, pallor, blood pressure and pulse)
- Thyroid enlargement or any nodules
- Breast lump or secretion from nipples or puckering of skin over breast
- Check for hirsutism
- Abdominal mass
- Any vaginal infection or abnormal discharge, if yes, take high vaginal swab
- Check for cervical erosion or cervicitis and offer pap smear
- Uterine enlargement, mobility and forniceal tenderness
- Ovarian enlargement and fixity
- Nodularity in pouch of Douglas.

■ TESTS

Female tests are performed to evaluate three principles axes: ovaries, tubes and uterus. Subsequent evaluation should be conducted in a systematic, cost-effective and expeditious manner. The pace and extent of evaluation should take into account the couples preferences, patient's age, duration of infertility and unique features in medical history and physical examination **(Flow chart 1)**.

Ovarian Factor

Establish Ovulation

Ovulatory dysfunction leads to irregular menstrual cycles. A regular menstrual cycle in a woman strongly suggests ovulation. However, objective measures are warranted in infertile female. Historically, basal body temperature (BBT) measurement was used to assess ovulation. Although a biphasic BBT provides presumptive evidence of ovulation, monophasic or uninterpretable BBT is also common in ovulatory patients. It is no longer considered best or preferred method to check ovulation.[3]

Another home ovulation test, which is easily available, is urinary luteinizing hormone (LH) kit. LH surge appears one or two days prior to ovulation. Positive predictive values for follicular collapse within 24 or 48 hours after positive urine LH testing have been noted to be 73% and 92% respectively.[4] However, false positive LH surge could occur in 7% of cases.

Single test, which provides reliable and objective measure of ovulatory function, is serum progesterone done in mid luteal phase. It retrospectively confirms ovulation and it is day specific. Values more than 3.0 ng/mL might be presumptive of ovulation whereas values greater than 10 ng/mL is suggestive of normal "in phase" endometrial histology. However, the criterion is not reliable as corpus luteum progesterone production is pulsatile and it varies by sevenfold within hours.[2]

Endometrial biopsy and dating is another test to evaluate ovulation. This test lacks accuracy and precision and cannot differentiate between fertile and infertile female. Hence, it is abandoned.[5]

If above method fails, patient can be subjected to serial transvaginal sonography (TVS) to check for follicular growth. Many centers prefer calling patient on day 12 of cycle to check for follicular dominance, endometrial thickness and cervical mucus. A follicle of more than 16 mm with endometrium more than 7 mm and presence of cervical mucus suggests normal follicular growth with normal serum estradiol levels. It does add to costs and requires expertise, but it is confirmatory test.

Flow chart 1 First visit workup

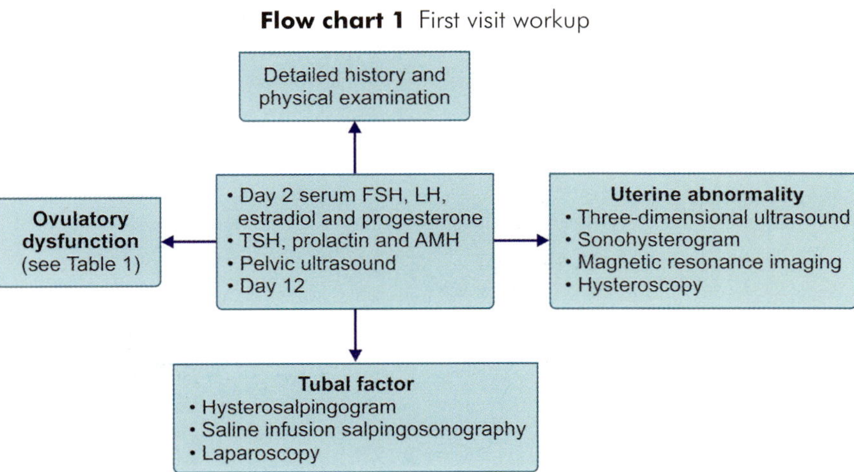

Establish cause for Anovulation

Anovulatory patients should be subjected to estimation of day 3 hormones follicle-stimulating hormone (FSH), LH and estradiol **(Table 1)**. Along with this, other endocrine abnormality, which may cause ovulatory dysfunction, should be check for thyroid abnormality and hyperprolactinemia. Polycystic ovarian disorder is the most common cause of anovulation. It can be diagnosed by reversed FSH:LH ratio with normal estrogen levels. These patients may be hyperandrogenic. Testing of serum testosterone, dehydroepiandrosterone sulfate (DHEAS) is advocated. Other causes of anovulation can be hypogonadotropic hypogonadism (low FSH, low estradiol) and ovarian failure (high FSH, low/normal estradiol). Hypogonadotropic hypogonadism will respond to gonadotropins replacement therapy whereas patients with ovarian failure should be offered donor eggs.

Ovarian Reserve Testing

Ovarian reserve is defined as the number and quality of remaining follicles and oocytes in both ovaries at a given age. Decline in follicle number relates to occurrence of irregular cycles and menopause, while quality decay is suggestive of decreasing fertility. With advancing age, quality deteriorates first followed by quantity.

Tests required to assess ovarian reserve includes day 2/3 serum FSH, estradiol, antral follicular count (AFC) and anti-Müllerian hormone (AMH).

Follicle-stimulating hormone is an indirect marker of ovarian reserve. It is suggestive of quality of eggs too. Higher the FSH, poorer is the quality of eggs. FSH is downregulated by estradiol. Both hormones should be evaluated together.

Unlike FSH, antral follicle count is a direct ovarian reserve marker. Antral follicles of 2–6 mm are counted in early follicular phase. A low AFC may range from 3 to 10. Low AFC indicates low ovarian reserve.[6]

Another direct marker for ovarian reserve is serum AMH. It is a dimeric glycoprotein produced only by ovaries in women. AMH expression starts from granulose cells of primary follicle and becomes strongest in pre-antral and small antral follicles (gonadotropin independent). Its value is relatively consistent all through the menstrual cycle, so it can be tested on any day. AMH is undetectable in menopausal women and does not appear to be regulated by FSH.

It can be used to detect low and high responders in IVF cycle. AMH less than 1 ng/mL is found to be associated with poor response to ovarian stimulation, poor embryo quality and poor pregnancy outcome in an IVF cycle. AMH levels more than 4 ng/mL is associated with high responders to ovarian stimulation. It has been suggested as a predictor for ovarian hyperstimulation syndrome.[7]

Tubal Factor

In vitro fertilization was initially used for tubal factor infertility. Tubal occlusion and tubal adhesions

Table 1 Changes in serum concentrations of sex hormones in women of childbearing age group with conditions causing female infertility

Hormones	Normal values	Serum levels in conditions causing infertility			
		Hypothalamic/ pituitary failure (WHO I)	PCOS (WHO II)	Ovarian failure (WHO III)	Hyperprolactine-mia
Day 3 FSH	<10 IU/L	Decreased	Normal	Increased	Normal
Day 3 LH	<10 IU/L	Decreased	Normal or increased	Increased	Normal
LH:FSH ratio	About 1:2	Normal	Reversed	Normal	Normal
Day 3 estradiol	<50 pmol/L	Decreased	Normal	Decreased	Decreased
DHEAS	2–10 nmol/L	Normal	Increased	Normal	Normal
Testosterone	1–3 nmol/L	Normal	Increased	Normal	Normal
Prolactin	15–20 ng/mL	Normal	Normal or increased	Normal	Increased

Abbreviations: DHEAS, dehydroepiandrosterone sulfate; FSH, follicle-stimulating hormone; LH, luteinizing hormone; PCOS, polycystic ovary syndrome; WHO, World Health Organization
Source: Hargreave TB, Mills JA. Investigating and managing infertility in general practice. BMJ. 1998;316:1438-41.

accounts for 25% of causes of female infertility. Hydrosalpinx accounts for 30% of all tubal diseases. Major causes for tubal disease are pelvic inflammatory disease, endometriosis, previous surgeries, abdominal tuberculosis in the developing countries and corneal or large subserous fibroids. It is important to obtain tubal status before proceeding for any ART procedures. Our ability to assess tubal status is limited to tubal patency and peritubal adhesions. Tube testing can be bypassed in case patient needs IVF for other reasons (severe male factor, age more than 39 years, grade 4 endometriosis, poor ovarian reserve).

Hysterosalpingography

It is a radiographic evaluation of Fallopian tubes. It is an outpatient procedure, performed postmenstrual day 7–9 to ensure absence of pregnancy and facilitate maximum uterine cavity assessment due to thin proliferative endometrium. It also reduced the chance of false positivity as thick endometrium in secretory phase of cycle can mimic cornual block. Under premedication (atropine and analgesics), cervix is cannulated either with metal cannula or silicon catheter, and nonionic radiopaque dye is passed thru it. We usually perform it under fluoroscopic guidance to minimize dye usage and radiation exposure. Contraindications to hysterosalpingography (HSG) are suspected pregnancy, active pelvic infection and history of contrast allergy (rarely seen with nonionic dye). Uterine cavity, tubal architecture and patency, hydrosalpinx and level of tubal block can be assessed.

It is a slightly painful procedure, tolerated well by most patients. Pain can be reduced by using silicon HSG cannula.[8] If not available, pediatric Foley's no. 8 works well. Intracervical block has also shown to reduce pain.[9] Patients with real low pain threshold can be posted for procedure under general anesthesia. Not to forget, it will add to cost and will demand daycare.

Post HSG infections can occur in 0.3–3.1% of patients.[10] It is advisable to give prophylactic doxycycline for 2 weeks postexposure to reduce this risk.[11] Cornual or proximal tubal block are usually due to tubal spasm or collection of debris or minimal adhesion due to chlamydial infection. Fluoroscopic tubal cannulation can be offered in such cases with vagal block. In proximal block cases, mostly remaining tube functions normally. Distal tubal block is suggestive of more severe damage to function of tube and most of the times it is not correctable with surgery. Such a patient should be offered IVF.

Sensitivity and specificity of HSG are 65% and 83% respectively. It is more specific in detecting distal when compared to proximal block. It has high correlation (95%) with laparoscopy.[12]

Saline Infusion Salpingosonography

It is ultrasonography combined with uterine instillation of saline. It is also an outpatient procedure done postmenstrually. However, saline infusion salpingo-sonography (SIS) has advantages of avoiding the use of ionizing radiation and the risk of iodine allergy. Compared to HSG, SIS also has greater sensitivity and specificity for detecting intrauterine pathologies and enables concomitant visualization of the ovaries and the myometrium.[13] However, one cannot distinguish unilateral or bilateral tubal patency. In a systematic review comparing efficacy of SIS with HSG, it was inferred that SIS was associated with a 10% rate of false occlusion and 7% of false patency compared to 13% and 11% respectively with HSG.[14]

Laparoscopy

Patients with suspected pelvic pathology, unexplained infertility, significant tubal disease requiring treatment and doubtful HSG findings. Along with chromopertubation, it is considered as gold standard for evaluating tubal patency. An advantage over HSG/SIS includes possibility to evaluate peritoneal factors like pelvic endometriosis, adhesions and simultaneously correct pathology. Disadvantages are cost, requirement of expertise, and need for general anesthesia requiring admission.

Uterine Factor

Congenital uterine malformations, endometrial polyp, submucosal fibroid, Asherman's syndrome and uterine septum are though not very common; yet they are significant causes for female infertility and if not treated, they do affect ART outcome.

Body of Uterus

Transvaginal sonography: It is an inexpensive, easily available, easy and well tolerable procedure giving immense information regarding all—uterus, tubes and ovaries.

It is a first-line investigation, which should be offered to all female patients. A mid cycle ultrasound can actually tell us about complete anatomy and physiology of patient. Apart from checking folliculogenesis, uterine cavity abnormality like endometrial polyp/adhesions or submucosal fibroid are better made out in mid cycle scan.

Specificity of ultrasonographic detection of hydrosalpinx is over 99%.[15]

Saline hysterosonography: Saline infusion through cervix while performing TVS can help in delineating cavity. It is especially helpful in differentiating endometrial polyp/fibroid from endometrial hyperplasia when in doubt. It has a high sensitivity from 78% to 100% and high specificity from 71% to 91%. It is more accurate than TVS and HSG.[16]

Three-dimensional ultrasound: It is an emerging technology with great promise. It offers more rapid and reproducible image acquisition as well as enhanced visualization and post-processing capabilities. Its main applications include assessment of uterine congenital anomalies, intrauterine pathology, tubal patency, polycystic ovaries, ovarian follicular monitoring and endometrial receptivity.[17] It should ideally be done in luteal phase of menstrual cycle.

Magnetic resonance imaging of pelvis: Magnetic resonance imaging should be offered specially to patients with suspicion of congenital abnormalities of uterus. It is also most sensitive modality for detecting endometriosis and fibroid mapping before planning surgery. It is as accurate as laparoscopy, noninvasive but costly investigation.[18]

Hysteroscopy: Hysteroscopy is a gold standard in diagnosing pathology of endometrial cavity, tubal ostia and endocervical canal. It allows direct visualization of cavity. However, it is the most costly and most invasive method of evaluation of uterine cavity. Contraindications to hysteroscopy are viable intrauterine pregnancy, active pelvic infection (including genital herpes infection) and known cervical or uterine cancer. Diagnostic hysteroscopy is an office procedure and does not require admission and anesthesia.

Endometrial biopsy: Synchronous development of the endometrium (to achieve a receptive state) and of the embryo is essential for successful implantation and ongoing pregnancy. Acute or chronic endometritis may be the cause for recurrent implantation failure. Female genital tuberculosis causing endometritis is one of the most common causes for female infertility in developing countries. Mere presence of tubercle bacilli on the endometrial surface has been found to affect fertility. These bacillary infestations bring an inflammatory change in an endometrium and produces harmful cytokines, which are responsible for implantation failure. A study conducted by Choudhary et al. (2010) including 217 cases of unexplained infertility, recurrent abortions, ectopic pregnancy and mild endometriosis, showed 44.5% of patients had endometrial involvement of tuberculosis.[19] After treatment, pregnancy rate went up to 37.4%. We routinely take endometrial biopsy to rule out on day 1 of menses as pregnancy will be ruled out and it will be easy to negotiate cervical canal. It is subjected to histopathology, AFB smear and Bactec culture.

Cervical Factor

Postcoital test: It evaluates the adequacy of cervical mucus at late follicular phase, and its interaction with sperm. It was a traditional method for identifying cervical factor and indirectly a male factor. Abnormalities of cervical mucus production or sperm/mucous interaction will rarely be a sole cause for infertility. It has poor inter- and intra-observer variability. It should not be part of routine fertility testing.[2]

◼ REFERENCES

1. National, regional, and global trends in infertility prevalence since 1990: A systematic analysis of 277 health surveys. WHO survey, December 2012.
2. Thonneau P, Marchand S, Tallec A, et al. Incidence and main causes of infertility in a resident population of three French regions. Hum Reprod. 1991;6:811-6.
3. The practice committee of the American Society of Reproductive Medicine. Diagnostic evaluation of an infertile female: a committee opinion. Fertil Steril. 2012;98:302-7.
4. Miller PB, Soules MR. The usefulness of a urinary LH kit for ovulation prediction during menstrual cycles of normal women. Obstet Gynecol. 1996;87(1):13-7.
5. Coutifaris C, Meyers ER, Guzick DS, et al. Histological dating of times endometrial biopsy is not related to fertility status. Fertil Steril. 2004;82:1264-72.
6. Practice committee opinion of ASRM: Testing and interpreting measures of ovarian reserve: a committee opinion. Fertil Steril. 2012;98(6):1407-15.
7. Polyzos N, Tournaye H, Guzman L, et al. Predictors of ovarian response in women treated with corifollitropin alfa for in vitro fertilization/intracytoplasmic sperm injection Fertil Steril. 2013;100(2):430-7.
8. Mansour R, Nada A, El-Khayat W, et al. A simple and relatively painless technique for hysterosalpingography, using a thin catheter and closing the cervix with the vaginal speculum: a pilot study. Postgrad Med J. 2011;87(1029):468-71.
9. Chauhan MB, Lakra P, Jyotsna D, et al. Pain relief during hysterosalpingography: role of intracervical block. Arch Gynecol Obstet. 2013;287(1):155-9.
10. Stumpf PG, March CM. Febrile morbidity following hysterosalpingography: identification of risk factors and recommendation for prophylaxis. Fertil Steril. 1980;33:487-92.
11. ACOG Committee on Practice Bulletins-Gynecology. ACOG practice bulletin no. 104: antibiotic prophylaxis in gyneco-logical procedures. Obstet Gynecol. 2009;113:1180-9.

12. Robabeh M, Roozbeh T. Comparison of hysterosalpingography and laparoscopy in infertile Iranian women with tubal factor. Ginekol Pol. 2012;83(11):841-3.
13. Acholonu UC, Silberzweig J, Stein DE, et al. Hysterosalpingography versus sonohysterography for intrauterine abnormalities. JSLS. 2011;2:471-4.
14. Sarah Maheux-Lacroix, Amélie Boutin, Lynne Moore, et al. Hysterosalpingosonography for diagnosing tubal occlusion in subfertile women: a systematic review protocol. Syst Rev. 2013;2:50.
15. Guerriero S, Ajossa S, Lai MP, et al. Transvaginal ultrasonography associated with color Doppler energy in the diagnosis of hydrosalpinx. Hum Reprod. 2000;15:1568-72.
16. Grimbizis GF, Tasolakidis D, Mikos T, et al. A prospective comparison of transvaginal ultrasound, saline infusion sonohysterography, and diagnostic hysteroscopy in evaluation of endometrial pathology. Fertil Steril. 2010;94:2720-5.
17. Grigore M, Mare A. Applications of 3-D ultrasound in female infertility. Rev Med Chir Soc Med Nat Iasi. 2009;113(4):1113-9.
18. Steinkeler JA, Woodfield CA, Lazarus E, et al. Female infertility: a systematic approach to radiologic imaging and diagnosis. Radiographics. 2009;29(5):1353-70.
19. Choudhary RG, Paine SK, Bhattacharyajee B, et al. Infestation of endometrium by Mycobacterium tuberculosis bacilli-cause of reproductive failure. Al Ameen J Med Sci. 2010;3(4):322-31.

6 Ultrasound and Doppler in Infertility

Sonal Panchal, Narendra Malhotra, Jaideep Malhotra, Chaitanya Nagori

INTRODUCTION

Continuous complex hormonal changes occurring during the menstrual cycle result into cyclical morphological changes and vascular changes in ovaries and uterus, and these are the basis of reproductive function in human. Transvaginal ultrasound (US) is the modality of choice to study these changes. The accuracy of diagnosis and monitoring of infertility treatments such as ovulation induction has greatly increased because of the availability of sophisticated US technology and equipment.

MONITORING OF TREATMENT CYCLES IN PATIENTS WITH INFERTILITY

The purpose of monitoring in stimulated cycles:
- To evaluate ovarian response to stimulation in terms of the number and size of ovarian follicles
    - To identify exaggerated response
    - To identify poor response
- To decide the correct time of human chorionic gonadotropin (hCG) and intrauterine insemination (IUI) or ovum pick-up.

EARLY PROLIFERATIVE SCAN

The ovarian response can be assessed by a baseline or an early proliferative scan. Ovary is quiescent at this stage and so only antral follicles are visualized on this scan in the ovaries. This scan is done preferably on day 2–3 of the cycle. At this time estrogen, progesterone, follicle-stimulating hormone (FSH) and luteinizing hormone (LH) all the hormones are at baseline levels. Early antral follicles (1–2 mm) are the first follicular structures that may be visualized on US. Number of antral follicle count (AFC) in the ovary on this scan decides the ovarian reserve and may therefore help to plan the stimulation protocol.

Commonly used morphological US markers for deciding the stimulation protocol are:

- AFC
- Ovarian volume
- Mean ovarian diameter and size
- Ovarian stromal blood flow.

Number of antral follicles, measuring 2–10 mm in diameter, correlates well with the female's age, ovarian reserve and ovarian response to gonadotropin stimulation. Normal AFC in one ovary ranges from 5 to 10. AFC less than six correlates well with reduced ovarian reserve and poor response to ovarian stimulation, with positive predictive value of 75%. Total AFC more than 21 could lead to the decision to adjust the gonadotropin dose in trying to prevent a hyper-response leading to ovarian hyperstimulation syndrome.

Ovarian volume is a poor predictor of number of oocytes obtained in an in vitro fertilization (IVF) cycle. The mean ovarian diameter significantly correlated with age, day 3 FSH, day 3 LH and day 3 estradiol.

Measurement of ovarian stromal flow in early follicular phase is related to subsequent ovarian response in IVF treatment. Ovarian stromal peak systolic velocity (PSV) after pituitary suppression may be predictive of ovarian responsiveness and outcome of IVF treatment. Therefore, Doppler of ovaries on baseline scan can be helpful to decide stimulation protocol.

Undetectable basal ovarian stromal blood flow in at least one ovary is related to low ovarian reserve in infertile women undergoing in vitro fertilization and embryo transfer (IVF-ET). Ovarian stromal PSV was the most important single independent predictor of ovarian response in patients with normal basal serum FSH level. Patients with PSV more than or equal to 10 cm/sec had significantly higher median number of mature oocytes and higher clinical pregnancy rates. Ovarian stromal blood flow velocity after 2–3 weeks of pituitary suppression is a true representative of baseline ovarian blood flow and predictive of ovarian responsiveness and outcome of IVF treatment.[7] Endometrial thickness of less than or equal to 5 mm indicates adequate down regulation in IVF cycles.

While scanning for ovulation monitoring is a continuous process and cannot be confined to certain days. Before day 5 of the cycle, selection of the dominant follicle occurs. Between 5 days and 7 days, dominance of the follicle becomes apparent. Follicle, i.e. 10–12 mm in size is known as a dominant follicle, and it is this follicle that is most likely to grow to become a mature follicle. It is interesting to know that often first largest follicle on baseline scan is not the dominant follicle. A normal growth rate of a healthy follicle is approximately 2 mm/day and reaches a size of 18–24 mm **(Fig. 1A)** by the time of ovulation.

■ PREOVULATORY SCAN

Follicular Assessment

B-mode Features of a Mature Follicle

The follicular diameter is measured when the follicle is seen as a rounded structure on US image. Two to three measurements must be taken perpendicular to each other and the mean measurement is taken as follicular diameter. The follicle shape may become ellipsoid, if pressure is applied by the transvaginal probe on the follicle and therefore scans should be done with only optimum pressure applied by the probe. When there is multifollicular development, shape of follicles change from round to polygonal, due to pressure effect from adjacent follicles. In such follicles the follicular volume assessment may be more reliable instead of a single diameter.

A mature follicle is 16–18 mm (Fig. 1A). A follicular size of 17–18 mm is for gonadotropin stimulated cycle, whereas for clomiphene citrate (CC) stimulated cycles minimum size of 18–20 mm is required. A good quality follicle has thin walls, regular round shape and no echogenicity in the lumen. A thin hypoechoic halo surrounding the follicle and cumulus-like shadow in the follicle appears approximately 36 hours before rupture in response to initiation of LH surge. A flimsy irregular line is seen inside the follicle parallel to the wall about 6–10 hours before rupture **(Fig. 1B)**.

Doppler Features of a Mature Pre-hCG Follicle

Maturation of follicle and endometrium, ovulation and luteinization is a process of multiple biochemical, morphological and vascular changes. Vascular changes may therefore reflect the hormonal changes and combining Doppler to B-mode scans may help to understand the hormonal changes occurring during the menstrual cycle in response to stimulation. Perifollicular vascularity of dominant follicle starts developing as early as 8th day of the cycle when follicle reaches 10 mm in diameter. Resistance index (RI) of these vessels is reported as 0.54 ± 0.04. Perifollicular RI starts falling two days prior to ovulation and reaches its nadir of 0.44 ± 0.04 at ovulation and then with gradual rise reaches a peak in mid-luteal phase. Just prior to eruption, the vascularity surrounding the follicle increases along with the increase in its flow velocity. The mean changes in PSV, follows the mean rise in LH by approximately 12 hours. PSV increases 29 hours before the time of follicular rupture and continues

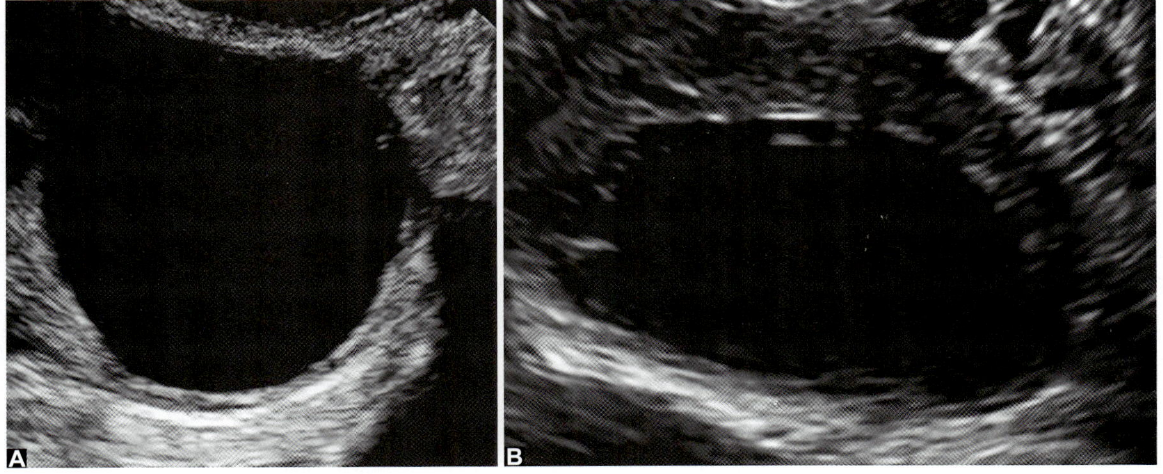

Figs 1A and B Preovulatory follicle on B-mode, a few hours before rupture

for at least 72 hours after corpus luteum is formed. When mature, on color Doppler, the follicle shows blood vessels covering at least 3/4th of the follicular circumference **(Fig. 2)**. Chui et al. graded the follicular flow on the day of oocyte collection as grade 1–4 when in a single cross area slice the flow covered less than 25%, 25–50%, 50–75% and more than 75% of follicular circumference. The conception was related to grade 3–4 vascularity.

On pulse Doppler when these blood vessels show an RI of 0.4–0.48 and PSV of more than 10 cm/sec, it indicates a mature preovulatory follicle **(Fig. 3)**. A marked increase in the PSV around the follicle, in the presence of a relatively constant pulsatility index (PI), could be a sign of follicle maturity and impending ovulation.

Implications of Flow Parameters on Ovum Quality

Ovarian flow correlates well with oocyte recovery rates and hence may be useful in determining the most appropriate time to administer hCG to optimize recovery rate. Oocytes from severely hypoxic follicles are associated with high frequency of abnormalities of organization of chromosomes on metaphase spindle and may lead to segregation disorders and catastrophic mosaics in embryo.

Higher RI indicates higher resistance flow to the follicle (perifollicular blood flow) meaning lower flow during diastolic phase and so reduced phasic oxygen supply to the ovum. Lower PSV again indicates lower blood supply and hence ovum hypoxia. It has been quoted in a study by Nargund et al. that embryos produced by fertilization of the ova obtained from the follicles which had a perifollicular PSV of less than 10 cm/sec, are less likely to be grade I embryos and also have higher chance of chromosomal malformations. In the same study it has been shown that the probability of developing a grade 1 or 2 embryo is 75% if PSV was more than 10 cm/sec, 40% if PSV was less than 10 cm/sec, 24% if there was no perifollicular flow.

Our unpublished data of more than 1,000 IUI cycles has shown that when the perifollicular RI more than 0.53 and PSV less than 9 cm/sec, 12 hours before hCG injection, the conception rates were only 8.3% and 10% respectively as compared to 32.8% and 28.2% respectively and individually when perifollicular RI less than 0.50 and PSV more than 11 cm/sec.

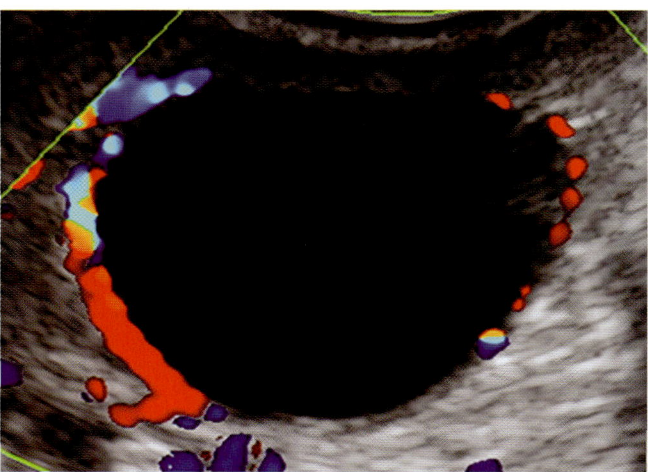

Fig. 2 Preovulatory follicle with vascular ring surrounding the follicle

Volume Ultrasound Parameters of Mature Pre-hCG Follicle

Although it is possible to assess the follicular flow as expressed by the PSV and perifollicular color map, 3D power Doppler (PD) provides more detailed quantitative information about the ovarian vascularization and perifollicular blood flow.

On 3D the follicular volume of 3–7.5 cc has been found to be optimum **(Fig. 4)**. It has been shown that in IVF-ET cycles, follicles with mean follicular diameter of 12–24 mm are associated with optimal rates of oocyte recovery, fertilization and cleavage. This corresponds to the follicular volumes of between 3 mL and 7 mL. The accuracy of 3D US measurement of follicular volume was better when compared to the standard 2D techniques by comparing the volume of aspirates from

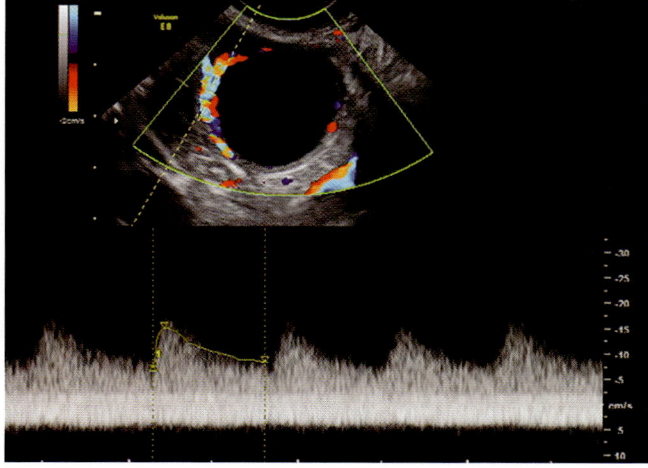

Fig. 3 Preovulatory follicle with pulse Doppler showing low resistance flow

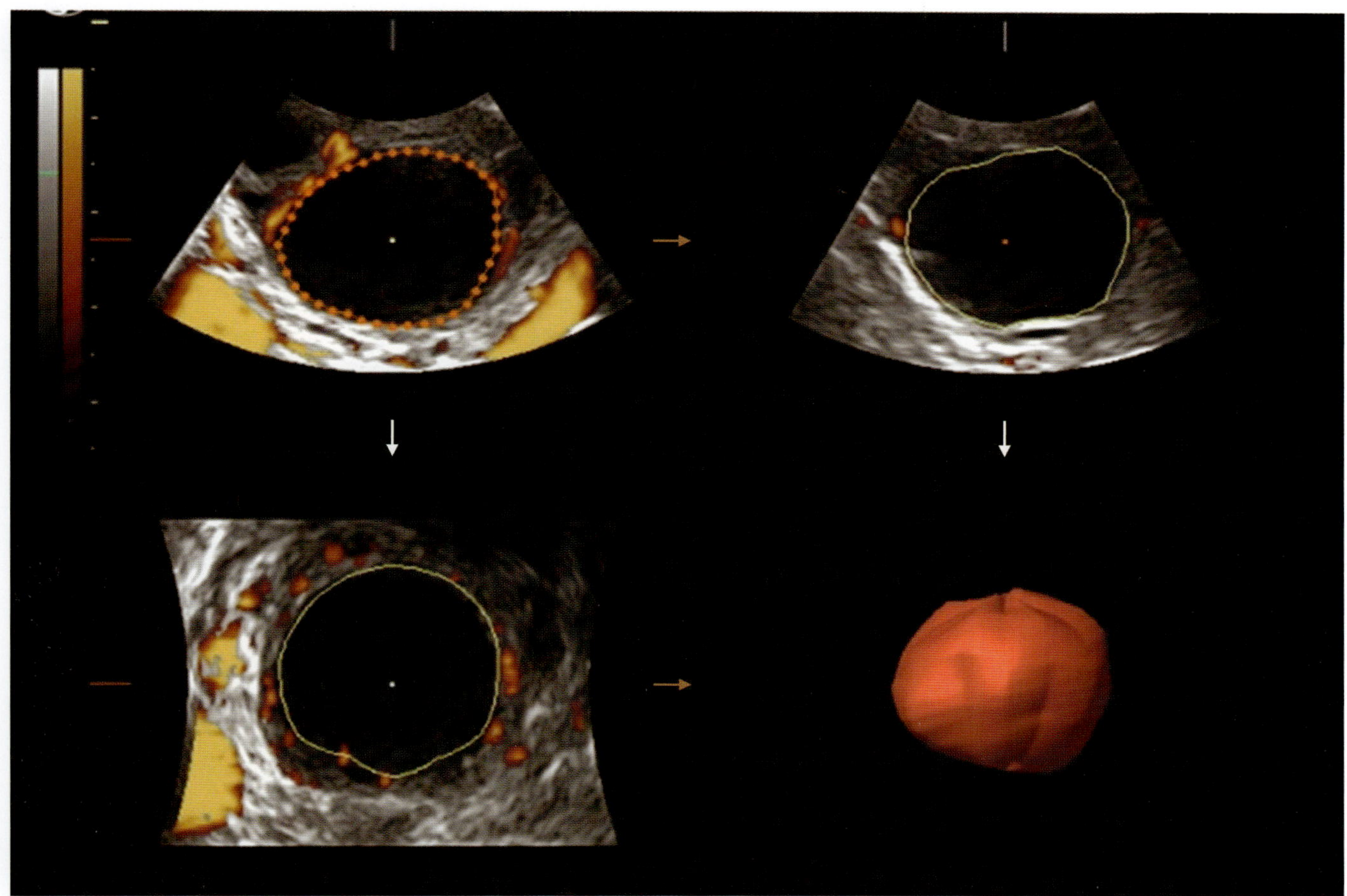

Fig. 4 3D model of a follicle generated using VOCAL software, which is utilized for manual delineation of ovarian follicle at different desired angle to 180° and this gives follicular volume

individual follicles with the limits of agreement between aspirates and calculated volume was + 3.47 to – 2.42 for 2D measurements as compared to + 0.96 to – 0. 43 when calculated by 3D US using VOCAL. However, the follicles of less than 10 mm in diameter, cannot be assessed accurately by 3D US as the limits of agreement are too wide in this range.

Feichtinger et al. in their study have shown presence of cumulus in follicles more than 15 mm by 3D US. Follicles without visualization of cumulus in all three planes are less likely to contain mature oocytes. Appearance of the intrafollicular cumulus-like structure by 3D US **(Fig. 5)** was correlated with the recovery rate of the mature oocytes. A significant correlation was found between the number of detected cumuli and the number of retrieved oocytes (P < 0.0001), mature oocytes (P < 0.0001) and number of fertilized oocytes (P < 0.0001). We, in our study of 500 IUI cycles, have been able to identify the cumulus in 94.6% of cases in conception cycles and in 53% of non-conception

cycles. It has also been suggested that the follicles containing oocytes capable to produce a pregnancy have a perifollicular vascular network more uniform and distinctive **(Figs 6A and B)**.

Quantification of PD information within a 3D model of an ovarian follicle **(Fig. 7)** can be performed using the "histogram facility" **(Fig. 8)**. Three indices of vascularity can be generated: the vascularization index (VI), which represents the ratio of PD information within the total dataset relative to both color and gray information; the flow index (FI), which is proportional to the PD signal intensity; and the vascularization flow index (VFI), which reflects a combination of the two. In our study, we have found perifollicular VI of between 6 and 20 and perifollicular FI more than 35 as most optimum. 68.4% of patients conceived when the VI was between 6 and 18 and 50% when it was between 18 and 20. With FI beyond 27, the conception rates rose consistently. A study by Kupesic and Kurjak shows that when the ratio of follicular volume

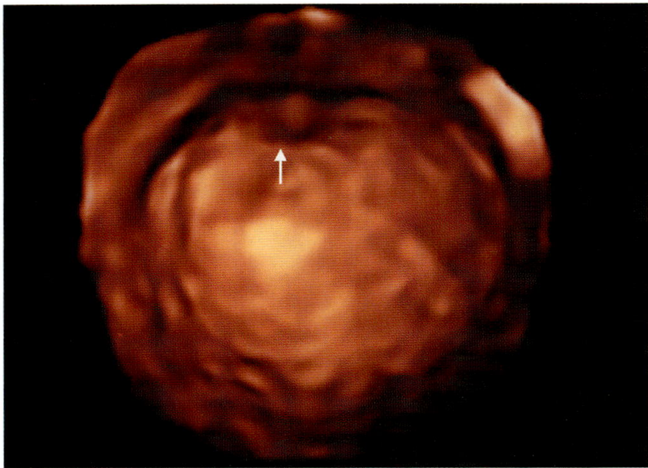

Fig. 5 Cumulus oophorus in preovulatory follicle on a 3D model of a preovulatory follicle

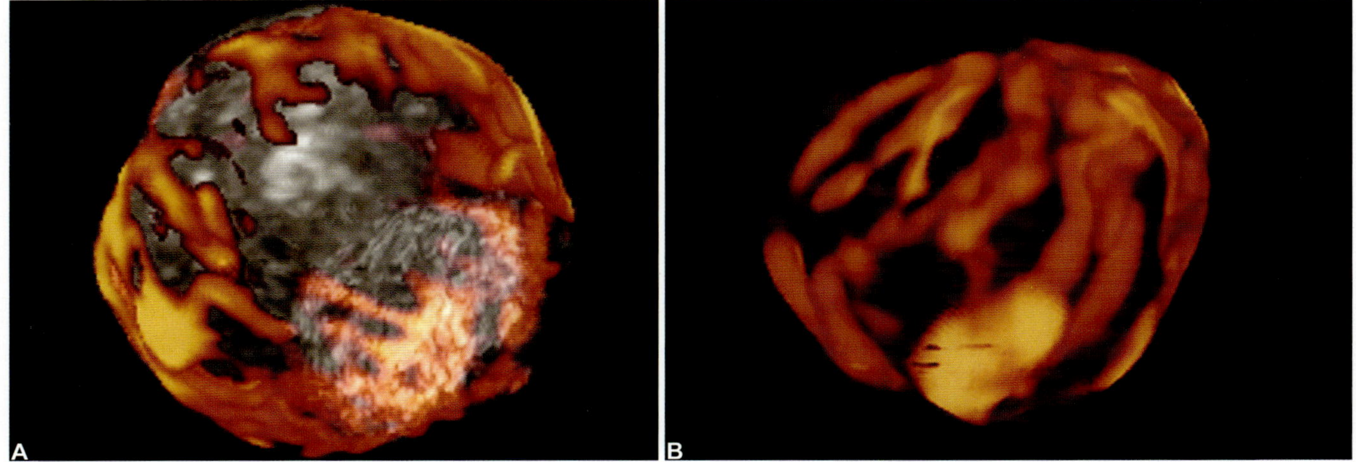

Figs 6A and B Power Doppler angiography of a preovulatory follicle demonstrating a uniform and distinctive perifollicular vascularity

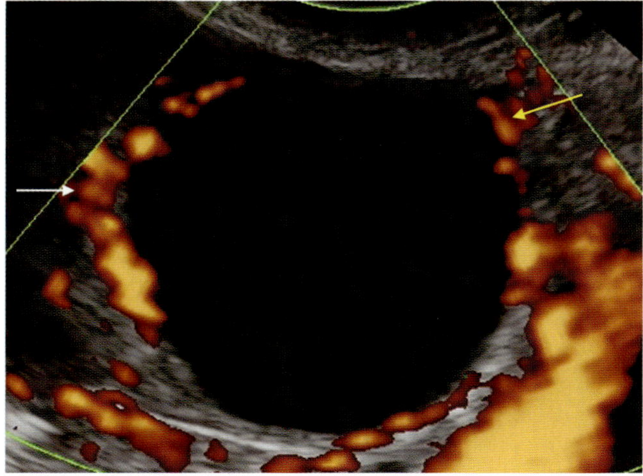

Fig. 7 True perifollicular vessel (yellow arrow), not a perifollicular vessel (white arrow)

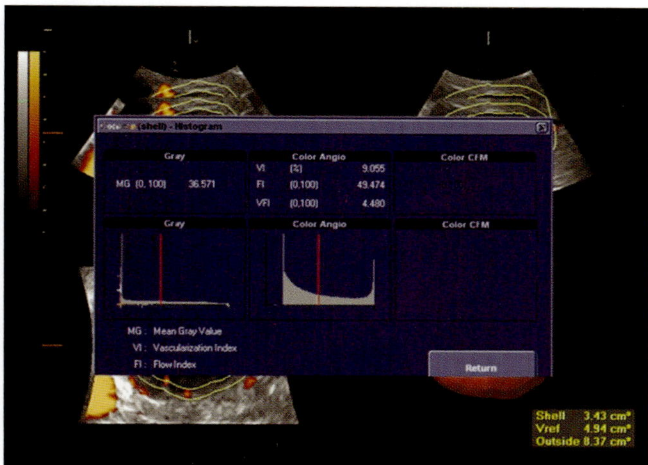

Fig. 8 Histogram for perifollicular flow giving values of 3D vascular indices, vascular index (VI), flow index (FI) and vascular flow index (VFI)

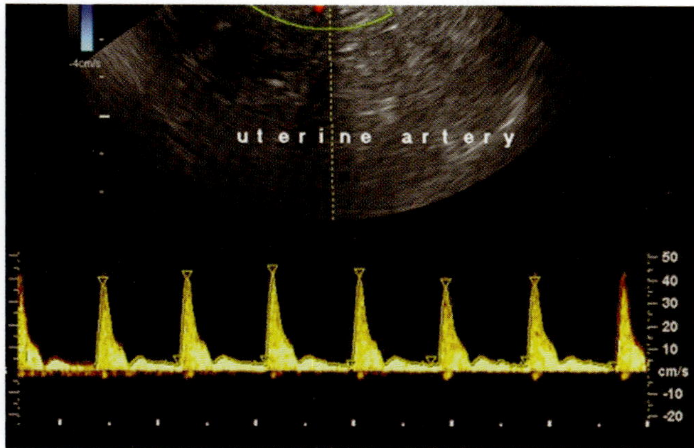

Fig. 9 Preovulatory uterine artery waveform

to blood flow index (FV/FI) is between 0.4 and 0.6 the pregnancy rates are 39%, if more than 0.6, it is 52% and when less than 0.4 is only 21%.

The above data from different studies indicate that even when the follicle appeared mature according to the 2D US and color and pulse Doppler parameters, the pregnancy rates were significantly better, when 3D and 3D PD assessment was added for decision making.

Recently introduced software, SonoAVC (Automatic Volume Calculation; GE Medical Systems), has been used to provide automated measurements of follicle size from the stored 3D datasets **(Fig. 9)**. SonoAVC is a software program designed to provide automatic volume calculations of fluid-filled areas. It is either incorporated into the US machine or installed on a personal computer for offline analysis of the datasets acquired by any US machine of the same manufacturer. SonoAVC identifies and quantifies hypoechogenic regions within a 3D dataset and provides automatic estimation of their absolute dimensions, mean diameter and volume. While this technique has been proven to be more reproducible and valid in measuring follicular diameter and volume than conventional 2D US method and may have implications for improving the work flow within an IVF center, timing final follicle maturation and oocyte retrieval on the basis of such automated measures does not appear to improve the clinical outcome of assisted reproductive technology (ART).

Endometrial Evaluation

Implantation has been weakest link in the success of infertility treatment. Endometrium is a receptor organ for majority of the hormones involved in fertility and therefore study of its morphology and vascularity is thought to explain the mysteries of implantation failure. US assessment of the endometrium is important in the analysis of factors that affect embryo implantation.

B-mode Features of Endometrium with Good Receptivity

Endometrial thickness is less than 5 mm in early follicular phase and slightly more echogenic than the myometrium. It grows at a rate of 1–2 mm/day. Endometrial thickness can be correlated with the rise in oestradiol. It grows to a thickness of 10–12 mm at ovulation and becomes multilayered or trilaminar. Though relationship of endometrial thickness to histological dating is controversial. Endometrial growth does not differ significantly in stimulated and non-stimulated cycles. However in CC stimulated cycle, the endometrial thickness may be less in the days immediately after CC is taken because of its antiestrogenic effect. But during late proliferative phase, endometrial thickness increases at a faster rate than in spontaneous cycles as it escapes from the antiestrogenic effect and effect of increased estrogen due to multifollicular growth. But in gonadotropin stimulated cycles the endometrial thickness is greater than in spontaneous cycles. On transvaginal sonography (TVS) an endometrial thickness of 6 mm is considered minimum that is required on the day of ovulation or on the day of hCG trigger for a successful outcome, although 8 mm is generally considered optimum. Even when pregnancy occurs with endometrial thickness of 6–8 mm on the day of hCG, the rates of preclinical miscarriage (biochemical pregnancy) and clinical miscarriage were 21.9% and 15.6% respectively, as compared to 0% and 12.9% respectively when endometrial thickness was more than 8 mm. Endometrial thickness has more negative predictive value for implantation. In healthy endometrium, the endometrio-myometrial interface is always seen as a clear hypoechoic halo surrounding the whole endometrium **(Figs 10A and B)**. Breach or irregularity of endometrio-myometrial junction may be an indication of unhealthy endometrium and therefore poor receptivity.

Morphology of the endometrium is as important as thickness of the endometrium. Popularly multilayered endometrium is considered a desired endometrial pattern. Endometrium starts becoming trilaminar from 6 days before LH surge. Morphologically the endometrium is graded as the best, grade A, when it is a triple line endometrium with the intervening area as hypoechoic as the anterior myometrium. The echogenicity is attributed to the development of multiple vessels penetrating in the endometrium producing multiple tissue interfaces and due to glycogen storage in the endometrial columnar epithelium **(Fig. 11)**. The endometrium is graded as intermediate or grade B **(Fig. 12)** when it is multilayered or triple line with hypoechoic intervening area. In grade C or the most unfavorable endometrium would be a homogeneous isoechoic endometrium **(Fig. 13)**.

Doppler Features of Receptive Endometrium

There are several reports by different groups that agree on the fact that implantation rates can be more correlated to the vascularity of the endometrium rather than the

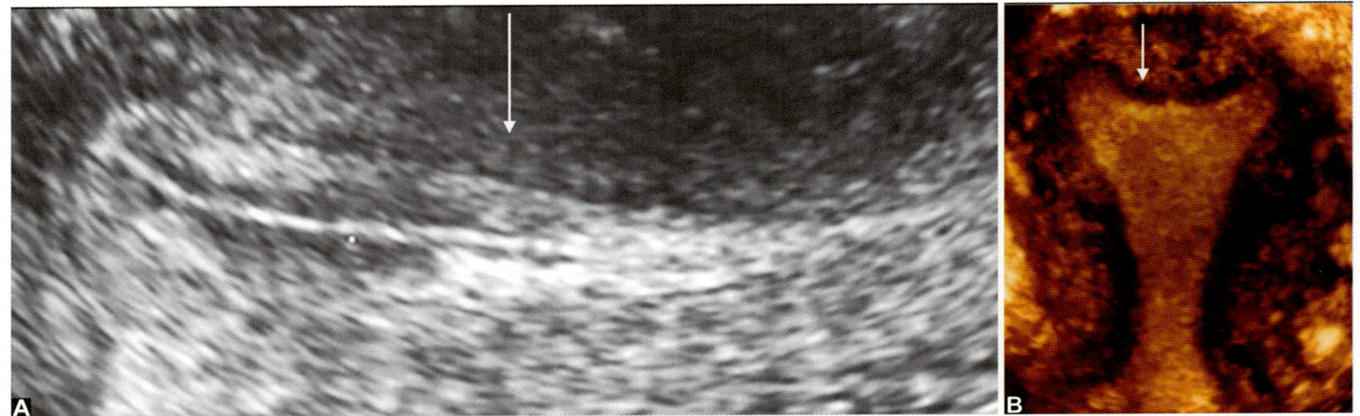

Figs 10A and B Endometrio-myometrial junction

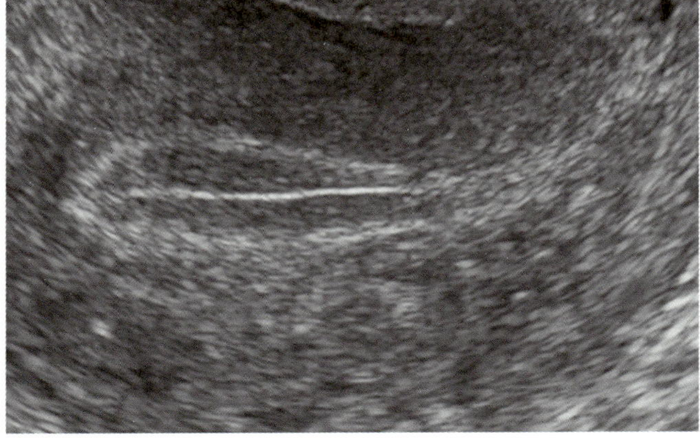

Fig. 11 Most receptive endometrium grade A—multilayered

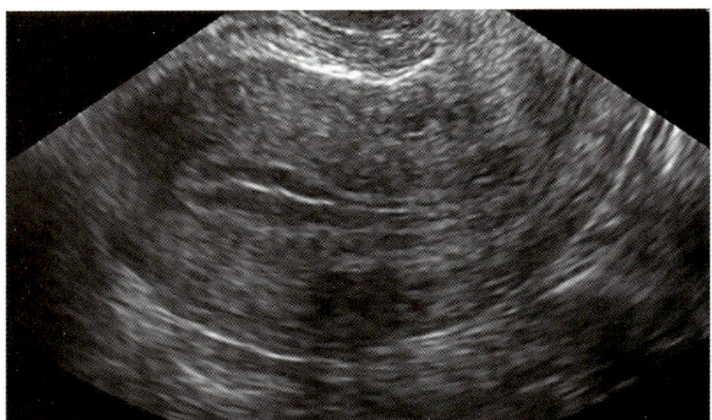

Fig. 12 Multilayered endometrium grade B—intermediate

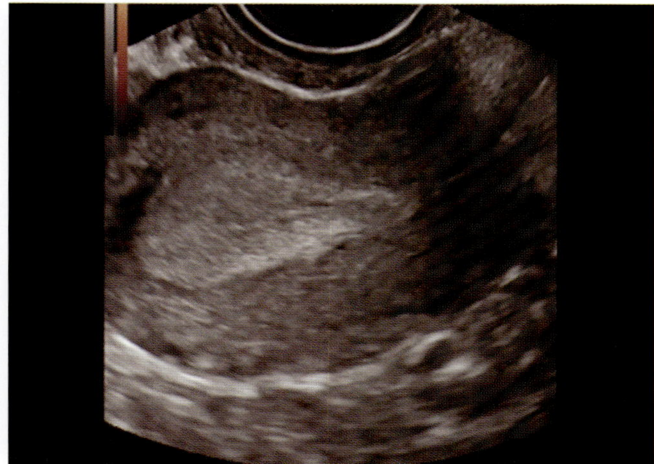

Fig. 13 Isoechoic homogeneous grade C endometrium

thickness and morphology of the endometrium. Segmental uterine artery perfusion demonstrates significant correlation with hormonal and histological markers of uterine receptivity, reaching the highest sensitivity for subendometrial blood flow. The proliferative phase flow is thought to be due to vasodilatory effect of estrogen and the secretory phase vascularity can be attributed to serum progesterone levels. Blood flow in the uterine vascular bed can be correlated to the estrogen or progesterone ratio.

But the endometrial neoangiogenesis differ in natural and stimulated cycles. In stimulated cycles, there may be 35% decrease in endometrial and subendometrial vascularity.

Endometrial and subendometrial vascular flow increases to its maximum 3 days prior to ovulation and then decreases until fifth postovulatory day due to probably vasodilatation of subepithelial capillary plexus leading to stromal edema. On color Doppler, the endometrium that has vascularity in zone 3 and 4 or in subendometrial and endometrial layers **(Fig. 14)** has been reported to have a high degree of endometrial receptivity. The zones of vascularity are defined according to Applebaum as:

- *Zone 1*: When the vascularity on PD is seen only at endometrio-myometrial junction.
- *Zone 2*: When vessels penetrate through the hyperechogenic endometrial edge.
- *Zone 3*: When it reaches intervening hypoechogenic zone.
- *Zone 4*: When vessels reach the endometrial cavity.

The pregnancy rates related to the zones of vascular penetration during IVF were 26.7% for zone 1, 36.4% for zone 2 and 37.9% for zone 3. Another comparative study

has also shown similar results with pregnancy rates for zone 1, zone 2, zone 3 and zone 4 were 5.2%, 28.7%, 52% and 74% respectively.

Zaidi et al. found that absence of flow in the endometrial and subendometrial zones on day of hCG indicate minimal chance for a successful implantation. In our unpublished data of more than 1,000 IUI cycles, when color Doppler studies were done 12 hours before hCG injection, we have found only 7.3% pregnancy rates for zone 1 and 13.4% for zone 2 vascularity. The conception rates with zone 3 and 4 the pregnancy rates were comparable and were 35.8 and 38.3% respectively.

While the reported correlation between vascularity in the endometrium and subendometrium and pregnancy rates is controversial, it has been concluded in two studies that no difference was found in patients with good prognosis for cycle outcome, but in patients with poor embryo quality, better endometrial vascularity seemed to improve the cycle outcome. The vessels that reach the endometrium covering at least 5 mm^2 area of the endometrium are reported to be a good prognostic factor. The pulse Doppler of these arteries indicating RI of between 0.6 and 0.8 and PI of between 1.1 and 2.3 has also been reported to be a good prognostic factor **(Fig. 15)**.

Uterine Artery Doppler

Uterine artery usually shows a moderate to high resistance flow and shows variations in resistance according to phase of the cycle, but also is affected by age. The RI of the uterine artery flow is 0.88 ± 0.04 till day 13 of the 28 day menstrual cycle. Pulse Doppler analysis of the uterine artery waveform is also reported to be predictive of endometrial receptivity with its PI less than 3.2 being desirable **(Fig. 9)**. Several authors have shown that the optimum uterine receptivity was obtained when average PI of the uterine artery was between 2 and 3 on the day of transfer or on the day of hCG. Coulam et al. and Cacciatore et al. have also reported that no pregnancy was achieved after when uterine artery PI was above 3.3 in an IVF program. Tsai and colleagues evaluated the prognostic value of uterine perfusion on day of hCG for IUI cycles and showed that no pregnancy occurred when the PI of ascending branch of uterine artery was more than 3. Fecundity rate was 18% when PI was less than 2 and 19.8% when PI was between 2 and 3. In our unpublished data of more than 1,000 IUI cycles, when color Doppler studies were done 12 hours before hCG injection, we have found no conceptions when uterine artery PI more than 3.5. The hypothesis is that the high resistance blood flow in the uterine artery may lead to higher resistance flow in endometrial vessels

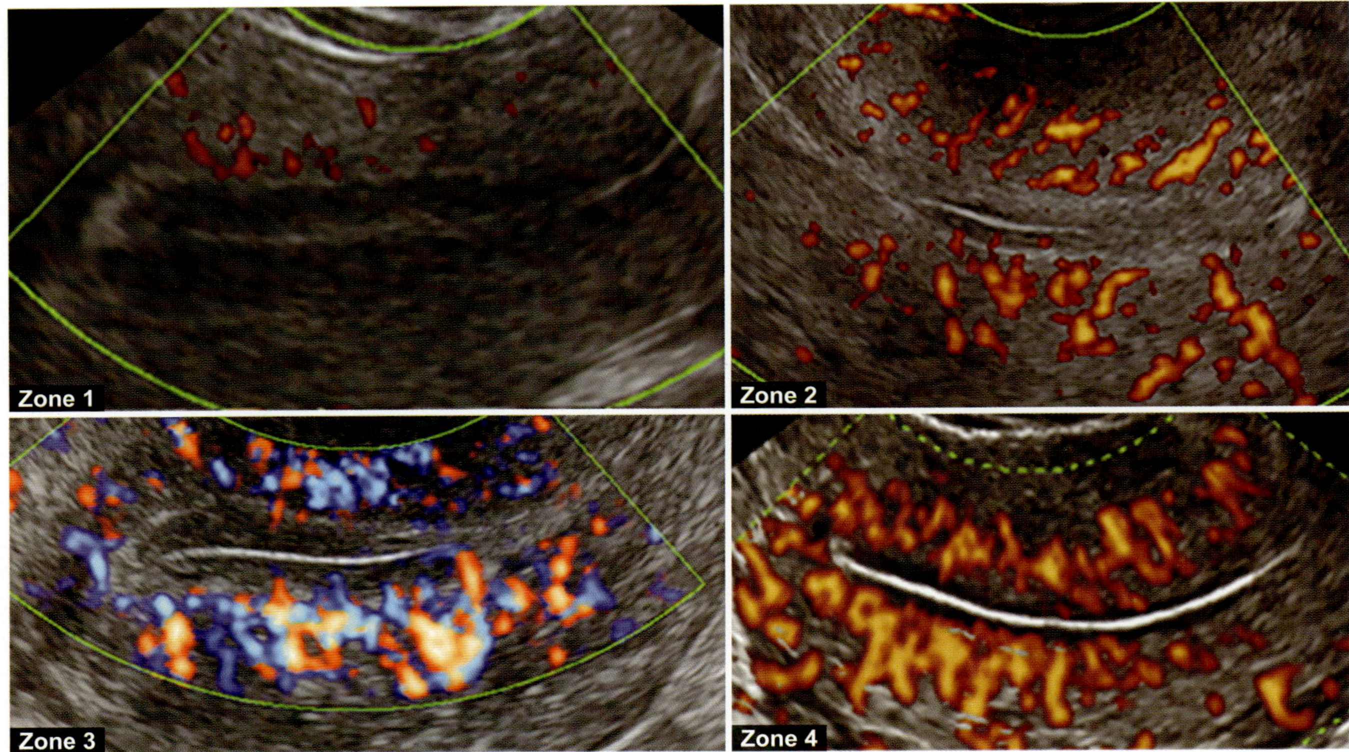

Fig. 14 Endometrial vascularity zones (Zone 1–4)

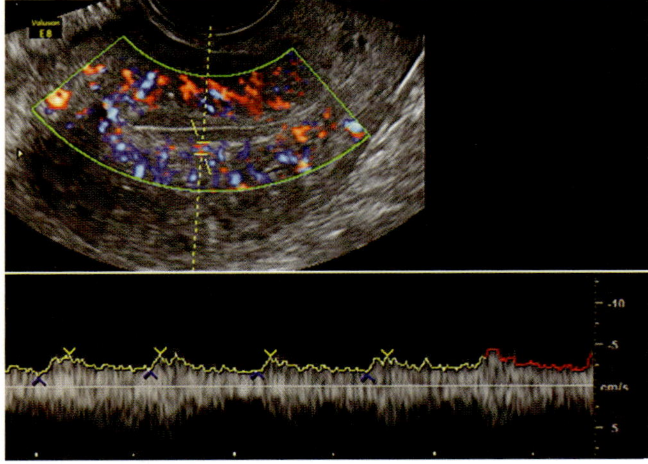

Fig. 15 Pulse Doppler of endometrial vascularity

and inadequate endometrial oxygenation and causes low implantation rates.

3D and 3D Power Doppler Features of Good Endometrial Receptivity

The correlation of IVF outcome with 3D US volume of the endometrium **(Fig. 16)** has been reported to be better than with endometrial thickness. It has been reported that pregnancy and implantation rates were significantly lower when endometrial volume is 1–2 mL. In a study of IVF population by our group, no pregnancy was observed in the group with endometrial volume of less than two on the day of hCG ovulation trigger. The pregnancy rates were 16.7%, 47% and 62% respectively when the endometrial volume was 2–3 cc, 3–5 cc and 5–7 cc respectively.

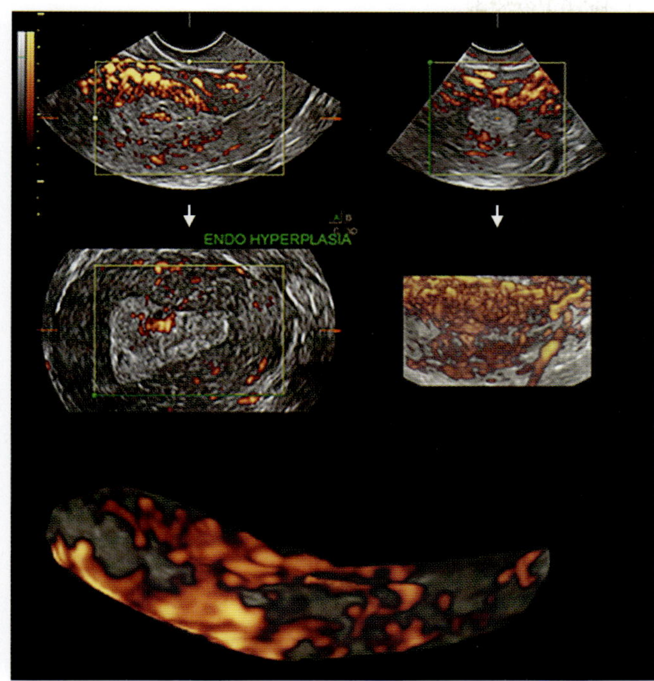

Fig. 16 Calculating endometrial volume by VOCAL software

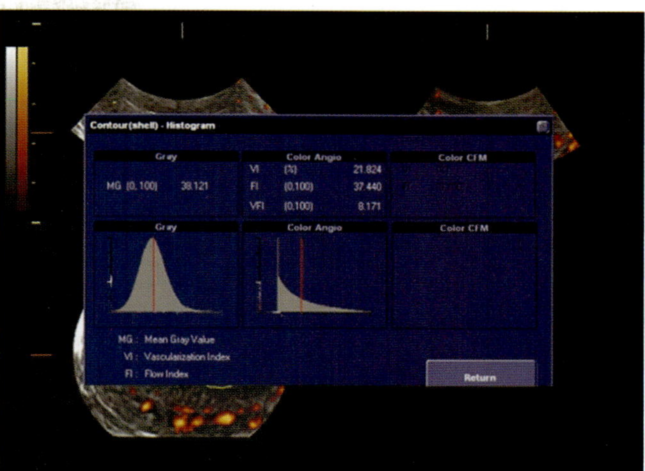

Fig. 17 Histogram of endometrium showing vascular index (VI), flow index (FI) and vascular flow index (VFI) values

While there is no consensus regarding the role of 3D PD indices (**Figs 17 and 18**) in predicting endometrial receptivity, a study by Kupesic et al., reported a sub-endometrial FI of less than 11 on the day of ET as a cutoff level for predicting poor implantation. No pregnancies occurred when FI was less than 11 and the conception group showed FI of 13.2 ± 2.2. Contrary to this, Ng et al. reported a low endometrial vascularizaton index (VI) and VFI in pregnant group on the day of oocyte retrieval and also a non-significant trend of higher implantation and pregnancy rates in patients with absent subendometrial and endometrial flow. This probably can be explained on the basis that hCG administration or LH peak causes increased uterine artery resistance and hence decrease in endometrial perfusion also on the day of oocyte retrieval. This also correlates with the observation made by Ng et al. which says that subendometrial vascularization flow indices are significantly lower in patients with uterine artery RI greater than or equal to 0.95. They concluded that number of embryos replaced and endometrial VFI were the only two predictive factors for pregnancy. Wu et al. reported that endometrial VFI was more reliable than VI and FI, and best prediction rate was achieved by VFI cutoff value of more than 0.24. As there are conflicting reports, the routine application of 3D PD indices for predicting endometrial receptivity in women undergoing assisted reproduction treatment currently is limited.

3D/4D ultrasound allows visualization of coronal plane of uterus and has been recommended by some researchers to identify the point of maximum implantation potential (MIP) within the endometrium while performing ET. Embryo transfers at the MIP were reported to be associated with good implantation and pregnancy rates. The MIP point is an intersection of two lines that are drawn parallel to both cornu on a mid-coronal section of uterus (**Fig. 19**). This was hypothesized as the MIP point, as this point of endometrium is in the trajectory line when the embryo falls into the uterus during the process of natural conception and is thought to be the thickest and having the greatest blood flow. Considering lack of universal availability of 3D US machine and limited evidence base on its advantage, 3D/4D US guided ET cannot be recommended for routine use.

Uterine Contractions

Endometrial wave like activity can be seen on US throughout the menstrual cycle and is highest in the periovulatory period and in 30–40% of spontaneous cycles its rate is 3–4 per minute. The contractions increase in frequency throughout the follicular phase to peak at four to five contractions per minute in the late follicular phase before reducing in frequency during the transition to luteal phase when the uterus essentially becomes quiescent. This pattern of contraction frequency has been suggested as being sex steroid dependent in that it parallels the rise in serum estradiol and the subsequent postovulatory increase in progesterone. The exact physiological benefit of such uterine activity is unknown but the propagation of contractions from the cervix toward the fundus

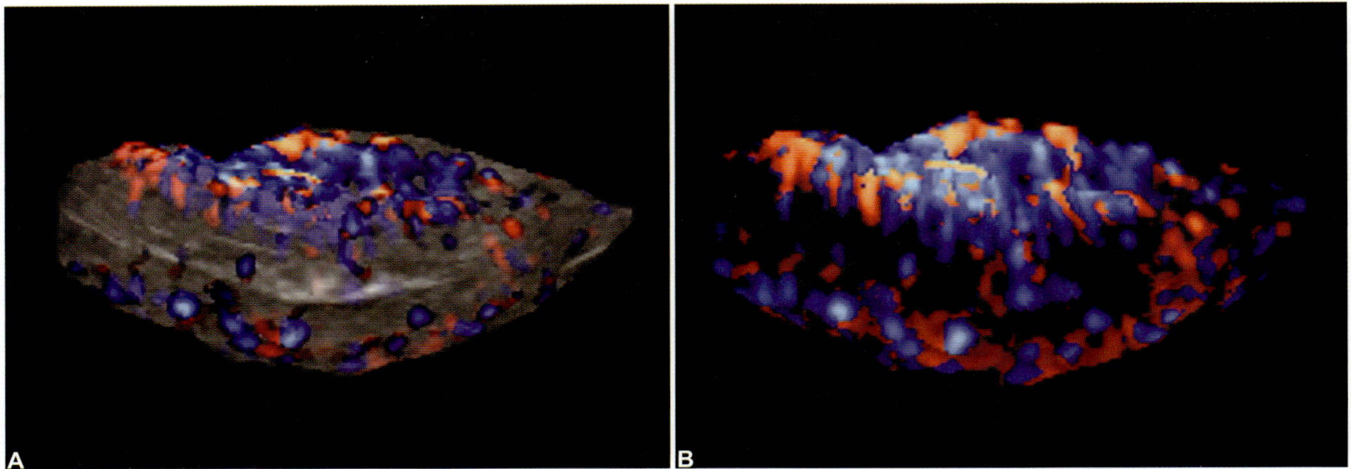

Figs 18A and B Glass body mode of endometrial 3D power Doppler vascularity

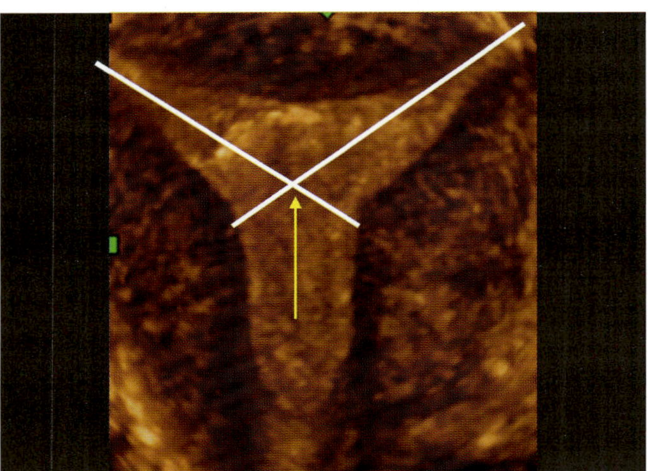

Fig. 19 Maximum implantation potential point

during the periovulatory period may favor the passage of spermatozoa through the uterus to the fallopian tubes. The relative quiescence during the luteal phase is more readily understandable and has been shown to occur during assisted reproduction treatment seven days following the administration of hCG at the time of blastocyst transfer. A contraction frequency of more than 5 per minute on the day of ET is associated with a very low implantation rate in comparison to one of three or less per minute (4% versus 21% respectively). Further studies have confirmed this negative association of symmetrical contractions with the chances of pregnancy following assisted reproduction. Early administration of vaginal progesterone decreases the contraction frequency at the time of ET but this has yet to be shown to significantly increase the conception rates.

Secretory Phase Evaluation

Ovulation is characterized by a blurring of the follicular borders, the appearance of intrafollicular echoes **(Fig. 1B)** and the appearance of free fluid in the pouch of Douglas. Ovulation results in collapse of the follicle with irregular contour followed by filling of its cavity with echogenic fluid, now called corpus luteum. Corpus luteum typically has variable appearances with ground glass echogenicity in lumen or lace like echogenicities **(Fig. 20A)** and has circumferential blood flow referred to as a "ring of fire" **(Fig. 21)**. Three to seven times increase in the blood flow is noted in the dominant ovary (ovary from which ovulation occurs) during the luteal phase. The flow is highest in the mid-luteal phase, which declines till menstruation in absence of conception.

Resistance index of the corpus luteum has been suggested as an adjunct to plasma progesterone assay as an index of luteal function. A healthy corpus luteum will show a vascular ring surrounding itself on color Doppler and on PD these vessels show RI 0.35–0.50, PI 0.70–0.80 and PSV 10–15 cm/sec **(Figs 22A and B)**. This resistance starts increasing on day 23 of the cycle in a non-conception cycle to RI 0.5–0.55. Based on these values, abnormal parameters indicate luteal phase problems like luteinized unruptured follicle or luteal phase defect.

Secretory changes are seen in the endometrium in the form of echogenicity of the endometrium, which starts from outside, proceeding to the central line making a ring sign of the endometrium **(Fig. 20B)**. Its thickness decreases by 0.5 mm on the day of LH surge and then increases by 2 mm in the luteal phase. It is due to postovulatory drop in serum estradiol concentration, that leads to increased resistance in uterine artery, 3 days after

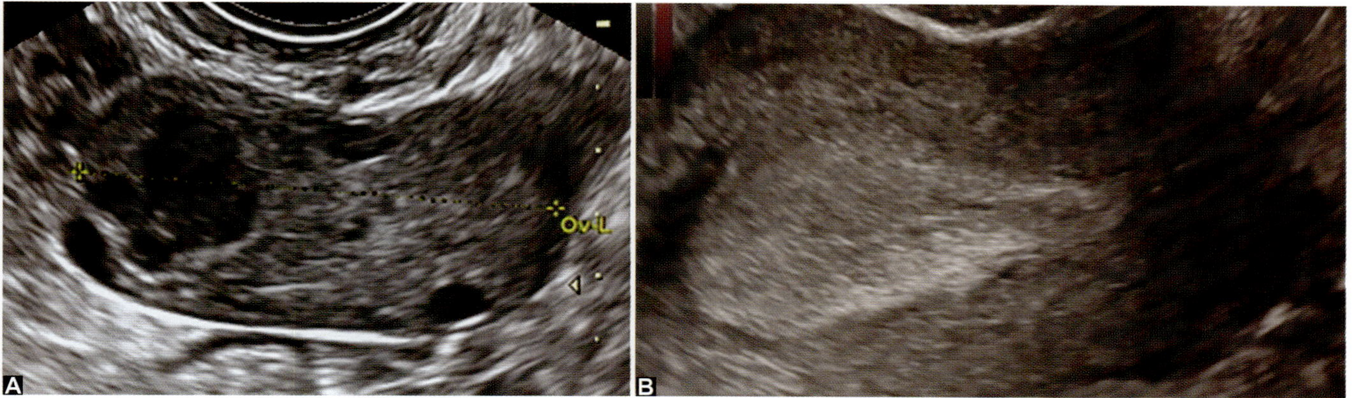

Figs 20A and B (A) Corpus luteum and (B) Secretory endometrium

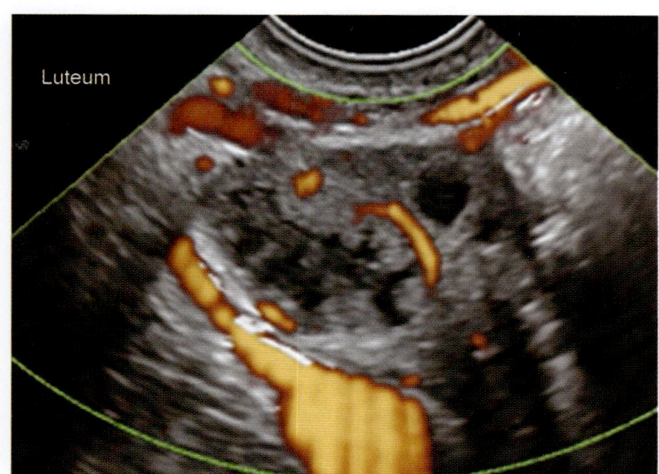

Fig. 21 A typical corpus luteum with vascularity around it

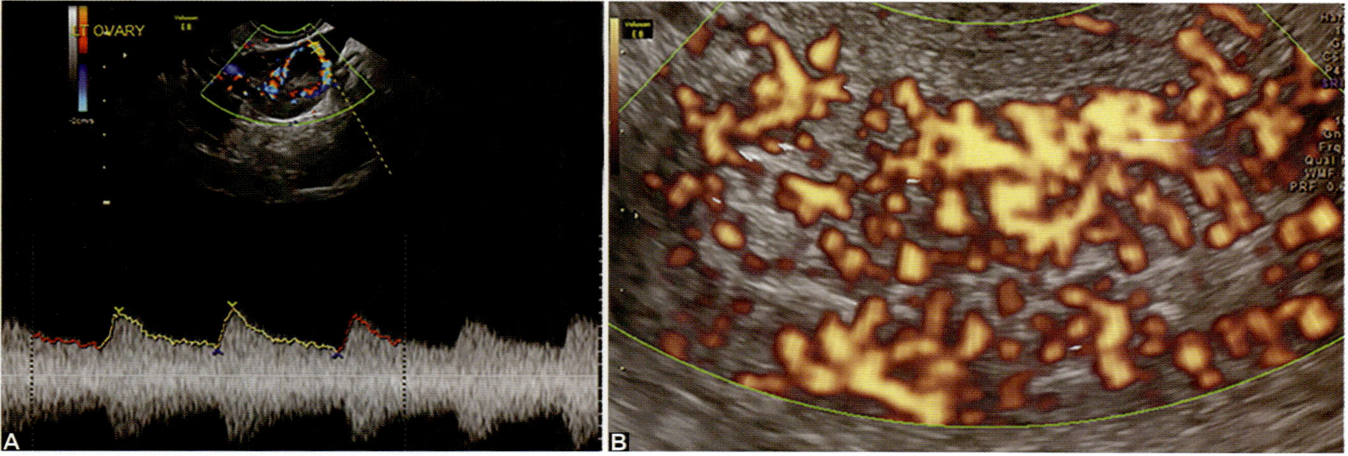

Figs 22A and B Corpus luteum (A) and endometrial Doppler (B) in secretory phase

LH peak with highest resistance on day 16. The uterine artery resistance then falls and reaches its lowest during the peak luteal function. Persistently low RI of uterine artery is maintained in the luteal phase, till menstruation.

Blood flow to the endometrium, which is by spiral arteries follow the similar pattern as the uterine arteries but show a lower resistance and lower velocity than the uterine arteries.

Posterior wall of the uterus also appears more echogenic in this phase due to acoustic enhancement by the endometrium due to fluid accumulation.

■ LUTEINIZED UNRUPTURED FOLLICLE

Rarely, ovulation fails to occur leading to a luteinized, unruptured follicle in which, despite the absence of follicular rupture and release of the oocyte, the unruptured follicle undergoes luteinization under the action of LH. US, but not the mid-luteal progesterone levels, aids in diagnosing this condition as there is normal production of progesterone.

On 2D, US shows persistent follicle with thick walls and progressive loss of cystic appearance which is difficult to differentiate from corpus luteum. Endometrium is thick and echogenic and no fluid is seen in POD. On Doppler perifollicular RI is 0.51–0.59, which is higher than normal and remains almost normal till the end of the cycle. Nondominant ovary also shows similar Doppler indices. Endometrium is echogenic but endometrial flow is absent **(Fig. 23)**.

Luteal Phase Defect

In this case, there is normal follicular development and ovulation with early secretory transformation of endometrium. On Doppler corpus luteum shows high resistance flow with RI: 0.58 + 0.04. Increased resistance is also seen in spiral arteries RI: 0.72 ± 0.06.

This is the case when luteal phase defect is due to insufficient corpus luteum (Figs 20A and B). But when luteal phase defect is due to insufficient progesterone receptors in the endometrium, the endometrial flow is normal but endometrium is thin, non-hyperechogenic and shows scanty vascularity **(Figs 24A and B)**.

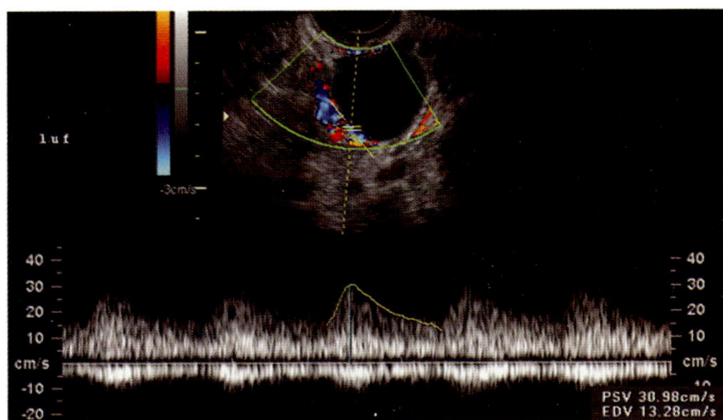

Fig. 23 Luteinized unruptured follicle: high resistance flow in luteinized unruptured follicle

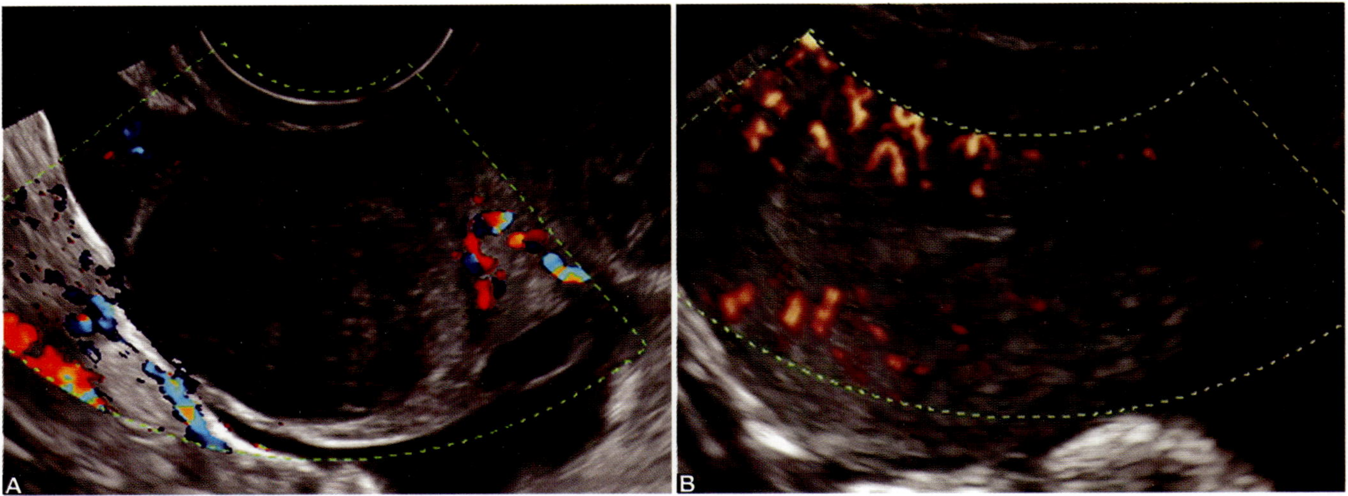

Figs 24A and B Possible luteal phase defect: decreased vascularity around corpus luteum and endometrial vascularity

Segmental uterine and ovarian artery perfusion demonstrates a significant correlation with histological and hormonal markers of uterine receptivity and may aid assessment of luteal phase defect.

■ CONCLUSION

Ultrasound is an excellent tool for cycle monitoring. Doppler helps to understand the hormonal changes occurring during the cycle. Volume assessment both for follicle and the endometrium, are much more reliable parameters than follicular diameter or endometrial thickness. The presence of cumulus can be confirmed by 3D US increases the surety of the presence of a mature ovum in the follicle. The 3D PD gives idea about the global vascularity of follicle and endometrium. Though larger studies and standardization of US parameters and settings are required to establish more precise values for follicular and endometrial VI, FI and VFI, the results are fairly promising. We can hope to understand the follicular and endometrial physiological status better with these parameters and achieve better pregnancy rates with ART procedures and reduce the span of unexplained infertility.

■ KEY POINTS

- Transvaginal ultrasound is the modality of choice to study these changes.
- Follicular tracking describes the serial ultrasonographic study of the ovary during the follicular phase of the menstrual cycle.
- Monitoring of a menstrual cycle should ideally start in early proliferative phase.
- A normal growth rate of a healthy follicle is approximately 2 mm per day and reaches a size of 18–24 mm by the time of ovulation.
- Follicular tracking is important during controlled ovarian stimulation as it is used as part of IVF treatment when multifollicular recruitment is desired.
- SonoAVC has been used to provide automated measures of follicle size and may have implications for the work flow within IVF centers.
- Commonly used markers of endometrial receptivity include endometrial thickness and endometrial pattern.
- Conception is unlikely in association with an endometrial thickness of 5 mm or less, although most centers would prefer to see it measure 8 mm or more prior to embryo transfer.
- While a trilaminar pattern is more frequently associated with conception, a homogenous, hyperechogenic endometrium lacking an echogenic central line has been shown to be associated with non-conception both in natural and assisted reproduction treatment cycles.
- Absent endometrial vascularity is a reliable negative marker of conception.
- Corpus luteum typically has variable appearances with ground glass echogenicity in lumen or lace like echogenicities and has circumferential blood flow referred to as a "ring of fire".
- The 3D power Doppler gives idea about the global vascularity of follicle and endometrium.
- While larger studies and standardization of ultrasound parameters and settings are required to establish more precise values for follicular and endometrial vascularity indices as measured by 3D ultrasound, the results are fairly promising.

■ BIBLIOGRAPHY

1. Andreotti RF, Thompson GH, Janowitz W, et al. Endovaginal and transabdominal sonography of ovarian follicle. J Ultrasound Med. 1989;8(10):555-60.
2. Applebaum M. The 'steel' or 'teflon' endometrium—ultrasound visualization of endometrial vascularity in IVF patients and outcome. Presented at The third World Congress of Ultrasound in Obstetrics and Gyneacolgy. Ultrasound Obstet Gynecol. 1993;3(Suppl 2):10.
3. Bakos O, Lundkvist O, Bergh T. Transvaginal sonographic evaluation of endometrial growth and texture in spontaneous ovulatory cycles—a descriptive study. Hum Reprod. 1993;8: 799-806.
4. Bald R, Hackeloer BJ. Ultraschall-darstellung verschiendener. Endometrium formen. In: Otto R, Jan FX (Eds). Ultraschall-diagnostik 1982. Stuttgart:Thieme; 1983:187.
5. Bourne TH, Athanasiou S, Bauer B. Ovulation and the periovulatory follicle. In: Bourne TH, Jauniaux E, Jurkovic D (Eds). Transvaginal Colour Doppler. Berlin: Springer-Verlag. 1995. pp. 119-30.
6. Bourne TH, Jurkovic D, Waterstone J, et al. Intrafollicular blood flow during human ovulation. Ultrasound Obstet Gynecol. 1991;1(1):53-9.
7. Boué J, Boue A, Lazar P. Retrospective and prospective epidemiological studies of 1500 karyotyped spontaneous human abortions. Teratology. 1973;12(1):11-26.
8. Cacciatore B, Simberg N, Fusaro P, et al. Transvaginal Doppler study of uterine artery blood flow in in vitro fertilization embryo transfer cycles. Fertil Steril. 1996;66(1):130-4.
9. Chein LW, Au HK, Chen PL, et al. Assessment of uterine receptivity by the endometrial-subendometrial blood flow distribution pattern in women undergoing in vitro fertilization-embryo transfer. Fertil Steril. 2002;78:245-51.
10. Coulam CB, Stern JJ, Soenksen DM, et al. Comparison of pulsatility indices on the day of oocyte retrieval and embryo transfer. Hum Reprod. 1995;10(1):82-4.
11. Dickey RP, Olar TT, Taylor SN, et al. Relationship of biochemical pregnancy to pre-ovulatory endometrial thickness and pattern in patients undergoing ovulation induction. Hum Reprod. 1993;8(2):327-30

12. Engmann L, Sladkevicius P, Agrawal R, et al. Value of ovarian stromal blood flow velocity measurement after pituitary suppression in the prediction of ovarian responsiveness and outcome of in vitro fertilization treatment. Fertil Steril. 1999;71(1):22-9.

13. Fanchin R, Righini C, de Ziegler D, et al. Effects of vaginal progesterone administration on uterine contractility at the time of embryo transfer. Fertil Steril. 2001;75(6):1136-40.

14. Fanchin R, Righini C, Olivennes F, et al. Uterine contractions at the time of embryo transfer alter pregnancy rates after in-vitro fertilization. Hum Reprod. 1998;13(7):1968-74.

15. Feichtinger W. Transvaginal three dimensional imaging for evaluation and treatment of infertility. In: Merz E (Ed). 3-D Ultrasound in Obstetrics and Gynecology. Philadelphia: Lippincott Williams & Wilkins; 1998. pp. 37-43.

16. Frattarelli JL, Levi AJ, Miller BT. A prospective novel method of determining ovarian size during in vitro fertilization cycles. J Assist Reprod Genet. 2002;19(1):39-41.

17. Gergely RZ, DeUgarte CM, Danzer H, et al. Three dimensional/ four dimensional ultrasound-guided embryo transfer using the maximal implantation potential point. Fertil Steril. 2005; 84(2):500-3.

18. Glock JL, Brumsted JR. Color flow pulsed Doppler ultrasound in diagnosing luteal phase defect. Fertil Steril. 1995;64:500-4.

19. Goswamy RK, Steptoe PC. Doppler ultrasound studies of the uterine artery in spontaneous ovarian cycles. Hum Reprod. 1988;3(6):721-6.

20. Hackelöer BJ, Fleming R, Robinson HP, et al. Correlation of ultrasonic and endocrinological assessment of human follicular development. Am J Obstet Gynecol. 1979;135(1):122-8.

21. Ijland MM, Evers JLH, Dunselman GAJ, et al. Endometrial wavelike movements during menstrual cycle. Fertil Steril. 1996;65:746-9.

22. Killam AP, Rosenfeld C, Battaglia FC, et al. Effect of estrogens on the uterine blood flow in oophorectomized ewes. Am J Obstet Gynecol. 1973;115(8):1045-50.

23. Kupesic S, Bekavac I, Bjelos D, et al. Assessment of endometrial receptivity by transvaginal color Doppler and three-dimensional power Doppler ultrasonography in patients undergoing in vitro fertilization procedures. J Ultrasound Med. 2001;20(2):125-34.

24. Kupesic S, Bekavac I, Bjelos D, et al. Assessment of endometrial receptivity by transvaginal color Doppler and three dimensional power Doppler ultrasonography in patients undergoing in vitro fertilization procedures. J Ultrasound Med. 2001;20(2):125-34.

25. Kupesic S, Kurjak A. Prediction of IVF outcome by three-dimensional ultrasound. Hum Reprod. 2002;17(4):950-5.

26. Kupesic S, Kurjak A. The assessment of normal and abnormal luteal function by transvaginal color Doppler sonography. Eur J Obstet Gynecol. 1997;72:83-7.

27. Kupesic S, Kurjak A. The assessment of normal and abnormal luteal function by transvaginal color Doppler sonography. Eur J Obstet Gynecol Reprod Biol. 1997;72:83-7.

28. Kupesic S, Kurjak A. Uterine and ovarian perfusion during the periovulatory period assessed by transvaginal color Doppler. Fertil Steril. 1993;60(3):439-43

29. Kupesić S, Kurjak A, Vujisic S, et al. Luteal phase defect: comparison between Doppler velocimetry, histological and hormonal markers. Ultrasound Obstet Gynecol. 1997;9: 105-12.

30. Kupesić S. The first three weeks assessed by transvaginal color Doppler. J Perinat Med. 1996;24(4):301-17.

31. Kurjak A, Kupesic-Urek S, Schulman H, et al. Transvaginal color flow Doppler in the assessment of ovarian and uterine blood flow in infertile women. Fertil Steril. 1991;56(5):870-5.

32. Kurjak A, Kupesic-Urek S. Infertility. In: Kurjak A (Ed). Transvaginal Color Doppler. Carnforth, UK: Parthenon Publishing; 1991. pp. 33-8.

33. Kwee J, Elting ME. Schats R, et al. Ovarian volume and antral follicle count for the prediction of low and hyper responders with in vitro fertilization. Reprod Biol Endocrinol. 2007;5:9.

34. Kyei-Mensah A, Maconochie N, Zaidi J, et al. Transvaginal three-dimensional ultrasound: reproducibility of ovarian and endometrial volume measurements. Fertil Steril. 1996;66(5):718-22.

35. Kyei-Mensah A, Zaidi J, Pittrof R, et al. Transvaginal three-dimensional ultrasound: accuracy of follicular volume measurements. Fertil Steril. 1996;65:371-6.

36. Lesny P, Killick SR, Tetlow RL, et al. Uterine junctional zone contractions during assisted reproduction cycles. Hum Reprod Update. 1998;4(4):440-5.

37. Luciano GN, Tarek AG. Ultrasonography and IVF. In: Botros RMB Rizk (Ed). Ultrasonography in Reproductive Medicine and Infertility, 1st edition. Cambridge University Press; 2010. pp. 193-201.

38. Merce LT, Barco MJ, Kupesic S, Kurjak A. 2D and 3D power Doppler ultrasound from ovulation to implantation. In: Kurjak A, Chervenak FA (Eds). Textbook of Perinatal Medicine. London: Parthenon Publishing; 2005.

39. Merce LT. Ultrasound markers of implantation. Ultrasound Rev Obstet Gynecol. 2002;2:110-23.

40. Mercé LT, Barco MJ, Bau S, et al. Are endometrial parameters by three-dimensional ultrasound and power Doppler angiography related to in vitro fertilization/embryo transfer outcome? Fertil Steril. 2008;89(1):111-7.

41. Mercé LT, Barco MJ, Bau S, et al. Prediction of ovarian response and IVF/ICSI outcome by three-dimensional ultrasonography and power Doppler angiography. Eur J Obstet Gynecol Reprod Biol. 2007;132(1):93-100.

42. Nargund G, Bourne T, Doyle PE, et al. Association between ultrasound indices of follicular blood flow, oocyte recovery and preimplantation embryo quality. Hum Reprod. 1996;11(1):109-13.

43. Nargund G, Doyle PE, Bourne TH, et al. Ultrasound derived indices of follicular blood flow before HCG administration and prediction of oocyte recovery and preimplantation embryo quality. Hum Reprod. 1996;11:2512-17.

44. Ng EH, Chan CC, Tang OS, et al. Comparison of endometrial and subendometrial blood flow measured by three-dimensional power Doppler ultrasound between stimulated and natural cycles in the same patients. Hum Reprod. 2004;19(10): 2385-90.

45. Ng EH, Chan CC, Tang OS, et al. Relationship between uterine blood flow and endometrial and subendometrial

blood flows during stimulated and natural cycles. Fertil Steril. 2006;85(3):721-7.

46. Ng EH, Chan CC, Tang OS, et al. The role of endometrial and subendometrial blood flows measured by three-dimensional power Doppler ultrasound in prediction of pregnancy during IVF treatment. Hum Reprod. 2006;21(1):164-70.

47. Niswender GD, Moore RT, Akbar AM, et al. Flow of blood to the ovaries of ewes throughout the estrous cycle. Biol Reprod. 1975;13(4):381-8.

48. Panchal SY, Nagori CB. Can 3D PD be a better tool for assessing the pre HCG follicle and endometrium? A randomized study of 500 cases. Presented at 16th World Congress on Ultrasound in Obstetrics and Gynecology. J Ultrasound Obstet Gynecol. 2006;28(4):504.

49. Poehl M, Hohlagschwandtner M, Doerner V, et al. Cumulus assessment by three-dimensional ultrasound for in vitro fertilzation. Ultrasound Obstet Gynecol. 2000;16:251-3.

50. Raine-Fenning N, Deb S, Jayaprakasan K, et al. Timing of oocyte maturation and egg collection during controlled ovarian stimulation: a randomized controlled trial evaluating manual and automated measurements of follicle diameter. Fertil Steril. 2010;94(1):184-8.

51. Raine-Fenning N, Jayaprakasan K, Clewes J. Automated follicle tracking facilitates standardization and may improve work flow. Ultrasound Obstet Gynecol. 2007;30(7):1015-8.

52. Rainne-Fenning NJ, Campbell BK, Kendall NR, et al. Quantifying the changes in endometrial vascularity throughout the normal menstrual cycle with three-dimensional power Doppler angiography. Hum Reprod. 2004;19:330-8.

53. Randall JM, Fisk MM, McTavish A, et al. Transvaginal ultrasonic assessment of endometrial growth in spontaneous and hyperstimulated menstrual cycles. Br J Obstet Gynaecol. 1989;96:954-9.

54. Salim A, Kurjak A, Zalud I. Ovarian Luteal flow in normal and abnormal early pregnancies. J Matern Fetal Invest. 1992;2:119.

55. Scheffer GJ, Broekmans FJ, Looman CW, et al. The number of antral follicles in normal women with proven fertility is best reflection of reproductive age. Hum Reprod. 2003;18(4):700-6.

56. Scholtes MC, Wladimiroff JW, van Rijen HJ, et al. Uterine and ovarian flow velocity waveforms in the normal menstrual cycle: a transvaginal study. Fertil Steril. 1989;52(6):981-5.

57. Smith B, Porter R, Ahuja K, et al. Ultrasonic assessment of endometrial changes in stimulated cycles in an in vitro fertilization and embryo transfer program. J In Vitro Fert Embryo Transf. 1984;1(4):233-8.

58. Soldevila PN, Carreras O, Tur R, et al. Sonographic assessment of ovarian reserve. Its correlation with outcome of in vitro fertilization cycles. Gynecol Endocrinol. 2007;23(4):206-12.

59. Steer CV, Campbell S, Tan SL, et al. The use of transvaginal color flow imaging after in vitro fertilization to identify optimum uterine conditions before embryo transfer. Fertil Steril. 1992;57(2):372-6.

60. Tsai YC, Chang JC, Tai MJ, et al. Relationship of uterine perfusion to outcome of intrauterine insemination. J Ultrasound Med. 1996;15(9):633-6.

61. Van Blerkom J, Antczak M, Schrader R. The developmental potential of human oocyte is related to the dissolved oxygen content of follicular fluid: association with vascular endothelial growth factor levels and perifollicular blood flow characteristics. Hum Reprod. 1997;12(5):1047-55.

62. Vlaisavljević V, Reljic M, Gavrić Lovrec V, et al. Measurement of perifollicular blood flow of the dominant preovulatory follicle using three-dimensional power Doppler. Ultrasound Obstet Gynecol. 2003;22:520-6.

63. Weissman A, Gotlieb L, Casper RF. The detrimental effect of increased endometrial thickness on implantation and pregnancy rates and outcome in an in vitro fertilization program. Fertil Steril. 1999;71(1):147-9.

64. Wittmack FM, Kreger DO, Blasco L, et al. Effect of follicular size on oocyte retrieval, fertilization, cleavage and embryo quality in in vitro fertilization cycles: a 6-year data collection. Fertil Steril. 1994;62(6):1205-10.

65. Wittmack FM, Kreger DO, Blasco L, et al. Effect of follicular size on oocyte retrieval, fertilization, cleavage and embryo quality in in vitro fertilization cycles: a 6-year data collection. Fertil Steril. 1994;62:1205-10.

66. Wittmack FM, Kreger DO, Blasco L, et al. Effect of follicular size on oocyte retrieval, fertilization, cleavage and embryo quality in in vitro fertilization cycles: a 6 year data collection. Fertil Steril. 1994;62(6):1205-10.

67. Wu HM, Chiang CH, Huang HY, et al. Detection of the sub-endometrial vascularization flow index by three-dimensional ultrasound may be useful for predicting pregnancy rate for patients undergoing in vitro fertilization-embryo transfer. Fertil Steril. 2003;79(3):507-11.

68. Yagel S, Ben-Chetrit A, Anteby E, et al. The effect of ethinyl estradiol on endometrial thickness and uterine volume during ovulation induction by clomiphene citrate. Fertil Steril. 1992;57(1):33-6.

69. Yang JH, Wu MY, Chen CD, et al. Association of endometrial blood flow as determined by modified colour Doppler technique with subsequent outcome of in-vitro fertilization. Hum Reprod. 1999;14(6):1606-10.

70. Zaidi J, Barber J, Kyei-Mensah A, et al. Relationship of ovarian stromal blood flow at the baseline ultrasound scan to subsequent follicular response in an in vitro fertilization program. Obstet Gynecol. 1996;88(5):779-84.

71. Zaidi J, Campbell S, Pittrof R, et al. Endometrial thickness, morphology, vascular penetration and velocimetry in predicting implantation in an in vitro fertilization program. Ultrasound Obstet Gynecol. 1995;6:191-8.

72. Zaidi J, Pittrof R, Shaker A, et al. Assessment of uterine artery blood flow on the day of human chorionic gonadotrophin administration by transvaginal colour Doppler ultrasound in an in vitro fertilization program. Fertil Steril. 1996;65:377-81.

Effect of Environment on Fertility

Sunita R Tandulwadkar, Sejal Naik

INTRODUCTION

A review of the literature on the determinants of fertility raises more questions than can be answered in the current state of knowledge. It has been known since years, high local temperature (tight clothing, hot water/steam bath, working with laptop putting on lap) reduces semen quality. Smoking and alcohol consumption produce not only subfertility in both male and female but also cause damage to exposed in utero fetus. Emotional or social stress is confounding factor in subfertility. Though, these social, occupational or emotional factors have great role in etiology of subfertility, in this chapter we have focused only in the environmental factors, and its effect on fertility, in a population that has been exposed. It is estimated that over 1,000 new chemicals are being introduced into the world every year, yet less than 5% have been investigated for their effect on reproduction. There is evidence that fertility rate, quality and quantity of semen in normal men are declining drastically over past few years. Though the hazardous effects of various environmental factors have been suspected, there is lack of priority to research on reproduction in basic biology, epidemiology and toxicology.[1-3]

Not only the topic has been largely ignored but it is complicated and difficult task to document any effect of compound. Moreover, it needs huge funding too, because of following issues:

Inability to perform randomized controlled trials (RCTs): RCTs is widely recognized as the gold standard in medical research, but use of such trials poses distinct challenges when studying toxicity. It would be unethical to deliberately expose individuals to potentially toxic chemicals.

Time-lag bias: The compound can have its devastating effects in the long term that are not immediately recognizable. This can be explained by our experience with DES, which has estrogenic potency comparable to that of estradiol. From the late 1940s onward, it was widely used during pregnancy, especially in the USA to prevent pregnancy complications. It is estimated that more than two million women were exposed to this drug. A RCT published in 1953 discovered that in utero exposure of DES to female fetuses led to a risk of developing clear cell adenocarcinoma some 15 years later.[4,5] While this particular risk is fortunately rare, DES-exposed girls have reproductive tract anomalies, and they subsequently have reduced fertility and increased rates of ectopic pregnancy, spontaneous abortion and preterm delivery.[5]

Phenotypic variations in response to toxic agent: There is variation in genetic vulnerability and phenotypic response, which can mask the compound's impact. For example, the toxicological experiments consistently find stronger effects of estrogens on females than males.[6] As their potency combined with exposure concentrations are lower than endogenous hormones, so, intake of phytoestrogen in Oriental populations, a strong effect seems unlikely.

Unpredictable dose-response mechanisms: Hormonal toxicants do not always respond according to the classic dose-response curve. If endocrine disrupting chemicals (EDCs) are hormonal mimickers, they probably act as "biphasic dose-response curve". For example, estradiol has negative feedback effect on gonadotropin-releasing hormone (GnRH) release until it reaches a critical concentration, at which it begins to increase the release of GnRH and thus luteinizing hormone (LH) surge that initiate ovulation. Thus in low dose, they may show effect but at higher concentration usually used to test for chemical toxicity, they may not show negative impact.[7]

Bio-accumulation of multiple compounds: Humans are exposed to thousands of compounds over a lifetime, and it is therefore difficult to sort out the relationship between a specific compound and a specific outcome. The Centers for Disease Control and Prevention has only evaluated 148 compounds through blood and urine analysis of the known 80,000 synthetic compounds in our environment.[8]

■ MECHANISM OF DAMAGE TO CELL

Any pathogen or compounds damages the cell by two ways:
1. Direct cell membrane damage, or
2. Damage to intracellular components.

Some compounds alter the normal communication pathways by mimicking or blocking them. Some EDCs are identified causing negative effect on reproduction by directly or indirectly displacing hormones.[9] These EDCs have been shown to have deleterious effects on animal and fish reproduction and can exact more influence than the genes they inherit.[10]

Some compounds damage the intracellular organelles and thus cell death. Few toxins have been identified to damage or incorporate into DNA of the cells and can transmit this genoenvironmental effect to offsprings.

■ COMMON COMPOUNDS DETRIMENTAL TO FERTILITY

Smoking, tobacco intake and alcohol have been clearly accepted as potential cause of poor sperm quality, increased abortion rate and multiple fetal abnormalities. Apart from these major environmental or habitual toxins, there are certain environmental compounds identified as harmful to reproductive function. Many compounds are now banned in many countries for their commercial use **(Table 1)**.

To understand environment and its effects on fertility in a better way, we have discussed its effects in three parts:
1. The seminal fluid (contains sperm).
2. The follicle (contains egg).
3. The amniotic sac (contains developing embryo).

Seminal Fluid

The seminal plasma acts as a chemical concentrator, increasing levels of various environmental toxicants in the fluid. Men having higher exposure to pesticides show higher level of pesticides in blood and semen, with low sperm counts and motility than men having low exposure.[11]

Demography

Study objectives: Two types of endpoint can be studied in male factor: semen quality and fertility as measured by the time taken to conceive (time to pregnancy, or TTP). TTP reflects the probability of conception for couples having unprotected intercourse. It is a functional measure of biological fertility at the level of the couple.[12] All are subject to large degrees of biological variation and/or measurement errors in interpretation of sperm concentration, motility and morphology. In addition, representative samples of the general population, which are so important for descriptive epidemiology, are unachievable as subjects are either candidate for semen donation, for vasectomy or from men with fertility-related problem.

Trend: A much-cited paper published in 1992 reviewed that worldwide there was 50% decline in mean concentration over 50 years from 113 million/mL to 66 million/mL and should be treated with great caution.[3] An attempt at a more rigorous analysis, they found the decline in sperm density, sperm motility and morphology to be much steeper in Europe than in America; studies from elsewhere were too sparse and diverse to draw confident conclusions.[13] The findings are compatible not only with a period effect but also with a birth cohort effect, men born in the 1940s having better quality semen than those born in the 1960s.[14]

Spatial variation: Based on the available evidence, sperm concentrations and TTP appear to be relatively high in New York and Finland and low in California and Northwestern Europe including Denmark and Britain.[15,16] Possible explanations include environmental pollution, and dietary changes involving macronutrients or micronutrients, or contaminants. Other possible factors could include an excess meat consumption, increasingly sedentary way of life, tight clothing, since raising the intratesticular temperature strongly affects the quality as well as the quantity of sperm—sufficient to cause reduced fertility in men.

Genetic factors/gene–environment interaction: Male fertility problems tend to aggregate in families,[17,18] infertile men have relatively few siblings, and their brothers have inferior semen quality.[2] A recent report reported the heritability of sperm concentration as 20%, sperm morphology was 41%, and that of chromatin stability was 68%. Exposure to a genotoxic agent would lead to some form of mutation; its survival in subsequent generations would depend on various factors. One of them is the extent

Table 1 Summary of common environmental toxic agents

Toxic agents	Source of exposure	Potential effects	How to reduce exposure
Phthalates	Plastic toys, shampoos, soaps, nail polish, medical devices, coating of timed released drugs, flooring, lacquers and varnishes	↑ Time to pregnancy, ↑ Anogenital distance (genital anomalies and low testicular volume)	Unavoidable
Pesticides	DDT, DDE, organochlorides (fruits, vegetables, flowers, air exposure)	↓ Fecundability, ↓ Success with IVF, ↓ Semen quality, ↑ Spontaneous abortion, ↑ Preterm birth, ↑ Small of gestational age fetus	Proper washing of raw food, use of organic products
Polychlorinated biphenyls	Dioxin like property, oils and lubricants, electrical insulators; exposure by contaminated food consumption	↓ Response to ovulation induction, ↓ Fecundability, ↓ Lactation, ↓ Sperm quality, ↑ Endometriosis, altered menstrual cycle	Avoid consumption of contaminated fish/food
Dioxin	Industrial activities, fires. In fatty meats, fish and dairy products	↑ Cancer, ↑ Birth defects, ↑ Endometriosis	Avoid fatty meats or other contaminated food
Polybrominated diphenyl ethers	Flame retardants in mattresses, furniture, pillows, carpets, electronic devices, TVs, DVD players, computers	Reproductive development disruption	Unavoidable
Bisphenols	Polycarbonate plastics, rigid water bottles, soda bottles and plastic food containers	Breast cancer, prostate changes	Avoid hard plastic bottles and food containers, but likely unavoidable
Heavy metals			
Lead	Paints, old pipes	↓ IQ in offspring, ↓ Semen quality/quantity, ↓ Spontaneous abortion, ↑ Time to pregnancy, ↑ Preterm labor	Avoid old paint and pressure treated lumber, limit certain fish consumption
Mercury	Old thermometers, large fish		
Chromium and arsenic	Pressure treated wood		

Abbreviations: DDT, dichlorodiphenyltrichloroethane; DDE, dichlorodiphenyldichloroethylene; IQ, intelligence quotient

to which it affects biological fertility. In case of severely affected genomic damage where end of reproductive life/sterility developed thus unable to transmit the disease to offspring. Gonadoblastoma, testicular dysgenesis syndrome and some childhood cancers have been associated with genetic transmission.

Some common substances affect male fertility are:

Estrogen: Exposure of developing male fetus to dietary phytoestrogens increases the risk of testicular cancer and cryptorchidism. In contrast to the marked impact on girls, boys exposed in utero to DES show relatively minor effects. They tend to have genital abnormalities such as cysts, urethral stenosis, cryptorchidism, risk of testicular cancer and hypospadias is raised.

Dibromochloropropane (DBCP), used for soil fumigation on fruit plantations, is a potent testicular toxin. High exposure causes permanent azoospermia. DBCP was banned in the late 1970s in the USA, although it is still used elsewhere.[19]

Dichlorodiphenyldichloroethylene (DDE): The stable breakdown product of DDT, can block the androgen receptor, as can certain other pesticides, and that some phthalates inhibit testosterone synthesis.

Lead and cadmium: No effect was seen below a blood level of lead about 44 µg/dL and, even in the occupational context, few men have higher exposures than this, in the economically developed world.[20,21]

Dioxin is known to lower serum testosterone and raised follicle-stimulating hormone and LH levels with occupational exposure. Vietnam veterans tended to have lower sperm concentrations, fewer morphologically "normal" cells, testicular cancer (seminoma) and many birth defects years after exposed to Agent Orange, a pesticide containing dioxin than non-Vietnamese. All these findings would relate to a period effect, following exposure of adult males as dioxin has a half-life of 6–11 years.

Follicular Environment

The study of follicular fluid became possible for studies demonstrating the presence of toxicants by process of IVF.[22-25] If toxicants are present in follicular fluid at the time of resumption of meiosis; the chromosome susceptibility is at its highest. The follicular toxicant concentrations are usually lower than the serum level, thus exposure beyond certain limit can only cause damage to oocyte. Moreover, the preovulatory oocyte is quiescent and poses second meiotic division as early as fertilization stage. Thus, more studies will be required to understand if there is any adverse impact on oocyte DNA.

Adverse effects of some common substances in follicular fluid:
- *DDE* failed fertilization,[22] reduce TTP. In one study, it shows no effect on TTP.[26]
- *Paracervical block (PCB)* reduces oocyte recovery, embryo cleavage rate,[25] increase pregnancy success, and reduce TTP. While, few studies demonstrated no relation with PCB exposure and TTP, miscarriage rate, stillbirth or subfertility.[26,27]
- *Lead* destroy oocytes, lead to follicular atresia, suppression of menarche, decreased circulating progesterone levels, oligomenorrhea in non-human primates.[28] The mechanism by which lead affect directly ovary or central neuroendocrine system in human is unknown. In some studies, it showed to raise spontaneous miscarriage rate,[29] but more recent study failed to demonstrate the same.[30]
- *Mercury:* Its levels have not been reported in follicular fluid, but mercury's effect on developing fetus in utero has been subject to a great deal of scrutiny.

Amniotic Sac Microenvironment

"Fragile fetus" is the term given by endocrinologist Howard Bern (US) to the vulnerable developing fetus in utero exposed to intrauterine insult and to toxic substances.

Mercury: It is a commonly found element with deposits in land as well as sea. And via contaminated food (fish) or by "coal mining", human get exposed. There is little evidence correlating mercury poisoning and infertility but its great concern is its effects on fetus. It passes through placenta and enters amniotic fluid. Inability of fetus to defecate or remove this heavy metal through liver (not fully functional liver) causes accumulation of mercury. Moreover, in utero urine is cycled from amniotic fluid into the developing fetus, nose and mouth, and back into the amniotic fluid. Importantly, the blood–brain barrier is more permeable during development and thus brain of fetus receives greater exposure than that of adult. The mercury exposure lowers cognitive core of child, higher exposure lead to neonatal central nervous system damage and even death. The current Food and Drug Administration recommendations are for women of childbearing age to avoid consuming fish containing more than 1 µg/g.

PCB: Children exposed to PCBs in utero by used of contaminated cooking oil, showed abnormal sperm motility, morphology and decreased ability to penetrate hamster eggs.

Estrogen: In form of dietary phytoestrogens or DES exposure, in utero exposure of female fetuses led to a risk of reproductive tract anomalies. DES exposure can cause clear cell adenocarcinoma some 15 years later. The girls subsequently have reduced fertility and increased rates of ectopic pregnancy, spontaneous abortion and preterm delivery.[5]

■ CLINICAL CONSIDERATION

The question regarding environmental exposure is to include during history taking especially about solvents, pesticides or heavy metals. The questions regarding their location of residence, food habits, amount of fish consumption, etc. Educate them about the potential toxicants and help them to avoid its exposure.

As no decontaminating method is scientifically proved effective, and concrete evidence on impact of EDCs are lacking, further studies are needed to elaborate our knowledge on this topic. The pharmaceuticals use of any drug needs to be proved safe before it consumed, while we allowing an "innocent until proven guilty" policy in environmental toxicant exposure is in question.

CONCLUSION

- Out of 80,000 suspected compounds in environment only few are identified as toxic for human.
- The study on toxicants is difficult because inability to conduct RCTs, long time-lag since exposure to effect, phenotypic variation in response, biphasic dose-response curve and accumulation of multiple toxic agents in humans.
- Toxicants can damage the cells by two ways: (1) direct cell membrane damage, or (2) damage to intracellular components.
- Certain toxicants are unavoidable like phthalates, polybrominated diphenyl ethers, bisphenols, etc.
- The seminal plasma acts as a chemical concentrator and has higher level of toxicants than in blood, thus, affecting more.
- Several evidence points toward genetic damage and impairment of the male reproductive system which could arise through male or female exposure. Possibly the Y chromosome is especially important as a target for mutation. A genetic etiology raises the possibility that additional health endpoints are also affected.
- Very few toxic agents found in follicular fluid, but it is potentially important as preovulatory egg is being exposed.
- Fetus in amniotic sac is not completely devoid of exposure to maternal toxins. Heavy metal like mercury has great detrimental effect on fetus beyond certain concentration in maternal blood.
- It is important to note while history taking, any exposure to chemicals, pesticides, certain drugs, anticarcinogens, radiation or high consumption on fish. As evidence are lacking in their concrete review on toxicants, one should be caution while counseling.
- There is emerged need to study in detail about the toxic compound to reproduction and human health.

REFERENCES

1. Nonaka K, Miura T, Peter K. Recent fertility decline in Dariusleut Hutterites: an extension of Eaton and Mayer's Hutterite fertility study. Hum Biol. 1994;66:411-20.
2. Auger J, Kunstmann JM, Czyglik F, et al. Decline in semen quality among fertile men in Paris during the past 20 years. N Engl J Med. 1995;332:281-5.
3. Carlsen E, Giwercman A, Keiding N, et al. Evidence for decreasing quality of semen during past 50 years. BMJ. 1992;305:609-13.
4. Dieckmann WJ, Davis ME, Rynkiewicz LM, et al. Does the administration of diethylstilbestrol during pregnancy have therapeutic value? 1953. Am J Obstet Gynecol. 1999;181:1572-3.
5. Goldberg JM, Falcone TF. Effect of diethylstilbestrol on reproductive function. Fertil Steril. 1999;72:1-7.
6. Committee on Toxicity of Chemicals in Food, Consumer Products and the Environment. Phytoestrogens and Health. London: Food Standards Agency, 2003. http://www.foodstandards.gov.uk/multimedia/pdfs/phytoreport0503, last accessed November 7, 2003
7. Welshons WV, Thayer KA, Judy BM, et al. Large effects from small exposures. I. Mechanisms for endocrine-disrupting chemicals with estrogenic activity. Environ Health Perspect. 2003;111:994-1006.
8. Sharpe RM, Fisher JS, Millar MM, et al. Gestational and lactational exposure of rats to xenoestrogens results in reduced testicular size and sperm production. Environ Health Perspect. 1995;103:1136-43.
9. Brevini TA, Zanetto SB, Cillo F. Effects of endocrine disruptors on developmental and reproductive functions. Curr Drug Targets Immune Endocr Metabol Disord. 2005;5:1-10.
10. Damstra T. Potential effects of certain persistent organic pollutants and endocrine disrupting chemicals on the health of children. J Clin Toxicol. 2002;40:457-65.
11. Younglai EV, Holloway AC, Foster WG. Environmental and occupational factors affecting fertility and IVF success. Hum Reprod Update. 2005;11:43-57.
12. Joffe M. Time to pregnancy: a measure of reproductive function in either sex. Asclepios Project. Occup Environ Med. 1997;54:289-95.
13. Swan SH, Elkin EP, Fenster L. The question of declining sperm density revisited: an analysis of 101 studies published 1934–1996. Environ Health Perspect. 2000;108:961-6.
14. Joffe M. Are problems with male reproductive health caused by endocrine disruption? Occup Environ Med. 2001;58:281.
15. Karmaus W, Juul S. European Infertility and Subfecundity Group. Infertility and subfecundity in population-based samples from Denmark, Germany, Italy, Poland and Spain. Eur J Public Health. 1999;9:229-35.
16. Joffe M. Lower fertility in Britain compared with Finland. Lancet. 1996;347:1519-20.
17. Lilford R, Jones AM, Bishop DT, et al. Case control study of whether subfertility in men is familial. BMJ. 1994;309:570-3.
18. Meschede D, Lemke B, Behre HM, et al. Clustering of male infertility in the families of couples treated with intra-cytoplasmic sperm injection. Hum Reprod. 2000;15:1604-8.
19. Goldsmith AJR. Dibromochloropropane: epidemiological findings and current questions. Ann N Y Acad Sci. 1997;837:300-6.

20. Bonde JP, Giwercman A. Occupational hazards to male fecundity. Reprod Med Rev. 1995;4:59-73.
21. Bonde JP, Joffe M, Apostoli P, et al. Sperm count and chromatin structure in men exposed to inorganic lead: lowest adverse effect levels. Occup Environ Med. 2002;59:234-42.
22. Younglai EV, Foster WG, Hughes EG, et al. Levels of environmental contaminants in human follicular fluid, serum, and seminal plasma of couples undergoing in vitro fertilization. Arch Environ Contam Toxicol. 2002;43:121-6.
23. Foster WG, Jarrell JF, Younglai EV, et al. An overview of some reproductive toxicology studies conducted at Health Canada. Toxicol Ind Health. 1996;12:447-59.
24. Jarrell J, Villeneuve D, Franklin C, et al. Contamination of human ovarian follicular fluid and serum by chlorinated organic compounds in three Canadian cities. CMAJ. 1993; 148:1321-7.
25. Trapp M, Baukloh B, Bhnet HG, et al. Pollutants in human follicular fluid. Fertil Steril. 1984;42:146-8.
26. Law DC, Klebanoff MA, Brock JW, et al. Maternal serum levels of polychlorinated biphenyls and 1,1-dichloro-2, 2-bis (p-chlorophenyl) ethylene (DDE) and time to pregnancy. Am J Epidemiol. 2005;162:523-32.
27. Axmon A, Rylander L, Stromberg U, et al. Polychlorinated biphenyls in serum and time to pregnancy. Environ Res. 2004;96:186-95.
28. Miller R, Bellinger D, Metals. In: Paul M, (Ed). Occupational and Environmental Reproductive Hazards: A Guide for Clinicians. Baltimore: Williams & Wilkins; 1993.
29. Rom WN. Effects of lead on the female and reproduction: a review. Mt Sinai J Med. 1976;43:542-52.
30. Murphy MJ, Graziano JH, Popovac D, et al. Past pregnancy outcomes among women living in the vicinity of a lead smelter in Kosovo, Yugoslavia. Am J Public Health. 1990;80:33-5.

Endoscopy in Infertility

8 Fertility Enhancing Laparoscopic Surgery

Sanjay Patel

INTRODUCTION

Conception is a complex and delicate process, which requires normal ovaries, tubo-ovarian relationship, tubal patency and a normal uterine cavity.

Anything that disturbs pelvic anatomy can lead to infertility. Even for assisted reproductive technologies (ART), normal pelvic anatomy, free from endometriosis, hydrosalpinx, uterine myomas etc. is crucial.

Advancements in minimally invasive techniques like hysteroscopy and laparoscopy have revolutionized treatment of infertility. These fertility-enhancing surgeries not only help in natural conception but also improves success rates after ART.

Fertility enhancing laparoscopic surgery can be classified mainly into four types of surgeries:
1. Tubal surgery
2. Endometriosis surgery
3. Myomectomy
4. Adenomyomectomy.

TUBAL SURGERY

Hysteroscopic Transcervical Tubal Cannulation

It is indicated in proximal tubal occlusion (PTO), 5F catheter along with obturator is inserted into the operating channel of the hysteroscope. The obturator is then removed, and tip of this catheter is curved and wedged against the tubal ostium. Dilute methylene blue dye may be injected. If dye is seen coming from the tube, patency is confirmed and the procedure is finished. If no dye is seen, then guidewire is introduced inside the catheter. The guidewire is advanced slowly through the uterotubal junction into the intramural portion of the tube into the isthmic portion. The guidewire is removed and the dilute dye is injected under laparoscopic observation. If dye is observed, the procedure is terminated. If there is resistance to passage of the guidewire or catheter, an attempt is made to mobilize the tube laparoscopically. If unsuccessful, patient is counseled for tubal surgery or in vitro fertilization (IVF) **(Figs 1A and B)**.

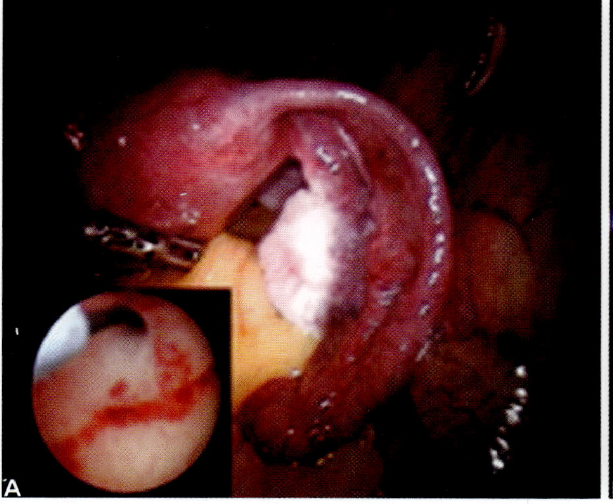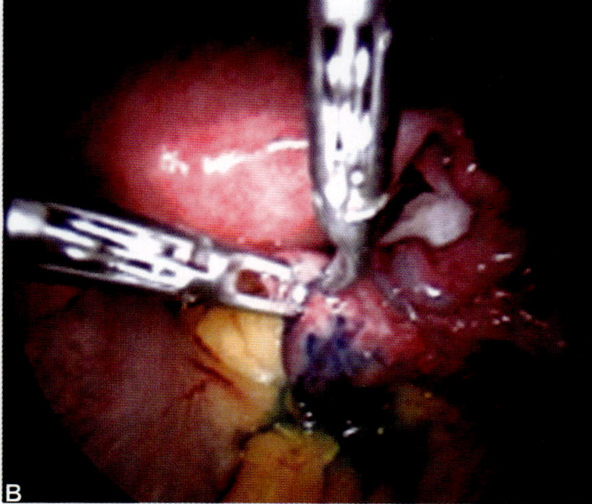

Figs 1A and B In vitro fertilization

Tubo-tubal Anastomosis

Before proceeding for the tubal reconstruction one must evaluate the inside of the tube, so as to confirm that the anastomosis is going to be fruitful or not. This involves salpingoscopy. Salpingoscopy allows direct inspection of tubal mucosa in the ampullary part. The degree of tubal mucosal damage is probably the major factor in establishing the prognosis of tubal surgery.

Brosen's Classification

Grade 1: Normal intraluminal findings with healthy major (primary) and minor (secondary) folds **(Fig. 2A)**.

Grade 2: Mucosal nuclear staining with methylene blue dye **(Fig. 2B)**.

Grade 3: Minimal flattening and minimal adhesions of endosalpinx **(Fig. 2C)**.

Grade 4: Moderate flattening of endosalpinx with intra-luminal adhesions **(Fig. 2D)**.

Grade 5: Severe flattening of mucosa with severe intra-luminal adhesions **(Fig. 2E)**.

We prefer to perform tubal microsurgery in salpingo-scopy Grade 1 or Grade 2 cases.

Types of Anastomosis

- Isthmo-isthmic anastomosis
- Isthmo-ampullary anastomosis
- Ampullo-ampullary anastomosis
- Tubocornual anastomosis.

Important surgical steps (Figs 3A to G)
- Total five ports are used (10 mm primary umbilical port, two 5 mm and two 3 mm ancillary ports)
- Distension of the proximal segment of the tube by transcervical chromopertubation to know the exact site of the block
- Excision of the pathological segment of the tube
- Make sure that the incision does not extend beyond the mesosalpinx
- Ensure the right-angled cut of the tubal ends for better alignment and approximation
- Free spillage of the dye
- Mesosalpinx is sutured first, using 6-0 polypropylene
- Thorough peritoneal irrigation with ringer lactate solution throughout the operation.

First layer, the mucosal-muscularis layer
- Most important is 6 o'clock position stitch
- To keep the knot outside the lumen, stitches are taken from outer to inner side on proximal end and vice versa on distal end

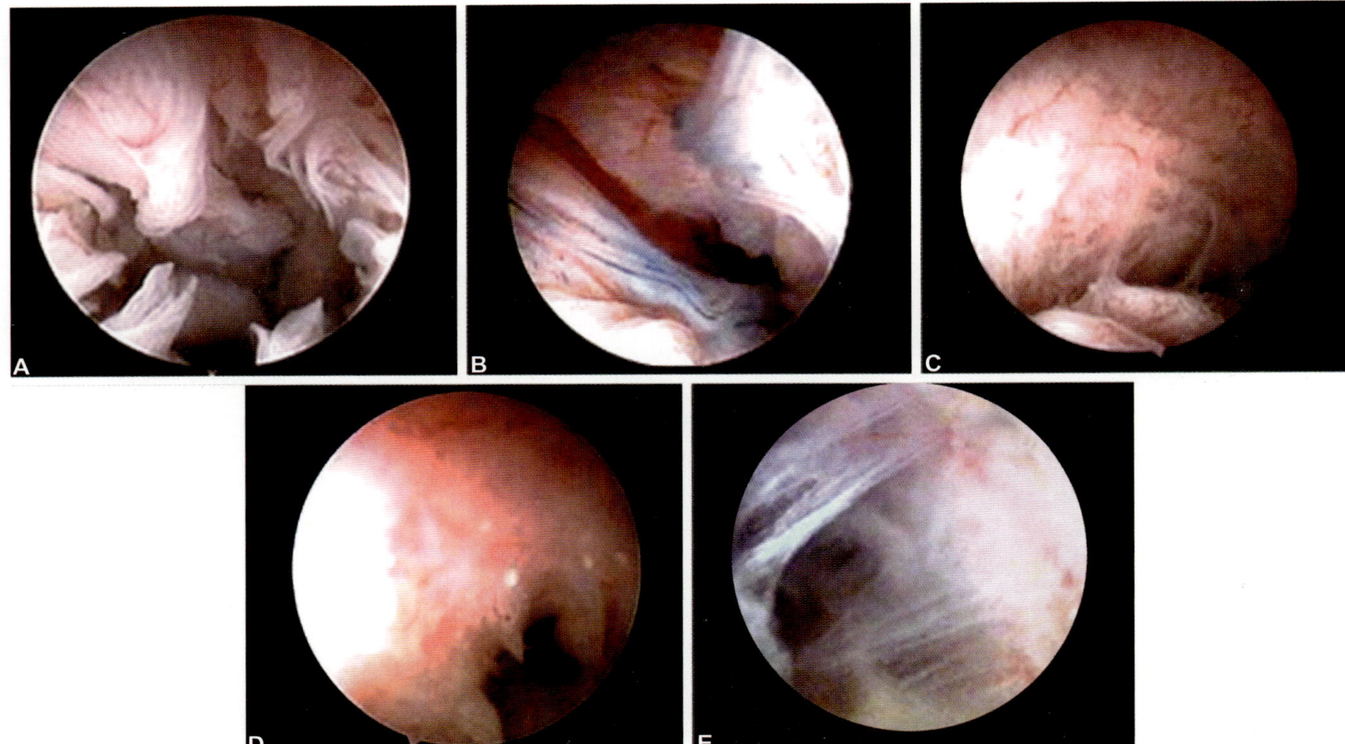

Figs 2A to E Brosen's grade classification

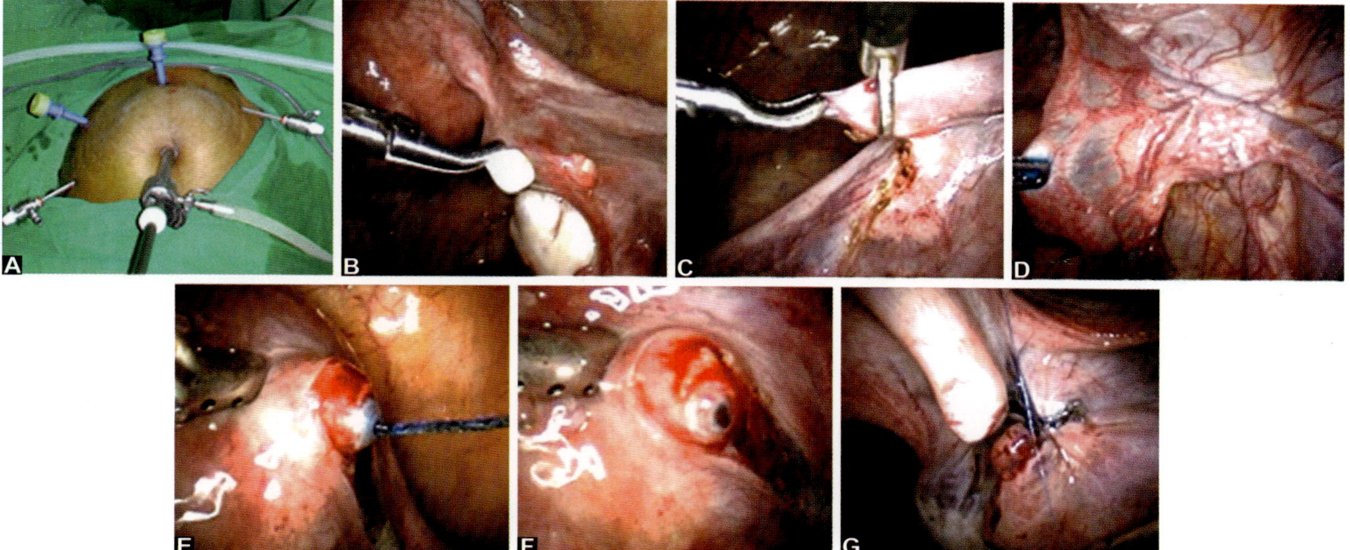

Figs 3A to G Surgical steps of in vitro fertilization

- Rest of the stitches are taken at 12, 3 and 9 o'clock positions in similar manner.
  Second layer, the sero-muscularis layer; sutured with 6-0 polypropylene **(Figs 4A to E)**.

Salpingo-ovariolysis and Fimbrioplasty

- Whenever possible, either the adhesions or ovarian ligaments are grasped instead of the ovarian cortex to reduce the trauma. Once the ovaries are lifted from the cul-de-sac and mobilized, the peritubal adhesions are removed.
- Agglutinated fimbrial folds are caused by avascular adhesions. They are grasped, stretched and cut with scissor (fimbrioplasty) **(Figs 5A to C)**.
- Never use thermal energy near Fallopian tube while doing salpingo-ovariolysis.
- After doing fimbrioplasty, one should do salpingoscopy. If salpingoscopy findings are Grade 3 or more, it is advisable to do salpingectomy and proceed for in vitro fertilization-embryo transfer (IVF-ET) **(Figs 6A to C)**.

Our Experience
Pregnancy rates were comparable with open tubal recanalization. Average surgical duration was 2 hours and 30 minutes. The average hospital stay was 2 days.

Case Type Versus Result

Out of the 436 successful surgeries, 331 (75.92%) conceived, including 14 cases of ectopic pregnancy (4.2%) (Tables 1 to 4).

■ ENDOMETRIOSIS SURGERY

Mainly three types of lesions are seen in endometriosis: red lesions (recent), black or powder burn lesions and while lesions (chronic). Endometriotic lesions are associated with neo-vascularity of surrounding tissue.

Surgical Management of Ovarian Endometriosis

- Ovary is most common site of endometriosis. Ovarian endometrioma is usually extraovarian. It develops due to inclusion of endometriotic tissue in ovary leading to chocolate cyst **(Fig. 7A)**.
- Surface fulguration of endometriotic lesions present on ovary should be done **(Fig. 7B)**.
- Chocolate cystectomy is preferred method over fulguration in ovaries having chocolate cyst. All fibrosed white lesions along with cyst wall should be removed. Attempt to preserve maximum amount of healthy ovarian tissue should be made **(Fig. 7C)**.
- Endometrioma should not be aspirated as it can lead to ovarian abscess **(Fig. 7D)**.
- Pouch of Douglas (POD) is usually gets obliterated due to adhesions between uterus, recto-sigmoid colon and ovarian endometriosis. Bilateral tubo-ovarian adhesions are also present. Attempts should be made to restore near normal anatomy **(Fig. 7E)**.
- Endometriotic tissue should be retrieved through trocar sleeve or should be kept in endobag and then retrieved **(Fig. 7F)**.

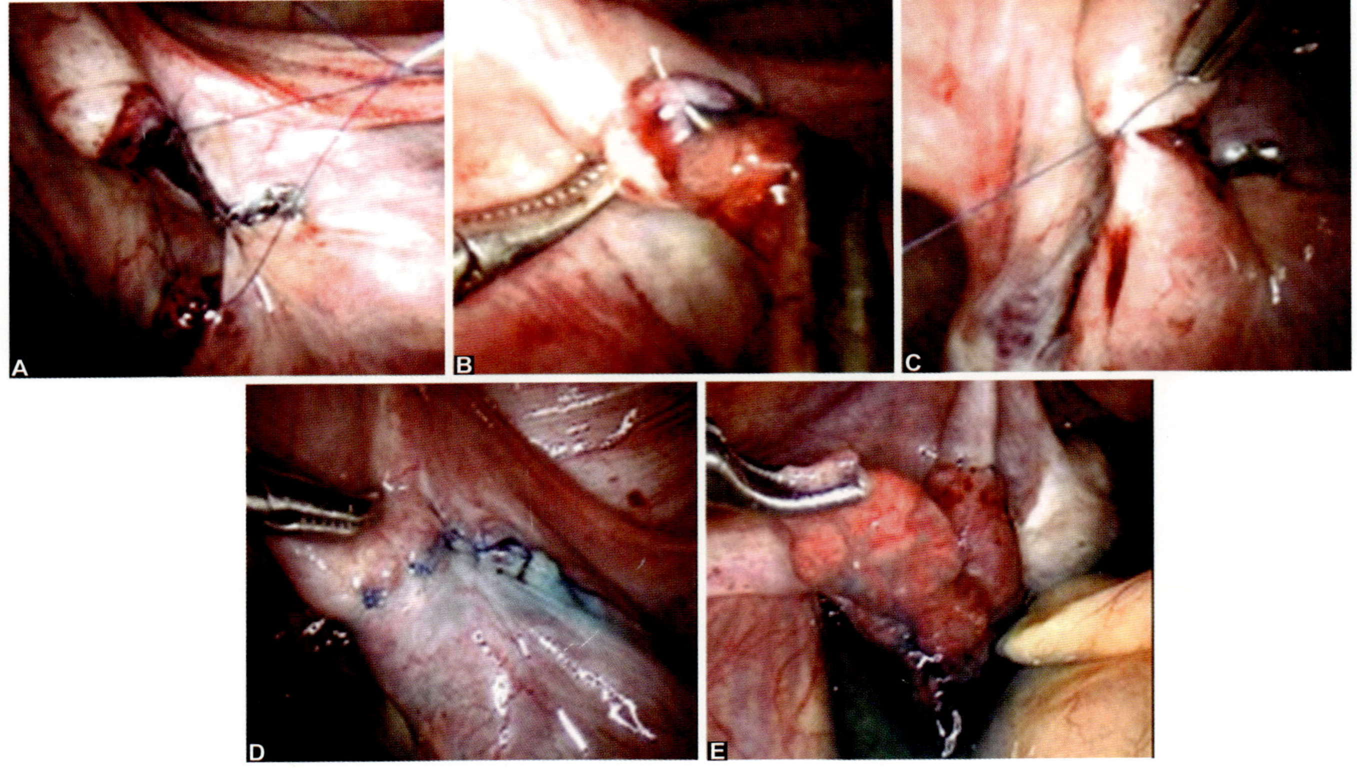

Figs 4A to E Sero-muscularis layer, sutured

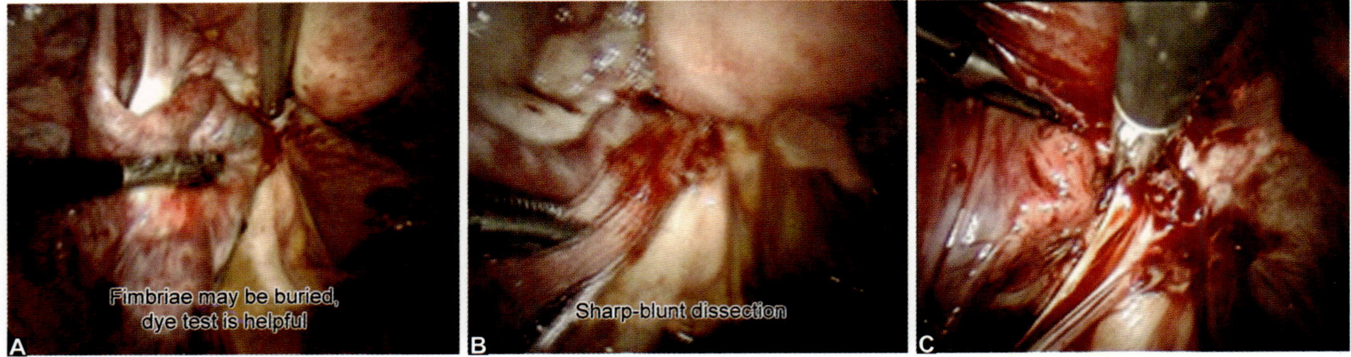

Figs 5A to C Fimbrioplasty, stretched and cut with scissor

- It should not be retrieved directly otherwise it will lead to port site endometriosis **(Fig. 7G)**.
- In cases of huge ovarian endometrioma, direct trocar entry should be done in the chocolate cyst and chocolate fluid should be drained by doing suction.

Suction cannula occasionally should be used for dissection **(Fig. 7H)**.
- Patient may present with acute abdomen due to rupture of ovarian endometrioma which requires urgent laparoscopic surgery **(Fig. 7I)**.

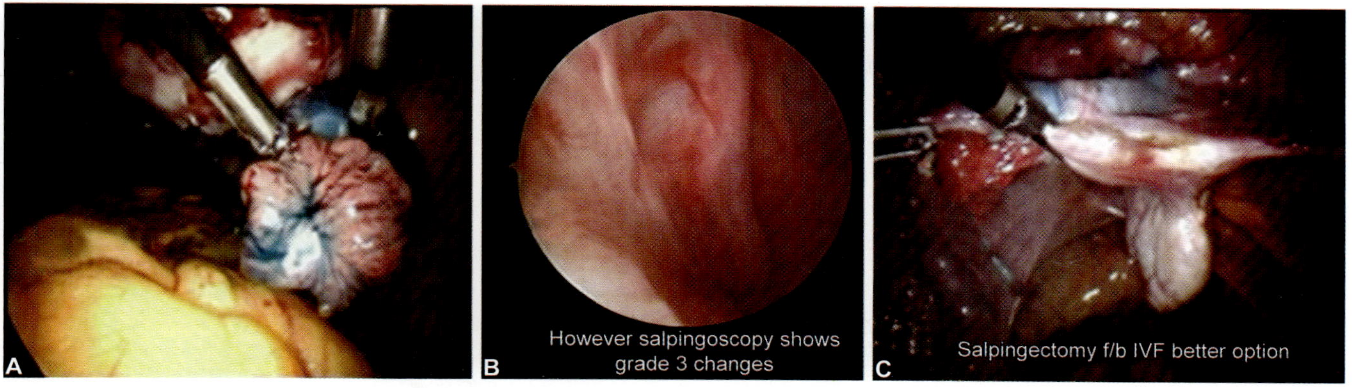

Figs 6A to C In vitro fertilization-embryo transfer

Table 1 Study from 1996 to 2006

Tubal ligation reversal	Tubal block due to pelvic inflammatory disease	Tubal block secondary to ectopic pregnancy	Failed tubal cannulation for proximal block	Total
299 (68.57%)	90 (20.64%)	16 (3.66%)	31 (7.11%)	436 cases

Table 2 Types of anastomosis

Bilateral	Unilateral	Incomplete (due to multiple blocks)	Total
324 (74.31%)	92 (21.1%)	20 (4.58%)	436 cases

Table 3 Types of anastomosis and its result

Types of anastomosis	Isthmo-isthmic	Isthmo-ampullary	Ampullo-ampullary	Juxtamural-isthmic	Juxtauterine-isthmic	Intramural-isthmic	Total
Total No.	186 (42.66%)	137 (31.42%)	57 (13.0%)	26 (5.96%)	12 (2.75%)	18 (4.13%)	436
Cases conceived	165 (88.7%)	119 (86.86%)	26 (45.61%)	13 (50%)	03 (25%)	5 (27.77%)	331 (75.92%)

Table 4 Types of cases

Type of cases	Tubal ligation reversal (N = 299)	Pathological tubes (N = 137)	Total (N = 436)
Cases conceived	266 (88.96%)	65 (47.45%)	331 (75.92%)

Surgical Management of Fallopian Tube in Endometriosis

- Tubo-ovarian adhesions along with hydrosalpinx may be present in patient having endometriosis. Due to fimbrial adhesions or external kinking of Fallopian tube or fibrosis, Fallopian tube may be having hydrosalpinx or hematosalpinx. Nodular lesions or puckering may be present in mesosalpinx **(Figs 8A to C)**.
- Salpingo-ovariolysis should be done; contour of the tube should be restored by sharp dissection. Endometriotic lesions near Fallopian tube or in mesosalpinx should be fulgurated taking of care of tubal blood supply **(Figs 8D and E)**.

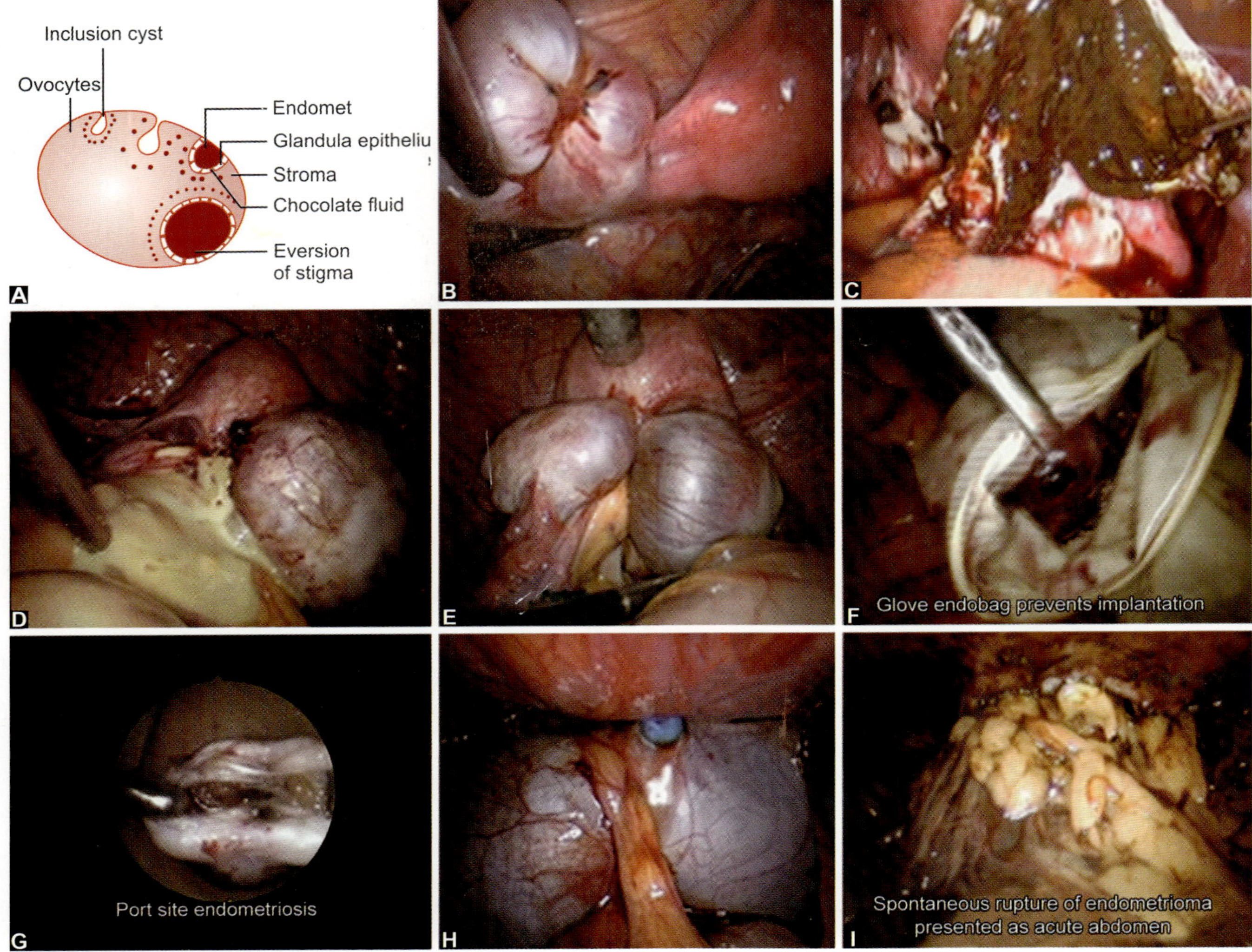

Figs 7A to I Surgical management of overian in endometriosis

Surgical Management of Uterus in Endometriosis

- Axis rotation of uterus occurs due to anterior or posterior compartment adhesions in endometriosis. Uterine vessels get displaced anteriorly due to adhesions between uterus and recto-sigmoid colon.
- There is apparent migration of bladder fold over the uterus, as uterus gets gradually adherent posteriorly to recto-sigmoid colon obliterating POD **(Figs 9A to C)**.
- Ureters also get displaced medially due to peritoneal puckering in endometriosis.
- Dissection with suction cannula should be done to restore near normal anatomy. Dense band of adhesions may require cut with scissor **(Figs 9D and E)**.

- Uterus may also be having adenomyosis or localized adenoma which needs surgical intervention.
- Cystoscopy should be done in anterior compartment adhesions to rule out bladder endometriosis **(Fig. 9F)**.
- If require, ureteric catheters should be placed peroperatively to identify ureters in cases of severe endometriosis.
- Spurt of urine should be check from both ureteric orifices to rule out injury to ureters in cases of surgery for severe posterior compartment endometriosis.
- Colorectal nodule should be excised by shaving technique. Colorectal integrity test should be done in every case by doing air enema test **(Figs 9G and H)**.

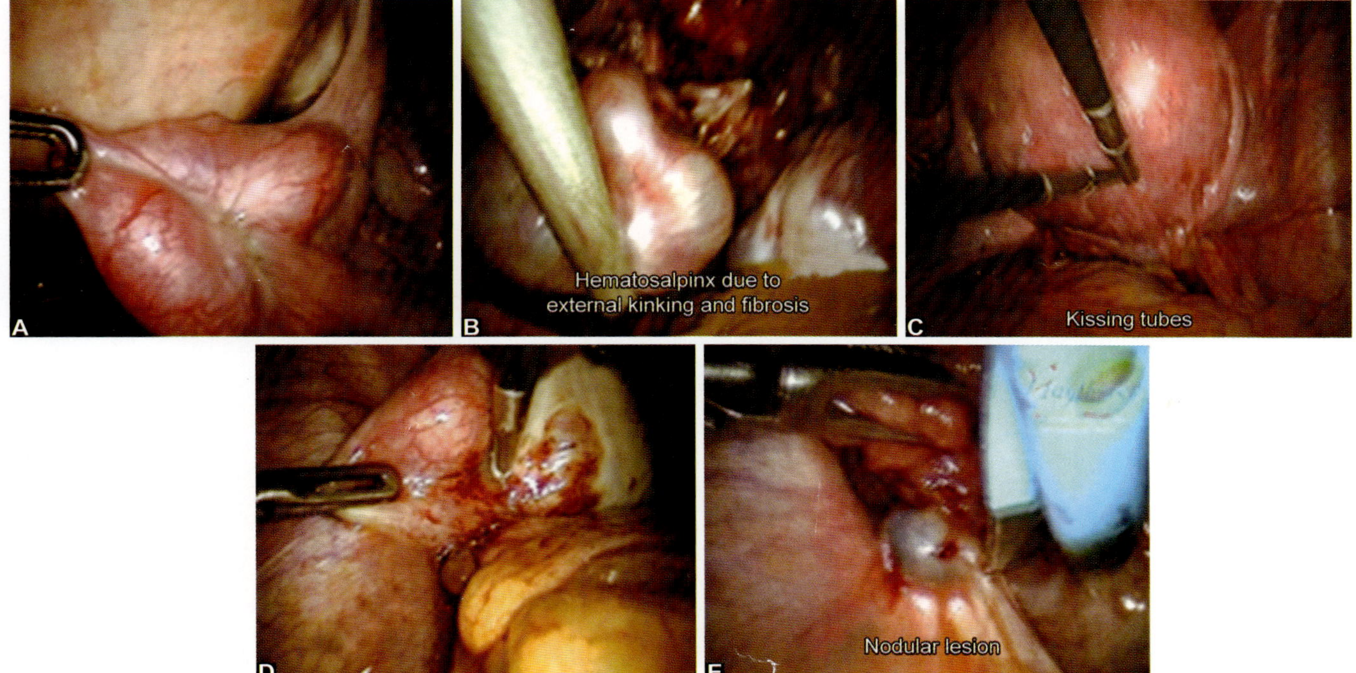

Figs 8A to E Surgical management of fallopian tube in endometriosis—mesosalpinx and tubal blood supply

Classification of Endometriosis at Our Institute

There is no role of gonadotropin-releasing hormone (GnRH) analogs preoperatively as it converts wet endometriosis into dry endometriosis making the surgery difficult **(Table 5)**.

■ LAPAROSCOPIC MYOMECTOMY

Preoperative sonography mapping should be done in every case regarding number, size and location of the fibroids.

If required, intraoperative sonography should also be done. Pitressin injection (1:200 mL dilution) should be injected in capsule of the fibroid before making incision.

- Incision should be made away from the cornual attachment of the Fallopian tube.
- Multiple myomas may also be removed through single incision on uterus **(Fig. 10A)**.
- In case of multiple fibroids, endobag should be introduced, and all fibroids excised should be kept in endobag during surgery and then retrieved at the end of the procedure **(Fig. 10B)**.
- Occasionally in situ morcellation is required in huge fibroid due to lack of space **(Fig. 10C)**.
- In case of associated broad ligament fibroid, retroperitoneal space should be opened, course of ureter identified and then one should proceed for myomectomy **(Fig. 10D)**.
- Myoma bed should be sutured in single or double layer depending on the depth. Angles of the incision should be secured properly. One can suture myoma bed by intracorporeal slip knot technique or barbed sutures. More important is not to leave any dead space, which can lead to weak scar. Formation of hematoma should be avoided in myoma bed otherwise it can invite infection and also leads to weak scar. Minimal amount of thermal energy should be used for hemostasis to prevent tissue necrosis in myoma bed.
- In case of cervical fibroid, postmyomectomy hysteroscopy should be done to check for patency of cervical canal.
- If required in huge or multiple fibroids, laparoscopic surgery should be converted into laparotomy **(Fig. 10E)**.

■ LAPAROSCOPIC ADENOMYOMECTOMY

- Adenoma is usually diagnosed on ultrasound but may be misdiagnosed as fibroid **(Fig. 11A)**.
- It appears as uncapsulated, heterogeneous anechoic areas. All these changes will be more pronounced if seen during menstruation.

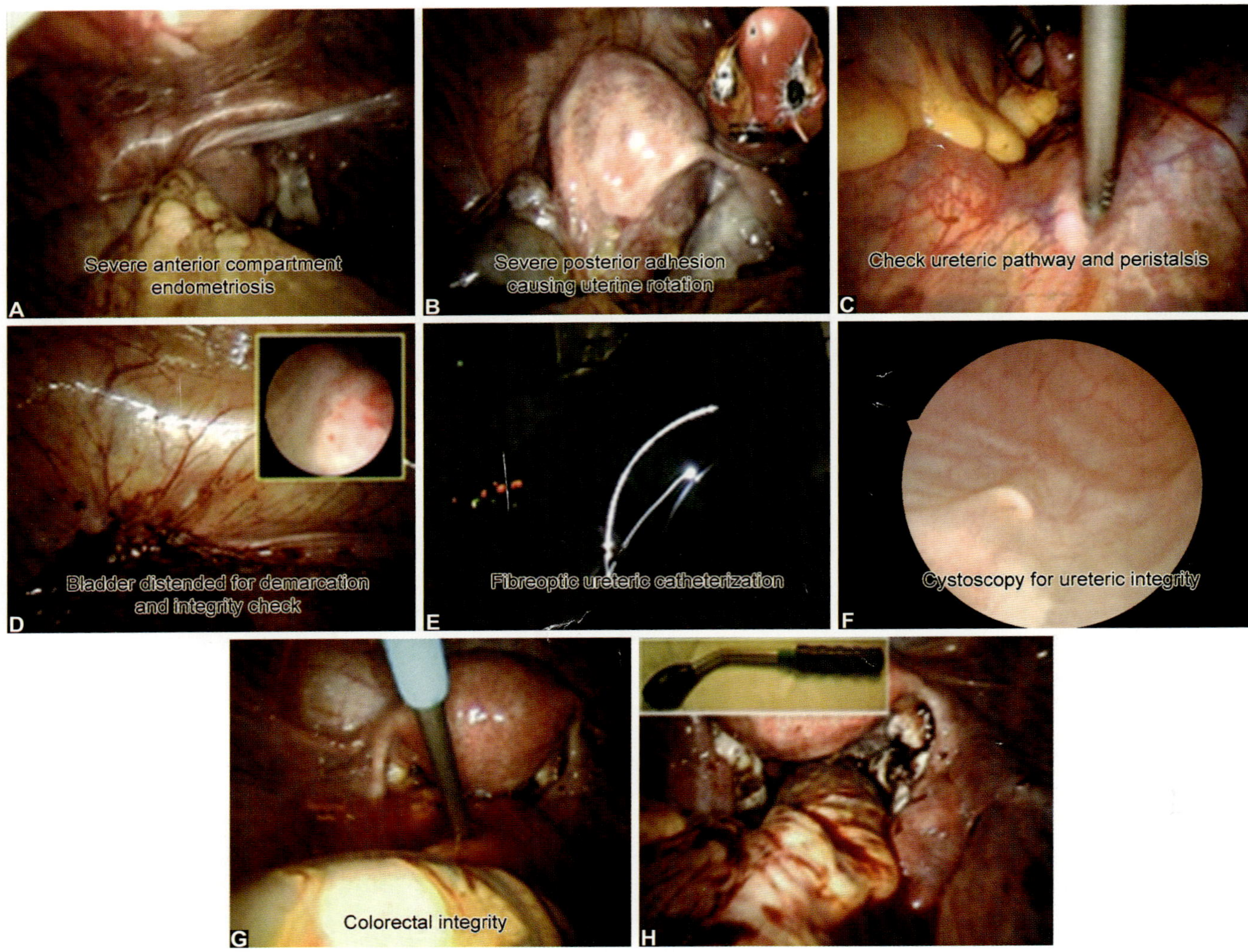

Figs 9A to H Surgical management of uterus in endometriosis

Table 5 Wet and dry endometriosis

Wet endometriosis	Dry endometriosis
Early disease	Long standing disease
Adhesive type of adhesions	Infiltrating type of adhesions
Recurrence rate of adhesions low as peritoneal injury preventable at first attempt	Recurrence rate high as peritoneal injury non-preventable
Easily separable	Difficult adhesiolysis
Good prognosis	Poor prognosis

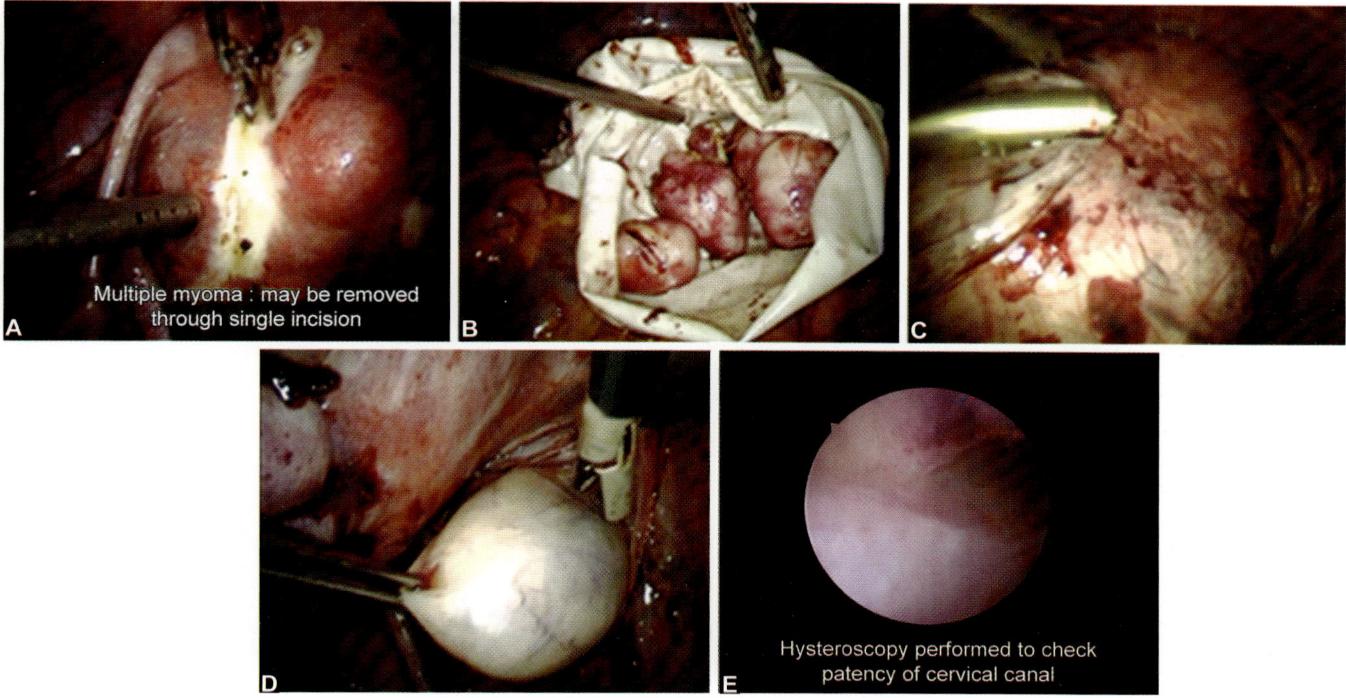

Figs 10A to E Laparoscopic myomectomy

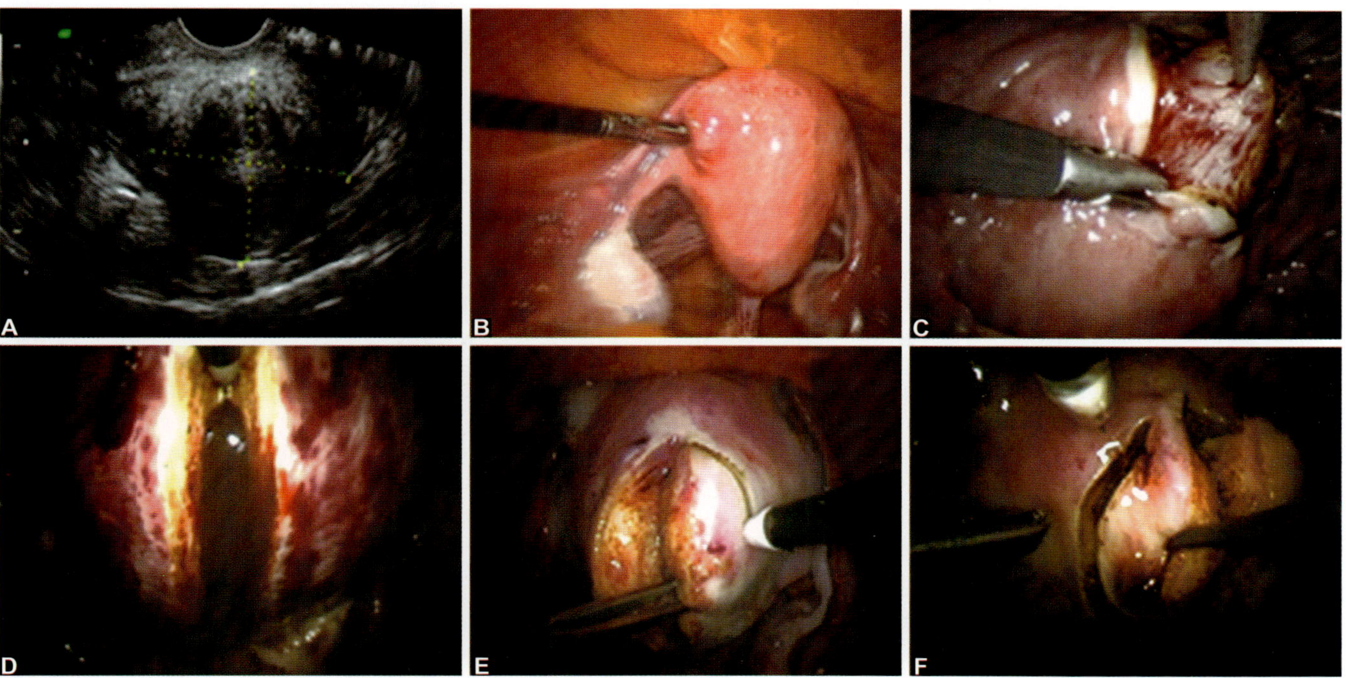

Figs 11A to F Laparoscopic adenomyomectomy

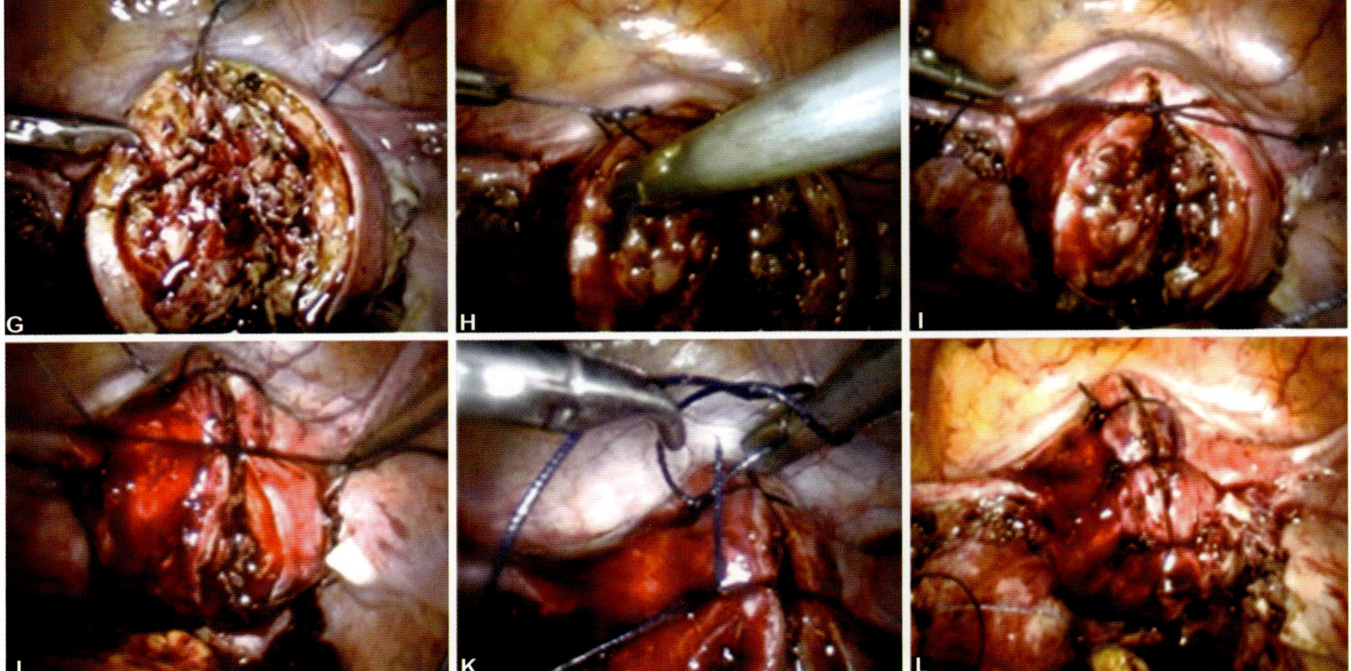

Figs 11G to L Laporoscopic adenomyonection

- Preoperative sonography mapping should be done in every case regarding number, size and location of the adenoma.
- There may be chocolate colored fluid collection in the myometrium (intramyometrial cyst). Adenomyosis/adenoma may coexist with endometriosis and fibroid **(Figs 11B to D)**.
- Resection of adenoma helps in improving the symptoms by reducing the uterine vascularity, thus improving pain, menorrhagia and fertility. As adenoma/adenomyotic tissue is tough, it is better to use monopolar pure cutting current than scissor. Too much smoke generated during use of monopolar current should be evacuated periodically.
- Elliptical strip excision would be better for adenoma resection than attempting enucleation as in fibroid. The aim of resection is to reduce tension in myometrium (similar to debulking surgery of benign SOL of brain without injuring vital areas of brain) **(Figs 11E and F)**.
- Adenoma bed should be sutured by intracorporeal slip knot technique **(Figs 11G to L)**.

Our Experience

So we advised to perform adenoma resection for improving fertility outcome up to Grade 2A cases (Tables 6 to 8 and Figs 12 to 14).

Table 6 Cases (Year 1996–2005)

Our series	Year 1996–2005
Localized adenoma	210 cases
Diffuse disease	46 cases
Total	256 cases

Table 7 Symptomatic improvements

Dysmenorrhea	92%	236 cases
Menstrual loss	84%	215 cases
Recurrence rate after 3 years	38%	97 cases

Note: Recurrence rate is higher in Grade II and Grade III.

Table 8 Pregnancy rates

Group	No. of cases
Localized adenoma	87 cases (37%)
Diffuse adenomyosis	20 cases (8%)

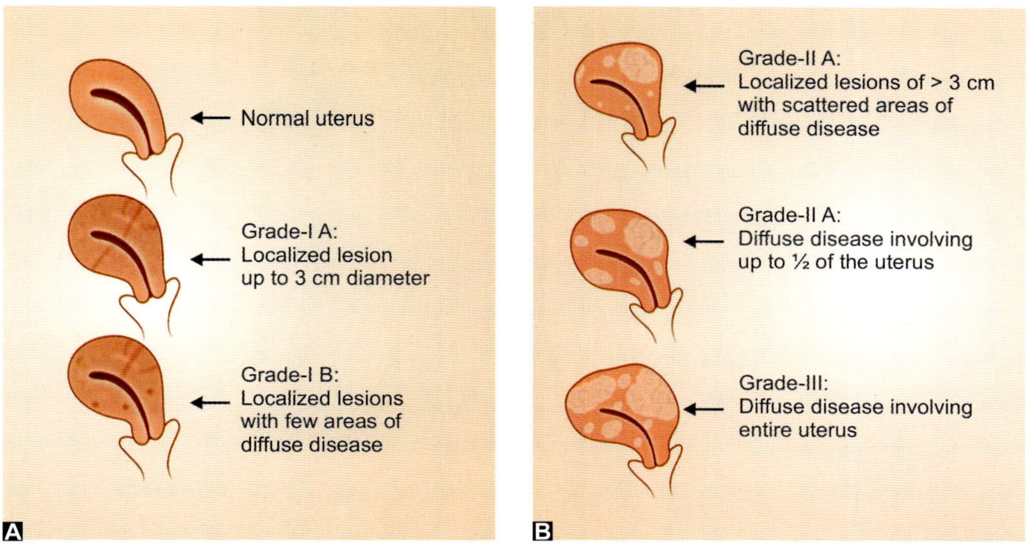

Figs 12A and B Dr Sanjay Patel's classification of adenomyosis

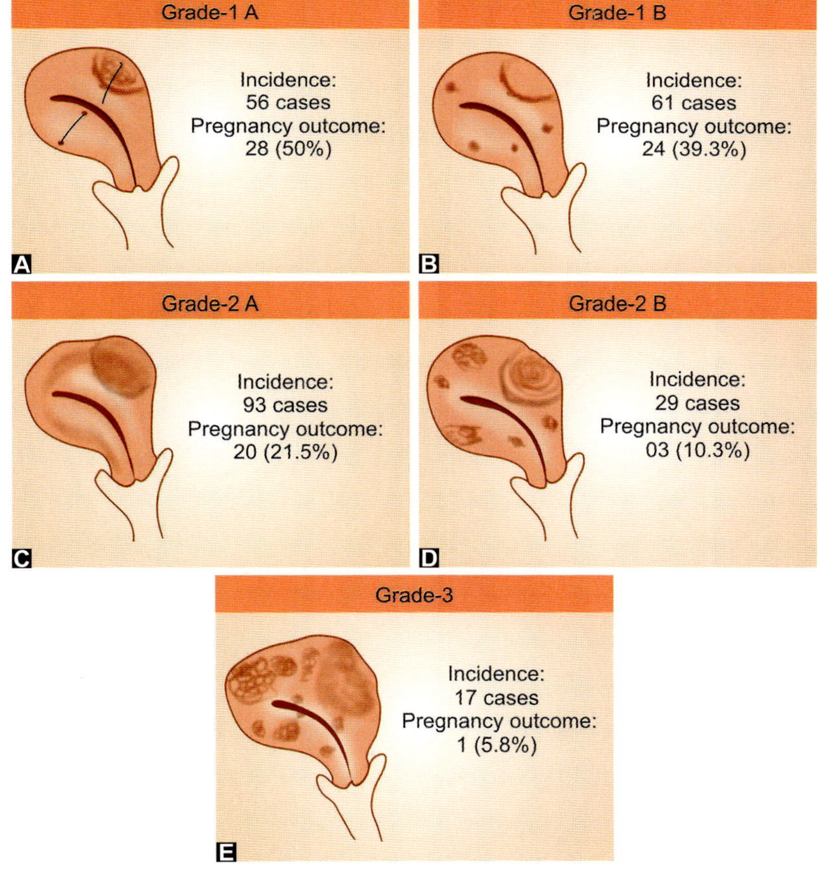

Figs 13A to E Fertility outcome grades

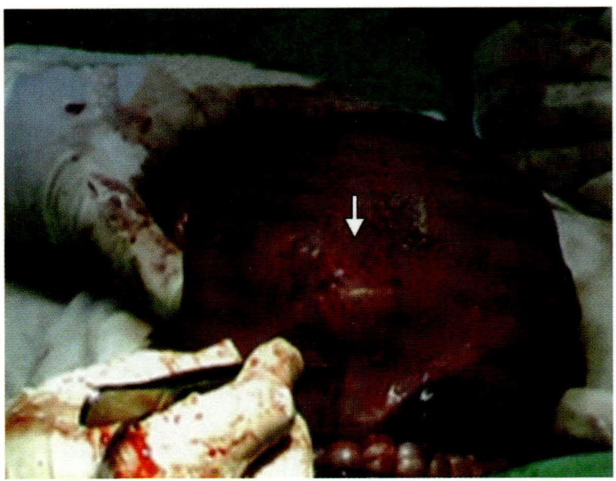

Fig. 14 Elective cesarean at 34 weeks for post adenomomectomy pregnancy

9

Fertility Enhancing Hysteroscopic Surgery

Rishma Pai, Hrishikesh Pai, Nandan Roongta

■ INTRODUCTION

Uterine abnormalities including congenital pathologies, polyps, submucous leiomyomata, intrauterine adhesions (IUAs), and chronic endometritis, have been found in 10–15% of women seeking treatment for fertility problems.[1] Also, multiple studies have identified that between 26% and 50% of patients who fail in vitro fertilization (IVF) have uterine abnormalities, suggesting that hysteroscopy could serve as a prognostic factor for the IVF outcome, especially in case of fibroids which distort the endometrial cavity.[2] Compared with hysterosalpingography (HSG), hysteroscopy is recognized as the "gold standard" test for identifying uterine abnormalities as it allows direct visualization of the uterine cavity.

However, the position of hysteroscopy in current fertility practice is under debate. In 2004, the Royal College of Obstetrics and Gynaecologists (RCOG) did not recommend hysteroscopy as an initial investigation unless clinically indicated, and it had categorized hysteroscopic treatment as a grade B recommendation in its evidence-based guidelines on fertility assessment and treatment. The same recommendation is reiterated by them in the 2013 guidelines,[1] as also by the European Society for Human Reproduction and Embryology.[3] A Cochrane Review 2013, states that "hysteroscopic myomectomy might increase the odds of clinical pregnancy in women with unexplained subfertility and submucous fibroids, but the evidence is at present not conclusive. The hysteroscopic removal of endometrial polyps suspected on ultrasound in women prior to intrauterine insemination (IUI) might increase the clinical pregnancy rate. More randomized studies are needed to substantiate the effectiveness of the hysteroscopic removal of suspected endometrial polyps, submucous fibroids, uterine septum or IUAs in women with unexplained subfertility or prior to IUI, IVF or intracytoplasmic sperm injection (ICSI)".[4] Hysteroscopic septoplasty, polypectomy and synechiolysis have all been established as the gold standard methods in patients with subfertility. It is advisable to perform a second-look hysteroscopy after correction of these pathologies to ensure their proper correction before embarking on a costly IVF program.

The role of the uterus in sperm migration, embryo implantation, and fetal nourishment is well established. As such, congenital uterine anomalies, acquired uterine lesions, and systemic disease may affect these functions adversely precluding a successful pregnancy. Also, a receptive endometrium is morphologically and functionally primed for blastocyst attachment. And so, pathological conditions like endometriosis, endocrine abnormalities, immunologic factors, thrombophilias, congenital and acquired anatomic factors may contribute to implantation failure, resulting in recurrent pregnancy loss or infertility.

The outcome of assisted reproductive technology (ART) depends mainly on the embryo quality and uterine environment among other factors. Evaluation of the uterine cavity is hence recommended to screen for pathologies like fibroids, polyps, adhesions, and uterine Müllerian abnormalities, which are commonly considered to have a negative impact on the ART cycle and then the pregnancy outcome.[5-7]

Comparing HSG and hysteroscopy for the purpose, studies report that HSG has a false positive rate of 15.6% and a false negative rate of 35.4%.[8,9] Hysteroscopic evaluation of uterine cavity for women with infertility has more recently become a routine procedure. It enables direct visualization of the cervical canal and the uterine cavity, as also offers assistance for the interpretation of uncertain findings from other diagnostic methods, and it permits the treatment of most benign intrauterine pathologies.[10] The technological advances and improvements in hysteroscopy, both diagnostic as well as operative, has significantly contributed to the better management of uterine surgeries. Proper instrumentation is essential in achieving a complication free optimal outcome.

At present, with the development of smaller diameter scopes with working channels and continuous flow systems, it is possible to treat several uterine, cervical and vaginal pathologies in an office setting without cervical dilatation and consequently without anesthesia or analgesia. Mechanical operative instruments (scissors, biopsy cup, grasper, corkscrew) have been for long time the only way to apply the "see and treat" procedure in the office setting. The advent of bipolar VersaPoint technology, with introduction of several types of 5 Fr electrodes, and usage of saline as a distention medium has increased the number of pathologies treated.[11,12]

■ ENDOMETRIAL POLYPS

Endometrial polyps **(Fig. 1)** are the most common pathological findings in hysteroscopy. The mechanism by which polyps may adversely affect fertility is also poorly understood but may be related to mechanical interference with sperm transport, embryo implantation, or through increased production of inhibitory factors such as glycodelin that can inhibit natural killer cell function. Tubocornual polyps, especially when bilaterally present and large, may preferentially interfere with oocyte or embryo transport. Moreover, they may protect (through a valve mechanism) against retrograde menstruation and possibly pelvic endometriosis. Polyps in the isthmic-cervical part of the uterus may preferentially interfere with sperm transport and may facilitate retrograde

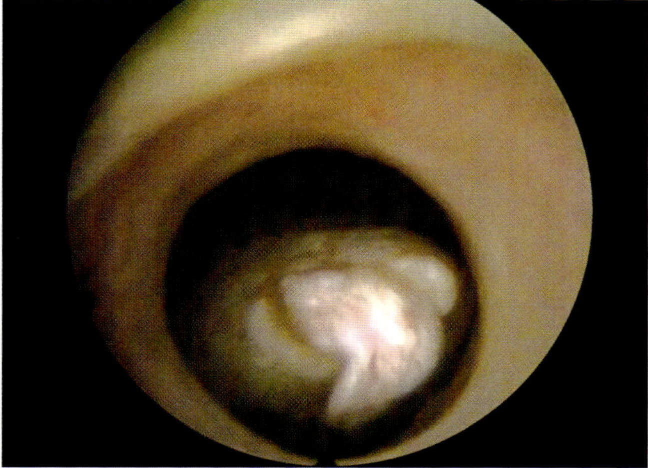

Fig. 1 Endometrial polyp: hysteroscopic view by means of a 1.6 mm diagnostic hysteroscope

Source: Muzii L, Bellati F, Pernice M, et al. Resectoscopic versus bipolar electrode excision of endometrial polyps: a randomized study. Fertil Steril. 2007;87(4):909-17.

menstruation through a similar valve mechanism. Endometrial polyps are identified by hysteroscopy in 16.5–26.5% of women with otherwise unexplained infertility. The rate is much higher (46.7%) in infertile women with endometriosis and lower (0.6–5%) in women with recurrent pregnancy loss. Some adenomatous polyps are associated with atypical or cystic endometrial hyperplasia, and rarely there can be malignant changes in the base. It is hence advisable to remove all endometrial polyps even, if they are asymptomatic.

Hysteroscopic Polypectomy

A causal relationship between endometrial polyps and infertility is not certain. Their removal prior to embarking upon ART may be justified, though limited evidence supports this practice. Resection of a polyp is easier than that of a fibroid. Grasping it with a grasper is usually sufficient to excise it, though at times cauterization of the base and extraction may be required. Sometimes transecting the base and removing the compressible mass through the cervix may be more convenient.

Office Technique

Office hysteroscopy is a safe, feasible, and effective tool for endometrial polypectomy, with a high rate of patient acceptability and a low recurrence rate of pathology.

Small polyps (<0.5 cm) should be removed using 5 Fr mechanical instruments (scissor and/or crocodile forceps). Cervical polyps have to be treated with scissors because of their fibrotic base. Larger polyps can be removed intact, with the VersaPoint Twizzle electrode, only if the internal cervical os size is wide enough for their extraction. Otherwise, they are sliced from the free edge to the base into 2–3 fragments, by the VersaPoint bipolar twizzle electrode, large enough to be pulled out through the uterine cavity using 5 Fr grasping forceps with teeth. For fundal polyps, the electrode can be bent by ~30° to cut the entire base without going too deep into the myometrium.

■ MYOMAS

Fertility outcomes are decreased in women with submucosal fibroids, and removal seems to confer benefit. Subserosal fibroids do not affect fertility outcomes, and removal does not confer benefit. Intramural fibroids appear to decrease fertility, but the results of therapy are unclear.[13]

Most myomas are asymptomatic masses detected occasionally during clinical or ultrasonographic evaluation. However, those that are not so, may be associated with menorrhagia or metrorrhagia, pelvic pain, and bladder and bowel dysfunction due to their pressure, infertility, and recurrent pregnancy loss. Approximately 5–10% of infertile patients have at least one myoma, and this is the sole etiologic factor in 1–2.4% of infertile women.[14]

Although the mechanism for the association between submucous myomas and infertility is not well understood, theories include changes in local vascular supply that deprive the implanted embryo of oxygen and nutrients; mechanical obstruction of the tube; or induction of inflammation or local biological factors that interfere with transport, implantation, or embryo development. The extent of such effects may depend upon the number, size, and distortion effect of the myomas.

Besides subfertility, large fibroids are also associated with other pregnancy complications, such as premature labor or abnormal fetal presentation. Submucous fibroids **(Fig. 2A)** may be also associated with other gynecologic symptoms such as pain, metromenorrhagia, or recurrent pregnancy loss.

Hysteroscopic Myomectomy

Classification of submucous myomas is based on the degree of the myoma within the cavity **(Fig. 2B)**: type 0 myomas are entirely intracavitary, type I myomas have more than 50% of the myoma within the cavity, and type II myomas have less than 50% of the myoma within the cavity.[15]

Retrospective and case-control studies demonstrate that submucosal and intramural myomas that protrude into the endometrial cavity are associated with a decreased pregnancy rate and implantation rate in patients who attempt to conceive spontaneously or who are undergoing IVF, and the pregnancy rate improves after their removal.

The current management of myomas for fertility preservation or enhancement is surgical removal either

Type	Intramural extension
0	None
I	<50%
II	>50%

Fig. 2B Classification of submucous myomas based on percentage of myoma within uterine cavity

Source: Cohen LS, Valle RF. Role of vaginal sonography and hysterosonography in the endoscopic treatment of uterine myomas. Fertil Steril. 2000;73(2):197-204.

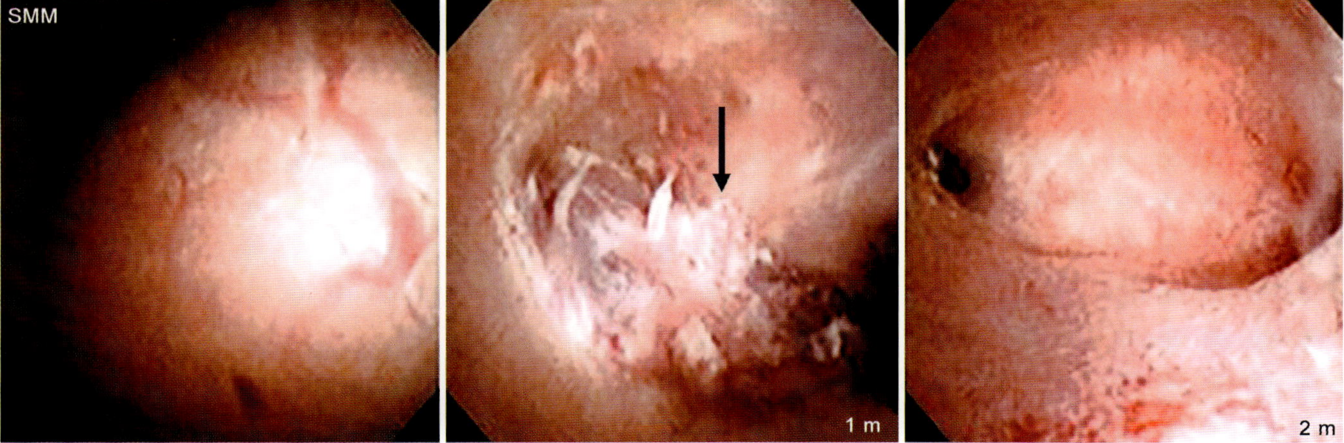

Fig. 2A Submucous myoma. In hysteroscopic surgeries for submucous myoma (SMM) subsequent office hysteroscopy demonstrates that the endometrial wound healing may take as long as 2 months. Arrow shows the site of resection of submucous myoma

Source: Yang JH, Chen MJ, Chen CD, et al. Optimal waiting period for subsequent fertility treatment after various hysteroscopic surgeries. Fertil Steril. 2013;99(7):2092-6.

by laparotomy, laparoscopy, or hysteroscopy. The goals of myomectomy include restoration of uterine morphology, return of normal menstrual function, and enhancement of fertility.

Several studies suggest an adverse effect in women undergoing IVF, particularly with large myomas (>4 cm), whereas others fail to show this association. Women with fibroids more than 4 cm required an increased number of cycles to obtain an ongoing pregnancy. At present, it has yet to be ascertained whether small myomas that minimally distort the uterine cavity reduce fertility potential. However, it is likely that as a submucous myoma gets bigger or invades further into the uterine layers, it will exert a more detrimental effect on fertility and will be more difficult to remove. The influence of myomas that do not distort the endometrial cavity on spontaneous or after ART conception remains controversial. However, if the woman has a pathologic medical background (e.g., history of recurrent miscarriage or early pregnancy loss) the removal of these lesions should always be recommended.[16]

Hysteroscopic access has revolutionized and significantly facilitated myomectomy for totally submucous myomas or those with an intramural component. Resectoscopic myomectomy is typically performed under general or spinal anesthesia, and the cervix is dilated. The uterus is distended by the use of an electrolyte-free, low-viscosity solution such as 1.5% glycine, 3% D-sorbitol, 5% mannitol, and cytosol, which is necessary for monopolar loop **(Fig. 2C)**. However, the recent development of a bipolar loop, bipolar scissors, and special morcellator to excise submucous myoma allows surgery to be performed in an electrolyte-rich media such as normal saline solution in selected cases.

Complication rates increase with increasing size and number of myomas. Up to 6.6% of women experience a complication of resectoscopic myomectomy that includes hemorrhage, cervical laceration, infection, uterine perforation, or fluid overload.

It has been observed that pregnancy rates after hysteroscopic myomectomy increase in direct proportion with increasing myoma size.

Office Technique

The intrauterine myomas usually are relatively avascular with whitish aspect and occasionally they have large blood vessels over the surface. The dimension limit for the office hysteroscopic myomectomy is 1.52 cm. A technique similar to polypectomy is applied in office to remove a submucosal myomas with the difference that, due to their higher tissue density, they have to be first divided into two half-spheres and then each of these is sliced and removed with the grasping forceps with teeth.

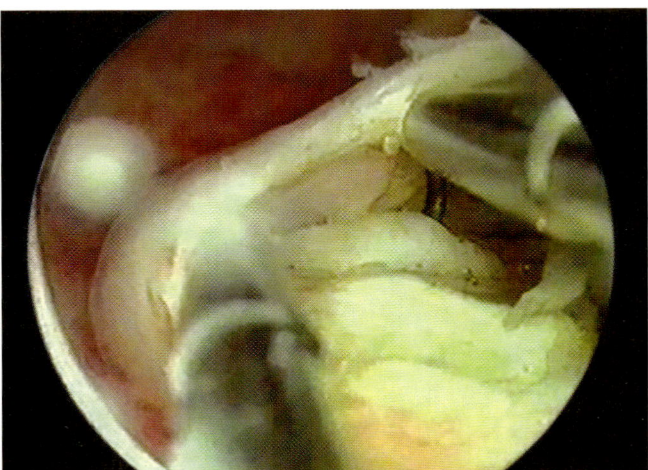

Fig. 2C Hysteroscopic excision of the intramural component of the myoma by slicing using electrosurgery

Source: Di Spiezio Sardo A, Mazzon I, Bramante S, et al. Hysteroscopic myomectomy: a comprehensive review of surgical techniques. Hum Reprod Update. 2008;14(2):101-19.

Particular attention has to be paid to the intramural part of the myoma, if present. First the myoma is gently separated from the capsule using mechanical instruments (grasping, forceps or scissor) to avoid any myometrial stimulation or damage of the surrounding healthy myometrium. Once the intramural section becomes submucosal then it is sliced with the VersaPoint Twizzle electrode. If there is an appreciable amount of the fibroid projecting into the myometrium it is safer to administer a course of gonadotropin-releasing hormone analogs for 2–3 months to decrease its size and reduce the vascularization.

A new hysteroscopic technique for the preparation of partially intramural myomas in the office setting (OPPIuM technique) was assessed to facilitate the subsequent resectoscopic or hysteroscopic myomectomy. It consists of an incision of the endometrial mucosa covering the myoma by means of 5 Fr scissors or the bipolar VersaPoint Twizzle electrode, along its reflection line on the uterine wall, up to the precise identification of the cleavage surface between the myoma and its pseudocapsule. Such a procedure is aimed at triggering the protrusion of the intramural portion of the myoma into the uterine cavity during the following menstrual cycles, thus allowing the subsequent total removal of the lesion via resectoscopic or hysteroscopic surgery more safely and quickly.

Myomas and Assisted Reproductive Techniques

The advent of ART and in particular of IVF has offered a useful tool for elucidating the impact of myomas on embryo implantation. However, because there still is no definite consensus on whether myomas affect the outcome, they should be removed before any attempt.[16]

Also considering the potential risk of failure, patients undergoing ART, especially those with unexplained infertility or with a history of recurrent implantation failures, need the best conditions before any treatment cycle.

Small myomas, being hormone-dependent benign tumors, have a high potential to grow and either become symptomatic or cause complications during natural or assisted conception and pregnancy. In the menstrual cycle itself, the induced ovarian hyperstimulation during ART, as well as pregnancy, in most cases will enlarge myomas.

Nevertheless, every situation and patient must to be judged separately; that is, management options must be biased toward the least risk of impairing fertility or of causing complications during pregnancy.

The use of large-diameter instruments such as resectoscopes, even in the presence of such small lesions, is not recommended because it requires cervical dilatation; local or general anesthesia; and an operating room with dedicated personnel, with correspondingly elevated health care costs. However, office hysteroscopy appears to be an excellent method for the treatment of such lesions.

■ SEPTATE UTERUS

A septate uterus results from failure of the partition between the two fused Müllerian ducts to resorb. The extent of the septum can involve part of the uterine cavity, or completely divide both the uterine cavity and the cervical canal into two equal or unequal parts. It sometimes happens that the septum extends almost to the endocervical canal and if the telescope is passed to one side of the septum the diagnosis can easily be missed. Although combining modalities can improve diagnostic accuracy, concurrent hysteroscopy and laparoscopy is the gold standard for diagnosing the septate uterus.

The septate uterus is the most common structural uterine anomaly seen among patients of subfertility or reproductive failure. Further, it may be associated with first- and second-trimester pregnancy loss and infertility. Such outcomes are thought to be a result of poor blood supply rendering the septum inhospitable to the implanting embryo; additionally scanning electron microscopy of endometrial septa demonstrates the morphological development of endometrial septal specimens to be suboptimal.

The association between septate uterus and endometriosis, as reported in some non-controlled studies, may explain the subfertility of at least some patients with septate uterus, but it requires further research.

Hysteroscopic Metroplasty (Figs 3A to C)

Until the introduction of operative hysteroscopy, division of uterine septa was performed by laparotomy. Hysteroscopy revolutionized and greatly simplified the management of the septate uterus.

Hysteroscopic metroplasty is typically performed under general or spinal anesthesia. Hysteroscopic division

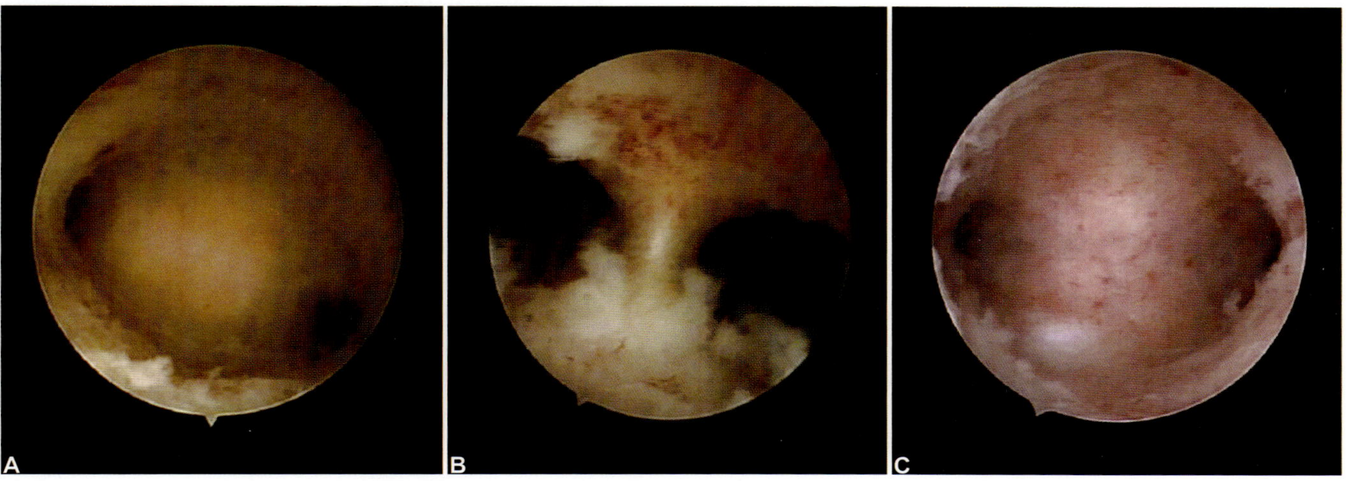

Figs 3A to C Septum. Images of hysteroscopy recordings

Source: Smit JG, Kasius JC, Eijkemans MJ, et al. The international agreement study on the diagnosis of the septate uterus at office hysteroscopy in infertile patients. Fertil Steril. 2013;99(7):2108-13.

of the uterine septum is performed using microscissors, electrosurgery, or laser, and it may be performed under ultrasonic or laparoscopic control. Although the reproductive outcomes after transabdominal and transcervical metroplasty are similar, the transabdominal approach is associated with significantly more complications, longer hospital stay, longer recovery period, and the obvious drawbacks of hysterotomy. For this reason hysteroscopic metroplasty is the current standard of care.

Published data comparing reproductive outcome before and after hysteroscopic metroplasty for septate uterus in women with recurrent miscarriage, have all shown significant improvement in pregnancy outcome. The miscarriage rate decreases from 88% before metroplasty to 14% after. Further, 80% of women will have a term livebirth after metroplasty compared with 3% before surgery. In the largest series published to date, 29.5% of women with otherwise unexplained infertility had a term livebirth after hysteroscopic metroplasty. Finally, IVF is less successful in women with a septate uterus compared with women who have undergone metroplasty. The RCOG guidelines (2013) however state that "Hysteroscopic metroplasty has not been shown to increase pregnancy rates in women with infertility who have a septate uterus".[1]

Office Technique

During office hysteroscopy the septum is progressively cut, starting from the proximal part, equidistantly from the anterior and the posterior uterine wall. The decision to stop the incision of the septum is taken when significant bleeding was observed, as well as pinkish tissue is seen. Office hysteroscopic metroplasty, in awake patients, can alert the surgeon as soon as the muscular tissue is reached by the incision, causing the patient pain. There are no pain fibers in uterine septa. Using these criteria we can avoid the need for concurrent laparoscopy. In that instant the metroplasty must be stopped regardless of the length of the septum left. This makes possible the prevention of unnecessary damage to the myometrium.

■ INTRAUTERINE ADHESIONS

The obliteration of the uterine cavity secondary to trauma to the uterine body was described in 1950 as Asherman's syndrome. In 1989, the American Fertility Society classified IUAs from stage I to III based on the extent and type of adhesions and the menstrual pattern **(Table 1)**.

The European Society of Hysteroscopy (ESH) and European Society of Gynecological Endoscopy (ESGE) in 1995 developed a classification system based only on the

Table 1 American Fertility Society classification of intrauterine adhesions, 1988

Extent of cavity involved	<1/3	1/3–2/3	>2/3
	1	2	4
Type of adhesions	Filmy	Filmy and dense	Dense
	1	2	4
Menstrual pattern	Normal	Hypo-menorrhea	Amenorrhea
	0	2	4
Prognostic classification		*HSG[a] score*	*Hysteroscopy score*
Stage I	(Mild)	1–4	
Stage II	(Moderate)	5–8	
Stage III	(Severe)	9–12	

Source: Yu D, Wong YM, Cheong Y, et al. Asherman syndrome: one century later. Fertil Steril. 2008;89(4):759-79.
[a]All adhesions should be considered dense.

type and extent of adhesions seen during hysteroscopic treatment. The clinical symptoms were not included **(Table 2)**.

An injury or insult to the endometrium is generally the primary cause for adhesion of the myometrium to the opposing uterine wall, leading to IUAs. The most such injury is uterine curettage to the vulnerable gravid uterus. Uterine infection can also cause IUAs, and in particular genital tuberculosis, is associated with uterine cavity obliteration in more than half of the cases.

Hysteroscopy, the gold standard for the diagnosis, identifies IUA in 3–16% of women before their first IVF attempt. Hysteroscopy identified IUA in 7–21.8% of women with recurrent pregnancy loss.

The reproductive outcomes of women with IUAs are generally poor. Subfertility in patients with IUAs may be caused by complete or partial occlusion of the tubal ostia, uterine cavity, or the cervical canal, preventing the migration of sperm or the implantation of the embryo. Severe destruction of the endometrium may also lead to defective or absent implantation. Of the pregnancies that occurred in cases of untreated IUAs, the rates of spontaneous abortion and preterm deliveries were significantly increased.

Hysteroscopic Synechiolysis (Fig. 4)

Women with amenorrhea who are found to have IUAs should be offered hysteroscopic adhesiolysis because this

Table 2 European Society of Gynecological Endoscopy classification of intrauterine adhesions (1995 version)

Grade	Extent of intrauterine adhesions[a]
I	*Thin or filmy adhesions*
	Easily ruptured by hysteroscope sheath alone
	Cornual areas normal
II	*Singular dense adhesion*
	Connecting separate areas of the uterine cavity
	Visualization of both tubal ostia possible
	Cannot be ruptured by hysteroscope sheath alone
IIa	*Occluding adhesions only in the region of the internal cervical os[b]*
	Upper uterine cavity normal
III	*Multiple dense adhesions*
	Connecting separate areas of the uterine cavity
	Unilateral obliteration of ostial areas of the tubes
IV	*Extensive dense adhesions with (partial) occlusion of the uterine cavity*
	Both tubal ostial areas (partially) occluded
Va	*Extensive endometrial scarring and fibrosis in combination with grade I or grade II adhesions*
	With amenorrhea or pronounced hypomenorrhea
Vb	*Extensive endometrial scarring and fibrosis*
	In combination with grade III or grade IV adhesions[b] with amenorrhea

Source: Yu D, Wong YM, Cheong Y, et al. Asherman syndrome: one century later. Fertil Steril. 2008;89(4):759-79.
[a]From findings at hysteroscopy and hysterography
[b]Only to be classified during hysteroscopic treatment.

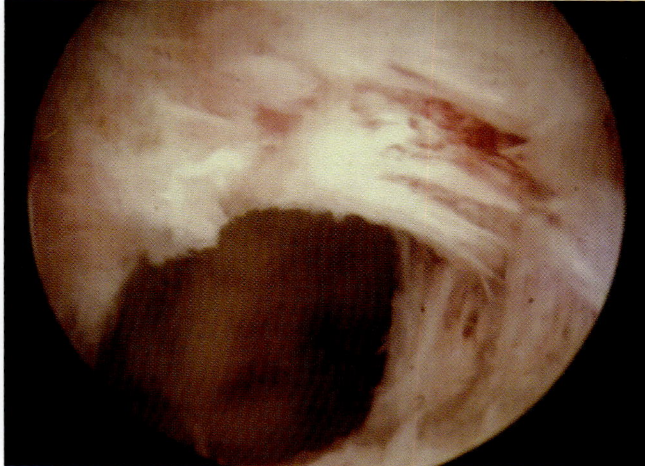

Fig. 4 Synechiae. Adhesions bands in the anterior and left lateral side wall of the uterine cavity

Source: Yu D, Wong YM, Cheong Y, et al. Asherman syndrome: one century later. Fertil Steril. 2008;89(4):759-79.

is likely to restore menstruation and improve the chance of pregnancy.[17]

The blind lysis of adhesions by curettage can cause trauma to the basal layer of the endometrium and may promote adhesion reformation. Hysteroscopic adhesiolysis can be performed using forceps, scissors, or knife electrode.

The occurrence of postoperative new IUA significantly affects subsequent reproductive outcome. Office hysteroscopy is an easy and effective procedure to separate these newly formed IUAs, as long as it is done within 2 weeks after surgery. To reduce the chance of recurrent IUA, the use of hormone therapy (estrogen with or without a progestin), intrauterine stents, intrauterine devices, and antibiotics have been advocated. There is no evidence to support the use of these adjuvant measures.[18]

The overall pregnancy rate following treatment of IUA is approximately 30–75%. The gestational outcome among those with a normal uterus has been identical irrespective of the pretreatment extent. The mean term live birthrate of the six published series of hysteroscopic adhesiolysis in infertile women using various techniques is 33%. The rates of first- and second-trimester pregnancy loss in these series were 11% and 14%, respectively. A correlation between the extent of uterine adhesions and subsequent pregnancy outcome following therapy has been observed in the largest study that classified IUAs. This study reported a term pregnancy rate of 81.3% among women with mild disease, 66.0% among women with moderate disease, and 31.9% of those with severe disease.[19]

Office Technique

Intrauterine synechiae can be treated by using bipolar electrodes and grasping forceps to cut them in the middle. Most authors recommend using cold non-energized instruments such as 5F scissors to minimize thermal trauma to normal endometrium. Adhesiolysis, no data has yet demonstrated one technique superior to another.

■ KEY POINTS

- There is scarce evidence on the effectiveness of hysteroscopic surgery in subfertile women as first-line treatment before spontaneous or medical-assisted conception, as well as first-line screening in all subfertile women.
- Hysteroscopic resection of submucous myomas that distort the endometrial cavity gives good results in cases opting for ART.
- Women with amenorrhea who are found to have intrauterine adhesions should be offered

hysteroscopic adhesiolysis because this is likely to restore menstruation and improve the chance of pregnancy.

- In patients with at least two failed cycles of ART, diagnostic hysteroscopy and, if necessary, operative hysteroscopy is mandatory to improve reproductive outcome.
- Operative office hysteroscopy in subfertile women is a powerful tool for the diagnosis and treatment of intrauterine pathologies. It is a simple, safe, reproducible, effective, quick, well-tolerated and low-cost surgical procedure because no operating room is necessary.

■ REFERENCES

1. National Collaborating Centre for Women's and Children's Health. Fertility: assessment and treatment for people with fertility problems. London (UK): National Institute for Health and Clinical Excellence (NICE); 2013 Feb. 63 p. (Clinical guideline; no. 156).
2. Gianaroli L, Racowsky C, Geraedts J, et al. Best practices of ASRM and ESHRE: a journey through reproductive medicine. Fertil Steril. 2012;98(6):1380-94.
3. Crosignani PG, Rubin BL. Optimal use of infertility diagnostic tests and treatments. The ESHRE Capri Workshop Group. Hum Reprod. 2000;15(3):723-32.
4. Bosteels J, Kasius J, Weyers S, et al. Hysteroscopy for treating subfertility associated with suspected major uterine cavity abnormalities. Cochrane Database Syst Rev. 2013;1: CD009461.
5. Lasmar RB, Barrozo PR, Parente RC, Lasmar BP, et al. Hysteroscopic evaluation in patients with infertility. Rev Bras Ginecol Obstet. 2010;32(8):393-7.
6. Alanís Fuentes J, Pérez Ramírez Mde L. Hysteroscopy used in infertility. Diagnosis and therapy. Ginecol Obstet Mex. 2008;76(11):679-84.
7. El-nashar IH, Nasr A. The role of hysteroscopy before intracytoplasmic sperm injection (ICSI): a randomized controlled trial. Fertil Steril. 2011;96(3):S266.
8. Taşkın EA, Berker B, Ozmen B, et al. Comparison of hysterosalpingography and hysteroscopy in the evaluation of the uterine cavity in patients undergoing assisted reproductive techniques. Fertil Steril. 2011;96(2):349-52.
9. Cunha-Filho JSL, de Souza CAB, Salazar CC, et al. Accuracy of hysterosalpingography and hysteroscopy for diagnosis of intrauterine lesions in infertile patients in an assisted fertilization programme. Gynaecol Endosc. 2001;10:45-8.
10. Rama Raju GA, Shashi Kumari G, Krishna KM, et al. Assessment of uterine cavity by hysteroscopy in assisted reproduction programme and its influence on pregnancy outcome. Arch Gynecol Obstet. 2006;274(3):160-4.
11. Bettocchi S, Achilarre MT, Ceci O, et al. Fertility-enhancing hysteroscopic surgery. Semin Reprod Med. 2011;29(2):75-82.
12. Bettocchi S, Ceci O, Nappi L, et al. Operative office hysteroscopy without anesthesia: analysis of 4863 cases performed with mechanical instruments. J Am Assoc Gynecol Laparosc. 2004;11(1):59-61.
13. Pritts EA, Parker WH, Olive DL, et al. Fibroids and infertility: an updated systematic review of the evidence. Fertil Steril. 2009;91(4):1215-23.
14. Taylor E, Gomel V. The uterus and fertility. Fertil Steril. 2008;89(1):1-16.
15. Parker WH. Uterine myomas: management. Fertil Steril. 2007;88(2):255-71.
16. Bettocchi S, Siristatidis C, Pontrelli G, et al. The destiny of myomas: should we treat small submucous myomas in women of reproductive age? Fertil Steril. 2008;90(4):905-10.
17. Myers EM, Hurst BS. Comprehensive management of severe Asherman syndrome and amenorrhea. Fertil Steril. 2012;97(1):160-4.
18. Yang JH, Chen MJ, Chen CD, et al. Optimal waiting period for subsequent fertility treatment after various hysteroscopic surgeries. Fertil Steril. 2013;99(7):2092-6.
19. Yu D, Li TC, Xia E, et al. Factors affecting reproductive outcome of hysteroscopic adhesiolysis for Asherman's syndrome. Fertil Steril. 2008;89(3):715-22.

10

Pilot Hysteroscopy before ART

Nandita Palshetkar, Hrishikesh Pai, Nandan Roongta

■ INTRODUCTION

Uterine factors represent only 2–3% of infertility, but intrauterine lesions are much more common in infertile women (40–50%). These lesions can interfere with spontaneous fertility and can compromise pregnancy rates in assisted reproduction. Exploration of the uterine cavity is actually one of the basic explorations in infertility workup.[1] Classically, hysterosalpingography (HSG).[2,13] and transvaginal sonography (TVS) are most commonly used for this purpose. Hysteroscopy is known as the gold standard procedure for uterine cavity assessment and is a valuable diagnostic and therapeutic modality in the management of infertility, with a changing role as it replaces some of the conventional tests, and also as in certain scenarios, it is being replaced by some of the newer methods.

The word 'Pilot' when used as an adjective implies something that is serving as a guide to a full-scale operation. Hysteroscopy is quick, safe and well-tolerated. Therefore, it has become an excellent tool for the diagnostic and therapeutic infertility workup, and whether done as an office procedure or under anesthesia, it is frequently advised as a routine procedure prior to in vitro fertilization/intracytoplasmic sperm injection (IVF/ICSI) treatment. But after repeated implantation failure in IVF cycles, the uterine cavity should be re-evaluated by hysteroscopy as this practice has been demonstrated to improve pregnancy rates.

According to the "Best practices of ASRM and ESHRE"[3] in December 2012, "*Multiple studies have identified that between 26% and 50% of patients who fail IVF have uterine abnormalities, suggesting that hysteroscopy could serve as a prognostic factor for the IVF outcome, especially in the case of fibroids which distort the endometrial cavity (Bozdag et al., 2008; Sunkara et al., 2010). Specific hysteroscopic interventions have been reported to significantly improve the pregnancy rate (Demirol and Gurgan, 2004)."*

However, the benefit of the systematic use of hysteroscopy in the initial assessment of infertility remains unclear and the exploration of the uterine cavity in the initial assessment of infertility should ideally be based on a noninvasive method like HSG, 3-dimensional (3-D) ultrasonography, MRI or hysterosonography.[9]

■ GENERAL CONSIDERATIONS

Hysteroscopy allows direct visualization of the utero-cervical canal and endometrial assessment, and is thus considered as the gold-standard reference test.[4-6] The availability of the newer small caliber systems enables one to diagnose and treat a range of uterine pathologies effectively and safely in one sitting on an outpatient basis without any need for cervical dilatation or general anesthesia.

- Hysteroscopy should be performed after a careful history and physical examination as well as utilization of adjunctive preoperative tests. It is preferable to do TVS before the hysteroscopy to evaluate the size and direction of the uterus and to rule out any adnexal pathology.
- All hysteroscopies should be planned so as to avoid conception cycles.
- General anesthesia is desirable for medical indications, for those who request it and for operative interventions.

Indications

- Any abnormality seen on HSG or TVS
- History of previous instrumental intervention or uterine scarring
- History of recurrent miscarriages
- History of recurrent IVF failures.

Absolute Contraindications

- Pelvic infection
- Uterine bleeding
- Patient's refusal.

Relative Contraindications

- A grossly distorted pelvic anatomy
- Suspected pelvic infection
- Anticipated technical difficulty.

The Procedure

The hysteroscope is introduced slowly through the cervix and into the uterine cavity under video monitoring, avoiding contact with the mucosa with the aid of saline distension. The initial step at hysteroscopy is to identify the uterine cavity and ostia and to evaluate the right and left cornu, fundus, anterior and posterior walls, and lateral walls for specific lesions, as well as to evaluate the overall contour of the uterine cavity. A biopsy is taken before withdrawing the scope so that tissue could be sent for histopathology or TB culture, if required. The endocervical canal is also then carefully evaluated. The histopathology can be used to diagnose an out-of-phase endometrium, endometritis, neoplastic lesion, etc. The sample can also be used to co-culture the embryos that are produced in subsequent treatment cycles.

Distension Media

If energy sources are not used, as for example surgery carried out with scissors, any standard irrigating fluid such as normal saline, Ringer's lactate or 5% glucose can be used. When monopolar energy source is to be used for techniques like use of a resectoscope, 1.5% glycine or sorbitol is preferred. Normal saline can be used safely with bipolar energy source and that is one of its advantages. Liquid media have the advantage of being cleared from time to time by aspiration or by flushing.

Instruments

Rigid instruments are still preferred because they are sturdy, reliable and offer a good vision. The conventional resectoscope works satisfactorily to perform most hystero-scopic surgeries conveniently. However, scissors are preferred whenever possible as resection or adhesiolysis can be carried out without the use of electric current which is helpful in preventing a decrease in vascularity of the endometrium which would happen after the use of energy sources.

■ DIAGNOSTIC HYSTEROSCOPY PRIOR TO ART

Despite advances in the field of artificial reproductive techniques over the past 20 years, implantation rates per embryo transferred still remains low, at about 15–20%. The two key factors in question for this problem are the quality of the embryo and the receptivity of the uterus. Though uterine receptivity cannot be fully evaluated, some uterine factors can be assessed by TVS (endometrial thickness, pattern and blood flow in the uterine and subendometrial arteries), and also some by hysteroscopy.

Hysteroscopy Assesses

- Fibroids
- Endometrial polyp
- Asherman's syndrome
- Uterine anomaly
    - Septate uterus
    - Bicornuate uterus
    - Arcuate uterus
    - Unicornuate uterus

One of the main priorities in future research should become the development of a guideline with exact definitions of what should be judged as an intrauterine abnormality. Hysteroscopy-guided biopsies of polypous-like structures might clarify the definition of a polyp. Moreover, hysteroscopy features of a septate uterus might be compared with a HSG or 3-D ultrasound image to make its hysteroscopic diagnosis clear. Through such research, the exact difference between intrauterine pathology and physiological variations of a normal uterine cavity should become universal.

The place of routine hysteroscopy in the management of infertile women without other diagnosed or doubtful intrauterine pathologies is still a matter of debate.[10-12] With the invention of the miniature hysteroscope, it is possible to perform hysteroscopy in an office setting for diagnostic indications and certain therapeutic interventions.

The two main problems that argue against the case of hysteroscopy are: first, it is an invasive procedure, and second, there is still an ongoing debate about the real significance of the observed intrauterine pathology on fertility. The European Society of Human Reproduction and Embryology (ESHRE) guidelines[8] indicate hysteroscopy to be unnecessary, unless it is for the confirmation and treatment of doubtful intrauterine pathology. On the other hand, many patients are diagnosed with conditions during hysteroscopy that were not found during the previous tests of HSG or USG. Studies also indicate that such intrauterine abnormalities may be a cause for failure of IVF-ET and therefore hysteroscopy should be part of the infertility workup for all patients, prior to undergoing IVF treatment to minimize implantation failures.

"Fertility Effect" of Diagnostic Hysteroscopy

Just as with HSG, it has been shown that improved spontaneous pregnancy rates are seen following diagnostic hysteroscopy. Distension of the uterine cavity might clear any debris, casts, mucus plugs, filmy adhesions, and thus help. It was also found that a deliberate local injury to the endometrium with sampling devices doubled the clinical pregnancy rates in patients with history of repeated IVF attempt failures undergoing repeated IVF. And also that the expression of several genes was modulated by biopsy-induced local injury; prominent among which was the upregulation of bladder transmembranal protein (UPIb). The ensuing inflammatory response is apparently beneficial for embryo implantation by improving uterine receptivity. Pregnancy outcome was positively correlated with MIP-1B (macrophage inflammatory protein 1B) and TNF-alpha expression, and the number of macrophages/dendritic cells.

Advantages of Pre-ART Office Hysteroscopy[14]

- The procedure is minimally invasive, and unlike traditional hysteroscopy it can be performed in an office-based gynecological practice with no need for hospitalization, cervical dilatation, or anesthesia.
- The procedure has a very low technical failure rate.
- The procedure gives the ability to visualize the entire lower genital tract (vaginoscopy, cerviscopy). Abnormalities, such as cervical stenosis, large nabothian cyst, or cervical polyp, may need treatment before ART to ensure easy Embryo Transfer.
- The procedure gives reliable visual assessment of the uterine cavity. Abnormalities, such as endometrial polyp, submucous myoma, or intrauterine adhesions, may need surgical interference before ART to improve the pregnancy rates and also to save the patient additional costs, especially in cases with recurrent failures.
- The procedure takes only a few minutes and patient compliance was very high. No speculum or tenaculum needs to be used minimizing discomfort to the patient. The ability of the patients to interact while performing the procedure increases their understanding and acceptability.
- The patient being awake makes pain a safeguard against complications, such as faulty introduction or perforation. Likewise, as entry into the uterine cavity is made under vision, the risk of perforation is minimal. Normal saline used as a distention medium avoids the problem of fluid imbalance.

■ HYSTEROSCOPY IN CASES OF REPEATED IVF FAILURES[15,16]

Most IVF Units currently use hysteroscopy as a second-level investigation, only in selected patients with repeated implantation failures and abnormal findings on ultrasonography.

The most consistent factor for predicting pregnancy and implantation rates in patients undergoing IVF-ET is the quality of the embryos. However, the significance of embryo quality in determining pregnancy and implantation rates should not be considered apart from other factors, including endometrial receptivity and uterine integrity. Endometrial integrity is the only variable that can be studied on a large scale by using hysteroscopy and endometrial biopsy. Important unsuspected intrauterine abnormalities, such as chronic endometritis and adhesions, were found only on hysteroscopy. This fact highlights the importance of the use of hysteroscopy as second-level investigation independent of TVS examination. Hence, evaluation of uterine and endometrial integrity by hysteroscopy is valuable and should be performed in all patients who have repeated IVF-ET failure after transfer of good-quality embryos.[17]

■ OPERATIVE HYSTEROSCOPY

Hysteroscopic correction of uterine anomalies and lesions is the best possible manner to maintain normal uterine anatomy and function thereby restoring fertility.[7]

Hysteroscopy has several advantages over open or laparoscopic surgery in that it has a low morbidity, decreased hospitalization time and absence of hysterotomy. Hysteroscopic septoplasty, polypectomy and synechiolysis are now established methods in patients with subfertility. It is advisable to perform a second-look hysteroscopy after correction of these pathologies to ensure their proper correction before embarking on a costly IVF program.

Endometrial Biopsy and Polypectomy

Endometrial abnormalities include polypoid endometrium, corrugated/rough endometrium, pale/edematous endometrium, atrophic endometrium, endometritis, mixed distribution of blood vessels and glandular openings, neovascularization, endometrial ridges and focal elevations.

Persistent benign-looking raised lesions can be subgrouped as polypoid, corrugated and edematous. Most of these pathologies contribute to infertility and/or IVF failure and can be diagnosed with hysteroscopy. Patients with poor grade of luteal phase endometrium (consisting of pinpoint glandular openings and thinner blood vessels) resulted in fewer clinical pregnancies in their attempts to conceive.

A reddish appearing endometrium in which the white openings of the glands produce a strawberry-like pattern is characteristically seen in endometritis and is due to the significantly increased vascularity. Hysteroscopic diagnosis of endometritis is highly specific (93.2%). Appropriate hormonal or antimicrobial treatment following hysteroscopic diagnosis of endometritis has been shown to improve clinical pregnancy rates following natural or assisted conception. Hysteroscopy can aid in diagnosing genital tuberculosis (TB) not only by taking a biopsy and culture assessment with polymerase chain reaction (TB-PCR), but also simply by assessing the "look" of the endometrium. The finding of endometrial micropolyps at fluid hysteroscopy has been shown to be a marker for chronic endometritis. Sequelae of old infection would include atrophic endometrium and scarring as in Asherman syndrome.

The impact of polyps on infertility is mainly dependent of their size and location **(Figs 1A and B)**.

Polyps may cause infertility by virtue of their location thereby causing mechanical block (e.g., tubo cornual polyp), by their association with endometriosis, or by expression of the enzyme aromatase. Polyp removal appeared to improve fertility and increase pregnancy rates in previous infertile women with no other reason to explain their infertility, regardless of the size or number of the polyps.

Biopsy is easily carried out with use of a biopsy instrument or grasper, or curettage of the cavity. This will identify polyps as well as luteal phase dysfunction, endometritis, or rarely an infertile patient's malignancy. Resection of a polyp is easier than that of a fibroid. Grasping it with a grasper is usually sufficient to excise it, though at times cauterization of the base and extraction may be required. Sometimes transecting the base and removing the compressible mass through the cervix may be more convenient.

Uterine Myomas

Leiomyomata are the most common tumors of the uterus, occurring most commonly in women of reproductive age, particularly in their 30s and 40s. The impact of fibroids on fertility depends on the parameters of location, number, and size. Types of leiomyomata include subserosal, intramural, and submucosal varieties. Submucous myomas, by virtue of their mass effect and inhospitable surface area for nidation, have been clearly associated with infertility and with pregnancy loss. These myomas appear as rounded masses that bulge to varying extents into the endometrial cavity, and the overlying endometrium may be atrophic, congested, ulcerated, or hemorrhagic. Because of their intracavitary location, submucosal fibroids may be effectively removed via a hysteroscopic approach **(Figs 2A and B)**.

However, large myomas which only produce a subtle deformation of the cavity can be difficult to recognize. Additionally, large myomas, even though easily recognizable, can be very difficult to treat.

Preoperative evaluation with ultrasonography can improve our ability to diagnose and treat the condition

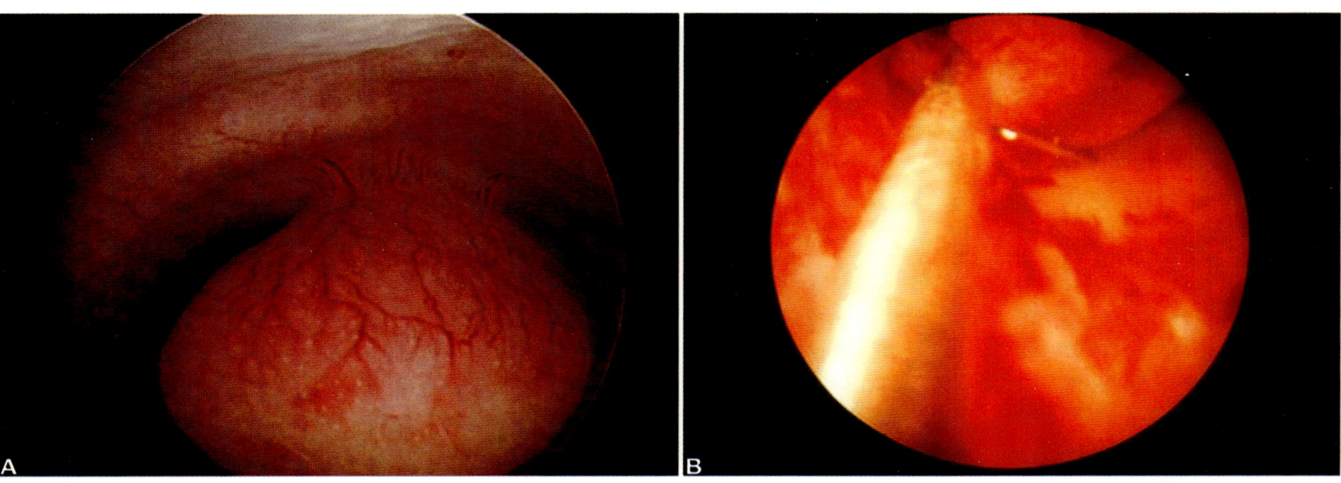

Figs 1A and B (A) Pedunculated endometrial polyp; (B) Dividing pedicle of polyp

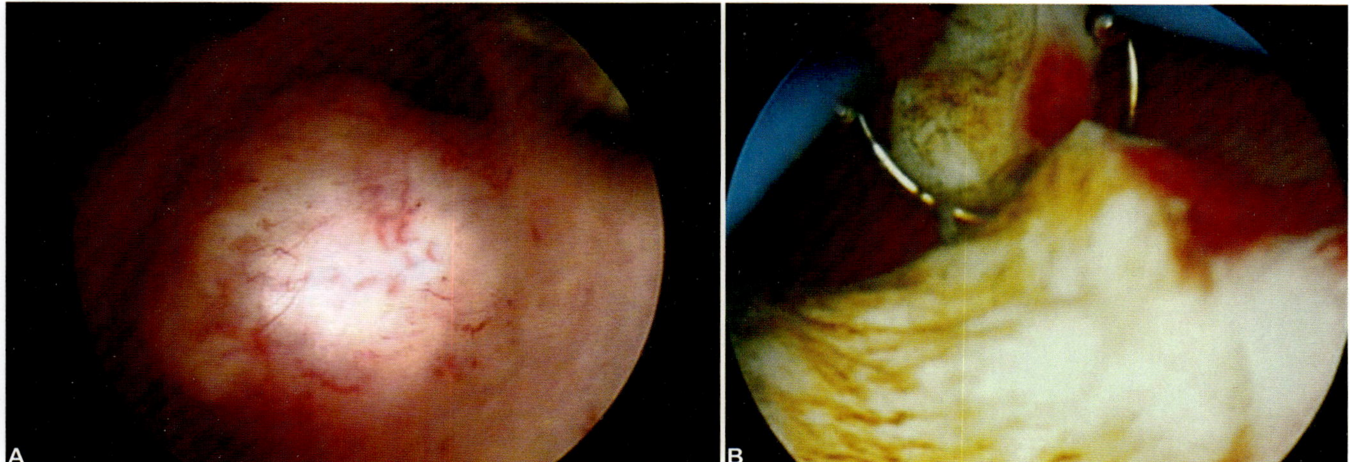

Figs 2A and B (A) Submucosal leiomyoma; (B) Resection of a sessile submucous leiomyoma using a cutting loop

appropriately. Myomas can be removed effectively with a resectoscope if they have more than 50% of their volume inside the contour of the uterine cavity. Usually treatment of intrauterine myomas with gonadotropin-releasing hormone (GnRH) agonists prior to hysteroscopic resection is beneficial. GnRH agonists will reduce the myoma volume approximately 50% in most, but not all, cases. It is important to recognize that the uterine volume would also be reduced and that the uterus would be hypoestrogenic and therefore more susceptible to perforation, even in the premenopausal woman, who has been treated with GnRH agonists. Resectoscopic myomectomy is a highly effective procedure, but fraught with potential hazards with respect to uterine injury from the electrosurgical energy, perforation of the uterus, bleeding, infection, and most importantly, serious complication as a result of fluid overload. The upper range of uterine size when performing procedures such as myomectomy should be approximately 8–12 cm of depth, depending on the surgeon's experience, and only extremely knowledgeable and experienced surgeons should attempt myomectomies larger than 5 cm. Despite the inherent risks of hysteroscopic myomectomy, the advantages of hysteroscopic resection include the avoidance of laparotomy and a uterine incision, as well as the avoidance of a need for a later cesarean section and avoidance of the creation of tubo-ovarian adhesions. Overall, this is considered an excellent procedure if performed by skilled surgeons.

Asherman's Syndrome

Intrauterine adhesions have been reported in 7–25% of infertile women, although the incidence is probably less today than historically. The pathophysiology involves damage to the stratum basalis and bridging of denuded uterine walls with variable cavity obliteration.

Symptoms associated with intrauterine adhesions include hypomenorrhea, amenorrhea as a result of endometrial destruction, cyclic pain, infertility possibly as a result of sperm migration disruption, tubal ostia obstruction, or impairment of blastocyst implantation. Recurrent abortions have been reported because of decreased uterine size or insufficient endometrium, and abnormal placentation may result in a defective stratum basalis.

Predisposing factors to intrauterine adhesions include an antecedent pregnancy, which is found approximately 90% of the time, with 70% being postabortal and 20% being postpartum. Uterine trauma from curettage at surgery increases the probability of adhesions. It is felt that infection plays an important role in the development of intrauterine adhesions although its role is still somewhat controversial. Tuberculous endometritis is an etiologic infection, and patients with congenital abnormalities, such as DES, may be at higher risk.

Based on their severity and nature Asherman syndrome can be classified as mild (flimsy and composed of endometrial tissue only), moderate (fibromuscular tissue covered with endometrium) and severe (composed of fibromuscular tissue only and partially/totally occluding the uterine cavity).

Hysteroscopy permits the classification of the extent of the disease and most importantly allows one to lyse the adhesions under vision, making it a safe surgery. Treatment involves removal or division of the adhesions (**Figs 3A and B**) with an endoscope, endoscope sheath, curettes, scissors, cautery, resectoscope, or neodymium-YAG laser. Use of energy sources, especially in

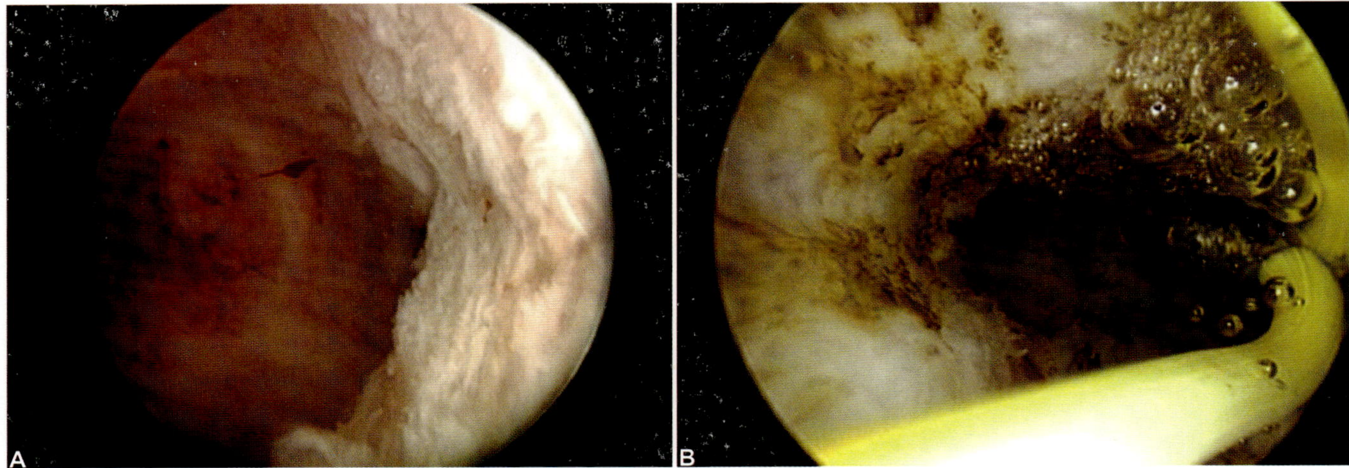

Figs 3A and B (A) Left lateral wall adhesions; (B) Resection of adhesions with an L-shaped electrode

inexperienced hands, is to be kept at minimum because the energy source itself can lead to surrounding tissue damage and further fibrosis.

It is controversial whether patients should receive prophylactic antibiotics or postoperative estrogen, or use of an intrauterine device or Foley catheter. Complications specific to adhesiolysis include recurrent adhesion formation, extensive endometrial damage and perforation of the uterus, which happens particularly while operating near the cornual area. The surgical management of intrauterine adhesions is reported to be very effective, with pregnancy rates above 80% among patients treated for mild to moderate disease.

Congenital Uterine Abnormalities

It has been reported that 5–10% of infertile women who are evaluated hysteroscopically are found to have congenital uterine abnormalities. Comprehensive infertility evaluation is necessary prior to concluding that a congenital uterine anomaly is a cause of infertility. Intravenous pyelogram should be performed to rule out associated renal anomalies.

The American Fertility Society Classification of congenital uterine anomalies has five major groupings which are hypoplastic/agenic, unicornuate, didelphis, bicornuate, or septate. The true clinical relevance of the mild to moderate uterine cavity anomalies is unclear. A higher incidence of arcuate, septate and subseptate uteri was reported in women with history of recurrent miscarriages. Moreover, a higher incidence of mid-trimester abortions, preterm deliveries and low live-birth rates following assisted conception treatments were reported in women with uterine malformations. Metroplasty for a T-shaped uterus and infantile or

hypoplastic uterus in women with recurrent miscarriages has also been shown to increase live birth rates. No treatment is needed for uterus didelphis or unicornuate uterus.

Postoperative hysterosalpingogram at 2 months can evaluate the results prior to patients attempting pregnancy.

Septate Uterus

With an incidence of 2–3% in the general population, uterine septation represents the most common Müllerian fusion defect. Clinical sequelae of this condition may include infertility, spontaneous pregnancy loss in the first or second trimester, or late-trimester pregnancy complications. However, pregnancy outcome in the presence of a septum depends on the site of embryo implantation in a particular cycle. This may explain the situation in which a woman with a septate uterus might encounter recurrent pregnancy loss even after having delivered a term infant.

Hysteroscopic septoplasty **(Figs 4A and B)** has been demonstrated to decrease significantly the risk for spontaneous abortion in women with septate uteri, and surgical therapy is indicated in patients with known uterine septi and a history of recurrent spontaneous abortions.

However, if the presenting complaint is only infertility without any history of miscarriages then the indication is less straightforward. It is reasonable to consider surgical management in some infertile patients with uterine septi because septoplasty may maximize the chance of having a live birth by decreasing the associated risks for spontaneous abortion and preterm labor. The hysteroscopic approach to septum resection is often

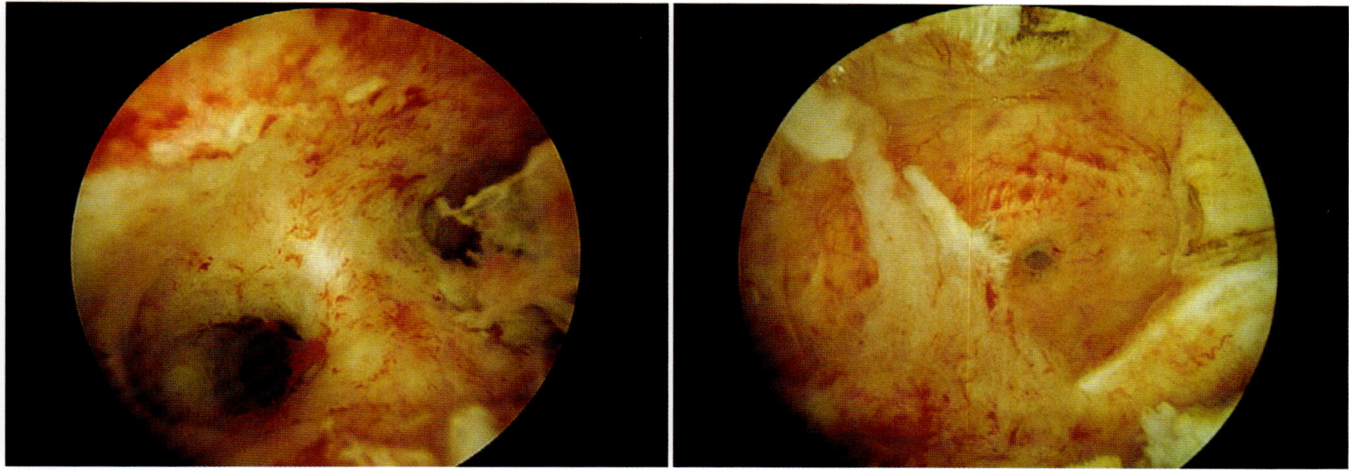

Figs 4A and B (A) Uterine septum; (B) After septoplasty

performed with microscissors, the resectoscope, or laser. The coaxial bipolar electrode surgical system is particularly advantageous in this setting as it enables one to operate in a crystalloid distention medium, and has been successfully applied toward hysteroscopic septum resection.

Proximal Tubal Occlusion

Proximal tubal occlusion can be diagnosed by HSG and confirmed at laparoscopy. In clinical situations when obstruction seems to be persistent, selective hydrotubation performed hysteroscopically can help diagnose and/or overcome these occlusions. Current technology also allows for tubal catheterization and possibly falloposcopy helping evaluation of the Fallopian tubes.

Contraindications to tubal catheterization include active pelvic infection or uterine bleeding, allergic reaction to local anesthetic agents, extensive uterine synechiae or submucous myomata, or other significant medical disease. There are low complication rates for this procedure. Laparoscopic assistance is sometimes required in order to completely cannulate the Fallopian tube.

■ OTHER INDICATIONS

- *Sperm migration test*: To assess the survival of spermatozoa in the upper genital tract
- Removal of intrauterine foreign bodies
- Gamete intrafallopian transfer and zygote intra-fallopian transfer
- Hysteroscopic tubal cannulation
- Abortion

- Abnormalities of the cervix
- Unexplained infertility
- Women of advanced reproductive age
- Multiple previous IVF attempt failures.

■ CONCLUSION

- Hysteroscopy is the gold standard in evaluating and treating certain important uterine pathologies that can contribute to infertility and/or IVF failure by providing suboptimal conditions for the implanting embryo. It is clearly more sensitive and specific for endometrial abnormalities. Evidence suggests that such endometrial pathologies lead to fewer pregnancies and more miscarriages whereas their correction is associated with a higher chance of clinical pregnancy and reduced risk of miscarriages.
- Used either alone or along with other modalities for evaluation like endometrial biopsy, hysterosalpingo-graphy (HSG), transvaginal sonography (TVS), saline contrast sonography (SCS) or sonohysterography, magnetic resonance imaging, and simultaneously performed laparoscopy, hysteroscopy has helped improve the success rates in ART cycles.
- Conventionally hysteroscopy was performed before a treatment cycle, but now evidence suggests that it can be performed safely and effectively in the early phase of the ovarian hyperstimulation cycle, with added benefits to the patient.
- Cost-effective analysis indicates that hysteroscopy as a universal screening test even before the first IVF cycle is well justified even in a population where there is only a 10% prevalence of uterine pathologies. However, the issue is still a matter of debate.

- But in cases of repeated IVF failures there is consensus as to the beneficial effects of diagnostic with operative hysteroscopy, and the endometrial assessment which could detect otherwise undiagnosed pathologies especially endometritis and adhesions.

■ REFERENCES

1. Ait Benkaddour Y, Gervaise A, Fernandez H. Which is the method of choice for evaluating uterine cavity in infertility workup? J Gynecol Obstet Biol Reprod. 2010;39(8):606-13.
2. Streda R, Mardesic T, Kult D, et al. The diagnostic value of hysterosalpingography in the diagnosis of tubal disease. Ceska Gynekol. 2009;74(1):18-21.
3. Elif Aylin Taşkın, Bülent Berker, Batuhan Özmen, et al. Comparison of hysterosalpingography and hysteroscopy in the evaluation of the uterine cavity in patients undergoing assisted reproductive techniques. Fertil Steril. 2011;96(2):349-52.
4. Gianaroli L1, Racowsky C, Geraedts J, et al. Best practices of ASRM and ESHRE: a journey through reproductive medicine. Fertil Steril. 2012;98(6):1380-94.
5. Margit Dueholm, Erik Lundorf, Estrid S, et al. Evaluation of the uterine cavity with magnetic resonance imaging, transvaginal sonography, hysterosonographic examination, and diagnostic hysteroscopy. Fertil Steril. 2001;76(2):350-7.
6. Lasmar RB, Barrozo PR, Parente RC, et al. Hysteroscopic evaluation in patients with infertility. Rev Bras Ginecol Obstet. 2010;32(8):393-7.
7. Pansky M, Feingold M, Sagi R, et al. Diagnostic hysteroscopy as a primary tool in a basic infertility workup. JSLS. 2006;10(2): 231-5.
8. Alanís Fuentes J, Pérez Ramírez Mde L. Hysteroscopy used in infertility. Diagnosis and therapy. Ginecol Obstet Mex. 2008;76(11):679-84.
9. Akmal El-Mazny, Nermeen Abou-Salem, Walid El-Sherbiny, et al. Outpatient hysteroscopy: a routine investigation before assisted reproductive techniques? Fertil Steril. 2011;95(1): 272-6.
10. Banerjee K. Pre-IVF hysteroscopy—is it a must? Fertile Steril. 2008;90:S447-8.
11. El-nashar IH, Nasr A. The role of hysteroscopy before intra-cytoplasmic sperm injection (ICSI): a randomized controlled trial. Fertil Steril. 2011;96(3):S266.
12. Crosingnani RG, Rubin BL. Optimal use of infertility diagnostic tests and treatments: The ESHRE Capri Workshop Group. Hum Reprod. 2000;15:723-32.
13. Milki AA, Mooney SB. Does Hysteroscopy Immediately Prior to Stimulation Affect IVF Outcome? Fertil Steril. 2000;74(3):S212.
14. Bozdag G, Aksan G, Esinler I, et al. What is the role of office hysteroscopy in women with failed IVF cycles? Reprod Biomed Online. 2008;17:410-5.
15. Demirol A, Gurgan T. Effect of treatment of intrauterine pathologies with office hysteroscopy in patients with recurrent IVF failure. Reprod Biomed Online. 2004;8:590-4.
16. Flávio G Oliveira, Vicente G Abdelmassih, Michael P Diamond, et al. Uterine cavity findings and hysteroscopic interventions in patients undergoing in vitro fertilization–embryo transfer who repeatedly cannot conceive. Fertil Steril. 2003:80(6): 1371-5.
17. Campo R, Gordts S, Brosens I. Minimally invasive exploration of the female reproductive tract in infertility. Reprod Biomed Online. 2002;4(Suppl 3):40-5.

Endocrinology and Stimulation Protocols

11

Genetic Markers of Ovarian Response

Giulia Brigante, Manuela Simoni

OVARIAN RESPONSE

Ovarian response could be defined as the endocrine and follicular reaction to stimulation.[1] In cases of chronic anovulation, ovulation can be achieved by means of clomiphene and human chorionic gonadotropin (hCG), or follicle stimulating hormone (FSH) and/or hCG, followed or not by intrauterine insemination.

In women undergoing controlled ovarian hyperstimulation (COH), there is a high variability of the clinical outcome and, in particular, two opposite situations should be avoided—on one hand, poor ovarian response and on the other hand, ovarian hyperstimulation syndrome (OHSS).[2] Thus, it is of high clinical relevance to identify predictive factors of ovarian response that will enable clinicians to set up the best schemes of ovulation induction and ovarian stimulation, in order to optimize pregnancy rate without complications and to avoid failure of the clinical treatment. Ovarian monitoring by ultrasonography or screening for endocrine and genetic characteristics could be currently used as predictive approaches, but actually treatment parameters are still entrust to the clinical experience and personal feelings of the physician.[1]

Many efforts have been made in order to improve assisted reproductive technology (ART) success rate and reduce complications. The ovarian response to COH is associated to well-known individual features, such as ovarian reserve, chronological age, anti-Müllerian hormone (AMH) levels, ovarian volume, ovarian Doppler score and smoking habits.[3] A combination of four of such factors [baseline serum FSH, body mass index (BMI), age, antral follicular count] was assessed in an algorithm to calculate the exact FSH dose for each single woman candidate to assisted reproduction.[4] However, none of these approaches seems to be completely successful. Probably, individual differences in COH response that cannot be justified by these known factors are linked to genetic variability among subjects. Discovering the genetic variants associated with ovarian response to gonadotropins is an important step toward individualized pharmacogenetics protocols of ovarian stimulation. To date, an individualized ovarian stimulation treatment designed on genetic predictive factors is still missing.

GENETIC ASPECTS

Genetic variability among subjects is probably the main cause of individual drug response; the effects of a pharmacological therapy administered uniformly to a population can vary in terms of clinical response, side effects and adverse events. Pharmacogenetics is the science that describes the relationship between genetic variability and drug response.

The human genome is 99.9% identical in all individuals. More than 90% of the genetic variability is caused by the presence of single nucleotide polymorphisms (SNPs). The remaining 10% is due to insertions, deletions, tandem repeats and microsatellites. A genetic variation is defined as an SNP when it is common in a specific population, by definition a polymorphism occurs in more than 1% of individuals belonging to the same group, while a mutation is rare, with a frequency less than 1%.[3] A minority of SNPs occurs in exons (protein coding regions of a gene), the remaining are intronic. SNPs can modify gene function by changing biochemical properties of the gene product (protein) or by modifying the activity of the promoter, or altering the stability/metabolism/degradation of mRNA, resulting in a larger or smaller amount of protein.[5]

A study approach to test response to gonadotropins is to assess genetic variations for association to a medical condition. If an association is present, a variant will be seen more often than expected by chance in a population carrying the trait. Such analyses are based on a chromosomal property called "linkage disequilibrium", for which DNA variants located close to each other tend to be observed together more frequently than two variants located further apart. Considering this, human genome can be subdivided in haplotype blocks. Haplotypes are combinations of alleles observed in a population and determined by the SNP combination in a given genome sequence. Therefore, haplotype blocks could be used as marker regions in genome-wide association studies as they are mapped in online databases such as HapMap or NCBI **(Fig. 1)**.

Different genes have been studied in relation to the characteristics of normal ovarian cycle and to the individual response to COH. Considering physiology, luteinizing hormone (LH) (encoded by *LHB gene*) and FSH (*FSHB gene*) are glycoproteins produced by the pituitary under gonadotropin releasing hormone (GnRH) pulsatile stimulation. Glycoprotein hormones are heterodimers consisting of a common alpha (α) subunit and a specific beta (β) subunit which determines receptor specificity. FSH and LH act on the gonads and are essential for reproduction and sexual development. In women, FSH stimulates the maturation of the follicular granulosa cells and the production of estrogens, while LH induces the theca interna cells to produce androgens and leads to maturation of the follicle, ovulation and maintenance of the corpus luteum, contributing to progress of the ovarian cycle. Gonadotropins act by binding their receptors localized in the gonads, the FSH receptor (*FSHR* gene) and LH/hCG receptor (*LHCGR gene*). Both receptors belong to the superfamily of G protein-coupled receptors.

GENOMIC STRUCTURES

The human FSHB is a single-copy gene of 4,262 base pairs located on chromosome 11p13. The LHB and hCG beta (hCG β) subunit genes span over a complex gene cluster, including one copy of LHB and six copies of human CGB.[6] They are located in contiguity in a shared genomic region 45,165 base pairs long at position 19q13.32.[7] The structural similarity of the glycoprotein heterodimeric hormones forecasted the homology in the extracellular domain of their receptors.[8] The *FSHR gene* consists of ten exons and nine introns. Exons 1–9 encode the extracellular domain, while exon 10 encodes the transmembrane and intracellular domains and the C-terminal portion of the extracellular domain.[9] The *LHCGR gene* consists of 11 exons and 10 introns. The first 10 exons and part of the last exon encode the extracellular domain of the receptor while the transmembrane and intracellular domains are encoded by the remaining part of the last exon.[10] These similarities suggest a possible phylogenetic relationship between FSHR and LHCGR **(Figs 2 and 3)**.[8]

GENETIC POLYMORPHISMS AND OVARIAN RESPONSE TO GONADOTROPINS

Ovulation Induction and Controlled Ovarian Stimulation

In in vitro fertilization (IVF) programs, exogenous FSH is administered for ovarian stimulation of multiple follicles. Numerous studies have been carried out to evaluate individual variability in the ovarian response to

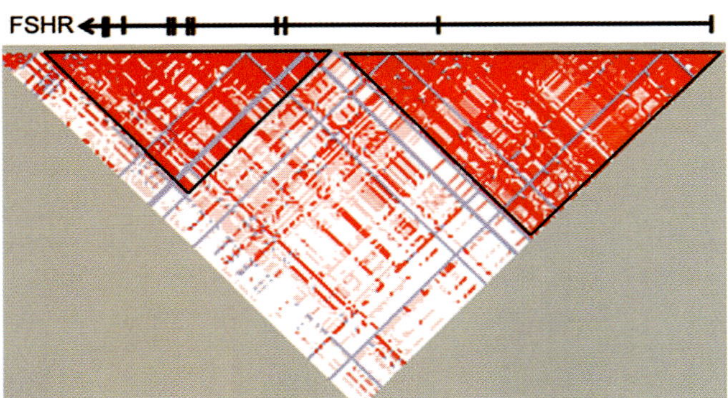

Fig. 1 *FSHR gene* (NCBI Ref. Seq. NG_008146.1) mapped on HapMap. The black triangles indicate linkage disequilibrium blocks

Source: International HapMap Project. [online] Available from http://hapmap.ncbi.nlm.nih.gov/ [Accessed July 2013]

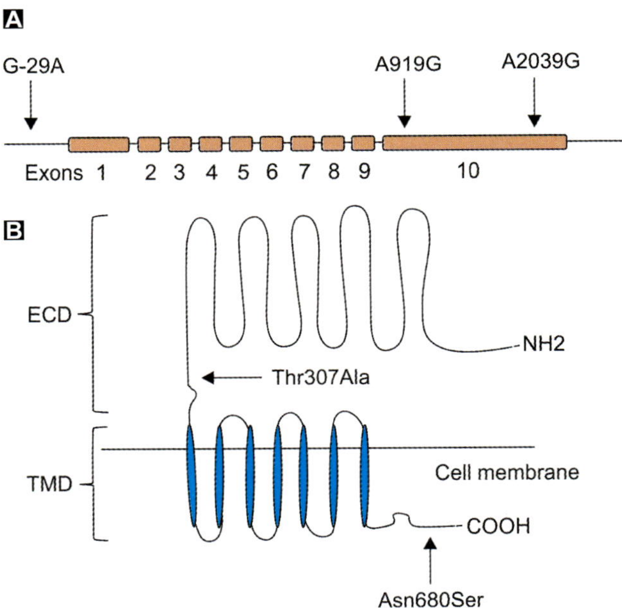

Figs 2A and B Schematic model of *FSHR* gene (A) and protein (B). The position of the single nucleotide polymorphisms considered in this article is shown

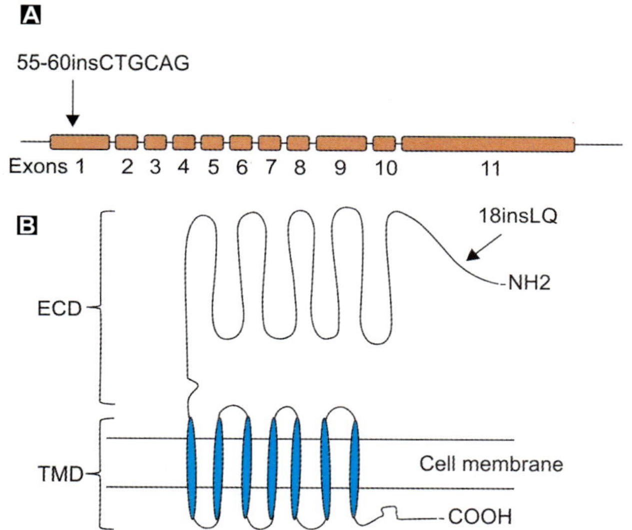

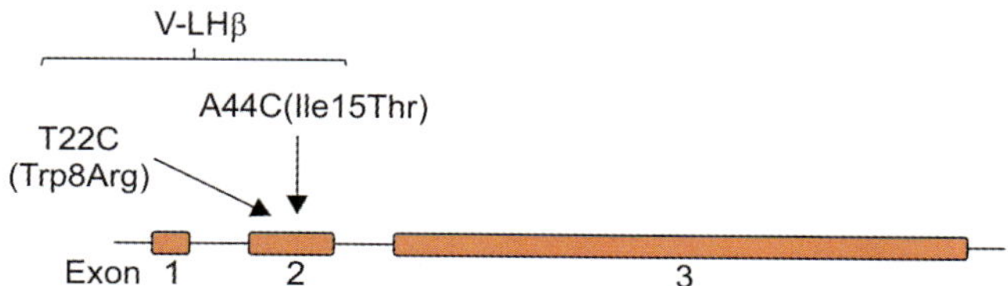

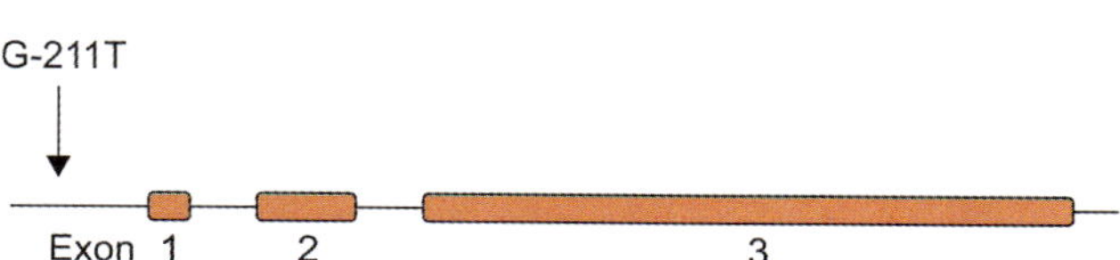

Figs 3A and B Schematic model of *LHCGR* gene (A) and protein (B). The position of the single nucleotide polymorphism considered in this article is shown

Fig. 4 Schematic model of *LHB* gene. The position of the single nucleotide polymorphisms considered in this article is shown

Fig. 5 Schematic model of *FSHB* gene. The position of the single nucleotide polymorphism considered in this article is shown

gonadotropins, using different markers—hormonal (FSH, AMH), functional (*antral follicle count*) or genetic.

At present, the FSH dosage for a single patient candidate to IVF is individualized taking into account parameters of ovarian reserve. A high variability in ovarian response to exogenous FSH can be observed and this variability is only in part explained by known individual factors, for example, the presence of a polycystic ovary syndrome (predisposing to a high response) or ovarian aging (associated with a low response).[3] Some studies have been conducted to determine how FSHR SNPs can affect the necessary FSH dosage, independently and in association with already known clinical features, and to know in advance the optimal FSH dose for each patient. Changing gonadotropin dose during ovarian stimulation according to the number of recruited follicles and estradiol concentration on days 7–8 is problematic. Increasing the dose often results in a heterogeneous cohort of follicles because large follicles continue to grow while the FSH threshold of non-growing small follicles will be passed. On the other side, decreasing the dose could result in a diffuse follicle atresia and poor oocyte quality.[3]

Considering pathophysiology, possible genetic markers of ovarian response could be mutations or different SNPs combination in the genes coding for LH, LHCGR, FSH, FSHR and finally, estrogen receptors.

A common variant of the β subunit of LH (v-LH), consisting of the double amino acid change Trp8Arg and Ile15Thr in the protein **(Fig. 4)**,[11] is characterized by an additional sulphonated sugar at asparagine (Asn)-13.[12] This SNP, especially present in North European women,[11] affects FSH sensitivity and the ovarian response to FSH. For example, in a study conducted on 204 women classified as normogonadotropic, 21 heterozygotes for v-LH and one homozygote were identified. The FSH dose necessary for an adequate response was significantly correlated with the presence of the variant, so that women homozygous or heterozygous required higher doses than normal controls.[13]

Concerning the LHCGR, the more frequently investigated SNP consists of the presence or absence of two amino acids at position 18 in exon 1 **(Fig. 3)**. There seems to be a correlation between this SNP and breast cancer and high serum levels of estrogen. No studies on a possible correlation with ovarian response have been conducted so far.[14]

Considering FSHB, a low number of SNPs, mainly within non-coding regions, has been identified **(Fig. 5)**. Recently, a strong effect of the SNP-211G>T in the *FSHB* gene promoter on transcription of the FSH beta subunit and serum FSH levels was found in men.[15] The same SNP was studied in 365 normally cycling women undergoing ART, the presence of T allele, i.e. showing lower promoter activity and FSH levels in men, was associated with higher FSH serum levels in the follicular phase and lower progesterone levels in the luteal phase.[16] However, in a recent study involving 193 women, FSH concentrations were significantly lower in carriers of T allele, when stratified by the FSHR genotype.[17] Thus, women carriers of the T allele did not show the age-related increase of serum FSH observed in GG homozygotes, confirming the importance of FSHB genotype when FSH levels are evaluated as a marker of ovarian reserve.[17]

To date, the *FSHR* gene is the most studied genetic factor in relation to COH. Despite some discordance,[18] there is sufficient evidence to state that genetic variations in FSHR have a role in COH outcome. In fact, the importance of mutations in the FSHR gene in ovarian response has been confirmed by various well-designed clinical studies.[19,20] Considering the 2010 SNPs discovered on FSHR, five are located in exon 10, at codons 307, 329, 524, 665 and 680. Only four of these cause an amino acid substitution.[5] Ala665Thr and Arg524Ser are not well-characterized with respect to frequency and ethnic distribution, while more information is available about the prevalence of Ala307Thr and Ser680Asn.[5] These have been correlated with an altered response to FSH.[21,22] The two codons codifying for the amino acids 307 and 680 are in linkage disequilibrium, i.e. during recombination they are linked to each other in a way that does not follow a casual pattern. This generates four allelic variants, which are found with a specific frequency in a given population. Therefore, if one SNP occurs at one site, the nucleotide at the second site is usually exchanged as well, resulting in the two most common allelic variants, Ala307/Ser680 and Thr307/Asn680, the latter representing about 55% of the alleles in the Caucasian population.[19] Each allelic variant can be found in homozygosity or in heterozygosity. Exon 10 encodes the intracellular and the transmembrane domains, and the C terminal end of the extracellular domain of the FSHR, therefore, it is involved in signal transduction, but it is not fundamental for ligand binding.[5] Residue 307 is located in the region that connects the hormone-binding domain to the transmembrane domain and that varies among three glycoprotein hormone receptors. Residue 680 is located in another region that is highly variable in these receptors, the C terminal region of the intracellular domain **(Fig. 2)**.[5]

There is no difference in the fertility potential in women carrying Ala307/Ser680 or Thr307/Asn680. The similar frequency of these two SNPs in the human species implies that both are compatible with normal fertility and no evolutionary advantage is clearly evident at this point of human evolution.[3] Anyway, these SNPs influence the dynamics of normal ovarian cycle, which is characterized by a discrete FSH "threshold"; serum concentrations of FSH have to be higher than a certain level to maintain follicle growth, otherwise follicles become atretic. Duration of FSH increase is more important than magnitude in determining how many follicles will

mature. FSH also promotes differentiation and growth of granulosa cells in tertiary follicles, induces the production of estradiol and aromatase, and the acquisition of LH receptors.[3] Greb et al. studied the dynamics of menstrual cycle in 29 eumenorrheic women carrying homozygous Ser680 or homozygous Asn680 genotype. LH levels were similar in two groups, while Ser680/Ser680 women showed higher FSH levels both in late luteal and in follicular phase. Luteal levels of estradiol, progesterone and inhibin A decreased earlier in the Ser680/Ser680 women and this was correlated to a longer length of the follicular phase, while dynamics of luteolysis were similar. These women show a significantly longer duration of the menstrual cycle (medium values of 29.3 days vs. 27.0 days). No significant differences in estradiol levels during follicular phase could be demonstrated suggesting that in Ser680/Ser680 women higher FSH levels are necessary to reach the same estradiol levels.[3] Estradiol production of granulosa cells depends on the availability of androgen substrate, which is LH-dependent and FSH stimulates the expression of LH receptors.[23] It is possible that FSHR in Ser680/Ser680 women could be less effective in inducing LH receptors or aromatase expression. However, more studies are necessary to verify this hypothesis. Follicular maturation was affected only before the selection of the dominant follicle, but its growth was similar, as soon as the dominant follicle was selected.[3]

Women with a homozygous genotype Ser680 require a higher dose of exogenous FSH to obtain the same estradiol levels of women who are homozygote Asn680 or heterozyogte.[20] These data are supported by another study demonstrating that the same FSH dose implies much lower estradiol levels in homozygote Ser680 women compared to homozygote Asn680 women.[24] On the other hand, no significant difference was found between the two groups regarding the number of follicles, retrieved oocytes, fertilization rate and embryo score. It is still unknown whether the SNP Ser680 might have an effect on pregnancy rate since data are discordant and do not provide sufficient strength to obtain conclusive results.[14] Regarding the FSHR 680Ser variant, it should be highlighted that the only clinical trial on this gene variant and COH outcome conducted so far confirmed the previous findings of an Asn680Ser SNP effect, indicating that lower FSH sensitivity of 680Ser homozygote carriers can be overcome by higher FSH doses.[24] Finally, a recent meta-analysis of different European studies, confirmed the role of the 680Ser variant in poor responses during COH treatment.[20]

The polymorphism G/A in position-29 of the FSHR gene can also modulate ovarian response to gonadotropin administration.[5] Recent in vitro studies showed that the A allele at position-29 is associated with a reduced transcriptional activity. Moreover, a study conducted on 50 women undergoing an IVF cycle demonstrated that women with AA genotype required higher doses of FSH, had lower estradiol levels the day before hCG administration, produced less follicles and showed a lower number of retrieved oocytes.[25] The poor ovarian response observed in patients with AA genotype in position-29 could depend on a reduced expression of the receptors on granulosa cells.[14] Nevertheless, further larger studies are necessary to confirm this finding.[14]

Estrogens are directly involved in follicle growth, maturation and oocyte release. Thus, estrogen receptor genes (ESR) are good candidates for evaluating SNPs in relation to COH response. Estradiol binds two intracellular receptors, receptor α (ERα) and receptor β (ERβ), encoded respectively by *ESR1* and *ESR2* genes. ESR1 is on chromosome 6, whereas ESR2 is on chromosome 14.[26] Georgiu et al. examined SNPs of ESR1 after using PvuII and BstUI restriction enzymes in 100 Greek women candidates for IVF. The authors found that Pp and PP genotypes of PvuII showed a higher follicle/oocyte number ratio, if compared to pp genotype; the PP genotype was also associated with a lower pregnancy rate, so they suggested that these different alleles might also affect embryo implantation during IVF-embyo transfer. However, PvuII and BstUI markers of ESR1 were related neither to the overall number of follicles nor to oocytes obtained during COH.[26]

Sundarrajan et al. examined Korean women and confirmed the findings regarding pregnancy rate, but found that PP carriers showed lower number of follicles and oocytes, smaller follicle size and lower number of embryos retrieved during COH, in addition to higher estrogen levels at the end of COH cycle. In this study, patients did not differ from fertile controls as for the frequency of PvuII SNP, suggesting that different alleles do not cause infertility, but could have an effect on the quality of follicles and oocytes.[27] None of these studies presented data about ovarian hyperstimulation syndrome (OHSS).

De Castro et al. found no correlation of ESR1 PvuII markers and poor or high response, estrogen levels, number of oocyte or follicles obtained during COH in Spanish women. Moreover, they found no association of ESR2 gene with poor or high response to gonadotropins.[28] The same group proposed that COH outcome could be influenced by the interaction of several genes, in a multifactorial model.[28] They found evidence of an interaction among FSHR, ESR1 and ESR2 in relation to COH outcome, in particular, the association between FSHR Ser680, ESR1 PvuII p and *39G ESR2 was linked to

a low response to COH, even in heterozygous women. An association with COH outcome of ESR1 and ESR2 or of CYP19 aromatase allelic form was not found so far.[28]

In another study, the same loci are analyzed in relation to pituitary suppression with triptorelin, a GnRH agonist, in 213 premenopausal women. This is a good model to study the regulation of estrogens production via CYP19 aromatase, because a part of treated women presents only partial estrogen suppression after GnRH agonist treatment.[28] They found out that the C allele of the rs10046 marker of the CYP19 aromatase locus is associated with poor pituitary suppression and a higher number of days to reach pituitary suppression, if compared with T allele carriers.[28]

In summary, the literature does not report univocal results about the role of ESR1 and ESR2 or of CYP19 aromatase allelic variants in determining response to COH. It is probable that response to COH is influenced by several clinical and genetic factors, acting together in a polygenic model. More studies are necessary to clarify the interaction between different SNPs of different genes.

Ovarian Hyperstimulation Syndrome

Ovarian hyperstimulation syndrome (OHSS) is an iatrogenic condition caused by stimulation with gonadotropins in IVF cycles. The basis of OHSS is mainly identified in an exaggerated ovarian response to gonadotropin administration, but other factors such as low BMI, young age, high estradiol or interleukins levels, renin-angiotensin system activation and vascular endothelial growth factor (VEGF) expression could be associated to OHSS.[29]

A relatively low degree of ovarian hyperstimulation is considered normal in women undergoing ovulation induction and mild OHSS occurs with an incidence between 3% and 6% of all stimulated cycles, even though it is not a condition with clinical relevance. Severe OHSS occurs in about 0.1–5% of all cycles and its clinical feature mainly consists of increased permeability of the ovarian capillary vessels resulting in transfer of fluids into the abdominal cavity.[29] An ovarian hypersensitivity to gonadotropins has been suggested but the clear association of OHSS with high hormone concentrations is not constant and was never demonstrated. A few studies addressed the association between OHSS and SNPs in FSHR or *LHCGR* genes since they are direct targets of gonadotropins, but no consistent correlation was found. Since some cross-interaction between FSHR and heterologous ligands of the pituitary glycoprotein hormone family at high concentrations has been suggested,[30] the pathogenesis of OHSS could indeed be associated to FSHR-mediated signals. In fact, some rare activating mutations of *FSHR* gene result in a predisposition to OHSS.[30] However, mutations in the FSHR are rare in OHSS and SNPs could rather be involved. In a recent review, SNPs on *FSHR* gene associated to OHSS are listed;[23] the Asn680 FSHR genotype has been associated with severity of iatrogenic OHSS in a study performed on 37 French patients undergoing IVF, while the Ser680 variant occurred significantly more often in women who develop iatrogenic OHSS. In another study, the FSHR SNP Ala307 was associated with risk of iatrogenic OHSS and with low amount of FSH required for ovarian stimulation among 50 Indian patients undergoing IVF. However, the number of patients investigated so far is too limited to draw any conclusion and a clear correlation between the FSHR SNPs and the risk of OHSS has not been demonstrated. Anyhow, in a limited number of studies, it clearly appears that the identification of the genetic profile of the FSHR prior to ovarian stimulation could permit a treatment that is safer for patients, reducing fearsome complications such as severe OHSS. The current scientific opinion supports the hypothesis that a combination of several other factors such as VEGF, the renin-angiotensin system and interleukins may have a strategic role in the pathogenesis of OHSS, but the exact mechanism remains unclear.[23]

CONCLUSION AND FUTURE PERSPECTIVES

Pharmacogenetics is rapidly changing our approach to drug therapy, allowing the individualized treatment of patients depending on their genetic background. During the last two decades, the scientific understanding about the role of SNPs in the modulation of reproductive functions and in a variety of pathological conditions has been improved. In silico technologies such as online SNPs databases or softwares for linkage disequilibrium block analysis gave a strong contribution to the development of accurate genome-wide association studies in cohorts of reproductive anomalies or cancer patients.

A genetic SNP may alter tissue and cellular response to glycoproteins hence being one of the most important regulators of hormonal activity at target level. Evidence indicates that SNPs in gonadotropins and their receptor are most probably not associated with modifications in ovarian reserve. Conversely, SNPs of the FSHR seem to alter the response of recruitable follicles to FSH. To date, the common SNP Asn680Ser mostly in linkage disequilibrium with Ala307Thr is a well-established determinant of response to FSH in IVF program. In women, in vivo results suggest that Ser680 genotypes is a factor of major "resistance" to FSH stimulation resulting in a higher FSH serum levels, thus leading to prolonged duration of the menstrual cycle, although its role in vitro remains to be determined.

Until present only the Asn680Ser polymorphism of the FSHR gene shows a strong association with ovarian function and this suggests that the polymorphisms in exon 10 could be used as a marker to predict ovarian response to exogenous FSH in women with normal ovarian function.[14]

This aspect needs to be considered in patients undergoing COH because some women could be at risk of ovarian hyperstimulation due to an excessive stimulation by FSH. For other SNPs described until present such as -29G/A FSHR, -211G/T of FSHB subunit and SNPs regarding LH or estrogens and their receptors, further studies are necessary before a clear definition of their clinical role can be established.

Including genetic markers in an extended algorithm to choose the gonadotropin dose might improve ovarian stimulation success and reduce side effects. However, such approach requires clinical validation and well-controlled multicenter, longitudinal studies should be performed to acquire the necessary evidence. Since genetic testing is a relatively simple and inexpensive procedure, its usefulness to optimize ovarian stimulation should be carefully assessed (**Box 1**).

Box 1 Genetic testing to optimize ovarian stimulation

- Genetic variations in FSHR have a role in controlled ovarian hyperstimulation outcome: the common polymorphism Asn680Ser, mostly in linkage disequilibrium with Ala307Thr, is the only well established determinant of response;
- Ser680 genotype is a factor of "resistance" to FSH stimulation resulting in a higher FSH serum levels;
- In IVF programs, women with a homozygous genotype Ser680 require a higher dose of exogenous FSH to obtain the same estradiol levels;
- The genetic profile of FSHR prior to ovarian stimulation could permit a safer treatment, reducing risk of OHSS.

■ REFERENCES

1. Fauser BC, Diedrich K, Devroey P, et al. Predictors of ovarian response: progress towards individualized treatment in ovulation induction and ovarian stimulation. Hum Reprod Update. 2008;14:1-14.
2. de Castro F, Morón FJ, Montoro L, et al. Pharmacogenetics of controlled ovarian hyperstimulation. Pharmacogenomics. 2005;6:629-37.
3. Greb RR, Behre HM, Simoni M. Pharmacogenetics in ovarian stimulation—current concepts and future options. Reprod Biomed Online. 2005;11:589-600.
4. Olivennes F, Howles CM, Borini A, et al. Individualizing FSH dose for assisted reproduction using a novel algorithm: the CONSORT study. Reprod Biomed Online. 2009;18:195-204.
5. Gromoll J, Simoni M. Genetic complexity of FSH receptor function. Trends Endocrinol Metab. 2005;16:368-73.
6. Henke A, Gromoll J. New insights into the evolution of chorionic gonadotrophin. Mol Cell Endocrinol. 2008;291:11-9.
7. Nagirnaja L, Rull K, Uusküla L, et al. Genomics and genetics of gonadotropin beta-subunit genes: Unique FSHB and duplicated LHB/CGB loci. Mol Cell Endocrinol. 2010;329: 4-16.
8. Ascoli M, Fanelli F, Segaloff DL. The lutropin/choriogonadotropin receptor, a 2002 perspective. Endocr Rev. 2002;23(2): 141-74.
9. Simoni M, Gromoll J, Nieschlag E. The follicle-stimulating hormone receptor: biochemistry, molecular biology, physiology, and pathophysiology. Endocr Rev. 1997;18:739-73.
10. Atger M, Misrahi M, Sar S, et al. Structure of the human luteinizing hormone-choriogonadotropin receptor gene: unusual promoter and 5′ non-coding regions. Mol Cell Endocrinol. 1995;111:113-23.
11. Nilsson C, Jiang M, Pettersson K, et al. Determination of a common genetic variant of luteinizing hormone using DNA hybridization and immunoassays. Clin Endocrinol (Oxf). 1998;49:369-76.
12. Manna PR, Joshi L, Reinhold VN, et al. Synthesis, purification and structural and functional characterization of recombinant form of a common genetic variant of human luteinizing hormone. Hum Mol Genet. 2002;11:301-15.
13. Alviggi C, Pettersson K, Longobardi S, et al. A common polymorphic allele of the LH beta-subunit gene is associated with higher exogenous FSH consumption during controlled ovarian stimulation for assisted reproductive technology. Reprod Biol Endocrinol. 2013;11:51.
14. La Marca A, Papaleo E, Alviggi C, et al. The combination of genetic variants of the FSHB and FSHR genes affects serum FSH in women of reproductive age. Hum Reprod. 2013;28:1369-74.
15. Grigorova M, Punab M, Ausmees K, et al. FSHB promoter polymorphism within evolutionary conserved element is associated with serum FSH level in men. Hum Reprod. 2008;23:2160-6.
16. Schüring AN, Busch AS, Bogdanova N, et al. Effects of the FSH-β-subunit promoter polymorphism -211G->T on the hypothalamic-pituitary-ovarian axis in normally cycling women indicate a gender-specific regulation of gonadotropin secretion. J Clin Endocrinol Metab. 2013;98:E82-6.
17. La Marca A, Sighinolfi G, Argento C, et al. Polymorphisms in gonadotropin and gonadotropin receptor genes as markers of ovarian reserve and response in in vitro fertilization. Fertil Steril. 2013;99:970-8.
18. Genro VK, Matte U, De Conto E, et al. Frequent polymorphisms of FSH receptor do not influence antral follicle responsiveness to follicle-stimulating hormone administration as assessed by the Follicular Output RaTe (FORT). J Assist Reprod Genet. 2012;29:657-63.
19. Simoni M, Nieschlag E, Gromoll J. Isoforms and single nucleotide polymorphisms of the FSH receptor gene: implications for human reproduction. Hum Reprod Update. 2002;8:413-21.
20. Moròn FJ, Ruiz A. Pharmacogenetics of controlled ovarian hyperstimulation: time to corroborate the clinical utility of FSH receptor genetic markers. Pharmacogenomics. 2010;11: 1613-8.
21. Sudo S, Kudo M, Wada S, et al. Genetic and functional analyses of polymorphisms in the human FSH receptor gene. Mol Hum Reprod. 2002;8:893-9.
22. Achrekar SK, Modi DN, Desai SK, et al. Follicle-stimulating hormone receptor polymorphism Thr307Ala is associated with variable ovarian response and ovarian hyperstimulation syndrome in Indian women. Fertil Steril. 2009;91:432-9.
23. Casarini L, Pignatti E, Simoni M. Effects of polymorphisms in gonadotropin and gonadotropin receptor genes on reproductive function. Rev Endocr Metab Disord. 2011;12: 303-21.
24. Behre HM, Greb RR, Mempel A, et al. Significance of a common single nucleotide polymorphism in exon 10 of the follicle-stimulating hormone (FSH) receptor gene for the ovarian response to FSH: a pharmacogenetic approach to controlled ovarian hyperstimulation. Pharmacogenet Genomics. 2005;15:451-6.
25. Achrekar SK, Modi DN, Desai SK, et al. Poor ovarian response to gonadotrophin stimulation is associated with FSH receptor polymorphism. Reprod Biomed Online. 2009;18:509-15.
26. Georgiou I, Konstantelli M, Syrrou M, et al. Oestrogen receptor gene polymorphisms and ovarian stimulation for in-vitro fertilization. Hum Reprod. 1997;12:1430-3.
27. Sundarrajan C, Liao W, Roy AC, et al. Association of oestrogen receptor gene polymorphisms with outcome of ovarian stimulation in patients undergoing IVF. Mol Hum Reprod. 1999;5:797-802.
28. de Castro F, Morón FJ, Montoro L, et al. Human controlled ovarian hyperstimulation outcome is a polygenic trait. Pharmacogenetics. 2004;14:285-93.
29. Nastri CO, Ferriani RA, Rocha IA, et al. Ovarian hyperstimulation syndrome: pathophysiology and prevention. J Assist Reprod Genet. 2010;27:121-8.
30. Dieterich M, Bolz M, Reimer T, et al. Two different entities of spontaneous ovarian hyperstimulation in a woman with FSH receptor mutation. Reprod Biomed Online. 2010;20:751-8.

12

Physiology of Follicular Phase

Ubaldi F, Cimadomo D, Capalbo A, Rienzi L

■ INTRODUCTION

The ovary is a structure shaped like an almond, covered by a capsule known as tunica albuginea made of thick connective tissue. A mesothelium, called germinal epithelium, surrounds and covers it. Ovarian follicles are found in the cortex and the so-called helicine arteries constitute a highly vascular medulla. The follicles, made up of differentiated epithelial cells, surround the germ cells. A constant bidirectional communication between the germinal and the somatic compartments of this unique structure throughout folliculogenesis is pivotal for the oocyte to reach maturity and acquire developmental competence. In the ovary, particularly around the edges of the cortex, many primordial follicles are visible. Fewer follicles (namely those recruited for maturation) at subsequent stages of development can also be found within the ovary from menarche to menopause. Strikingly, the number of female germ cells sharply decreases from 6 million in the developing fetus, to 300,000 primordial follicles at birth, among which no more than 500 will be selected to become a mature oocyte. These numbers subtend the strict selection of follicles that the ovary elicits throughout life until depletion of the ovarian reserve. Folliculogenesis at all its stages hereafter described, is a highly regulated process, essential to sustain oocyte growth and maturation toward and beyond ovulation.

■ THE SAGA OF PRIMORDIAL GERM CELLS

Primordial germ cells (PGCs) are the first cells of the future ovary, the predecessors of the oocytes, whose process of formation includes several stages. PGCs develop under the influence of signals, such as bone morphogenetic proteins (BMPs), during gastrulation[1] (when the embryo differentiates into the three layers: ectoderm, mesoderm and endoderm) and become recognizable in the posterior rim of the embryonic disk. From here, they move in the yolk sac and in the region of the allantois, then, through an ameboid movement, via the connective tissue of the hindgut, they reach the genital ridge. In this phase, the expression of a gene called *Stella* allows retention of pluripotency and escape from a somatic fate.[2] During this journey, the cells multiply rapidly, and those cells which end up in inappropriate locations, die, while the survivors reach the primitive gonad and cluster together in the so-called germ cell cysts (or nests). Once PGCs reach the primitive gonad, a first phase of genetic reprograming will take place. In particular, a general demethylation will occur, by the end of which only 7% of the whole genome would be methylated (which is a significantly low percentage if compared to the 70–80% of embryonic stem cells and somatic ones). Within the germ cell cysts, PGCs continue to divide by mitosis and differentiate into oogonia. Noticeably, in their absence, the gonad degenerates into cord-like structures, suggesting the pivotal role of oogonia in its organogenesis.[3] Oogonia proliferate, meanwhile also mesenchymal cells in the early ovaries will grow in number and surround them, giving origin to the primordial follicles. Within them the oocytes are enclosed in a layer of flattened squamous follicular cells. The formation of primordial follicles stands for the beginning of the long process of folliculogenesis.

Hormonal Regulation of Folliculogenesis During the Menstrual Cycle

Once a woman reaches sexual maturity at puberty and until menopause, cyclically-produced hormones will accurately control folliculogenesis and the events subsequent to ovulation. The main players are the follicle stimulating hormone (FSH) and the luteinizing hormone (LH), both produced by the pituitary gland. The former triggers follicle development in the very first phase of the menstrual cycle. Follicular growth results in rising of estrogen levels, due to their production by follicular cells themselves. This increasing level of estrogen, in a negative feedback fashion, is responsible for suppression of a further secretion of FSH from the pituitary gland. At the same time, also inhibin, a second hormone produced from the follicle, will be released to further lower FSH levels. Estrogen rising level is also responsible for LH mid-cycle surge. This event causes the rupture of the follicle at its last stage of development (Graafian follicle) and, consequently, ovulation. LH is also involved in luteinization of the ruptured follicle to form the corpus luteum, a transitory endocrine organ. Corpus luteum secretes progesterone and estrogen. The former exerts a negative feedback on the pituitary gland inhibiting a further release of LH. If fertilization would not occur, corpus luteum will degenerate in the so-called corpus albicans and progesterone levels will fall, resulting in menstruation. Estrogen levels will also precipitate, thus triggering a new wave of FSH production. New follicles will be recruited to mature and a new cycle will begin.

Primordial Follicle

Primordial germ cells migrate into the developing gonad early in embryogenesis, and differentiate into oogonia. These oogonia proliferate by mitosis. Some of these enlarge and develop into larger cells called primary oocytes and enter meiosis. This happens between 3 months and 8 months of gestation. In all mammals, peak numbers of germ cells are observed around the time of the mitotic to meiotic transition. In vivo results suggest that the rapid proliferation of oogonia may be associated with germ cells loss. From their peak number, around 6 million by the 20th week of gestation, the number of germ cells sharply decreases with two main periods of high germ cell loss—the pachytene stage of meiosis in oocytes and the formation of the primordial follicles. As a consequence, the number of germ cells enclosed in primordial follicles at birth surprisingly decreases at 90% in women; this process is called "attrition".[4] Formation of primordial follicles subtends the ability of oocytes to detach from the nests and associate with a layer of ovarian epithelial cells, known as granulosa cells. They are small, normally found close to the outer edge of the cortex and contained in a poorly vascularized layer under the tunica albuginea. Interestingly, primordial follicles appear to provide protection from atresia and a women's reproductive lifespan is determined by their number in the ovary.[5] During the primordial-primary oocyte transition, the shape of the follicle changes from a layer of flat to cuboid granulosa cells. Soon after, the oocyte will arrest the machinery for meiotic division, remaining suspended in prophase I until sexual maturity, while growing in size. In particular, the combined effect of several biochemical processes maintains low levels of CDK1 activity, so that

resumption of meiosis cannot take place.[6] Noteworthy, the initial recruitment of quiescent primordial follicles into the growing pool starts in fetal life, but it is continuously carried out postnatally until depletion of the ovarian reserve (to almost 1,000 primordial follicles) at the time of menopause; on an average, by that time, just 1% (around 300–500) of the initial peak number of germ cells would have escaped atresia and reached the ovulatory state.[7]

The TGF-β Protein Family

The follicle must be considered as a unique structure. The oocyte undertakes an active role in its own growth regulation, but there is an essential interdependence of the gamete and granulosa cells on paracrine communication, ultimately aimed to follicle growth. TGF-β superfamily enrolls several secreted growth factors involved in this intercommunication. In particular, these proteins mediate primordial follicle formation and transition through different stages of folliculogenesis, as well as a variety of processes during embryonic development, from differentiation to apoptosis. Mainly, they cover upstream roles in either paracrine or autocrine signaling cascades. Growth differentiation factors (GDFs) and BMPs are the most important components of this family. In particular, GDF9 and BMP15 are two oocyte-secreted factors playing pivotal roles in the intercommunication between the oocyte itself and the somatic counterparts of the follicle. Their absence determines increased follicle atresia and subfertility.[8] Another important subgroup within TGF-β protein family are activins. These molecules are part of a signaling pathway interconnecting the pituitary gland to the ovary via the FSH production. Activins determine FSH receptor's expression in granulosa cells and consequently, synergize with FSH in the regulation of granulosa cell's proliferation and differentiation. Their function is counteracted by inhibin, the antagonistic endocrine regulator produced by granulosa cells. Anti-Müllerian hormone (AMH) is a further component of this family of proteins to be expressed by granulosa cells.[9] AMH is a suppressor of initial follicle growth currently used as a marker of female fertility, in particular of the quality of ovarian follicle pool, since its levels decline in adult women as the follicle reserve becomes depleted.

Primary Follicle

During the prolonged prophase of meiosis I, while nuclear maturation is arrested at the diplotene stage, the primary oocytes synthesize a glycoprotein coat, cortical granules and accumulate ribosomes, glycogen, lipids, and mRNA that will later direct the synthesis of proteins required for early embryonic development. As the oocyte faces this process of maturation, which does not occur until sexual maturity, the follicle around it changes its conformation. Granulosa cells, which are surrounded by the basement membrane, change their structure from flat to cuboidal. Under the mediation of the transcription factor FIGLα, the glycoproteins zona pellucida (ZP)1, ZP2 and ZP3 are recruited to the deposition and assembly of the zona pellucida, an extracellular matrix polymer. Despite the creation of this barrier, not only the fundamental contact between granulosa cells and the oocyte is maintained, but it becomes even more apparent. In the meanwhile, stromal cells would be recruited to the formation of a further layer outside the basement membrane, named theca (the Greek word for "box"). Theca cells together with granulosa cells constitute the two somatic components of the follicle. These kinds of cells, besides providing structural support to the follicle, play some exclusive roles in follicle growth within the ovary; they, once acquired LH responsiveness, are the main producers of steroidogenic precursors for estrogen synthesis in granulosa cells. Furthermore, androstenedione, which is LH-dependent, is derived from theca cells and acts in granulosa cells to cytodifferentiate the response to FSH. Each follicle wave is preceded by a rise in serum FSH concentration and FSH-sensitive follicles respond to this increase by forming a cohort of growing follicles. When the oocyte is recruited to leave the resting pool and acquire the ability to resume meiosis, granulosa cells proliferate creating a double layer that marks the passage to a secondary follicle. Noteworthy, only one of the maturing follicles completes the maturation process each month, while the rest degenerate into atretic follicles. The whole process takes about 3 months.

Secondary Follicle

The primary follicle will develop into a secondary follicle. A transition regulated by the oocyte-specific transcription factor NOBOX. A secondary follicle is very similar to a primary one, except that it is larger, surrounded by more follicular cells and characterized by small accumulations of fluid in the intracellular spaces, called follicular fluid (a nutritive fluid for the oocyte). In particular, granulosa cells keep proliferating to form 3–6 layers, while the oocyte nears its maximum dimensions. In the meanwhile, cavities filled with follicular fluid, probably derived from blood flowing through thecal capillaries, start to form. It has been proposed that these cavities could be formed by cell death (as for the blastocysts, where programed cell death of inner ectodermal cells creates a cavity),

since the occasional presence of dead granulosa cells in healthy follicles. These foci, then, slowly coalesce to a unique follicle antrum. The rate of follicular antrum expansion and fluid accumulation varies among different follicles, particularly among the so-called dominant and subordinate ones.[10] This transition from a pre-antral to an antral follicle is concomitant with the morphological and functional distinction between two subsets of granulosa cells—mural granulosa cells, lining the follicle wall and mainly responsible of steroidogenesis, and cumulus cells, in intimate association with the oocyte. Cumulus cells possess highly specialized transzonal cytoplasmic projections which penetrate through the ZP and form gap junctions at their tips with the oocyte, forming an elaborate structure called the cumulus oocyte complex (COC).[11] In fact, there is a deep bidirectional communication between the oocyte and the cumulus cells, which are essential for oocyte viability and developmental competence, particularly since the metabolic support they provide. Intercellular channels consist of connexons, hexameric structures whose monomers are proteins named connexins; each cell provide one connexon that then docks end-to-end to the others provided from the cells surrounding it.[12] Different gap junctions are built on different connexins composition resulting in a variable permeability, strictly dependent on size, molecular charge of the molecule to be imported and intracellular environment (pH, cations concentration, protein kinases activity). Mainly, granulosa cells use gap junctions to provide the oocyte with amino acids, glucose and ribonucleosides. In fact, in this phase, the accumulation of mRNAs, ribosomes and polypeptides by the oocyte is crucial to later development. Furthermore, signals for oocyte meiotic maturation travel via gap junctional communication. All these evidences together convey the importance of this bidirectional communication in maintaining the oocyte in the appropriate differentiated state. However, there is no clear evidence of a link between mutations in connexin-encoding genes and infertility, it seems that the strength of coupling cumulus-granulosa cells correlates with IVF success rates.[13] Importantly, also the surrounding theca differentiates into two distinct layers, the theca interna (rounded cells that secrete androgens and follicular fluid) and a more fibrous theca externa.

In the absence of an LH surge, the dominant follicle starts to regress and triggers the recruitment of a new wave of growing follicles. On the contrary, if this stimulus occurs, it marks the end of folliculogenesis and triggers a cascade of signals that lead to final maturation, meiotic resumption and finally ovulation of the oocyte.

Graafian Follicle

Final maturation is characterized by chromosomes condensation and nucleus disassembly (germinal vesicle breakdown). At the time of ovulation, the first meiotic division is completed and the first polar body is expelled, but the oocyte is arrested again at metaphase II (MII) stage. Meiosis will be resumed only with fertilization. It is important to underline that interruption of the physical link between oocyte and follicle cells itself has been shown to trigger meiosis resumption.[14] The mature COC contains a secondary oocyte, arrested at MII after extrusion of the first polar body, and the tightly linked cumulus cells. In order for ovulation to occur properly, cumulus expansion should take place. In particular, actin assembles in microfilaments causing a massive remodeling of the cytoskeleton, and hyaluronic acid is secreted determining mucification of the cumulus cells and ultimately disconnecting the transzonal projections. The signals triggering these periovulatory events are mainly gonadotropins or epidermal growth factors-like peptides. Cumulus cells in ovulating COC start synthesizing prostaglandins thanks to COX2 enzymatic activity. In fact, this enzyme has been proposed as part of a molecular clock setting the proper species-specific timing for ovulation. Instead, hyaluronic acid, a pivotal component of the extracellular matrix, is produced using glucose as substrate (which is the reason for an increase in both glucose uptake and glycolytic activity in this phase).[15] Interestingly, the absence of cumulus matrix components is causative of reduced fertility or sterility.[16]

At this stage of folliculogenesis, the oocyte has completed its maturation inside the follicle environment, and is ready to be expelled from the ovary through ovulation. It is noteworthy that mature oocytes are transcriptionally silent and will keep this inactivity until zygote genome activation occurring at day 3 postfertilization.[17] Silencing, in particular, is due to mechanisms such as histone deacetylation[18] and chromatin structure condensation.[19] Oocyte transcriptional inactivity is another solid evidence of its dependence from the surrounding metabolically-active and transcriptionally-active somatic cells.

Ovulation

The LH surge determines a massive increase in cyclic adenosine monophosphate (cAMP) levels in cumulus cells, while these decrease in the oocyte, thus eliciting resumption of meiosis. At the same time, gap junctions will undergo phosphorylation and, together with COC expansion, will cause disruption of the intercommunication within the complex. In the meanwhile, proteases degrade the basement membrane and cause thinning of the follicular apex by disrupting extracellular membrane layers. Theca cells and immune cells enter the antral space, while granulosa cells differentiate into luteal cells. Also, angiogenesis takes place. Ultimately, ovulation occurs due to vascular changes, increasing pressure inside the follicle and digestion of the follicle walls. The oocyte, still surrounded by a group of loosely-linked mucified cumulus cells, known as corona radiata, is expelled in the ampulla of the oviduct. Importantly, cumulus matrix is critical for both oocyte capture and oviductal transport. In fact, oocyte capture depends on adhesion between the infundibular epithelium and COC matrix, while oviductal transport seems to be improved in the presence of cumulus cells with respect to denuded oocytes. Noticeably, impairment of these processes is related to ectopic pregnancies and/or infertility.[20] Once ovulation has occurred, the oocyte can be fertilized. If fertilization would not occur within a defined window of time, aging processes would begin, thus determining impairment of oocyte developmental competence. In particular, these processes include mithocondrial dysfunctions and cytoskeletal abnormalities leading to membrane and cortical changes. After ovulation has occurred, granulosa cells left within the ovary start to accumulate lipids, proteins and pigments, thus generating a structure known as corpus luteum.

Corpus Luteum

The corpus luteum is a temporary endocrine gland that is maintained due to LH, prolactin and estradiol. After ovulation, the ruptured follicle collapses into a blood clot (corpus hemorrhagicum) which then forms the corpus luteum. The granulosa cells enlarge, and become vesicular, folded, and are then called granulosa lutein cells. These cells begin to secrete mainly progesterone. The spaces between the folds are filled with theca interna cells, which also enlarge, become glandular, and are known as theca lutein cells. They are responsible for the secretion of both estrogen, which inhibits FSH, and relaxin, which relaxes the fibrocartilage of the pubic symphysis. If pregnancy does not occur, then the corpus luteum degenerates into the corpus albicans, and levels of estrogen and progesterone fall, allowing release of FSH and LH. On the contrary, if pregnancy does occur, the syncytiotrophoblasts of the placenta releases human chorionic gonadotropin (hCG) that would prevent both FSH and LH production from the hypothalamus-pituitary axis, and the corpus luteum persists.

Corpus Albicans

In case fertilization would not occur, the corpus luteum would collapse forming a pale structure known as corpus albicans. The cellular elements degenerate and are phagocytosed. Fibrous tissue is left behind. The structure will then shrink and eventually form a small visible scar on the side of the ovary.

■ CONCLUSION

The follicle is an ideal form of intercommunication and interdependence between somatic cells and the oocyte. This plastic structure, formed at the very beginning of the process would drive the female gamete toward ovulation and beyond, providing structural support, protection, metabolites and contemporarily evolving with it throughout all the phases of oocyte maturation. All the molecular processes and the cascades of events occurring within the different compartments of the follicle itself are aimed at the acquisition and maintenance of oocyte developmental competence. The establishment of pregnancy could be achieved only via a sublime coordination of endocrine, paracrine, immune and metabolic stimuli. Any impairment of the process of folliculogenesis is a detrimental event that could irreversibly affect oocyte developmental competence.

■ FUTURE PERSPECTIVES

In the last decade, the dogma of a fixed and finite number of fertilization-competent oocytes in the ovarian reserve has been challenged by few astonishing papers claiming the existence within the ovary of the so-called oogonial stem cells (OSCs), generating oocytes, as it happens in the male reproductive system where spermatogonial stem cells support sperm production in adult testes.[21] In particular, a study published in 2009 claims the feasibility of isolation, in vitro culture and transplantation of OSCs in mice leading in vivo to the production of ovulated eggs that after fertilization would result in viable offspring.[22] If such a breakthrough would be certified as effective and in particular applicable also to humans, it will definitely revolutionize our current perception of the ovary and bring about a great improvement in assisted reproductive technology (ART). This is especially relevant for patients undergoing cryopreservation of ovarian cortical tissue.

Currently, ovarian cortical tissue cryopreservation is an important possibility for women affected by malignant cancers to preserve their fertility. It is proposed for those women who will undergo antitumoral therapies compromising the ovarian reserve or the menstrual cycle hormonal regulation. The patients will undergo laparoscopy, the ovarian tissue will be fragmented and all the different fragments will be then cryopreserved. After thawing, the patient could eventually undergo an orthotopic autotransplantation of the tissue. A second fascinating possibility after thawing is the so-called in vitro maturation (IVM). This technique is based on the isolation of primordial follicles from the cryopreserved ovarian tissue and their maturation at specific environmental conditions and in appropriate culture media. The mature oocytes thus obtained will then be used in conventional ART. Unfortunately, this technique is still experimental and needs a strict standardization in order to be approached clinically. Currently, IVM has been employed mainly in animal models in order to investigate the physiology of folliculogenesis. Many molecules involved in its regulation have been identified, while others are still unknown. In future, the identification of molecules, such as transcription factors, directly involved in the regulation of folliculogenesis and potentially in oocyte developmental competence, could provide us with methods, other than conventional hormonal stimulation, to trigger oocyte growth and ovulation.

All the techniques described here represent promising improvements in the scenario of ART that may introduce new technical, clinical and ethical issues in the next years, and should be deeply studied and considered.

■ REFERENCES

1. Lee WS, Yoon SJ, Yoon TK, et al. Effects of bone morphogenetic protein-7 (BMP-7) on primordial follicular growth in the mouse ovary. Mol Reprod Dev. 2004;69(2):159-63.
2. Lange UC, Saitou M, Western PS, et al. The fragilis interferon-inducible gene family of transmembrane proteins is associated with germ cell specification in mice. BMC Dev Biol. 2003;3:1.
3. Merchant-Larios H, Centeno B. Morphogenesis of the ovary from the sterile W/Wv mouse. Prog Clin Biol Res. 1981;59B: 383-92.
4. Reynaud K, Driancourt MA. Oocyte attrition. Mol Cell Endocrinol. 2000;163(1-2):101-8.
5. Abir R, Orvieto R, Dicker D, et al. Preliminary studies on apoptosis in human fetal ovaries. Fertil Steril. 2002;78(2): 259-64.
6. Solc P, Schultz RM, Motlik J. Prophase I arrest and progression to metaphase I in mouse oocytes: comparison of resumption of meiosis and recovery from G2-arrest in somatic cells. Mol Hum Reprod. 2010;16(9):654-64.
7. Oktem O, Oktay K. The ovary: anatomy and function throughout human life. Ann N Y Acad Sci. 2008;1127:1-9.
8. Galloway SM, McNatty KP, Cambridge LM, et al. Mutations in an oocyte-derived growth factor gene (BMP15) cause increased ovulation rate and infertility in a dosage-sensitive manner. Nat Genet. 2000;25(3):279-83.
9. Visser JA, Themmen AP. Anti-Müllerian hormone and folliculogenesis. Mol Cell Endocrinol. 2005;234(1-2):81-6.

10. Rodgers RJ, Irving-Rodgers HF. Formation of the ovarian follicular antrum and follicular fluid. Biol Reprod. 2010;82(6):1021-9.
11. Albertini DF, Combelles CM, Benecchi E, et al. Cellular basis for paracrine regulation of ovarian follicle development. Reproduction. 2001;121(5):647-53.
12. Kidder GM, Vanderhyden BC. Bidirectional communication between oocytes and follicle cells: ensuring oocyte developmental competence. Can J Physiol Pharmacol. 2010;88(4): 399-413.
13. Wang HX, Tong D, El-Gehani F, et al. Connexin expression and gap junctional coupling in human cumulus cells: contribution to embryo quality. J Cell Mol Med. 2009;13(5):972-84.
14. Pincus G, Enzmann EV. The comparative behavior of mammalian eggs in vivo and in vitro: I. the activation of ovarian eggs. J Exp Med. 1935;62(5):665-75.
15. Russell DL, Salustri A. Extracellular matrix of the cumulus-oocyte complex. Semin Reprod Med. 2006;24(4):217-27.
16. Irving-Rodgers HF, Rodgers RJ. Extracellular matrix in ovarian follicular development and disease. Cell Tissue Res. 2005;322(1):89-98.
17. Dobson AT, Raja R, Abeyta MJ, et al. The unique transcriptome through day 3 of human preimplantation development. Hum Mol Genet. 2004;13(14):1461-70.
18. Borsuk E, Milik E. Fully grown mouse oocyte contains transcription inhibiting activity which acts through histone deacetylation. Mol Reprod Dev. 2005;71(4):509-15.
19. De La Fuente R, Viveiros MM, Burns KH, et al. Major chromatin remodeling in the germinal vesicle (GV) of mammalian oocytes is dispensable for global transcriptional silencing but required for centromeric heterochromatin function. Dev Biol. 2004;275(2):447-58.
20. Russell DL, Robker RL. Molecular mechanisms of ovulation: co-ordination through the cumulus complex. Hum Reprod Update. 2007;13(3):289-312.
21. Johnson J, Canning J, Kaneko T, et al. Germline stem cells and follicular renewal in the postnatal mammalian ovary. Nature. 2004;428(6979):145-50.
22. Zou K, Yuan Z, Yang Z, et al. Production of offspring from a germline stem cell line derived from neonatal ovaries. Nat Cell Biol. 2009;11(5):631-6.

13

Progesterone in Follicular Phase during Controlled Ovarian Stimulation

Sunita R Tandulwadkar, Sejal Naik

INTRODUCTION

Controlled ovarian stimulation for in vitro fertilization-embryo transfer (IVF-ET) induces dramatic changes in the hormonal profile of the menstrual cycle. Stimulated IVF cycles are different from natural cycles in supraphysiological estrogen levels in follicular phase and rapid change in estrogen and progesterone levels following egg retrieval.

However, premature LH surges, caused by the modulatory actions of 5–10 times higher levels of estradiol induced by gonadotropins, have led to premature luteinization, premature rise in progesterone level in late follicular phase.

Before the introduction of GnRH analogs in ART cycles, detection of premature endogenous LH surges was a constant concern because it occurred when follicular development was still uncompleted and had some deleterious effects on oocyte quality and on the implantation rate. Detection of plasma progesterone was considered to detect partial luteinization of granulosa cells. The current use of GnRH analogs (agonist and antagonist) by suppressing the release of endogenous gonadotropins from pituitary has decreased the incidence of premature LH surge.[1]

Despite the use of GnRH analogs, subtle increases in serum progesterone levels beyond an arbitrarily defined threshold value have been observed at the end of the follicular phase in COS cycles for IVF. Although, the frequency of elevated serum progesterone levels varies, incidence is as high as 35% (5–35%) of stimulated cycles in individuals treated with GnRH agonist and 38% of with GnRH antagonist.[2-5]

This 'premature luteinization' term used to describe increased levels of serum progesterone is misleading as it is occurring in presence of GnRH analogs (under low serum LH concentration).[6] This is different to luteinisation, the process by which the ovarian follicle transforms into a corpus luteum through vascularization, follicular cell hypertrophy, and lipid accumulation. There are many factors regulating the luteinization, granulosa cells exiting from the cell cycle, and it is controlled by intracellular signaling pathways, cell adhesion factors, intracellular cholesterol and oxysterols, and perhaps progesterone itself as a paracrine or intracrine regulator.[7]

There has been debate regarding the origins, clinical significance and the "cut-off"/threshold level of elevated progesterone concentrations seen in plasma during the late follicular phase of cycles of ovarian stimulation.

IMPACT OF PROGESTERONE ON PREGNANCY

Several studies suggest that there is no association between progesterone levels and pregnancy.[2,3,8-10] The meta-analysis,[11] found no relationship and dismissed the importance of raised follicular-phase progesterone concentration (RFPPC) on pregnancy outcomes. Several large programs have provided strong evidence that RFPPC is associated with impaired expected pregnancy rates.[5,12-17]

However, the results are conflicting because of the different GnRH analogs administered and the different "cut-off" levels that were used to define "high" progesterone serum levels. The majority of studies that failed to demonstrate an association between serum progesterone levels and pregnancy rate used a threshold value of 0.9 ng/mL, which was mostly chosen arbitrarily. Bosch E et al., in 2010, demonstrated significantly better ongoing pregnancy rates with lower progesterone level on the day of human chorionic gonadotropin (hCG) administration compared with those having higher levels. They also showed that this difference in ongoing pregnancy rates and number of oocytes retrieved was significant at the threshold value of 1.5 ng/mL of progesterone.[18]

IMPACT OF PROGESTERONE ON OOCYTES AND ENDOMETRIUM

The mechanism by which these subtle increases in serum progesterone may impact on pregnancy rates is unclear, with data suggesting that it may impair endometrial receptivity rather than oocyte quality.[17,19]

Many authors[20,21] had studied the effect of high progesterone on oocytes donors and oocytes recipients programs, and they did not find any detrimental effect on oocyte performance with raised progesterone value in terms of number oocytes obtained, fertilization rate, cleavage rate, blastocyst formation, number of embryos cryopreserved, implantation rate, pregnancy rate or miscarriage rate. This study suggests that the negative impact of high progesterone level in late follicular phase of IVF cycles may be due to a detrimental effect on endometrial receptivity, rather than on the oocyte-embryo factor.

A progesterone rise during the late follicular phase has been considered a negative predictive factor for clinical outcome in both GnRH agonist[3,22,23] and GnRH antagonist protocols.[5,24] Whatever the underlying mechanism for early rise in serum progesterone levels, it induces both advanced endometrial histological maturation[25] and differential endometrial gene expression.[26,27] This results in a change in the normal synchrony between the endometrium and oocyte/embryo.[28] When excessively disturbed, this asynchrony may reduce embryo implantation and pregnancy rates.

PATHOGENESIS

In spite the pathogenesis of progesterone elevation in COS is still poorly understood, several hypotheses have been suggested to explain it.

Elevation of Follicular LH Levels

Some authors related the elevated endogenous LH with that of progesterone level in follicular phase.[29] The pituitary desensitization induced by GnRH is incomplete; therefore, supraphysiological estradiol level causes LH secretion which could be sufficient to stimulate granulosa cells to produce progesterone although inadequate to trigger ovulation.[30]

Accumulation of hCG from hMG

It been suggested that serum accumulation of hCG arising from human menopausal gonadotropin (hMG) could be responsible for elevated progesterone level. Therefore, the use of rFSH instead of hMG has been regarded as beneficial. Contrarily, according to this hypothesis, the use of rFSH or human urinary FSH in which LH activity is negligible or practically absent should not provoke an increase on progesterone level.[31]

Increased LH Receptor Sensitivity of the Granulosa Cells to FSH

Ubaldi et al.[4] suggested that the subtle rise in progesterone may be related to an increased LH sensitivity of the granulosa cells of FSH-treated cycles. These high sensitivity is due to increased estradiol levels as well as to the increased number of follicles of more than 17 mm,[5,32] i.e. higher cumulative exposure to estradiol which, in conjunction with FSH, could be one of the mechanism for the premature increases in serum progesterone concentration.

Poor Ovarian Response with Increased LH Sensitivity

Premature luteinization is more prevalent in poor ovarian responders. Based on LH measurement and use of rFSH, Younis et al. suggested that elevated progesterone is not due to LH or hCG content of recombinant preparations; it is not necessarily an LH-dependent event and may be primarily related to an adversely affected cumulus-oocyte complex. This is still unclear whether the progesterone increase is related to some disruption of ovarian steroidogenic pathway induced by high FSH doses **(Fig. 1)**, or the early expression of an occult ovarian failure.[33]

"Cross Talk" between Ovaries and Adrenals

The luteinizing hormone receptors have been detected in the human adrenal cortex.[34] The activity of the adrenals is not influenced by the cyclic activity of the ovaries. It is clearly demonstrate that the adrenals constitute the main source of circulating progesterone during early follicular development,[35] whereas the ovaries provide most of the circulating progesterone during the late follicular phase. The data also demonstrate that adrenal steroidogenesis is influenced by ovarian action. The adrenocortical–ovarian crosstalk may be similar to that between the granulosa and the theca interna in which thecal progesterone synthesis is stimulated by the granulosa.[36-38]

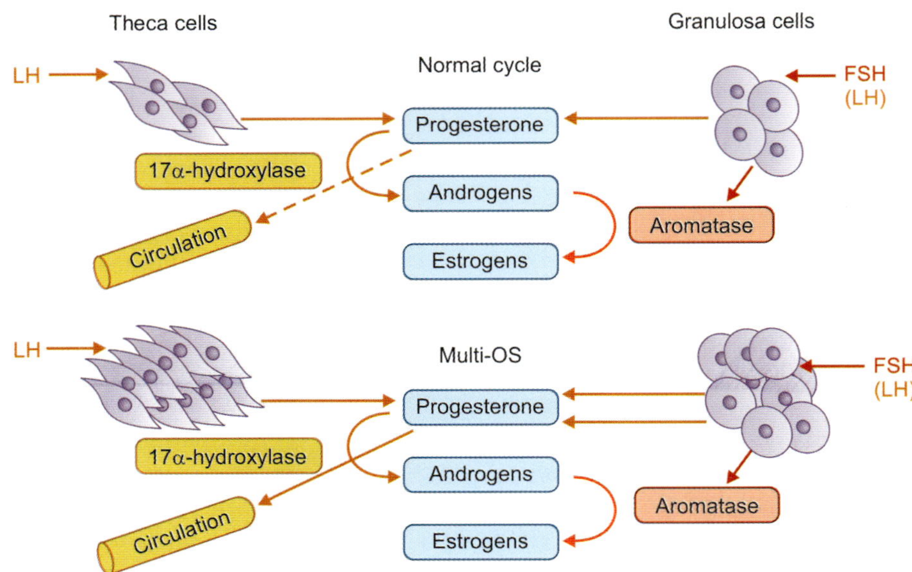

Fig. 1 Steroidogenesis during normal follicular phase and following ovarian stimulation

Multivariate Approach

The rise in progesterone level cannot be explained by luteinization of granulosa cells, since this occurs in the presence of GnRH analogs and, hence, low LH levels. Bosch E et al. performed a multivariate large scale study involving 4,000 IVF cycles.[18]

- They found significant positive correlation found between serum progesterone levels on the day of hCG administration and daily FSH dose.
- They observed patients with progesterone levels less than or equal to 1.5 ng/mL had a significantly lower incidence of ovarian hyperstimulation syndrome compared with more than 1.5 ng/mL.
- The results showed statistically significant correlation of occurrence of serum progesterone elevation with:
  – Higher the daily FSH dose
  – Serum estradiol level on the day of hCG
  – Number of oocytes collected.

To explain this complicated hormonal changes and effects, we first need to refresh our knowledge of hormonal profile in normal as well as stimulated cycles.

FOLLICULAR-PHASE PROFILE IN THE NORMAL CYCLE "TWO-CELL, TWO-GONADOTROPIN"

In brief, FSH acts on granulosa cells, promoting cell division and conversion of cholesterol to progesterone.[39] According to the two-cell, two-gonadotropin theory of estrogen biosynthesis,[40] progesterone is further metabolized to androgens by the thecal cells under the trophic influence of LH, and this step can only take place in the thecal cell compartment. Androgens are subsequently converted to estrogens through aromatization back in the granulosa cells.

Progesterone produced by the granulosa cells under FSH drive must pass to the vascularized thecal cell compartment to be catabolized to androgens. However, from here, steroids gain access to the general circulation as well as being metabolized in the normal steroid cascade. It is probable that the greater the LH drive to the thecal cells, the more progesterone catabolism to androgens will take place, leaving less progesterone to find its way into the general circulation. This can be summarized as follows: there are two sources of progesterone in the follicle, but only one step of further metabolism (catabolism of progesterone to androgens) which is driven by LH activity in thecal cells. A lack of LH drive to the thecal cells is therefore likely to leave more progesterone to find its way into the general circulation.[41]

PROFILES DURING OVARIAN STIMULATION

It can be predicted that an ovary with a large number of growing follicles, stimulated by maintained high FSH concentrations by dint of daily FSH injections, will produce and secrete more progesterone into the ovarian vein than a single follicle in the normal mid-follicular phase, with declining FSH concentrations. In the event of ovarian stimulation-induced multiple-follicle growth, the progesterone output to the periphery will be magnified in accord with the number of follicles and the FSH drive. This is likely to impact upon progesterone concentrations in the periphery and may influence endometrial development. Thus, the three major components to the degree of progesterone secretion from the ovaries will be: (1) the number of follicles (or granulosa cells), (2) the degree of trophic stimulus (FSH drive to granulosa cells), and (3) the degree of LH drive to thecal cells, which will encourage conversion of progesterone to androgens and estrogen.

The older studies that can be explained and support these findings are:

- GnRH antagonist cycles with high progesterone on the day of hCG administration required higher doses of FSH and a longer stimulation period than lower progesterone levels.[5] Therefore, the explanation proposed for early rise in progesterone level—that it results from an initial intense FSH stimulation, leading to increased granulosa cell steroidogenic activity—remains plausible.[5]
- The positive correlation between follicular phase progesterone levels and administered FSH dose, as well as with circulating FSH concentration.[32]
- Higher progesterone levels have been related to greater FSH administration in both GnRH agonist and antagonist cycles.[5,12]
- *The MERiT study:*[12] The Menotropin versus Recombinant FSH was used in IVF Trial, where, despite increases in oocyte production, the implantation rate was lower when progesterone levels were higher. The importance of balanced LH activity may also be reflected by the fact that there was higher incidence of elevated progesterone in the rFSH group versus the highly purified-hMG (HP-hMG) group.

CLINICAL IMPLICATIONS OF ELEVATED PROGESTERONE IN FOLLICULAR PHASE

It is important to establish whether there is evidence supporting the hypothesis that these elevations in progesterone concentration in COS are clinically significant and whether they can be predicted.

- High serum progesterone concentration on the day of hCG administration is a frequent event in cycles with both GnRH agonists and antagonists and, when observed, it is associated with a decreased pregnancy rate.[18] According to the hypothesis, those cases showing raised progesterone on the last stimulation day may have breached "normal" concentrations

some days beforehand, which may be responsible for advancement of endometrial maturation, leading to asynchrony with embryo development and a detrimental effect on implantation.

- Higher progesterone values showed lower embryo implantation rate in rFSH group. (HP-hMG, 24% versus 19%, not statistically significant; rFSH, 23% versus 11%, $P = 0.025$).[12]
- The effect more commonly seen in young women considered to be "ideal" (high-responding) patients, with a low body mass (associated with higher circulating FSH concentrations) and when "pure" FSH is used.
- By contrast, the hCG-driven LH activity in HP-hMG stimulation may offset the rise in progesterone by stimulating thecal cell activity toward the catabolism of progesterone to androgens and, thereafter, metabolism to estrogens in granulosa cells.
- The progesterone threshold concentration of 4 nmol/L in the MERiT study is equivalent to 1.26 ng/mL, which is similar to that used in the Bosch study (1.5 ng/mL, or 4.77 nmol/L), above which ongoing pregnancy rates fell.[18]
- Theoretically, the measurement of progesterone in each cycle may help to improve implantation rates and, ultimately, pregnancy outcomes. However, in the past poor reliability of assay methods at these low progesterone concentrations offered weak prospect of benefit.[39] More appropriate methods are now available.[42]
- The strategic approach in selection of dose and choice of FSH, examination of appropriate clinical and biochemical responses, cryopreservation of embryos and withheld embryo-transfer may prove beneficial in improving outcome by preventing, predicting and reacting to high progesterone levels on the day of hCG administration in stimulated ART cycles.

CONCLUSION

- Despite the use of GnRH analogs, subtle increases in serum progesterone levels beyond an arbitrarily defined threshold value at the end of the follicular phase in COS cycles for IVF is a common event with incidence is as high as 35% (5–35%) of stimulated cycles in individuals treated with GnRH agonist and 38% of with GnRH antagonist.
- High serum progesterone concentration on the day of hCG administration is associated with a decreased pregnancy rate. Authors rejected any negative effect on raised progesterone on oocytes or embryos. According to the hypothesis, those cases

showing raised progesterone on the last stimulation day may have breached "normal" concentrations some days beforehand, which may be responsible for advancement of endometrial maturation, leading to asynchrony with embryo development and a detrimental effect on implantation.

- The "two-cells, two-gonadotropins" theory better explains the pathogenesis and escaping of progesterone in circulation, when:
  - The number of follicles (or granulosa cells) are more
  - The higher degree of trophic stimulus (dose and duration of FSH administered, circulating concentration of FSH)
  - The lower degree of LH drive to thecal cells (use of "pure" FSH/low endogenous LH), which will encourage conversion of progesterone to androgens and estrogen.
- Using trend analysis, a serum progesterone level of 1.5 ng/mL (4.77 nmol/L) on the day of hCG administration was identified as the most appropriate threshold to define detrimental outcome of IVF/ICSI-ET cycles; beyond which implantation and ongoing pregnancy rate falls.
- This threshold value helps clinician to decide whether to continue to ET in a fresh cycle or cryopreserve the embryos and transfer in a subsequent frozen-thawed cycles.
- Alternatively, administering hCG at an earlier time point in the follicular phase, prior to progesterone elevation, might be beneficial in patients who have previously exhibited elevated progesterone levels after COS.
- This can also help choosing the type of gonadotropins used for COS.

■ REFERENCES

1. Fleming R, Adam AH, Barlow DH, et al. A new systematic treatment for infertile women with abnormal hormone profiles. Br J Obstet Gynaecol. 1982;89:80-3.
2. Edelstein MC, Seltman HJ, Cox BJ, et al. Progesterone levels on the day of human chorionic gonadotropin administration in cycles with gonadotropin-releasing hormone agonist suppression are not predictive of pregnancy outcome. Fertil Steril. 1990;54:853-57.
3. Silverberg KM, Burns Wn, Olive DL, et al. Serum progesterone levels predict success of in vitro fertilization/embryo transfer in patients stimulated with leuprolide acetate and human menopausal gonadotropins. J Clin Endocrinol Metab. 1991;73:797-803.
4. Ubaldi F, Smitz J, Bourgain C, et al. Premature luteinization in in vitro fertilization cycles using gonadotropin-releasing hormone agonist (GnRH-a) and recombinant follicle-stimulating hormone (FSH) and GnRH-a and urinary FSH. Fertil Steril. 1996;66:275-80.
5. Bosch E, Valencia I, Escudero E, et al. Premature luteinization during gonadotropin-releasing hormone antagonist cycles and its relationship with in vitro fertilization outcome. Fertil Steril. 2003;80:1444-9.
6. Legro RS, Ary BA, Paulson RJ, et al. Premature luteinisation as detected by elevated serum progesterone is associated with a higher pregnancy rate in donor oocyte in-vitro fertilization. Hum Reprod. 1993;8:1506-11.
7. Murphy BD. Models of luteinisation. Biol Reprod. 2000;63:2-11.
8. Check JH. Predictive value of serum progesterone levels for pregnancy outcome? Fertil Steril. 1993;62:1090-1.
9. Givens CR, Schriock ED, Dandekar PV, et al. Elevated serum progesterone levels on the day of human chorionic gonadotropin administration do not predict outcome in assisted reproduction cycles. Fertil Steril. 1994;62:1011-7.
10. Bustillo M, Stern JJ, Coulam CB. Serum progesterone at the time of human chorionic gonadotrophin does not predict pregnancy in in-vitro fertilization and embryo transfer. Hum Reprod. 1995;10:2862-7.
11. Venetis CA, Kolibianakis EM, Papanikolaou E, et al. Is progesterone elevation on the day of human chorionic gonadotrophin administration associated with the probability of pregnancy in in vitro fertilization? A systematic review and meta-analysis. Hum Reprod Update. 2007;13:343-55.
12. Andersen AN, Devroey P, Arce JC. Clinical outcome following stimulation with highly purified hMG or recombinant FSH in patients undergoing IVF: a randomized assessor-blind controlled trial. Hum Reprod. 2006;21:3217-27.
13. Check JH, Lurie D, Askari HA, et al. The range of subtle rise in serum progesterone levels following controlled ovarian hyperstimulation associated with lower in vitro fertilization pregnancy rate is determined by the source of manufacturer. Eur J Obstet Gynecol Reprod Biol. 1993;52:205-9.
14. Fanchin R, de Ziegler D, Taieb J, et al. Premature elevation of plasma progesterone alters pregnancy rates of in vitro fertilization and embryo transfer. Fertil Steril. 1993;59:1090-4.
15. Harada T, Yoshida S, Katagiri C, et al. Reduced implantation rate associated with a subtle rise in serum progesterone concentration during the follicular phase of cycles stimulated with combination of a gonadotrophin-releasing hormone agonist and gonadotrophin. Hum Reprod. 1995;10:1060-4.
16. Shulman A, Ghetler Y, Beyth Y, et al. The significance of an early (premature) rise of plasma progesterone in in vitro fertilization cycles induced by a "long protocol" of gonadotropin releasing hormone analogue and human menopausal gonadotropins. J Assist Reprod Genet. 1996;13:207-11.
17. Fanchin R, Hourvitz A, Olivennes F, et al. Premature progesterone elevation spares blastulation but not pregnancy rates in in vitro fertilization with coculture. Fertil Steril. 1997;68:648-52.
18. Bosch E, Labarta E, Crespo J, et al. Circulating progesterone levels and ongoing pregnancy rates in controlled ovarian stimulation cycles for in vitro fertilization: analysis of over 4000 cycles. Hum Reprod. 2010;25:2092-100.
19. Smitz J, Andersen AN, Devroey P, et al. Endocrine profile in serum and follicular fluid differs after ovarian stimulation with

HP-hMG or recombinant FSH in IVF patients. Hum Reprod. 2007;22:676-87.

20. Melo MA, Meseguer M, Garrido N, et al. The significance of premature luteinisation in anoocyte-donation programme. Hum Reprod. 2006;21:1503-7.

21. Soares SR, Troncoso C, Bosch E, et al. Age and uterine receptiveness: predicting the outcome of oocyte donation cycles. J Clin Endocrinol Metab. 2005;90:4399-404.

22. Schoolcraft W, Sinton E, Schlenker T, et al. Lower pregnancy rate with premature luteinization during pituitary suppression with leuprolide acetate. Fertil Steril. 1991;55:563-6.

23. Elnashar AM. Progesterone rise on the day of HCG administration (premature luteinization) in IVF: an overdue update. J Assist Reprod Genet. 2010;27:149-55.

24. Papanikolaou EG, Kolibianakis EM, Pozzobon C, et al. Progesterone rise on the day of human chorionic gonadotropin administration impairs pregnancy outcome in day 3 single-embryo transfer, while has no effect on day 5 single blastocyst transfer. Fertil Steril. 2009;91:949-52.

25. Saadat P, Boostanfar R, Slater CC, et al. Accelerated endometrial maturation in the luteal phase of cycles utilizing controlled ovarian hyperstimulation: impact of gonadotropin-releasing hormone agonists versus antagonists. Fertil Steril. 2004;82:167-171.

26. Labarta E, Martı́nez-Conejero JA, Alamá P, et al. Endometrial receptivity is affected in women with high circulating progesterone levels at the end of the follicular phase: a functional genomics analysis. Hum Reprod. 2011;26:1813-25.

27. Van Vaerenbergh I, Fatemi HM, Blockeel C, et al. Progesterone rise on HCG day in GnRH antagonist/rFSH stimulated cycles affects endometrial gene expression. Reprod Biomed Online. 2011;22:263-71.

28. Achache H, Revel A. Endometrial receptivity markers, the journey to successful embryo implantation. Hum Reprod Update. 2006;12:731-46.

29. Younis JS, Simon A, Laufer N. Endometrial preparation: lessons from oocyte donation. Fertil Steril. 1996;66:873-84.

30. Ubaldi F, Smitz J, Wisanto A, et al. Oocyte and embryo quality as well as pregnancy rate in intracytoplasmic sperm injection are not affected by high follicular phase serum progesterone. Hum Reprod. 1995;10:3091-6.

31. Mannaerts B, de Leeuw R, Geelen J, et al. Comparative in vitro and in vivo studies on the biological characteristics of recombinant human follicle-stimulating hormone. Endocrinology. 1991;129:2623-30.

32. Filicori M, Cognigni GE, Pocognoli P, et al. Modulation of folliculogenesis and steroidogenesis in women by graded mentrophin administration. Hum Reprod. 2002;17:2009-15.

33. Younis JS, Matilsky M, Radin O, et al. Increased progesterone/estradiol ratio in the late follicular phase could be related to low ovarian reserve in in vitro fertilization- embryo transfer cycles with a long gonadotropin releasing hormone agonist. Fertil Steril. 2001;76:294-99.

34. Pabon JE, Li X, Lei ZM, et al. Novel presence of luteinizing hormone/chorionic gonadotrophin receptors in human adrenal glands. J Clin Endocrinol Metab. 1996;81:2397-400.

35. Eldar-Geva T, Margalioth EJ, Brooks B, et al. The origin of serum progesterone during the follicular phase of menotrophin-stimulated cycles. Hum Reprod. 1998;13:9-14.

36. Makris A, Ryan JJ. Evidence for interaction between granulosa cells and theca in early progesterone synthesis. Endocr Res Comm. 1977;4:233-46.

37. Kotsuji F, Kamitani N, Goto K, et al. Bovine theca and granulosa interactions modulate their growth, morphology, and function. Biol Reprod. 1990;43:726-32.

38. Yada H, Hosokawa K, Tajima K, et al. Role of ovarian theca and granulosa cell interaction in hormone production and cell growth during the bovine follicular maturation process. Biol Reprod. 1999;61:1480-6.

39. Fleming R. Progesterone elevation on the day of hCG: methodological issues. Hum Reprod Update. 2008;14:391-2.

40. Moon YS, Tsang BK, Simpson C, et al. 17Beta-estradiol biosynthesis in cultured granulosa and thecal cells of human ovarian follicles: stimulation by follicle-stimulating hormone. J Clin Endocrinol Metab. 1978;47:263-7.

41. Richard F, Julian J. The source and implications of progesterone rise during the follicular phase of assisted reproduction cycles. Reprod Biomed Online. 2010;21:446-9.

42. Coucke W, Devleeschouwer N, Libeer JC, et al. Accuracy and reproducibility of automated estradiol-17beta and progesterone assays using native serum samples: results obtained in the Belgian external assessment scheme. Hum Reprod. 2007;22:3204-9.

Arveen Vohra, Kamini A Rao

14 Therapeutic Window for Luteinizing Hormone in Controlled Ovarian Stimulation

■ INTRODUCTION

The anterior pituitary secretes the major hormone releasing factors, follicle-stimulating hormone (FSH), luteinizing hormone (LH), thyroid-stimulating hormone (TSH), and adrenocorticotropic hormone (ACTH) along with growth hormone (GH) and prolactin. FSH and LH have markedly different functions in the control of ovarian physiology though secreted from common cells. The control of FSH and LH is through a combination of differential control of their synthesis and secretion by gonadotropin-releasing hormone (GnRH).

As an oocyte matures within a follicle, a myriad of complex hormonal events take place, particularly during the follicular phase. The two gonadotropins LH and FSH play distinct but complementary roles in ensuring follicular growth and ovulation. These two gonadotropins are active in the final weeks of the development of a mature surviving oocyte, with initiation of folliculogenesis occurring independently of gonadotropic stimulation. Secretion of LH and FSH in an orderly fashion is therefore crucial to the final development of a mature oocyte.

Although recent studies have facilitated better understanding of the LH and FSH hormone interrelation and effect on fertilization and implantation, there is still confusion on the usefulness of LH supplementation in controlled ovarian stimulation. Therefore, the use of recombinant human LH (r-hLH) in controlled ovarian hyperstimulation (COH) should be guided by a rationale that is based on the individualized patient profile and requirements. The concept of an LH therapeutic window has implications for the choice of LH supplementation in assisted reproduction technology (ART). Endogenous LH production is pulsatile and occurs in response to the pulsatile release of GnRH from the hypothalamus. The most physiological way to maintain LH concentrations is to utilize endogenous LH secretion.

■ PHYSIOLOGICAL ROLE OF LUTEINIZING HORMONE

Follicle-stimulating hormone and LH both are glycoproteins that share identical α-subunits along with TSH and placental human chorionic gonadotropin (hCG) differing only in the structure of their β-subunits, which confers receptor specificity. LH is required for the growth of preovulatory follicles, ovulation and luteinization of the dominant follicle. The LH receptor (*LHR*) gene is expressed in granulosa cells of human antral follicles throughout the follicular phase and is significantly associated with expression of the *CYP19a1* gene and with the corresponding follicular fluid concentrations of estradiol and progesterone. *LHR* gene is expressed in human granulosa cells from around a diameter of 5–6 mm and until ovulation. LHR expression peaks in granulosa cells just before initiation of the mid-cycle of gonadotropins and may affect human follicular development earlier than previously believed. In small antral follicles with a diameter of 3–10 mm, around 80% express LHR; exhibiting strong positive associations to estradiol, progesterone, anti-Müllerian hormone, and inhibin-B in the corresponding follicular fluid, suggesting that functional receptors are present on the granulosa cells[1] **(Fig. 1)**.

The FSH receptors are present over the granulosa cells. The ovarian thecal and granulosa cells are the principal sites of LH bioactivity, although LHRs are also present in extra-gonadal sites such as the uterus.[2] During the follicular phase of the menstrual cycle, LH induces androgen synthesis by theca cells that is essential for robust steroidogenesis; stimulates proliferation, differentiation, and secretion of follicular theca cells and also increases LHRs on granulosa cells. The preovulatory LH surge drives the oocyte into the first meiotic division and initiates luteinization of theca and granulosa cells.

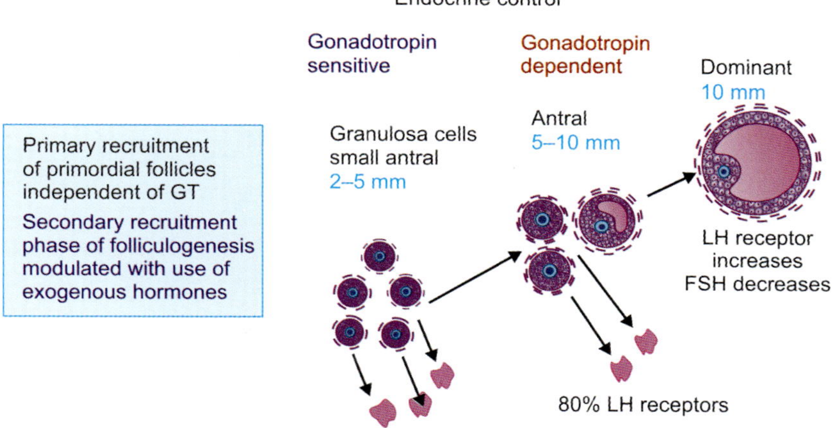

Fig. 1 LH receptors in different stages of folliculogenesis

The resulting corpus luteum produces high levels of progesterone and some estrogen.

Therapeutic LH Window

Luteinizing hormone in association with FSH is recommended for stimulating follicular development in women with severe LH and FSH deficiency with an endogenous serum LH concentration less than 1.2 IU/L. According to the threshold theory of LH in ovarian function, the ovarian follicle requires a minimal amount of LH for steroidogenesis (<1% of receptors attached by LH). There is also a ceiling beyond which excessively high concentrations of LH may actually suppress granulosa aromatase activity and inhibit cell growth. The LH ceiling is dependent on timing of the menstrual cycle but for optimal follicle development, this concentration is typically between 1.2 IU/L and 5 IU/L.[3]

The LH dependent phase of preovulatory follicular development proceeds normally only if LH is present at concentrations within the LH window, which is above the threshold level and beneath the ceiling value. The developing follicles have specific requirements for exposure to LH beyond which normal maturation ceases which gave rise to the concept of an "LH ceiling", meaning that each follicle would have an upper limit of stimulation. The LH ceiling may be higher in larger follicles and lower in smaller ones. As a consequence, an increasing LH concentration would promote leading follicle progression (being below its ceiling) and degeneration of secondary ones (by overcoming their ceiling). A dynamic interplay between LH secretion and receptor expression by different ovarian compartments governs the selection of dominant follicles. The small follicles in granulosa

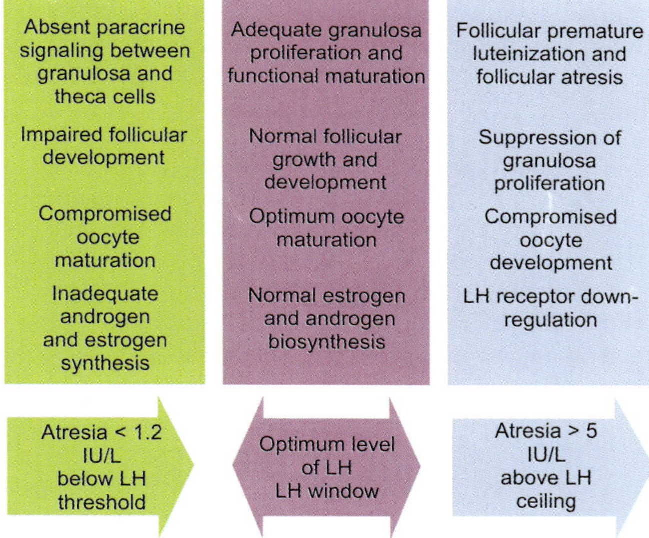

Fig. 2 Impact of different concentrations of LH on the menstrual cycle

cells do not express LHRs so LH may indirectly promote their degeneration. It should be recognized that the LH threshold evolves through the follicular cycle and conceptually should become higher as the follicles grow[4] **(Fig. 2)**.

The usefulness of exogenous LH in ovarian stimulation protocols in assisted reproduction continues to be controversial. Though there are no clear guidelines on when exactly LH needs to be added. It is critical that add-back LH is administered in appropriate patients as excess of LH can cause suppression of granulosa cells and follicular atresia.

Two-cell–Two-gonadotropin Concept

Follicle-stimulating hormone is essential for follicular recruitment and development, as well as for inducing many enzymes and hormones (e.g. aromatase, inhibin) that are subsequently controlled by LH and required for continued follicle maturation.[5] LH stimulates adenylate cyclase and cyclic AMP production resulting in mitochondrial cholesterol transport and steroidogenesis, essential events leading to oocyte maturation and ovulation.[6] Not only does LH play an important function in the periovulatory and ovulatory events within the ovary, but also LHRs have been identified in the human endometrium, raising the possibility that LH has a necessary function in implantation.[7]

Luteinizing hormone seems to play two roles during folliculogenesis. One is exerted in the theca compartment and consists of induction of androgen production. The second begins during the intermediate follicular phase, involves granulosa cells, and consists of inducing the local production of various molecules. These factors promote the growth of granulosa cells, which in turn regulate oocyte maturation. These two mechanisms are closely related and probably support each other. According to the so-called "spare receptor hypothesis", at a time when inhibin-B and IGF-1 are adequately secreted, androgen synthesis and release are optimal even with less than 1% of LHRs occupied.[3]

LH optimizes final stages of maturation. FSH stimulated estrogen production from the granulosa cells is dependent on LH stimulated androgen production by the theca cells. This is not fully functional till later part of antral development. Theca cells are characterized by expression of LHRs, 3β-hydroxy steroid dehydrogenase and CYP-P450c 17 essential for internalizing LDL cholesterol into mitochondria and thereby converting 21 carbons to androgens. The steroidogenic acute regulatory protein (StAR protein) is the primary regulator of production of androstenedione, which subsequently diffuses into granulosa cells to serve as an estrogen precursor. In the preovulatory follicle, cholesterol in theca cells arises from circulating lipoproteins and de novo biosynthesis.[8]

Granulosa cells express FSH receptors and CYP-450 aromatase to convert androgen substrate from theca into estrogens. Increased expression of aromatase indicates increased follicular maturity. Exclusive function of P450c 17 in theca cells and aromatase in granulosa cells is the basic principle of two-cell–two-gonadotropin theory.

Pure FSH treatment causes early development of follicle, but estradiol production is limited. Some aromatization occurs from the androgens of adrenal glands, but robust steroidogenesis is not possible.

Only dominant follicle with more FSH receptors, high aromatase activity and robust steroidogenesis is selected as dominant follicle. Following the mid-cycle LH surge, granulosa cell mitosis is blocked, and oocyte meiosis is resumed **(Fig. 3)**.

The best evidence for a critical role of LH in ovulation induction has come from studies evaluating pregnancy outcomes in women with hypogonadotropic hypogonadism (WHO class I). In the presence of low endogenous LH production, particularly among women with LH concentrations less than 1.2 mIU/mL, studies utilizing FSH alone for ovulation induction have found poor pregnancy outcomes.[9] Consequently, both FSH and LH supplementation appear to be critical for optimal follicular development, implantation and pregnancy. At the other extreme, elevated LH concentrations have likewise been associated with poor fertilization, poor implantation and detrimental effects on pregnancy rates. While insufficient LH results in inadequate steroidogenesis, excessive LH may suppress aromatase activity and inhibit cell growth. Taken together, this evidence supports the theory that a therapeutic window exists for LH, above or below which maximum reproductive outcomes may be negatively impacted.[6]

Luteinizing hormone administration may induce atresia of smaller follicles and the remaining larger follicles may represent those with greater reproductive competence. Improved endometrial receptivity may also be produced as implantation rates have been shown to positively correlate with increasing doses of LH.[10]

Nevertheless, whether the LH component of human menopausal gonadotropins (hMG) for ovarian stimulation is advantageous, disadvantageous or inconsequential to

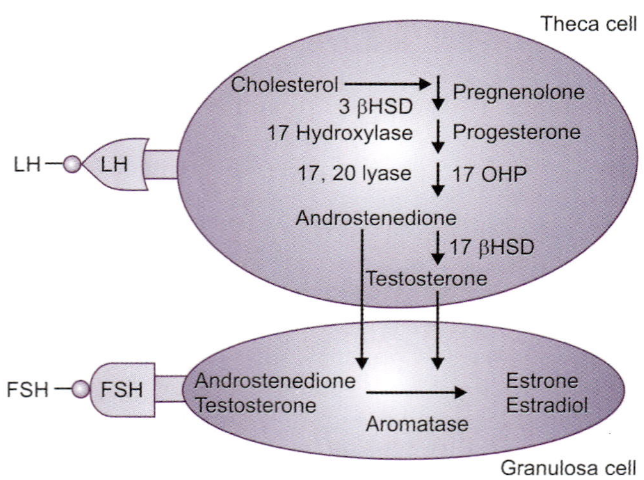

Fig. 3 Two-cell–two-gonadotropin theory

the ultimate outcome of interest, pregnancy rates, has been a matter of controversy.

■ LUTEINIZING HORMONE: DIFFERENT FORMS

It is clear that there is no absolute requirement for LH in the exogenous gonadotropin used for ovarian stimulation, but it has potential advantages in definable situations. Until recently, the only available source of exogenous LH activity has been hMG, a urine-derived preparation containing both FSH and LH, which comprises about 5% of the total protein content. LH activity can currently be derived from hMG preparations, urinary hCG, recombinant LH (rLH) and recombinant hCG.

Role of Human Menopausal Gonadotropins

Human menopausal gonadotropins are urinary-derived gonadotropins containing roughly equivalent amounts of LH and FSH bioactivity (approximately 75 IU of each). For many years, hMG was the only gonadotropin available. Despite their widespread use, there have been several proposed disadvantages of these compounds, including protein contamination leading to local allergic reactions and batch-to-batch inconsistencies, as well as supply limitations. Despite significant improvements in processing, different hMG preparations are subject to wide variation in LH quantity and bioactivity and with increased purification, more LH is lost. Thus, hCG is often added in an attempt to boost the LH bioactivity to meet the required LH activity range (FSH:LH ratio = 1:1) as stated in the pharmacopoeia. This may result in the end product having much more hCG than LH activity.

The Van Hell bioassay of hMG-only detects LH bioactivity and does not distinguish LH from hCG. Analysis of one hMG product (Menopur) showed that the content of hCG was more than 10 times higher than LH. Another analysis also showed that about 95% of the LHR bioactivity in one hMG product (Menopur) was attributed to hCG, with less than 5% contributed by pure LH.[11]

Owing to the controversial nature of the topic, in the past decade, five meta-analyses have contributed to the current understanding of the effect of hMG compared with FSH-only protocols on assisted reproduction outcomes.[12,13]

With regard to the type of pituitary downregulation, data showing that hMG cycles yield a 3–4% higher live birth rate than recombinant FSH (rFSH)-only cycles have come from trials utilizing long GnRH agonists.[13] In a single randomized controlled trial comparing hMG to rFSH while using a GnRH antagonist, Bosch et al. demonstrated

a 3% higher live birth rate in the hMG group. However, this finding was not significant as even though the similar increase in live birth rates is notable, the data on hMG use in GnRH antagonist cycles is too limited to make definitive conclusions.[14]

The studies have estimated that hMG protocols may provide a 3–4% but significant improvement in live birth rate compared with rFSH-only protocols when a long GnRH agonist protocol was utilized. While statistically significant, the clinical significance of this finding remains controversial. An important patient consideration has been that significantly fewer ampoules of gonadotropins were required among those receiving hMG as compared with rFSH-only protocols, resulting in a lower cost per live birth in the hMG group without compromising patient safety. With the potential for lower treatment costs, there seems to be a benefit to the inclusion of hMG in treatment protocols.[15]

Role of Recombinant Human LH

Recombinant human FSH (r-hFSH) replacement has been used in ovarian stimulation protocols since its approval in 1994. There is increasing interest in exploring the role of LH and its optimal use in relation to assisted reproduction. With the availability of rLH, stimulation protocols have incorporated its use in place of hMG. Pharmacodynamics' studies of rLH have shown it to have a similar volume of distribution, half-life and bioactivity to urinary products. These profiles have not differed whether rLH was administered SC or IM and have not been shown to affect FSH pharmacodynamics when coadministered. Since LH has a precise therapeutic window, the physician needs to have precise control over the activity of exogenous LH administered. rLH is analogous to endogenous LH and characterized by high purity, precision of dosing and consistency. When administered by subcutaneous injection, rLH has a terminal half-life of 24 hours. rLH is structurally and functionally analogous to endogenous human LH. In a RCT with patients with a suboptimal response to stimulation with a long GnRH agonist stimulation protocol that compared adding higher doses of r-hFSH versus adding rLH or hMG, those given rLH had higher live birth rates (40.7%) than those given hMG (18%). The rLH group also had higher implantation rates. The authors speculated that the differences between the two preparations could produce different biological effects in women who exhibit a suboptimal response to FSH and concluded that using rLH is justified if better outcomes can be achieved.[9,16,17]

While some advocate add-back LH to the mid-follicular phase in ovarian stimulation cycles, others deem add-back LH to be unnecessary, justifying that the small amount of LH present after downregulation is enough to sustain theca and granulosa cell stimulation.[18] However, supplementation with rLH has shown lower levels of cumulous cell apoptosis than treatment with FSH alone, possibly indicating improved oocyte quality in LH-supplemented cycles. The decreased granulosa cell apoptosis in the rLH group might be the result of lower levels of follicular fluid vascular endothelial growth factor; marker of maturity and quality of oocytes that is produced by granulosa and theca cells in response to FSH, LH, hCG and proliferative and apoptotic factors.[19,20]

The importance of LH supplementation in studies of ovulation induction has been shrouded by conflicting data. The best evidence for a critical role of LH in ovulation induction has come from studies evaluating pregnancy outcomes in women with hypogonadotropic hypogonadism. In the presence of low endogenous LH production, particularly among women with LH concentrations less than 1.2 mIU/mL, studies utilizing FSH alone for ovulation induction have found poor pregnancy outcomes.[9] Consequently, both FSH and LH supplementation appear to be critical for optimal follicular development, implantation and pregnancy.[21]

On the other hand, elevated LH concentrations have been associated with poor fertilization, poor implantation and detrimental effects on pregnancy rates. While insufficient LH results in inadequate steroidogenesis, excessive LH may suppress aromatase activity and inhibit cell growth. Taken together, this evidence supports the theory that a therapeutic window exists for LH, above or below which maximum reproductive outcomes may be negatively impacted.[6]

The larger randomized controlled trials have been published on the use of rLH supplementation from day 6 in long agonist protocols and rLH supplementation from day 1 of stimulation in antagonist protocols. These trials have failed to document that serum LH concentrations during stimulation or the addition of rLH have overall clinical benefits in terms of higher pregnancy rates. However, LH concentrations were related to end points like duration of stimulation, gonadotropin consumption, number of oocytes retrieved, estradiol and preovulatory progesterone rises in many studies. This suggests many highly significant associations, but no association with the key end point—pregnancy. The overall conclusion is that, irrespective of protocols, circulating LH concentration is a predictor of various important parameters. Data suggests that like hMG, rLH results in higher estradiol concentrations and decreased usage of rFSH, but it does not demonstrate convincing evidence that rLH improves pregnancy outcomes over rFSH alone.[14,22]

There are several possible explanations for why there may be demonstrable evidence of benefit with hMG but not when utilizing rLH. First, the studies performed to date utilizing rLH have had much smaller patient populations. Secondly, the studies evaluating rLH represented a much more heterogeneous group than those evaluating hMG. Thirdly, rLH and hMG may differ in their biological activity due to differences in LH glycosylation patterns and because of the addition of hCG in hMG. Finally, because of the fixed ratio of LH:FSH found in hMG, any addition of LH is coincident to the addition of FSH. Finally, due to its cost, studies have estimated that rLH may add 45% to the cost of ovarian stimulation despite the reduction in rFSH use.

Role of hCG in the Mid to Late Follicular Phase

Luteinizing hormone and hCG are structurally quite similar and bind to the same receptors. However, their β-subunits are different. The two hormones differ in the composition of their carbohydrate moieties that, in turn, affects bioactivity and half-life. Except for the CTP on the β-subunit of hCG (amino acids 113–145), the two hormones share more than 85% sequence homology. Relative to hLH, the serum half-life of hCG is more than twofold greater. hCG is more stable with slower plasma metabolic clearance rate. hCG has a higher binding affinity to the LHR, with 1 IU hCG having biological activity approximately 6–8 times greater than 1 IU LH. After subcutaneous injection, hCG exhibits a longer serum half-life, thus leading to the possibility of significant accumulation over time.[10]

hCG/hMG may Induce LH Receptor Internalization

A recent study comparing stimulation with hMG versus r-hFSH in women undergoing IVF/intracytoplasmic sperm injection treatment found statistically significantly reduced expression of LHR messenger RNA in ovarian granulosa cells in the hMG group, which was associated with altered expression of genes and proteins involved in steroidogenesis in preovulatory granulosa cells.[23]

These studies show that hCG is not equivalent to LH and there are effects at the level of LHR internalization, which may explain why there is 'tolerance' or a lack of effect. Finally, it is known that there is a LH ceiling associated with the use of rLH. Hugues et al. established that in World Health Organization type II anovulatory women undergoing follicular stimulation, this LH ceiling was more than 60 mcg or 1,325 IU rLH/day when these women showed atresia of non-dominant follicles, elevated progesterone concentrations and reduced clinical pregnancy rates.[24]

The role of hCG as a supplement to FSH in the late follicular phase, in long and short agonist and antagonist protocols has been reviewed in a recent meta-analysis of nine studies. From the four treatment strategies defined in the analysis, hCG supplementation in the GnRH antagonist group was associated with a non-significant benefit in clinical pregnancy rate. A pilot study which compared the effect of hCG supplementation exclusively in GnRH antagonist cycles, found comparable rates of oocyte yield and pregnancy in the hCG and control groups, but a reduction in FSH consumption in the former. Four randomized trials demonstrated that the use of hCG in the mid-follicular phase could significantly reduce FSH dosage without a reduction in pregnancy rates and may represent a decrease in stimulation-associated costs. However, these studies were not powered to detect pregnancy or live birth rates as primary end points.[18]

The current evidence suggests that hCG or LH in the mid to late follicular phase can support continued follicular progression and estradiol production in the face of partial or complete FSH withdrawal. The potential advantage of this protocol is the consumption of less FSH for ovarian stimulation, potentially leading to a cost saving. However, convincing cost analyses of mid-cycle hCG protocols are lacking. The data shows mid-cycle hCG to be equivalent to FSH protocols and no advantages to outcomes have been reported. Before widespread use, larger studies are needed to evaluate pregnancy and live birth rates.[25]

■ ROLE OF LH IN ASSISTED REPRODUCTIVE TECHNOLOGY

Exogenous LH and ART Outcome in Unselected Population

There is no evidence that supplementation with LH activity is necessary in an unselected IVF population, it may yet be beneficial in select subgroups of patients who usually need high doses of FSH.

A meta-analysis of four randomized controlled trials comparing r-HFSH and hMG treatment in normogonadotropic patients undergoing a GnRH, a long protocol failed to show any statistically significant difference in the ongoing pregnancy rates and live birth rate. In a meta-analysis utilizing GnRH antagonist, an increase in peak estradiol concentrations and a higher number of mature oocytes but no benefit in implantation and pregnancy rates is noted.[26]

Another meta-analysis of RCT comparing r-hFSH versus r-hFSH plus rLH ovarian stimulation showed that for unselected patients undergoing ART there is no difference between the two treatments in live birth rate and does not recommend adding LH to unselected patients (age <35 years). However, the authors mentioned that their conclusion should be interpreted with caution, as it was not statistically significant.[27]

Hence, the present evidence is insufficient to prove that LH administration in unselected groups is associated with any significant improvement in the IVF/ICSI outcome parameters like implantation and pregnancy rates, when compared with r-hFSH only stimulation.[18]

Exogenous LH and ART Outcome in Selected Population

Severe Endogenous LH Deficiency

Luteinizing hormone polymorphism contributes to severe endogenous LH deficiency. The *LHR* gene is known to carry as many as 282 single-nucleotide polymorphisms (SNPs). A common genetic LHβ variant (v-βLH) owing to the alterations in two polymorphic base changes in the β-subunit gene leading to changes in the amino acid sequence, Trp8Arg and Ile15Thr, has been identified. It was earlier thought to be an immunological anomalous LH form.[28]

The shorter half-life of v-βLH may be linked to the presence of extra glycosylation signal into the β-subunit that could lead to an addition of second oligosaccharide to Asn13 of the β-protein. It has been found that there is more potency of the overall LH activity of v-βLH at the receptor site; however, its duration is shorter in vivo. Previous clinical trials conducted to determine the impact of this variant on reproductive health reported its association with ovulatory disorders, premature ovarian failure, hyperprolactinemia, luteal insufficiency, menstrual disorders, endometriosis and infertility. A few studies have noted low response in some women following ovarian stimulation, resulting in a greater need for r-hFSH (>2,500 IU) due to the presence of v-βLH. Based on the findings, the researchers suggest the potential of v-βLH as a marker of ovarian responsiveness to r-hFSH. This role of v-βLH, if validated with further research, could facilitate clinicians in identifying patients requiring exogenous LH addition during ovarian stimulation.[29]

Hypogonadotropic hypogonadism (WHO class I) impairs pituitary neuroendocrine function that results in abnormally low LH and FSH concentrations. Such patients typically have amenorrhea with small ovaries having follicles in arrested development due to the lack of effective hypothalamic–pituitary activity. These women do not have sufficient endogenous LH for optimal follicular growth and steroidogenesis when treated with FSH alone and will typically benefit from FSH and LH for optimal follicular development.

Hypophysectomized animal studies and studies in hypogonadotropic hypogonadism women confirm that r-hFSH increases follicular growth in a dose-dependent manner, but is ineffective in stimulating synthesis of estradiol due to the extremely low or near-undetectable endogenous LH concentrations. The role of LH in hypophysectomized women and in women with isolated gonadotropin deficiency has been reviewed and concluded that although r-hFSH increases the growth of multiple ovarian follicles, serum LH, androstenedione and estradiol concentrations remain low or show only negligible increase.[6,16,21]

The reviews confirm that LH is physiologically essential for estradiol synthesis and that replacement to above the minimal threshold concentration is necessary in women with inherent gonadotropin insufficiency.

Severe LH Deficiency due to Suppression by GnRH Analogs in ART

Women treated with GnRH analogs (agonists or antagonists) during ovarian stimulation in IVF, may similarly experience severely reduced LH and FSH concentrations due to over suppression of endogenous LH and FSH pituitary secretion. In some patients, the suppressed baseline LH concentrations may reach levels seen in hypogonadotropic hypogonadism women (i.e. <1.2 IU/L). However, not every patient undergoing ovarian stimulation requires exogenous LH replacement, as endogenous production of small amounts of LH may remain sufficient for theca cell function. The studies show poorer outcomes among those patients who have a lower LH concentration or a sharper fall in LH from baseline concentrations and in patients whose endogenous LH is low after GnRH agonist treatment.[30]

A randomized trial in oocyte donors that compared r-hFSH versus r-hFSH combined with rLH in an antagonist protocol showed a significantly higher metaphase-II oocyte count, fertilization rates, grade 1 embryos and implantation rates, in recipients whose embryos originated from donors receiving added rLH than in donors receiving GnRH antagonist and r-hFSH alone. Future research is required to lend further support to the use of adjuvant rLH in patients on antagonist ovarian stimulation protocols.[31]

There may be a role for other biomarkers, for example, LH polymorphisms such as the v-LHβ in further identifying LH-deficient patients.[28] Another way to identify the severely LH-deficient patient is to look at the ovarian response to FSH stimulation. Supplementation of LH may benefit selected women with LH deficiency and suboptimal ovarian response during ART as measured by clinical end points such as estradiol concentrations and follicular development. The evidence for addition of rLH to rFSH in antagonist protocols for ovarian stimulation is still being accumulated and more research is needed.

However, we must remember that early overexposure of LH in ovarian stimulation can result in premature follicle luteinization of small follicles and follicular atresia leading either to cycle cancellation due to follicle maturation arrest or to poor-quality oocytes, all of which translates into severely compromised outcomes.

Poor Responders

Poor ovarian reserve is estimated to occur in around 26% of the ART procedures. Evidence indicates that rLH and r-hFSH co-administration in these patients may help in improving ongoing pregnancy rates in poor responders and women of advanced age.[14,20,32]

On the contrary, some recent studies concluded that there is an insufficient evidence to validate the effectiveness of rLH in subjects with poor response undergoing ART.[33]

Some clinicians use a short GnRH agonist or microflare protocol in some of their older or poor-responder patients. There is substantial evidence of a benefit of adding rLH to women who have a poor response to ovarian stimulation, including poor response in a previous cycle; and a suboptimal ovarian response with suboptimal follicular progression in a current cycle by day 6–8.[20]

Patients at Risk of Hyporesponse during Ovarian Stimulation

In an ongoing COH cycle, there is a group of patients who, after using suppressive GnRH analogs (either agonists or antagonists), develop severe LH deficiency and exhibit a suboptimal ovarian follicular response by day 6–8. A review defines this suboptimal ovarian response as: (1) having no follicle more than 10 mm by day 6, (2) low estradiol concentration less than 200 pg/mL by day 6 and (3) poor progression or slowing of follicle growth, i.e. previously 1–2 mm progression/day slowing to less than 2 mm in 3 days. There is an opportunity in this group of patients to salvage the ongoing cycle through rLH supplementation. When compared with increasing r-hFSH dose, adding rLH on day 8 was associated with a better cumulative implantation rate (14.2 versus 10.5) and cumulative pregnancy rate (37.2 versus 29.3).[20,34,35]

There are recommendations for the use of LH supplementation in the ongoing cycle for patients with a history of prior poor response and patients who exhibit a suboptimal response during long agonist ovarian stimulation protocols. There is a possibility to optimize the ovarian response in both these patient groups through the addition of rLH.[20,34] Thus, LH supplementation seems appropriate for poor responders where it restored the follicular and endometrial milieu and improves the cycle outcome.

Advanced Reproductive Age

A recent systemic review and meta-analysis concluded that the inclusion of rLH to FSH stimulation enhanced the clinical pregnancy and implantation rates in ART cycles in patients aged greater than or equal to 35 years. Similar results were reported in many other randomized trials. Similarly, a Cochrane review reiterated the usefulness of rLH in poor responders and advanced aged women at risk of spontaneous miscarriage.[14,15,30,32]

A retrospective observational study evaluating ART patients undergoing stimulation with an antagonist procedure reported clinical pregnancy success of 36% for patients aged more than 38 years treated with r-hFSH and rLH compared with 19.1% for those stimulated with r-hFSH and hMG. An open-label randomized controlled study found that rLH is beneficial in improving the implantation rate in women aged from 36 to 39 years, but not so in those younger than 36 years of age. This might be due to the fact that the serum androgen levels decline steeply with age, as does the response to FSH stimulation. Change in LHRs of theca cells with age renders ovaries less sensitive to LH. Hence, exogenous LH administration enhances follicular androgen production followed by its aromatization to estrogen. It also controls progesterone production by granulosa cells, which is also FSH dependent **(Fig. 4)**.

Based on these clinical studies and personal clinical experience, starting adjuvant rLH on either day 1 of stimulation or day 6–8 may be beneficial in patients older than 35 years in long agonist or antagonist protocol ovarian stimulation. Monitoring of the response to add-back LH will depend on clinical tests and equipment available. The monitoring of follicular progression, estradiol concentrations and endometrial thickness as a clinical measure of LH response is suggested.[14,15]

FSH/LH Ratio

Day-3 gonadotropin and estradiol testing is typically included in the evaluation of ovarian reserve and the prediction of response to ovarian stimulation. Several

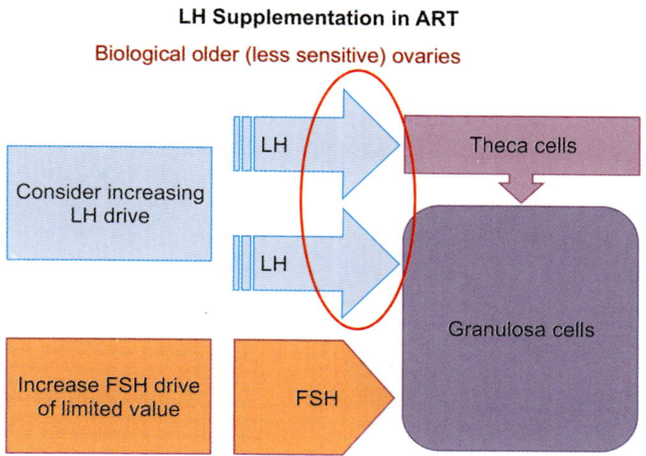

Fig. 4 Change in LH receptors of ovaries with advancing age

authors have proposed utilizing the basal FSH:LH ratio as a predictor of ovarian response and ART success. Some did not find any differences in outcomes between patients with an FSH:LH ratio greater than 3:1 versus those less than 3:1. This is in contrast to several other retrospective studies which have shown significantly better outcomes in patients with an FSH:LH ratio less than 3:1, with more oocytes retrieved, more metaphase-II oocytes, higher fertilization rates and increased pregnancy rates. Orvieto et al. retrospectively evaluated patients with FSH:LH ratios of more than 2:1 and less than 3:1 who had undergone treatment with two assisted cycles, once with an hMG-only protocol and once with rFSH-only protocol. When the hMG cycles were compared with rFSH cycles, the hMG cycles resulted in significantly higher peak estradiol, a higher oocyte maturity rate, better embryos, a higher implantation rate and a higher clinical pregnancy rate. However, these studies are retrospective, and there is no randomized controlled data to demonstrate if the use of LH is beneficial for patients with an elevated FSH:LH ratio. More research is required to determine if pre-cycle testing can yield predictors that identify patients most likely to benefit from additional exogenous LH.[36]

Polycystic Ovary Syndrome

The detrimental impact of this endocrinological disorder, which is linked to hypersecretion of LH and ovulatory dysfunction, is attributed to increased LH levels. Studies have found that such women are associated with poor fertilization, oocyte quality and embryo quality, which could be due to underlying mechanisms such as androgen excess induced by LH. However, contrary to previous belief, it was later demonstrated that hyperinsulinemia and not LH hypersecretion plays a vital role in polycystic ovary syndrome pathogenesis. Adding LH in this scenario would lead to ovarian hyperstimulation syndrome and hence LH should be avoided.[37] In practice, individual patient response should be assessed and LH may be added in hyporesponders or severely downregulated patients with caution.

Exogenous LH Supplementation in Asian Population

There are wide variations in ovarian response in patients so the treatment regimes tailored to individual patient phenotypes and based on sound paracrine principles are more likely to achieve positive outcomes. Asian assisted reproduction practitioners make use of both long agonist and antagonist protocols for ovarian stimulation. Published literature on the beneficial effects of exogenous LH in patients with previous suboptimal response or low baseline serum LH concentrations is more extensive in long agonist protocols.[20,34]

The recommendations based on literature review and expert opinion regarding exogenous LH apply mainly to the use of GnRH agonists **(Table 1)**. The evidence for addition of rLH to r-hFSH in antagonist protocols for ovarian stimulation is inconclusive and future studies are awaited.[18]

Dose and Timing of Initiation of r-hLH

The dose of r-hLH in hypogonadotropic hypogonadism patients as stated in the summary of product characteristics for r-hLH is 75 IU combined with 150 IU of r-hFSH, i.e. a 2:1 ratio of FSH to LH. In patients undergoing ART with prevention of LH surge using GnRH analogs, most of the published studies on the combination of rLH and r-hFSH in suboptimal responders used rLH doses of 75–150 IU daily combined with r-hFSH doses of 300–375 IU. While this dose is sufficient in hypogonadotropic patients, it is unclear if higher doses are optimal in assisted reproduction patients. The studies of normal assisted reproduction populations have failed to clearly demonstrate the ideal LH dose.

Studies suggest that a small percentage of women may require up to 225 IU of rLH/day subcutaneously, but high dose of rLH is also found to be immunogenic and well tolerated. To achieve an optimal benefit, Ramaraju et al. also suggest a dose of 75 IU/day of rLH for supplementation with r-hFSH.[35]

The widely used dosage is a ratio of 2:1 for FSH:LH, i.e. 150 IU:75 IU starting on day 1 or day 6 of stimulation, especially in hypogonadotropic hypogonadism patients and is an appropriate dose to drive follicular development, estradiol production and endometrial development. A study showed that the administration of rLH (75 IU/day for 4 days), 1 day before the beginning r-hFSH stimulation, offers some benefits in terms of clinical pregnancies when compared with the patients undergoing stimulation with r-hFSH alone.[18]

The timing of initiation of rLH in ovarian stimulation is inconsistent in practice. In some protocols, patients start on rLH from day 1 of stimulation and for others patients start on days 6–8. Currently, there is no evidence supporting either day 1 or day 6–8 for starting rLH. However, theoretically there may be a benefit to start patients on day 1 if a clinician wants to maximize the benefit of increased ovarian androgen production even

Table 1 Consensus on recommended use of luteinizing hormone (LH) in Asian women undergoing long gonadotropin-releasing hormone agonist protocols

Patient category	Indication
Substantial evidence of benefit of r-LH in addition to r-FSH	Known poor responders (oocyte count <4 in previous cycle)
	Mid-follicular (day 6) suboptimal response on long agoinst:
	1. No follicles > 10 mm
	2. Estradiol < 200 pg/mL
	3. Endometrial thickness < 6 mm
Some evidence of benefit of r-LH in addition to r-FSH	Age >35 years started on ovarian stimulation with either the long agonist or antagonist protocol
Further research needed to determine benefit of r-LH	Biomarkers, e.g. variant LH
	Low baseline serum LH < 1.2 IU/L
	Low antral follicle count
	Low anti-Müllerian hormone

though the cost may increase. LH supplementation from day 1 may increase circulating androgen concentrations, which in combination with FSH can act synergistically to promote FSH receptor mRNA expression, follicular development and steroidogenesis.[16-18]

Studies have also fortified that rLH in combination with FSH is better than hMG with FSH. This might be due to excessive or inconsistent LH activity from the hCG component in hMG that may affect oocyte maturation in the latter half of the ovarian stimulation cycle, giving rise to the differences in numbers of oocytes retrieved and success of pregnancy.

Concluding from the accumulated data, 75 IU LH is sufficient to develop follicles, estradiol and endometrial growth in even the most profoundly LH-suppressed patients. Further studies are required to determine if higher doses are beneficial or detrimental to follicular development and the endometrium.

■ CONCLUSION

The synergistic yet complex LH and FSH interactions are imperative for adequate follicular development, ovulation and endometrial advancement. According to the LH threshold concept, there is a minimum and maximum effective dose for LH. The LH therapeutic window is best observed in two patient groups, namely hypogonadotropic hypogonadism patients or LH polymorphism and patients who are profoundly suppressed by downregulation with either GnRH agonists or antagonists in ART. It is now recognized that with GnRH analog protocols in ovarian stimulation, levels of LH bioactivity in some patients (e.g. age >35 years) may be reduced to below the threshold and they may benefit from adjuvant rLH.

The best predictive factor for need of exogenous LH in ART is a prior poor or suboptimal response to ovarian stimulation. There is increasing evidence that age is an important marker of deficient LH bioactivity in women undergoing ART, with multiple studies showing benefit in women aged above 35 years. Another patient demographic that may benefit from adjuvant rLH in addition to r-hFSH are poor responders and women who exhibit suboptimal ovarian response during ovarian stimulation. These recommendations mostly apply to GnRH agonist protocols where there is substantial evidence for the use of adjuvant rLH.

Current evidence supports the use of hMG to improve outcomes in long GnRH agonist cycles. Data on using LH or hMG in GnRH antagonist cycles is currently limited, but substantial biological plausibility exists for LH supplement use in these cycles. This is due to the profound and rapid LH suppression that occurs at a time in follicle development dominated by LH activity. There is insufficient evidence to make definitive conclusions on the need for exogenous LH activity in GnRH antagonist cycles or the benefit of rLH and hCG protocols. The use of both rLH and hCG to supplement ovarian stimulation may be associated with a substantial increase in stimulation cost and therefore more studies are needed to establish benefit both in terms of outcomes and cost effectiveness.

The research in hypogonadotropic patients suggests that 75 IU of LH has demonstrable biological activity. However, studies have not established an optimal dose of LH or an optimal ratio of FSH:LH supplementation to maximize assisted reproduction outcomes. It is possible that such doses or ratios are patient specific and should be adjusted based on patient response to stimulation. Further research is indicated for development of variable FSH:LH ratio in drugs.

In conclusion, the importance of LH in the biological process of follicular development and oocyte maturation should not be forgotten. Biomarkers to ascertain women who are in need of exogenous LH need to be sought. Future research should focus on the benefits and cost effectiveness of rLH and hCG; and methods for identifying patients who are most likely to benefit from LH supplementation, either with pre-stimulation or intra-stimulation parameters.

■ MESSAGE BOX

There is a dilemma regarding the usefulness of LH supplementation in controlled ovarian stimulation despite growing understanding of the LH and FSH interrelation and their effects on fertilization and implantation. The use of r-hLH in COH should be guided by a rationale that is based on the individualized patient profile. The use of LH has been recommended in older patients (>35 years) as about 15–20% of women have less sensitive ovaries with increasing age. Poor responders, those with deeply suppressed endogenous LH like hypogonadotropic hypogonadism and patients with LH suppression during ART benefit from rLH supplementation. Hypo-responders where FSH and AFC is considered adequate at the start of the stimulation cycle seem to respond better with the addition of rLH. SNPs of LH-receptors should be considered in such patients. Further research is needed to identify adequate dosing, cost efficacy, need for rLH and hCG supplementation in different patient profiles for maximum benefit during controlled ovarian stimulation.

■ REFERENCES

1. Jeppesen JV1, Kristensen SG, Nielsen ME, et al. LHR gene expression in human granulosa cells. J Clin Endocrinol Metab. 2012,97(8):E1524-31.
2. McGee EA, Hsueh AJ. Initial and cyclic recruitment of ovarian follicles. Endocr Rev. 2000;21:200-14.
3. Chappel SC, Howles C. Reevaluation of the roles of luteinizing hormone and follicle stimulating hormone in the ovulatory process. Hum Reprod. 1991;6:1206-12.
4. Balasch J, Fábregues F. Is luteinizing hormone needed for optimal ovulation induction? Curr Opin Obest Gyncol. 2002;14(3):265-74.
5. Hillier SG. Gonadotropic control of ovarian follicular growth and development. Mol Cell Endocrinol. 2001;179:39-46.
6. Shoham Z. The clinical therapeutic window for luteinizing hormone in controlled ovarian stimulation. Fertil Steril. 2002;77(6):1170-7.
7. Shemesh M. Actions of gonadotrophins on the uterus. Reproduction. 2001;121:835-42.
8. Melmed S, Polonsky KS, Larsen PR, Kronenberg HM (Eds). Williams Textbook of Endocrinology, 12th edition. Philadelphia: Saunders Elsevier; 2011.
9. O'dea L, O'brien F, Currie K, et al. Follicular development induced by recombinant luteinizing hormone (LH) and follicle-stimulating hormone (FSH) in anovulatory women with LH and FSH deficiency: evidence of a threshold effect. Curr Med Res Opin. 2008;24:2785-93.
10. Filicori M. Use of luteinizing hormone in the treatment of infertility: time for reassessment? Fertil Steril. 2003;79:253-5.
11. van de Weijer BH, Mulders JW, Bos ES, et al. Compositional analyses of a human menopausal gonadotrophin preparation extracted from urine (menotropin). Identification of some of its major impurities. Reprod Biomed Online. 2003;7:547-57.
12. Al-Inany HG, Abou-Setta AM, Aboulghar MA, et al. Efficacy and safety of human menopausal gonadotrophins versus meta-analysis recombinant FSH: a meta-analysis. Reprod BioMed Online. 2008;16:81-8.
13. Coomarasamy A, Afnan M, Cheema D, et al. Urinary hMG versus recombinant FSH for controlled ovarian hyperstimulation following an agonist long down-regulation protocol in IVF or ICSI treatment: a systematic review and meta-analysis. Hum Reprod. 2008;23:310-5.
14. Bosch E, Labarta E, Crespo J, et al. Impact of luteinizing hormone administration on gonadotropin-releasing hormone antagonist cycles: an age-adjusted analysis. Fertil Steril. 2011; 95:1031-6.
15. Hill MJ, Levens ED, Levy G, et al. The use of recombinant luteinizing hormone in patients undergoing assisted reproductive techniques with advanced reproductive age: a systematic review and meta-analysis. Fertil Steril. 2012;97(5):1108-14.e1.
16. Recombinant human luteinizing hormone (LH) to support recombinant human follicle-stimulating hormone (FSH) induced follicular development in LH- and FSH-deficient anovulatory women: a dose-finding study. The European Recombinant Human LH Study Group. J Clin Endocrinol Metab. 1998;83(5):1507-14.
17. Ferraretti AP, Gianaroli L, Magli MC, et al. Exogenous luteinizing hormone in controlled ovarian hyperstimulation for assisted reproduction techniques. Fertil Steril. 2004;82(6): 1521-6.
18. Wong PC, Qiao J, Ho C, et al. Current opinion on use of luteinizing hormone supplementation in assisted reproduction therapy: an Asian perspective. Reprod Biomed Online. 2011;23(1):81-90.
19. Ruvolo G, Bosco L, Pane A, et al. Lower apoptosis rate in human cumulus cells after administration of recombinant luteinizing hormone to women undergoing ovarian stimulation for in vitro fertilization procedures. Fertil Steril. 2007;87(3):542-6.
20. Pezzuto A, Ferrari B, Coppola F, et al. LH supplementation in downregulated women undergoing assisted reproduction with baseline low serum LH levels. Gynecol Endocrinol. 2010;26(2):118-24.
21. Shoham Z, Smith H, Yeko T, et al. Recombinant LH (lutropin alfa) for the treatment of hypogonadotrophic women with profound LH deficiency: a randomized, double-blind, placebo-controlled, proof-of-efficacy study. Clin Endocrinol. 2008;69:471-8.
22. Andersen AN. Lack of association between endogenous LH and pregnancy in GnRH antagonist protocols. Reprod Biomed Online. 2011;23:692-94.
23. Grondahl ML, Borup R, Lee YB, et al. Differences in gene expression of granulosa cells from women undergoing controlled ovarian hyperstimulation with either recombinant follicle-stimulating hormone or highly purified human menopausal gonadotropin. Fertil Steril. 2009;91:1820-30.
24. Hugues JN, Soussis J, Calderon I, et al. On behalf of the Recombinant LH Study Group. Does the addition of recombinant LH in WHO group II anovulatory women over-responding to FSH treatment reduce the number of developing follicles? A dose-finding study. Hum Reprod. 2005;20:629-35.
25. Filicori M, Cognigni GE, Gamberini E, et al. Efficacy of low-dose human chorionic gonadotropin alone to complete controlled ovarian stimulation. Fertil Steril. 2005;84:394-401.
26. Baruffi R, Mauri AL, Petersen C, et al. Recombinant LH supplementation to recombinant FSH during induced ovarian stimulation in the GnRH-antagonist protocol: a meta-analysis. Reprod BioMed Online. 2007;14:14-25.
27. Kolibianakis EM, Kalogeropoulou L, Griesinger G, et al. Among patients treated with FSH and GnRH analogues for in vitro fertilization, is the addition of recombinant LH associated with the probability of live birth? A systematic review and meta- analysis. Hum Reprod Update. 2007;13:445-52.
28. Alviggi C, Clarizia R, Pettersson K, et al. Suboptimal response to GnRH a long protocol is associated with a common LH polymorphism. Reprod Biomed Online. 2009; 18(1):9-14.
29. Mafra FA, Bianco B, Christofolini DM, et al. Luteinizing hormone beta-subunit gene (LH beta) polymorphism in infertility and endometriosis-associated infertility. Eur J Obstet Gynecol Reprod Biol. 2010;151(1):66-9.
30. Humaidan P, Bungum L, Bungum M, et al. Ovarian response and pregnancy outcome related to mid-follicular LH levels in women undergoing assisted reproduction with GnRH agonist down-regulation and recombinant FSH stimulation. Hum Reprod. 2002;17(8):2016-21.

31. Acevedo B, Sanchez M, Gomez JL, et al. Luteinizing hormone supplementation increases pregnancy rates in gonadotropin-releasing hormone antagonist donor cycles. Fertil Steril. 2004;82:343-7.

32. Hill MJ, Levy G, Levens ED. Does exogenous LH in ovarian stimulation improve assisted reproduction success? An appraisal of the literature. Reprod Biomed Online. 2012;24(3):261-71.

33. Bosdou JK, Venetis CA, Kolibianakis EM, et al. The use of androgens or androgen-modulating agents in poor responders undergoing in vitro fertilization: a systematic review and meta-analysis. Hum Reprod Update. 2012;18(2):127-45.

34. De Placido G, Alviggi C, Perino A, et al. Italian Collaborative Group on Recombinant Human Luteinizing Hormone. Recombinant human LH supplementation versus recombinant human FSH (rFSH) step-up protocol during controlled ovarian stimulation in normogonadotrophic women with initial inadequate ovarian response to rFSH. A multicentre, prospective, randomized controlled trial. Hum Reprod. 2005;20:390-6.

35. Raju GA, Teng SC, Kavitha P, et al. Combination of recombinant follicle stimulating hormone with human menopausal gonadotrophin or recombinant luteinizing hormone in a long gonadotrophin-releasing hormone agonist protocol: a retrospective study. Reprod Med Biol. 2012;11:129-33.

36. Orvieto R, Meltzer S, Rabinson J, et al. Does day 3 luteinizing-hormone level predict IVF success in patients undergoing controlled ovarian stimulation with GnRH analogues? Fertil Steril. 2008;90:1297-300.

37. Rekha PS. Is LH necessary in ovulation induction? In: Desai S, Parihar M, Allahabadia G (Eds). Infertility: Principles and Practice. India: BI Publications Pvt Ltd; 2004. p. 5.

15 Stimulation Protocols for ART

Padma Rekha Jirge

INTRODUCTION

Controlled ovarian stimulation (COS) for *in vitro* fertilization (IVF) comprises of three important aspects—ovarian stimulation, pituitary suppression and ovulation triggering. Assisted reproductive technology (ART) has evolved over the past three decades in all these three aspects resulting in improvement in both efficacy and safety of treatment. This chapter looks at the various stimulation strategies to optimize the success rate in IVF in good or poor responders. Ovarian stimulation strategies in women with polycystic ovary syndrome (PCOS) have been discussed in a subsequent chapter.

The factors such as age of the woman, etiology of infertility, BMI and ovarian reserve are taken into consideration while choosing the most appropriate protocol for COS. Availability of choice in the stimulants and gonadotropin-releasing hormone (GnRH) analogs used for COS, and development of robust methods for assessing the ovarian reserve such as anti-Müllerian hormone and antral follicle count to predict ovarian response are some of the important milestones in the field of ART over the past two decades.

The primary aim of ovarian stimulation in IVF is to recruit an adequate cohort of follicles and consequently egg yield. It is understood that the follicles need to exceed the follicle-stimulating hormone (FSH) sensitivity threshold to be recruited during ovarian stimulation.[1] The factors influencing the number of antral follicles attaining FSH sensitivity include the size of the primordial follicle pool and factors promoting or controlling follicular growth and survival such as members of the transforming growth factor β family.[2] Further, the two cohorts of follicles observed in standard cycles of ART represent phenomena under different control mechanisms. Age appears to have no impact upon the initial response cohort, while insulin resistance promotes the size of this cohort. In contrast, the secondary cohort representing the follicles attaining FSH sensitivity on a daily basis is negatively influenced by age but unaffected by insulin resistance.[3]

OVARIAN STIMULATION

Even though IVF cycles were performed in natural cycles in the initial years, there is now a consensus that COS with gonadotropins is necessary to maintain the success rates in the recent years. The choice of gonadotropins includes urinary preparations such as human menopausal gonadotropins (hMG) [containing an equal amount of FSH and luteinizing hormone (LH)], highly purified hMG (hp-hMG), or highly purified urinary FSH (hp-uFSH) and recombinant FSH (rFSH). rFSH provides a reliable source of FSH with batch-to-batch consistency, a constant supply to meet the ever increasing demand and makes fine adjustments in the dose possible when necessary. Despite the concerns of a negative impact of profound suppression of LH when rFSH, which has no LH activity, is used for COS;[4] initial studies suggested a better clinical outcome with rFSH.[5] However, its efficacy in terms of improving ongoing pregnancy rate and live birth rate has remained controversial. Further comparison of hMG and rFSH as ovarian stimulants found no difference in the clinical outcomes except a reduction in the total requirement of gonadotropin with hMG.[6] A recent meta-analysis has reported a better live birth rate with hp-hMG.[7] The beneficial effect of hMG on oocyte maturation and embryo quality is attributed to the LH activity present in it or the difference in the isoforms of FSH.[8] The most recent Cochrane Database Review comparing different FSH preparations, including more than 9,000 women concluded that any substantive differences in efficacy or safety between rFSH and urinary FSH preparations is unlikely to be identified with further research.[9] Further, a cost-effective analysis has shown that highly purified urinary FSH is more cost effective compared to rFSH with similar live birth rates.[10] Hence, the choice of FSH preparation should include consideration for the availability and the cost factor. Both highly purified FSH/hMG preparations and rFSH are administered subcutaneously and does not require a daily visit to the doctor. Availability of recombinant LH has led to attempts to use it in routine clinical practice in protocols using rFSH for ovarian stimulation. However, the evidence at present does not show an improvement in pregnancy or live birth rate and its routine use cannot be recommended.[11,12]

Corifollitropin alfa is a long acting hybrid molecule of rFSH devoid of any LH activity, with a half-life of 65 hours. A single injection is sufficient to replace the first 7 days of daily injections. Corifollitropin alfa in combination with daily GnRH antagonist seems to be an alternative for daily rFSH injections in normal responder patients undergoing ovarian stimulation in IVF/intracytoplasmic sperm injection (ICSI) treatment cycles.[13] Limited availability, and cost factors have precluded its widespread use.

Gonadotropin-releasing Hormone Analogs

Gonadotropin-releasing hormone analogs, both agonists and antagonists, have played a vital role in improving both efficacy and safety of IVF. Their primary role remains prevention of premature rise in LH, which occurs due to a supraphysiological levels of estradiol (E2) in COS in up to 20% of COS cycles. GnRH agonists have been used for pituitary downregulation since 1980s. It is also understood that in addition to pituitary downregulation, and consequent reduction in the incidence of cycle cancelation, they improve the number of oocytes retrieved due to their role in recruitment of follicles. The antagonists do not influence the follicle recruitment as they do not have the flare-up effect of agonists and have proven to be a safer alternative in women with PCOS who are hyper-responders. In the current scenario, where the emphasis is on individualized protocols, various protocols incorporating the analogs are in use, and they will be reviewed in the following section:

Gonadotropin-releasing Hormone Agonist Long Protocol

The most widely used protocol in good responders has been the long protocol **(Fig. 1)**.[14] In addition to the aforementioned benefits, scheduling the IVF cycles becomes convenient without compromising the results. The downregulation commences in mid-luteal phase (day 21–24) of the cycle prior to ovarian stimulation and continues along with stimulation till the day of hCG.[15] Most often, agonists are administered as daily intranasal spray or subcutaneous injections. Injections are preferred to nasal spray in tropical countries in view of the common problem of nasal allergies and stability of the molecules. Depot preparation offers a convenient single dose with prolonged effect; however, they increase the duration of stimulation and the total FSH requirement. Once the downregulation is achieved (usually in 10–14 days)

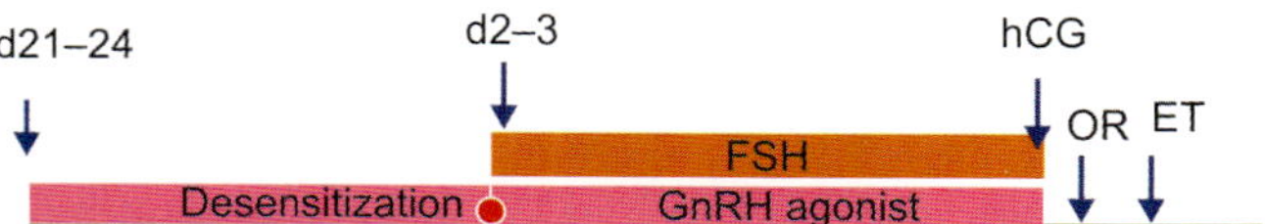

Fig. 1 Schematic representation of long agonist protocol

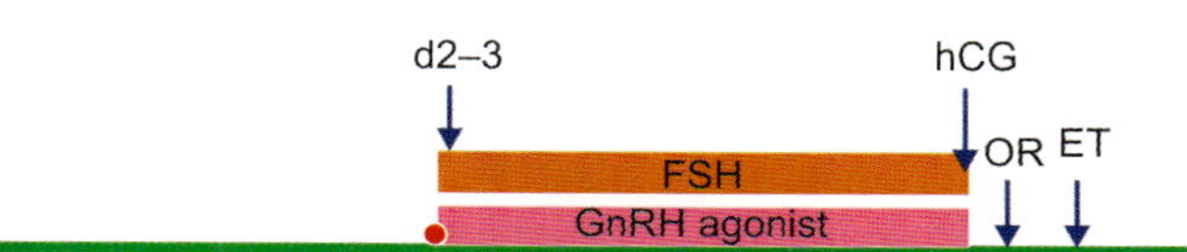

Fig. 2 Schematic representation of short agonist protocol

confirmed by ultrasonography and low serum LH, E2 and progesterone levels, stimulation is initiated with either hMG or rFSH. The standard starting dose used is 225 IU and any changes effected after 5–6 days of stimulation in correlation with the ovarian response as assessed by TVS and/or endocrine parameters. The average duration of stimulation is 9–10 days and ovulation trigger is administered when at least three leading follicles are of 18 mm diameter.

Short Agonist (Flare-up) Protocol

Any modifications of long protocol are usually applied in the clinical scenario of poor responders. The profound suppression achieved with long protocol adds to the difficulty in stimulating ovaries in women with poor ovarian reserve and to the total dose of gonadotropins required for ovarian stimulation, and thus to the cost of treatment without improving the outcome. In the short protocol, the daily GnRH agonist administration is commenced from day 2–3 of the treatment cycle in conjunction with the FSH, so that the patient benefits from the initial flare-up of endogenous FSH and LH that may "jump start" the follicles, in addition to the action of exogenous gonadotropin **(Fig. 2)**.[16] The daily dose of FSH is 300–450 IU. Higher doses do not improve the oocyte yield or clinical outcome. The use of short protocol does not adversely affect the outcome when compared to long agonist or antagonist protocols in poor responders. Other variations of agonist protocols including ultra-short or stop agonist protocol are not widely used as they are not very effective in preventing the premature luteinization of follicles.

Antagonist Protocols

Antagonists act by competitive inhibition of GnRH receptors on gonadotrophs. Their effect is immediate in comparison to agonists, and they have a relatively short half-life. They have been used under all the clinical scenario of good, poor or excessive ovarian response. The various protocols used are either single dose (3 mg) cetrorelix administered on day 5 of stimulation, multiple dose fixed protocol (0.25 mg of cetrorelix or ganirelix daily from day 5 till the day of ovulation trigger) or multiple dose flexible protocol, where day of commencing antagonist administration depends on the follicular diameter and serum E2 concentrations. Current evidence shows that in good responders there is no difference in the live birth rate whether antagonist or agonist is used. However, the duration of treatment and gonadotropin requirement is reduced with antagonist treatment.[17] Reduction in number of oocytes retrieved in antagonist cycles and its impact on cumulative pregnancy rate including both fresh and frozen-thawed cycles is unknown at present. The clinical outcome with antagonist protocols is comparable to short agonist protocol in poor responders **(Fig. 3)**.[18] It is a safer alternative to agonist protocol in hyper-responders as it reduces the risk of ovarian hyperstimulation syndrome (OHSS) in this subgroup of women.[17]

Mild or Minimal Stimulation IVF

Over the past decade, efforts have been made to introduce more patient friendly options of ovarian stimulation for poor responders and reduce the cost of treatment in both good and poor responders. This has led to exploration of various protocols under the broad title of mild stimulation.

Mild stimulation protocols use oral ovulogens alone or more commonly in combination with FSH and antagonist. Use of clomiphene citrate (CC) throughout follicular phase with late start of FSH is increasingly used in clinics offering mild stimulation IVF. Continuous use of CC serves the dual purpose of recruitment of follicles as well as prevention of premature rise in LH. Such a protocol necessitates vitrification of all embryos followed by transfer in a subsequent cycle. The low numbers of oocytes, increased risk of cancellation, and need for accepting a low pregnancy rate per started cycle and need for more completed cycles to achieve similar PR to conventional IVF are some of the important limitations of mild stimulation IVF.[19]

■ CONCLUSION

Controlled ovarian stimulation is an integral part of IVF and has contributed to the improved clinical outcome in IVF. Use of gonadotropins to influence the oocyte yield necessitates use of GnRH analogs to prevent premature rise in LH due to supraphysiological rise in E2. Agonists have been in use for over three decades now and in the recent years, antagonists have proven to be invaluable in prevention of clinically significant OHSS associated with IVF. The use of mild stimulation protocols is limited at present due to a low pregnancy rate in comparison to conventional protocols.

■ REFERENCES

1. Baird DT. Factors regulating the growth of the pre-ovulatory follicle in sheep and humans. J Reprod Fertil. 1983;69:343-52.
2. Hussein MR. Apoptosis in the ovary: molecular mechanisms. Hum Reprod Update. 2005;11:162-77.
3. Fleming R, Deshpande N, Traynor I, et al. Dynamics of FSH-induced follicular growth in subfertile women: relationship with age, insulin resistance, oocyte yield and anti-Mullerian hormone. Hum Reprod. 2006;21(6):1436-41.
4. Fleming R, Rehka P, Deshpande N, et al. Suppression of LH during ovarian stimulation effects differ in cycles stimulated with purified urinary FSH and recombinant FSH. Hum Reprod. 2000;15:1440-5.
5. Daya S. Updated meta-analysis of recombinant follicle-stimulating hormone (FSH) versus urinary FSH for ovarian stimulation in assisted reproduction. Fertil Steril. 2002;77(4):711-4.
6. Al-Inany H, Aboulghar MA, Mansour RT, et al. Ovulation induction in the new millennium: recombinant follicle-stimulating hormone versus human menopausal gonado-tropin. Gynecol Endocrinol. 2005;20(3):161-9.
7. Coomarasamy A, Afnan M, Cheema D, et al. Urinary hMG versus recombinant FSH for controlled ovarian hyperstimulation following an agonist long down-regulation protocol in IVF or ICSI treatment: a systematic review and meta-analysis. Hum Reprod. 2008;23(2):310-5.

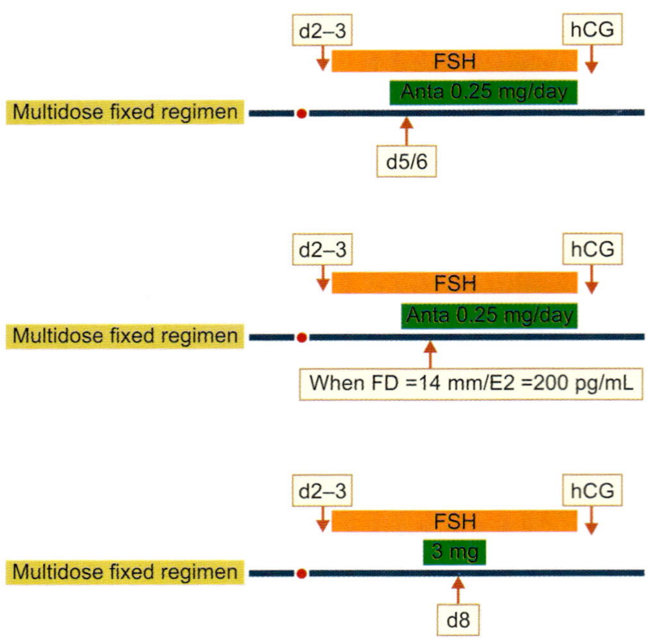

Fig. 3 Schematic representation of antagonist protocols

8. Selman HA, Santo M, Sterzik K, et al. Effect of highly purified urinary follicle-stimulating hormone on oocyte and embryo quality. Fertil Steril. 2002;78:1061-7.

9. van Wely M, Kwan I, Burt AL, et al. Recombinant versus urinary gonadotrophin for ovarian stimulation in assisted reproductive technology cycles. Cochrane Database Syst Rev. 2011;(2):CD005354.

10. Gerli S, Bini V, Favilli A, et al. Clinical efficacy and cost-effectiveness of HP-human FSH (Fostimon®) versus rFSH (Gonal-F®) in IVF-ICSI cycles: a meta-analysis. Gynecol Endocrinol. 2013;29(6):520-9.

11. Franco JG Jr, Baruffi RL, Oliveira JB, et al. Effects of recombinant LH supplementation to recombinant FSH during induced ovarian stimulation in the GnRH-agonist protocol: a matched case-control study. Reprod Biol Endocrinol. 2009;7:58.

12. Bosch E, Labarta E, Crespo J, et al. Impact of luteinizing hormone administration on gonadotropin-releasing hormone antagonist cycles: an age-adjusted analysis. Fertil Steril. 2011;95(3):1031-6.

13. Mahmoud Youssef MA, van Wely M, Aboulfoutouh I, et al. Is there a place for corifollitropin alfa in IVF/ICSI cycles? A systematic review and meta-analysis. Fertil Steril. 2012;97(4): 876-85.

14. Macklon NS, Stouffer RL, Giudice LC, et al. The science behind 25 years of ovarian stimulation for in vitro fertilization. Endocr Rev. 2006;27:170-207.

15. Balasch J. GnRH agonist protocols: which one to use? In: Shoham Z, Jacobs HS, Howles CM (Eds). Female Infertility Therapy: Current Practice. London, UK: Martin Dunitz Ltd; 1998. pp. 89-203.

16. Loutradis D, Vomvolaki E, Drakakis P. Poor responder protocols for in-vitro fertilization: options and results. Curr Opin Obstet Gynecol. 2008;20:374-8.

17. Al-Inany HG, Youssef MA, Aboulghar M, et al. Gonadotrophin-releasing hormone antagonists for assisted reproductive technology. Cochrane Database Syst Rev. 2011;(5):CD001750.

18. Kyrou D, Kolibianakis EM, Venetis CA, et al. How to improve the probability of pregnancy in poor responders undergoing in vitro fertilization: a systematic review and meta-analysis. Fertil Steril. 2009;91(3):749-66.

19. Revelli A, Casano S, Salvagno F, et al. Milder is better? Advantages and disadvantages of "mild" ovarian stimulation for human in vitro fertilization. Reprod Biol Endocrinol. 2011;9:25.

16 | Stimulation Protocols for Polycystic Ovarian Syndrome in ART

Padma Rekha Jirge

INTRODUCTION

Polycystic ovarian syndrome (PCOS) is the most common cause of anovulatory infertility.[1] Majority of women with PCOS conceive with clomiphene, aromatase inhibitors or superovulation with gonadotropins with or without intrauterine insemination (IUI). However, a proportion of women with PCOS need to undergo assisted reproductive technique (ART) either because they fail to achieve pregnancy with simpler forms of treatment or because of presence of concomitant factors necessitating in vitro fertilization (IVF).[2] Even though IVF effectively has reduced the risk of high order multiple pregnancies, the risk of ovarian hyperstimulation syndrome (OHSS) still remains real. PCOS ovaries contain a larger cohort of follicle-stimulating hormone (FSH) sensitive follicles compared to normal responders.[3] In addition, in women with insulin resistant PCOS, antral follicles maintain their FSH sensitivity longer than controls before proceeding to atresia, leading to an enlarged stockpile and excessive responses to exogenous FSH.[4] Administration of any dose of FSH higher than the threshold of such ovaries leads to recruitment of a large cohort of follicles, and hence an increased risk of OHSS. Hence, any stimulation protocol used for IVF in the context of PCOS should incorporate measures to improve the safety of treatment to prevent OHSS without compromising the pregnancy outcome.

OVARIAN STIMULATION IN IVF

Choosing the effective starting dose of FSH plays a crucial role in influencing the ovarian response in PCOS. Rotterdam criteria are the most widely used method for the diagnosis of PCOS.[5] Increasingly, anti-Müllerian hormone (AMH) is being used as marker for diagnosing PCOS and to choose the appropriate ovarian stimulation regime.[6] Factors such as age, BMI and clinical response in a previous IVF cycle are taken into consideration while choosing the initial dose of gonadotropin. It is a common practice to start ovarian stimulation with a lower than normal dose of FSH, i.e. 150 IU in non-obese women with PCOS and modify the dose based on the clinical response. However, obesity may necessitate commencing the stimulation with higher doses of 200–225 IU.[7]

Most widely used gonadotropin preparation for ovarian stimulation in PCOS is recombinant FSH (rFSH). This provides the advantages of batch-to-batch consistency and making minute adjustments in the dose feasible. Even though, it is believed that use of rFSH is beneficial because of lack of luteinizing hormone (LH) in it, in a condition associated with high basal LH, there is no clinical evidence to substantiate that FSH is better than human menopausal gonadotropin (hMG). There appears to be no difference in the pregnancy rate between hMG, urinary and rFSH. However, a reduction in possible OHSS is attributed to the use of rFSH.[8]

Transvaginal ultrasonography is the mainstay of cycle monitoring in those undergoing IVF. However, as serum E2 concentration is a good predictor of OHSS, endocrine monitoring is necessary to improve the safety of IVF in women with IVF.

PREVENTION OF PREMATURE LUTEINIZATION

One of the drawbacks of controlled ovarian stimulation with multiple follicular developments is the occurrence of premature luteinization of follicles. Gonadotropin-releasing hormone (GnRH) agonists have been successfully used for more than three decades to effectively reduce the incidence of premature luteinization. However, the role of GnRH agonists in enhancing the risk of OHSS by increasing the size of the recruited follicular cohort is now well understood, and hence their use is abandoned in the context of PCOS.[9] It is now almost a universal practice to incorporate GnRH antagonist into

IVF protocols in PCOS.[10-12] Most widely used protocols involve a lower commencing dose of rFSH followed by assessment of ovarian response on day 5 of the stimulation by transvaginal sonography. In multiple dose flexible protocol, GnRH antagonist is administered daily from day 5 or 6 until and inclusive of the day of ovulation triggers.[13] Cetrorelix or ganirelix are the two available antagonists and are administered subcutaneously at a daily dose of 0.25 mg. However, a single dose protocol may also be used, wherein a single 3 mg dose of antagonist is administered on 7th or 8th stimulation day. For individuals in whom the development of follicles does not qualify for oocyte retrieval 96 hours subsequent to a 3 mg cetrorelix injection, a further 0.25 mg of antagonist is administered on a daily basis until the day of human chorionic gonadotropin (hCG) administration.[14] Once 2–3 follicles reach a diameter of 18 mm, ovulation trigger is administered followed by ovum pickup 36 hours later.

Certain strategies are used in conjunction with antagonist protocols to improve the cycle outcome and reduce the risk of OHSS in women with PCOS. These are discussed in the following sections:

■ PRETREATMENT

Use of antagonist protocols in IVF has brought forth the problem of suboptimal synchronization of follicles during stimulation. In an effort to overcome this, oral contraceptive pills (OCP) and more recently, natural estrogens and synthetic progesterone have been used as "pretreatment" to influence the endogenous steroid dynamics. OCP used to aid in scheduling of the cycle, primarily inhibit FSH secretion. A combined OCP is administered from cycle day 2–3 daily for 15–21 days. Recent evidence shows that OCP pretreatment in antagonist cycles may be detrimental to the cycle outcome.[15-17] Limited evidence shows that pretreatment with natural estrogens improves follicle synchronization in antagonist treated cycles.[18] Micronized estradiol is administered daily for 10 days, commencing 10 days prior to presumed menses in a twice daily dose of 2 mg. Norethisterone 10–15 mg/day is the most commonly used synthetic progesterone as pretreatment, for scheduling the cycle and it acts by suppression of basal LH secretion. No data is available on any impact on cycle outcome when progesterone is used as pretreatment in antagonist cycles. However, they are shown to be beneficial in agonist cycles.[17] Stimulation usually is commenced after a five day washout period for OCP and synthetic progesterone and a shorter wash out period of 1–2 days may be sufficient when natural estrogen is used, to achieve an ideal basal FSH and LH levels.[19]

■ METFORMIN AS AN ADJUVANT WITH GONADOTROPINS IN IVF

The role of metformin in women with PCOS undergoing IVF is not well understood. However, the available evidence suggests that metformin given for 4–6 weeks prior to IVF, in a divided daily dose of 1000–1500 mg, metformin use is associated with a better yield of mature oocytes, reduction in the number of small follicles, an improvement in fertilization and pregnancy rates. In addition, a reduction in the follicular fluid levels of insulin-like growth factor has been documented.[20] A study involving women who needed coasting, metformin co-treatment reduced the days of coasting and achieved lower peak E2 levels. Both these parameters had a positive impact on fertilization and pregnancy rate.[21] Reduction in the number of small follicles may contribute to a reduction in the incidence of OHSS.

■ OVULATION TRIGGER

Human chorionic gonadotropin—either 250 µg of recombinant hCG or 10,000 IU of urinary hCG is the most widely used ovulation trigger, when the leading follicle diameter reaches 18 mm. However, it is known that hCG triggers a cascade of events resulting in early onset OHSS in those at a high risk of developing this complication. American Society for Reproductive Medicine (ASRM) practice committee has suggested certain guidelines to identify those at high risk of OHSS and those who may benefit by avoiding hCG administration, i.e. those with rapidly increasing E2 levels, peak E2 more than 2,500 pg/mL and emergence of a large number of intermediate sized follicles.[22] In such women, administration of GnRH agonist as ovulation trigger is an effective alternative to achieve oocyte maturation.[23-27] Single subcutaneous dose of triptorelin 0.2 mg or leuprolide 1 mg is used for this purpose. It is important to note that GnRH agonist leads to severe compromise in luteal phase events. Hence, freeze all policy or single embryo transfer with intense luteal phase management with both estrogen and progesterone supplementation and consideration for small bolus doses of hCG, all need to be considered for rescuing the luteal phase and safe management of the clinical situation.[28] This also necessitates availability of a robust embryo-freezing program in the unit.

■ COASTING

Coasting is a strategy of withholding gonadotropin administration while continuing GnRH agonist, resulting in a drop in the serum estradiol and consequently risk of OHSS.[29] Coasting acts by reducing the vascular endothelial growth factor levels. It is considered when serum E2 concentration reaches greater than 3,000 pg/mL or when more than 10 follicles are growing in each ovary, with the leading follicular diameter of 16–18 mm. hCG is administered once E2 level falls below 3,000 pg/mL. The reported duration of coasting has ranged from 1 day to 11 days.[30] Coasting in antagonist treated cycles has been attempted and is shown to have no detrimental impact on cycle outcome.[31] However, there is some evidence that coasting for more than 4 days may lead to a reduction in the fertilization and pregnancy rates.[32]

IN VITRO MATURATION OF OOCYTES

It has been long realized that ovarian stimulation with gonadotropins increases the risk of OHSS. Use of GnRH agonists further worsens this risk. Prior to the availability of antagonists for clinical use, *in vitro* maturation (IVM) provided a safe alternative to conventional gonadotropin stimulation. IVM involves retrieval of immature oocytes and maturing them in culture media usually containing small amounts of FSH and hCG, for 24–48 hours following oocyte retrieval. Intracytoplasmic sperm injection (ICSI) is the most common procedure used to fertilize in vitro matured oocytes, even though IVF is found to be effective too. IVM can be done in a natural cycle without any ovarian stimulation.[33] However, priming with small doses of FSH[34] or hCG[35] or a combination of the two[36] and retrieval 36 hours later are also frequently used. When FSH is used, 75–150 IU is administered for 3–6 days from day 3 and transvaginal ultrasound monitoring is performed to rule out development of any dominant follicle. Oocyte retrieval is performed 3–4 days after the last dose of FSH. hCG is administered depending on endometrial thickness and day of the cycle (day 9–14) and oocyte retrieval is performed 36 hours later. When hCG priming is used, it is common to find a combination of metaphase II, metaphase I and germinal vesicle oocytes. Metaphase II oocytes are treated with conventional IVF or ICSI, and embryo transfer is performed in the usual manner. Immature oocytes are cultured for 24–48 hours to achieve maturation and subsequently ICSI is performed. Resulting embryos can then be cryopreserved for future use. IVM necessitates skills to retrieve eggs form small follicles, ability to identify small cumulus-oophorus-complex, novel culture system for IVM of immature oocytes. Lower pregnancy rates, lower fertilization rate and concerns regarding health of offspring have been the limitations of IVM. Repeated failures of conventional IVF, a very-high risk of clinically significant OHSS may still necessitate IVM for some women undergoing IVF.

CONCLUSION

Ovarian stimulation for IVF in women with PCOS is challenging, as the ovarian response is not predictable. Starting with a lower than normal dose of FSH and use of antagonists instead of agonists have reduced the risk of OHSS, but by no means eliminated. Incorporation of antagonists into stimulation protocol improves the safety of ovarian stimulation in women with PCOS as unlike agonists, antagonists do not have any impact on the follicular recruitment. Coasting for a short duration and use of GnRH agonist instead of hCG for ovulation trigger are other measures to minimize the risk of early onset OHSS. However, GnRH agonist trigger necessitates either freezing of all embryos or intense management and rescue of luteal phase with a combination of estrogen and progesterone supplement, and at times, small boluses of hCG in addition. Even though, routine use of metformin for ovulation induction in PCOS is not recommended, its use in IVF may improve the pregnancy outcome. IVM eliminates the risk of OHSS completely when performed on unstimulated ovaries. Its application has remained limited with the advent of antagonists and other strategies mentioned above. With the use of AMH to identify hyper-responders, the stimulation strategies used for women with PCOS is now being extended for all excessive responders. At present, key to successful outcome in women with PCOS undergoing IVF remains highly individualized management.

REFERENCES

1. Balen AH, Conway GS, Kaltsas G, et al. Polycystic ovary syndrome: the spectrum of the disorder in 1741 patients. Hum Reprod. 1995;10:2107-11.
2. Homburg R. The management of infertility associated with polycystic ovary syndrome. Reprod Biol Endocrinol. 2003;1:109.
3. Van der Meer M, Hompes P, de Boer J, et al. Cohort size rather than follicle-stimulating hormone threshold levels determines ovarian sensitivity in polycystic ovary syndrome. J Clin Endocrinol Metab. 1988;83:423-6.
4. Fleming R, Deshpande N, Traynor I, et al. Dynamics of FSH-induced follicular growth in subfertile women: relationship with age, insulin resistance, oocyte yield and anti-Mullerian hormone. Hum Reprod. 2006;21(6):1436-41.
5. Rotterdam ESHRE/ASRM-Sponsored PCOS Consensus Workshop Group. Revised 2003 consensus on diagnostic criteria and long-term health risks related to polycystic ovary syndrome. Fertil Steril. 2004;81(1):19-25.
6. Lauritsen MP, Bentzen JG, Pinborg A, et al. The prevalence of polycystic ovary syndrome in a normal population according to the Rotterdam criteria versus revised criteria including anti-Mullerian hormone. Hum Reprod. 2014;29(4):791-801.

7. Kolibianakis E, Zikopoulos K, Albano C, et al. Reproductive outcome of polycystic ovarian syndrome patients treated with GnRH antagonists and recombinant FSH for IVF/ICSI. Reprod Biomed Online. 2003;7(3):313-8.

8. Al-Inany HG, Abou-Setta AM, Aboulghar MA, et al. Efficacy and safety of human menopausal gonadotrophins versus recombinant FSH: a meta-analysis. Reprod Biomed Online. 2008;16(1):81-8.

9. Hughes E, Collins J, Vandekerckhove P. Gonadotrophin-releasing hormone analogue as an adjunct to gonadotropin therapy for clomiphene-resistant polycystic ovarian syndrome. Cochrane Database Syst Rev. 2000;(2):CD000097.

10. Elkind-Hirsch KE, Webster BW, Brown CP, et al. Concurrent ganirelix and follitropin beta therapy is an effective and safe regimen for ovulation induction in women with polycystic ovary syndrome. Fertil Steril. 2003;79:603-7.

11. Fatemi HM, Doody K, Griesinger G, et al. High ovarian response does not jeopardize ongoing pregnancy rates and increases cumulative pregnancy rates in a GnRH-antagonist protocol. Hum Reprod. 2013;28(2):442-52.

12. Nelson SM, Yates RW, Lyall H, et al. Anti-Müllerian hormone-based approach to controlled ovarian stimulation for assisted conception. Hum Reprod. 2009;24(4):867-75.

13. Mansour RT, Aboulghar MA, Serour GI, et al. The use of gonadotropin-releasing hormone antagonist in a flexible protocol: a pilot study. Am J Obstet Gynecol. 2003;189(2):444-6.

14. Olivennes F, Belaisch-Allart J, Emperaire JC, et al. Prospective, randomized, controlled study of in vitro fertilization-embryo transfer with a single dose of a luteinizing hormone-releasing hormone (LH-RH) antagonist (cetrorelix) or a depot formula of an LH-RH agonist (triptorelin). Fertil Steril. 2000;73:314-20.

15. Kolibianakis EM, Papanikolaou EG, Camus M, et al. Oral contraceptive pill pretreament on ongoing pregnancy rates in patients stimulated with GnRH antagonists and recombinant FSH for IVF. A randomized controlled trial. Hum Reprod. 2006;21:352-7.

16. Rombauts L, Healy D, Norman RJ, On behalf of the Orgalutran Scheduling Study Group. A comparative randomized trial to assess the impact of oral contraceptive pretreatment on follicular growth and hormone profiles in GnRH antagonist-treated patients. Hum Reprod. 2006;21:95-103.

17. Smulders B, van Oirschot SM, Farquhar C, et al. Oral contraceptive pill, progestogen or estrogen pre-treatment for ovarian stimulation protocols for women undergoing assisted reproductive techniques. Cochrane Database Syst Rev. 2010; 20(1):CD006109.

18. Fanchin R, Cunha-Filho JS, Schonauer LM, et al. Coordination of early antral follicles by luteal estradiol administration provides a basis for alternative controlled ovarian hyper-stimulation regimens. Fertil Steril. 2003a;79:316-21.

19. Cédrin-Durnerin I, Bständig B, Parneix I, et al. Effects of oral contraceptive, synthetic progestogen or natural estrogen pre-treatments on the hormonal profile and the antral follicle cohort before GnRH antagonist protocol. Hum Reprod. 2007;22(1):109-16.

20. Stadtmauer LA, Toma SK, Riehl RM, et al. Metformin treatment of patients with polycystic ovary syndrome undergoing in vitro fertilization improves outcomes and is associated with modulation of the insulin-like growth factors. Fertil Steril. 2001;75:505-9.

21. Stadtmauer LA, Toma SK, Riehl RM, et al. The impact of metformin on ovarian stimulation and outcome in coasted patients with polycystic ovary syndrome undergoing in-vitro fertilization. RBM Online. 2002;5:112-6.

22. The Practice Committee of the American Society for Reproductive Medicine (ASRM): Ovarian hyperstimulation syndrome. Fertil Steril. 2008;90:S188-S193.

23. Griesinger G, Diedrich K, Devroey P, et al. GnRH agonist for triggering final oocyte maturation in the GnRH antagonist ovarian hyperstimulation protocol: a systematic review and meta-analysis. Hum Reprod Update. 2006;12:159-68.

24. Orvieto R, Rabinson J, Meltzer S, et al. Substituting HCG with GnRH agonist to trigger final follicular maturation–a retrospective comparison of three different ovarian stimulation protocols. Reprod Biomed Online. 2006;13:198-201.

25. Engmann L, DiLuigi A, Schmidt D, et al. The use of gonadotropin-releasing hormone (GnRH) agonist to induce oocyte maturation after cotreatment with GnRH antagonist in high-risk patients undergoing in vitro fertilization prevents the risk of ovarian hyperstimulation syndrome: a prospective randomised controlled study. Fertil Steril. 2008;89:84-91.

26. Griesinger G, Schultz L, Bauer T, et al. Ovarian hyperstimulation syndrome prevention by gonadotropin-releasing hormone agonist triggering of final oocyte maturation in a gonadotropin-releasing hormone antagonist protocol in combination with a 'freeze-all' strategy: a prospective multicentric study. Fertil Steril. 2011;95:2029-33.

27. Kol S, Humaidan P. GnRH agonist triggering: recent developments. Reprod Biomed Online. 2013;26:226-30.

28. Humaidan P, Papanikolaou EG, Kyrou D, et al. The luteal phase after GnRH-agonist triggering of ovulation: present and future perspectives. Reprod Biomed Online. 2012;24:134-41.

29. Mansour R, Aboulghar M, Serour G, et al. Criteria of a successful coasting protocol for the prevention of severe ovarian hyperstimulation syndrome. Hum Reprod. 2005;20:3167-72.

30. Delvigne A, Rozenberg S. A qualitative systematic review of coasting, a procedure to avoid ovarian hyperstimulation syndrome in IVF patients. Hum Reprod Update. 2002;8:291-6.

31. Farhi J, Ben-Haroush A, Lande Y, et al. In vitro fertilization cycle outcome after coasting in gonadotropin-releasing hormone (GnRH) agonist versus GnRH antagonist protocols. Fertil Steril. 2009;91:377-82.

32. Moreno L, Diaz I, Pacheco A, et al. Extended coasting duration exerts a negative impact on IVF cycle outcome due to premature luteinization. Reprod Biomed Online. 2004;9:500-4.

33. Cha KY, Han SY, Chung HM, et al. Pregnancies and deliveries after in vitro maturation culture followed by in vitro fertilization and embryo transfer without stimulation in women with polycystic ovary syndrome. Fertil Steril. 2000;73:978-83.

34. Mikkelsen AL, Andersson AM, Skakkebaek NE, et al. Basal concentrations of oestradiol may predict the outcome of in-vitro maturation in regularly menstruating women. Hum Reprod. 2001;16:862-7.

35. Chian RC, Buckett WM, Tulandi T, et al. Prospective randomized study of human chorionic gonadotrophin priming before immature oocyte retrieval from unstimulated women with polycystic ovarian syndrome. Hum Reprod. 2000;15:165-70.

36. Lin YH, Hwang JJ, Huang LW, et al. Combination of FSH priming and HCG priming for in-vitro maturation of human oocytes. Hum Reprod. 2003;18:1632-6.

17 GnRH Agonists and Antagonists in Assisted Reproduction

Pratap Kumar

■ INTRODUCTION

In vitro fertilization (IVF) involves a sequence of highly coordinated steps beginning with controlled ovarian hyperstimulation with exogenous gonadotropins, followed by retrieval of oocytes from the ovaries under transvaginal ultrasound guidance, fertilization in the laboratory, and transcervical transfer of embryos into the uterus. The ideal ovarian stimulation regimen for IVF should have a low cancelation rate, minimize drug costs, risks and side effects, require limited monitoring for practical convenience and maximize singleton pregnancy rates. Luteinizing hormone (LH) levels can rise prematurely without control and hence ovulation may occur before oocyte pickups are done or there may be premature luteinization and poor implantation. Moreover, evidence indicates that increased LH exposure during early follicular development may be detrimental and predispose to lower pregnancy rates. Hence, the importance of understanding the role of gonadotropin-releasing hormone (GnRH) analogs with agonist and antagonist protocol for better outcome.

■ EXOGENOUS GONADOTROPIN STIMULATION AFTER DOWNREGULATION WITH A LONG-ACTING GnRH AGONIST: LONG PROTOCOLS

The introduction of long-acting GnRH agonists in the late 1980s revolutionized the approach to ovarian stimulation in assisted reproductive technology (ART) by providing the means to downregulate endogenous pituitary gonadotropin secretion, and thereby prevents a premature LH surge during exogenous gonadotropin stimulation. Adjuvant treatment with a GnRH agonist eliminated the need for frequent serum LH measurements and assuaged fears of premature luteinization, which previously had necessitated cancelation of approximately 20% of all IVF cycles before oocyte retrieval. Because fewer than 2% of cycles are complicated by a premature LH surge after downregulation with a GnRH agonist, stimulation could continue until follicles were larger and more mature. Clinical trials subsequently demonstrated that egg yields and pregnancy rates were significantly higher than in cycles stimulated with exogenous gonadotropins alone.[1] Moreover, GnRH agonist treatment offered the welcome additional advantage of scheduling flexibility, allowing programs to coordinate cycle starts for groups of women simply by varying the duration of GnRH agonist suppression. Not surprisingly, the long protocol quickly became the preferred ovarian stimulation regimen for all forms of ART.

Disadvantages

Gonadotropin-releasing hormone agonist treatment sometimes blunts the response to subsequent gonadotropin stimulation and increases the dose and duration of gonadotropin therapy required to stimulate follicular development. The combined costs of the additional gonadotropins and the agonist itself increase the total cost of treatment.

Nevertheless, because GnRH agonists have more advantages than disadvantages, the long protocol has remained the standard ovarian stimulation regimen in ART cycles for well more than a decade.

In the typical cycle, GnRH agonist treatment begins during the mid-luteal phase, approximately 1 week after ovulation, at a time when endogenous gonadotropin levels are at or near their nadir and the acute release of stored pituitary gonadotropins in response to the agonist, known as the "flare effect" is least likely to stimulate a new wave of follicular development.[2] Treatment may also begin in the early follicular phase, but the time required to achieve pituitary downregulation is longer and the prevalence of cystic follicles is higher. Gonadotropin stimulation also yields more follicles and oocytes when agonist treatment begins during the luteal phase, possibly because LH-stimulated androgen production and circulating androgen levels are more effectively suppressed throughout folliculogenesis. Because the egg yield is greater, the number of embryos available is also increased. Consequently, the probability of having an optimal number of embryos for transfer and excess embryos for cryopreservation is greater. GnRH agonist treatment may be scheduled to begin on cycle day 21 (assuming a normal cycle of approximately 28 days duration).

The two GnRH agonists in common use are leuprolide acetate (administered by subcutaneous injection) and nafarelin acetate (administered by intranasal spray). Elsewhere, buserelin acetate (administered by subcutaneous injection or intranasal spray) and triptorelin (administered subcutaneously) are also commonly used, and all appear equally effective. For leuprolide, the usual treatment regimen begins with 1.0 mg daily for approximately 10 days or until the onset of menses or gonadotropin stimulation, decreasing to 0.5 mg daily thereafter until human chorionic gonadotropin (hCG) administration. For nafarelin, the initial dose is typically 400 µg twice daily, decreasing to 200 µg when stimulation begins. In women who respond poorly to stimulation using the standard daily GnRH agonist treatment regimens, decreasing the doses of agonist by half or more or discontinuing agonist treatment early (after 5 days of gonadotropin stimulation) or completely (when stimulation begins) helps to improve response and overall results **(Fig. 1)**.[3]

Ideally, effective GnRH agonist-induced suppression of serum estradiol levels (less than approximately 40 pg/mL) and ovarian follicular activity (baseline transvaginal ultrasound examination revealing no follicular cysts larger than 10–15 mm in diameter) should be documented before gonadotropin stimulation begins. Even when GnRH agonist treatment begins during the mid-luteal phase, some women may require longer durations of treatment to achieve suppression or may

develop a follicular cyst.[4] Although the outcomes observed in completed cycles may be similar in women with and without baseline cysts, cycle cancelation rates are higher and the total dose of gonadotropins required is generally greater in those with cysts.[5]

Overall, the weight of available evidence suggests that women who require longer durations of GnRH agonist treatment to achieve suppression or who develop cysts are more likely to respond poorly to gonadotropin stimulation; those who do are understandably less likely to succeed. The initial dose of exogenous gonadotropins used to stimulate ovarian follicular development after GnRH agonist-induced downregulation should be tailored to the needs of the individual woman. Typical starting doses range between 225 IU and 300 IU of urinary follicle-stimulating hormone (uFSH), recombinant FSH (rFSH), or urinary menotropins (human menopausal gonadotropin or hMG) daily, depending on age, the results of ovarian reserve testing, and the response observed in any previous superovulation or IVF cycles. Either a "step-up" (beginning with a low dose, increasing as necessary based on response) or "step-down" (beginning with a higher dose, decreasing as necessary based on response) may be used, but the latter approach is generally preferred.

Concerns persist that GnRH agonist treatment may suppress endogenous LH levels below those necessary for normal follicular development in at least some women. Because only about 1% of LH receptors must be occupied to support normal follicular steroidogenesis, the low levels of LH secretion after downregulation with a GnRH agonist are sufficient to meet the need in most women stimulated with uFSH or rFSH alone.[6] However, LH concentrations also may be inadequate in those who are more profoundly suppressed. Indeed, LH levels are markedly suppressed (less than 1 IU/L) in many who are treated only with FSH, and in such cycles, the dose and duration of gonadotropins required are higher and peak

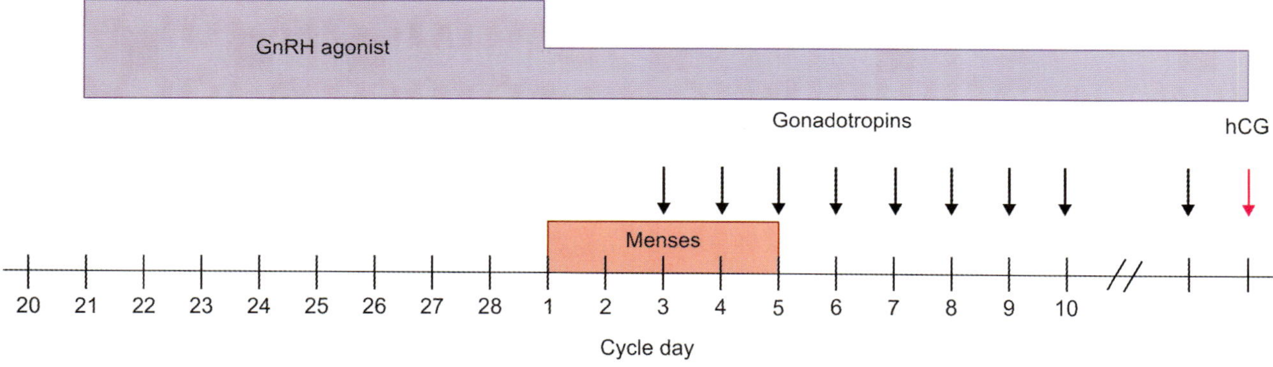

Fig. 1 Long protocol

estradiol levels are lower; the numbers of oocytes and embryos may also be reduced. Other evidence suggests that fertilization, implantation, and pregnancy rates may be adversely affected when LH levels are extremely low.[7] The evidence indicates that there may be a subgroup of eugonadotropic women that could benefit from supplemental hMG or rLH during ovarian stimulation.

Monitoring the Cycle

The response to stimulation is monitored with serial measurements of serum estradiol and transvaginal ultrasound imaging of ovarian follicles. The first serum estradiol level usually is obtained after 3–5 days of stimulation to determine whether the chosen dose of gonadotropins requires adjustment. Thereafter, serum estradiol concentrations and ovarian scans are obtained every 1–3 days, based on the quality of the response and the need to evaluate the impact of any further adjustments in the dose of gonadotropin treatment. Most women require a total of 9–10 days of stimulation. In general, the goal is to have at least two follicles measuring 17–18 mm in mean diameter, ideally accompanied by a few others in the 14–16 mm range, and a serum estradiol concentration that is consistent with the overall size and maturity of the cohort (approximately 200 pg/mL per follicle measuring 14 mm or greater). Typically, endometrial development is also monitored during stimulation by measuring the endometrial thickness. Although multiple studies have examined the prognostic value of endometrial thickness and echotexture in ART cycles, the issue remains controversial. Many have suggested that results are best when endometrial thickness measures 8–9 mm or greater and poor when the endometrium is less than 6–7 mm in thickness or appears homogeneous on the day of hCG administration.[8] However, numerous others have failed to observe any clear correlation between endometrial thickness or appearance and outcomes. Once the targeted thresholds of response are met, hCG (5,000–10,000 IU) is administered to induce final follicular maturation.

High Responders

Occasionally, stimulation generates an exaggerated follicular response, characterized by massive ovarian enlargement, extremely large numbers of follicles of all sizes, and markedly elevated serum estradiol concentrations (>3,000 pg/mL). Under such circumstances, the risk for the ovarian hyperstimulation syndrome (OHSS) is substantially increased and may lead to cycle cancelation.

Canceling the cycle and starting a new using a more conservative stimulation regimen may ultimately decrease overall costs and maximize the chances for success. The prognosis for high responders in subsequent cycles is generally very good.

Poor Responders

The challenges presented by "poor responders" are far greater. Poor responders include women in whom a previous cycle yielded three or fewer oocytes or was canceled because of observations of three or fewer follicles 16 mm or greater, a single dominant follicle, or a peak serum estradiol less than 500 pg/mL. In such women, a more aggressive or alternative stimulation regimen is warranted and there are several options from which to choose:

- The long protocol, beginning with higher doses of gonadotropin stimulation
- Decreasing the doses of GnRH agonist or discontinuing agonist treatment immediately before or soon after gonadotropin stimulation begins
- A short follicular phase GnRH agonist treatment regimen using a standard or microdose "flare" protocol
- Using a GnRH antagonist instead of a long-acting agonist
- Sequential treatment with clomiphene citrate and exogenous gonadotropins.

Sequential Stimulation with a GnRH Agonist and Exogenous Gonadotropins the "Short" or "Flare" Protocols

In a typical standard short protocol, leuprolide acetate (1.0 mg daily) is administered on cycle days 2–4, continuing thereafter at a reduced dose (0.5 mg daily) and gonadotropin stimulation (150–450 IU daily) begins on cycle day 3. Later adjustments in the dose of gonadotropin stimulation, if needed, are based on response and indications for hCG. Administration is the same as in the long protocol (described previously). The standard flare protocol generally improves follicular response and lowers cycle cancelation rates in poor responders, although pregnancy and live birth rates remain relatively low.[9] Decreased scheduling flexibility is one distinct disadvantage of the flare protocol, unless the onset of menses is controlled by preliminary treatment with an oral contraceptive. The standard flare treatment regimen also is commonly associated with significant increases in serum progesterone and androgen levels, presumably resulting from late corpus luteum rescue which may have adverse effects on oocyte quality and fertilization and on pregnancy rates. The "ultrashort" GnRH agonist protocol is a variation of the short protocol in which an agonist is administered for 3 days to stimulate the flare response but then discontinued; treatment proceeds with exogenous gonadotropins alone. As might be expected, premature LH surges are more prevalent than in cycles stimulated with the standard short or long protocols because downregulation of endogenous gonadotropin secretion requires longer-term agonist treatment. The ultrashort GnRH agonist stimulation protocol yields results inferior to those obtained with the short and long protocols and is seldom employed.

■ STIMULATION WITH EXOGENOUS GONADOTROPINS WITH ADDITION OF A GnRH ANTAGONIST

The relatively recent introduction of GnRH antagonists into clinical practice has provided another option for ovarian stimulation in ART. GnRH antagonists, being more complex than agonists, act through a completely different mechanism for inhibiting gonadotropin secretion. GnRH antagonists bind competitively to GnRH receptors preventing the action of endogenous GnRH pulses on the pituitary. Not only the secretion of gonadotropins is decreased within hours of antagonist administration, but in addition no flare-up effect occurs. Moreover, discontinuation of GnRH-antagonist treatment results in rapid and predictable recovery of the pituitary-gonadal axis as the pituitary receptor system remains intact.

In contrast to the agonists, antagonist treatment is highly dose dependent, relying on the balance between endogenous GnRH present and antagonist administered. Most importantly, within 6–8 hours of administration, any imminent LH surge is blocked. The first generation of GnRH antagonists, besides binding to pituitary receptors, could in addition bind to GnRH receptors in mast cells resulting in granulation and histamine release, consequences that impeded their use in assisted reproductive technologies for almost a decade. This, until recently, downregulation in IVF was accomplished almost exclusively with the use of GnRH agonists.

Advantages

- The duration of treatment for an antagonist is substantially shorter than for an agonist
- Since its only purpose is to prevent a premature endogenous LH surge and its effects are immediate, antagonist treatment can be postponed until later in follicular development (after 5–7 days of gonadotropin stimulation), after estradiol levels are already elevated, thereby eliminating the estrogen deficiency symptoms that can emerge in women treated with an agonist
- Because any suppressive effects that agonists may exert on the ovarian response to gonadotropin stimulation are also eliminated, the total dose and duration of gonadotropin stimulation required may be decreased
- By eliminating the flare effect of agonists, GnRH antagonists avoid the risk of stimulating development of a follicular cyst
- The risk of severe ovarian hyperstimulation associated with the use of antagonists appears lower than with agonists.

Disadvantages

- When administered in small daily doses, strict compliance with the prescribed treatment regimen is essential
- Low levels of LH observed during agonist treatment are usually sufficient to support normal follicular steroidogenesis when uFSH or rFSH is used for stimulation, the even lower concentrations in women treated with an antagonist may not be sufficient however
- There is evidence to suggest that pregnancy rates in antagonist treatment cycles may be modestly lower than in cycles using agonists in the long protocol, possibly because GnRH antagonists may influence the mitotic programing of cells involved in folliculogenesis, blastomere formation and endometrial development. But carefully choosing the timing of antagonists does not really bring down the pregnancy rates.

The two GnRH antagonists available for clinical use, ganirelix and cetrorelix, are equally potent and effective. For both, the minimum effective dose to prevent premature LH surge is 0.25 mg daily, administered subcutaneously.[10] Either of the antagonists can be administered in a series of small daily doses (0.25 mg). The treatment protocol can be fixed to begin after 5–6 days of gonadotropin stimulation or tailored to the response of the individual, starting treatment when the lead follicle reaches approximately 13–14 mm in diameter. Alternatively, a single larger dose of cetrorelix (3.0 mg) will effectively prevent an LH surge for 96 hours. If given on day 6–7 of stimulation, the interval of effective suppression will encompass the day of hCG administration in most women (75–90%); the remainder may receive additional daily doses (0.25 mg) as needed, ending on the day of hCG treatment. The single-dose antagonist treatment regimen also may be withheld until the lead follicle reaches 13–14 mm in diameter **(Fig. 2)**.[10]

Overall, the total dose and duration of gonadotropin stimulation required, peak serum estradiol levels, and the number of follicles and oocytes were also lower in antagonist cycles.

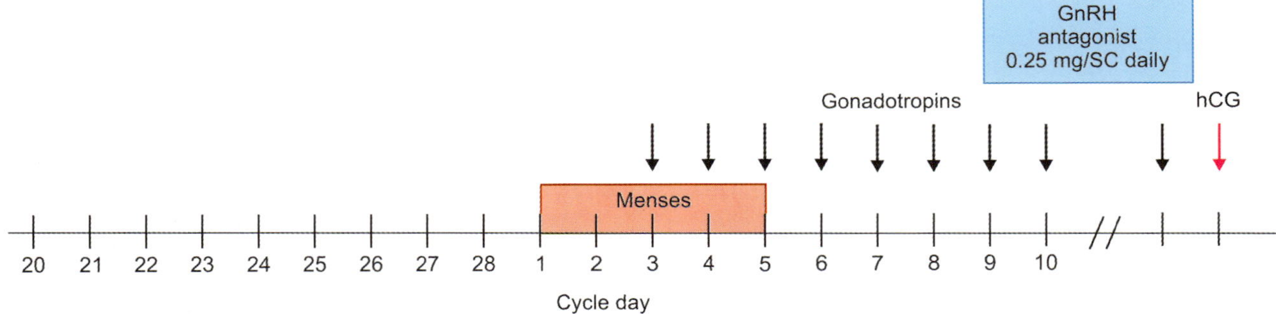

Fig. 2 Antagonist protocol

The explanation for the modestly lower pregnancy rates observed in antagonist treatment cycles is not clear. It is possible, but unlikely, that GnRH antagonists may have adverse effects on oocytes, embryos, or the endometrium. It seems more likely that early results simply reflected inexperience and will improve with time and further refinements in the treatment regimen. Many of the advantages originally envisioned for GnRH antagonists already have been realized. Whether antagonists will ultimately replace agonists and become standard in ART stimulation regimens is still uncertain, but antagonists have been viewed as holding particular promise for women with polycystic ovary syndrome and those who respond poorly to stimulation after treatment with an agonist. The antagonist treatment regimens currently in use also have potential disadvantages for women with polycystic ovary syndrome. Their tonically elevated LH levels will remain high until antagonist treatment begins. Consequently, LH levels can rise prematurely, particularly if antagonist treatment is withheld until the lead follicle reaches 14 mm or more. Moreover, evidence indicates that increased LH exposure during early follicular development may be detrimental and predispose to lower pregnancy rates.

In theory, pretreatment with an oral contraceptive might prove quite useful by suppressing LH and androgen levels before stimulation begins, decreasing exposure during early follicular development and the risk of rising LH levels before antagonist treatment begins. Preliminary oral contraceptive suppression and later antagonist treatment may also help to limit the follicular response to gonadotropin stimulation while preserving the option to use an agonist to trigger final oocyte maturation. An earlier start to antagonist treatment may offer similar advantages. These and other considerations simply serve to illustrate that GnRH antagonists are not a panacea and may not even be the best choice for women with polycystic ovary syndrome.

Poor responders are another group for which GnRH antagonists may have particular value because antagonist treatment eliminates any suppressive effects that the long-acting agonists may have on follicular response and can prevent the premature LH surges commonly observed in women stimulated with gonadotropins alone.

Review of Literature

Over the last two decades, GnRH agonists have been used in ovarian stimulation protocols in ART in combination with gonadotropins to prevent a premature LH surge. The concept of suppressing gonadotropins by competitive receptor blockage rather than through pituitary desensitization with its inevitable flare-up is compelling. Controlling the endogenous LH surge by GnRH antagonists may increase the efficiency both in unstimulated and clomiphene citrate cycles.

Twenty-one randomized controlled trials (RCTs) have been studied which included 3,865 participants. The study design was similar to ours, and the patient characteristics such as age, body mass index, duration of infertility, basal FSH levels were comparable. After pooling the data from all the included studies, the following observations were made. The number of oocytes retrieved was consistently smaller in women treated with GnRH antagonist, which was in good agreement with the smaller cohort of growing follicles, the lower amount of gonadotropin used and the shorter duration of stimulation. There was a statistically significant reduction in pregnancy rates in GnRH antagonist group. This reduction occurred despite the transfer of an equivalent number of good quality embryos in both group being transferred. However, there was reduction in incidence of OHSS.[11]

It has been recognized that there was a consistent trend in favor of GnRH agonists whether in terms of oocytes retrieved, number of good quality embryos obtained or the clinical pregnancy rates.

Sonographic delineation of follicle size is crucial as hCG is best administered once follicles reach 15–18 mm in size. Studies done have shown that the probability of retrieving a mature oocyte was higher in 18–20 mm follicles and lower in those less than 11 mm. In one of the studies done previously, results showed that on the day of hCG administration, there were fewer number of follicles in the antagonist group as compared to the agonist group.[12] In our study too, we found significantly lower number of follicles in the antagonist group. This may be partly explained by the shorter mean duration of treatment and lower dose of hMG administration in subjects treated with antagonists. Pooled data from a number of studies done previously have showed that on the day of oocyte pick-up, less oocytes were retrieved in the antagonist arm, and this lead to less embryos available for transfer. However, the number of embryos transferred was concerning the risk of OHSS a statistically significant reduction in its incidence with the antagonist protocol as compared to the long protocol has been described. A recent review confirmed that there is a statistically significant reduction in the incidence of severe OHSS with the antagonist protocol, and even of the interventions to prevent it (e.g. coasting, cancelation).[11]

However, another recently published meta-analysis based on the analysis of 22 published RCTs, compared the effectiveness of GnRH agonist and GnRH antagonists in IVF with respect to the probability of live birth per patient randomized, and concluded that the probability of live birth between agonists and antagonists was not significantly different.[13] These results are in disagreement with the ones exposed in the review mentioned before.[11] Despite the theoretical advantages of GnRH antagonists, their use was hampered due to the results obtained in a Cochrane review, which indicated a trend toward slightly lower implantation and pregnancy rates for the GnRH antagonist treatment group compared to those in the GnRH agonist group. Various theories have been put forth to explain the lower pregnancy rates observed in antagonist cycles, but consensus has not yet been reached. The uptake of GnRH antagonists has been slow and a great number of ovarian stimulation cycles are still performed in GnRH agonist long protocols. This means that clinicians are less trained to use antagonists and need to overpass the learning curve to reach similar outcomes. It has been suggested that GnRH antagonist is an inhibitor of the cell cycle by decreasing the synthesis of growth factors and, therefore, compromising the mitotic program of follicles, embryo blastomere and endometrium.[14] This mechanism of action might be a reason for the poorer pregnancy outcome. It has been clearly demonstrated that premature luteinization (defined as elevation of serum progesterone the day of hCG administration) during GnRH antagonist IVF-embryo transfer cycles is a frequent event that is associated with lower pregnancy and implantation rates.[15]

We should take into account that GnRH antagonists as compared with GnRH agonists have been usually prescribed in patients with a worse prognosis, who are older, poor responders and have performed more IVF cycles. It hence follows the worse results in terms of clinical outcome. In order to optimize the cycle outcome when antagonists are used, several strategies have been classically proposed, such as pretreatment with an oral contraceptive (OC) to allow greater control over patient response rate and to avoid follicular asynchrony. Some authors have proposed the need of developing flexible antagonists regimens designed for individual patients.[16] Serum progesterone must be controlled during the ovarian stimulation cycle in order to avoid premature luteinization. Regarding the effect of GnRH antagonists on human endometrium, Simón et al. studied the gene expression profile on the endometrium of women undergoing ovarian stimulation for oocyte donation, and observed that the endometrial development after GnRH antagonist mimics the natural endometrium more closely than after GnRH agonist.[17]

We may assume that the significant reduction of severe OHSS together with the reduction in the amount of gonadotropins and the much shorter duration of analog treatment could have a direct impact on reduction of the cost of the cycle in favor of the antagonist regimen. However, it should be noted that the cost effectiveness should be estimated by cost per pregnancy rather that the cost per cycle.

■ CONCLUSION

There has been a consistent trend in favor of GnRH agonists in terms of number of follicles, mature oocytes and pregnancy rates in subfertile couples seeking IVF/intracytoplasmic sperm injection. However, in the recent past since there is a better understanding of GnRH antagonist protocol which is a short and simple protocol with significant reduction in incidence of severe OHSS and amount of gonadotropins used seem to be a good alternative.

■ REFERENCES

1. Daya S. Gonadotropin releasing hormone agonist protocols for pituitary desensitization in in vitro fertilization and gamete intrafallopian transfer cycles. Cochrane Database Syst Rev. CD001299, 2000.

2. Meldrum DR, Wisot A, Hamilton F, et al. Timing of initiation and dose schedule of leuprolide influence the time course of ovarian suppression. Fertil Steril. 1988;50:400-2.

3. Faber BM, Mayer J, Cox B, et al. Cessation of gonadotropin-releasing hormone agonist therapy combined with high-dose gonadotropin stimulation yields favorable pregnancy results in low responders. Fertil Steril. 1998;69:826-30.

4. Meldrum D. GnRH agonists as adjuncts for in vitro fertilization. Obstet Gynecol. 1989;44:314-6.

5. Goldberg JM, Miller FA, Friedman CI, et al. Effect of baseline ovarian cysts on in vitro fertilization and gamete intrafallopian transfer cycles. Fertil Steril. 1991;55:319-23.

6. Balasch J, Vidal E, Penarrubia J, et al. Suppression of LH during ovarian stimulation: analysing threshold values and effects on ovarian response and the outcome of assisted reproduction in down-regulated women stimulated with recombinant FSH. Hum Reprod. 2001;16:1636-43.

7. Gordon UD, Harrison RF, Fawzy M, et al. A randomized prospective assessor-blind evaluation of luteinizing hormone dosage and in vitro fertilization outcome. Fertil Steril. 2001;75:324-31.

8. Noyes N, Liu HC, Sultan K, et al. Endometrial thickness appears to be a significant factor in embryo implantation in in-vitro fertilization. Hum Reprod. 1995;10:919-22.

9. Karande V, Morris R, Rinehart J, et al. Limited success using the "flare" protocol in poor responders in cycles with low basal follicle-stimulating hormone levels during in vitro fertilization. Fertil Steril. 1997;67:900-3.

10. The Ganirelix Dose-Finding Study Group, A double-blind, randomized, dose-finding study to assess the efficacy of the gonadotropin-releasing hormone antagonist ganirelix (Org 37462) to prevent premature luteinizing hormone surges in women undergoing ovarian stimulation with recombinant follicle stimulating hormone (Puregon). Hum Reprod. 1998;13:3023-31.

11. Al-Inany HG, Abou-Setta AM, Aboulghar M. Gonadotrophin releasing hormone- antagonist for assisted conception (review). The Cochrane Library. 2009;19;(3):CD001750.

12. Badrawi A, Al-Inany H, Hussein M, et al. Agonist versus antagonist in ICSI cycles: a randomized trial and cost effectiveness analysis. Middle East Fertil Soc J. 2005;10(1):49-54.

13. Kolibianakis EM, Collins J, Tarlatzis BC, et al. Among patients treated for IVF with gonadotrophins and GnRH analogues, is the probability of live birth dependent on the type of analogue used? A systematic review and meta-analysis. Hum Reprod Update. 2006;12(6):651-71.

14. Hernández ER. Embryo implantation and GnRH antagonists: the Rubicon for GnRH antagonists. Hum Reprod. 2000;15:1211-16.

15. Bosch E, Valencia I, Escudero E, et al. Premature luteinization during gonadotropin-releasing hormone antagonist cycles and its relationship with in vitro fertilization outcome. Fertil Steril. 2003;80:1444-9.

16. Felberbaum RE, Diedrich K. Gonadotrophin-releasing hormone antagonists: will they replace the agonists? RBM Online. 2002;6(1):43-53.

17. Simon C, Oberye J, Bellver J, et al. Similar endometrial development in oocyte donors treated with either high- or standard-dose GnRH antagonist compared to treatment with a GnRH agonist or in natural cycles. Hum Reprod. 2005;20(12):3318-27.

Monitoring Ovarian Stimulation

Madhuri Patil

INTRODUCTION

Conventional fertility treatment often involves ovulation induction, which is more likely to be successful if the preovulatory follicular diameter is 18–24 mm[1] and whilst follicles smaller than 18 mm are capable of producing metaphase II oocytes; fertilization is only 60% of the lead follicular group.[2]

Drugs used for ovulation induction, induce the follicular growth by initiating, augmenting or modulating the hormonal and gametogenic response of the ovary to overcome natural follicular selection process to increase the number of oocytes available for fertilization. Improvements in the efficiency of ovulation induction included the use of recombinant hormones, the daily monitoring of hormone concentrations and high-definition vaginal transducers and use of three-dimensional (3D) transvaginal ultrasound for monitoring the follicular and endometrial growth.

Accurate measurement of follicular size is important and is used to monitor natural and induced cycles and to time the administration of human chorionic gonadotropin (hCG) to promote oocyte maturation prior to timed intercourse, intrauterine insemination (IUI) or oocyte retrieval. Inappropriately, early or delayed induction of oocyte maturation may result in an unexpectedly high proportion of immature oocytes or postmature oocytes with suboptimal fertilization rate and embryogenesis.

The nonassisted reproductive technology cycle aim at monofollicular development as compared to an assisted reproductive technology (ART) cycle, which aims at multifollicular development. The protocols used are different in anovulatory and ovulatory cycles.

Accurate measurement of all follicles especially in multifollicular development is very important and essential to and is associated with a higher follicle to oocyte ratio at oocyte retrieval and a reduction in the number of immature oocytes. Obtaining higher number of mature oocytes is associated with better embryogenesis, and thus has a higher chance of pregnancy.

WHY MONITOR OVULATION INDUCTION CYCLES?

The monitoring process is intended to enable the physician to choose the most suitable protocol to obtain best possible outcome and trying to avoid complications. It involves studying the patients initial parameters, monitor ovarian response to ovulation induction and diagnose complications and success of treatment **(Table 1)**.

HOW DO WE MONITOR THE OVULATION INDUCTION CYCLE?

The ovary holds the key to all stimulation strategies as the response is dependent on the number of recruitable follicles, their sensitivity to and the bioavailability of follicle-stimulating hormone (FSH). It is only the secondary recruitment phase of folliculogenesis and selection of ovulatory follicles that can be modulated with the use of exogenous hormones **(Fig. 1)**.

ASSESSMENT OF OVARIAN RESERVE

Before ovulation induction especially with gonadotropins, it is important to identify those women who are poor responders due to diminished ovarian reserve and have a low pregnancy rates and require high dose of FSH, and those women who are hyper-responders and therefore have an excessive response with high incidence of ovarian hyperstimulation syndrome (OHSS) and at oocyte retrieval (OR) have large number of immature oocytes.

Ovarian reserve test (ORT) predicts response to ovarian stimulation and also identify women of relatively young

Table 1 Reasons for monitoring ovulation induction cycle

Why monitor OL cycles?		
Patient's initial parameters	**Ovarian response to ovulation induction**	**Completion of therapy**
• **Base line scan- TRO** Ovarian or Uterine pathology, AFC • **Base line hormonal profile-** Ovarian reserve, FSH: LH ratio, androgen excess, thyroid profile and hyperprolactenemia • **Choose appropriate stimulation regimen to** prevent OHSS, multiple pregnancy and predict response to ovarian stimulation	• Confirmation of **downregulation** after GnRH agonist • Determine **response** to drug • Determine the **dose** and length of GT TX • Determine optional **time** for hCG administration • Detect **ovulation** • Time **OR** • Identify—**poor responders** and women at **risk OHSS**	• **Diagnose complication of OI** 1. Premature lutenization 2. LUF 3. Endogenous LH surge 4. Retention/Functional cyst • **Confirm pregnancy** • **TRO multiple pregnancy** • **TRO** late onset **OHSS**

Abbreviations: AFC, antral follicle count; FSH, follicle-stimulating hormone; LH, luteinizing hormone; OHSS, ovarian hyperstimulation syndrome; GnRH, gonadotropin-releasing hormone; GT, gonadotropin; LUF, luteinized unruptured follicle

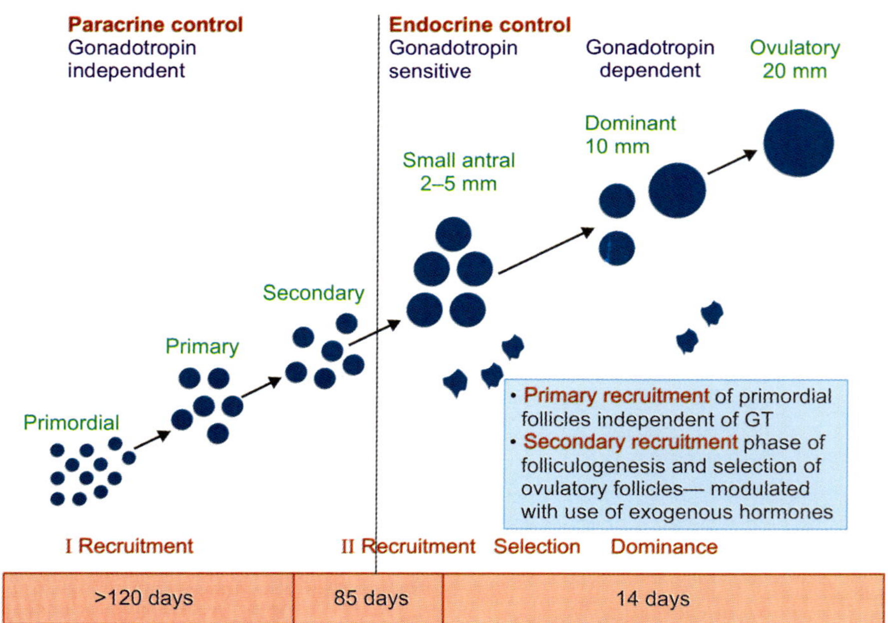

Fig. 1 Recruitment of follicles from the primordial pool

age with diminished reserve, and those around the mean age at which natural fertility on average is lost (41 years) but still have adequate ovarian reserve. ORTs include age, biochemical testing [FSH, anti-Müllerian hormone (AMH), inhibin B, estradiol (E2)], clomiphene citrate challenge test (CCCT), exogenous FSH ovarian reserve test (EFORT) and ultrasound [AFC (antral follicle count), ovarian volume and ovarian blood flow] **(Flow chart 1)**. It is most efficiently done by assessing, the AFC, AMH and FSH levels.

Prediction ovarian response accurately enables clinician to choose the right protocol to optimize the outcome and prevent complications like OHSS and multiple pregnancies. At one extreme of the response spectrum we can identify women who are at risk of OHSS where we can use gonadotropin-releasing hormone (GnRH) antagonists[3] with GnRH agonist trigger before oocyte retrieval.[4] This will not only minimize the risk of this potentially fatal complication, but also completely eliminate it by adopting freeze-all embryos policy.

Flow chart 1 Assessment of ovarian reserve

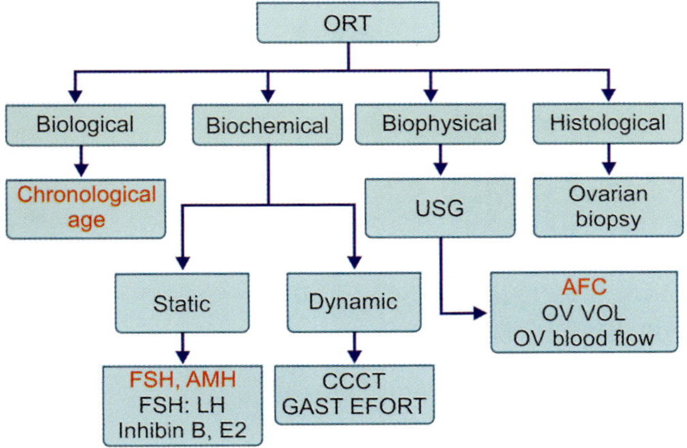

Abbreviations: ORT, ovarian reserve test; FSH, follicle-stimulating hormone; AMH, anti-Müllerian hormone; LH, luteinizing hormone; E2, estradiol; USG, ultrasonography; CCCT, clomiphene citrate challenge test; GAST, GnRH agonist stimulation test; EFORT, exogenous FSH ovarian reserve test

For potential poor responders, one could use a flare strategy because of its reduced treatment burden and ability to capitalize on endogenous luteinizing hormone (LH) activity, in accordance with recent studies supporting a beneficial role of LH in older women.[5] But one needs to remember that most ORTs are adequate in predicting ovarian response, but fail to predict the occurrence of pregnancy.

■ OVARIAN RESERVE TEST

Age

With aging, there is decrease in both oocyte number, quality and fertility but age per se can be a poor determinant of female fertility, since there is wide range in the relationship between ovarian reserve and age.

Biochemical Test

To predict ovarian response to ovarian stimulation and to individualize the starting dose of exogenous gonadotropin or the need for exogenous LH, various hormonal tests have been suggested. These include FSH, AMH and E2 levels. Though the standard first-line investigation to assess ovarian function is measuring FSH, it has a much lower correlation with primordial follicle counts and follicular recruitment rates and has limited ability to diagnose ovarian dysfunction, including polycystic ovarian syndrome (PCOS). Today AMH is considered to be the best marker for prediction of ovarian reserve and response with a strong linear relationship of AMH with AFC in predicting ovarian reserve.

Basal FSH

Basal FSH is the indirect measure of the size of follicle cohort and is regulated by inhibins, activins, E2 and follistatins.[6] Early-follicular phase fluctuations are reflection of balance between ovarian steroid and peptide inhibition and the hypothalamo-pituitary drive during the period just before the selection of dominant follicle. High FSH therefore does not reflect aging oocytes, it is just that fewer are produced.

Multiple cutoff values above 10 IU/L (10–20 IU/L) demonstrate high specificity (83–100%) but poor sensitivity (10–80%) for predicting poor response to stimulation (<2–3 follicles or <4 retrieved oocytes).[7] Using similar cutoff values the sensitivity for predicting pregnancy is very low.[8] High FSH levels have not been associated with an increased risk of aneuploidy in pregnancies resulting from in vitro fertilization (IVF).[9,10] Although FSH rises with increasing reproductive age, it remains unknown whether high FSH levels in women of reproductive age predict an earlier onset of menopause.[11] Elevated day 3 FSH is a heterogeneous group, which could be either due to true reduced ovarian reserve, presence of heterophilic antibodies or FSH receptor polymorphism in patients with otherwise normal ovaries.

Pregnancy rates significantly higher (P < 0.05) in women with normal FSH in those aged under 36 years compared to those aged over or equal to 36 years. Consistently elevated FSH concentrations confer a poor prognosis,[12] a single elevated FSH value in women under 40 years of age may not predict a poor response to stimulation or failure to achieve pregnancy.[12] FSH does not diagnose poor ovarian reserve until high thresholds are reached.[13]

Limited evidence suggests that women with fluctuating FSH levels should not wait for the "ideal" cycle, wherein the FSH concentration is normal, to undergo IVF stimulation.[14,15] Thus, a basal FSH level has limited utility as a screening test.[7,13,16]

A single FSH value has very limited reliability because of intercycle and intracycle variability (particularly if it is not elevated).

Elevated day 3 FSH/LH ratio due to low LH concentrations predicts reduced ovarian response and is associated with inferior outcome in IVF treatment cycles and may be used as an additional predictor for decreased ovarian response.

Estradiol

As a test of ovarian reserve, basal E2 on day 2, 3, or 4 of the menstrual cycle has poor intercycle and intracycle reliability. Very low predictive accuracy, both for poor response or excessive response and therefore basal E2 alone should not be used to screen for ovarian reserve. The test has value only as an aid to correct interpretation of a "normal" basal serum FSH value. Elevated day 2 E2 values (>75–80 pg/mL) indicates an inappropriately advanced stage of follicular development, consistent with ovarian aging or simply reflect the presence of functional ovarian cysts. No relationship has also been found between serum E2 levels and pregnancy rates.[17] Thus, the use of day 2, E2 value for prediction of ovarian reserve is still debatable.[18]

Inhibin B

Inhibin B concentrations decline before rise in basal FSH levels and therefore is an earlier markers of a reduction in ovarian reserve.[19] Normal day 3 inhibin B value is greater than 45 pg/mL. Early follicular phase elevation is followed by decrease before another brief peak after LH surge. Low levels associated with poor response, high cancelation rate and overall reduction in pregnancy rate.

Using 45 pg/mL as threshold for low ovarian reserve, it has specificity between 64% and 90% and sensitivity between 40% and 80%. The positive productive value (PPV) of inhibin B is generally low (19–22%) and the negative productive value (NPV) is high (95–97%) in general IVF populations.[20,21] In populations at high risk for decreased ovarian reserve, PPV can be as high as 83%.[22] The odds ratio for a clinical pregnancy (basal serum inhibin >45 pg/mL vs <45 pg/mL) was 6.8 (CI 1.8–25.6). It has a better predictor for cancelation than ovarian response and is influenced by the amount of fat in an individual with lower levels in obese women.[23]

Anti-Müllerian Hormone

Maximal expression of AMH occurs in preantral and small antral follicles and this expression disappears in maturing preovulatory follicles. It affects the transition from resting primordial follicles into growing follicles.[24-27]

The levels of AMH remain relatively consistent within and between menstrual cycles in both normal young ovulating women and in women with infertility.[28-31] The true individual cycle fluctuation of AMH is only about 11%.

The reference range for AMH values is given in **Table 2**.

For hyperresponse, the optimal cutoff value of 3.36 ng/mL has a sensitivity of 90.5% (95% CI 69.6–98.5) and specificity of 81.3% (95% CI 75.8–86.0).[32] Sensitivity

Table 2 Reference ranges for anti-Müllerian hormone

Ovarian fertility potential	ng/mL
Optimal fertility	4–6.8
Satisfactory fertility	2.2–4
Low fertility	0.3–2.2
Very low/undetectable	0.0–0.3
High level	>6.8
	? suspicion of Polycystic Ovarian Disease/Granulosa cell tumors

and specificity of AFC and AMH for prediction of high ovarian response were 89% and 92% for small AFC and 93% and 78% for AMH at the cutoff values of greater than or equal to 16 and greater than or equal to 34.5 pmol/L, (4.86 ng/mL) respectively. On the other hand, for prediction of poor response, the optimum cutoff value for AMH is 0.99 ng/mL and the post-test probability was highest at cutoff levels of 0.59 ng/mL.

Dynamic Test

Clomiphene Citrate Challenge Test

Women with elevated day-10 FSH levels after administration of clomiphene citrate (CC) from day 5 to 9 may demonstrate diminished ovarian reserve. It has a value in unmasking poor responders to controlled ovarian stimulation (COS), who would not have been detected by basal FSH screening alone. It was also observed that abnormal test is associated with a reduced chance of pregnancy.

Exogenous FSH Ovarian Reserve Test

Increment of inhibin B and E2 is a normal response after 24 hours of administration of 300 IU of FSH on day 3 of the menstrual cycle. EFORT has not been tested outside the ART population[33] and hence, the results cannot be extrapolated to predict the fertility potential of the general population. False positive prediction may hamper the use of this test if a high level of detection is needed and patients are refused IVF on the basis of the test result.

Inhibin B increment in the EFORT has best discriminative potential for hyperresponse receiver operating characteristic area under the curve (ROC-AUC 0.92). Whereas E2 increment in EFORT, CCCT, and basal FSH at different cutoff levels were of less clinical relevance compared with inhibin B increment in the EFORT at the cutoff level of 130 ng/L for prediction of hyperresponse.[34]

Clomiphene citrate challenge test appeared to have the best discriminative potential for poor response,

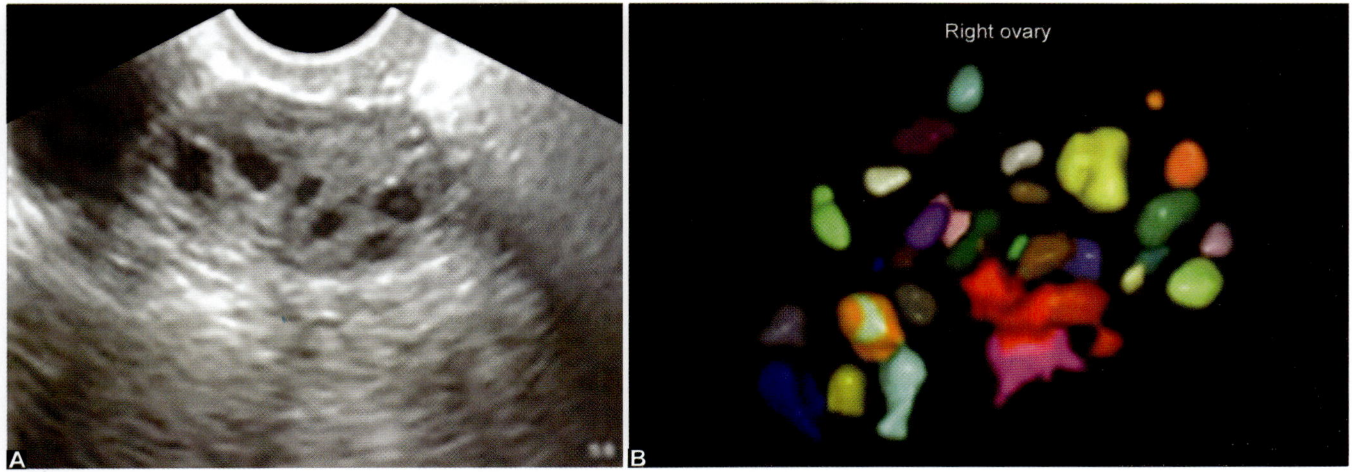

Figs 2A and B Antral follicle count

as expressed by the largest ROC-AUC (0.88) followed by inhibin increment in EFORT. Whereas E2 and inhibin B increment in EFORT and basal FSH at different cutoff levels were of less clinical relevance compared with CCCT at the cutoff level of 18 IU/L, which has 85% positive predictive value.[34]

Biophysical Tests

Antral Follicle Count

Size of antral follicles (2–5 mm) cohort is proportionally related to primordial follicle pool and it decreases with age. An AFC of less than five is a good marker to predict poor ovarian response to COS in assisted reproduction programs. There could be some intercycle variability in the AFC and 71% of variation is due to intrasubject examination and only 29% is due to individual cycle variation.

Antral follicle count can be done either using the two-dimensional (2D), 3D or four-dimensional (4D) ultrasonography (USG) [Sono-automated volume count (Sono-AVC)-hypoechoic aspect of the ultrasound display is inverted to demonstrate fluid-filled areas within the 3D dataset]. Sono-AVC is the best model in predicting the number of oocytes retrieved with a retrieval rate of 60%. AFC is good predictors of response but not of pregnancy. Optimum cutoff value of AFC for poor response is less than or equal to 10 but the post-test probability was highest at cutoff levels of less than 8 **(Figs 2A and B)**.[35]

The optimum cutoff value for hyperresponse of AFC is greater than or equal to 14 with a sensitivity of 82% and specificity 89% to predict OHSS **(Fig. 3)**.

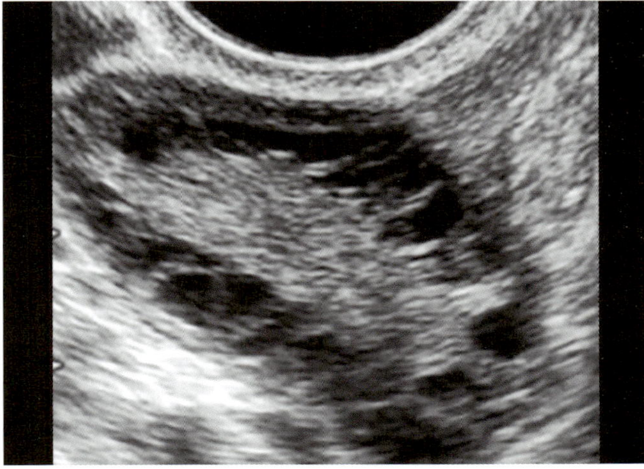

Fig. 3 Antral follicle count of more than 14

Ovarian volume **(Figs 4A and B)** also correlates with number of growing follicles, but not with number of oocytes retrieved.[36] It was also observed that women with small ovaries with a volume of less than 3 cm³ have a very high cancelation rate of IVF.[37] 3D ultrasound allows more precise in calculation of ovarian and stromal volumes. Again the predictive value for pregnancy by measuring the ovarian and stromal volume is limited (1.0–1.4).[38,39]

Prediction of response to COS with color and power Doppler can be done using the stromal flow index (FI) and peak systolic velocity (PSV).

When the stromal FI[40] was less than 11 low response was seen as against normal response with FI between 11 and 14 and a hyperresponse when FI was more than 15.

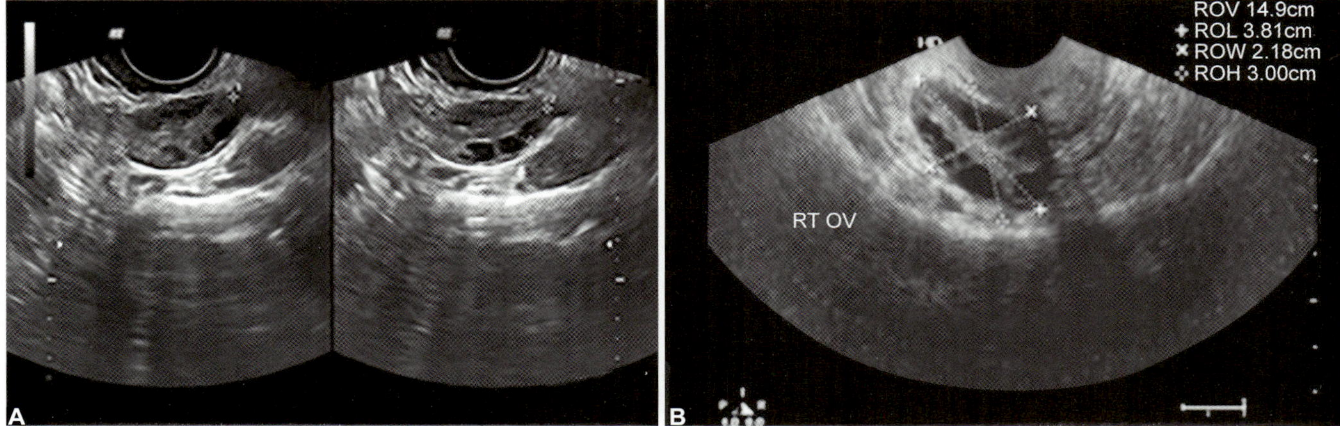

Figs 4A and B Ovarian volume

Low stromal PSV in the early follicular phase predicts poor responders and an increased stromal PSV with unchanged resistance predicts increased risk of OHSS.

Uterine artery resistance index (RI) and PSV may also predict the response. Lower uterine artery RI and higher PSV has high incidence of OHSS as against a uterine artery RI of more than 0.79, which is indicative of poor response and higher requirement of gonadotropin dose.

Limitations of ovarian blood flow:
- Not much decrease until late forties.
- No data indicating reliability and reproducibility of measurements.
- Low sensitivity and specificity.
- Systematic review of seven studies has reported the predictive capacity of ovarian vascular flow parameters for ovarian response to be low.

Ovarian Biopsy

Not a useful routine test of ovarian reserve[41] as it is invasive and possesses unknown future adverse effects. Moreover, it is not a reliable test to assess effect of reproductive aging on fertility, as follicular distribution in the ovarian cortex is extremely heterogeneous, thus ovarian biopsy sample is not representative of the actual follicular pool, and therefore unlikely to add any new information.

Ovarian reserve testing allows us to choose individualized COS protocols based on the age, AFC and AMH. The dose can be further amended according to the body mass index (BMI).

Monitoring Ovulation Induction Cycle

Follicle tracking, involves the serial assessment of follicle number and size by transvaginal ultrasound (TVS) is commonly employed to assess the response to ovarian stimulation. Normally, a 2D ultrasound is used to identify and then systematically scroll through an ovary, measuring each follicle in turn. Till date there is no consensus as to how many measurements should be taken or how they are best performed but a single measurement is less reliable than two or three measures.[42] During COS, using gonadotropin the presence of numerous follicles of different sizes makes such an assessment difficult as the clinician has to identify each and every follicle individually and measure it only once. The validity and reliability of such measurements are likely to reduce as the number of follicles increases.

Follicular monitoring is today a pivotal investigation in both infertility evaluation and treatment. It is the gold standard to document ovulation, follicular development and growth, corpus luteum integrity and endometrial growth and character. Ovulation induction involves administration of either oral ovulogens or gonadotropins to enhance fertility. These drugs cause a supraphysiological increase in serum FSH either indirectly as with oral ovulogens or directly as with gonadotropins leading to the recruitment of a larger cohort of follicles. To time, the intercourse, IUI or oocyte retrieval, we need to trigger ovulation at a particular diameter of the growing follicle for optimal outcome. Moreover, ovulation induction can be associated with multiple gestation, OHSS and torsion of ovary. Monitoring of the ovarian function, especially when the woman is administered ovulation induction drugs becomes mandatory. The monitoring can be done either by ultrasound or bioassay of hormones.

Ultrasound Monitoring

Ultrasound provides information on uterine and adnexal pathology, ovarian morphology, ovarian reserve and blood flow, endometrial thickness, morphology, thickness and blood flow, follicular growth and timing to trigger ovulation and feasibility of oocyte retrieval.

Color Doppler provides qualitative information, while power Doppler signal can provide quantitative information.[43,44] In combination with 3D ultrasound, PD offers a tool with which one may not only demonstrate but also quantify total endometrial and regional uterine blood flow.[45,46]

Monitoring Ovarian Response to Ovulation Induction Agents

Ultrasound assessment of follicular growth was first introduced in 1979 when Hackelöer and Robinson[1] described a linear relationship between follicle size and circulating E2 levels. Since then, TVS scan has been used to routinely monitor follicular growth in natural cycles, in ovulation induction programs, and during controlled ovarian hyperstimulation (COH) for ART cycles. TVS is the method of choice because of better visualization and accuracy, though at times a transabdominal scan (TAS) may be required in special situations especially if ovary placed high in the pelvis and not visualized on a TVS.

The monitoring is different for a timed intercourse, IUI and ART cycle and also for a natural, COS and oral ovulation induction cycle.

During the natural cycle, a cohort of small antral follicles (2–5 mm in diameter) appears in the ovary early in the proliferative phase which is selected 80–90 days prior from the primordial follicular pool. As FSH levels rise in the early follicular phase, further growth of the follicles occurs. Decline of FSH in the late follicular phase, which is physiological, allows the selection of the single most sensitive follicle to continue to develop. The follicle, which will be selected to become dominant, will depend on the FSH and LH receptor content of the granulosa cells. The follicle, which has developed maximum receptors for FSH and LH in response to FSH, will continue to grow, while the other follicles will undergo apoptosis and atresia. Once the leading follicle reaches a diameter of approximately 14 mm, the daily growth rate is between 1.5 mm and 2.0 mm until reaching a diameter of 18–24 mm, when ovulation occurs **(Flow chart 2)**.

Thus, in a natural cycle, monitoring provides information on whether the menstrual cycles is ovulatory or anovulatory. It can also identify delayed ovulation despite normal cycle length (28–30 days), short luteal phase, assess hormonal (P4) competence and support. It also provides information about the endometrial growth and characteristic. It can also diagnose luteal phase abnormalities like luteinized unruptured follicle (LUF).

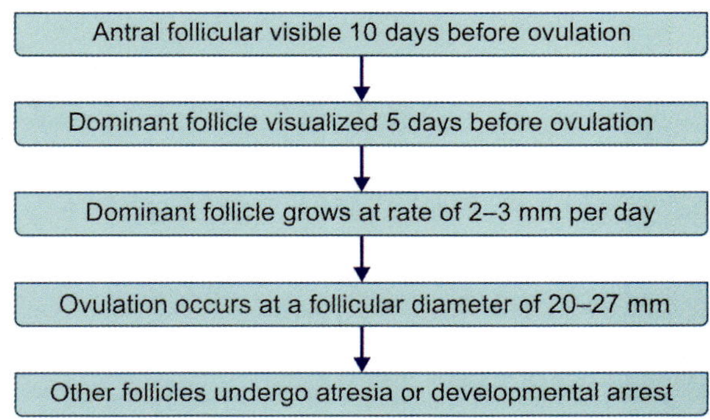
Flow chart 2 Monitoring a natural cycle

In natural cycles, serum E2 levels correlate with follicle size, while the contribution of small atretic follicles to the steroidal milieu is negligible.

In a natural cycle, the first scan can be done either on day 9 or 10 of the menstrual cycle after the baseline scan on day 2 or 3. Till the follicles reach 14 mm, the scans can be repeated every 48 hours, but once dominance is established and the follicle is 14 mm, the scan is repeated every 24 hours. This is essential to determine the exact time of ovulation as the follicle can rupture at any time one the follicle becomes more than 16 mm. In these patients if IUI is done once the follicular rupture is documented, pregnancies have occurred and so the importance of daily monitoring.

Characteristic ultrasound appearance at the time of ovulation includes diminution in the follicle size or sudden collapse of the follicle, blurring of the follicle borders, which become crenated, and appearance of intrafollicular echoes, which are more isoechogenic with respect to surrounding ovary **(Fig. 5)** and presence of a small amount of free fluid in the pouch of Douglas (POD) **(Fig. 6)**. Thereafter, an irregular, slightly cystic structure representing the corpus luteum shrinks throughout the luteal phase of the cycle until luteolysis occurs before menses.

The role of ovulation-inducing agents for IVF is to disturb this normal relationship by increasing the amounts of FSH available to follicles other than the dominant follicles and thus to increase the total number of follicles that reach the preovulatory stage. When oral ovulogens are used we have fewer dominant follicles as compared to gonadotropin cycles.

Baseline scan on day 2 or 3 is essential before initiation of any ovulation induction therapy to **(Fig. 7)**:
- Identify morphology of ovary and adnexal abnormalities—ovarian cyst, hydrosalpinx.

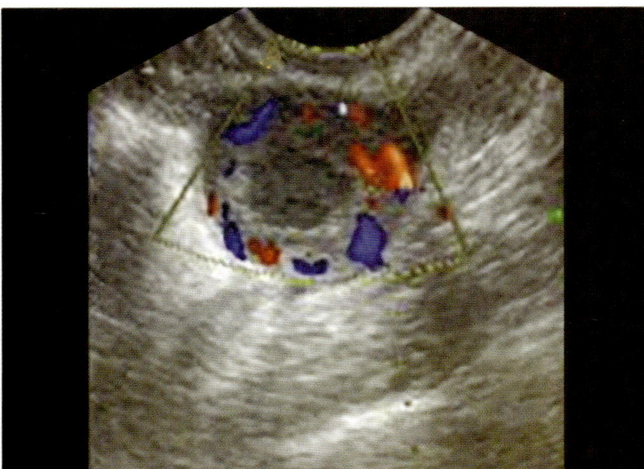

Fig. 5 Corpus luteum with increased peripheral blood flow

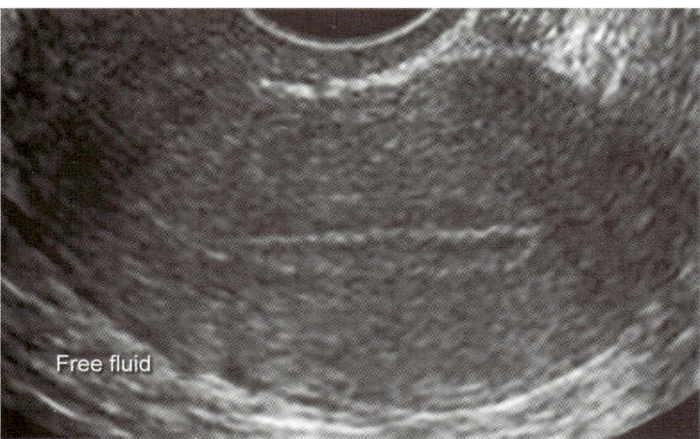

Fig. 6 Free fluid in the pouch of Douglas

- Assess the ovarian reserve.
- Identify uterine abnormalities—myoma, adenomyosis, polyps, intrauterine adhesions, endometrial abnormalities, congenital anomalies.
- Decide the stimulation protocol for adequate response.

As selection of dominant follicle occurs early in follicular phase, ovulation induction drugs initiated within 3 days of menstrual cycle if **(Fig. 8)** the follicular size is less than 10 mm, there is absence of ovarian cyst, endometrial thickness less than 6 mm and E2 levels are less than 50 pg/mL and progesterone level is less than 1.5 ng/mL. The dose of drugs used should be tailored to each individual.

Ultrasound scanning is useful in monitoring the response to oral ovulogens like CC, tamoxifen and aromatase inhibitors in anovulatory women. TVS is usually performed 4–5 days after the last dose of the oral ovulogen and then every other day till the follicle is 14 mm and then daily until a follicle of approximately 20 mm in diameter is seen. Ovulation trigger is given with either recombinant hCG 250 µg subcutaneous or urinary hCG 5,000 IU intramuscular (IM) or GnRH agonist 1 mg subcutaneous **(Flow chart 3)**.

Ovulation induction with gonadotropins overcomes the normal feedback mechanism that allows for physiological unifollicular ovulation causing growth of a cohort of follicles at various stages of development. For an IUI cycle only a maximum of two or three follicles are required to prevent OHSS and multiple pregnancies. To prevent these complications gonadotropin use requires close monitoring with ultrasound and E2 levels **(Fig. 5)**. In ovulation induction cycles, a baseline ultrasound scan is performed to exclude functional ovarian cysts, as well as other pelvic pathologies. Monitoring is usually carried out using TVS on day 4 of treatment and then on day 7 and then depending on the follicular diameter the scans are repeated either daily or on alternate days. The dose of exogenous gonadotropins is adjusted according to the response. If two leading follicles (>18–20 mm) are seen, hCG should be administered. IUI is done 36 hours after the hCG injection.

When gonadotropins are used for COS in ART **(Flow chart 4)**, the monitoring is more stringent due to multifollicular development. When measuring large number of follicles, the interobserver variation in measurement is larger than the intraobserver variation and therefore follicular tracking is more accurate when each scan is performed by the same clinician.[47]

The gonadotropins are initiated after a baseline scan on day 2 or 3 is normal and the first scan after initiation of gonadotropins is done on fourth day. Further adjustment of gonadotropin dose depends on serial USG findings and E2 levels as follows:

Change in the dose depending on the USG for follicular tracking:
- If on day 4:
  - Number of follicles less than four dose increased by 37.5/75 IU.
  - Number of follicles greater than eight dose reduced by 37.5/75 IU.
- If on day 7:
  - Rate of growth—less than 1.5–3 mm/day and less than four follicles which are less than 12 mm in size dose increased by 37.5/75 IU.
  - Rate of growth greater than 1.5–3 mm/day and number of follicles greater than 10 which are greater than 12 mm in size decrease the dose by 37.5/75 IU.

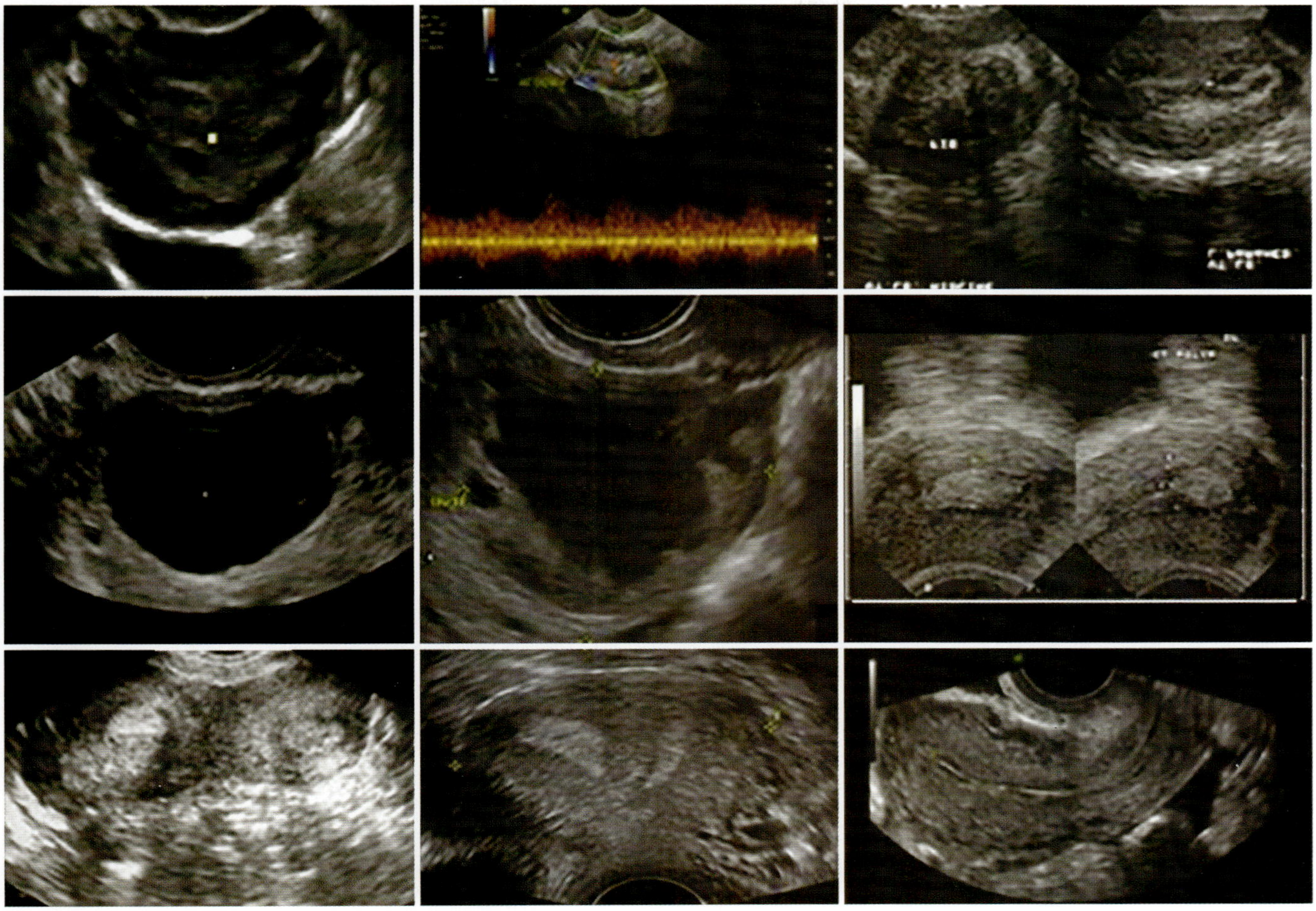

Fig. 7 Baseline scan before ovulation induction triple rule-out (TRO) pathology

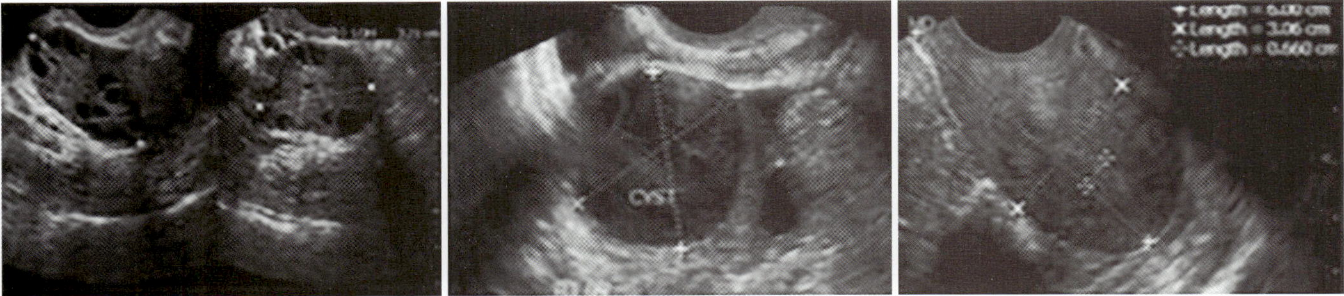

Fig. 8 Criteria for initiation of ovulation induction drugs

Once dominance is achieved the follicular growth is approximately 1.5–3 mm/day. So, we continue the same dose if follicular growth is 1.5–3 mm/day. Thereafter, the dose is increased or decreased depending on rate of growth and number of dominant follicles along with E2 levels.

Monitoring of preovulatory follicles with follicle diameters has limitation to predict oocyte quality. Although the follicle growth pattern may be a predictive indicator of the oocyte quality,[48] it is difficult to identify each follicle changes in multiple ovarian follicle growth induced by the gonadotropin stimulation.

Flow chart 3 Monitoring a timed intercourse (TI) or intrauterine insemination (IUI) cycle

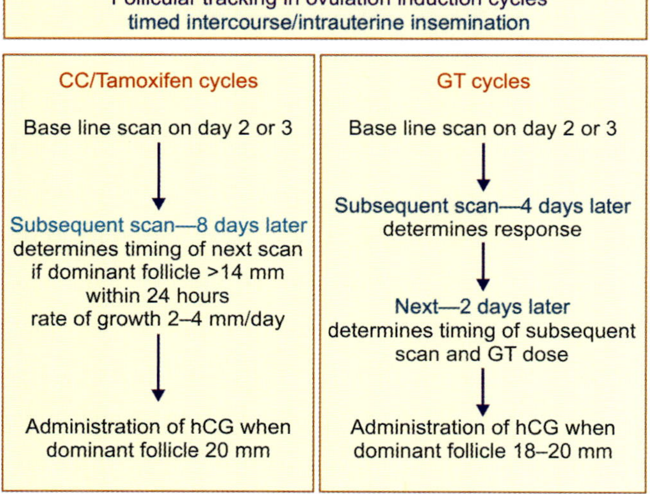

Abbreviations: CC, clomiphene citrate; GT, gonadotropin; hCG, human chorionic gonadotropin

Flow chart 4 Monitoring an assisted reproductive technology cycle

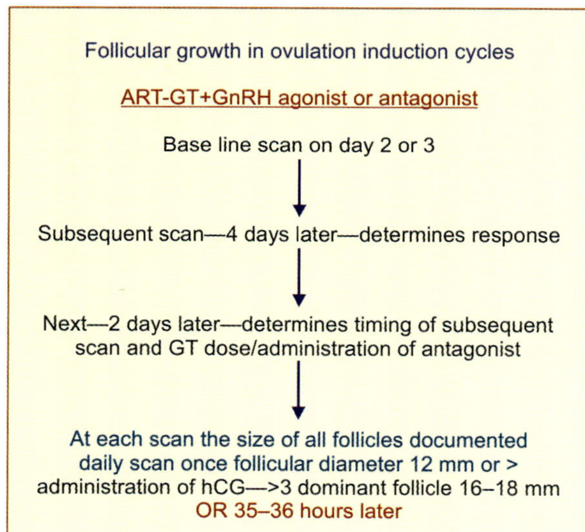

Abbreviations: ART, assisted reproductive technology; GT, gonadotropin; GnRH, gonadotropin-releasing hormone; hCG, human chorionic gonadotropin

Transvaginal ultrasound performed by an experienced operator and the daily measurements of serum E2 concentrations may have limited value in predicting the success of the cycle or the risk of OHSS. Probably hormonal monitoring along with ultrasound is required only in cases where there is a poor response or hyperresponse. It is also required in those cases who are undergoing frozen embryo transfer (FET) in a natural cycle. Usually the serum E2 concentrations are proportional to the amount of LH in the gonadotropin preparation used, it is lower in only FSH cycles as compared to those where human menopausal gonadotropin (hMG) is administered.

It is not only the follicular size but the follicular volume also matters, when it comes to oocyte quality and fertilization rate. Wittmaack et al.[49] reported enhanced fertilization and cleavage rates in oocytes coming from follicles with a volume greater than 1 mL but found no difference in embryo quality, concluding that once fertilization is achieved, follicle diameter has no significant effect on embryo developmental potential.

Oocytes obtained from follicles less than 16 mm had lower incidence of nuclear maturation and have lower developmental rates. On the other hand, oocytes obtained from larger follicles had higher rates of developmental potential, this suggested that hCG administration should be postponed until follicle diameter is at least 18 mm.

Color Doppler Studies of Ovarian Circulation

Using color Doppler one can detect the vascularity of the ovarian stroma, follicular surface and corpus luteum. PD analysis is an indirect indication of "health" of the follicle and possibly developmental competence of the corresponding oocyte. Follicular vascularization is closely related to oocyte oxygenation[50] and the initiation and maintenance of follicular growth depends on development of perifollicular microvascular network and intrafollicular hypoxia can have an effect on mitochondrial function and chromosomal organization in oocytes and early embryos.

Thus, quantitative and qualitative assessment of perifollicular flow allows more accurate assessment of follicular competence **(Figs 9A to D)**. Follicles that have more than 75% of their surface perfused, ovarian stromal PSV of more than 10 cm/s and RI of less than 0.4–0.48 contain mature oocytes of satisfactory quality and result in better grade of embryos.

Balakier and Stronell[51] found a positive correlation between perifollicular peak velocity and follicular size while Oyesanya[52] reported a positive correlation between oocyte recovery rate and follicular vascularity.

Perifollicular blood flow (PFBF) grading:
- *Grade 1:* Blood flow less than 25% of the follicle's circumference.
- *Grade 2:* Blood flow greater than or equal to 25% but less than 50%.

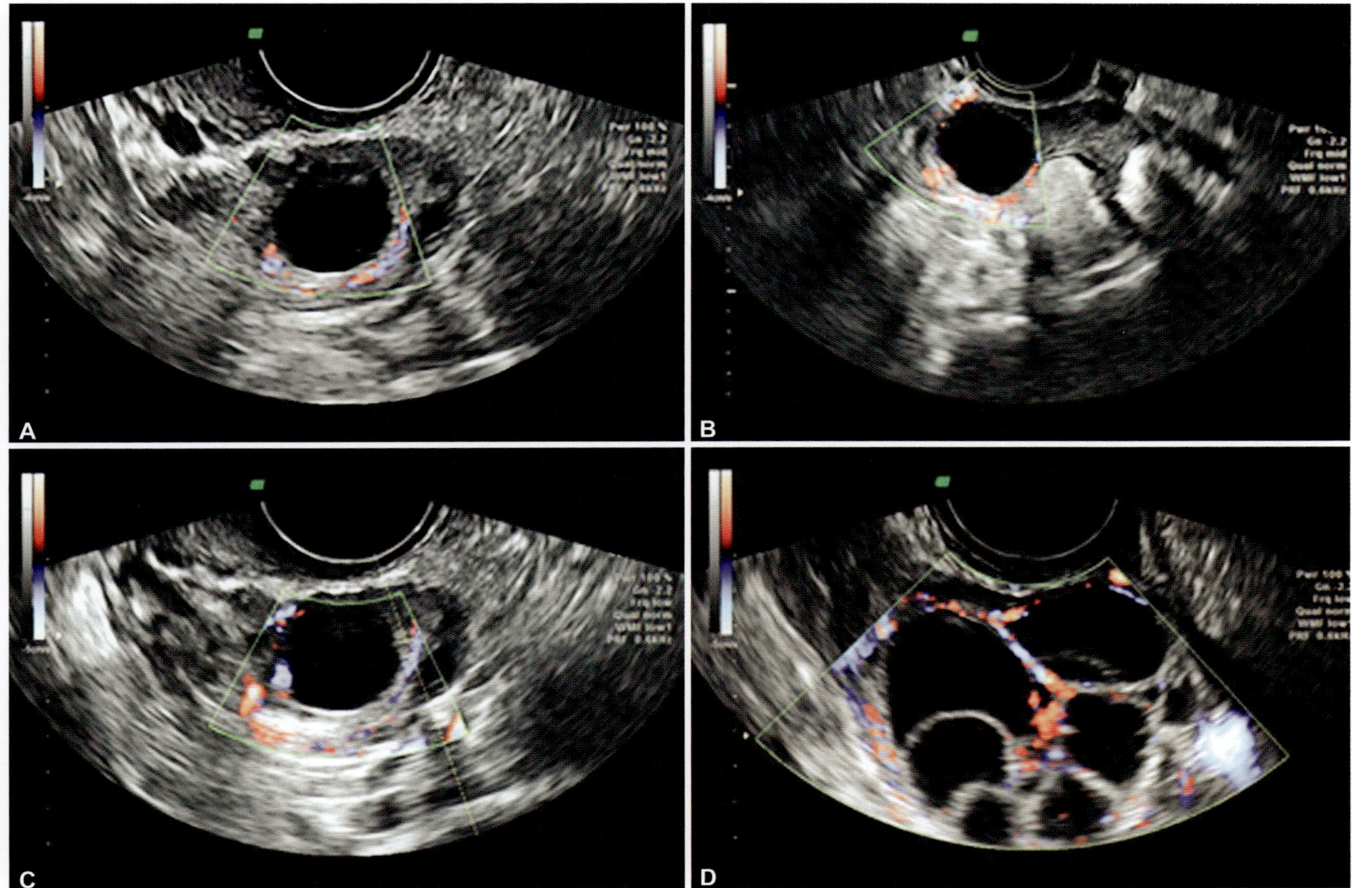

Figs 9A to D Perifollicular blood flow. (A and B) Less than 50% perfused; (C and D) Greater than 75% perfused

- *Grade 3:* Blood flow greater than 50% but less than 75%.
- *Grade 4:* Blood flow greater than or equal to 75%.

The pregnancy rate in cycles where the embryos transferred came from follicles graded 3–4 was significantly higher than in cases where transferred embryos came from either class 1–2 or "mixed" group (1-2-3-4) follicles (34.7% vs 18%). It was also observed that the oocytes aspirated from poorly vascularized follicles presented a higher incidence of triploidy and lower oocyte retrieval fertilization and implantation rates. Van Blerkom[50] confirmed a significantly higher incidence of aneuploidy and spindle defects in the less vascularized group of oocytes.

The PFBF characteristics measured by color Doppler images are related to the intrafollicular oxygen content and vascular endothelial growth factor (VEGF) concentration, and oocytes from severely hypoxic follicles were associated with high frequencies of abnormalities in the organization of the chromosomes on the metaphase spindle. The best predictors of IVF outcome are the ovarian FI using 3D ultrasound and power Doppler angiography (PDA) on the hCG day and the transfer of grade 1 embryos.[53]

Rising PSV with steady low RI suggests that the follicle is close to rupture (Follicular PSV goes as high as 45 cm/s before an hour of ovulation). Whereas steady or decreasing PSV with rising RI suggests that the follicle is proceeding toward LUF. It was also observed that fertilization of a follicle with PSV of less than 10 cm/s, have high chances of embryo being chromosomally abnormal.

Doppler in the secretory phase gives an idea about the function of corpus luteum. Usually the RI of the corpus luteum is between 0.35 and 0.50. In luteal phase deficiency (LPD), RI is 0.58 ± 0.04, PI is 0.70–0.80 and PSV is between 10 and 15.

Luteal Phase Doppler (Fig. 10)

In the mid-luteal phase, the spiral artery RI is 0.48–0.52, uterine artery PI is 2.0–2.5 and uterine artery PSV is 15–20. Increased resistance to uterine blood flow in the mid-luteal phase is an important contributing factor in some cases of infertility. When PI is used as the measure of impedance, it was found that a PI of less than 3.0[54] or less than 3.34[55] was more favorable for pregnancy. No difference was found in uterine or ovarian artery PI between pregnant and nonpregnant women, but there was a nonsignificant increase in uterine receptivity when the uterine artery PI was in the range of 2.0–2.99 on the day of embryo transfer.[56] It was also seen that RI was found to be significantly lower at the time of oocyte collection in women who achieved a pregnancy.[57] In a recent study, Ng and colleagues performed 3D ultrasound power Doppler one day after LH surge in women undergoing FET in natural or clomiphene-induced cycles. These investigators found that endometrial thickness, endometrial volume, endometrial pattern, uterine PI, uterine RI, and endometrial and subendometrial 3D power Doppler flow indices were similar between the nonpregnant and pregnant groups.[58] They concluded that measurement of uterine artery blood flow should not be part of routine IVF practice. It was also emphasized in this study that the age of women was the only predictive factor for pregnancy. Early secretory transformation of endometrium is a feature of LPD.

Effect of Ovarian Stimulation Drugs on PFBF

- *Clomiphene citrate*: Clomiphene citrate administration reduces the ovarian and, specifically, the perifollicular

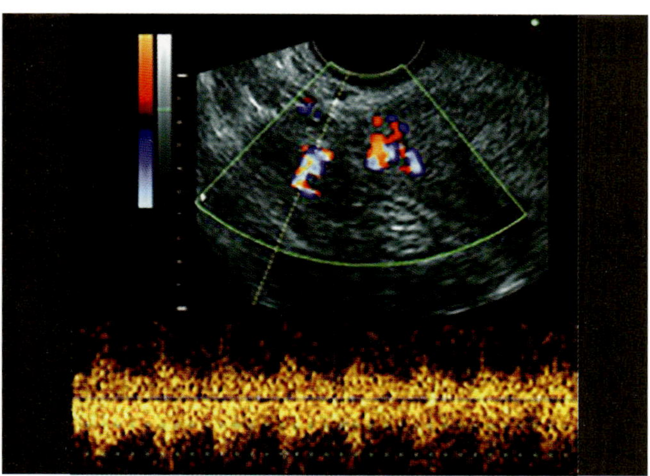

Fig. 10 Doppler of corpus luteum

vascularization.[59] In one study, it was noted that PCOS patients who ovulate on metformin treatment, the ovarian blood flow is similar to those observed in healthy women.[59]

- *Letroz:* Does not alter PFBF.
- *Gonadotropins:* LH activity in urinary gonadotropins is associated with greater than PFBF as compared to recombinant FSH. In the group with high PFBF, the clinical pregnancy rate was higher in women treated with urinary gonadotropins as compared to those treated with recombinant FSH (P < 05), although the numbers are small.[60]

Perifollicular Blood Flow and ART Results

High-grade ovarian PFBF in the early follicular phase during IVF is associated with both high-grade PFBF in the late follicular phase and a higher clinical pregnancy rate. In an oocyte donation cycle, women who received embryos originating from oocytes developed in well-vascularized follicles had a statistically higher pregnancy rate than women who received embryos deriving from oocytes grown in more poorly vascularized follicles (34% vs 13.7%).[61] It was also observed that poor responders had significantly higher uterine and perifollicular Doppler flow resistances. Moreover, it was noted that the pregnancy rate per cycle was significantly higher in normoresponders (26%) than poor responders (6%).[62]

Ultrasound Assessment of the Endometrium

Successful implantation depends on a close dialog between a good quality embryo and the receptive endometrium. Synchronization between endometrial and embryo development is an essential prerequisite for successful implantation and therefore monitoring endometrial changes during ovulation inductions is important. These changes are a reliable bioassay of the patient's estrogenic status and correlate with plasma E2 and P4 levels. Ultrasound examination of the endometrium provides a noninvasive method to evaluate endometrial receptivity during ART cycle.[63] Different ultrasound parameters that can be evaluated to determine the endometrial receptivity include endometrial thickness, endometrial pattern, endometrial volume **(Figs 11A to C)**, Doppler study of uterine arteries and endometrial blood flow. Endometrial thickness and pattern have low positive predictive value and specificity for ART outcome.[63,64] Minimum volume of 2.0–2.5 mL is essential to achieve a pregnancy.[65,66] Endometrial volume measured on the day of hCG administration especially by 3D USG was statistically significantly higher in the pregnant group.

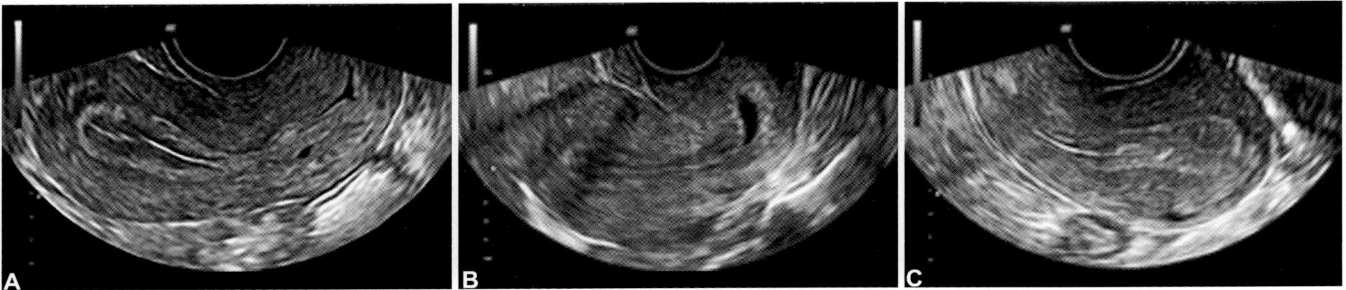

Figs 11A to C Endometrial pattern and thickness

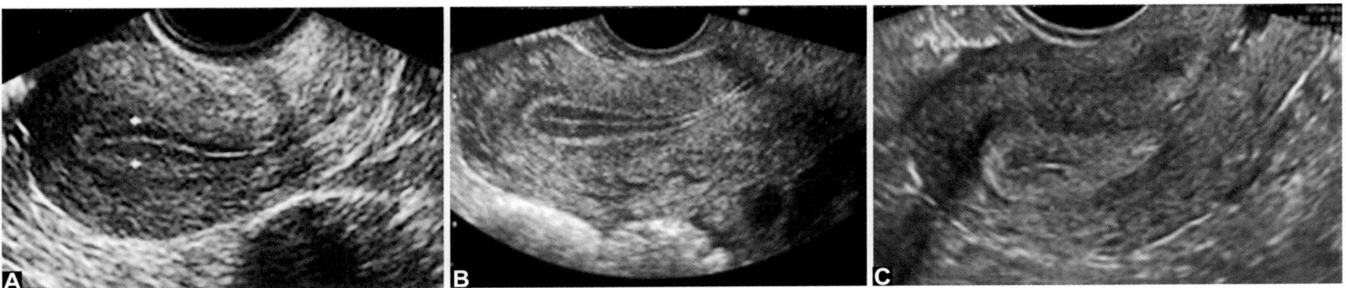

Figs 12A to C Morphology of endometrium in the different phases of menstrual cycle. (A) Early proliferative phase; (B) Late proliferative phase; (C) Following ovulation

The endometrium undergoes cyclic morphological as well as histological changes throughout the menstrual cycle. During menstruation, the endometrium appears as a thin echo that gradually thickens throughout the proliferative phase to reach the typical periovulatory trilaminar appearance. After ovulation, the rise in circulating progesterone induces stromal edema and growth of spiral arterioles, resulting in increased echogenicity of the thick secretory endometrium.

The morphology of the endometrium in the different phases of menstrual cycle is illustrated below **(Figs 12A to C)**:

- Early proliferative phase—translucent and thin on either side of mid-line echo.
- Late proliferative phase—increase in thickness with hyporeflective area in the center.
- Following ovulation—shrinks in thickness, becomes dense echogenic on either side of mid-line echo.

Endometrial Receptivity Markers

Conventional markers
- Thickness
- Morphology
- Uterine artery flow
- Peristalsis.

Newer markers
- Three-dimensional endometrial volume.
- Three-dimensional endometrial configuration.
- Three-dimensional endometrial vascularity quantification.

Many clinicians have reported no difference in endometrial thickness between pregnant and nonpregnant women,[67,68] while others have observed a positive correlation between endometrial thickness and pregnancy outcome.[69,70] Zhang and coauthors found that increased endometrial thickness was associated with improved treatment outcome, but the association was dependent on patient age, duration of ovarian stimulation, and embryo quality.[71] On the contrary, Richter and colleagues found that the higher clinical pregnancy and live birth rates associated with increasing endometrial thickness were independent of the effects of patient age and embryo quality.[72] A meta-analysis demonstrated that endometrial thickness is a better negative than positive predictor of implantation.[64] Different studies have proposed different endometrial thickness cutoff levels for successful implantation to occur: greater than or equal to 6 mm,[67] greater than or equal to 10 mm,[70] and greater than or equal to 13 mm.[73] There have been no reports of adverse effects of a thickened endometrium on implantation, pregnancy, or miscarriage rates in IVF.[74]

An association also has been noted between the ultrasound endometrial texture, echogenic patterns and serum hormonal (E2 and progesterone) levels.[73] In IVF cycles, a preovulatory, echogenic, and homogeneous pattern has been associated with premature rise in progesterone levels, probably due to high LH levels in the early proliferative phase or premature secretion of LH especially in the antagonist flexible protocol.[67,57] This is due to the presence of high E2 levels, which are related to multifollicular development. Endometrial hyperechogenicity prior to ovulation is a poor prognostic factor for pregnancy **(Fig. 13A)**.[75,76] On the other hand, women with a triple-line pattern on the day of oocyte retrieval conceived in 80.0% of cases **(Fig. 13B)**.[77]

The endometrial pattern with an outer hyperechogenic and inner hypoechogenic layer on the day of oocyte retrieval had predictive value on IVF treatment.[63] Homogeneous and hyperechogenic sonographic endometrial pattern had a predictive value of 100% for a nonconceptional cycle, whereas multilayered endometrium was visualized in conception cycles.[78]

The endometrial thickness and pattern also provide useful information in FET or oocyte donation cycles in which the endometrium is supplemented with estrogen and progesterone. A minimal endometrial thickness of 6 mm is required before embryo replacement for pregnancy to be achieved.[79,80] In a study published by El-Toukhy et al.[81] an endometrial thickness of 9–14 mm on the day of progesterone supplementation in an FET cycle was found to be associated with higher implantation and pregnancy rates compared with an endometrial thickness of 7–8 mm. They reported lowest pregnancy rates when the endometrial thickness was either less than 7 mm or more than 14 mm.

Endometrial Volume

The minimum endometrial volume, which is associated with pregnancy is 1.59 mL when calculated by 3D ultrasound, but most pregnancies occur in volumes of 2–13 mL. Calculation of endometrial volume is particularly useful in cases of synechiae, adenomyosis and uterine anomalies to predict the outcome of treatment.

Endometrial and subendometrial volume increases rapidly during the follicular phase and then remains almost unchanged during the luteal phase.[82]

Ultrasound parameters, which indicate a good receptive endometrium include:

- Endometrial morphology, which shows a "triple-line" pattern.
- Endometrial thickness of 8–14 mm.
- Uterine vascularity: Mean uterine artery PI between 2 and 3, and uterine artery PSV 15–20 cm/s.
- Presence of subendometrial and endometrial flow.
- Higher subendometrial VI, FI and vascularization flow index (VFI) was observed on the day of hCG in the conception group.
- Endometrial volume of greater than 2 mL has a significantly higher pregnancy rates.

Persisting presence of endometrial fundocervical waves after hCG administration has lower pregnancy rates. Normally, these are seen till administration of hCG and later the wave direction switch occurs to cervicofundal. With this pattern of endometrial wave switch there is a higher the likelihood of pregnancy.[83] Less than three peristaltic contractions of the subendometrial myometrium at every 2 minutes interval on the day of hCG administration is associated with poor implantation rate. High E2 levels in COS cycles are associated with more peristalsis, which negatively correlates with implantation.

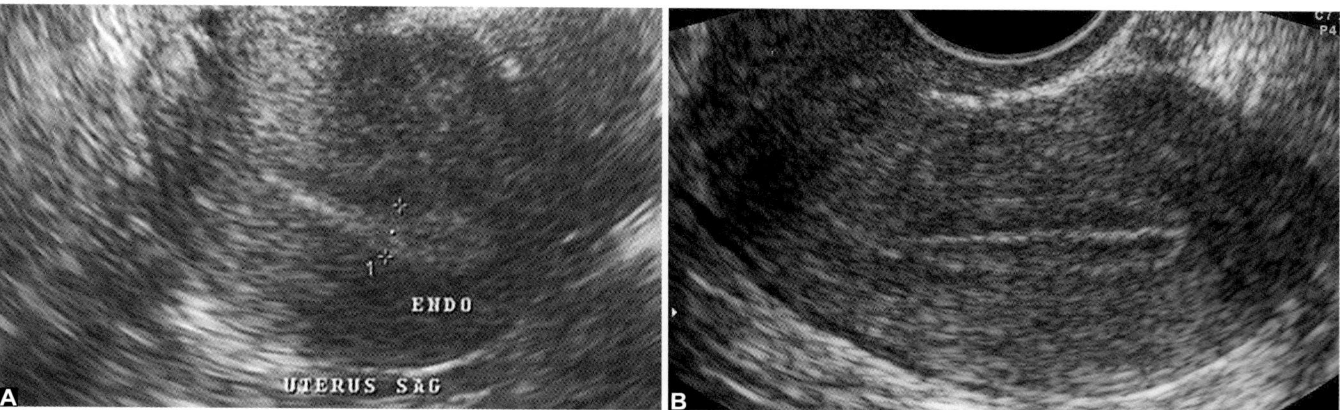

Figs 13A and B (A) Hyperechogenic; (B) Triple-line pattern on the day of oocyte retrieval

Number and type of wave form during the menstrual cycle:

- *Follicular phase:* 4–5 uterine contractions per minute retrograde.
- *Luteo-follicular transition:* 2–3 uterine contractions per minute antegrade.
- *Luteal phase:* Less than 2.5 uterine contractions per minute.

Presence of high frequency uterine contractions on the day of embryo transfer negatively affect IVF–ET outcome. If frequency of contractions is less or fall, the clinical pregnancy rate rises.[84]

Recently pulsed Doppler and 3D color and power Doppler studies have been applied to evaluate endometrial receptivity by the uterine and endometrial blood flow status.

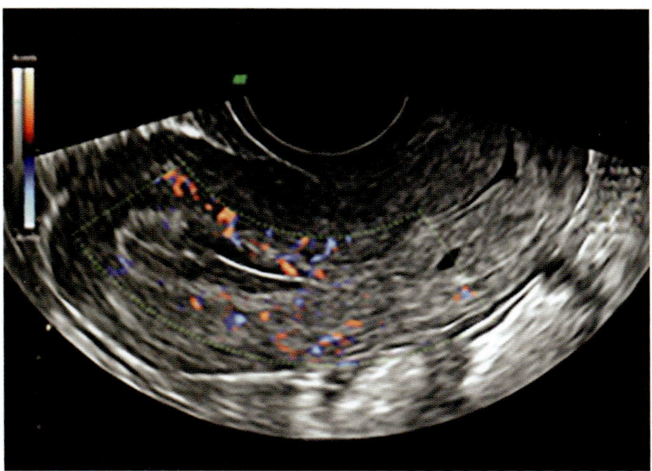

Fig. 15 Endometrial blood flow

Endometrial and Subendometrial Vascularity

A good blood supply to the endometrium is usually considered as an essential requirement for implantation. Assessment of endometrial blood flow adds a physiological dimension to the anatomical ultrasound parameters.

When power Doppler is combined with 3D, it gives a better idea about the blood supply to the whole endometrium and the subendometrial region (5 mm). However, the role of endometrial and subendometrial blood flow **(Figs 14 and 15)** in IVF outcomes remains controversial though endometrial or subendometrial blood flow was seen to be significantly higher in pregnant patients.[85-87]

Endometrial and subendometrial vascularity indices are high throughout follicular phase, peak value is reached 3 days before ovulation and reduce to a nadir 5 days after ovulation and then increase again during the luteal phase.[88] This reduction in endometrial perfusion from the late follicular phase through to the early luteal phase may be an important marker for endometrial receptivity. Hypoxia in the endometrium has been shown to have a beneficial role for implantation as the expression of VEGF is upregulated by hypoxia[89] and relatively low oxygen tension was present during the time of implantation on day 5–6.[90]

Percentage change in endometrial and subendometrial blood flow between evaluations done on the days of hCG and embryo transfer would probably help in predicting the success of an ART cycle.

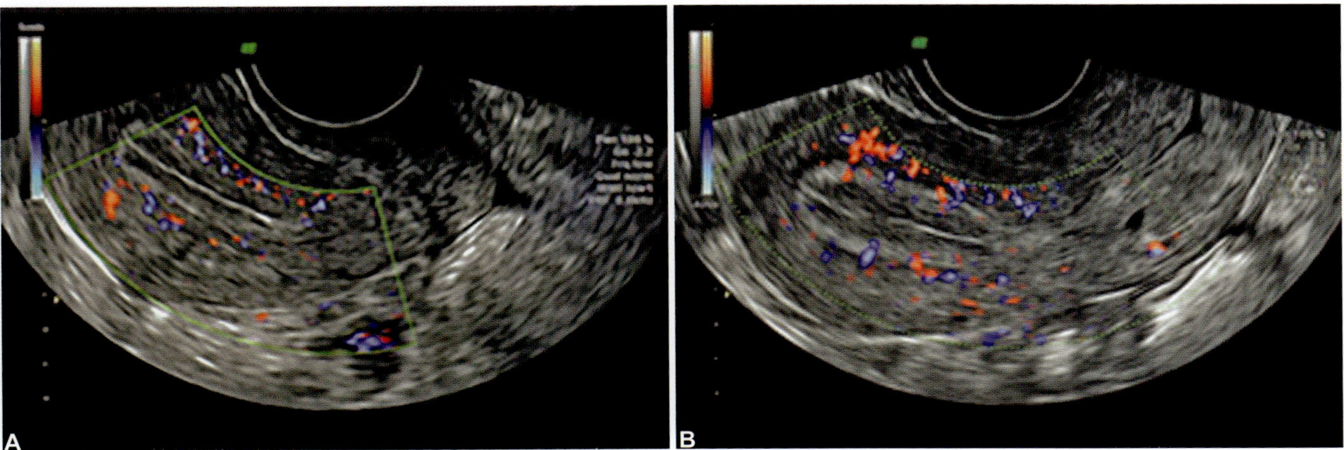

Figs 14A and B Subendometrial blood flow

It was observed that subendometrial FI was significantly higher in pregnant cycles while subendometrial VI and VFI were similar between pregnant and nonpregnant patients.[85] Another study demonstrated that subendometrial VFI was significantly higher in the pregnant group and was superior to endometrial volume, sub-endometrial VI and FI in predicting the outcome.[86] Endometrial VI, FI and VFI were also found to be significantly higher in pregnant cycles.[87] A marked reduction in endometrial and subendometrial VI and VFI and a modest reduction in endometrial and subendometrial FI was seen in COS cycles.

Endometrial microvascular blood flow, which is determined by an intrauterine laser Doppler technique in the early luteal phase of the cycle preceding an IVF cycle, has been shown to be predictive of pregnancy and is superior to other conventional parameters predicting endometrial receptivity.[91] The chance of pregnancy was significantly higher in women with endometrial tissue blood flow of at least 29 mL/minute per 100 g of tissue than in women with lower values.

Endometrial and subendometrial blood flow on the days of hCG and embryo transfer was not predictive of pregnancy following IVF treatment but would give an idea about the endometrial receptivity.

Endometrial Blood Flow Quantification

Endometrial blood flow quantification is done using the 3D power Doppler with Virtual Organ Computer-aided Analysis (VOCAL). It is shell-imaging, which is used to define and quantify the power Doppler signal within the endometrial and subendometrial regions producing indices of their relative vascularity.

Endometrial Vascularization Using 3D Power Doppler

Endometrial vascularization is calculated by measuring the vascular index (VI), FI, vascular FI and flow vessel quotient.

- Vascularization index reflects number of vessels in volume of tissue and is calculated by dividing the number of color voxels by total number of voxels.
- Flow index reflects the amount of blood flow and is calculated by dividing the sum of color intensities by number of color voxels.
- VFI reflects vessel presence and blood flow and is calculated by dividing the sum of color intensities by total voxels.
- Flow vessel quotient (FVQ) is calculated by dividing FI by VI (FI/VI).

We can use these indices in predicting the occurrence of pregnancy.
- No pregnancy, if VI less than 1.0.
- No pregnancy, if FI less than 31.
- No pregnancy, if VFI less than 0.25.

Endometrial and subendometrial vascularity (VI/FI/VFI) significantly less (P ≤0.003) in patients with low volume endometrium, but not in those with thin endometrium.[92] It is also significantly lower in stimulated cycle than that in the natural cycle.[93] CC reduces endometrium vascularity as compared to letrozole. In COS cycles, endometrial blood flow was negatively affected by E2 concentration.[94] Hyperresponders tended to have low VI/VFI on 2 days after hCG administration and also had a higher incidence of having absent endometrial and subendometrial blood flow. Luteal phase vascularity was also altered in high responders.[93]

Endometrial Vascularity in Special Situations

Fibroids
Endometrial and subendometrial 3D power Doppler flow indices were similar in patients with and without small intramural fibroids.[95]

Hydrosalpinx
Patients in the hydrosalpinx group had significantly lower endometrial and subendometrial VI and VFI.

Unexplained Infertility
Endometrial and subendometrial vascularity significantly less during mid-late follicular phase irrespective of E2 or P concentration and endometrial morphometry.

Repeated Miscarriage
Patients with live birth had significantly higher endometrial VI and VFI and subendometrial VI, FI and VFI, when compared with those who had a miscarriage. Among all the vascular indices only endometrial VI was significantly associated with the chance of live birth with an odds ratio of 1.384 [95% confidence interval (CI) 1.025 – 1.869, P = 0.034]. In FET cycles, patients with live birth had significantly high endometrium VFI, SE VI and VFI than those with miscarriage. So, we can conclude that endometrial and subendometrial vascularity was significantly higher in pregnant patients with live birth following stimulated IVF and FET treatment than in those who suffered a miscarriage.[96]

Correlation of Endometrial and Subendometrial Blood Flow to Pregnancy Rate in ART

Endometrial and subendometrial blood flow on the days of hCG and on the day of embryo transfer and the percentage change in endometrial and subendometrial blood flows between these 2 days were not predictive of pregnancy in ART cycles.[91] It is just prognostic and not predictive index in ART cycles.

Maintenance of Records during Monitoring of an Ovulation Induction Cycle

For optimal outcome of infertility treatment, monitoring of the ovarian response in COH cycles should be plotted in a chart. Follicular growth recorded on especially these designed charts allows us to see at a glance all the relevant characteristics of the cycle.

These include:

- Date and day of cycle
- Number of developing follicles in each ovary
- Dynamics of follicular growth
- Endometrial thickness
- Type of ovulation regimen
- Quantity of medication used
- Baseline hormone levels
- Estradiol, if required in the proliferative phase
- Estradiol and P4 on the day of hCG
- Any change in the dose and hormonal evaluation done also noted
- Date and time of administration of hCG.

Follicles can occasionally be confused with other pelvic structures, but they can be differentiated by rotating the transducer 90°. If the structure is a vessel, it will then elongate, acquiring a tubular shape. The internal iliac artery can easily be identified by its arterial pulsations, while a hydrosalpinx generally has a less regular shape.

Ultrasound after oocyte retrieval and before embryo transfer can also identify fluid in the endometrial cavity **(Fig. 16)** and is usually associated with poor prognosis. It could be present due to excessive cervical mucus that ascends into the endometrial cavity, fluid reflux from a hydrosalpinx, subclinical uterine infection and abnormal endometrial development.

Presence of persistent fluid accumulation at the time of embryo transfer warrants freezing of all embryos and transfer in a subsequent cycle.

Uterine Artery Blood Flow

There have been conflicting reports in the literature regarding the usefulness of the application of color Doppler ultrasound for monitoring and predicting pregnancy outcome of IVF cycles. It was observed that uterine blood flow is a poor reflection of subendometrial blood flow during stimulated and natural cycles, and its

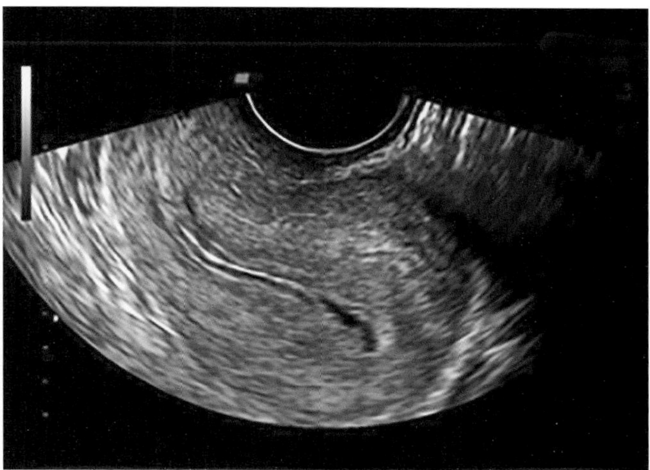

Fig. 16 Fluid in the uterine cavity

measurement cannot reflect endometrial blood flow during stimulated cycles.[94]

Several studies used the PI as the measure of impedance and determined that a PI of less than 3.0[55] or less than 3.34[68] was more favorable for pregnancy. More recently, Steer and coauthors found similar results in women undergoing FET in a downregulated hormonally prepared cycle.[97] In contrast, other researchers found that uterine artery PI did not significantly change until the midluteal phase. No difference was found in uterine or ovarian artery PI between pregnant and nonpregnant women, but there was a nonsignificant increase in uterine receptivity when the uterine artery PI was in the range of 2.0–2.99 on the day of embryo transfer.[57] Other investigators used RI and found that it was significantly lower at the time of oocyte collection in women who achieved a pregnancy.[58] In a recent study, Ng and colleagues performed 3D ultrasound power Doppler one day after LH surge in women undergoing FET in natural or clomiphene-induced cycles. The age of women was the only predictive factor for pregnancy. Endometrial thickness, endometrial volume, endometrial pattern, uterine PI, uterine RI, and endometrial and subendometrial 3D power Doppler flow indices were similar between the nonpregnant and pregnant groups.[94] Currently, measurement of uterine artery blood flow should not be part of routine IVF practice.

Uterine arterial blood flow was lower in CC stimulated cycles during the periovulatory period than those in the spontaneous menstrual cycles,[98] and also demonstrated that uterine vascular impedance during the day of ovulation was lower in the conception cycles, while there were no differences between conception and nonconception cycles in the luteal phase.[99]

*Tridimensional Automated USG for
Monitoring COS Cycles*

Two-dimensional TVS is typically performed to monitor follicle growth in ovulation induction cycles and to determine the optimal time for administration hCG. 2D only provides the size of the follicle unlike 3D, which also provided the volume. The automated measurement of follicular size in 3D using a software program that identifies and quantifies hypoechoic regions within a 3D dataset might provide an objective, fast, valid and reliable standard for follicular measurements. Each different volume is separately color coded, making Sono-AVC an ideal tool for studying follicular development in response to ovarian stimulation (**Fig. 17**).

An AVC software program is commercially available and it provides an automatic estimation of their absolute volumes, calculating back from each volume to a mean diameter of a perfect sphere.[100]

It has been shown that the follicular volumes measured and calculated with the AVC are in accordance with the aspirated volumes[101] and that they also provide more accurate data than traditional 2D measurements.[102]

Besides that, 3D AVC took less time for follicular diameter measurement (data not shown) than the 2D measurement method, with no interobserver variability. The shorter examination time and objective follicle diameter measurement associated with 3D AVC, combined with reduced exposure to ultrasound due to the acquisition of 3D data,[103] may confer clinical benefits to patients and guarantee the quality standards.

Some investigators have shown that the number of follicles between certain volumes correlates with the number of oocytes retrieved as well as their subsequent developmental competence after fertilization.[49,104]

It was also seen that the oocyte yield is best when the cohort of follicles lies between 16 mm and 22 mm; fewer oocytes are retrieved if the cohort of follicles is below or above this range.[105]

It would be useful to further research whether the data gathered using 3D AVC may lead to better criteria for determining the optimal time of hCG administration, fertilization rate and embryo development.

Monitoring Abnormal Response

Ultrasound is also useful in monitoring abnormal response to ovulation induction, which includes premature lutenization, LUF, endogenous LH surge, poor response, hyperstimulation, presence of retention or functional cyst and ovarian torsion.

Premature Luteinization (Fig. 18)

Follicles less than 15 mm with echoes are seen and these correlates with high P4 levels in follicular phase. It is due to premature and suboptimal LH surge resulting in progesterone production but no ovulation, oocyte maturation without follicular rupture. It is associated with poor quality oocytes and embryos with endometrium, which is out of phase; thus, reducing the implantation rate.

Luteinized Unruptured Follicle (Fig. 19)

Diagnosed when dominant follicle is still apparent 48 hours after administration of hCG or LH surge. The size of the

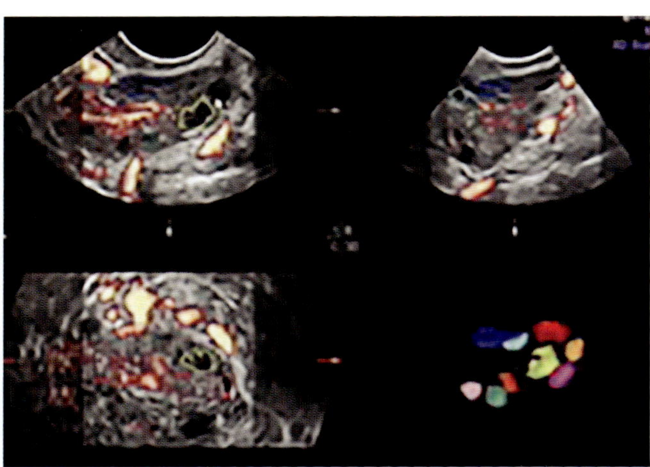

Fig. 17 Three-dimensional follicular monitoring using sono-automated volume count

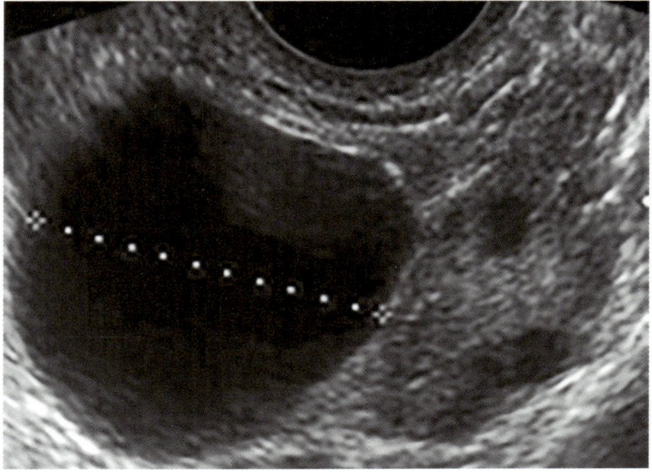

Fig. 18 Premature luteinization

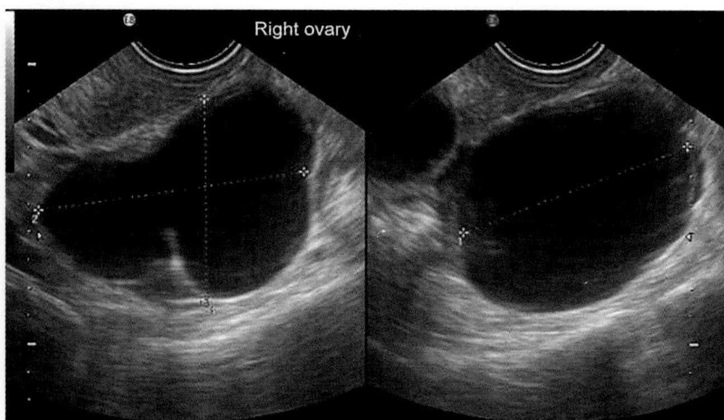

Fig. 19 Luteinized unruptured follicle

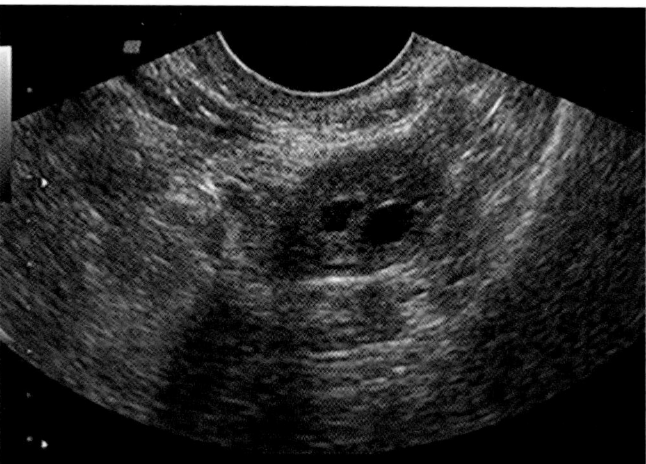

Fig. 20 Poor response

follicle may reach 34–36 mm and have internal echoes. It is due to insufficient strength of LH surge to induce follicular rupture but sufficient to induce oocyte maturation.

Endogenous LH Surge

It is seen on ultrasound as premature rupture of follicles at diameter of less than 16–17 mm. It is associated with compromised oocytes and embryo quality as a result of exposure to inappropriate LH levels. Thus, requires extensive endocrine monitoring and be prevented with use of GnRH agonist or antagonist.

Poor Response (Fig. 20)

Poor response can be predicted by estimating the baseline AFC and ovarian volume (<3–4 antral follicles and volume <3 mL). At times the AFC may be normal but the women may not respond to gonadotropin for various reasons, so presence of less than 2–3 follicles on ultrasound on day 7 of ovulation induction with gonadotropins also suggests poor response.

Ovarian Hyperstimulation Syndrome (Fig. 21)

Ultrasound is essential for prevention, diagnosis and monitoring of OHSS. Judicial use of TVS for follicular monitoring while inducing ovulation with gonadotropins remains critical for prevention of OHSS. TVS is also used to monitor the ovarian volume, keep record of number of follicles and corpus luteum and their size, diagnose ascites and pleural effusion when monitoring for the progress of OHSS. Ultrasound can also be used to guide paracentesis of the ascites or pleural effusion in cases, which develop severe respiratory distress to avoid trauma to ovaries or other abdominal structures.

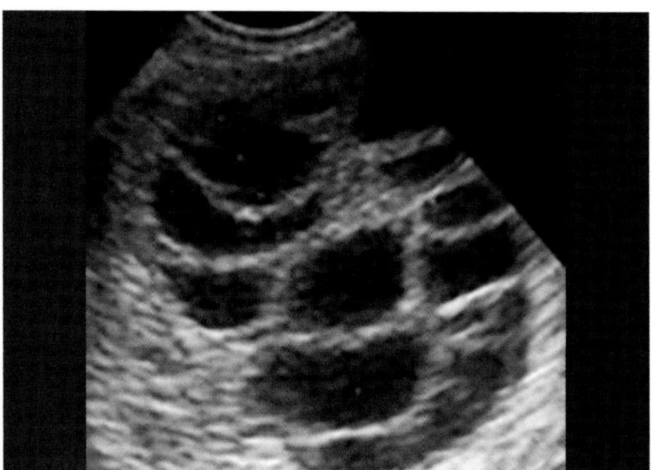

Fig. 21 Ovarian hyperstimulation syndrome

Functional Cyst (Fig. 22)

Functional cyst is diagnosed by the presence of cyst at prestimulation baseline scan on day 2 or 3 of the menstrual cycles following GnRH agonist administration for downregulation. It is characterized by sharp edges and anechogenic contents and is due to the initial FSH surge, which occurs after commencement of GnRH agonist in a long downregulation cycle. Presence of a functional cyst requires either cancelation of cycle or an ultrasound-guided aspiration of the cyst before commencing ovulation induction.

Persistent/Retention Cyst (Fig. 23)

Presence of cyst at baseline scan suggests a follicle from previous cycle or a persistent corpus luteum. It may

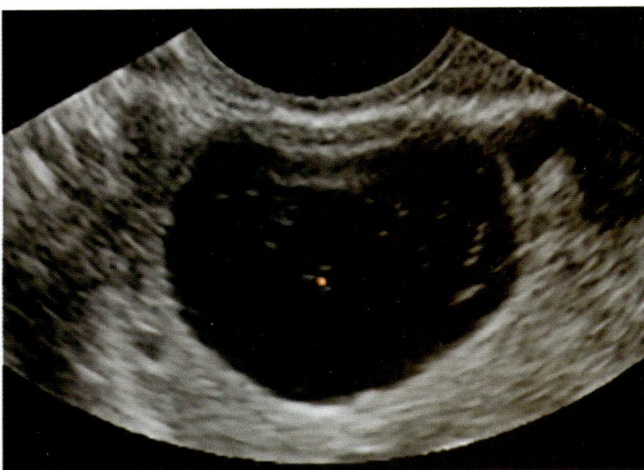

Fig. 22 Functional cyst

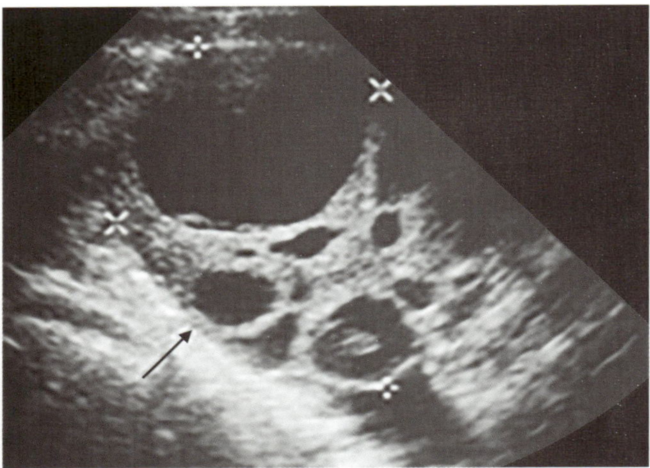

Fig. 23 Persistent or retention cyst

result due to growth of the smaller follicles following hCG trigger. No drugs are administered for ovulation induction in the presence of a retention cyst. It is followed ultrasonographically and if persistent may require medical or surgical treatment.

Hormonal Monitoring

Fertility is associated with marked daily changes in hormone output especially E2, LH and progesterone. Any pattern that shows no changes from day-to-day denotes infertility and estimation of these hormones during ovulation induction may prove useful. Evaluation of hormonal values can predict both ovarian reserve as well as ovarian response.

Hormonal Monitoring in an Ovulation Induction Cycle

Ovulation induction without the use of gonadotropins and GnRH analogs is easy and occasionally requires measurement of E2 levels depending on response endometrial thickness and number and size of follicles. Estimation of LH in these cycles allows us to precisely identify the time of ovulation and therefore is used in natural cycles and oral ovulogen cycles. But with the use of gonadotropin and GnRH analogs in ART cycles both E2 and LH are monitored more often. We very well know that premature LH surge can impair the development of the oocyte and affect its fertilizing ability it needs to be detected. A premature LH surge can occur with high levels of E2 in mid-follicular phase. This could be due to use of estrogen in early part of follicular cycle, development of large number of follicles resulting in high E2 especially in cycles where GnRH analogs are not used.

Serum LH

Relationship between follicle size and the serum E2 level is not sufficiently strong to predict the LH surge confidently on the basis of only one variable, but it has been observed that LH surge is unlikely to occur before the follicle diameter has reached 15 mm and/or the serum E2 level has reached 164 pg/mL. LH levels should be measured daily once the follicle reaches 15–16 mm to determine the LH surge and exact time of ovulation. The mean peak value of LH is 97 U/L/24 hour with a standard deviation is equal to 78 U/L. The LH surges that result in ovulation are extremely variable in configuration, amplitude and duration.

Luteinizing hormone surge can be detected by measuring:
1. Serum LH levels.
2. Metabolites of LH in urine using urinary LH detection kits. Urinary hormone metabolites accurately reflect LH and correspond to serum patterns and thus a high predictive value for detecting ovulation. Detection of LH surge by urinary LH test may have false-negative results, when:
   - Peak levels are 40 IU/L
   - Women have surges of 10 hours in duration
   - Diluted urine is tested.

In a study by Lloyd et al. showed that when LH kits alone were used to time IUI:

- Thirty-six percent of inseminations were timed incorrectly
- Fifteen percent of women had already ovulated.

Serum Estradiol Levels

By day 5–8 of the menstrual cycle, aromatase activity begins in granulosa cells of follicles larger than 6–8 mm, with the dominant follicle producing more E2 than other follicles in the cohort.[106-110]

To best reflect the ovarian response to stimulation and provide an efficient flow of information, gonadotropins generally are administered in the evening, typically between 5:00 PM and 8:00 PM, and serum E2 measurements are obtained early in the morning. Results usually are available for review by midday, and change in the dose and duration of gonadotropins can be done. Follicles less than approximately 10 mm in mean diameter produce relatively little measurable estrogen and larger follicles secrete progressively more as they grow and approach maturity. Usually, E2 levels rise at a constant exponential pace, doubling approximately every 2–3 days over the days before peak follicular development is achieved. A shallower or steeper slope of increase suggests the need to increase or decrease the level of stimulation. In contrast to a natural cycle, the linear relationship between follicle size and E2 measurements is lost due to the presence of many developing follicles that contribute to the circulating E2. In the natural ovulatory cycle, E2 levels peak between 200 pg/mL and 400 pg/mL just before the LH surge. Comparable levels of E2 should be expected in GT-stimulated cycles, for each mature follicle observed. In a COS cycle, one must also consider the number and size of smaller follicles and their lesser but collective contributions to the serum E2 concentration apart from the large follicles when measuring E2 levels. Cycle fecundability increases with serum E2 levels; unfortunately, so do the risks of multiple pregnancy and ovarian hyperstimulation and this is due to multifollicular development, making more oocytes available for fertilization. With existing COS regimens, best results are generally obtained when E2 concentrations peak between 500 pg/mL and 1,500 pg/mL; pregnancies are uncommon at levels below 200 pg/mL.

Normal follicular growth correlates with E2 measurements and therefore it can be measured to modulate the dose of gonadotropins in the following manner.

Initial dose changed after 4–5 days depending on E2 levels:

- If rise greater than 100% then the dose is reduced by 75 IU.
- If rise less than 50% then the dose is increased by 75 IU.
- If rise between 50–100% then same dose is maintained. Plateauing or decreasing levels require cancelation of the cycle.

Progesterone

Progesterone levels are done on day 2 of the menstrual cycle before COS is initiated and on the day of hCG. Elevated progesterone (PE) is associated with endometrial asynchrony and subsequently low pregnancy rates, though the pathophysiology of pre-hCG progesterone rise and its impact on pregnancy outcomes remain inconclusive as no randomized controlled trial (RCTs) are available. But Chu-Chun Huang et al. studied 1,784 IVF/ICSI cycles and concluded that clinical pregnancy rate was significantly decreased in women with longer durations of serum progesterone elevation, independent of the protocol used and the ovarian response.[111]

Despite the use of GnRH analogs, a subtle preovulatory rise in the serum progesterone concentration before the administration of hCG for final oocyte maturation still occurred in 5–30% of COS cycles.[112-114]

An inverse correlation was observed between the clinical pregnancy rate and the duration of preovulatory progesterone elevation and not the absolute progesterone value on the day of hCG administration. It was also noticed that these patients tend to be younger with better reserve and have lower baseline FSH levels.[115]

Progesterone elevation on the day of hCG administration is associated with a significantly decreased probability of pregnancy after fresh embryo transfer in women undergoing ovarian stimulation using gonadotropins and GnRH analogs for IVF but not after transfer of frozen-thawed embryos originating from that cycle. The corresponding number needed to harm (NNH) is 10, which means that for every 10 patients with PE, three instead of four pregnancies should be expected.

It was also observed that E2 levels on the day of hCG appear to be increased in the presence of PE. In addition, there was some evidence that PE is associated with an increase in the total amount of FSH used for ovarian stimulation but not the length of stimulation. Freezing embryos and transferring them in a subsequent frozen-thawed cycle (the "freeze-all" strategy) has been proposed as a way to bypass impaired endometrial receptivity,[116,117] and it is also considered to be the most frequently used method for managing PE.[118]

It was also observed that prolongation of follicular phase is associated with a higher incidence of premature secretory changes on the day of oocyte retrieval in cycles stimulated with recombinant follicle-stimulated hormone (rFSH) and GnRH antagonists.[119]

Cancelation of Ovarian Stimulation Cycles

The definite indication for cancellation of cycle is poor follicular growth and E2 levels of less than 100 pg/mL on day 5–6 of COS. The possible indication for cancelation may be presence of an adnexal cyst secondary to GnRH agonist used in a long protocol, risk of OHSS, occurrence of an endogenous LH surge or a steady decline in E2 levels and poor ovarian response.

Monitoring a Frozen Embryo Transfer Cycle

Natural Cycle Frozen Embryo Transfer

In ovulatory patients, FET is commonly performed during a natural cycle.[120] The natural cycle offers the advantages of utilizing the natural physiological process of endometrial preparation for implantation, and decreases medical intervention as compared with hormone replacement cycles. These advantages make natural cycle frozen embryo transfer a good option as against a hormone replacement therapy (HRT) cycle. In a natural cycle, synchronization between the endometrium and the frozen embryos is done by detecting the day of ovulation. The day of spontaneous ovulation in the natural cycle corresponds to the day of egg retrieval in the "fresh" IVF cycle. Thawing and transferring of embryos is scheduled according to the stage at which embryos were frozen.

The disadvantage of a natural cycle FET is that detection and documentation of ovulation may require numerous monitoring visits even in women with regular menstrual cycles. Furthermore, the date of embryo transfer cannot be planned in advance, a difficulty for centers that do not operate 7 days a week.

Patient monitoring prior to FET in a natural cycle consists of serial blood and ultrasound testing until the detection of ovulation.[121] Alternatively, hCG can be given for trigger in the presence of a mature follicle and satisfactory endometrial development. This may simplify the monitoring process by decreasing the visits to the clinic, the time and expense involved with hormone testing and USG for documentation of ovulation.

Because ovulation is a must, only patients with regular ovulatory cycles can be included in NC–FET programs.[122]

Detection of Ovulation

Patients were monitored form day 9 of the menstrual cycle after a baseline USG on day 2 with evaluation of E2 and P4.

Criteria for ovulation detection in a natural cycle without administration of hCG included: (1) fall in serum estradiol concentration compared with the previous test; (2) detection of ovulation surge with fall in LH levels; (3) rise in serum progesterone concentration greater than 1.5 ng/mL; and (4) disappearance or typical change in the shape of the lead follicle.

Patients in whom hCG trigger was given for ovulation USG scans were done from day 9 until the criteria for ovulation triggering by hCG were met. Criteria for hCG administration included: (1) visualization of a leading follicle greater than 18 mm in diameter by TVS; (2) serum estradiol concentration greater than 200 pg/mL; and (3) serum progesterone concentration less than 1 ng/mL.

Hormone Replacement Therapy Cycle FET

In an HRT cycle, the endometrium is artificially prepared with exogenous steroids (estrogen and progesterone), with or without pituitary suppression by GnRH agonists.[121-123]

In the Cochrane review published in 2008, comparing the above treatment regimens, it was concluded that at the present time there is insufficient evidence to support the use of one intervention in preference to another.[124]

Monitoring Luteal Phase

What do women want to know after treatment with ovulation induction medication taken either for a timed intercourse, IUI or ART cycle is whether there is a pregnancy, whether it is in the right place, is it normal and is it going to continue normally.

The most important hormones monitored for this in the luteal phase is progesterone and β-hCG.

Luteal Phase

During the luteal phase, the increased values of progesterone and E2 play an important role in the maintenance of the low FSH and LH levels. During the luteal phase, the frequency of GnRH pulses decreases, while the amplitude increases[125] due to the high progesterone and E2 concentrations.[126,127] Gonadotropin secretion is also suppressed by E2 and progesterone and this action is possibly mediated via an increase in β-endorphin activity in the hypothalamus.[128]

What we measure normally in the luteal phase is day 21 progesterone level in a 28-day menstrual cycle, which will detect ovulation and adequacy of the luteal phase. In irregular cycles test may be performed later in the cycle and repeated weekly until the next menstruation. Progesterone has a pulsatile release, thus single level may not be useful unless elevated. Values of 10 ng/mL or more are suggestive of normal progesterone production.

The capacity of the corpus luteum to produce progesterone is closely related to the extent of its vascular network.[129-132] Corpus luteum angiogenesis is controlled by local secretion of growth factors[133] viz VEGF.[134-136]

The relation of blood flow indices in the corpus luteum measured by transvaginal color Doppler USG and hormone profiles were studied; the velocity and the impedance indices of the blood flow were both associated with the P/E2 ratio in spontaneous and CC cycles, while the blood flow indices and the P/E2 ratio were not correlated in COH cycles.[137]

Progesterone is responsible for endometrial decidualization, decreases smooth muscle contractility, decreases prostaglandin (PG) formation and immune responses (inhibitsT-lymphocyte-mediated tissue rejection).

Luteal-follicular Transition

During the passage from the luteal to the next follicular phase, an increase, or "intercycle rise", in serum FSH concentrations occurs. FSH starts to increase 2–3 days before the onset of the menstrual period[138] remains elevated during the early follicular phase and returns to the basal value in mid-follicular phase.[139,140]

In absence of pregnancy, there is a gradual but significant decline in the levels of inhibin A, E2 and progesterone takes place[141,142] which is responsible for the intercycle rise of FSH that starts in late luteal phase.

Controlled ovarian stimulation cycle, which aims to mature several FSH sensitive antral follicles during IVF/ICSI treatment using gonadotropins in an GnRH agonist or antagonist protocol result in multi-folliculogenesis. After hCG trigger all these follicles are converted into corpora lutea after release of oocyte in a timed intercourse or IUI cycle or after oocyte retrieval in an ART cycle. Several corpora lutea created produce large amount of progesterone and E2. If there is a pregnancy, the hCG produced by the chorionic villi will rescue the corpus luteum to support early pregnancy.

Luteoplacental shift occurs at 7–8 pregnancy week. Dominant ovary volume and vascularization decrease throughout the 1st trimester as placenta and gestational sac grow continuously.

It was seen that the luteal activity significantly increased for the first week of pregnancy in a COS cycle. It was also observed that the placental development maybe delayed/disturbed after COH and probably this is the cause for the adverse outcome after fresh embryo transfer following COS cycle. Therefore, today many clinicians are freezing all the embryos to be transferred in the subsequent natural or hormone replacement treatment cycle to improve the outcome.

Monitoring Early Pregnancy after Ovulation Induction

Prediction of pregnancy is the outcome desired by every patient who conceives during fertility treatment. However, this has been found to be uniformly difficult due to multiple factors.

A clinical pregnancy is confirmed by elevated concentrations of hCG, progesterone levels and observation of the gestational sac with TVS and later by appearance of yolk sac, the fetal pole and cardiac activity. The location of the gestational sac is essential to establish the viability of the pregnancy.

A single progesterone measurement in early pregnancy is useful test for discriminating between viable and nonviable pregnancies. A low progesterone value early in the pregnancy especially in presence of a positive β-hCG in patients presenting with bleeding, pain and inconclusive ultrasound results can rule out a viable pregnancy.[143]

Eighty-one percent of women undergoing IVF report highest level of psychological stress at the stage of the pregnancy test and waiting for the result.[144] The time between the first pregnancy test and confirmation of a viable intrauterine pregnancy (IUP) by ultrasound can also be emotionally stressful, with 46% of patients reporting this waiting time as being extremely or very stressful.[145] Stress and anxiety can then result in poor treatment outcome.

The maternal age, day 14 β-hCG concentration and the day 16 β-hCG concentration were found to be strong predictors of successful pregnancy continuation. The difference in age between those pregnancies that were ongoing and those that were not was strongly significant (P = 0.0005), as was the difference within the day 14 and day 16 β-hCG concentrations (P < 0.001). This significance indicates that these variables may be predictive of implantation success.

The rate of rise in β-hCG after implantation through to early pregnancy has been established,[146,147] and this concentration of β-hCG soon after implantation has been shown to have a direct correlation with pregnancy outcome.[148-151] Prior studies have also related outcome to both single β-hCG concentrations as well as multiple serial measurements.[152-161]

At times, despite a positive β-hCG, the pregnancy of unknown location (PUL) on ultrasound. This may be because we are performing the ultrasound too early (before β-hCG is 1,000 mIU/mL or too late in cases where the pregnancy has failed or due to altered anatomy, it is too difficult to visualize the pelvic structures or the pregnancy is too bad to be seen.

In such cases, it is important to diagnose an ectopic pregnancy as early as possible in order to initiate treatment. A slow rise in β-hCG and steady decrease in the progesterone levels is suggestive of an ectopic pregnancy.

An absolute single serum hCG level had the lowest diagnostic value, while strategies using serum hCG ratios, either alone or incorporated in logistic regression models, showed reasonable diagnostic performance for EP.

In the presence of PUL, one has to balance fears of mistakenly treating IUP against missing a "life-threatening ectopic". In such instances, it inevitably leads to overdiagnosis of ectopic pregnancy and employment of "preventative" management strategies. This may at times harm a normal IUP.

The majority of women with PUL (50–70%) have a spontaneously resolving pregnancy with serum hCG levels declining to undetectable levels. Such a pregnancy can either be a failed IUP or a resolved EP, as the location of the pregnancy remains undetermined. In some women, the pregnancy duration is simply too short to allow its visualization on the initial scan. Follow-up scans in combination with rising serum hCG levels will eventually demonstrate an IUP. In 7–20% of women with a PUL, an ectopic pregnancy is eventually diagnosed and these women can be treated either with laparoscopic surgery or medical therapy with systemic methotrexate (MTX). Only a minority of women will have a persisting PUL, defined as an inconclusive TVS in combination with a rise or plateau in serial serum hCG levels. The optimal management for persisting PUL is not known. Systemic MTX as well as expectant management are reported to be successful.[162]

We also need to differentiate patients with pathological pregnancy that will resolve spontaneously from those with pathological pregnancy necessitating active therapeutic intervention and those with an early normal IUP.

Future research involving progesterone test to explore its relation with β-hCG may help in predicting outcomes and calculate post-test probabilities for the whole range of progesterone and β-hCG values.

Monitoring FET Cycle

Success of FET depends greatly on synchronization between development of the endometrium and the frozen-thawed embryo. To achieve synchronization, one can use a hormone replacement cycle or a natural cycle.

Natural cycle does not require medication but requires more careful and regular monitoring of the cycle. This is done with ultrasound monitoring of follicular development with detection of LH surge and progesterone rise to identify the optimal time of endometrial receptivity. But if rise in LH goes undetected, it may result in an undetected rise in progesterone, which could result in the period of receptivity being advanced so that by the time of FET, the optimal period for implantation has passed.

Luteinizing hormone surges trigger ovulation within 36–48 hours later and ovulation initiates an endocrine shift from estrogen to progesterone. Window of implantation is anywhere between 5 and 7 days after ovulation. Identification of the onset of the LH surge makes it possible to estimate the moment of ovulation and thus the window. One can determine the mid-cycle LH rises in either urine or blood and ovulation can also be triggered with an injection of hCG in an unstimulated cycle. This ultrasound-based ovulation induction of the dominant follicle can be supplemented with LH monitoring to detect unexpected LH rises and therefore prevent FET being performed too late. Probably monitoring a natural cycle by transvaginal USG and LH will improve the results of FET as detection of the window of implantation is more accurate when both parameters are used. Testing LH levels in blood is much better as appearance of LH surges in urine lags several hours behind the appearance of the LH surge in blood.[163,164]

In an HRT cycle, the endometrium is prepared with hormonal support (estrogen and progesterone) prior to FET. HRT cycle requires very little monitoring, which reduces the burden on both patients and clinics.

■ DISCUSSION

To ensure safe clinical practice, and prevent OHSS and multiple pregnancies, it is important to monitor treatment response carefully by serial ultrasound scans and serum E2 and LH levels. Evaluating serum progesterone may help in improving the success rate of ART treatment.

Baseline ovarian USG is prudent between consecutive cycles of stimulation with exogenous gonadotropin. In the absence of any significant residual ovarian cysts or gross enlargement, treatment can begin again immediately without need for an intervening rest cycle. Higher cycle fecundability and cumulative pregnancy rates have been observed in consecutive treatment cycles than with alternating cycles of stimulation and no treatment.[165,166] When baseline USG reveals one or more residual ovarian cysts, it is usually best to briefly postpone further treatment. Stimulation cycles in the presence of ovarian cysts are less often successful,[167] possibly because newly emerging follicles can be difficult to distinguish from regressing cystic follicles, leading to errors in interpretation. Although many believe that suppressive therapy with a cycle of oral contraceptives helps regression of residual ovarian cysts, there is no evidence that such treatment is more successful than observation alone.

Studies of endometrial growth in exogenous gonadotropin-induced ovulatory cycles suggest that ultrasonographic measurements of endometrial thickness have great value. Cycle fecundity increases with endometrial thickness, which correlates with serum E2 concentrations.[168] Few pregnancies result from cycles in which endometrial thickness is less than approximately 7 mm on the day of hCG when treated with ovulation induction drugs.[168-171]

Previously, monitoring of ovarian function was based mainly on measuring serum E2 concentrations, and results were interpreted in relation to the success rate and development of OHSS. More over previously it was thought that complications were not dependent on monitoring but on the stimulation protocol.[172] Today, we know that monitoring as a whole cannot prevent the complications but helps us to identify patients at risk of developing these complications and thus modify our protocols. In ART cycles, the goal is to retrieve mature oocytes and this goal cannot be reached by measuring estrogen only, since the maturity of the oocyte is closely associated to the size of the follicle, a parameter, which can accurately be measured by ultrasound. In addition to the size of the follicles, it has been shown that the best bioassay for serum estrogen concentration, and also a major factor in the implantation process is the endometrial thickness and its ultrasonographic texture, a parameter which, again, can adequately be measured by ultrasound. Thus, ultrasound is accurate for it to be used alone in monitoring ovulation induction therapy for both in vivo and IVF by successfully measuring endometrial thickness and size of ovarian follicles. Follicular growth, uterine measurements, and endometrial thickness correlated strongly with E2 concentrations (P < 0.0001). Endometrial thickness on the day of hCG administration was significantly thicker (P < 0.01) in conception compared with nonconception

cycles, whereas no significant differences were observed in serum E2 concentrations.

The chance of achieving pregnancy predicted by uterine artery Doppler and PFBF in women whose PI values were higher than 3.26 and 1.08 was very low, with a sensitivity of 1.00 and specificity of 0.59 and 0.82, respectively. The data provided evidence for an association between utero-ovarian perfusion and reproductive outcome following IVF treatment.[173] The ovarian volume, follicular volume, vascularization index, FI and VFI were significantly greater in the pregnant group. 3D USG and power Doppler angiography allow for an easier ovarian assessment in IVF cycles.[174]

Estradiol measurement may provide additional information in predicting OHSS or poor response, which requires cycle cancelation, though avoidance of E2 and LH assay may simplify the IVF protocols. Monitoring by both ultrasound and E2 levels is important in those women, who are at risk of developing OHSS. Evaluation of E2 level during monitoring will help us in deciding between hCG and GnRH agonist for ovulation trigger.

Apart from the selection of trigger we could use certain preventive measures like coasting, intravenous albumin or hydroxyethyl starch solution and cryopreservation of all embryos with transfer in the subsequent cycle.

Ovulation induction cycles with gonadotropin, which do not use GnRH analogs premature LH rise or luteinization may occur. These cycles require more stringent monitoring with ultrasound, serum LH and progesterone along with E2 in order to accurately time hCG administration or detect ovulation in an non-ART cycle.

In ovulation induction cycles, which use GnRH analogs monitoring by ultrasound alone is sufficient and will simplify the treatment and its cost and also increase the patient's convenience. Measuring serum estrogen levels will not add significantly to efficacy or safety of the treatment.

■ SUMMARY

- Monitoring helps the physician to choose the most suitable protocol, to obtain best possible outcome avoiding complications.
- Baseline USG provides valuable information on ovarian morphology and allows choosing appropriate stimulation regimen to prevent OHSS and multiple pregnancies and helps in predicting patient's response to ovarian stimulation.
- Antral follicle count and AMH are equally accurate predictors of high ovarian response to COS and allow

us to identify the patients who are at increased risk of OHSS.

- Relationship between AFC and AMH concentrations is more reliable than that observed with FSH, inhibin B and estradiol on cycle day 3.
- Basal FSH should not be used as a screening tool but instead used to counsel patients appropriately regarding the realistic chance of conception and aiding determination of appropriate gonadotropin dose.
- Induction of ovulation and IVF protocols can be monitored successfully by measuring endometrial thickness and size of ovarian follicles.
- Ultrasonography monitoring of follicular growth is the most important tool in assessment of progress in ovarian stimulation and improves chance of safe and effective treatment with various ovulation induction agents.
- Ultrasonography also allows diagnosis of disorders and complications of ovulation induction.
- Ultrasound is accurate for it to be used alone in monitoring ovulation induction therapy for both in vivo and IVF by successfully measuring endometrial thickness and size of ovarian follicles and correlates strongly with serum E2 concentrations.
- Estradiol measurement may provide additional information in predicting OHSS or poor response.
- Evaluation of E2 along with ultrasound monitoring in women with risk of developing OHSS, helps in choosing the trigger for ovulation and luteal phase support.
- Monitoring luteal phase helps confirm ovulation, luteal function and pregnancy.
- Pregnancy can be documented by evaluation of β-hCG 15 days after ovulation or by ultrasound 20 days post-ovulation when β-hCG is 1,000 mIU/mL, an end point desired of tracking ovulation.
- Monitoring OI cycles adds to the common pool of information, which increases our knowledge and understanding of human reproduction.

■ REFERENCES

1. Hackeloer BJ, Fleming R, Robinson HP, et al. Correlation of ultrasonic and endocrinologic assessment of human follicular development. Am J Obstet Gynecol. 1979;135: 122-8.
2. Rosen MP, Shen S, Dobson AT, et al. A quantitative assessment of follicle size on oocyte developmental competence. Fertil Steril. 2008;90:684-90.
3. Al-Inany HG, Youssef MA, Aboulghar M, et al. Gonadotrophin-releasing hormone antagonists for assisted reproductive technology. Cochrane Database Syst Rev. 2011:CD001750.
4. Devroey P, Polyzos NP, Blockeel C. An OHSS-free clinic by segmentation of IVF treatment. Hum Reprod. 2011;26: 2593-7.
5. Hill MJ, Levens ED, Levy G, et al. The use of recombinant luteinizing hormone in patients undergoing assisted reproductive techniques with advanced reproductive age: a systematic review and meta-analysis. Fertil Steril. 2012;97: 1108-14.e1.
6. te Velde ER, Pearson PL. The variability of female reproductive ageing. Hum Reprod Update. 2002;8(2):141-54.
7. Esposito MA, Coutifaris C, Barnhart KT. A moderately elevated day 3 FSH concentration has limited predictive value, especially in younger women. Hum Reprod. 2002;17:118-23.
8. Scott RT Jr, Elkind-Hirsch KE, Styne-Gross A, et al. The predictive value for in vitro fertility delivery rates is greatly impacted by the method used to select the threshold between normal and elevated basal follicle-stimulating hormone. Fertil Steril. 2008;89:868-78.
9. Thum MY, Abdalla HI, Taylor D. Relationship between women's age and basal follicle-stimulating hormone levels with aneuploidy risk in in vitro fertilization treatment. Fertil Steril. 2008;90:315-21.
10. Massie JA, Burney RO, Milki AA, et al. Basal follicle-stimulating hormone as a predictor of fetal aneuploidy. Fertil Steril. 2008;90:2351-5.
11. Soules MR, Sherman S, Parrott E, et al. Executive summary: Stages of Reproductive Aging Workshop (STRAW). Fertil Steril. 2001;76:874-8.
12. Roberts JE, Spandorfer S, Fasouliotis SJ, et al. Taking a basal follicle-stimulating hormone history is essential before initiating in vitro fertilization. Fertil Steril. 2005;83:37-41.
13. Bancsi LF, Broekmans FJ, Mol BW, et al. Performance of basal follicle-stimulating hormone in the prediction of poor ovarian response and failure to become pregnant after in vitro fertilization: a meta-analysis. Fertil Steril. 2003;79:1091-100.
14. Jayaprakasan K, Campbell B, Hopkisson J, et al. Establishing the intercycle variability of three-dimensional ultrasonographic predictors of ovarian reserve. Fertil Steril. 2008;90(6):2126-32.
15. Abdalla H, Thum MY. Repeated testing of basal FSH levels has no predictive value for IVF outcome in women with elevated basal FSH. Hum Reprod. 2006;21:171-4.
16. Jain T, Soules MR, Collins JA. Comparison of basal follicle-stimulating hormone versus the clomiphene citrate challenge test for ovarian reserve screening. Fertil Steril. 2004;82:180-5.
17. Scott RT, Toner JP, Muasher SJ, et al. Follicle-stimulating hormone levels on cycle day 3, are predictive of in vitro fertilization outcome. Fertil Steril. 1989;51(4):651-4.
18. Bukulmez O, Arici A. Assessment of ovarian reserve. Curr Opin Obstet Gynecol. 2004;16(3):231-7.
19. Seifer DB, Scott RT Jr, Bergh PA, et al. Women with declining ovarian reserve may demonstrate a decrease in day 3 serum inhibin B before a rise in day 3 follicle-stimulating hormone. Fertil Steril. 1999;72(1):63-5.
20. Muttukrishna S, McGarrigle H, Wakim R, et al. Antral follicle count, anti-mullerian hormone and inhibin B: predictors of ovarian response in assisted reproductive technology? BJOG. 2005;112(10):1384-90.

21. Seifer DB, MacLaughlin DT, Christian BP, et al. Early follicular serum mullerian-inhibiting substance levels are associated with ovarian response during assisted reproductive technology cycles. Fertil Steril. 2002;77:468-71.

22. McIlveen M, Skull JD, Ledger WL. Evaluation of the utility of multiple endocrine and ultrasound measures of ovarian reserve in the prediction of cycle cancellation in a high-risk IVF population. Hum Reprod. 2007;22:778-85.

23. Tinkanen H, Bläuer M, Laippala P, et al. Correlation between serum inhibin B and other indicators of the ovarian function. Eur J Obstet Gynecol Reprod Biol. 2001;94(1):109-13.

24. Laven JS, Mulders AG, Visser JA, et al. Anti-Mullerian hormone serum concentrations in normoovulatory and anovulatory women of reproductive age. J Clin Endocrinol Metab. 2004;89(1):318-23.

25. Weenen C, Laven JS, Von Bergh AR, et al. Anti-Mullerian hormone expression pattern in the human ovary: potential implications for initial and cyclic follicle recruitment. Mol Hum Reprod. 2004;10:77-83.

26. Durlinger ALL, Kramer P, Karels B, et al. Control of primordial follicle recruitment by anti-Mullerian hormone in the mouse ovary. Endocrinology. 1999;140:5789-96.

27. Lee MM, Donahoe PK. Mullerian inhibiting substance: a gonadal hormone with multiple functions. Endocr Rev. 1993;14:152-64.

28. Fanchin R, Taieb J, Lozano DH, et al. High reproducibility of serum anti-Mullerian hormone measurements suggests a multi-staged follicular secretion and strengthens its role in the assessment of ovarian follicular status. Hum Reprod. 2005;20:923-7.

29. Tsepelidis S, Devreker F, Demeestere I, et al. Stable serum levels of anti-Mullerian hormone during the menstrual cycle: a prospective study in normo-ovulatory women. Hum Reprod. 2007;22:1837-40.

30. La Marca A, Stabile G, Artenisio AC, et al. Serum anti-Mullerian hormone throughout the human menstrual cycle. Hum Reprod. 2006;21:3103-7.

31. Hehenkamp WJ, Looman CW, Themmen AP, et al. Anti-Mullerian hormone levels in the spontaneous menstrual cycle do not show substantial fluctuation. J Clin Endocrinol Metab. 2006;91:4057-63.

32. Lee TH, Liu CH, Huang CC, et al. Serum anti-Müllerian hormone and estradiol levels as predictors of ovarian hyperstimulation syndrome in assisted reproduction technology cycles. Hum Reprod. 2008;23(1):160-7.

33. Bukman A, Heineman MJ. Ovarian reserve testing and the use of prognostic models in patients with subfertility. Hum Reprod Update. 2001;7:581-90.

34. Kwee J, Schats R, McDonnell J, et al. The clomiphene citrate challenge test versus the exogenous follicle-stimulating hormone ovarian reserve test as a single test for identification of low responders and hyperresponders to in vitro fertilization. Fertil Steril. 2006;85:1714-22.

35. Jayaprakasan K, Campbell B, Hopkisson J, et al. A prospective, comparative analysis of anti-Müllerian hormone, inhibin-B, and three-dimensional ultrasound determinants of ovarian reserve in the prediction of poor response to controlled ovarian stimulation. Fertil Steril. 2010;93(3):855-64.

36. Tomas C, Nuojua-Huttunen S, Martikainen H, et al. Pretreatment transvaginal ultrasound examination predicts ovarian responsiveness to gonadotrophins in in-vitro fertilization. Hum Reprod. 1997;12:220-3.

37. Sharara FI, McClamrock H.D. High E2 levels and high oocyte yield are not detrimental to in vitro fertilization outcome. Fertil Steril. 1999;72:401-5.

38. Syrop CH, Wilhoite A, Van-Voorhis BJ. Ovarian volume: a novel outcome predictor for assisted reproduction. Fertil Steril. 1995;64:1167-71.

39. Lass A, Skull J, McVeigh E, et al. Measurement of ovarian volume by transvaginal sonography before ovulation induction with human menopausal gonadotrophin for in-vitro fertilization can predict poor response. Hum Reprod. 1997;12:294-7.

40. Kupesic S, Kurjak A. Predictors of in vitro fertilization outcome by three-dimensional ultrasound. Hum Reprod. 2002;17(4):950-5.

41. Lambalk CB, de Koning CH, Flett A, et al. Assessment of ovarian reserve. Ovarian biopsy is not a valid method for the prediction of ovarian reserve. Hum Reprod. 2004;19:1055-9.

42. Duijkers IJ, Louwe LA, Braat DD, et al. One, two or three: how many directions are useful in transvaginal ultrasound measurement of ovarian follicles? Eur J Obstet Gynecol Reprod Biol. 2004;117:60-3.

43. Amso NN, Watermeyer SR, Pugh N, Quantification of power Doppler energy, its future potential. Fertil Steril. 2001;76: 583-7.

44. Jun WS, Lee KH, Koo K, et al. A straightforward algorithm for the quantification of power Doppler signals. Invest Radiol. 2002;37:343-8.

45. Fleischer AC. New developments in the sonographic assessment of ovarian, uterine and breast vascularity. Semin Ultrasound CT MR. 2001;22:42-9.

46. Raine-Fenning NJ, Campbell BK, Clewes JS, et al. The reliability of virtual organ computer-aided analysis (VOCAL) for the semiquantification of ovarian, endometrial and sub-endometrial perfusion. Ultrasound Obstet Gynecol. 2003;22: 633-9.

47. Eissa MK, Hudson K, Docker MF, et al. Ultrasound follicle diameter measurement: an assessment of inter observer and intra observer variation. Fertil Steril. 1985;44:751-4.

48. Nayudu PL. Relationship of constructed follicular growth patterns in stimulated cycles to outcome after IVF. Hum Reprod. 1991;6:465-71.

49. Wittmaack FM, Kreger DO, Blasco L, et al. Effect of follicular size on oocyte retrieval, fertilization, cleavage, and embryo quality in in vitro fertilization cycles: a 6-year data collection. Fertil Steril. 1994;62:1205-10.

50. Van Blerkom J. Can the developmental competence of early human embryos be predicted effectively in the clinical IVF laboratory? Hum Reprod. 1997;12:1610-4.

51. Balakier H, Stronell RD. Color Doppler assessment of folliculogenesis in in vitro fertilization patients. Fertil Steril. 1994;62:1211-6.

52. Oyesanya OA, Parsons JH, Collins WP, et al. Prediction of oocyte recovery rate by transvaginal ultrasonography and color Doppler imaging before human chorionic

gonadotropin administration in in vitro fertilization cycles. Fertil Steril. 1996;65:806-9.

53. Mercé LT, Bau S, Barco MJ, et al. Assessment of the ovarian volume, number and volume of follicles and ovarian vascularity by three-dimensional ultrasonography and power Doppler angiography on the hCG day to predict the outcome in IVF/ICSI cycles. Hum Reprod. 2006;21:1218-26.

54. Steer CV, Campbell S, Tan SL, et al. The use of transvaginal colour flow imaging after in vitro fertilization to identify optimum uterine conditions before embryo transfer. Fertil Steril. 1992;57:372-6.

55. Coulam CB, Stem IJ, Soenksen DM, et al. Comparison of pulsatility indices on the day of oocyte retrieval and embryo transfer. Hum Reprod. 1995;10:82-4.

56. Tekay A, Martikainen H, Jouppila P. Blood flow changes in uterine and ovarian vasculature, and predictive value of transvaginal pulsed colour Doppler ultrasonography in an in vitro fertilization programme. Hum Reprod. 1995;10:688-93.

57. Serafini P, Batzofin J, Nelson J, et al. Sonographic uterine predictors of pregnancy in women undergoing ovulation induction for assisted reproductive treatments. Fertil Steril. 1994;62:815-22.

58. Ng EHU, Chan CCW, Tang OS, et al. The role of endometrial and subendometrial vascularity measured by three-dimensional power Doppler ultrasound in the prediction of pregnancy during frozen-thawed embryo transfer cycles. Hum Reprod. 2006;21:1612-7.

59. Palomba S, Orio F, and Zullo F. Ovulation induction in women with polycystic ovary syndrome. Fertil Steril. 2006;86:S26-7.

60. O'Leary AJ, Griffiths AN, Evans J, et al. "Perifollicular blood flow and pregnancy in superovulated intrauterine insemination (IUI) cycles: An observational comparison of recombinant follicle-stimulating hormone (FSH) and urinary gonadotropins." Fertil Steril. 2009;92(4):1366-8.

61. Borini A, Maccolini A, Tallarini A, et al. Perifollicular vascularity and its relationship with oocyte maturity and IVF outcome. Ann N Y Acad Sci. 2001;943:64-7.

62. Battaglia C, Genazzani AD, Regnani G, et al. Perifollicular Doppler flow and follicular fluid vascular endothelial growth factor concentrations in poor responders. Fertil Steril. 2000;74:809-12.

63. Turnbull LW, Lesny P, Killick SR. Assessment of uterine receptivity prior to embryo transfer: a review of currently available imaging modalities. Hum Reprod Update. 1995;1:505-14.

64. Friedler S, Schenker JG, Herman A, et al. The role of ultrasonography in the evaluation of endometrial receptivity following assisted reproductive treatments: a critical review. Hum Reprod Update. 1996;2:323-35.

65. Yaman C, Ebner T, Sommergruber M, et al. Role of three-dimensional ultrasonographic measurement of endometrium volume as a predictor of pregnancy outcome in an IVF-ET program. A preliminary study. Fertil Steril. 2000;74:797-801.

66. Zollner U, Zollner KP, Specketer MT, et al. Endometrial volume as assessed by three-dimensional ultrasound is a predictor of pregnancy outcome after in vitro fertilization and embryo transfer. Fertil Steril. 2003:80;1515-7.

67. Coulam CB, Bustillo M, Soenksen DM, et al. Ultrasonographic predictors of implantation after assisted reproduction. Fertil Steril. 1994;62:1004-10.

68. Ayustawati, Shibahara H, Obara H, et al. Influence of endometrial thickness and pattern on pregnancy rates in in vitro fertilization-embryo transfer. Reprod Med Biol. 2002;1:17-21.

69. Gonen Y, Casper RF, Jacobson W, et al. Endometrial thickness and growth during ovarian stimulation: a possible predictor of implantation in in-vitro fertilization. Fertil Steril. 1989;52:446-50.

70. Check JH, Nowroozi K, Choe J, et al. The effect of endometrial thickness and echo pattern on in vitro fertilization outcome in donor oocyte-embryo transfer cycle. Fertil Steril. 1993;59: 72-5.

71. Zhang X, Chen CH, Confino E, et al. Increased endometrial thickness and embryo implantation, based on 1,294 cycles of in vitro fertilization with transfer of two blastocyst-stage embryos. Fertil Steril. 2007;87:53-9.

72. Richter KS, Bugge KR, Bromer JG, et al. Relationship between endometrial thickness and embryo implantation, based on 1,294 cycles of in vitro fertilization with transfer of two blastocyst-stage embryos. Fertil Steril. 2007;87:53-9.

73. Rabinowitz R, Laufer N, Lewin A, et al. The value of ultrasonographic endometrial measurement in the prediction of pregnancy following in vitro fertilization. Fertil Steril. 1986;45:824-8.

74. Dietterich C, Check JH, Choe JK, et al. Increased endometrial thickness on the day of human chorionic gonadotropin injection does not adversely affect pregnancy or implantation rates following in vitro fertilization-embryo transfer. Fertil Steril. 2002;77:781-6.

75. Sher.G, Herbert C, Maassarani, G, et al. Assessment of the late proliferative phase endometrium by ultrasonography in patients undergoing in-vitro fertilization and embryo transfer. Hum Reprod. 1991;6:232-7.

76. Fanchin R, Righini C, Ayoubi JM, et al. New look at endometrial echogenicity, objective computer-assisted measurements predict endometrial receptivity in in-vitro fertilization-embryo transfer. Fertil Steril. 2000;74:274-81.

77. Järvelä IY, Sladkevicius P, Kelly S, et al. Evaluation of endometrial receptivity during in-vitro fertilization using three-dimensional power Doppler ultrasound. Ultrasound Obstet Gynecol. 2005;26(7):765-9.

78. Ueno J, Oehninger S, Brzyski RG, et al. Ultrasonographic appearance of the endometrium in natural and stimulated in vitro fertilization cycles and its correlation with outcome. Hum Reprod. 1991;6:901-4.

79. Abdalla HI, Brooks AA, Johnson MR, et al. Endometrial thickness: a predictor of implantation in ovum recipients. Hum Reprod. 1994; 9: 363-5.

80. Shapiro H, Cowell C, Casper RF. Use of vaginal ultrasound for monitoring endometrial preparation in a donor oocyte program. Fertil Steril. 1993;59:1055-8.

81. El-Toukhy T, Coomarasamy A, Khairy M, et al. The relationship between endometrial thickness and outcome of medicated frozen embryo replacement cycles. Fertil Steril. 2008;89:832-9.

82. Jokubkiene L, Sladkevicius P, Rovas L, et al. Assessment of changes in volume and vascularity of the ovaries during the normal menstrual cycle using three-dimensional power Doppler ultrasound. Hum Reprod. 2006;21:2661-8.

83. IJland MM, Hoogland H J, Dunselman G A, et al.. Endometrial wave direction switch and the outcome of in vitro fertilization. Fertil Steril. 1999;71(3):476-81.

84. Fanchin R, Righini C, Olivennes F, et al. Uterine contractions at the time of embryo transfer alter pregnancy rates after in-vitro fertilization. Hum Reprod. 1998;13(7):1968-74.

85. Kupesic S, Bekavac I, Bjelos D, et al. Assessment of endometrial receptivity by transvaginal color Doppler and three-dimensional power Doppler ultrasonography in patients undergoing in vitro fertilization procedures. J Ultrasound Med. 2001;20:125-34.

86. Wu HM, Chiang CH, Huang HY, et al. Detection of the subendometrial vascularization flow index by three-dimensional ultrasound may be useful for predicting the pregnancy rate for patients undergoing in vitro fertilization-embryo transfer. Fertil Steril. 2003;79:507-11.

87. Mercè LT, Barco MJ, Bau S, et al. Are endometrial parameters by three-dimensional ultrasound and power Doppler angiography related to in vitro fertilization/embryo transfer outcome? Fertil Steril. 2008;89:111-7.

88. Raine-Fenning NJ, Campbell BK, Kendall NR, et al. Quantifying the changes in endometrial vascularity throughout the normal menstrual cycle with three-dimensional power Doppler angiography. Hum Reprod. 2004;19:330-8.

89. Sharkey AM, Day K, McPherson A, et al. Vascular endothelial growth factor expression in human endometrium is regulated by hypoxia. J Clin Endocrinol Metab. 2000;85:402-9.

90. Graham CH, Postovit LM, Park H, et al. Adriana and Luisa Castellucci award lecture 1999: role of oxygen in the regulation of trophoblast gene expression and invasion. Placenta. 2000;21:443-50.

91. Jinno M, Ozaki T, Iwashita M, et al. Measurement of endometrial tissue blood flow: a novel way to assess uterine receptivity for implantation. Fertil Steril. 2001;76:1168-74.

92. Ng EH, Yeung WS, Ho PC. Endometrial and sub endometrial vascularity are significantly lower in patients with endometrial volume 2.5 ml or less. Reprod Biomed Online. 2009;18:262-8.

93. Ng EHY, Chan CCW, Tang OS, et al. Comparison of endometrial and subendometrial blood flow measured by three-dimensional power Doppler ultrasoud between stimulated and natural cycles in the same patients. Hum Reprod. 2004;19:2385-90.

94. Ng EHY, Chan CCW, Tang OS, et al. The role of endometrial and subendometrial blood flows measured by three-dimensional power Doppler ultrasoud in the prediction of pregnancy during IVF treatment. Hum Reprod. 2006;21: 164-70.

95. Ng EH, Naveed F, Lau EY, et al. A randomized double-blind controlled study of the efficacy of laser-assisted hatching on implantation and pregnancy rates of frozen-thawed embryo transfer at the cleavage stage. Hum Reprod. 2005;20(4): 979-85.

96. Ng EHY, Chan CCW, Tang OS, et al. Endometrial and subendometrial vascularity is higher in pregnant patients with livebirth following ART than in those who suffer a miscarriage. Hum Reprod. 2007;22(4):1134-41.

97. Steer CV, Tan SL, Dillon D, et al. Vaginal color Doppler assessment of uterine artery impedance correlates with immunohistochemical markers of endometrial receptivity required for the implantation of an embryo. Fertil Steril. 1995;63:101-8.

98. Nakai A, Yokota A, Koshino T, et al. Assessment of endometrial perfusion with Doppler ultrasound in spontaneous and stimulated menstrual cycles. J Nippon Med Sch. 2002;69: 328-32.

99. Yokota A, Nakai A, Oya A, et al. Changes in uterine and ovarian arterial impedance during the periovulatory period in conception and nonconception cycles. J Obstet Gynecol Res. 2000;26:435-40.

100. Raine-Fenning N, Jayaprakasan K, Clewes J, et al. Sono AVC: a novel method of automatic volume calculation. Ultrasound Obstet Gynecol. 2008;31:691-6.

101. Raine-Fenning N, Jayaprakasan K, Clewes J, et al. Establishing the validity of a new technique that facilitates automated follicular volume measurement. Ultrasound Obstet Gynecol. 2007;30:393.

102. Raine-Fenning N, Jayaprakasan K, Chamberlain S, et al. Automated measurements of follicle diameter: a chance to standardize? Fertil Steril. 2009;91(suppl. 4):1469-72.

103. Jayaprakasan K, Campbell BK, Clewes JS, et al. Three-dimensional ultrasound improves the interobserver reliability of antral follicle counts and facilitates increased clinical work flow. Ultrasound Obstet Gynecol. 2008;31:439-44.

104. Ectors FJ, Vanderzwalmen P, Van Hoeck J, et al. Relationship of human follicular diameter with oocyte fertilization and development after in-vitro fertilization or intracytoplasmic sperm injection. Hum Reprod. 1997;12:2002-5.

105. Shmorgun D, Hughes E, Mohide P, et al. Prospective cohort study of three- versus two-dimensional ultrasound for prediction of oocyte maturity. Fertil Steril. 2010;93(4):1337-4.

106. Mikhail G. Sex steroids in blood. Clin Obstet Gynecol. 1967;10:29-39.

107. Baird D, Fraser IS. Concentration of oestrone and oestradiol in follicular fluid and ovarian venous blood of women. Clin Endocrinol. 1975;4:259-66.

108. McNatty KP, Baird DT, Bolton A, et al. Concentration of oestrogens and androgens in human ovarian venous plasma and follicular fluid throughout the menstrual cycle. J Endocrinol. 1976;71:77-85.

109. Hillier SG, Reichert LE Jr, Van Hall EV. Control of preovulatory follicular estrogen biosynthesis in the human ovary. J Clin Endocrinol Metab. 1981;52:847-56.

110. Chikazawa K, Araki S, Tamada T. Morphological and endocrinological studies on follicular development during the human menstrual cycle. J Clin Endocrinol Metab. 1986;62:305-13.

111. Huang CC, Lien YR, Chen HF, et al. The duration of pre-ovulatory serum progesterone elevation before hCG administration affects the outcome of IVF/ICSI cycles. Hum Reprod. 2012;27(7):2036-45,.

112. Melo MA, Meseguer M, Garrido N, et al. The significance of premature luteinization in an oocyte-donation programme. Hum Reprod. 2006;21:1503-07.

113. Segal S, Glatstein I, McShane P, et al. Premature luteinization and in vitro fertilization outcome in gonadotropin/gonadotropin-releasing hormone antagonist cycles in women with polycystic ovary syndrome. Fertil Steril. 2009;91:1755-9.

114. Elnashar AM. Progesterone rise on the day of HCG administration (premature luteinization) in IVF: an overdue update. J Assist Reprod Genet. 2010;27:149-55.

115. Venetis CA, Kolibianakis EM, Bosdou JK, et al. Progesterone elevation and probability of pregnancy after IVF: a systematic review and meta-analysis of over 60 000 cycles. Hum Reprod Update. 2013;19(5):433-57.

116. Aflatoonian A, Oskouian H, Ahmadi S, et al. Can fresh embryo transfers be replaced by cryopreserved-thawed embryo transfers in assisted reproductive cycles? A randomized controlled trial. J Assist Reprod Genet. 2010;27:357-63.

117. Shapiro BS, Daneshmand ST, Garner FC, et al. Evidence of impaired endometrial receptivity after ovarian stimulation for in vitro fertilization: a prospective randomized trial comparing fresh and frozen–thawed embryo transfer in normal responders. Fertil Steril. 2011;96:344-8.

118. Shapiro BS, Daneshmand ST, Garner FC, et al. Embryo cryopreservation rescues cycles with premature luteinization. Fertil Steril. 2010;93:636-41.

119. Kolibianakis EM, Bourgain C, Papanikolaou, et al. Prolongation of follicular phase by delaying hCG administration results in a higher incidence of endometrial advancement on the day of oocyte retrieval in GnRH antagonist cycles. Hum Reprod. 2005;20(9):2453-6.

120. Byrd W. Cryopreservation, thawing, and transfer of human embryos. Semin Reprod Med. 2002;20:37-43.

121. al-Shawaf T, Yang D, al-Magid Y, et al. Ultrasonic monitoring during replacement of frozen/thawed embryos in natural and hormone replacement cycles. Hum Reprod. 1993;8:2068-74.

122. Dal Prato L, Borini A, Cattoli M, et al. Endometrial preparation for frozen–thawed embryo transfer with or without pretreatment with gonadotropin-releasing hormone agonist. Fertil Steril. 2002;77:956-60.

123. Gelbaya TA, Nardo LG, Hunter HR, et al. Cryopreserved–thawed embryo transfer in natural or down-regulated hormonally controlled cycles: a retrospective study. Fertil Steril. 2006;85:603-9.

124. Ghobara T, Vandekerckhove P. Cycle regimens for frozen–thawed embryo transfer. Cochrane Database of Syst Rev. 2008;(1):CD003414.

125. Filicori M, Santoro N, Merriam GR, et al. Characterization of the physiological pattern of episodic gonadotropin secretion throughout the human menstrual cycle. J Clin Endocrinol Metab. 1986;62:1136-44.

126. Soules MR, Steiner RA, Clifton DK, et al. Progesterone modulation of pulsatile luteinizing hormone secretion in normal women. J Clin Endocrinol Metab. 1984;58:378-83.

127. Nippoldt TB, Reame NE, Kelch RP. The roles of estradiol and progesterone in decreasing luteinizing hormone pulse frequency in the luteal phase of the menstrual cycle. J Clin Endocrinol Metab. 1989;69:67-76.

128. Wehrenberg WB, Wardlaw SL, Frantz AG. beta-Endorphin in hypophyseal portal blood: variations throughout the menstrual cycle. Endocrinology. 1982;111:879-81.

129. Niswender GD, Reimers T J, Diekman MA. Blood flow: a mediator of ovarian function. Biol Reprod. 1976;14(1):64-81.

130. Miyazaki T, Tanaka M, Miyakoshi K, et al. Power and colour Doppler ultrasonography for the evaluation of the vasculature of the human corpus luteum. Hum Reprod. 1998;13:2836-41.

131. Niswender GD, Juengel JL, Silva PJ, et al. Mechanisms controlling the function and life span of the corpus luteum. Physiol Rev. 2000;80:1-29.

132. Jarvela IY, Niinima¨ki M, Martikainen H, et al. Ovarian response to the human chorionic gonadotrophin stimulation test in normal ovulatory women: the impact of regressing corpus luteum. Fertil Steril. 2007;87:1122-30.

133. Hazzard TM, Stouffer RL. Angiogenesis in ovarian follicular and luteal development. Baillieres Best Pract Res Clin Obstet Gynaecol. 2000;14:883-900.

134. Sugino N, Kashida S, Takiguchi S, et al. Expression of vascular endothelial growth factor and its receptors in the human corpus luteum during the menstrual cycle and in early pregnancy. J Clin Endocrinol Metab. 2000;85:3919-24.

135. Wulff C, Dickson SE, Duncan WC, et al. Angiogenesis in the human corpus luteum: simulated early pregnancy by HCG treatment is associated with both angiogenesis and vessel stabilization. Hum Reprod. 2001;16:2515-24.

136. Wulff C, Wilson H, Rudge JS, et al. Luteal angiogenesis: prevention and intervention by treatment with vascular endothelial growth factor trap(A40). J Clin Endocrinol Metab. 2001;86:3377-86.

137. XIE HN, Hata K, Manabe A, et al. Associations between Doppler ultrasound-derived luteal blood flow indices and function hormonal profile in spontaneous and stimulated cycles. J Med Ultrasonics. 2001;28:139-46.

138. Miro F, Aspinall LJ. The onset of the initial rise in follicle-stimulating hormone during the human menstrual cycle. Hum Reprod. 2005;20:96-100.

139. Mais V, Cetel NS, Muse KN, et al. Hormonal dynamics during luteal-follicular transition. J Clin Endocrinol Metab. 1987;64:1109-14.

140. Messinis IE, Koutsoyiannis D, Milingos S, et al. Changes in pituitary response to GnRH during the luteal-follicular transition of the human menstrual cycle. Clin Endocrinol (Oxf). 1993;38:159-63.

141. Roseff SJ, Bangah ML, Kettel LM, et al. Dynamic changes in circulating inhibin levels during the luteal- follicular transition of the human menstrual cycle. J Clin Endocrinol Metab. 1989;69:1033-9.

142. Groome NP, Illingworth PJ, O'Brien M, et al. Measurement of dimeric inhibin B throughout the human menstrual cycle. J Clin Endocrinol Metab. 1996;81:1401-5.

143. Verhaegen J, Gallos ID, van Mello NM, et al. Accuracy of single progesterone test to predict early pregnancy outcome in women with pain or bleeding: meta-analysis of cohort studies. BMJ. 2012;345:e6077.

144. Yong P, Martin C, Thong J. A comparison of psychological functioning in women at different stages of in-vitro fertilization treatment using the mean affect adjective check list. J Assist Reprod Genet. 2000;17:553-6.

145. Hammarberg K, Astbury J, Baker H. Women's experience of IVF: a follow-up study. Hum Reprod. 2001;16:374-83.

146. Chung K, Sammel M, Coutifaris C, et al. Defining the rise of serum HCG in viable pregnancies achieved through use of IVF. Hum Reprod. 2006;21:823-8.

147. Lohstroh PN, Overstreet JW, Stewart DR, et al. Hourly human chorionic gonadotropin secretion profiles during the peri-implantation period of successful pregnancies. Fertil Steril. 2007;87:1413-8.

148. Qasim SM, Callan C, Choe JK. The predictive value of an initial serum beta human chorionic gonadotropin level for pregnancy outcome following in-vitro fertilization. J Assist Reprod Genet. 1996;13:705-8.

149. Poikkeus P, Hiilesmaa V, Tiitinen A. Serum HCG 12 days after embryo transfer in predicting pregnancy outcome. Hum Reprod. 2002;17:1901-5.

150. Urbancsek J, Hauzman E, Fedorcsak P, et al. Serum human chorionic gonadotropin measurements may predict pregnancy outcome and multiple gestation after in-vitro fertilization. Fertil Steril. 2002;78:540-2.

151. Kumbak B, Oral E, Karlikaya G, et al. Serum oestradiol and beta-HCG measurements after day 3 or 5 embryo transfers in interpreting pregnancy outcome. Reprod BioMed Online. 2006;13:459-64.

152. Yamashita T, Okamoto S, Thomas A, et al. Predicting pregnancy outcome after in-vitro fertilization and embryo transfer using estradiol, progesterone, and human chorionic gonadotropin [beta]-subunit. Fertil Steril. 1992;58:373-7.

153. Guth B, Hudelson J, Higbie J, et al. Predictive value of hCG level 14 days after embryo transfer. J Assist Reprod Genet. 1995;12:13-4.

154. Chen CD, Ho HN, Wu MY, et al. Paired human chorionic gonadotropin determinations for the prediction of pregnancy outcome in assisted reproduction. Hum Reprod. 1997;12:2538-41.

155. Bjercke S, Tanbo T, Dale P, et al. Human chorionic gonadotrophin concentrations in early pregnancy after in-vitro fertilization. Hum Reprod. 1999;14:1642-6.

156. Homan G, Brown S, Moran J, et al. Human chorionic gonadotropin as a predictor of outcome in assisted reproductive technology pregnancies. Fertil Steril. 2000;73:270-4.

157. Papageorgiou TC, Leondires MP, Miller BT, et al. Human chorionic gonadotropin levels after blastocyst transfer are highly predictive of pregnancy outcome. Fertil Steril. 2001;76:981-7.

158. Zayed F, Ghazawi I, Francis L, et al. Predictive value of human chorionic gonadotropin in early pregnancy after assisted conception. Arch Gynecol Obstet. 2001;265:7-10.

159. Alahakoon TI, Crittenden J, Illingworth P. Value of single and paired serum human chorionic gonadotropin measurements in predicting outcome of in-vitro fertilisation pregnancy. Aust N Z J Obstet Gynaecol. 2004;44:57-61.

160. Sutton-Riley JM, Khanlian SA, Byrn FW, et al. A single serum test for measuring early pregnancy outcome with high predictive value. Clin Biochem. 2006;39:682-7.

161. Porat S, Savchev S, Bdolah Y, et al. Early serum chorionic gonadotropin in pregnancies after in-vitro fertilization: contribution of treatment variables and prediction of long-term pregnancy outcomes. Fertil Steril. 2007;88:82-9.

162. Condous G, Okaro E, Bourne T. The conservative management of early pregnancy complications: a review of the literature. Ultrasound Obstet Gynecol. 2003;22:420-30.

163. Frydman R, Testart J, Feinstein, et al. Interrelationship of plasma and urinary luteinizing hormone preovulatory surge. J Steroid Biochem. 1984;20(2):617-9.

164. Park SJ, Goldsmith LT, Skurnick JH, et al. Characteristics of the urinary luteinizing hormone surge in young ovulatory women. Fertil Steril. 2007:88(3):684-90.

165. Diamond MP, DeCherney AH, Baretto P, et al. Multiple consecutive cycles of ovulation inductions with human menopausal gonadotropins. Gynecol Endocrinol. 1989;3:237-40.

166. Silverberg KM, Klein NA, Burns WN, et al. Consecutive versus alternating cycles of ovarian stimulation using human menopausal gonadotrophins. Hum Reprod. 1992;7:940-4.

167. Akin JW, Shepard MK. The effects of baseline ovarian cysts on cycle fecundity in controlled ovarian hyperstimulation. Fertil Steril. 1993;59:453-5.

168. Shoham Z, Di Carlo C, Patel A, et al. Is it possible to run a sucessful ovulation induction program based solely on ultrasound monitoring? The importance of endometrial measurements. Fertil Steril. 1991;56:836-41.

169. Dickey RP, Olar TT, Taylor SN, et al. Relationship of endometrial thickness and pattern to fecundity in ovulation induction cycles: effect of clomiphene citrate alone and with human menopausal gonadotropin, Fertil Steril. 1993;59(4):756-60.

170. Reuter KL, Cohen S, Furey L, et al. Sonographic appearance of the endometrium and ovaries during cycles stimulated with human menopausal gonadotropin. J Reprod Med. 1996;41:509-14.

171. Isaacs JD Jr, Wells CS, Williams DB, et al. Endometrial thickness is a valid monitoring parameter in cycles of ovulation induction with menotropins alone. Fertil Steril. 1996;65(2):262-6.

172. Klopper A, Aiman J, Besser M. Ovarian steroidogenesis resulting from treatment with menopausal gonadotropin. Eur J Obstet Gynecol Reprod Biol. 1974;4:25-30.

173. Ozturk O, Bhattacharya S, Saridogan E, et al. Role of utero-ovarian vascular impedance: predictor of ongoing pregnancy in an IVF-embryo transfer programme. Reprod Biomed Online. 2004;9:299-305.

174. Mendez Lozano DH, Fraydman N, Levaillant JM, et al. The 3D vascular status of the follicle after hCG administration is qualitatively rather than quantitatively associated with its reproductive competence. Hum Reprod. 2007;22:1095-9.

19 — Ovulation Trigger

Fessy Louis T

INTRODUCTION

When we give exogenous human chorionic gonadotropin (hCG), it substitutes the endogenous luteinizing hormone (LH) surge to induce final stages of oocyte maturation in ovarian stimulation protocols for in vitro fertilization (IVF). As a prelude to ovulation, which usually occurs within 38–42 hours of the intramuscular administration of a dose of hCG (usually 10,000 U) to women who have undergone controlled ovarian stimulation (COS), the egg begins a process known as meiosis (also known as reduction division or maturational division). Here, the egg, which to this point contains 46 chromosomes (23 pairs aligned in a spiral arrangement), sets out to halve its number of chromosomes from 46 to 23. Human oocytes are arrested at the prophase of the first meiotic division and are held in this arrest by the surrounding mural granulosa cells.[1] The endogenous LH surges or the exogenous hCG triggers the resumption of meiosis in the fully grown oocyte. The meiotic process is usually completed within 24–36 hours. Survival of the human species is totally dependent on the orderly occurrence of meiosis so that subsequent fertilization of the mature egg by a mature spermatozoon (which has also undergone meiosis to halve its number of 23 chromosomes) will result in the propagation of a chromosomally normal embryo (euploid embryo) with precisely 46 chromosomes (the normal human genomic make-up).

HUMAN CHORIONIC GONADOTROPIN

Human chorionic gonadotropin has been the universal trigger of final oocyte maturation for decades in assisted reproductive technology (ART) due to structural and biological similarities with LH as both molecules bind to the same receptor, the LH/hCG receptor.[2] hCG belongs to the same glycoprotein family as follicle stimulating hormone (FSH), LH and thyroid stimulating hormone (TSH). All members of this family share the same α subunit, but have different β subunit. Due to the extensive homology in molecular structure and amino acid sequence, both hCG and LH are capable of stimulating the same hormonal receptor. The main difference between hCG and LH is the prolonged half-life of hCG. This is due to the delayed degradation of the molecule attributed to the presence of a distinct C-terminal sequence in the β subunit. This long half-life results in a prolonged luteotropic effect of hCG when administered at mid-cycle and can lead to a false positive pregnancy test if hCG is administered during luteal phase. hCG derived from urine is being used for the last 50 years to induce the final oocyte maturation and ovulation triggering in infertility treatment. The ovulatory surge has two basic functions: (1) final oocyte maturation and (2) ovulation including the transition to form a functioning corpus luteum. It is established that the ovulatory dose of hCG induces dramatic changes in gene expression of the preovulatory follicle somatic compartment including the gonadotropin receptors, steroidogenic genes and epidermal growth factors.[3] After an initial attenuation of the gonadotropin receptor expression, the LH receptor mRNA reappears 36 hours after ovulation induction in preparation for the luteal phase, as shown recently in the primate preovulatory follicles.

The consented doses of hCG administered vary between 5,000 and 10,000 IU when urinary hCG is used and 250 and 500 μg when recombinant hCG is used. The half-life of hCG is significantly longer than that of LH, > 24 hours versus 60 minutes[4,5] facilitating ovarian hyperstimulation syndrome (OHSS) due to the sustained luteotropic activity and the production of vascular permeability mediators.[6,7] Even if frank OHSS is not diagnosed, luteal ovarian over stimulation is a significant source of physical discomfort during the luteal phase, increasing the treatment burden of the patient.[8] A standard bolus of hCG has been shown to induce a significant histological advancement of the endometrium, which could negatively affect the receptivity.[9] Thus, the ovulatory bolus of hCG increases the physical discomfort of the patient during the luteal phase, increases the risk of OHSS and might hamper implantation.

When hCG should be Administered?

Optimal criteria when to inject hCG remain yet to be defined, although on an empirical and arbitrary basis it is common practice to administer hCG when 2–3 leading follicles of 17–20 mm are present in ultrasound. Theoretically, hCG be timed according to estradiol (E2) hormone assessment and/or sonographic findings. The usage of gonadotropin-releasing hormone (GnRH) agonist during ovulation stimulation in IVF has made the timing of hCG administration easy because its use prevents the spontaneous LH surge and premature ovulation.

In a randomized trial for patients stimulated for IVF using short agonist protocol, in the group in which hCG was delayed for 24 hours after two leading follicles had reached 17 mm, pregnancy rate was significantly lower, but the cumulus oocyte complexes retrieved were similar in both the groups, even though the sample sizes were small.[10] But in a large randomized control trial of long GnRH agonist protocol for IVF, when leading follicle had reached 18 mm and two other follicle reached 14 and hCG was given on the same day and in another two groups delayed for 24 and 48 hours, the oocytes retrieved, fertilization and pregnancy rates were similar.[11]

Time Interval between hCG and Follicular Rupture

Time duration between the administration of 6,000 IU IM hCG and follicular rupture was examined by serial scans in patients undergoing ovulation induction with clomiphene citrate.[12] This was a prospective study and hCG was administered when the leading follicle reached a mean diameter of 18 mm. Follicle rupture was observed after a mean 38.3 hours. In a similar randomized study by Fischer et al. observed a mean time to ovulation of 40.4 hours with a broad range of less than 36–48 hours after patients receiving either 10,000 IU IM or 500 IU IV hCG after ovarian stimulation with clomiphene citrate.

Time Interval between hCG and Oocyte Retrieval

When will the oocyte retrieval be done after hCG administration? If oocyte retrieval is scheduled too early after hCG administration, a larger proportion of oocytes will be in germinal vesicle (GV) or metaphase I stage, whereas a delayed retrieval might result in premature

ovulation or oocyte over ripens and thus a decrease in the number of cumulus oocyte complexes retrieved. This depends on the time frame at which hCG becomes bioavailable at a sufficient concentration to trigger final oocyte maturation, and this depends on the route of administration and the speed of absorption.

In GnRH agonist protocol for ovarian stimulation, when oocyte retrieval was analyzed in a randomized study following 10,000 IU hCG, the number of metaphase II oocytes were significantly lower in 35-hour group. But it was better and similar in the 36- and 37-hour groups. Also the fertilized oocytes were significantly lower in the 35-hour group. The authors suggested that oocyte retrieval should not be attempted before 36 hours. But in another larger non-randomized observational study by Nargund et al. when oocyte retrieval after 10,000 IU hCG was compared in three groups of 33–36 hours, 36–38 hours and 38–41 hours, the number of oocytes retrieved per follicle punctured and fertilization rates were similar in all the three groups. Based on the current available data it can be concluded that oocyte retrieval can be scheduled with a larger time window of 34–40 hours till larger adequately powered randomized studies are available to evaluate the pregnancy rates associated with different time interval of oocyte retrieval following hCG administration.[13]

Minimal Effective Dose of hCG

In standard IVF, the available evidence indicates that 5,000 IU and 10,000 IU of hCG are equally effective for triggering final oocyte maturation. In an RCT by Wikland et al. found no difference in terms of oocyte yield, fertilization rates and pregnancy rates when either 5,000 or 10,000 IU were used.[12] In an another randomized trial published in 1987, when hCG was administered for IVF, oocyte recovery was significantly less in 2,000 IU group compared to 5,000 IU and 10,000 IU groups.[14] Bioavailability of hCG appears to be lower in women with higher body weight. Empirical clinical practice is to use a dose of 10,000 IU hCG instead of 5,000 IU in obese women. Larger randomized clinical trials are needed to effectively predict the effect of increased body weight in obese women and effect of hCG.

Route of hCG Administration

Since subcutaneous injections can be performed by the patients themselves and are better tolerated, it is now predominantly used nowadays. Also present data available tells when 10,000 IU hCG is used its results are similar in both intramuscular and subcutaneous routes. When serum hCG levels were analyzed 24 hours after subcutaneous and intramuscular administration of hCG 5,000 IU for women undergoing ovulation induction, the levels were similar in both the groups.[15] But in patients undergoing IVF when hCG 5,000 IU and 10,000 IU were administered both intramuscular and subcutaneous routes, serum concentration was higher in intramuscular group in 5,000 IU category, but in 10,000 IU category serum levels were similar in both intramuscular and subcutaneous groups.[16]

Recombinant hCG

There have been widespread uses of urinary hCG for several decades. However, as a urinary derived preparation, it has some disadvantages such as vast amount of urine required for getting the highest purity, the possible contamination with other proteins and batch-to-batch inconsistency, which leads to variations in clinical results among patients and also within the same patients in different cycles. Subcutaneous recombinant hCG has been recently introduced for final follicular maturation and ovulation induction in infertile women undergoing ART. Recombinant hCG preparations are derived from genetically engineered Chinese hamster ovary cells through recombinant DNA technology. This product is purified by repeated chromatographic steps to produce a high specific activity which makes the drug free from urinary contamination and suitable for subcutaneous injection and self administration with lower local reactions and higher tolerability. It has been reported that the inconsistency and low bioavailability of urinary preparations of hCG might result in lack of retrieved oocytes or empty follicle syndrome which is due to some difficulties through production, packaging and storage process of the drug and also rapid clearance of the drug by liver. Recently, the high purity and batch-to-batch consistency of recombinant preparations provide an effective and well tolerated alternative for urinary derived agents in IVF cycles.[17]

In some randomized trials administration of 250 µg rhCG rather than 5,000 or 10,000 IU uhCG improved oocyte quality.[18] Contrary to aforementioned studies, in some previous randomized trials no superiority was found in administration of recombinant hCG to urinary hCG in fertilization, implantation and pregnancy rates.[19] The incidence of OHSS as a serious complication of this treatment was comparable between groups. Current available data tells recombinant hCG shows equivalent efficacy to urinary hCG in terms of the number of oocytes per aspirated follicles in selected patients undergoing intracytoplasmic sperm injection (ICSI). However, 500 µg rhCG seems to be more advantageous than the lower dose in this indication. Larger randomized trials are needed to generalize this strategy.

GnRH Agonist Triggering of Final Oocyte Maturation

In IVF/ICSI patients co-treated with a GnRH antagonist, a bolus of GnRH agonist (GnRHa) may be administered as an alternative to hCG for final oocyte maturation **(Fig. 1)**. This ovulation trigger concept was previously shown to stimulate effectively final oocyte maturation and ovulation, as GnRH agonist displaces the GnRH antagonist from the GnRH receptor, inducing an initial activation (flare-up) of LH and FSH, similar to that of the natural cycle prior to down-regulation of the receptor.[20] However, the profile and duration of the GnRHa-induced surge of gonadotropins are significantly different and shorter than those of the natural cycle, contrasted by the sustained LH-like activity induced by hCG trigger. This leads to a luteal phase insufficiency with very low LH levels after the GnRHa trigger and malfunctioning corpus luteum.[21]

Previously, the use of a GnRHa trigger in IVF/ICSI cycles followed by only a standard luteal phase support resulted in implantation failure and a high early pregnancy loss rate. However, modifying the luteal phase support by adding a bolus of 1.500 IU hCG on the

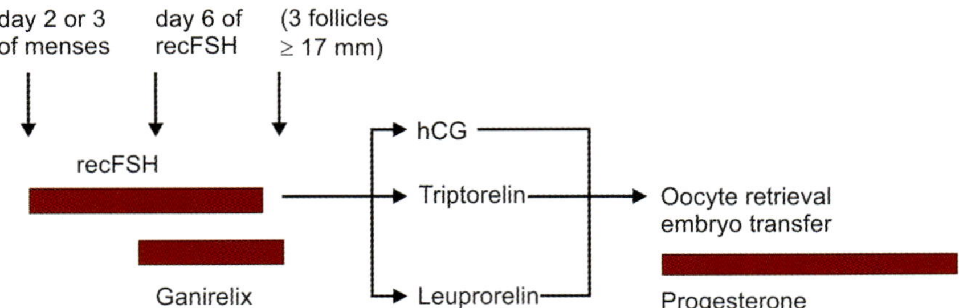

Fig. 1 Oocyte maturation

day of oocyte retrieval significantly reduced the early pregnancy loss rate and tended to increase the ongoing pregnancy rate when compared with hCG trigger.[22] Although non-significant, the difference in reproductive outcome was in favor of hCG trigger by 7%, and it was suggested further studies to optimize the luteal phase support after GnRHa trigger while maintaining a low risk of OHSS. Importantly, no OHSS was seen after GnRHa trigger despite supplementation with a small bolus of hCG, contrasted by an OHSS rate of 2% seen after hCG trigger.[23] Intensive luteal phase support with E2 and progesterone only in OHSS high-risk patients triggered with a bolus of GnRHa was originally described by Babayof et al.[24] No OHSS case was reported, however, at the cost of a disappointingly low reproductive outcome. The same intensive luteal phase support protocol with E2 and progesterone was given by Engmann et al.,[25] but reported low ongoing pregnancy rates. Recently, it was suggested that patients need to be stratified according to the E2 level on the day of trigger if intensive luteal phase support with E2 and progesterone only is to be used. Thus, OHSS risk patients with E2 levels more than 4,000 pg/mL may be supplemented during the luteal phase with intensive E2 and progesterone only, whereas patients with E2 levels less than 4,000 pg/mL should receive a dual trigger (GnRHa + 1,000 IU hCG) as well as intensive luteal phase support with E2 and progesterone.[26] Different types of luteal phase support have been evaluated in order to overcome the low pregnancy outcome in GnRH agonist triggering, including progesterone only, progesterone with estradiol, low dose hCG. It is yet not fully elucidated what constitutes the optimal luteal phase support after agonist triggering.

Regarding OHSS incidence, an overview of observational, uncontrolled trials on agonists triggering in high-risk patients for developing OHSS suggested that GnRH agonist triggering reliably prevents its incidence. This has been confirmed recently from randomized controlled studies in a Cochrane meta-analysis. Furthermore, in patients at risk for developing OHSS, GnRH agonist triggering has been combined with cryopreservation of all embryos or oocytes, those can be transferred in a subsequent cycle with good clinical pregnancy rates. Also by this OHSS can be completely avoided with very good cumulative pregnancy rates. So GnRh agonist triggering is also recommended in oocyte donors with GnRH antagonist protocol, in whom luteal phase support is not needed.

Recombinant LH

The most natural compound with which to trigger final oocyte maturation and with an expected low incidence of OHSS would have been LH. Thus, when recombinant LH (rLH) was introduced, a clinical trial was performed to explore the efficacy of rLH to trigger ovulation in a long GnRHa down-regulation protocol. Doses differing between 5,000 IU and 30,000 IU were explored. However, apart from the significant increase in cost of treatment, a low implantation rate was seen after only one bolus of rLH to trigger ovulation, moreover, a disappointingly high OHSS rate (12%) was reported.[27]

■ MESSAGE

> A bolus of 5.000–10.000 IU hCG has been successfully used for decades in assisted reproduction technology (ART) as a substitute for the endogenous LH surge to induce final oocyte maturation prior to oocyte retrieval. Then there are issues of the type, route, dose and timing of hCG administration. Agonist trigger in patients at high risk for OHSS with GnRH antagonists stimulation protocol has revolutionized our ability to eliminate OHSS. Although there is some debate concerning the clinical outcome of these cycles, aggressive luteal support and large number of frozen embryos in these cycles results in excellent per-oocyte retrieval pregnancy rates.

■ REFERENCES

1. Eppig JJ, Vivieros. Regulation of mammalian oocyte maturation. In: Leung, Adashi (Eds). The Ovary. Amsterdam: Elsevier Academic press; 2004. pp. 113-29.
2. Kessler MJ, Reddy MS, Shah RH, et al. Structures of N-glycosidic carbohydrate units of human chorionic gonadotropin. J Biol Chem. 1979;254:7901-8.
3. Xu F, Stouffer RL, Muller J, et al. Dynamics of the transcriptome in the primate ovulatory follicle. Mol Hum Reprod. 2011;17:152-65.
4. Yen SS, Llerena O, Little B, et al. Disappearance rates of endogenous luteinizing hormone and chorionic gonadotropin in man. J Clin Endocr Metab. 1968;28:1763-7.
5. Damewood MD, Shen W, Zacur HA, et al. Disappearance of exogenously administered human chorionic gonadotropin. Fertil Steril. 1989;52:398-400.
6. Delvigne A, Rozenberg S. Epidemiology and prevention of ovarian hyperstimulation syndrome (OHSS): a review. Hum Reprod Update. 2002;28:559-77.
7. Papanikolaou EG, Pozzobon C, Kolibianakis EM, et al. Incidence and prediction of ovarian hyperstimulation syndrome in women undergoing gonadotropin-releasing hormone antagonist in vitro fertilization cycles. Fertil Steril. 2006;85:112-20.

8. Cerrillo M, Rodriguez S, Mayoral M, et al. Differential regulation of VEGF after final oocyte maturation with GnRH agonist versus hCG: a rationale for OHSS reduction. Fertil Steril. 2009;91:1526-8.

9. Fanchin R, Peltier E, Frydman R, et al. Human chorionic gonadotropin: does it affect human endometrial morphology in vivo? Semin Reprod Med. 2001;19:31-5.

10. Clark L, Stanger J, Brinsmead M. Prolonged follicle stimulation decreases pregnancy rates after in vitro fertilization. Fertil Steril. 1991;55:1192-4.

11. Tan SL, Balen A, el Hussein E, et al. A prospective randomized study of the optimum timing of human chorionic gonadotropin administration after pituitary desensitization in in vitro fertilization. Fertil Steril. 1992;57:1259-64.

12. Andersen AG, Als-Nielsen B, Hornnes PJ, et al. Time interval from human chorionic gonadotropin (hCG) injection to follicular rupture. Hum Reprod. 1995;10:3202-5.

13. Nargund G, Reid F, Parsons J. Human chorionic gonadotropin-to-oocyte collection interval in a superovulation IVF program. A prospective study. J Assist Reprod Genet. 2001;18:87-90.

14. Abdalla HI, Ah-Moye M, Brindsen P, et al. The effect of the dose of human chorionic gonadotropin and the type of gonadotropin stimulation on oocyte recovery rates in an in vitro fertilization program. Fertil Steril. 1987;48:958-63.

15. Sills ES, Drews CD, Perloe M, et al. Periovulatory serum human chorionic gonadotropin (hCG) concentrations following subcutaneous and intramuscular non recombinant hCG use during ovulation induction: a prospective, randomized trial. Fertil Steril. 2001;76:397-9.

16. Wikland M, Borg J, Forsberg AS, et al. Human chorionic gonadotropin self-administered by the subcutaneous route to induce oocyte maturation in an in vitro fertilization and embryo transfer programme. Hum Reprod. 1995;10:1667-70.

17. Penarrubia J, Balasch J, Fabregues F, et al. Recurrent empty follicle syndrome successfully treated with recombinant human chorionic gonadotropin. Hum Reprod. 1999;14(7): 1703-6.

18. The European Recombinant Human Chorionic Gonadotropin Study Group. Induction of final follicular maturation and early luteinization in women undergoing ovulation induction for assisted reproduction treatment-recombinant hCG versus urinary hCG. The European Recombinant Human Chorionic Gonadotropin Study Group. Hum Reprod. 2000;15(7): 1446-51.

19. Madani T, Mohammadi Yeganeh L, Ezabadi Z, et al. Comparing the efficacy of urinary and recombinant hCG on oocyte/follicle ratio to trigger ovulation in women undergoing intracytoplasmic sperm injection cycles: a randomized controlled trial. J Assist Reprod Genet. 2013;30:239-45.

20. Gonen Y, Balakier H, Powell W, et al. Use of gonadotropin-releasing hormone agonist to trigger follicular maturation for in vitro fertilization. J Clin Endocrinol Metab. 1990;71:918-22.

21. Casper RF, Yen SS. Induction of luteolysis in the human with a long-acting analog of luteinizing hormone-releasing factor. Science. 1979;205:408-10.

22. Humaidan P, Bungum L, Bungum M, et al. Rescue of corpus luteum function with peri-ovulatory hCG supplementation in IVF/ICSI GnRH antagonist cycles in which ovulation was triggered with a GnRH agonist: a pilot study. Reprod Biomed Online. 2006;13:173-8.

23. Humaidan P, Ejdrup BH, Westergaard LG, et al. 1,500 IU human chorionic gonadotropin administered at oocyte retrieval rescues the luteal phase when gonadotropin-releasing hormone agonist is used for ovulation induction: a prospective, randomized, controlled study. Fertil Steril. 2010;93:847-54.

24. Babayof R, Margalioth EJ, Huleihel M, et al. Serum inhibin A, VEGF and TNF alpha levels after triggering oocyte maturation with GnRH agonist compared with hCG in women with polycystic ovaries undergoing IVF treatment: a prospective randomized trial. Hum Reprod. 2006;21:1260-5.

25. Engmann L, DiLuigi A, Schmidt D, et al. The effect of luteal phase vaginal estradiol supplementation on the success of in vitro fertilization treatment: a prospective randomized study. Fertil Steril. 2008;89:554-61.

26. Griffin D, Benadiva C, Kummer N, et al. Dual trigger of oocyte maturation with gonadotropin-releasing hormone agonist and low-dose human chorionic gonadotropin to optimize livebirth rates in high responders. Fertil Steril. 2012;97:1316-20.

27. European Recombinant LH Study Group. Human recombinant luteinizing hormone is as effective as, but safer than, urinary human chorionic gonadotropin in inducing final follicular maturation and ovulation in in vitro fertilization procedures: results of a multicenter double-blind study. J Clin Endocr Metab. 2001;86:2607-18.

Gamete Collection and Preparation

20 Oocyte Retrieval

Sunita R Tandulwadkar, Sejal Naik, Devika Chopra

■ INTRODUCTION

Recovery of oocytes from the ovary is a fundamental step of in vitro fertilization (IVF) treatment. Transvaginal ultrasound-guided oocyte retrieval (TVOR) during IVF treatment was first described in 1985. By virtue of its simplicity and effectiveness, it has gained widespread popularity and has now become the gold standard for IVF therapy. Nevertheless, despite the advantages, the aspiration needle may injure the adjacent pelvic organs and structures leading to serious complications. The most common complications are hemorrhage, trauma and injury of pelvic structures, and pelvic infection. However, there is wide variation in the way this common procedure is performed, with room for improvement through published guidelines. This chapter reviewed the most common technique of oocyte retrieval and its complications, summarized the recommendations made to minimize their occurrence, and raised some of the controversial issues related to the procedure.

The first human oocytes in vitro from ovarian tissue removed at laparotomy is ascribed to Gregory Pincus, and the same experience was repeated by Robert Edward. The need to retrieve individual oocytes by minimally invasive procedure was recognized by him and Patrick Steptoe, the only gynecologist operating with laparoscope came together to collaborate and ultimately to create the first child born as a result of in vitro fertilization and embryo transfer (IVF-ET).

Oocytes were collected by laparoscopy until the technology advances with ultrasound imaging allowed ovarian follicles to be clearly seen. By 1981, it was possible to retrieve oocytes by needling follicles with transabdominal ultrasound guidance. The method of oocytes recovery became simpler and less traumatic with vaginal scanners and became day-care procedure under sedation or light anesthesia.

■ PRIMARY ASSESSMENT

When the patient comes for the initial assessment of infertility, the clinician assesses the access of the ovaries via the transvaginal route using ultrasonography. This preliminary assessment enables the clinician to plan the route and technique of oocyte retrieval (transvesical, transuterine, etc.).

■ TECHNIQUES

Ultrasound-guided Method

- *Transvaginal method:* Ultrasound-guided oocyte recovery by vaginal route is now universal. It has very significant advantages: least invasive, simplicity of use, ease of learning, proximity of the transducer to the ovaries, patient acceptance, can be performed under short general anesthesia, an outpatient procedure and relatively few complications.
- *Transabdominal method:* The first recorded aspiration of oocytes from follicles under ultrasound guidance by Lenz and colleagues in 1981, and it was found that recovery rates were as good as those by laparoscopy, with fewer complications and easier ovarian access. It is performed when ovaries are inaccessible by the vaginal route like in frozen pelvis, bowel adhesions in pouch of Douglas, a very large fibroid uterus displacing the fundus and ovaries upward and, in Mayer-Rokitansky syndrome wherein the ovaries are upwardly displaced.
- *Transvesical method:* Transabdominal through urinary bladder approach.
- *Periurethral method:* Not used.

Laparoscopic Method

Laparoscopic method is now no longer being used for ovum pickup. It requires full general anesthesia. All visible follicles, even small ones, are aspirated. At completion of the recovery, the pouch of Douglas should be aspirated clear of all blood and flushing fluid; occasionally an oocyte may be found from the collected fluid.

Limitations: It is the procedure of the past, more invasive than vaginal aspiration, takes longer time, unexpected adhesions obscuring the ovary, endometriosis, bleeding and difficulty in recovery of oocytes, expensive and more morbid for the patient.

■ TIMING

Transvaginal ultrasound-guided oocyte retrieval is typically performed after controlled ovarian hyper-stimulation, where oocytes are pharmacologically stimulated to mature. When the ovarian follicles have reached a certain degree of development, induction of final oocyte maturation is performed, generally by an intramuscular or subcutaneous injection of human chorionic gonadotropin (hCG). TVOR is typically performed 34–36 hours after hCG injection, when the eggs are fully mature but just prior to rupture of the follicles.

■ EQUIPMENT

- Operating table and operating lights
- Ultrasonography machine with transvaginal probe
- Aspiration pump
- Aspiration needle (double lumen needle/single lumen needle)
- Heated block within a thermostat machine and a sterile non-toxic collection tube.

■ PROCEDURE (FIGS 1 TO 18)

A successful ART clinic requires a carefully designed operation theater complex dedicated for performing IVF, intracytoplasmic sperm injection and oocyte retrieval procedures. The entry into this complex is restricted for maintaining stringent sterile conditions. The complex should preferably have a double door system.

- The embryologist works in the IVF laboratory under laminar flow conditions wherein a Transferpettor pipette attached to a sterile tip, two 23 gauge needles for dissecting the blood clots, and a collection jar for disposing off the follicular fluid are kept.
- The washing area is always outside the laboratory. The surgeon as well as the embryologist washes their hands thoroughly with a non-soap, fragrance free, solution which has a germ inhibiting effect.
- The procedure of oocyte retrieval is performed under short general anesthesia preferably using anesthetics

like fentanyl and propofol so that the patient can be awoken shortly after the procedure is over and can be sent home within 2–3 hours after oocyte retrieval.

- The vulva and vagina are cleaned with lukewarm normal saline and are covered with sterile drapes.
- The procedure of oocyte retrieval is performed under ultrasonographic guidance. The sonography machine with two frequency head is used.
- The transvaginal ultrasonography probe is cleaned with 70% alcohol and cleaned 6–8 times with normal saline before use and is kept covered with sterile drape till its further use.
- The pressure of the aspiration pump is set to 100 mm Hg.
- The tubes in which the follicular fluid is aspirated are pre-warmed using a heat block. The heat block is set at a temperature higher than that of the body so that the tubes remain at body temperature.
- A small amount of coupling gel is used to cover the end of the probe and the probe is then covered with a disposable probe cover. The air within the probe cover should be removed. The needle guide is attached to the probe.
- Either the single or double lumen needle can be used for aspiration. The cork end of the aspiration needle is attached to the aspiration tube. The connection from the aspiration pump is also fitted to it.
- To maintain the temperature of the follicular fluid, the tubes are always kept in a heat block.
- The vaginal transducer is introduced and the pelvis is scanned thoroughly to confirm, the position, number of follicles and the accessibility of the ovaries. The uterus and the endometrial thickness can also be assessed.
- The needle is then removed from its sheath and is flushed with follicular flushing media. The needle is partially inserted into the needle guide and the probe is manipulated on such a way that the ovaries are just above the probe.
- Continuous rotator movement of the needle is necessary while aspirating the follicle to ensure the successful retrieval of an egg from the follicle.
- The aspiration is started from one side of the ovary and the follicles are aspirated serially till the surgeon reaches the other side.
- Once all the fluid from one follicle is aspirated, side to side movement of the probe is performed to ensure that the follicular fluid is completely aspirated and to decide which follicle needs to be aspirated next.
- The needle tip is thrust usually 1 cm within the follicle so that there is uniform intrafollicular suction pressure. It is preferable to enter the follicle from its base rather than the side wall.

- Usually it is possible to keep the needle within the ovary and aspirate all the follicles using a single puncture in the ovary. The ovary is reassessed before one move to the other side and then the similar procedure is performed on the other side.
- After 2–3 follicles are aspirated, the tube is changed. The tube is capped tightly and is kept in the heat block. The tubes are sent to the embryologist in the adjacent laboratory while been placed in the heat block so as to maintain the temperature of the tube.
- The procedure of oocyte retrieval is performed in dimmed light to prevent exposure of the oocyte to external light source.
- Once embryologist receives the tube, follicular fluid is poured in pre-warmed petri dishes. The fluid is carefully scanned for oocyte-cumulus complexes (OCCs) under low-power magnification using stereo microscope. The oocytes are then picked up by the Transferpettor tip and are placed in the outer well of the two-well dish. The two-well dish is kept in the working incubator so that the temperature of the collected oocytes is maintained. The OCCs are washed several times in the outer well of the two-well petri dish. In case of blood clots, 23 gauge needles are used to tease the OCCs free from the clots.
- The oocytes are then checked for maturity after incubation for a few hours.
- When all the follicles are empty, the transducer is withdrawn. Usually the blood loss is minimal. It should be rechecked by inserting a speculum and any trickle of blood can be controlled using pressure.

■ COMPLICATIONS

Overall, transvaginal oocyte retrieval is a safe procedure, with a low rate of major complications, generally less than 0.5%.

The aspiration needle may injure the adjacent pelvic organs and can lead to serious complications. The most common complications are hemorrhage, trauma and injury of pelvic structures and pelvic infection. Other complications described include adnexal torsion, rupture of endometriotic cysts, anesthetic and even vertebral osteomyelitis. In the last two decades, several reports have described the complications associated with this technique, and tried to address the risk factors and safety issues **(Table 1)**.

Potential injuries from transvaginal aspiration include bleeding, infection and injury to surrounding intra-abdominal structures including the intestine, uterus, Fallopian tubes or vessels.

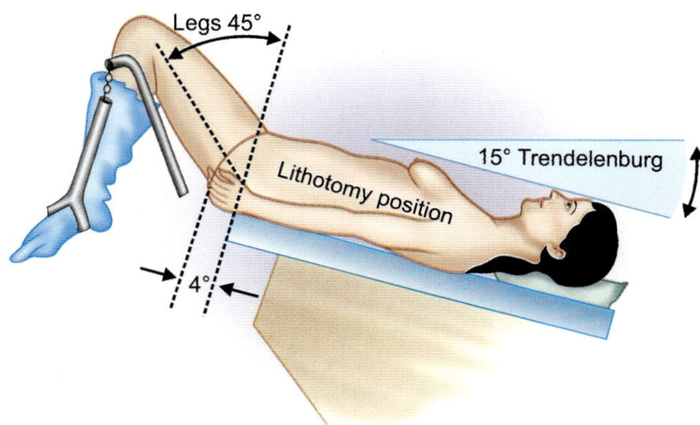

Fig. 1 Positioning of the patient for oocyte retrieval

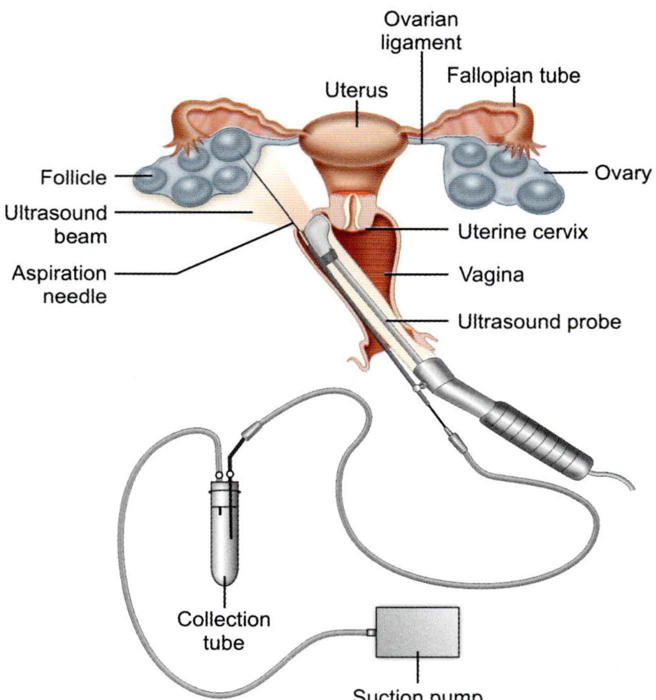

Fig. 2 Assembly for oocyte retrieval

Table 1 Major complications associated with transvaginal oocyte retrieval

Complication	Incidence (%)
Infection	0.06–0.24
Bleeding	0.03–0.24
Bowel injury	0.04

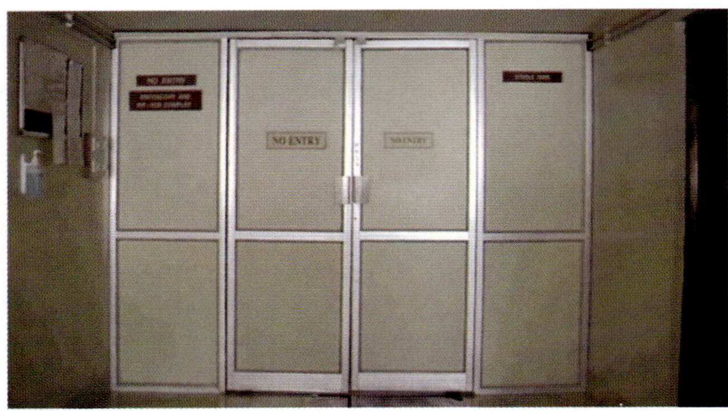

Fig. 3 Operation theater complex

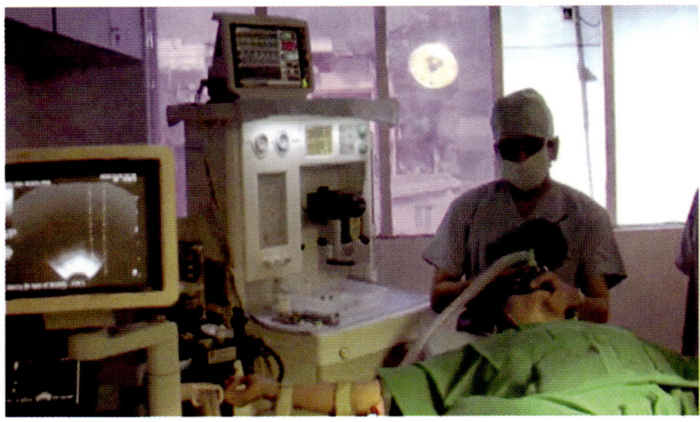

Fig. 6 Procedure under short general anesthesia

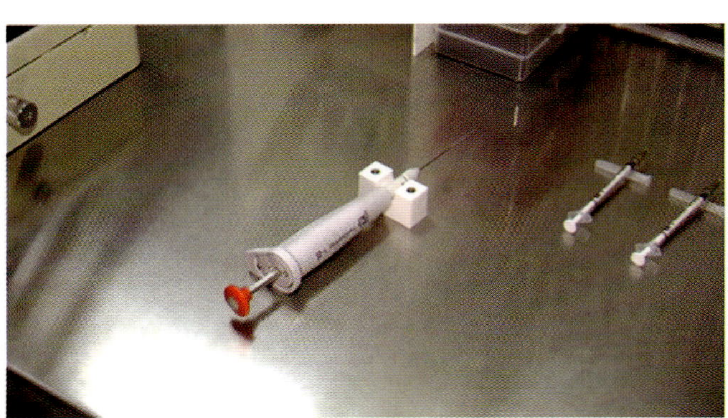

Fig. 4 Transferpettor

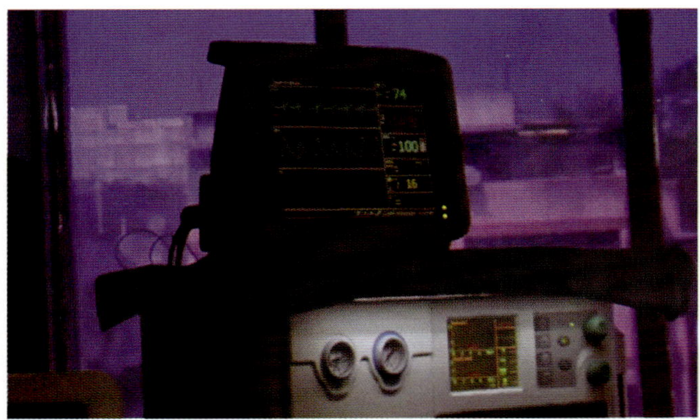

Fig. 7 Anesthesia machine

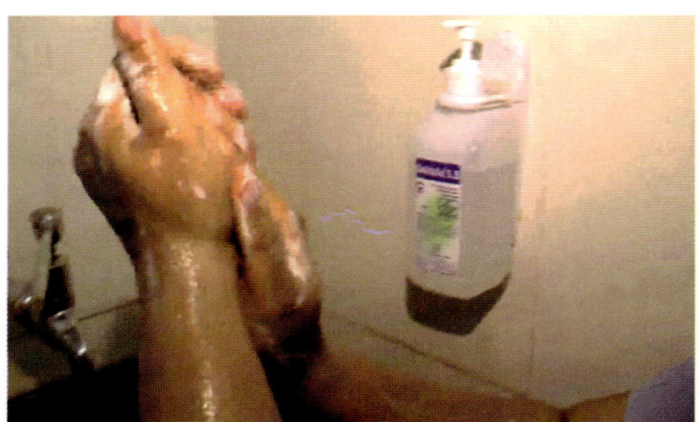

Fig. 5 Washing hands

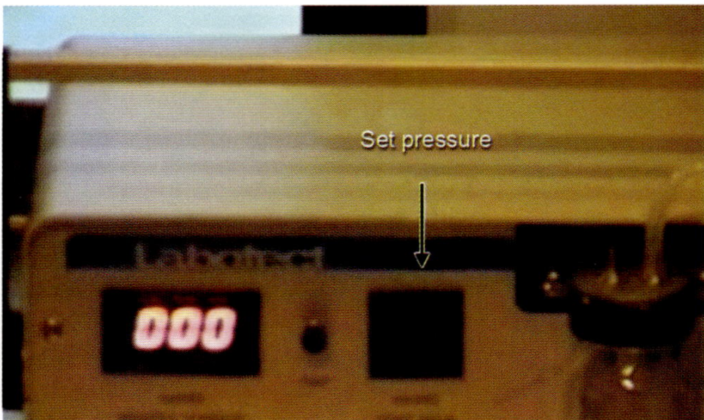

Fig. 8 Aspiration pump

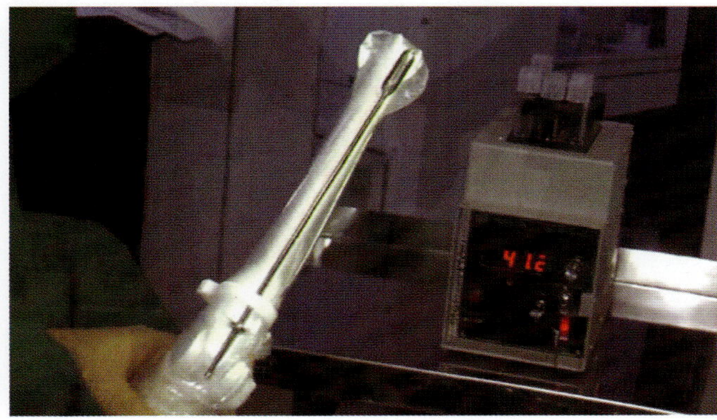

Fig. 9 Transvaginal probe with cover and needle guide

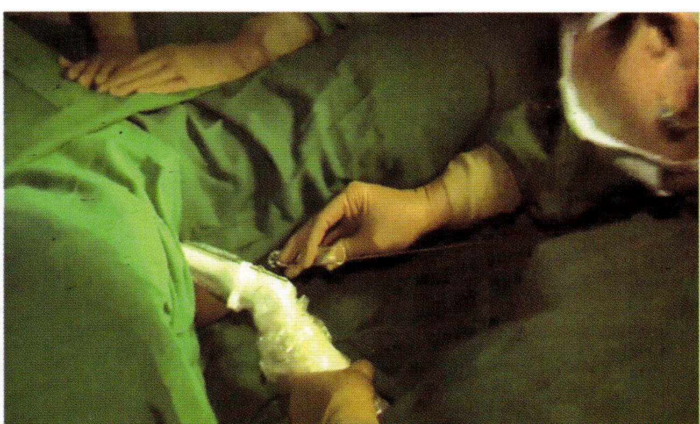

Fig. 11 Flushing media aspirated into needle

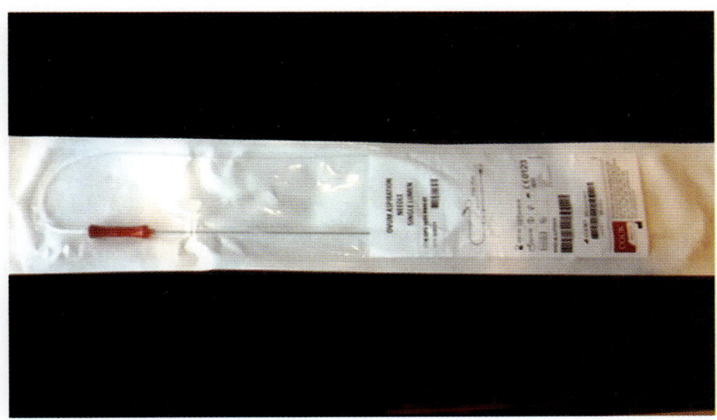

Fig. 10 Aspiration needle

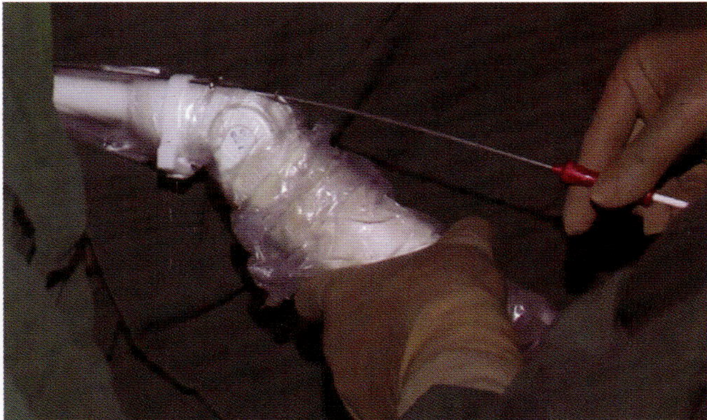

Fig. 12 Rolling of needle to ensure follicle aspiration

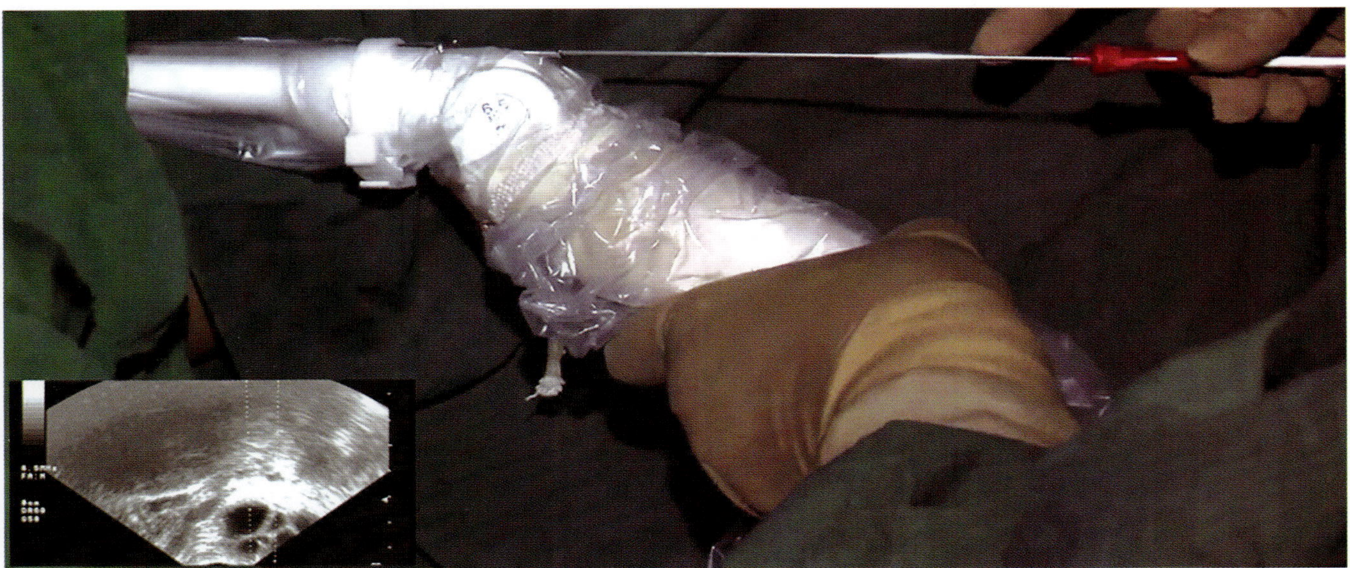

Fig. 13 Side-to-side movement of probe to ensure follicle aspiration

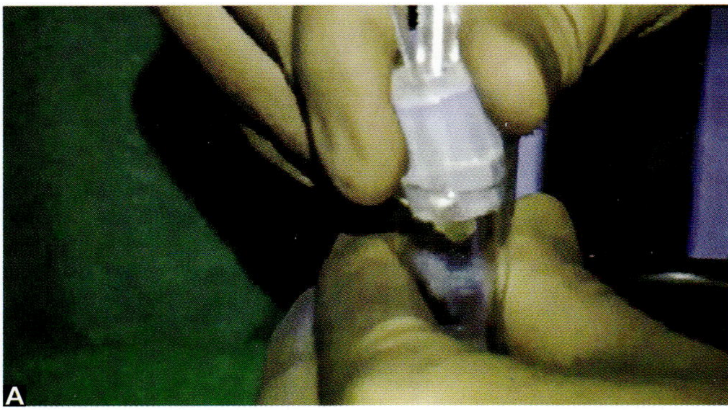
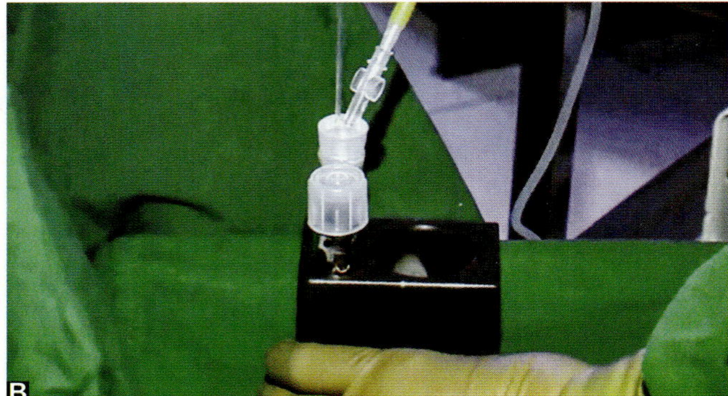

Figs 14A and B Changing cork from one tube after aspiration of 2–3 follicles

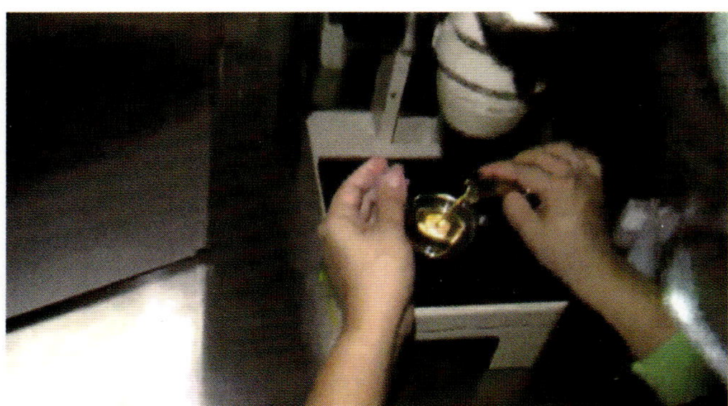

Fig. 15 Pouring follicular fluid in pre-warmed petri dish

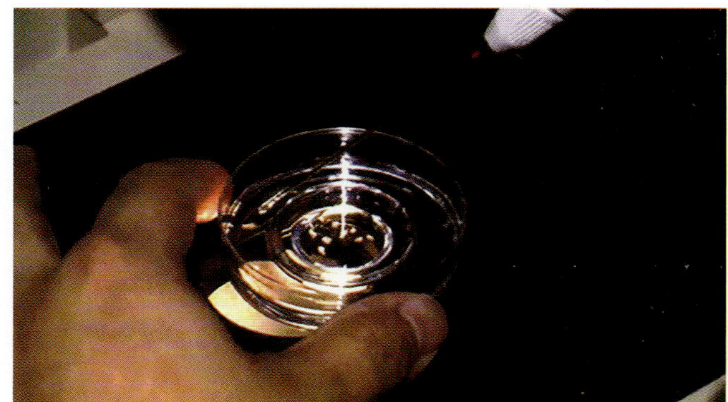

Fig. 17 Transfer of oocyte-cumulus complexes from outer to inner well

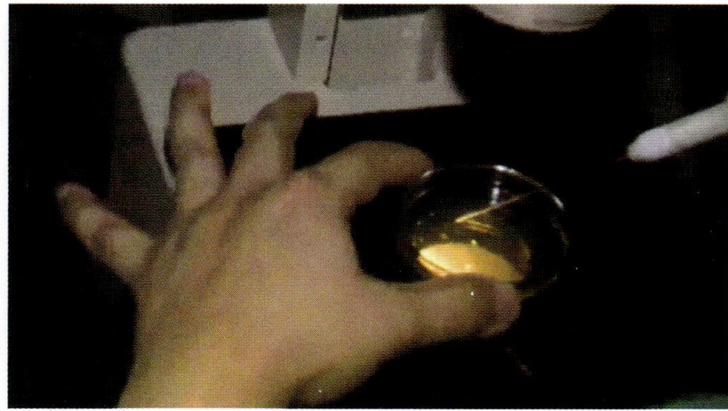

Fig. 16 Collecting oocyte-cumulus complexes with Transferpettor

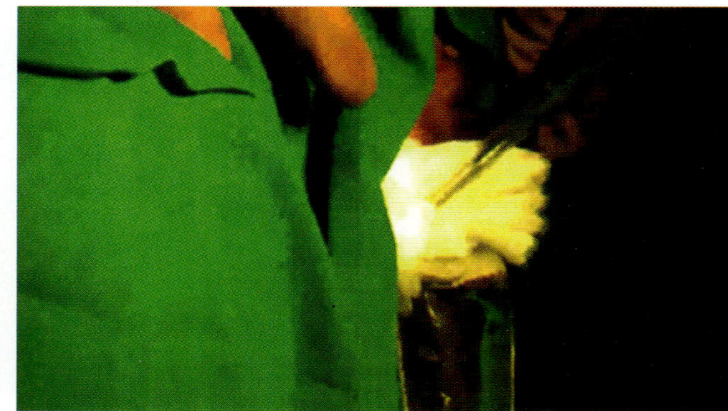

Fig. 18 Checking for PV bleeding

Injection of hCG as a trigger for ovulation confers a risk of ovarian hyperstimulation syndrome, especially in women with polycystic ovary syndrome who have been hyperstimulated during previous assisted reproduction cycles.

Additional complications may result from the administration of intravenous sedation or general anesthesia. These include asphyxia caused by airway obstruction, apnea, hypotension and pulmonary aspiration of stomach contents.

Propofol-based anesthetic techniques result in significant concentrations of propofol in follicular fluid. As propofol has been shown to have deleterious effects on oocyte fertilization (in a mouse model), some authors have suggested that the dose of propofol administered during anesthesia should be limited, and also that the retrieved oocytes should be washed free of propofol.

CONCLUSION

Oocyte retrieval is a crucial procedure in ART cycle. Vaginal ultrasound has undoubtedly been the greatest advance in ability that enables the surgeon to visualize the pelvic organs and making oocyte recovery safe and less painful. To summarize, the skill of oocyte retrieval requires practice and the results obtained in an ART cycle depend upon the procedure followed.

Oocyte Evaluation and Preparation

Sonal Vaidya

INTRODUCTION

With millions of oocytes being retrieved in the assisted reproductive technology (ART) cycles performed over the world, and with the ever increasing demand of achieving optimal livebirth rates, the ART clinics with the help of the guidelines provided by the regulatory bodies are ensuring that all the processes involved are monitored stringently. Tough the demand for higher success rates are the main driving force behind all the quality control (QC) procedures, the reduction in the multiple pregnancy rates thus avoiding the complications and unnecessary financial burden are equally important; thereby making the ability to select the best embryo(s) for transfer mandatory. In some countries, there are legal restrictions in the number of embryos transferred as well as number of oocytes inseminated.

The embryo selection begins from evaluation of oocytes, sperms and continues to the cleavage stage embryos and blastocysts. The methods deployed for selecting the most viable embryo for transfer involves the morphological grading of gametes and embryos and now involves the proteomic and biochemical analysis as well. This chapter will discuss the oocyte evaluation, the first step in analyzing the potential of the oocyte in formation of the viable embryo and will further proceed to discuss the stepwise preparation of the oocytes for fertilization.

THE OOCYTE

The oocyte is the largest cell of our body measuring up to 120–160 μm. The oocyte comprises of double layered zona pellucida (ZP) which is an acellular matrix composed of sulfated glycoproteins. It has been demonstrated that the ZP plays distinct roles during fertilization and embryo development.[1] The main function of ZP is however to prevent polyspermy[2,3] and to protect the integrity of the embryo.[4,5] The outer layer of the zona is thicker while the inner layer, though being thinner is more resilient.[6]

Generally speaking, in humans the thickness of the zona normally varies from 18 μm to 22 μm.[7-9] The zona however varies in the population of the oocytes retrieved from one individual and also with the varying stages of the embryonic development.[8]

While the ZP acts as a protecting layer around the oocyte, the ooplasm is packed with several important organelles like the meiotic spindle, the mitochondria, the endoplasmic reticulum, the Golgi apparatus—all ensuring that the fertilized oocyte is well equipped to result in a livebirth as the sperm that fertilizes the egg contributes the least cytoplasmic contents for the developing embryo. It is a well-known fact that only a limited number of oocytes reach ovulation stage and thereby a chance to develop into a baby. These oocytes are around a few million in number at the fetal stage, reduce to a few thousand till puberty while only one ovulates each cycle.[10-12] Since the oocytes are already recruited in the ovary at the fetal stage itself, their limited number, and the adverse effect of the environmental factors on their quality over the period of time make them the most precious entities of the ART clinics.

The polar body is a sign of a mature oocyte. It is oval in shape. The polar body, the ooplasm as well as the ZP are assessed for analyzing the oocyte quality (addressed later in this chapter).

Typically in an ART cycle, the ovaries are stimulated with various drugs to produce more number of oocytes. These oocytes are retrieved 36–40 hours following a human chorionic gonadotropin (hCG) trigger, the procedure being labeled as ovum pick-up (OPU). The trigger is administered on the day when the cohort containing maximum numbers of follicles reach the size of 18 mm. This ensures that around 80% of the oocytes retrieved are mature.

Needless to say that following an OPU procedure, around 10% immature oocytes and around 10% atresic oocytes maybe retrieved as stimulation regimes may produce the population of oocytes that are not synchronous in development. The oocytes that are retrieved during an OPU procedure are referred to as the oocyte-cumulus-complex (OCC) as the cumulus and corona cells engulf the oocytes. The mature oocyte is haploid as it has already completed its first meiotic division and is arrested in the metaphase II stage. Therefore a single oval polar body (~15 μm in diameter) is visible in the perivitelline space **(Fig. 1)**. However, the polar body is not easily identified due to the surrounding layers of cumulus cells. The retrieved oocytes are thus graded for their maturity status depending upon the layers of cumulus cells and the tightness of the corona cells. The gradual expansion of the cumulus and the corona cells is dependent on the follicle stimulating hormone in natural cycles; but this may be disturbed by the exogenous gonadotropins administered in the stimulated cycles, and hence may not truly correlate with the nuclear maturity status of the retrieved oocyte **(Fig. 2)**.

Oocyte Grading

The oocytes retrieved are graded as follows:

Grade I

Grade I oocytes have not undergone germinal vesicle breakdown, i.e. these are still diploid being arrested in the diplotene stage of meiosis I. The germinal vesicle

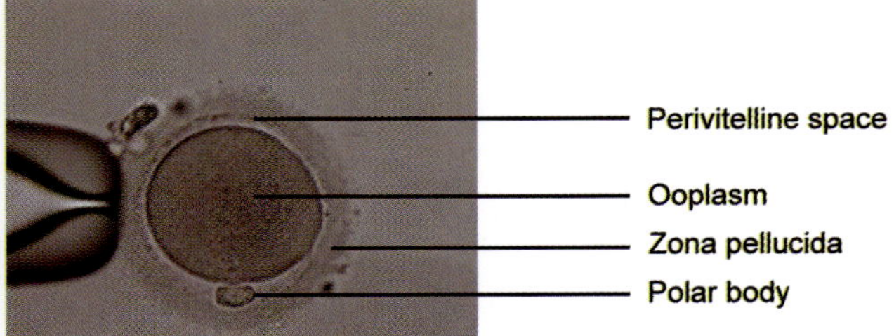

Fig. 1 Denuded oocyte approximately 39 hours post-hCG trigger prior to intracytoplasmic sperm injection

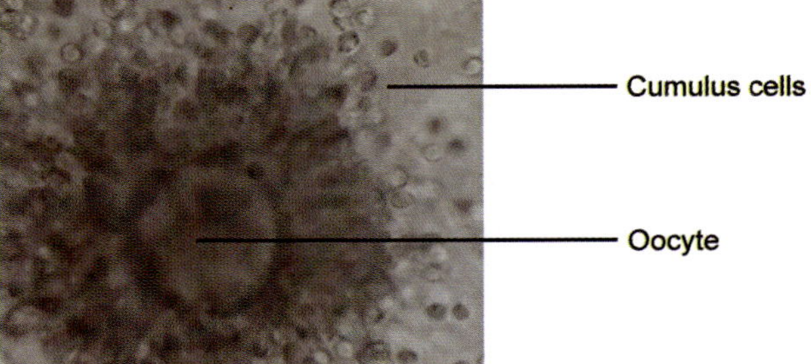

Fig. 2 A mature oocyte retrieved 36 hours post-hCG trigger (immediately after the ovum pick-up)

is distinctly visible following removal of cumulus cell layers (denudation). Corona cells are tightly packed thus giving an oocyte a dark appearance while the cumulus is scanty. These oocytes are generally retrieved from small follicles of less than 10 mm size. These oocytes need to be matured in vitro before insemination. However, very few pregnancies are reported so far **(Figs 3A to D)**.[13-15]

Grade II

The grade II oocyte reveals germinal vesicle breakdown but the polar body is yet to be extruded. The corona and the cumulus cells are still tightly packed. Such oocytes if inseminated immediately, may show absent or delayed fertilization **(Figs 4A and B)**.

Grade III

Grade III oocytes are mature oocytes, the polar body is already extruded. The oocyte is arrested in metaphase II. Polarization microscopy reveals that within grade III oocytes, the meiotic spindle fibers may still extend in the ooplasm making it necessary for culture of such oocytes for a few more hours before proceeding with intracytoplasmic sperm injection (ICSI). The corona cells are less tightly packed imparting light appearance to the oocytes and the cumulus cells are abundant **(Figs 5A to C)**.

Grade IV

These oocytes are the ovulatory oocytes. These are arrested at metaphase II. The corona cells appear as "sun burst" while the cumulus cells are fully expanded and abundant **(Figs 6A to C)**.

Grade V

Cumulus is gelatinous and mucified and the corona cells have begun to degenerate. The cumulus cells are seen as dark clusters while the corona cells appear dark and tight. They are thought to arise from the delayed hCG administration **(Fig. 7)**.

■ OOCYTE ABNORMALITIES

Around 3% of the retrieved oocytes though mature may display certain variations from the normal morphology. The degree and severity of variations in oocytes largely dictate the success rate of the given cycle. The oocytes with absent or ruptures zonae, empty zonae or severely vacuolated are simply discarded. Following are a few oocyte abnormalities that are seen within the population of the oocytes retrieved:

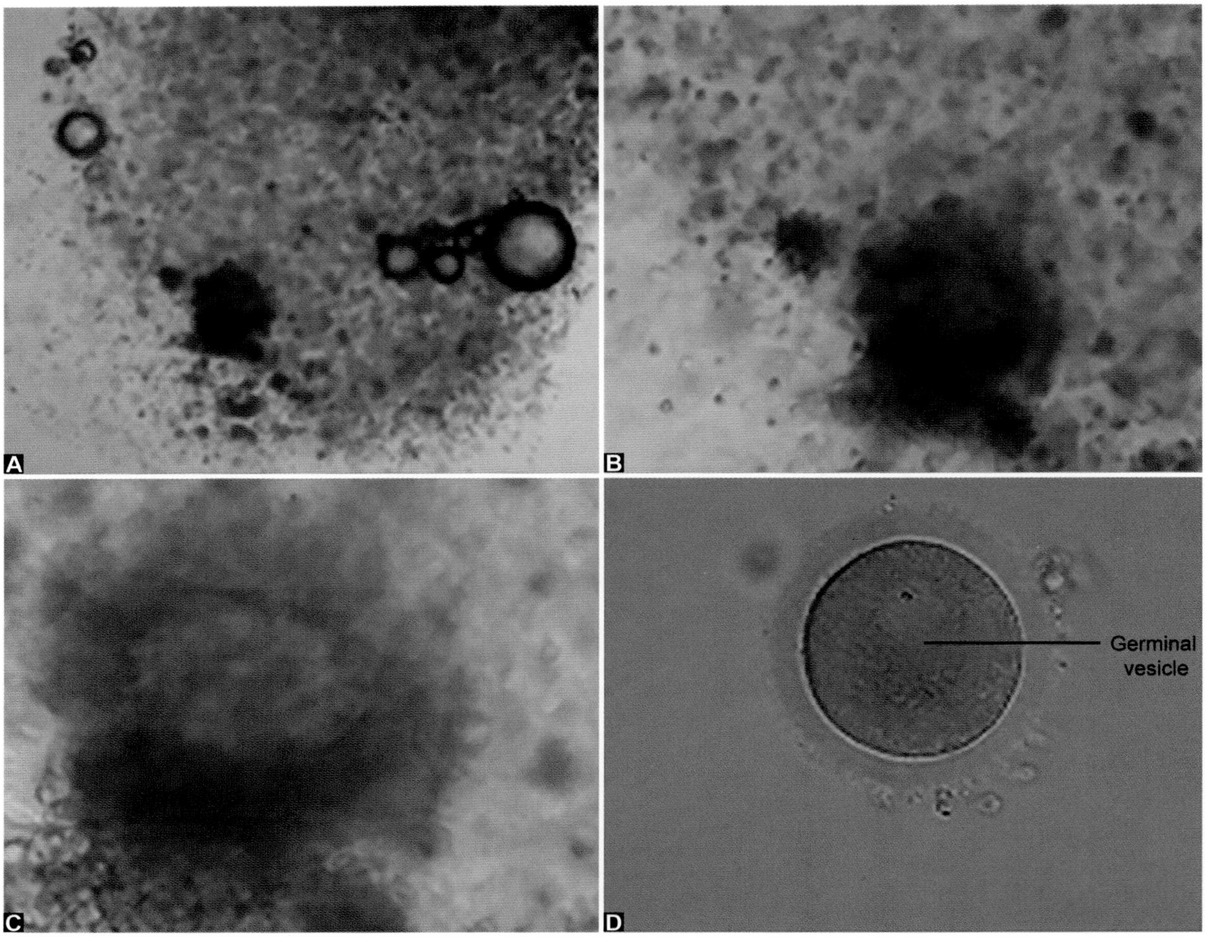

Figs 3A to D (A) Immature oocyte post-OPU as seen at 40x magnification; (B) The oocyte of Figure C as seen at 100x magnification; (C) The oocyte of Figure C as seen at 200x magnification; (D) The oocyte of Figure C as seen after denudation at 200x magnification

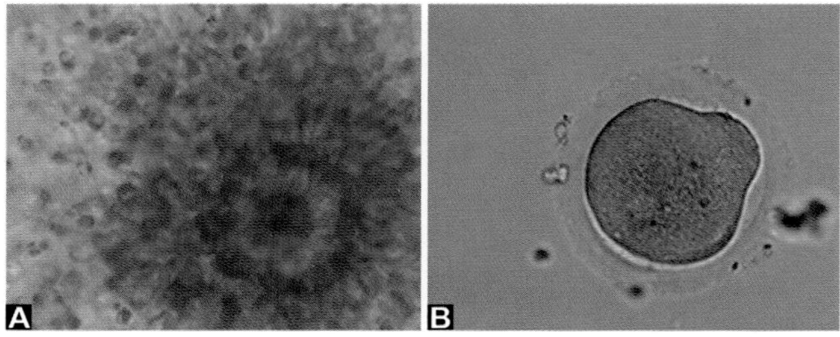

Figs 4A and B (A) The oocyte as seen at 100x magnification; (B) The oocyte as seen after denudation at 200x magnification—polar body is being extruded

- *Zona pellucida anomalies:* Distorted, elliptical, thinner or thicker than usual **(Figs 10A and B)**.[16-20]
- *First polar body anomalies:* Fragmented, elongated, flattened, very large or small in size **(Figs 9A to C)**.[21-24]
- *Ooplasm anomalies:* Nonuniform granularity, aggregation of smooth endoplasmic reticulum, centrally dark, refractile bodies, vacuoles, retracted ooplasm **(Figs 8A to C, 11 to 16)**.[19,20,25-27]

Distorted oocytes have been associated with higher incidences of aneuploidy[28,29] and therefore also indicate reduction in the fertilization and implantation rates.[30]

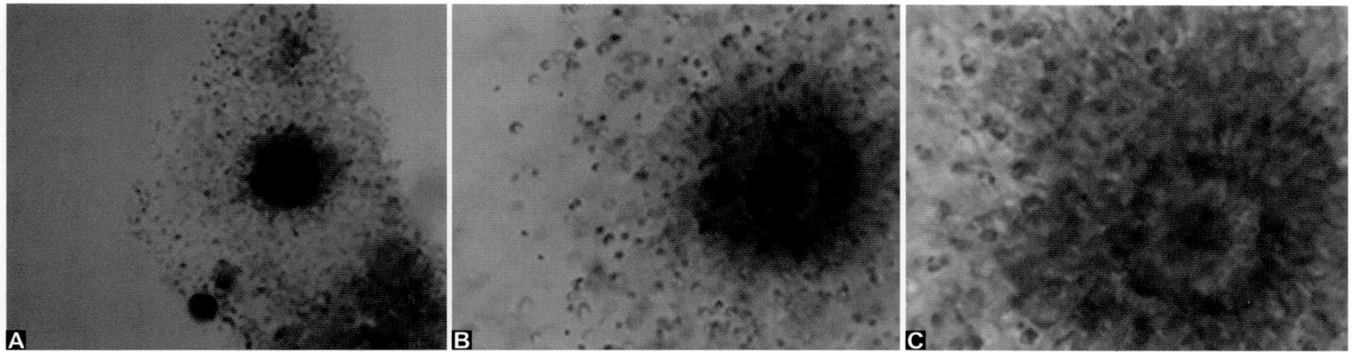

Figs 5A to C (A) Grade III oocyte at 40x magnification; (B) Oocyte at 100x magnification; (C) Oocyte at 200x magnification

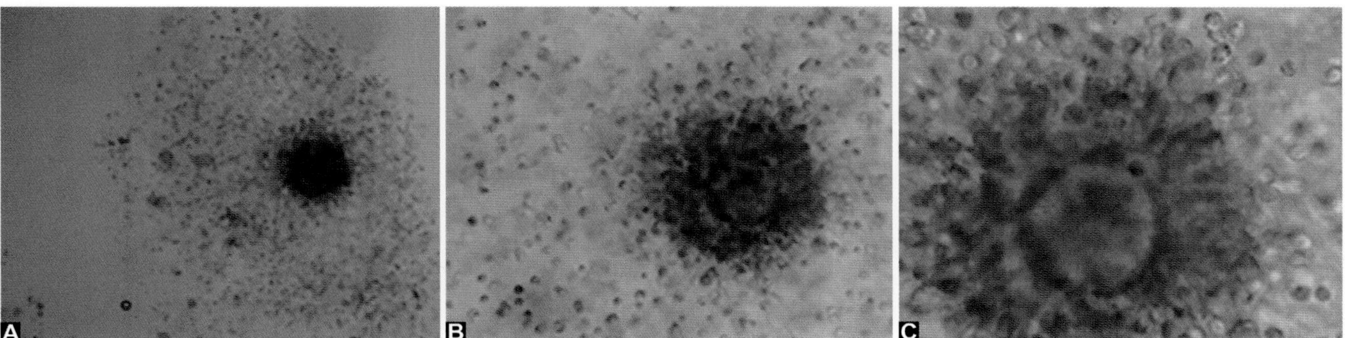

Figs 6A to C (A) Grade IV oocyte at 40x magnification; (B) Oocyte at 100x magnification; (C) Oocyte at 200x magnification

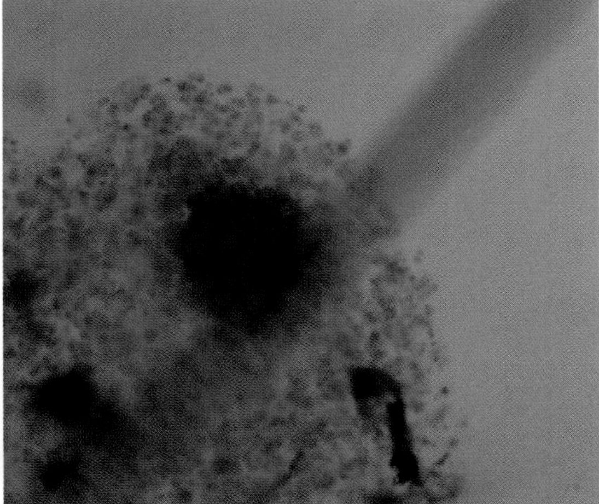

Fig. 7 Grade V oocyte at 40x magnification

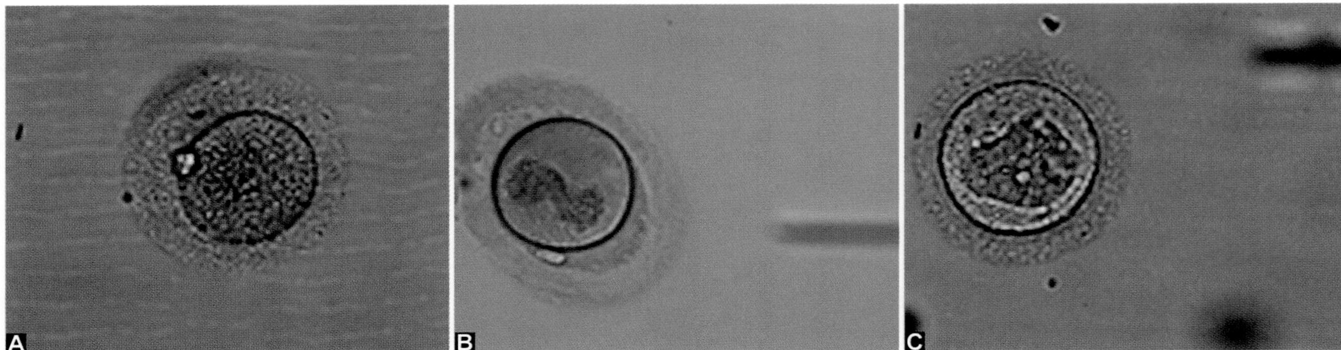

Figs 8A to C Varying degrees of granularity

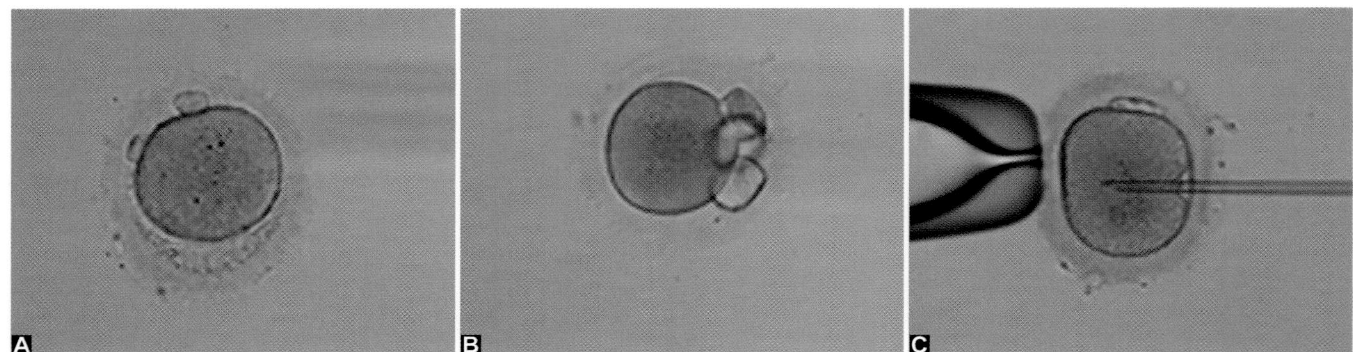

Figs 9A to C (A) Oocyte with two polar bodies; (B) Polar body (PB) large and severely fragmented; (C) Elongated PB

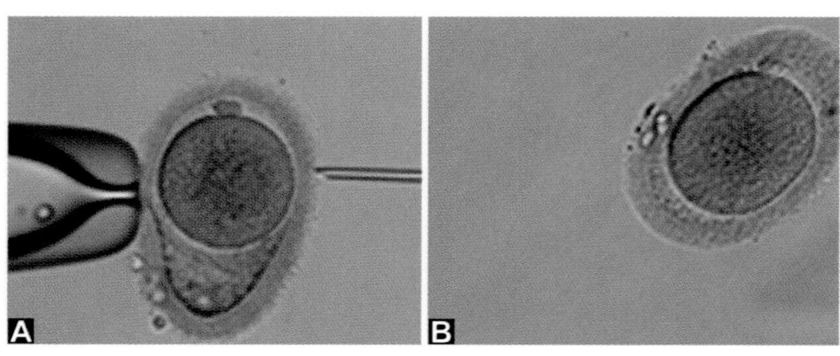

Figs 10A and B (A) Elliptical zona; (B) Elliptical oocyte

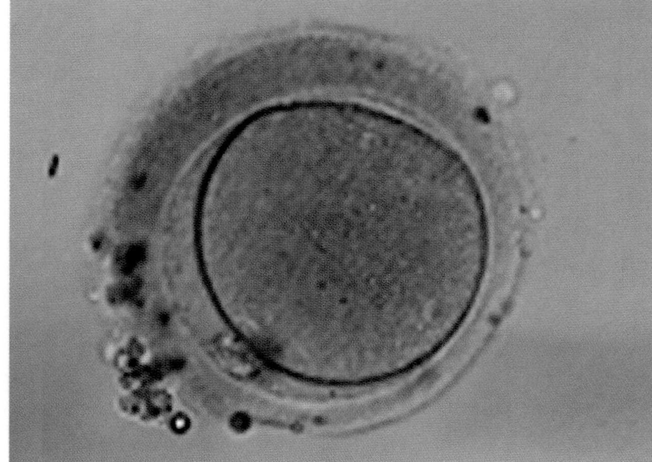

Fig. 11 Large oocyte

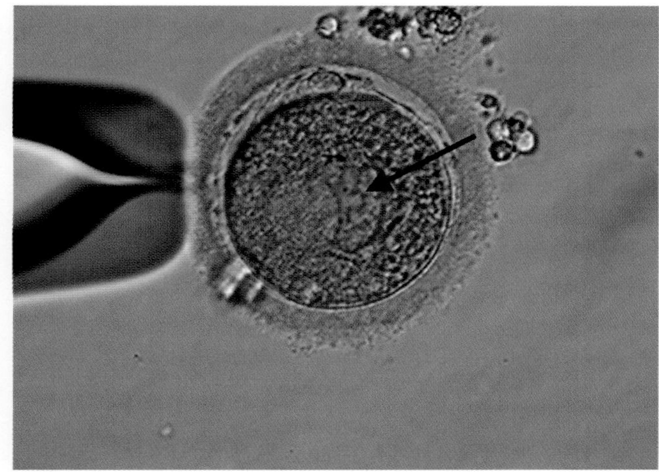

Fig. 12 Oocyte with smooth endoplasmic reticulum aggregation

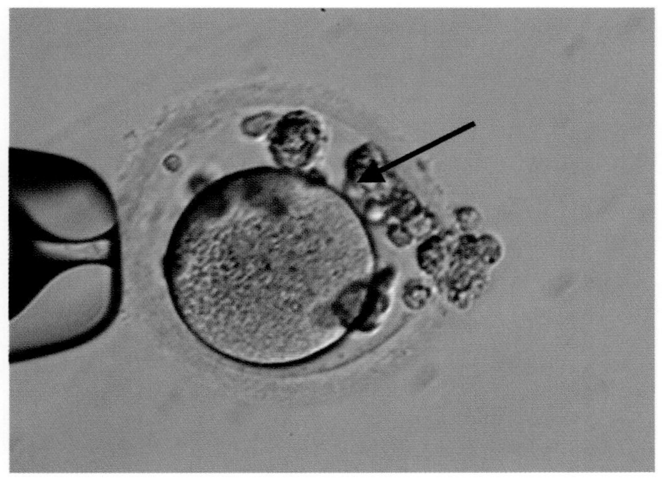

Fig. 13 Granular perivitelline space

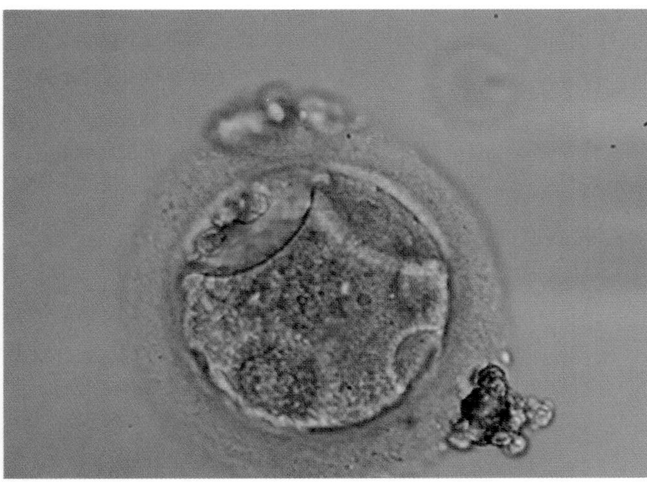

Fig. 14 Vacuolated

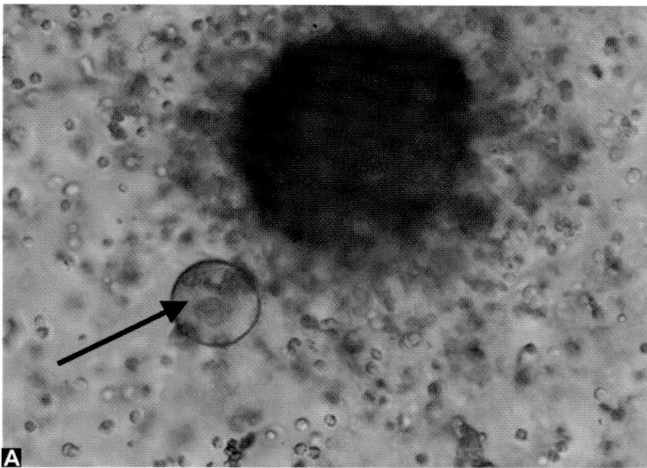

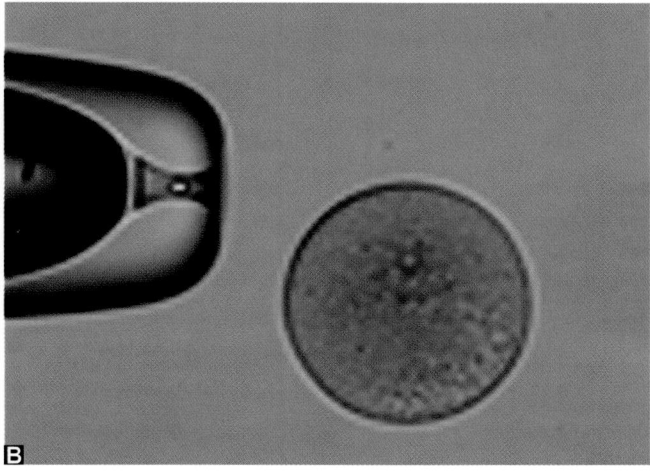

Figs 15A and B (A) Oocyte slipped cumulus; (B) Same oocyte after denudation

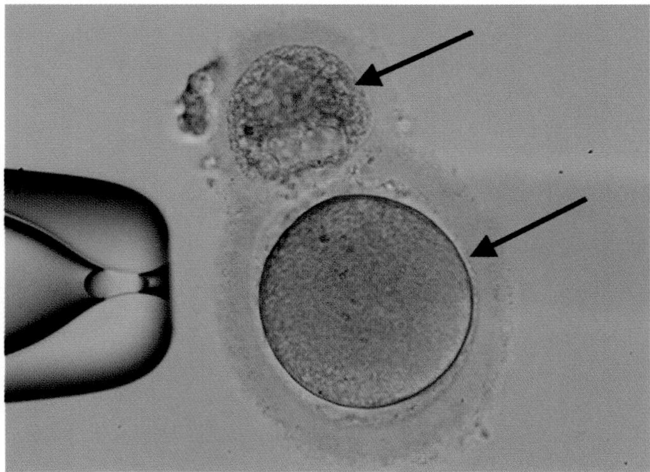

Fig. 16 Two oocytes in one single zona

Appendix

Preparation for Ovum Pick-up (Day 1)

- The center well dish (for collecting oocytes after OPU), the four-well dish (for culturing the embryos) and the adequate number of 60 mm Petri dish (for scanning the follicular fluid containing OCCs) are put in the laminar flow for off gassing of the volatile organic compounds (VOCs) for at least 24 hours.
- The 60 mm Petri dishes are kept for pre-warming at 37°C for at least 1 hour prior to the OPU so that the OCCs within the follicular fluid are not subjected to temperature shock.
- All the dish bases are pre-labeled with the patient's unique identification number and full name along with the specifications of the medium that each well contains.
- The center well dish is prepared with the oocyte wash medium, overlaid with a thin layer of culture oil and kept for gassing in the pre-mixed gaseous (5% O_2, 6% CO_2, balance nitrogen) incubator.
- The culture dishes are also prepared according to the number of oocytes expected to be retrieved and depending upon whether the oocytes will be further inseminated by IVF or ICSI.
- Little amount of extra medium of each kind is kept in the CO_2 incubator for gassing which may be required in subsequent days of oocyte-embryo culture.
- Checking and noting down the expiry of each medium is done. Care is taken not to use the medium kept in the CO_2 incubator for more than 7 days as the proteins in the medium degenerate to ammonium deteriorating the quality of the oocytes and embryos.

    *All the dishes prepared prior to the OPU day contain bicarbonate buffer for maintaining stable pH and are overlaid with culture oil to prevent evaporation and thereby maintain osmolarity of the medium.

Preparation for Ovum Pick-up (Day 0)

- The microscope stages are heated to 37°C.
- The follicular flush buffer containing 2 µ/mL heparin to prevent coagulation in blood stained aspirates and HEPES [4-(2-hydroxy-ethyl)-1-piperazineethanesulphonic acid] buffer to maintain pH is used during aspiration. This buffer is devoid of human serum albumin; it results in bubbling thereby causing fluctuations in the pH and therefore its usage in the flush media should be avoided. This buffer is pre-warmed to 37°C for 1–2 hours before OPU.
- The sterile test tubes are pre-warmed to 37°C for at least 1 hour before OPU.
- The syringes for dissecting the blood clot if any attached to the cumulus are kept ready.
- A sterile tip for picking up the OCCs is attached to the pipette.
- A container to discard the scanned follicular fluid is kept handy.

- Extra tissue papers to wipe off any spillage are also kept in handy.
- The identification of the patient and the respective dish are noted on the relevant documents.
- The informed consent forms with couples' signatures are verified.
- Room temperature is adjusted to around 25°C.
- Room lighting is kept to a minimal level.
- The follicular fluid aspirated in pre-warmed tubes is poured into the pre-warmed 60 mm Petri dish and scanned for presence of OCCs under stereo-zoom microscope with heated stage.
- The OCCs are picked up by the sterile tip and transferred to the outer well of the center well dish. This process continues till all the OCCs aspirated are collected.
- The remainder follicular fluid is discarded.
- Each OCC is washed several times to wash off the flush buffer as HEPES within the flush buffer is known to irreversibly alter the ionic channels and therefore is known to be embryotoxic. The OCCs are cleaned of any blood clots and finally collected in the inner well of the center well dish and transferred immediately in the incubator supplied with pre-mixed calibrated gaseous mixture and adjusted to 37°C for 3–4 hours till insemination in case of IVF or denudation in case of ICSI. In this period, the oocytes attain cytoplasmic maturation.
- The temperature is maintained to 37°C at each step as the meiotic spindles of the oocytes are extremely sensitive to the temperature.
- The semen either from the partner or from the donor as the case maybe, is processed and the post wash analysis of the sample is noted.

Preparation of Oocytes for In Vitro Fertilization (Day 0)

- The oocytes are then transferred to the four-well dish. Care is taken to place maximum of six oocytes per well.
- The concentration of the sperm suspension is adjusted to get 80,000–100,000 sperms per oocyte.
- The calculated number of sperms are released around the oocytes and the dish is either kept for short incubation (for 6 hours) or for long incubation (for 18–20 hours) to achieve fertilization.

Preparation of Oocytes for Intracytoplasmic Sperm Injection (Day 0)

- The OCCs are subjected to enzymatic and mechanical processing for denudation. The enzymatic processing includes exposure of OCCs to hyaluronidase enzyme (80 IU) for less than a minute; while the mechanical process involves serial washing of the oocytes (at least 2–3 washes) with 170 µ and finally 140 µ pipettes for complete denudation.
- Denudation facilitates better visualization and manipulation of the oocytes during ICSI.

- Culturing of the denuded oocytes for one hour before manipulation is advisable.
- ICSI dish is prepared around eight drops of oocyte wash medium (3–5 µL droplets each) with the central drop of 10% PVP (Polyvinylpyrrolidone). The drops are overlaid with pre-equilibrated culture oil and the dish is kept at 37°C for 1 hour.
- Alignment of the holding and the injection pipettes, loading and selection of normal sperms, assessment of each oocyte is followed by injection of all mature oocytes which are then cultured further for 16–18 hours, at which point these injected oocytes undergo fertilization check.

◼ CONCLUSION

Oocytes are one of the most important entities in any ART program as they hold key factors for normal development of the embryo. Their limited number, sensitivity to the temperature fluctuations as well as the adverse effects on their morphology correlating to the advanced maternal age has made their culture a challenging aspect to embryologists all over the world. ART clinics are constantly striving for better understanding of the molecular events during folliculogenesis, ovulation and fertilization in order to achieve optimal fertilization rates. Still due to the involvement of many factors working intricately to facilitate growth of a mature egg, the goal seems to be far-fetched. Developments in the culture media, QC procedures implemented in the ART clinics, continues assessment of the fertilization, cleavage and implantation rates of a given laboratory, together contribute to improve the success rate of the ART clinic.

◼ REFERENCES

1. Dean J. Biology of mammalian fertilization: role of the zona pellucida. J Clin Invest. 1992;89(4):1055-9.
2. Bungum M, Bungum L, Humaidan P, et al. A prospective study, using sibling oocytes, examining the effect of 30 seconds versus 90 minutes gamete co-incubation in IVF. Hum Reprod. 2006;21(2):518-23.
3. Sun QY. Cellular and molecular mechanisms leading to cortical reaction and polyspermy block in mammalian eggs. Microsc Res Tech. 2003;61(4):342-8.
4. Shen Y, Stalf T, Mehnert C, et al. High magnitude of light retardation by the zona pellucida is associated with conception cycles. Hum Reprod. 2005;20(6):1596-606.
5. Paz G, Amit A, Yavetz H. Case report: pregnancy outcome following ICSI of oocytes with abnormal cytoplasm and zona pellucida. Hum Reprod. 2004;19(3):586-9.
6. Bertrand M, Van der Bergh M, Englert Y. Does zona pellucida thickness influence the fertilization rate? Hum Reprod. 1995;10(5):1189-93.
7. Dirnfeld M, Shiloh H, Bider D, et al. A prospective randomized controlled study of the effect of short coincubation of gametes during insemination on zona pellucida thickness. Gynecol Endocrinol. 2003;17(5):397-403.
8. Gabrielsen A, Lindenberg S, Petersen K, et al. The impact of the zona pellucida thickness variation of human embryos in pregnancy outcome in relation to suboptimal embryo development. A prospective randomized controlled study. Hum Reprod. 2001;16(10):2166-70.
9. Gabrielsen A, Bhatnager PR, Petersen K, et al. Influence of zona pellucida thickness of human embryos on clinical pregnancy outcome following in vitro fertilization treatment. J Assist Reprod Genet. 2000;17(6):323-8.
10. Hseuh AJ, Billig H, Tsafriri A. Ovarian follicle atresia: a hormonally controlled apoptotic process. Endocrine Rev. 1994;15(6):707-24.
11. Hirshfield AN. Development of follicles in the mammalian ovary. Int Rev Cytol. 1991;124:43-101.
12. Zhang K, Pollack S, Ghods A, et al. Onset of ovulation after menarche in girls: a longitudinal study. J Clin Endocrinol Metab. 2008;93(4):1186-94.
13. Albuz FK, Sasseville M, Lane M, et al. Simulated physiological oocyte maturation (SPOM): a novel in vitro maturation system that substantially improves embryo yield and pregnancy outcomes. Hum Reprod. 2010;25(12):2099-3011.
14. Cha KY, Han SY, Chung HM, et al. Pregnancies and deliveries after in vitro maturation culture followed by in vitro fertilization and embryo transfer without stimulation in women with polycystic ovary syndrome. Fertil Steril. 2000;73(5):978-83.
15. Fadini R, Mignini Renzini M, Guarnieri T, et al. Comparison of the obstetric and perinatal outcomes of children conceived from in vitro or in vivo matured oocytes in in vitro maturation treatments with births from conventional ICSI cycles. Hum Reprod. 2012;27(12):3601-8.
16. Ebner T, Shebl O, Moser M, et al. Developmental fate of ovoid oocytes. Hum Reprod. 2008;23(1):62-6.
17. Balaban B, Urman B, et al, Comparison of the obstetric and perinatal outcomes of children conceived from in vitro or in vivo matured oocytes in in vitro maturation treatments with births from conventional ICSI cycles, Human Reproduction, 1998; 13(12):3431-3.
18. Esfandiari N, Ryan EA, Gotlieb L, et al. Successful pregnancy following transfer of embryos from oocytes with abnormal zona pellucida and cytoplasm morphology. Reprod Biomed Online. 2005;11(5):620-3.
19. Ebner T, Moser M, Tews G. Is oocyte morphology prognostic of embryo developmental potential after ICSI? Reprod Biomed Online. 2006;12(4):507-12.
20. Balaban B, Urman B. Effect of oocyte morphology on embryo development and implantation. Reprod Biomed Online. 2006;12(5):608-15.
21. Ebner T, Yaman C, Moser M, et al. Prognostic value of first polar body morphology on fertilization rate and embryo quality in intracytoplasmic sperm injection. Hum Reprod. 2000;15(2):427-30.
22. Ebner T, Moser M, Sommergruber M, et al. First polar body morphology and blastocyst formation rate in ICSI patients. Hum Reprod. 2002;17(9):2415-8.

23. Kuliev A, Cieslak J, Verlinsky Y. Frequency and distribution of chromosome abnormalities in human oocytes. Cytogenet Genome Res. 2005;111(3-4):193-8.

24. Ebner T, Moser M, Yaman C, et al. Elective transfer of embryos selected on the basis of first polar body morphology is associated with increased rates of implantation and pregnancy. Fertil Steril. 1999;72(4):599-603.

25. Wang Q, Sun Q. Evaluation of oocyte quality: morphological, cellular and molecular predictors. Reprod Fertil Devel. 2006;19(1):1-12.

26. Wallbutton S, Kasraie J. Vacuolated oocytes: fertilization and embryonic arrest following intra-cytoplasmic sperm injection in a patient exhibiting persistent oocyte macro vacuolization—Case report. J Assist Reprod Genet. 2010;27(4):183-8.

27. Franco Jr JG, Baruffi RL, Mauri AL, et al. Significance of large nuclear vacuoles in human spermatozoa: implications for ICSI. Reprod Biomed Online. 2008;17(1):42-5.

28. Palermo GD, Takeuchi T, Rosenwaks Z, et al. Technical approaches to correction of oocyte aneuploidy. Hum Reprod. 2002;17(8):2165-73.

29. Djalali M, Rosenbusch B, Wolf M, et al. Cytogenetics of unfertilized human oocytes. J Reprod Fertil. 1988;84(2): 647-52.

30. Vialard F, Lombroso R, Bergere M, et al. Oocyte aneuploidy mechanisms are different in two situations of increased chromosomal risk: older patients and patients with recurrent implantation failure after in vitro fertilization. Fertil Steril. 2007;87(6):1333-9.

22 Semen Analysis and Evaluation of Sperm

Daniel Franken

■ SEMEN ANALYSIS

Despite controversy regarding the clinical value of semen analysis, male fertility investigation still relies on a standardized analysis of the semen parameters. This is especially true for infertility clinics in both developing and developed countries. The new World Health Organization (WHO, 2010) manual for the examination and processing of human semen is a great improvement on the previous editions. The most important change in the manual is the use of evidence-based publications as references to determine cut-off values for normality. Apart from these changes, the initial evaluation and handling methods remain in most instances the same as in the fourth edition of the manual, i.e. sample collection, initial macroscopic examination and initial microscopic investigation.

The Wet Preparation

The initial step in the investigation of human semen focuses on the wet preparation, which provides preliminary information on the sperm concentration, motility and general appearance of the sample. The preparation is made with undiluted semen from a specific semen volume and cover slip area. The wet preparation is used to determine the dilution of semen required to allow accurate measurement of the sperm concentration. For example, 6 μL of well-mixed semen is placed on a clean microscope slide and covered with a cover slip (18 mm × 18 mm). This gives the preparation a depth of about 20 μm. Examination of this wet preparation should begin as soon as the "flow" in the preparation has ceased.

The wet preparation also allows insight into the following.

Azoospermia and Severe Oligozoospermia

If there are no or only very few spermatozoa in the wet preparation it should be noted in the sample record form. If no motile spermatozoa or only a few spermatozoa were found in the wet preparation, the sample should be centrifuged (WHO, 2010), and the pellet examined under the microscope (40x objective, phase contrast optics).

- *Sperm motility* is the first aspect of sperm function that should be assessed immediately to avoid temperature interference or dehydration.
- Sperm aggression and agglutination
- Presence of other cells and debris
- *No debris* is a very unusual situation, some debris is typical, but moderate contamination with debris is not necessarily abnormal.
- *Red blood cells* (erythrocytes) should not be found in semen, although a few can be present without indicating pathology.
- *Epithelial cells* (squamous, cubic and transitional) are usual in semen in low numbers. Increased presence is not related to any specific functional impairment or presence of infection.
- *Round cells* are often seen in semen, and it is important that leukocytes are differentiated from immature gametes or large cell bodies (usually without nucleus) with cytoplasm exfoliated from the seminiferous epithelium of the testis. Also cells of prostatic origin appear round in the ejaculate. If there are more than one million round cells/mL, counted in the Neubauer chamber (at the same time as sperm concentration is determined), a special method for detection of leukocytes should be used to determine the presence of "inflammatory cells".
- *Bacteria and protozoa* are usually not present in semen.

Sperm Concentration

The wet preparation is used to estimate the concentration, and select the most appropriate dilution. It is recommended to use 6 μL semen covered with an 18 mm × 18 mm cover slip. Duplicate wet preparations are prepared to ensure reliable and accurate sperm concentrations.

Neubauer counting procedures are often thought to be time consuming, especially in a busy andrology unit. In these cases, the less accurate Makler sperm counting chamber is recommended. The choice of the counting chamber is solely dependent on the reason why a sperm count is needed. In cases where research studies depend on accurate counts the Neubauer counting chamber is recommended.

The correct volume of semen is well mixed with the corresponding diluent volume and loaded into the chamber of the improved Neubauer counting chamber. The sperm concentration (10^6 per mL semen) is calculated by dividing the number of spermatozoa counted in the counting chambers, with a factor depending on the dilution and the number of squares counted. The total sperm number (10^6 per ejaculate) is the product of ejaculate volume and sperm concentration. It is important to remember that counting is done until 200 sperm are recorded. For example; for 1 + 4 (1:5) dilutions, using grids 4, 5 and 6, the concentration $C = (N/n) \times (1/20) \times 5$ spermatozoa per nL = $(N/n) \times (1/4)$ spermatozoa/nL (or 10^6 per mL of semen). That is where N = number of sperm counted, and n = number of rows counted.

The lower reference limit for sperm concentration is 15×10^6 spermatozoa per mL (5th centile, 95% CI 12–16 $\times 10^6$).[1]

Sperm Motility

A major change from previous editions is in the categorization of sperm motility. It is now recommended that spermatozoa should be categorized as:

- *Progressive motility (PR):* Spermatozoa moving actively, either linearly or in a large circle, regardless of speed.
- *Non-progressive motility (NP):* All other patterns of motility with an absence of progression, e.g. swimming in small circles, the flagellar force hardly displacing the head, or when only a flagellar beat can be observed.
- *Immotile (IM):* No movement.

These new values of assessment replaces the previous grades, i.e. a, b, c or d.

Sperm motility within semen should be assessed as soon as possible after liquefaction of the sample, preferably at 30 minutes, but in any case within 1 hour, following ejaculation, to limit the deleterious effects of dehydration, pH or changes in temperature on motility. The procedure may be performed at room temperature or at 37°C with a heated microscope stage, but should be standardized for each laboratory. The lower reference limit for total motility (PR + NP) is 40% (5th centile, 95% CI 38–42). The lower reference limit for PR is 32% (5th centile, 95% CI 31–34).[1]

Sperm Vitality

Vitality testing assesses the membrane integrity of spermatozoa and is indicated in cases for samples that with less than 40% progressive motile spermatozoa. The test methodology is simple and entails a one-step procedure using a eosin-nigrosin staining technique.[2] This test can provide a check on the motility evaluation, since the percentage of dead cells should not exceed (within sampling error) the percentage of immotile spermatozoa. The percentage of viable cells normally exceeds that of motile cells. Vitality should be recorded as soon as possible after liquefaction of the semen sample to prevent observation of deleterious effects of dehydration or of changes in temperature on vitality.[1]

The lower reference limit for vitality (membrane-intact spermatozoa) is 58% (5th centile, 95% CI 55–63).[1]

Sperm Morphology

Sperm morphology is regarded as possibly the most consistent sperm variable that appears to be related to in vitro fertilization (IVF) success. This observation has therefore a very important clinical and diagnostic role to play in the structured management of infertile couples. However, the value of sperm morphology as predictor of a man's fertilizing potential has often been challenged due to different classification systems. Several factors are responsible for this technical variation including differences in the methods used to prepare and stain specimens, differences in proficiency among technicians and inherent differences in classification criteria and methods.[3,4] By the strict application of certain criteria of sperm morphology, relationships between the percentage of normal forms and various fertility endpoints (time-to-pregnancy), pregnancy rates in vivo and in vitro have been established,[3,4] which may be useful for the prognosis of fertility.[1] Observations on spermatozoa recovered from the female reproductive tract, especially in postcoital endocervical mucus[5] and also from the surface of the zona pellucida[6,7] have helped to define the appearance of potentially fertilizing (morphologically normal) spermatozoa. Previous studies have indicated that training courses assist laboratory technicians to maintain the technical skills obtained during hands-on training sessions.

■ EVALUATION OF SPERM AND SPERM FUNCTION

Sperm Zona Pellucida Binding

Sperm zona pellucida binding assays currently used include the hemizona assay (HZA),[8] and a competitive intact zona pellucida-binding test.[9] Both bioassays have the advantage of providing an internally controlled homologous test for sperm binding to the zona pellucida, comparing populations of fertile and infertile spermatozoa in the same assay.

A unique feature of the human zona pellucida is its sperm selection capacity for morphologic normal sperm.[4] This phenomenon opens a possible sperm selection technique for intracytoplasmic sperm injection (ICSI) therapy, since sperm binding to human zona pellucida is highly selective for double-stranded DNA. Sperm with single stranded or denatured DNA bind less or do not bind at all to the zona pellucida, probably because of defects of motility and, more especially, morphology. In a previous study,[9] the percentage of sperm with double-stranded DNA was correlated with the percentage normal sperm in semen as well as after preparation. Furthermore, the proportion of double-stranded DNA sperm is significantly higher in motile sperm following preparation compared to ejaculated sperm. Thus, during fertilization under IVF or in vivo conditions, sperm with abnormal DNA will have much lower chance of binding or penetrating the zona pellucida of oocytes since most of them will be excluded by the sperm-zona pellucida binding process.[7] Moreover, the proportion of zona pellucida-bound spermatozoa with normal DNA is on average more than 90%, and very few sperm with abnormal DNA were found to bind the zona pellucida even in men with high percentage of DNA damaged sperm in semen.

It is well documented that these assays provide important evidence on the recognition event leading to fertilization.[10] The HZA has been introduced as a diagnostic test for the binding of human spermatozoa to the human zona pellucida to predict sperm fertilization potential under in vitro conditions.[10] The assay predicts pregnancy in the IVF/intrauterine insemination (IUI) setting with high sensitivity and negative predictive value in couples with male infertility.

Overall, patients with an HZI of less 30% had a significantly lower pregnancy rate compared to patients with an HZI of more than 30% [11.1% versus 40.6% respectively; p <0.05; relative risk for failure to conceive: 1.5 (confidence interval 1.2–1.9)]. The HZA is not routinely used in the clinical setting, but provides useful information especially during counseling couples before allocating them into IUI or IVF therapy.[8]

Acrosome Reaction

In clinical assisted reproductive programs, assessment of patients to be treated by either standard IVF or ICSI is mostly decided on the semen analysis results. Patients with normal semen analysis usually undergo standard IVF, and those with moderately to severely abnormal semen usually undergo ICSI. However, some patients with unexplained infertility with normal semen analysis may have subtle sperm defects that cannot be predicted by standard semen analysis.[11,12] Cases have been identified with normal semen parameters, including normal morphology, with impaired acrosomal response to the zona pellucida.[11,12]

In a previous study, we reported on 20 cases that were categorized according to the male's poor response to the zona induced acrosome reaction (ZIAR), i.e. men showing poor ZIAR results namely ZIAR less than 15% acrosome reacted sperm after exposure to zona pellucida. These men were then prospectively randomized to have their sibling oocytes inseminated with standard IVF or ICSI during the diagnostic cycle. One hundred eighty-two metaphase II oocytes were aspirated from 11 of the 20 cases. On the day of the aspiration, retrieved oocytes were randomly and, in most cases, equally divided and then treated by standard IVF procedure (n = 84) and ICSI (n = 98) in the same cycle. The fertilization results of the diagnostic cycle of metaphase II oocytes for IVF and ICSI were 4% and 68% respectively (p ≤0.001). Failed fertilization can be the consequence of oocyte anomalies (intrinsic or ovarian stimulation-derived), sperm defects (in quality and/or quantity) and/or technical factors.[11]

DNA Integrity

Fragmented sperm DNA can have severe consequences for couples undergoing assisted reproduction therapy, since spermatozoa with impaired DNA are capable of fertilizing oocytes.[13] Depending on the amount of DNA damage, embryo development can be affected and thus result in embryonic death.[14,15] Consequently, embryos formed with damaged DNA can also develop to full term. Therefore, fertilization of oocytes by ICSI may have far-reaching consequences for the offspring if the impairment is transferred to the germ line.

In recent years, to understand the fertilization process better and to improve fertility diagnostics, scientists and clinicians have become interested in apoptosis and DNA integrity.[16] Apoptosis is the controlled disassembly of cells from within and is characterized by changes in the phospholipid content of the plasma membrane outer leaflet.[17] One has to distinguish between physiological and nonphysiological apoptosis. The physiological cell death refers to apoptosis that is a planned and programmed event of which DNA fragmentation is one of the last steps. Contrary, nonphysiological cell death cannot be named apoptosis as it is not programmed and planned by the cell; it is due to other external events. Yet, one of the features is also DNA fragmentation. However, in order to trigger this DNA fragmentation, the apoptotic pathway by activating pro-apoptotic factors, such as Bax or Bak, and the downregulation of anti-apoptotic factors, such as Bcl-2, is not executed. Therefore, there exists a clear distinction between apoptosis and necrosis. During apoptosis, the cell shrinks due to dehydration, in necrotic cases the cells and mitochondria are swelling and the plasma membrane is disintegrating. DNA fragmentation appears in both processes. Sakkas et al.[17] reported a high percentage of fragmented sperm DNA linked to a high expression of apoptosis markers in semen samples with low spermatozoa concentration and high percentage of abnormal sperm (Henkel personal communications). The origin of DNA fragmentation is possibly caused by oxidative stress,[18,19] abortive apoptosis,[20] improper DNA packaging and ligation,[21] chemotherapy and radio-therapy,[22] environmental and occupational toxicants.[23]

A clear distinction should be made between apoptotic DNA fragmentation, and DNA fragmentation caused by ROS produced either by leukocytes or by the sperm cells.[24] The non-apoptotic sperm has a positive and significant correlation with the fertilization outcome. On the other hand, the impact of apoptosis as determined by clear apoptotic markers on sperm fertilizing capacity was described by previous studies as rather low. Infertile men with moderate and severe teratozoospermia, the spermatozoa with apparently normal morphology present in the motile fractions after swim-up technique may have DNA fragmentation.[25] The DNA fragmentation of morphologically normal sperm negatively impacts embryo quality, and probability of pregnancy in ICSI cycles.

Increased sperm DNA damage is enhanced among infertile compared with fertile men and with poor semen quality. Damage DNA sperm are closely related with sperm head abnormalities, possibly due to incomplete sperm chromatin condensation. Furthermore, motility and morphology were negatively related to DNA fragmentation index. Moreover, the grade of DNA damage increases with the number of abnormal parameters, i.e. concentration, motility, and normal morphology in a sample, and is most severe in patients with oligoasthenoteratozoospermia. Sperm DNA damage was correlated with IVF and ICSI outcome during a meta-analysis; the pooled results of IVF outcomes indicated that the clinical pregnancy rate, but not the fertilization rate decreased significantly for patients with high degree of sperm DNA damage compared with those with low degree of sperm DNA damage. Henkel et al.,[25] concluded that DNA fragmentation, as determined by the TUNEL (terminal deoxynucleotidyl transferase dUTP nick-end labeling) assay, is predictive for pregnancy in IVF. This implies that spermatozoa with DNA fragmentation can still fertilize an oocyte, but that when paternal genes are activated further embryonic development is discontinued, resulting in failed pregnancy.[25]

Perspectives

The role and contribution of sperm morphology in the diagnosis of the male infertility must be regarded as a first step to get valuable clinical information for the consulting clinician or scientist. It is well accepted that while basic semen analysis will stay as the cornerstone of the male investigation and most likely in WHO (2010) format, careful training and continuous quality control are of great importance to get reliable reports. The basic semen analysis should be complemented with sperm functional tests to give more information on the pathophysiology of spermatozoa. These tests could include the robust standardized methods, systems for training staff and ongoing quality control; and rigorous examination of the clinical outcomes. As of today the basic semen analysis should be regarded as the first level of the diagnostic approach. Emphasis should be on the quality of the sperm morphology reports since it plays a vital role in the forthcoming therapy. The andrological investigation should also be included as second level of approach, i.e. sperm functional tests that include genetic evaluation. For example, the ICSI setting provides a unique arena to evaluate sperm dysfunctions at a cellular and molecular level. Furthermore, the future of semen analysis will focus on the application and advanced methodologies, such as microarrays (to analyze the transcriptome of sperm), proteomics (identify specific biomarkers), glycomics, and metabolomics (analyses of breakdown components released in vivo or in vitro).

■ REFERENCES

1. World Health Organization. WHO laboratory manual for the processing of human semen, 5th ed. Geneva: World Health Organization; 2010.
2. Björndahl L, Soderlund I, Kvist U. Evaluation of the one-step eosin-nigrosin staining technique for human sperm vitality assessment. Hum Reprod. 2003;18:813-6.
3. Eggert-Kruse W, Reimann-Anderson J, Rohr G, et al. Clinical relevance of sperm morphology assessment using strict criteria and relationship with sperm-mucus interaction in vivo and in vitro. Fertil Steril. 1995;63:612-24.
4. Kruger TF, Menkveld R, Stander FS, et al. Sperm morphologic features as a prognostic factor in in vitro fertilization. Fertil Steril. 1986;46:1118-23.

5. Menkveld R, Stander FS, Kotze TJ, et al. The evaluation of morphological characteristics of human spermatozoa according to stricter criteria. Hum Reprod. 1990;5:586-92.

6. Liu DY, Baker HG. Morphology of spermatozoa bound to the zona pellucida of human oocytes that failed to fertilize in vitro. J Reprod Fertil. 1992;94:71-84.

7. Menkveld R, Franken DR, Kruger TF, et al. Sperm selection capacity of the human zona pellucida. Mol Reprod Dev. 1990;30:346-52.

8. Burkman LJ, Coddington CC, Franken DR, et al. The hemizona assay (HZA): development of a diagnostic test for the binding of human spermatozoa to human hemizona pellucida to predict fertilization potential. Fertil Steril. 1988;49:688-97.

9. Liu DY, Baker HG. Human sperm bound to the zona pellucida have normal nuclear chromatin as assessed by acridine orange fluorescence. Hum Reprod. 2007;22:1597-602.

10. Franken DR, Burkman LJ, Oehninger SC, et al. The hemizona assay using salt stored human oocytes: evaluation of zona pellucida capacity for binding human spermatozoa. Gamete Res. 1989;22:15-26.

11. Franken DR, Esterhuizen A, Oehninger SC. Diagnostic impact of the zona pellucida induced acrosome reaction in an assisted reproductive programme. Embryo Talk. 2007;2:3-9.

12. Liu DY, Baker HG. Disordered zona pellucida-induced acrosome reaction and failure of in vitro fertilization in patients with unexplained infertility. Fertil Steril. 2003;79:74-80.

13. Henkel R, Hajimohammad M, Stalf T, et al. Influence of deoxyribonucleic acid damage on fertilization and pregnancy. Fertil Steril. 2004;81:965-72.

14. Qiu J, Hales BF, Robaire B. Damage to rat spermatozoal DNA after chronic cyclophosphamide exposure. Biol Reprod. 1995;53:1465-73.

15. Seli E, Gardner DK, Schoolcraft WB, et al. Extent of nuclear DNA damage in ejaculated spermatozoa impacts on blastocyst development after in vitro fertilization. Fertil Steril. 2004;82:378-83.

16. Sakkas D, Moffatt O, Manicardi GC, et al. Nature of DNA damage in ejaculated human spermatozoa and the possible involvement of apoptosis. Biol Reprod. 2002;66:1061-7.

17. Henkel R, Franken DR. DNA Fragmentation: Its impact on human reproduction. J Reprod Stem Cell Biotechnol. 2001;2:88-108.

18. Agarwal A, Saleh RA. Role of oxidants in male infertility: rational, significance and treatment. Urol Clin N Am. 2002;29:817-27.

19. Henkel R, Kierspel E, Hajimohammad M, et al. DNA fragmentation of spermatozoa and ART. Reprod Biomed Online. 2003;7:477-84.

20. Rodriguez I, Ody C, Araki K, et al. An early and massive wave of germinal cell apoptosis is required for the development of functional spermatogenesis. EMBO J. 1997;16:2262-70.

21. McPherson SM, Longo FJ. Localization of DNAse I-hypersensitive regions during rat spermatogenesis: stage dependent patterns and unique sensitivity of elongating spermatids. Mol Reprod Dev. 1992;31:268-79.

22. Chatterjee R, Haines GA, Perera DMD, et al. Testicular and sperm DNA damage after treatment with fludarabine for chronic lymphocytic leukaemia. Hum Reprod. 2000;15:762-6.

23. Meeker JD, Barr DB, Hauser R. Human semen quality and sperm DNA damage in relation to urinary metabolites of pyrethroid insecticides. Hum Reprod. 2008;23:1932-40.

24. Henkel R, Hajimohammad M, Stalf T, et al. Influence of deoxyribonucleic acid damage on fertilization and pregnancy Fertil Steril. 2004;81:965-72.

25. Kasimanickam R, Pelzer KD, Kasimanickam V, et al. Association of classical semen parameters, sperm DNA fragmentation index, lipid peroxidation and antioxidant enzymatic activity of semen in ram-lambs. Theriogenology. 2006;65:1407-21.

23 Semen Collection and Preparation

Ashok Agarwal, Sejal Doshi

INTRODUCTION

Assisted reproductive technologies (ARTs) have been of great benefit to subfertile couples worldwide. Initially, such techniques solely targeted gynecologic causes of infertility. However, with increased understanding of the physiologic role spermatozoa play in zygote formation and embryo development, there has been a greater focus on andrological indications for infertility.[1-3] As a result, there has been a tremendous need to improve the current sperm processing and preparation methods used in ART.[2,4]

Ideally, such methods should be able to process large volumes of ejaculate to recover the maximum number of motile sperm. However, this should be performed in a manner that is gentle enough to prevent free radical formation and allow sperm to retain their function.[1,3,5] Furthermore, sperm processing techniques must be able to separate sperm from other components in the seminal plasma, which include epithelial cells, leukocytes, and bacterial contaminants.[1,6,7] Specifically, the World Health Organization recommends separating spermatozoa from the seminal plasma within one hour after ejaculation to prevent sperm damage from other cells in the semen.[8] Effective separation and timely collection of highly motile and functional sperm ensures that the offspring will carry the highest quality of genetic material provided by the male gamete.[9]

As of yet, no single method has been definitively proven to be more efficacious over another and thus, a wide variety of techniques are employed to obtain an optimal yield of functionally competent spermatozoa for ART.[3] First, though, a semen sample must be collected from the male partner in a manner that maximizes the quality and integrity of the sperm.

SEMEN COLLECTION

Ejaculated semen is preferably collected via masturbation after 2–4 days of sexual abstinence into a sterile, wide-mouthed container, which helps to minimize the risk of subsequent uterine infections.[2,6,10] Ejaculation contains two important components: semen emission and expulsion. Problems with either or both of these vital functions will affect sperm quantity and quality, requiring a change in the sperm collection method.[11] In that case, other methods of collection can be used such as spermicidal free condoms and electroejaculation. However, the latter form of collection is invasive and only used in some paraplegic patients with a spinal cord injury.[12]

Once collected from the patient, the sample is processed within 30–60 minutes after collection, liquefied, and mixed well. A drop of the sample is immediately placed on a clean, pre-warmed glass slide at 37°C with a cover slip.[2,13] Next, a macroscopic evaluation is completed in which the color, pH, and viscosity of the sample are reported. A microscopic examination is also conducted, which includes measuring the concentration, motility and morphology. The microscopic values are compared with those obtained after sperm preparation. Due to the time-sensitive nature of these measurements, it is crucial for the lab technologist to note when the semen sample was collected, delivered to the laboratory, and analyzed.[13]

Instructions to the Patient for Sperm Collection: Cleveland Clinic Protocol

- Patients are asked to refrain from sexual intercourse, masturbation, or any form of emission for at least 2–4 days prior to collection.
- A clean, sterile plastic specimen container is labeled with the patient's name, hospital number, date, and time of collection. It is placed into a specimen collection bag that is given to the patient before he enters the collection room. Non-sterile containers are not used because they may interfere with sperm activity and lead to inaccurate results.
- Patients are advised to refrain from using lubricants such as K-Y Jelly or Vaseline during collection because they can affect semen quality.

- The sample is collected by masturbation and ejaculated directly into the specimen container. The entire specimen is submitted because the first few drops of ejaculate contain the major portion of sperm. If some of the sample is lost during collection, the technologist accepting the specimen is notified.
- If the sample is collected on site, the technologist accepting the specimen asks the patient to provide picture identification (e.g. driver's license). He/she also inquires about the time since the patient's last ejaculation and whether the sample is complete or incomplete.
- If the specimen is collected at home, patients are asked to carry the sample container near the body so that the sample remains close to body temperature and deliver it to the laboratory within one hour of collection for best results.

■ COMMONLY USED MOVEMENT-BASED TECHNIQUES

The specific method used to process a semen sample for assisted reproduction is based on the initial sperm parameters, such as motility, concentration and morphology. Two movement-based techniques—swim-up and swim-down—are typically used when the male has normal sperm concentration and motility whereas the third technique—density gradient centrifugation—is used for samples containing mainly oligospermic, asthenozoospermic and teratozoospermic spermatozoa. The latter is the technique of choice in most andrology laboratories and ART programs worldwide,[11,14] but all three techniques are known for their efficacy in retrieving highly functional and competent spermatozoa.[2,15]

Swim-up

With this procedure, a cultured medium is placed over a pre-washed cell pellet that contains the liquefied semen sample. The medium includes nutrients for sperm growth, which attract healthy spermatozoa, drawing them up into the culture medium. The upper part of the culture layer is removed and analyzed for sperm that can be used for insemination.[6,16] Specifically, the spermatozoa that are the greatest distance from the pellet are the ones retrieved for ART because they have the greatest probability of being motile and morphologically competent. The efficacy of this technique depends on the initial motility of the sperm within the ejaculate and the concentration of the pellet as too many cell layers within the pellet can inhibit the movement of spermatozoa up into the culture medium.[2,14] Throughout this sperm processing technique,

sterile supplies are used, and the entire process, ideally, is completed by a single technologist.

Swim-up technique: Cleveland Clinic Protocol **(Fig. 1)**.

Prepare reagents: Bring sperm wash media to 37°C for 20 minutes in the incubator.

Handling of Patient Sample

- After collection, label the specimen container with the patient's name, hospital number, and time of collection.
- Label 15-mL sterile centrifuge tube(s) with the patient's name, hospital number, wash media and date.
- Label a 2-mL conical beaker for post-wash analysis.
- Remove a warmed tube of sperm wash media from the 37°C incubator and label with the patient's name and corresponding color code with the labeling tape.

Note: Color-code all paperwork, tubes, media and specimen container using one color for each patient.

Analysis and Processing of Patient Sample

- Allow the specimen to liquefy completely for 15–30 minutes in the incubator at 37°C before processing.
- Measure volume using a sterile 5–10 mL pipet.
- Transfer specimen from a plastic cup to a sterile 15-mL conical centrifuge tube. If specimen is more than 3 mL, split into two tubes.
- Gently mix the specimen with sperm wash media in a ratio of 1:4 by using a sterile pasteur pipet.
- Centrifuge the tubes at 1,600 rotations per minute (RPM) for 10 minutes.
- While the specimen is in the centrifuge, perform a pre-wash semen analysis.
  Note: While examining the specimen, pay particular attention to extraneous round cells, debris, and bacteria that may be present. If round cells are more than or equal to 5 per high power field, perform the Endtz test (>10^6 WBC/mL). A positive Endtz test result should be reported to the physician.
- Carefully aspirate the supernatant without disturbing the pellet and resuspend the pellet in 3 mL of fresh sperm wash media. Transfer the resuspended sample into two 15-mL sterile round bottom tubes using plastic pipettes.
- Centrifuge the tubes at 500 RPM centrifuge for 5 minutes.
- Incubate the tubes at a 45° angle for 1 hour for swim-up in a vertical rack in a 37°C incubator.
- After the incubation period, aspirate the entire supernatant from the round bottom tube. Use a pasteur pipet, with the tip placed at the pellet surface.

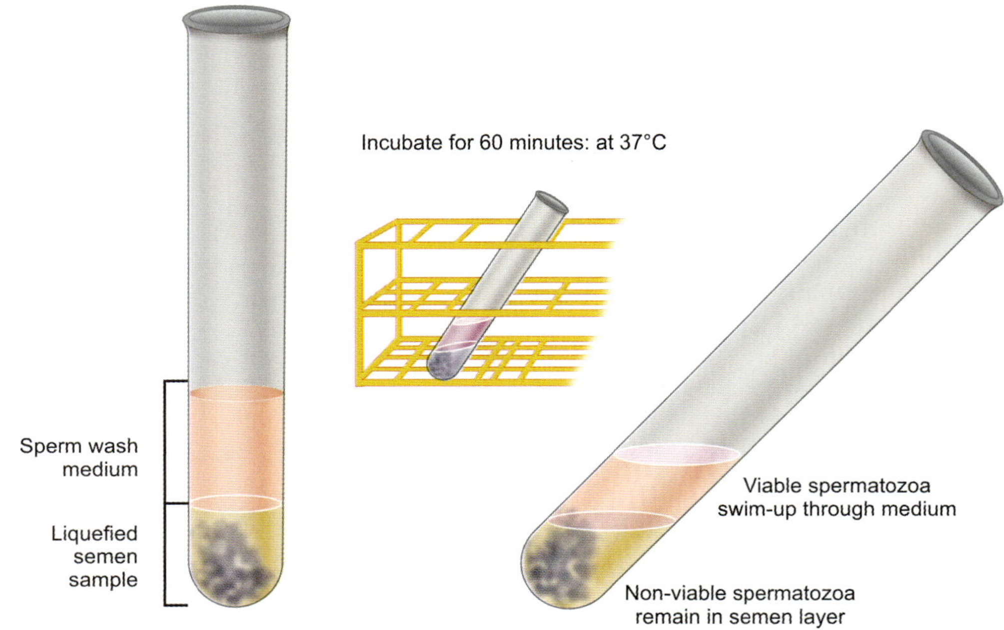

Fig. 1 Swim-up technique. During swim-up, functionally competent spermatozoa are attracted up into the culture medium. This portion of the medium is removed and analyzed for sperm that can be used for insemination. The functionally incompetent spermatozoa remain in the semen layer toward the bottom of the test tube

Source: Cleveland Clinic, Ohio, USA

- Pool supernatant from the two round bottom tubes into a single 15 mL conical centrifuge tube. Centrifuge the tube at 1,600 RPM for 7 minutes.
- Aspirate the supernatant from the top of the meniscus using a pasteur pipet.
- Resuspend the pellet in a volume of 0.5 mL sperm wash media using a 1-mL sterile pipet. Record the final volume.
- Remove a small well-mixed aliquot (~0.1 mL) and place in a labeled conical beaker for post-wash analysis.
- Place a drop of the specimen on a Microcell counting chamber to check for motile sperm cells.
- Check the pre-labeled tube containing the washed specimen to ensure it contains the patient's name and hospital number before giving it to the patient. The patient should be directed to the gynecologist for insemination.
- Perform post-wash semen analysis.

Advantages

- The swim-up technique is the simplest, quickest, and most cost-effective method for preparing sperm via migration.[2,14]
- This method allows for the retrieval of a clean fraction of highly motile sperm.[16]
- This technique also optimizes the surface area between the culture media and semen using round bottom tubes.[14]
- The use of several tubes with small volumes can also be used to further amplify the surface area and enhance the number of motile sperm recovered.[2]
- Spermatozoa after swim-up have higher DNA integrity than sperm prepared via density gradient centrifugation.[1]

Disadvantages

- If a highly concentrated pellet is used, then the motile sperm in the lower levels of the pellet are prevented from reaching the culture medium.[3,17]
- During the centrifugation steps, viable spermatozoa often come into close proximity to damaged components of the seminal plasma, leading to lipid peroxidation of the sperm plasma membrane.[14,17]
- The centrifugation steps involved in this method have been shown to produce reactive oxygen species (ROS).[3,18]

- The swim-up method is best for samples with high count and motility and is not effective for spermatozoa with abnormal semen parameters.[19]
- This technique normally yields a very low percentage of motile, morphologically competent sperm. However, this can be improved by avoiding the steps that involve washing and centrifugation.[16,18]
- Of all the spermatozoa used in the swim-up method, only 5–10% of sperm are actually recovered.[16,19]
- The swim-up technique decreases the percentage of sperm with intact chromatin because it increases the DNA fragmentation index (DFI) and leads to high DNA stainability (HDS)—a measure of immature chromatin.[1]

Swim-down Technique

In this technique, a liquefied semen sample is placed on a discontinuous bovine serum albumin medium, which becomes less concentrated from top to bottom. This pure medium has been shown to recover a higher number of spermatozoa as well as a higher percentage of sperm with forward progression than the medium used in the swim-up technique.[20] Once the sample is placed on top of the medium, the test tube is incubated at 37°C for one hour. During this time, the most motile sperm move downward into the gradient. Overall, this technique is much simpler and requires less equipment than most sperm preparation methods. However, studies have shown that the swim-down technique recovers spermatozoa with a much lower motility rate and has resulted in lower pregnancy rates after intrauterine insemination in comparison to the swim-up method.[21]

Density Gradient Centrifugation

This technique is based on the fact that morphologically normal and abnormal sperm have different densities. Specifically, a semen sample is pipetted on top of a density column and then centrifuged. At the end of centrifugation, each spermatozoon will migrate only to the position in the gradient where the density in the gradient column equals its own, and it will remain at this position.[19] Morphologically competent spermatozoa have a density of at least 1.10 g/mL where as immature, morphologically abnormal spermatozoa have a density between 1.06 g/mL and 1.09 g/mL.[22] Therefore, due to their higher density, the functionally viable spermatozoa form a pellet at the bottom of the test tube whereas the upper layers contain cellular debris, bacteria, leukocytes and abnormal spermatozoa. It is important to remove these upper layers immediately after centrifugation to prevent oxidative damage to the viable spermatozoa towards the bottom.[1,23]

Density gradients can be of two types: continuous or discontinuous. The former is the preferred method for normozoospermic samples in which the density gradually increases from top to bottom. Conversely, a discontinuous gradient—the more common type—requires layers of decreasing density to be placed on top of each other.[24] It is used when sperm counts and motility are suboptimal, which is usually the case in patients using ART. Typically, the density gradient medium of choice for this processing technique contains silane-coated silica particles because they allow for the most effective separation.[25] As with the first two movement-based techniques, sterile supplies must be used, and a single technologist ideally handles the patient specimen.

Density Gradient Centrifugation: Cleveland Clinic Protocol (Fig. 2)

Prepare reagents
- Bring all components of the density gradient medium (upper 47% and lower phase 90%) as well as semen samples to 37°C for 20 minutes in the incubator.
- Transfer 2-mL of the lower phase into a sterile conical bottom disposable centrifuge tube.
- Layer 2-mL of the upper phase on top of the lower phase using a transfer pipet. Slowly dispense the upper phase, lifting the pipet up the side of the tube as the level of upper phase rises. A distinct line separating the two layers will be observed. This two-layer gradient is stable for up to 2 hours.

Handling of patient sample
- After semen collection, check the specimen container to ensure it is labeled with the patient's name, hospital number and time of collection.
- Label 15-mL sterile centrifuge tubes with the patient's name, hospital number, wash media and date.
- Label a 2-mL conical beaker for post-wash analysis.
- Remove a warmed tube of sperm wash media from the 37°C incubator and label with the patient's name and corresponding color code with the labeling tape.

Note: Color-code all paperwork, tubes, media and specimen container using one color for each patient.

Analysis and processing of patient sample
- Allow the semen specimen to liquefy completely for 15–30 minutes in the 37°C incubator before processing.
- Measure volume using a sterile 5–10 mL pipet.
- Gently place up to 3 mL of liquefied semen onto the upper phase (leaving approx 0.1 mL in original

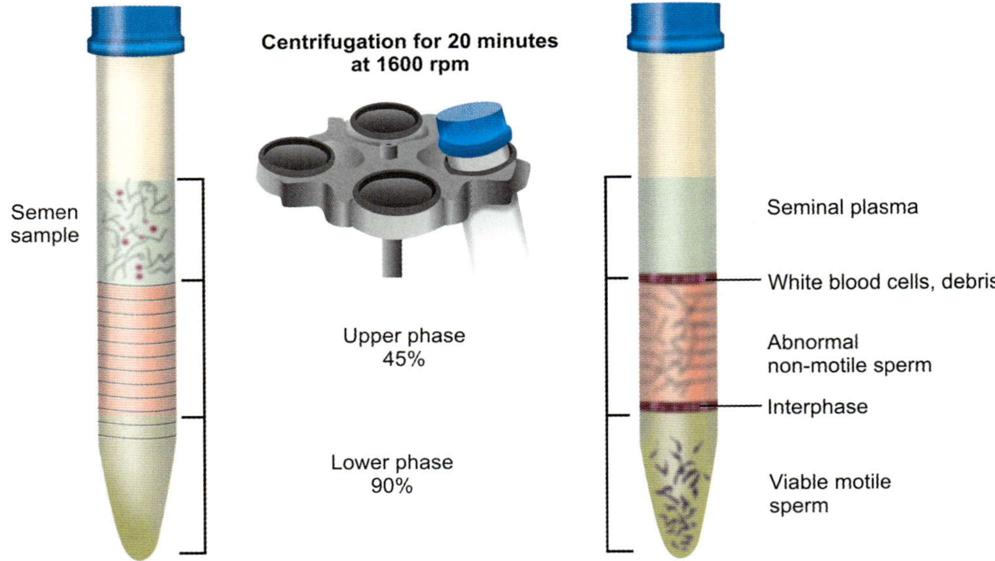

Fig. 2 Density gradient centrifugation. This figure illustrates how separation of functionally viable spermatozoa can be achieved from those that are non-viable based on their differing densities. Due to their higher density, the most viable spermatozoa form a cell pellet at the bottom. However, in comparison to these viable spermatozoa, the abnormal, non-motile sperm have a much lower density and therefore, remain higher-up in the test tube

Source: Cleveland Clinic, Ohio, USA

container for a pre-wash analysis). If volume is greater than 3 mL, it may be necessary to split the specimen into two tubes before processing.

- Centrifuge for 20 minutes at 1,600 RPM.
  Note: Occasionally, samples that do not liquefy properly remain too viscous to pass through the gradient. Increasing the centrifugal force up to but no more than 600 xg will help separate the sperm.
- While the specimen is in the centrifuge, perform pre-wash semen analysis.
  Note: While examining the specimen, pay particular attention to any extraneous round cells, debris and bacteria. If round cells are more than or equal to 5 per high power field, perform the Endtz test immediately. A positive Endtz should be reported to the physician.
- Remove the supernatant with a sterile transfer pipette to the level directly below the second layer.
- Using a transfer pipet, add 2–3 mL of sperm wash media and resuspend the pellet. Mix gently with pipet until the sperm pellet is in suspension.
- Centrifuge for 7 min at 1,600 RPM.
- Again, remove the supernatant from the centrifuge tube using a transfer pipet down to the pellet.
- Resuspend the final pellet in a volume of 0.5 mL using a 1-mL sterile pipet with sperm wash media. Record the final volume.

- Remove a small, well mixed aliquot (approximately 0.1 mL) and place it in a labeled conical beaker for a post-wash analysis.
- Place a drop of the specimen on a Microcell counting chamber to check for motile sperm cells. Check the pre-labeled tube containing the washed specimen to ensure it contains the patient's name and hospital number before giving it to the patient. The patient should be directed to the gynecologist for insemination.
- Perform post-wash semen analysis.

Advantages
- This technique allows for a higher retrieval of motile sperm in comparison to other migration techniques, such as swim-up.[16]
- It is easier to withdraw the supernatant without disturbing pellet.[14]
- With this technique, it is possible to create gradients with different densities, ensuring effective separation of spermatozoa from other cell types and debris.[19,26]
- In fresh semen samples, higher amounts of total motile sperm are retrieved after density gradient centrifugation than with swim-up.[18]
- In asthenozoospermic samples, there is a higher recovery of total motile sperm after density gradient centrifugation than after swim-up. This is significant

because most samples used in ART are from subfertile men with poor semen quality.[18]

- Cryopreserved samples prepared by the density gradient technique have increased longevity as well as a higher recovery of total motile sperm when compared to swim-up. This is especially useful in patients undergoing a vasectomy or chemotherapy who may want to cryopreserve their sperm for future use.[18,23]

Disadvantages

- Incubation of semen at room temperature or at 37°C after isolation by density gradient centrifugation may result in increased levels of sperm DNA fragmentation via apoptosis.[1,27]
- Repeated centrifugation in sperm preparation has been known to introduce iatrogenic damage within the spermatozoa and lead to the production of harmful free radicals.[1,16]
- It can take some time to produce good interphases between layers.[27]
- There is a risk of contamination with endotoxins.[16]

Conventional Sperm Preparation Techniques

Simple Wash and Resuspend

The simple wash and resuspend method is used mainly for samples with a good concentration of highly motile spermatozoa. Like the other techniques discussed thus far, the simple wash separates sperm from the seminal plasma, not only removing harmful contents from the seminal plasma but also concentrating sperm from the ejaculate.

In general, sperm washing is performed by mixing the ejaculate with an appropriate amount of protein-supplemented medium. The mixture is then centrifuged twice at 500 g, which causes spermatozoa pellets to form at the bottom of the test tube. The supernatant is aspirated, and the pellet is resuspended.

This method is not as efficacious as the swim-up technique, in recovering a high yield of functionally competent spermatozoa[28] because it is not a true separation technique—it only involves spinning and resuspending the sample in a medium. It is, however, easier *and less costly to perform*, so the decision to use it over swim-up or swim-down depends on semen parameters.

Glass Wool Filtration

In this procedure, a sperm sample is filtrated through densely compacted glass wool fibers.[29,30] Once filtration is complete, the sample is centrifuged to remove the spermatozoa from the functionally normal sperm cells. The main advantage of this technique is that it removes the majority of leukocytes, which are a major producer of ROS, from the semen sample.[15,31] Furthermore, it retrieves of a high number of total spermatozoa with good motility and can be performed directly from the ejaculated sample. However, the filtrate produced by this technique is not as clean as that produced by other sperm selection methods, since there are still remnants of cellular debris present in the sample after processing. Moreover, the raw glass wool fibers used in this method have a detrimental effect on spermatozoa in that they can induce apoptosis by disrupting the mitochondrial membrane potential and lead to caspase activation. Thus, glass wool filtration is not the method of choice in most andrology laboratories.[30]

Migration-Sedimentation

This technique is used in samples with poor motility. It utilizes the swim-up procedure but also relies on the natural downward movement of sperm due to gravity.[12] In this method, spermatozoa in Tea-Jondet test tubes swim-up from a ring-shaped well into a culture medium.[2,32] The sperm cells subsequently settle to the bottom through the central hole of the ring. The main advantage is that this form of sperm preparation is gentle and as a result, a minimal ROS are produced. Furthermore, this technique allows for a clean fraction of highly motile spermatozoa to be recovered. However, the main disadvantage is that it has a very low recovery rate and can only be used on normozoospermic samples, which is not optimal for most couples using assisted reproduction. Additionally, migration-sedimentation is quite costly due to the special test tubes that are required for the technique.[32]

Advanced Sperm Preparation Techniques

Magnetic Activated Cell Sorting

Magnetic activated cell sorting (MACS) is a preparation technique that separates spermatozoa based on their apoptotic properties. Typically during apoptosis, or programmed cell death, phosphatidylserine residues are translocated from the inner membrane to outer one of the spermatozoa. In particular, this processing technique requires a magnetic collection device, which contains superparamagnetic beads that are attracted to the antibodies of Annexin V, a cellular protein.[2,33] This protein has a strong attraction for phosphatidylserine residues located in the sperm membrane, but it cannot pass through an intact sperm membrane. Consequently, any binding of Annexin V to the spermatozoa, which in turn attracts the paramagnetic beads, signifies that the spermatozoa membrane has been compromised.[33] Furthermore, those spermatozoa that do not bind with Annexin V are associated with lower amounts of DNA damage, lower caspase activity, lower mitochondrial membrane disruption, higher motility, and higher oocyte penetration capacity.[34] Therefore, the main advantage of this technique is that it allows for separation of apoptotic spermatozoa from those that are functionally viable and non-apoptotic. Also, samples prepared by density gradient centrifugation followed by MACS recover spermatozoa have higher motility, higher viability, and lower expression of apoptotic markers. Furthermore, spermatozoa retrieved by MACS were associated with higher pregnancy rates than spermatozoa selected by density gradient centrifugation in oligoasthenozoospermic samples.[35] However, the main disadvantage is that the paramagnetic beads used in this process interfere with viability of sperm and are very difficult to detach from the spermatozoa because of their multiple connections to the sperm surface. As a result, the beads have the potential to be transmitted into the oocyte during insemination.[30,35]

Electrophoresis

This technique requires a microflow cell, which allows for the separation of mature spermatozoa from immature, dysfunctional sperm cells, leukocytes and other cell debris. In this method, functional spermatozoa pass through a polycarbonate membrane, which contain pores large enough to allow sperm cells to pass but small enough to prevent bigger cells such as leukocytes from doing so. Processing of spermatozoa via electrophoresis results in the recovery of highly motile sperm with good DNA integrity and morphology.[15] This method is also successful in isolating a higher quality of spermatozoa from testicular biopsies and cryopreserved samples. Furthermore, spermatozoa separated via electrophoresis are free of oxidative stress and undergo normal capacitation and zona pellucida binding.[2,15] However, due to the high cost of the equipment required for electrophoresis, this technique may not be the most suitable form of separation for every patient or andrology laboratory.[35]

Special Cases of Sperm Retrieval

Testicular Sperm Recovery

This technique involves the use of percutaneous needle biopsy to extract spermatozoa from the testes; it is usually performed in men with obstructive or nonobstructive azoospermia. Generally, sperm cells retrieved from the testes are used for intracytoplasmic sperm injection (ICSI)

because most spermatozoa salvaged from this location have no motility. However, the main disadvantage is that testicular sperm recovery is invasive, and sample from this location contains a variety of non-germ cells that must be separated from the functionally competent spermatozoa. Furthermore, testicular spermatozoa are often more fragile and have poorer motility than spermatozoa in ejaculated samples.[36]

Retrograde Ejaculation

In men with retrograde ejaculation, semen passes directly into the bladder instead of out through the urethra. As a result, very few spermatozoa are often in the ejaculate and hence, need to be recovered from the urine.[37] In order to obtain spermatozoa in such cases, patients are asked to urinate into a specimen cup without entirely emptying the bladder.[9] They are then asked to ejaculate and urinate again into another specimen cup containing 5–6 mL of culture medium, which allows for alkalinization of urine. After collection of urine, the sample should be prepared via density gradient centrifugation and the volume should be noted.[2,37] Overall, throughout this sperm processing technique sterile instruments must be used and handling of the patient specimen should be started and completed by a single technologist.

■ SALIENT POINTS

Overall, due to the increased use of assisted reproductive techniques to treat infertility, a variety of sperm processing techniques have become available for subfertile couples. The specific sperm preparation method should be chosen based on the initial sperm parameters of the patient, feasibility and cost to the patient. Continued research on sperm separation techniques can further enhance their safety and effectiveness, allowing for genetically robust offspring as well as improved pregnancy outcomes for ART.

■ REFERENCES

1. Jayaraman V, Upadhya D, Naryan PK, et al. Sperm processing by swim-up and density gradient is effective in elimination of sperm with DNA damage. J Assist Reprod Genet. 2012;29: 557-63.
2. Jameel T. Sperm Swim-up: a simple effective technique of semen processing for intrauterine insemination. J Pak Med Assoc. 2008;58(2):71-4.
3. Henkel RR, Schill WB. Sperm Preparation for ART. Reprod Biol Endrocinol. 2003;1:108-30.
4. Agnell NF, Mostafa HF, Rizk RMBR, et al. Intrauterine insemination. In: Rizk BRMB, Garcia-Velasco JA, Sallam HN, Makrigiannakis A (eds). Infertility and Assisted Reproduction. New York: Cambridge University Press; 2008. pp. 416-27.

5. Aitken RJ, Clarkson JS. Significance of reactive oxygen species and antioxidants in defining the efficacy of sperm preparation techniques. J Androl. 1998;9:367-76.

6. Safi J, Sharma RK, Agarwal A. Intrauterine Insemination. In: Seli E, (Ed). Infertility. Oxford, UK: Blackwell Publishing Ltd.; 2011. pp. 114-26.

7. Aitken RJ, Buckingham DW, Brindle J, et al. Analysis of sperm movement in relation to the oxidative stress caused by leukocytes in washed sperm preparations and seminal plasma. Hum Reprod. 1995;10:2061-71.

8. Sperm Preparation Techniques. In: Cooper TG, Aitken J, Auger J, et al. (Eds). World Health Organization Laboratory Manual for the Examination and Processing Human Semen. 5th edition. Switzerland: WHO Press; 2010. pp. 161-8.

9. Henkel R. Sperm preparation: state-of the-art—physiological aspects and application of advanced sperm preparation methods. Asian J Androl. 2012;14:260-9.

10. Jurema MB, Vieira AD, Bankowski B, et al. Effect of ejaculatory abstinence period on the pregnancy rate after intrauterine insemination. Fertil Steril. 2005;84(3):678-81.

11. Zhang XJ, Jeyendran RS. Sperm processing procedures for assisted reproductive technology. In: Rajasingam S Jeyendran (Ed). Sperm Collection and Processing Methods a Practical Guide. New York: Cambridge University Press; 2003. pp. 141-53.

12. Ohl DA, Sonksen J, Menge AC, et al. Electroejaculation versus vibratory stimulation in spinal cord injured men: sperm quality and patient preference. J Urol. 1997;157(6):2147-9.

13. Muller CH, Pagel ER. Recovery, isolation, identification, and preparation of spermatozoa from human testis. Methods Mol Biol. 2013;947:227-40.

14. Bjorndahl L, Mortimer D, Barratt CLR, et al. Sperm Preparation. A Practical Guide to Basic Laboratory Andrology. New York: Cambridge University Press; 2010. pp. 167-87.

15. Mortimer D. Sperm preparation techniques and iatrogenic failures of in vitro fertilization. Hum Reprod. 1991;6:173-6.

16. Ng FL, Liu DY, Baker HW. Comparison of Percoll, mini-Percoll and swim up methods for sperm preparation from abnormal semen samples. Hum Reprod. 1992;7:261-6.

17. Hammadeh ME, Kuhnen A, Amer AS, et al. Comparison of sperm preparation methods: effect on chromatin and morphology recovery rates and their consequences on the clinical outcome after in vitro fertilization embryo transfer. Int J Androl. 2001;24:360-8.

18. Allamaneni SS, Agarwal A, Rama S, et al. Comparative study on density gradients and swim-up preparation utilizing neat and cryopreserved spermatozoa. Asian J Androl. 2005;7(1):86-92.

19. Prakash P, Leykin L, Chen Z, et al. Preparation by differential gradient centrifugation is better than swim-up. In selecting sperm with normal morphology (strict criteria). Fertil Steril. 1998;69:772-6.

20. Gonzales GF, Pella RE. Swim down: a rapid and easy method to select motile spermatozoa. Arch Androl. 1993;30(1):29-34.

21. Suksomopogn S, Kunathikom S, Makemaharn O, et al. Comparison of sperm motility between the swim-up and swim-down methods. Siriraj Med J. 2001;53(5):269-99.

22. Oshio S, Kaneko S, Iizuk R, et al. Effects of gradient centrifugation on human sperm. Arch Androl. 1987;19(1):85-93.

23. Chen MJ, Bongso A. Comparative evaluation of two density gradient preparations for sperm separation for medically assisted conception. Hum Reprod. 1999;14:759-64.

24. Claassens O, Kaskar K, Coetzee K, et al. Comparison of motility characteristics and normal sperm morphology of human semen samples separated by percoll density gradient centrifugation. Arch Androl. 1996;36:127-32.

25. Soderlund B, Lundin K. The use of silane-coated silica particles for density gradient centrifugation in in-vitro fertilization. Hum Reprod. 2000;15:857-60.

26. Edelstein C, Pfaffinger D, Scanu AM. Advantages and limitations of density gradient ultracentrifugation in the fractionation of human serum lipoproteins: role of salts and sucrose. J Lipid Res. 1984;25:630-7.

27. Stevanto J, Bertolla RP, Barradas V, et al. Semen processing by density gradient centrifugation does not improve sperm apoptotic deoxyribonucleic acid fragmentation rates. Fertil Steril. 2008;90:889-90.

28. Falcone T. Assisted reproductive technology: laboratory aspects. In: Falcone T, Hurd W, (Eds). Clinical Reproductive: Medicine and Surgery. Philadelphia: Mosby Inc.; 2007. pp. 581-90.

29. Sauer R, Coulam CB, Jeyendran RS. Chromatin intact human sperm recovery is higher following glass wool column filtration as compared with density gradient centrifugation. Andrologia. 2012;1:248-51.

30. Grunewald S, Miska W, Miska G, et al. Molecular glass wool filtration as a new tool for sperm preparation. Hum Reprod. 2007;22(5):1405-12.

31. Sánchez R, Concha M, Ichikawa T, et al. Glass wool filtration reduces reactive oxygen species by elimination of leukocytes in oligozoospermic patients with leukocytospermia. J Assist Reprod Genet. 1996;13(6):489-94.

32. Tea NT, Jondet M, Scholler R. A migration-gravity sedimentation method for collecting motile spermatozoa from human semen. In: Harrison RF, Bonnar J, Thompson W, (Eds). In Vitro Fertilization, Embryo Transfer and Early Pregnancy. Lancaster: MTP Press Ltd.; 1984.pp.177-20.

33. Said TM, Agarwal A, Grunewald S, et al. Evaluation of sperm recovery following annexin V magnetic activated cell sorting separation. Reprod Biomed Online. 2006;13(3):336-9.

34. Lee TH, Liu CH, Shih YT, et al. Magnetic-activated cell sorting for sperm preparation reduces spermatozoa with apoptotic markers and improves the acrosome reaction in couples with unexplained infertility. Hum Reprod. 2010;25(4):839-46.

35. Miltenyi S, Muller W, Weichel W, et al. High gradient magnetic cell separation with MACS. Cytometry. 1989;11:231-8.

36. Esteves SC, Miyaoka R, Agarwal A. Sperm retrieval techniques for assisted reproduction. Int Braz J Urol. 2011;37(5):570-83.

37. Mahendran M, Leeton JF, Trounson AO. Non-invasive method of semen collection for successful artificial insemination in a case of retrograde ejaculation. Fertil Steril. 1981;36:243-47.

Micromanipulation

Micromanipulation: Instrument, Technique and ICSI Procedure

Sunita R Tandulwadkar, Susmitha Dulipalla, Chaithra SK

INTRODUCTION

Since the birth of the first test tube baby in 1978,[1] in vitro fertilization (IVF) has become a treatment procedure for certain types of infertility, including long-standing infertility due to tubal disease, endometriosis, unexplained infertility, or infertility involving male factor. However, couples with severe male factor infertility could not be helped by conventional IVF. Extremely low sperm counts, impaired motility, and poor morphology represent the main causes of failed fertilization in conventional IVF. The introduction of intracytoplasmic sperm injection (ICSI) has dramatically changed the management of severe male infertility.

The ICSI procedure is based on micromanipulation of oocytes and spermatozoa. Initially, partial zona dissection (PZD) was established to facilitate sperm penetration.[2,3] The barrier to fertilization represented by the zona pellucida was disrupted mechanically to allow the inseminated sperm cells direct access to the perivitelline space of the oocyte. Subzonal insemination (SUZI) was the next step in micromanipulation techniques. SUZI enabled the immediate delivery of several motile sperm cells into the perivitelline space by means of an injection pipette.[4] ICSI is even more invasive because a single spermatozoon is directly injected into the ooplasma, thereby crossing not only the zona pellucida but also the oolemma.

The first human pregnancies and births resulting from this novel assisted fertilization procedure were reported in 1992 by Palermo and colleagues. Thereafter, ICSI was found to be superior in terms of oocyte fertilization rate, number of embryos produced, and embryo implantation rate in male factor infertility. As a result, ICSI has been used successfully worldwide to treat infertility due to severe oligoasthenoteratozoospermia or azoospermia caused by impaired testicular function or obstructed ejaculatory ducts.

The main drawback of ICSI is the chance of selection of a sperm which otherwise would never be able to penetrate the oocyte because of its structural defects whose severity is related to increased incidence of chromosomal abnormalities.[5] Hence the introduction of ICSI has raised the concerns of increased risk of chromosomal abnormalities in infants born of this technique.[6]

To overcome this drawback, several techniques of sperm evaluation and selection were introduced like motile sperm organellar morphology examination (MSOME), sperm hyaluronic acid binding, sperm chromatin assessment tests, intracytoplasmic morphologically selected sperm injection (IMSI) techniques.

INDICATIONS OF INTRACYTOPLASMIC SPERM INJECTION

Indications for ICSI are not restricted to morphologically impaired spermatozoa but also include low sperm count and impaired kinetic quality of the sperm cells. The ICSI can also be used on spermatozoa from the epididymis or testis when there is an obstruction in the ejaculatory ducts. Azoospermia caused by testicular failure can be treated by ICSI if enough spermatozoa can be retrieved in testicular tissue samples. ICSI is indicated in PGD where contamination by sperm could affect the PCR based diagnosis, the likelihood of contamination is minimized by the use of ICSI. Following are the indications of ICSI.[7]

EJACULATED SPERMATOZOA

- Oligozoospermia
- Asthenozoospermia (caveat for 100% immotile spermatozoa)
- Teratozoospermia ($\leq$4% normal morphology using strict criteria—caveat for globozoospermia)
- High titers of antisperm antibodies
- Repeated fertilization failure after conventional in vitro fertilization.
- Autoconserved frozen sperm from patients with cancer in remission
- Ejaculatory disorders (e.g., anejaculation, retrograde ejaculation)

Epididymal Spermatozoa

- Congenital bilateral absence of the vas deferens
- Young syndrome
- Failed vasoepididymostomy
- Failed vasovasostomy
- Obstruction of both ejaculatory ducts.

Testicular Spermatozoa

- All indications for epididymal sperm
- Failure of epididymal sperm recovery because of fibrosis
- Azoospermia caused by testicular failure (maturation arrest, germ cell aplasia)
- Necrozoospermia.

■ EQUIPMENT AND MATERIALS

Manipulators

The aim of use of micromanipulators is to convert coarse movements into fine movements under magnification without affecting the viability of gametes handled.

Commercially available micromanipulators for ICSI include Eppendorf (Germany), Narishige (Japan), Integra RI (UK), Lieca-Eppendorf IMSI (Germany) and S-corporation (Japan).

There are two basic types of manipulation systems today, Motorized and Mechanical.

Motorized systems have come a long way since their introduction into the market. Narishige brand of manipulators are used in most of the ICSI workstations. These setups have a blend of motorized coarse movement with joystick and hydraulic fine movement translated through a separate joystick. The advantage of this system is that the joysticks are separate from the microscope and thus do not cause any movement of the specimen during manipulation. It offers good range of motion across a 300–400× field and very smooth movement. It permits to raise and lower tools without dramatic hand movement from the benchtop. Hand position on the benchtop is very comfortable when using the "drop down" joysticks. The disadvantage of this system is the hydraulic lines. If pinched in some way it may be impossible to fix on location. Additionally, these systems are not very portable and require a considerable amount of time to assemble and disassemble.

Research instruments (RI) produces completely mechanical systems. The RI system attaches entirely to the microscope; there are no lines or cords or plugs to deal with, and it provides a very clean and neat workstation. The course alignment of the manipulator is adjusted with small joysticks that protrude upright from the suspended arms off each side of the microscope. The fine movement joysticks hang down from the suspended arms. They have good three-dimensional movement across a 300–400× field; the joysticks are well oriented to the focus knobs of an inverted microscope. The RI system, once set, requires almost no course adjustment. There are levers on each side of the manipulator above the microscope stage that allow the micro tools to be raised and lowered within a fraction of an inch of the bottom of the manipulation plate. This manipulation system can be moved very easily without disassembly. The disadvantage is that you must move your hands from the benchtop to a position above the microscope stage to raise and lower glass tools. While this is seldom a problem, the "drop down" joysticks can translate some hand vibration to the manipulation plate and specimen (**Figs 1A to C**).

Optics

The optics employed should be sufficient to clearly visualize the ova, sperm and any components thereof. Micromanipulation is generally conducted using an inverted microscope between 200 and 400×, and therefore 10, 20, and 40× objectives are essential for setup and

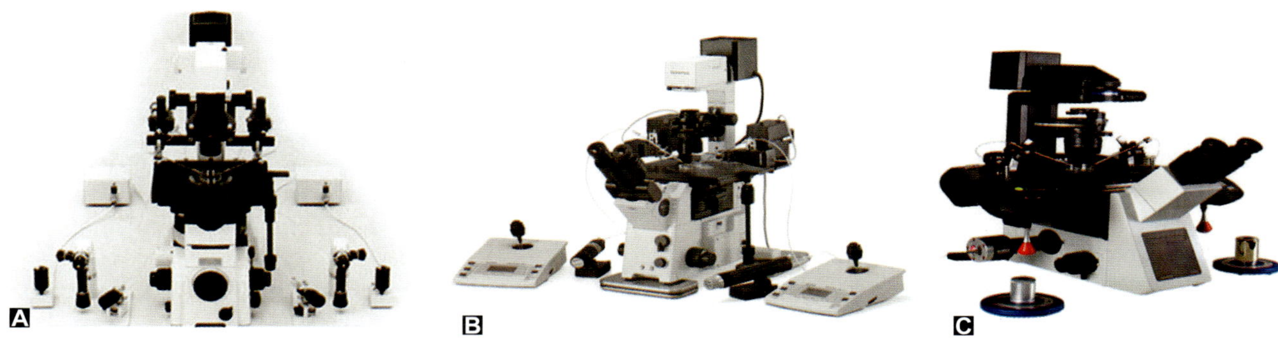

Figs 1A to C Micromanipulators. (A) Narishige: Japan; (B) Eppendorf: Germany; (C) Integra RI: UK

execution of the procedure. Phase contrast, differential interference contrast (DIC), or Hoffman modulation contrast can enhance the specimen image; Hoffman contrast is the popular choice for ICSI where plastic dishes are used. Easy, unobstructed movement between the focus adjustment and the objectives is desirable if a change in the objectives during manipulation is required. Look for inverted microscopes that have a 1.5×–2.0× slider just beyond the focus adjustment on the right side of the microscope; you can set the Hoffman condenser to 20 and the objective to 20× at the start of the manipulation session and with very little hand movement, the magnification increases 1.5×(300×) by simply pulling out the slider.

Stereomicroscope

Specimens should be quickly moved from the culture plate into the micromanipulation plate, manipulated, and then moved back again, to reduce the time held at room atmosphere. A stereomicroscope with a magnification range of 10 to 100× can be valuable for placing specimens into the micromanipulation plate. The "setup" station should be close to the micromanipulation workstation to avoid unnecessary chair movements **(Fig. 2)**.

Heated Stages

Heated stages are required to keep specimens at 37° C. There should be a heated stage on the micromanipulation microscope and on the setup stereomicroscope. Beware of hotspots on the stage that may exceed the critical threshold of specimens (greater than 38° C). Thermal cycling can be a problem with some stages; to achieve

a 37° C mean temperature the stage may actually cycle between 36 and 38° C.

Microsyringes, Tubing, and Tool Chucks

There are two basic types of microsyringe systems to choose from; those that require hydraulic movement of oil within the tubing that connects the glass micro tool to the microsyringe and those that simply contain air within the tubing. One of the control problems with the oil filled system is the potential for small air bubbles in the tubing which can compress and cause unexpected fluid movement in the glass micro tool, leading to disastrous results. Majority prefer air microinjector for holding the oocyte and oil microinjector for transferring the sperm. The type of tubing used to connect the microsyringe and the glass micro tools can be important. Soft tubing allows for too much expansion and ultimately a loss of control. Select a hard polyethylene tubing with little expansion capability. Tool chucks make the connection between the line and the glass microtool.

Glass Micro Tools

The other consideration with regard to glass micro tools is whether they should be straight or angled (30°). It is preferred to use angled pipettes because one can establish a clear focus on the horizontal section of the tool that provides a straight-on approach to the egg or embryo being manipulated.

Benchtop Incubators

To avoid cellular stress on the gametes, it is very important to maintain constant temperature, humidity, gas atmosphere for manipulation and culture. Hence bench-top incubators are to be placed next to the embryologist at the ICSI workstation so that the manipulation plates are quickly switched over to **(Fig. 3)**.

■ INTRACYTOPLASMIC SPERM INJECTION PROCEDURE

Sperm Collection and Processing Prior to Microinjection

Semen samples are collected by masturbation after ≥3 days of abstinence and allowed to liquefy for at least 20 minutes at 37°C before analysis. When the semen has a high viscosity, this can be reduced within three to five minutes by usually adding it to 2–3mL of HEPES buffered human tubal fluid (HTF-HEPES) containing 200 to 300 IU of chymotrypsin. Electroejaculation is applied to cases

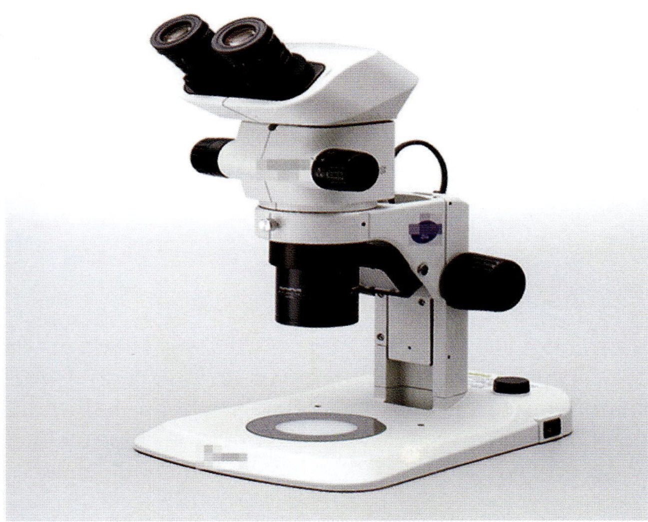

Fig. 2 Stereomicroscope

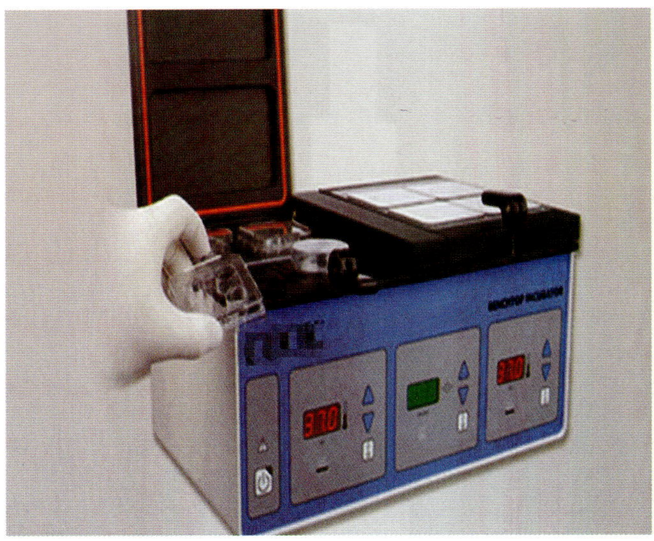

Fig. 3 Benchtop incubators

of spinal cord injury or psychogenic anejaculation. In case of irreparable obstructive azoospermia, a condition which is often caused by a congenital absence of the vas deferens (CABVD) and is associated with a cystic fibrosis gene mutation, spermatozoa are retrieved by microsurgical epididymal sperm aspiration (MESA) or percutaneous epididymal sperm aspiration (PESA). Azoospermic patients undergo testicular sperm retrieval either when the epididymal approach is unsuccessful because of impaired sperm production or transport, or in non-obstructive situations.

Sperm samples for ICSI are processed by density gradient centrifugation and or Swim up technique allowing an enrichment in number of motile and morphologically normal sperm needed for assisted reproduction. Only in cases of extreme oligozoospermic samples, i.e. when gradient centrifugation results in an insufficient yield of sperm cells for ICSI, simple washing of the sperm sample is performed to reduce the loss of sperm cells for injection. Epididymal and testicular samples are processed similarly to fresh semen and, when necessary, may be exposed to a motility enhancer (3.5 mM pentoxifylline) to allow selection of the most viable spermatozoa.

Sperm Selection for ICSI

Pentoxifylline

Sperm motility is the best indicator that both the functional (protective) plasma membrane and the metabolical processes are in place. Spermatozoa retrieved from the testis are in a different physiological state than sperm that have been transported through the epididymis. Many times these sperm (fresh or frozen-thawed) have extremely low motility or are immobile making it difficult to identify viable sperm for injection. Sperm motility can be stimulated with a variety of chemicals. One of the most commonly utilized chemicals for stimulating sperm motility is pentoxifylline. Pentoxifylline is a nonspecific inhibitor of phosphodiesterase that has stimulatory effect on sperm motility. The stimulatory effect is attributed to elevated intracellular levels of cyclic adenosine monophosphate (cAMP) via inhibition of its breakdown by cAMP phosphodiesterase. Pentoxifylline is also reported to enhance the acrosome reaction due to the increased levels of cAMP. Overstimulation of sperm with pentoxifylline can induce premature acrosome reaction. Therefore, this chemical should only be used on a limited basis in which no motile sperm can be readily identified.

Hypo-osmotic Swell Test

In cases where there is an absence of native of stimulated sperm motility, assessment of viability is essential. The hypo-osmotic swell test (HOST) is a simple viability test based on the semipermeability of the intact and physiologically functional plasma membrane. When sperms are exposed to hypo-osmotic conditions, an influx of water into the sperm results in an expansion of the cell volume. Cells that are viable will respond to the osmotic pressure of the external solution by attempting to attain equilibrium with the solution. If the solution is hyper-osmotic, the cell will shrink, if the solution is hypo-osmotic, the cell will swell.[8] When viable sperm are bathed in hypo-osmotic solution of 150 mOsmol for 30 minutes, the tails coil and the heads swell. Nonviable sperms will not undergo these changes. Therefore, this assay is effective in identifying viable non-motile sperm for ICSI use. Exposure of sperm for more than 120 minutes to a hypo-osmotic solution may be damaging and should be avoided. Once a viable sperm is identified, wash the sperm 2–3 times in your handling solution and then move them into the PVP solution before they are used for ICSI (**Fig. 4** and **Table 1**).

Morphologically Selected Sperm Injection

Conventional ICSI involves sperm selection at an optical magnification of approximately 400X. However, spermatozoa appearing morphologically normal at this magnification may carry various structural abnormalities at the subcellular level, which then remain undetected by the embryologist. MSOME is performed on an inverted microscope equipped with Normarski interference contrast optics, which allows observation at high

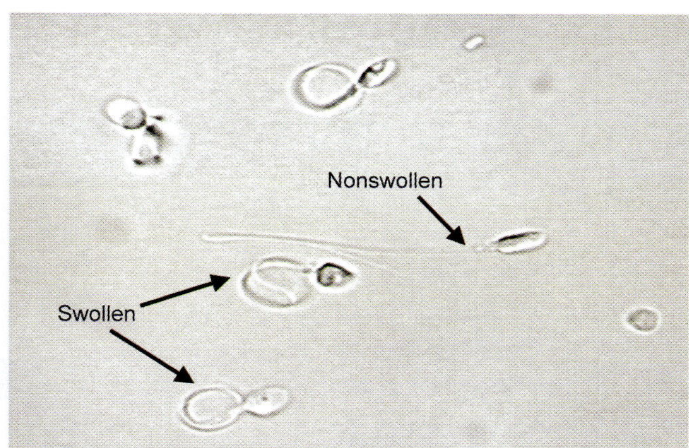

Fig. 4 Hypo-osmotic swell test of sperms

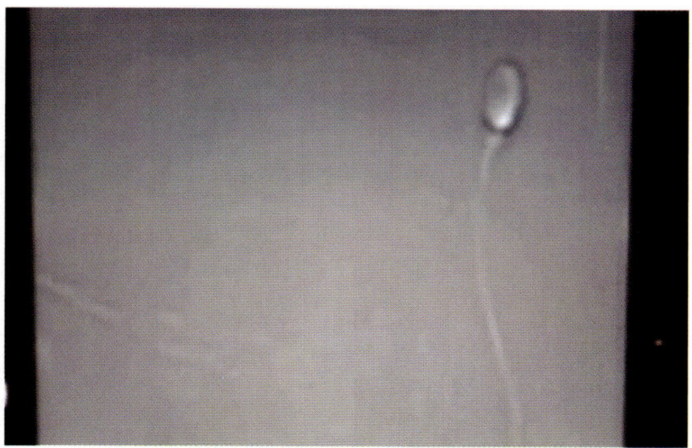

Fig. 5 Appearance of sperm in intracytoplasmic morphologically selected sperm injection (greater than 6000X)

magnification (greater than 6000X). This has led to the development of the intracytoplasmic morphologically selected sperm injection (IMSI) procedure.[9] The aim of this technology is to improve ICSI outcomes by selecting against sperm that have abnormalities that are associated with DNA damage **(Fig. 5 and Table 1)**.

Hyaluronic Acid-mediated Sperm Selections

Hyaluronic acid-mediated sperm selection is a novel and efficient technique that may alleviate potential problems related to ICSI fertilization with sperm of diminished maturity. Hyaluronic acid (HA) is a high molecular weight glycosaminoglycan and is the main component of the extracellular matrix of the cumulus oophorous **(Fig. 6 and Table 1)**. Spermatozoa that are able to permanently bind to HA in vitro are mature and have completed the spermiogenetic process of plasma membrane remodeling, cytoplasmic extrusion, and nuclear maturity. Hyaluronan bound (HB) sperm exhibit decreased levels of cytoplasmic inclusions, residual histones, and chromosomal aneuploidy, and an increased expression of the heat shock-related 70 kDa protein 2 (HspA2) chaperone protein. Bound sperm have also been shown to have a high density of HA receptors. In contrast, immature spermatozoa with deficient plasma membrane remodeling are not able to bind to HA as there is a deficiency in the zona and HA binding sites. These unbound and immature sperm have a high retention of creatine kinase, are associated with meiotic defects and possibly higher rates of aneuploidy. Sperm bound to HA have also been shown to have lower levels of DNA fragmentation and have a higher percentage of nuclear normalcy compared to those selected with traditional ICSI techniques. Overall, HB-sperm demonstrate

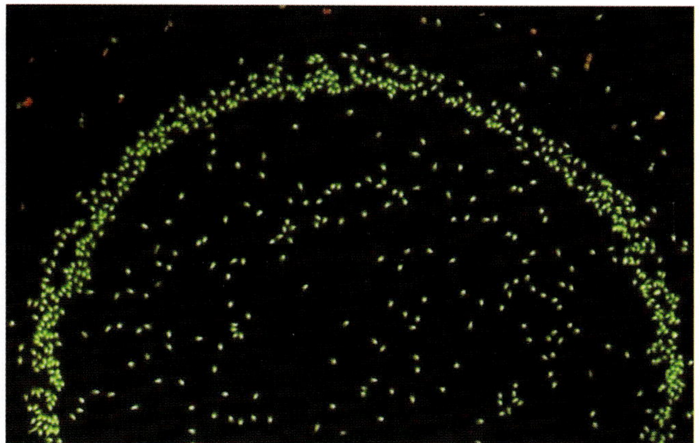

Fig. 6 Hyaluronic acid bound sperms

increased developmental maturity and enhanced levels of functional competence over their nonbinding counterparts.[10]

■ COLLECTION AND PREPARATION OF THE OOCYTES

After oocyte retrieval, oocytes are graded and incubated for more than four hours. Immediately prior to micromanipulation, the cumulus corona cells are removed by exposure to HTF-HEPES buffered medium containing 80 IU/mL of hyaluronidase (Type VIII, Sigma Chemical Co). The removal is necessary for observation of the oocyte and effective use of the holding and/or injecting pipette during micromanipulation. For final removal of the residual corona cells, the oocytes are repeatedly aspirated in and out of a hand drawn Pasteur pipette with an inner diameter of –200 μm. Each oocyte

Table 1 Methods of selecting sperms for intracytoplasmic sperm injection

Method	Advantages	Disadvantages
Standard ICSI selection	• Simple and inexpensive • Fastest method of sperm selection • Reduces manipulation time of oocytes and sperm	• Selection of sperm is based on motility and morphology, does not exclude spermatozoa with DNA damage
Morphologically selected sperm injection	• May increase implantation and pregnancy rates by selecting mature sperms	• Sperm selection can be time-consuming • Equipment cost can be prohibitive • Sperm selection should take place at room temperature to prevent DNA damage
HOST	• Simple and inexpensive test • Differentiates viable and non-viable sperm • May be able to differentiate degree of DNA fragmentation	• Time-consuming • Overexposure of sperm to hypo-osmotic conditions can affect viability • Can be difficult to use on frozen/thawed samples
Hyaluronic acid binding	• Assists in selecting mature sperm with normal morphology • Selects sperm with increased DNA integrity • May reduce rates of aneuploidy	• Difficulty micromanipulating sperm without using a viscous media • Sperm selection can be time-consuming • Relatively expensive

Abbreviation: HOST, hypo-osmotic swell test

is then examined under the microscope to assess the maturation stage and its integrity, metaphase II (MII) being assessed according to the absence of the germinal vesicle and the presence of an extruded polar body **(Fig. 7)**. The ICSI is performed only in oocytes that have reached this level of maturity.

It is essential that preparation of retrieved oocytes for ICSI must be carried out under tightly controlled conditions with a constant pH of 7.3 and stable temperature at 37° C. Fluctuations in temperature have been shown to be detrimental to the oocyte microtubular system, including reductions in spindle size, disorganization of microtubules within the spindle, and in some cases, even a complete absence of microtubules. Interference with spindle organization can cause chromosome disassociation, resulting in aneuploidy. For procedures which require extended periods outside of a low CO_2 incubator such as ICSI, it is important to maintain the appropriate pH using buffered culture media such as 4-(2-hydroxyethyl)-1-piperazineethane sulfonic acid (HEPES). The correct temperature can be maintained by properly equilibrating all media and by performing all manipulations on a heated stage. Also, covering all working media with equilibrated parafilm and mineral oil will prevent evaporation and minimize both temperature and pH shifts.

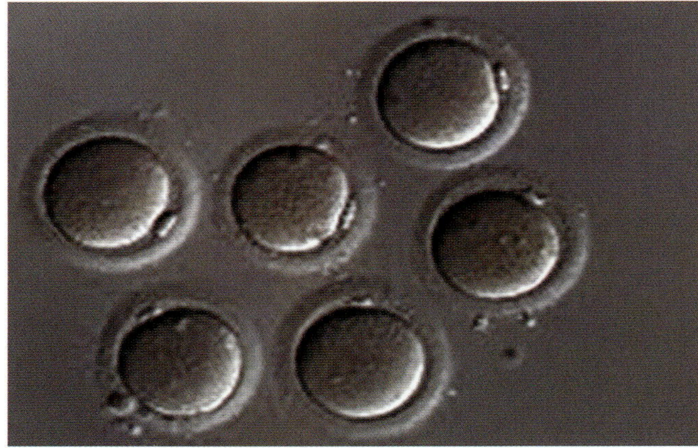

Fig. 7 Denuded metaphase II oocytes

PolScope

Integrity of the meiotic spindle in MII oocytes is crucial for normal fertilization and subsequent development. Therefore, it is thought that the morphology of the spindle may serve as a marker of oocyte quality.[11] A modification of the polarized light microscope "PolScope™," has been developed as a noninvasive instrument to view the meiotic spindle in living oocytes. The image of the spindle is based on the highly birefringent characteristic of the

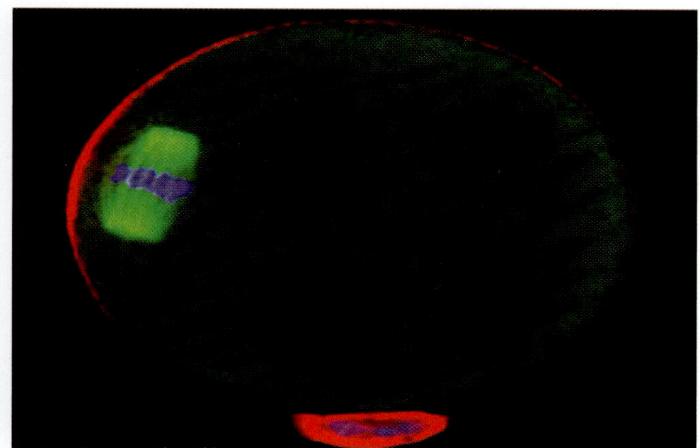

Fig. 8 Appearance of meiotic spindle through Polscope

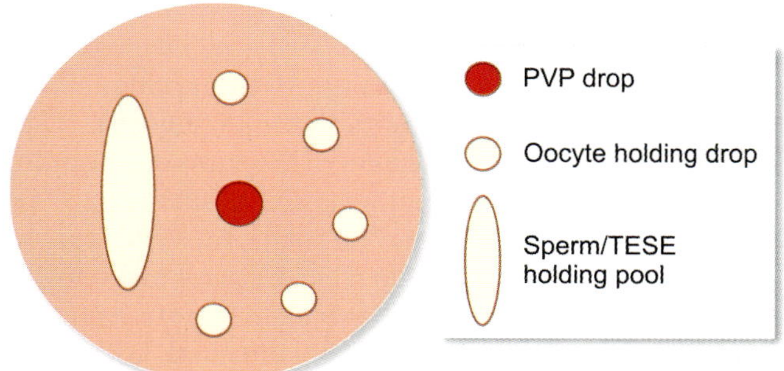

Fig. 9 Falcon injection dish

microtubule filaments under a polarization microscope. The presence of a birefringent spindle in human oocytes can predict not only a higher fertilization rate, but also greater embryo developmental competence.

So far, spindle imaging, in addition to the appearance of the first polar body, is an accurate indicator of oocyte maturity and can help to determine the timing of ICSI **(Fig. 8)**.[12]

Manipulation Plate Setup

- Label a Falcon 1006 plate with the identity and/or ownership of the specimen to be manipulated **(Fig. 9)**.
- Injection dishes are placed with small micro drops of 4–8 in the center of the plate of sufficient size to contain the specimens (5–10 µL). The drops are placed either in circular fashion with PVP in center or in parallel groups. Care is taken that the drops are not too close to the edge of the dish where manipulation is difficult. The drops are overlaid with 4–5 mL of mineral oil and placed in suitable incubators to equilibrate temperature.
- The micromanipulation plate setup should be performed at least 1 hour prior to manipulation so that temperature is equilibrated at 37° C.
- It is important that the drops be close together so they easily fit within the objective opening of the microscope stage.
- Prepare enough manipulation plates such that any given plate is only used once for a given patient or procedure. Care should be taken to keep plates warm. The time micro tools are exposed to air should be minimized when changing plates.
- If testicular sperms are to be used, on the left side of PVP drop, several drops are joined to form one long longitudinal drop where the sperm sample is placed for retrieval and then moved onto PVP for immobilization.

■ SETTING FOR THE MICROINJECTION

For the ICSI procedure itself, an inverted microscope equipped with micromanipulators and microinjectors should be available. Magnification capability of 200X and 400X is a prerequisite for precise procedures such as ICSI. A heating stage on the inverted microscope maintains the temperature at 37° C. Ambient temperature control is of vital importance for the survival of oocytes, which are very sensitive to a decrease in temperature that can cause irreversible damage to the meiotic spindle. Micromanipulators allow three-dimensional manipulation (coarse and fine movements) of the holding and injection pipette on the left-hand and right-hand sides, respectively. Microinjectors are used to either fix or release the oocyte with the holding pipette, or to aspirate and inject a spermatozoon with the injection pipette. The injectors can be filled with air or mineral oil. A micrometer controls the plunger. The whole setup is placed on a vibration-proof table to avoid possible interfering motion.[13]

Make sure that all parts are functioning smoothly before you begin the procedure. Insert holding and injecting pipettes parallel to the stage, tighten, check for alignment under lower magnification first and then at higher magnification. Check for the air bubbles in the tubing system. Adjust oil to the distal end of the pipette leaving a tiny gap of 5 mm for capillary action.

Immediately before injection, 1 µL of the sperm suspension is diluted with 4 µL of a 10% polyvinyl pyrrolidone solution (approximately 290 mOsm) in HTF-HEPES medium placed in the middle of the plastic Petri dish. It is necessary to use the viscous solution during the procedure in order to slow down the aspiration and prevent the sperm cells from sticking to the injection pipette. When there are <500000 spermatozoa per sample, the sperm suspension is concentrated in approximately 3 µL and transferred directly to the injection dish. Each oocyte is placed in a 5 µL droplet of medium surrounding the central drop containing the sperm suspension. HTF-HEPES medium supplemented with 6% Plasmanate® is used in the injection dish. The droplets are covered with lightweight paraffin oil. Spermatozoa are aspirated from the central droplet or the concentrated 3 µL sperm suspension drop, and transferred into the droplet containing PVP in order to remove debris and gain better aspiration control. The procedure is carried out on a heated stage fitted on a Nikon Diaphot inverted microscope at 400X using Hoffman Modulation Contrast optics. This microscope is equipped with two motor driven coarse control manipulators and two hydraulic micromanipulators. The micropipettes are inserted into a tool holder controlled by two IM-6 microinjectors.

SPERM IMMOBILIZATION

Although ICSI does not require any specific spermatozoa pretreatment, a gentle immobilization achieved through mechanical pressure is needed. This sperm immobilization is a membrane permeabilization process that may allow the release of a sperm cytosolic factor which activates the oocyte, and it has been demonstrated to improve fertilization rates.[14] When the immobilization procedure is performed in a standard fashion, spermatozoa are positioned at 90° to the tip of the pipette, which is then lowered gently to compress the sperm flagellum. The correctly immobilized sperm should maintain the shape of its tail **(Fig. 10)**. If during the process the latter is damaged or kinked, that spermatozoon is discarded and the procedure repeated with another sperm.

Owing to physiological differences in their membrane characteristics, a more aggressive technique is necessary when using epididymal and/or testicular spermatozoa that are considered immature. In fact, human spermatozoa undergo important modifications in the nuclear chromatin and several tail organelles during the epididymal transit. These modifications include the formation of disulfide bonds, a change in the membrane surface charge, a profound qualitative and quantitative modification in their lipid composition, and the absorption of specific proteins secreted by the epithelium of the epididymis. The lack of all these changes is associated with a decreased ability of epididymal sperm to bind and penetrate the oocyte. An alternative procedure is aggressive immobilization, where the sperm tail is rolled over the bottom of the Petri dish in a location posterior to

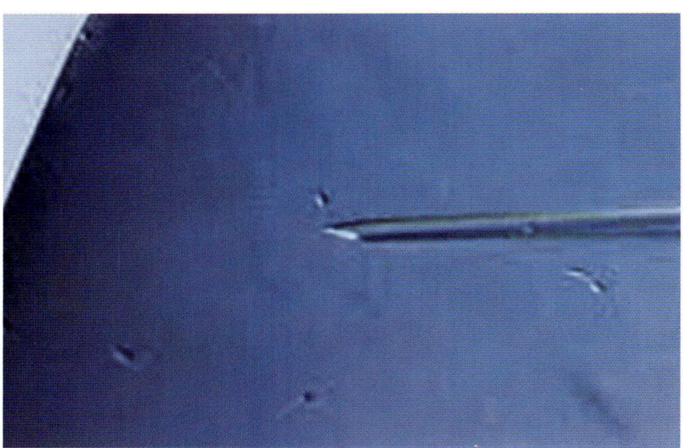

Fig. 10 Sperm immobilization

the midpiece. This induces a permanent crimp in the tail section, making it kinked, looped, or convoluted.

Although sperm immobilization is usually performed mechanically with the ICSI needle, laser-induced immobilization has also been described, resulting in identical fertilization rates.[15,16]

PENETRATION INTO THE OOPLASM

- The oocyte is held in place by the suction applied to the holding pipette. The inferior pole of the oocyte touching the bottom of the dish allows a better grip of the egg during the injection procedure.
- Position the polar body at 6 o'clock or 12 o'clock position to avoid damage to the meiotic spindle. The injection pipette is lowered and focused in accordance with the outer right border of the oolemma on the equatorial plane at 3 o'clock.
- The spermatozoon is then brought in proximity to the beveled opening of the injection pipette. The latter is pushed against the zona, permitting its penetration and thrusting forward to the inner surface of the oolemma. As the point of the pipette reaches the approximate center of the egg, a break in the membrane should occur. This is reflected by a sudden quivering of the convexities (at the site of invagination) of the oolemma above and below the penetration point, as well as the proximal flow of the cytoplasmic organelles and the spermatozoon back up into the pipette. These are then slowly ejected back into the cytoplasm, where the aspiration of the cytoplasm becomes an additional stimulus to activate the egg.
- To optimize the interaction with the ooplasm, the sperm cell should be ejected past the tip of the pipette to insure an intimate position among the

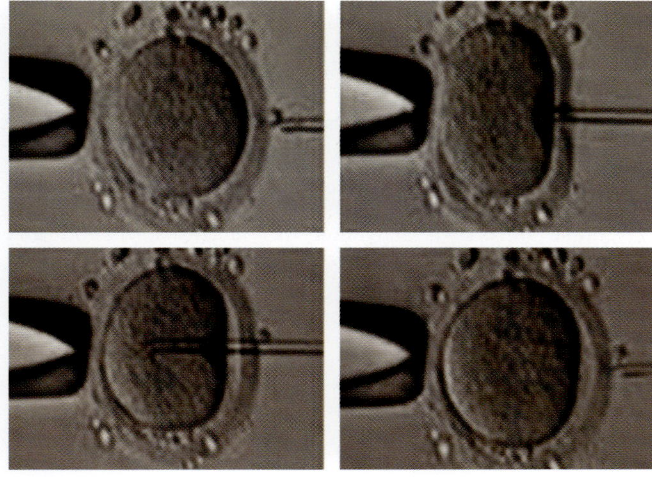

Fig. 11 Steps of intracytoplasmic sperm injection

organelles that will help to maintain the sperm in place while withdrawing the pipette. When the pipette is approximately at the center of the egg, some surplus medium is reaspirated with the result that the cytoplasmic organelles tighten around the sperm, thereby reducing the size of the breach produced during penetration.

- Once the pipette is removed, the breach area is observed, the order of the opening should maintain a funnel shape with a vertex into the egg . If the border of the oolemma becomes inverted, ooplasmic organelles can leak out.

After the completion of ICSI, the injected oocytes are placed in cleavage media and incubated to assess fertilization after 16–18 hours **(Fig. 11)**.

EVALUATION OF FERTILIZATION, EMBRYO DEVELOPMENT, CULTURE CONDITIONS, AND EMBRYO REPLACEMENT

Around 16–18 hours after injection, oocytes are analyzed with regard to the integrity of the cytoplasm as well as the number and size of pronuclei. First day cleavage is assessed 24 hours after fertilization, and the number and size of blastomeres recorded for each embryo. After an additional 24 hours, embryos are screened as to their need for assisted hatching.[17,18] At 72 hours after microinjection (the afternoon of day 3), those with good morphology are transferred into the uterine cavity or allowed for blastocyst culture or cryopreserved.

CONCLUSION

The ICSI procedure has been established as a reliable technique to overcome fertilization failure. The success rates of ICSI are largely independent of semen parameters making it a procedure of choice in severe male factor infertility and unexplained infertility. Complex techniques involved in the procedure is a limitation. Although many clinicians endorse ICSI for all to overcome fertilization failure, lack of long-term studies of children born of this technique is of concern and hence routine use is not advised.

REFERENCES

1. Steptoe PC, Edwards RG. Birth after the reimplantation of a human embryo. Lancet. 1978;2:366.
2. Cohen J, Malter H, Fehilly C, et al. Implantation of embryos after partial opening of oocyte zona pellucida to facilitate sperm penetration. Lancet. 1988;2:162.
3. Malter HE, Cohen J. Partial zona dissection of the human oocyte: a nontraumatic method using micromanipulation toassist zona pellucida penetration. Fertility and Sterility. 1989;51:139-48.
4. Laws-King A, Trounson A, Sathananthan H, Kola I. Fertilization of human oocytes by microinjection of a single spermatozoon under the zona pellucida. Fertility and Sterility. 1987;48: 637-42.
5. Carrell DT, Emery BR, Wilcox AL, et al. Sperm chromosome aneuploidy as related to male factor infertility and some ultrastructural defects. Arch Androl. 2004;50:181-5.
6. Van Steirteghem A, Bonduelle M, Devroey P, Liebaers I. Follow up of children born after ICSI. Hum Reprod Update. 2002;8: 111-16.
7. Review ESHRE Capri Workshop Group. Intracytoplasmic Sperm Injection (ICSI) in 2006: Evidence and Evolution. Hum Reprod. Update. 2007;13(6):515-52.
8. Stanger JD, Vo L, Yovich JL, Almahbobi G. Hypo-osmotic swelling test identifies individual spermatozoa with minimal DNA fragmentation. Reproductive Biomedicine Online. 2010; 21:474-84.
9. Antinori M, Licata E, Dani G, et al. Intracytoplasmic morphologically selected sperm injection: a prospective randomized trial. Reproductive Biomedicine Online. 2008;16:835-41.
10. Huszar G, Ozkavukcu S, Jakab A, Celik-Ozenci C, Sati GL, Cayli S. Hyaluronic acid binding ability of human sperm reflects cellular maturity and fertilizing potential: selection of sperm for intracytoplasmic sperm injection. Current Opinion in Obstetrics and Gynecology. 2006;18:260-67.
11. Rienzi L, Ubaldi F, Iacobelli M, Minasi MG, Romano S, Greco E. Meiotic spindle visualization in living human oocytes. Reproductive Biomedicine Online. 2005;10:192-98.
12. Rienzi L, Ubaldi F, Martinez F, et al. Relationship between meiotic spindle location with regard to the polar body position and oocyte developmental potential after ICSI. Hum Reprod. 2003;18:1289-93.

13. Joris H, Nagy Z, Van de Velde H, De Vos A, Van Steirteghem A. Intracytoplasmic sperm injection: laboratory set-up and injection procedure. Hum Reprod. 1998;13(Suppl 1):76-86.

14. Gomez-Torres MJ, Ten J, Girela JL, Romero J, Bernabeu R, De Juan J. Sperm immobilized before intracytoplasmic sperm injection undergo ultrastructural damage and acrosomal disruption. Fertility and Sterility. 2007;88:702-4.

15. Ebner T, Yaman C, Moser M, Sommergruber M, Hartl J, Tews G. Laser assisted immobilization of spermatozoa prior to intracytoplasmic sperm injection in humans. Hum Reprod. 2001;16:2628-31.

16. Montag M, Rink K, Delacretaz G, van der Ven H: Laser-induced immobilization and plasma membrane permeabilization in human spermatozoa. Hum Reprod. 2000;15:846-52.

17. Palermo GD, Alikani M, Bertoli M, et al: Oolemma characteristics in relation to survival and fertilization patterns of oocytes treated by intracytoplasmic sperm injection. Hum Reprod. 1996;11:172-76.

18. Nagy ZP, Liu J, Joris H, Devroey P, Van Steirteghem A. Time-course of oocyte activation, pronucleus formation and cleavage in human oocytes fertilized by intracytoplasmic sperm injection. Hum Reprod. 1994;9:1743-48.

25 Polarized Light Microscopy

Devika Chopra

INTRODUCTION

The identification of reliable markers for oocyte competence is an emerging concern in assisted reproduction. The knowledge of oocyte-related variables having a good prognostic value in predicting which embryo would implant and result in a pregnancy could allow selective insemination of oocytes and would limit the number of spare embryos.[1] The current level of knowledge of oocyte morphology is limited; it has been shown that cytoplasm and zona pellucida (ZP) appearance, as well as polar body (PB) morphology, may be helpful in assessing oocyte competence, but their reliability in identifying the real oocyte developmental potential is still poor.[2,3]

Polarized light microscopy (PLM) is a de novo non-invasive tool to analyze human oocytes as no cell fixation is needed and no detrimental effects are induced on the oocyte by the procedure. PLM allows the detection of anisotropic constituents of a cell (e.g. the microtubules of the meiotic spindle, the glycoproteins of the inner layer of the ZP), that once illuminated, produce light beams derived from polarized light. These beams are differentially slowed down by well-organized, anisotropic cell structures, and the birefringent signals that are generated may be measured as "retardance" by a specific computerized image-analysis system.[1,4]

This chapter has evaluated the use of PLM in assisted reproductive technology (ART) and provide an insight into its use on evaluating the oocyte competence and developmental potential.

POLARIZED LIGHT MICROSCOPY

Principle

By definition, polarization is the property of waves that is determined by the orientation of their oscillations. Birefringence, or double refraction, is the breakdown of a ray of light into two rays (a fast axis and a slow axis) when it passes through certain types of material (e.g. cellophane, calcite).[5] In relation to the fast axis, the progression of the light along the slow axis is slower. This effect occurs only if the structure of the material is anisotropic (directionally dependent). When entering the birefringent material, light is split into two beams and oscillates on both optical axes in phase. During the passage through the material, the two light beams are moving with different progressive speeds resulting in a phase shift. This phase shift (in nm) is called retardance and reflects the material's magnitude of birefringent power[5] **(Figs 1 and 2)**.

Over the last decade, polarization microscopy was introduced in ART laboratories for analyzing cellular components of oocytes, sperm and embryos. With improvements in computer technology, the real-time visualization of birefringent structures and the real-time calculation of polarization parameters is possible.[6] Several studies have evaluated the use of PLM in evaluating the developmental competence of the oocyte. This chapter has focused on the current status of PLM in the field of ART.

Use of Polarized Light Microscopy

Presence of the Meiotic Spindle

The first cellular organelle to be evaluated by PLM in the field of assisted reproduction was the meiotic spindle.[7] The meiotic spindle controls chromosomal movement through different stages of meiosis, and is involved in various functions that are essential for fertilization and early post-fertilization events. These include the responsibility for proper chromosome segregation and genomic stability after oocyte activation.[8] It has been suggested that defects in meiotic spindle formation can be associated with nondisjunction, which results in aneuploid gametes and aneuploid embryos.[8]

Spindle imaging raises new questions; should an oocyte that is without a germinal vesicle (GV) and with

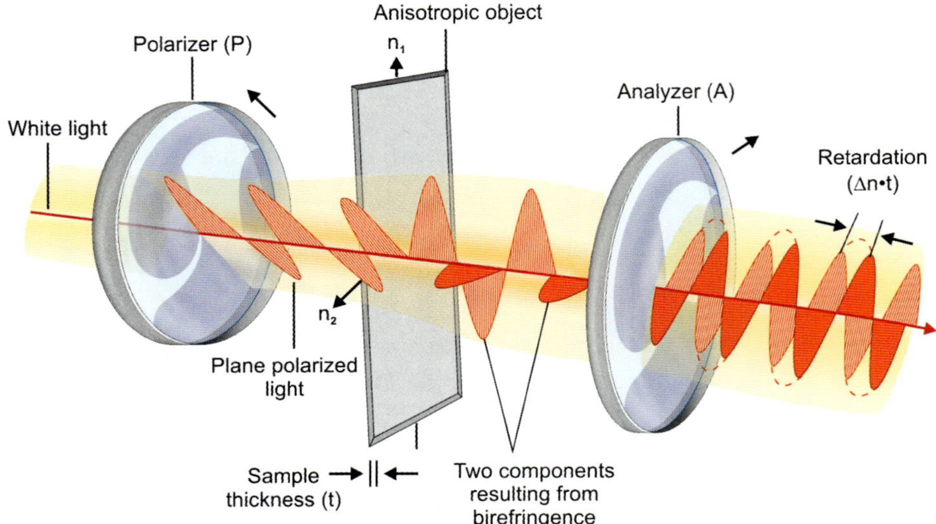

Fig. 1 Principle of polarized light microscopy. When polarized light passes through a birefringent object (meiotic spindle, inner layer of zona pellucida), it is broken down into two light phases (slow and fast). These waves when evaluated by an analyzer the difference in phase (phase shift in mm) between the two waves is called "retardance"

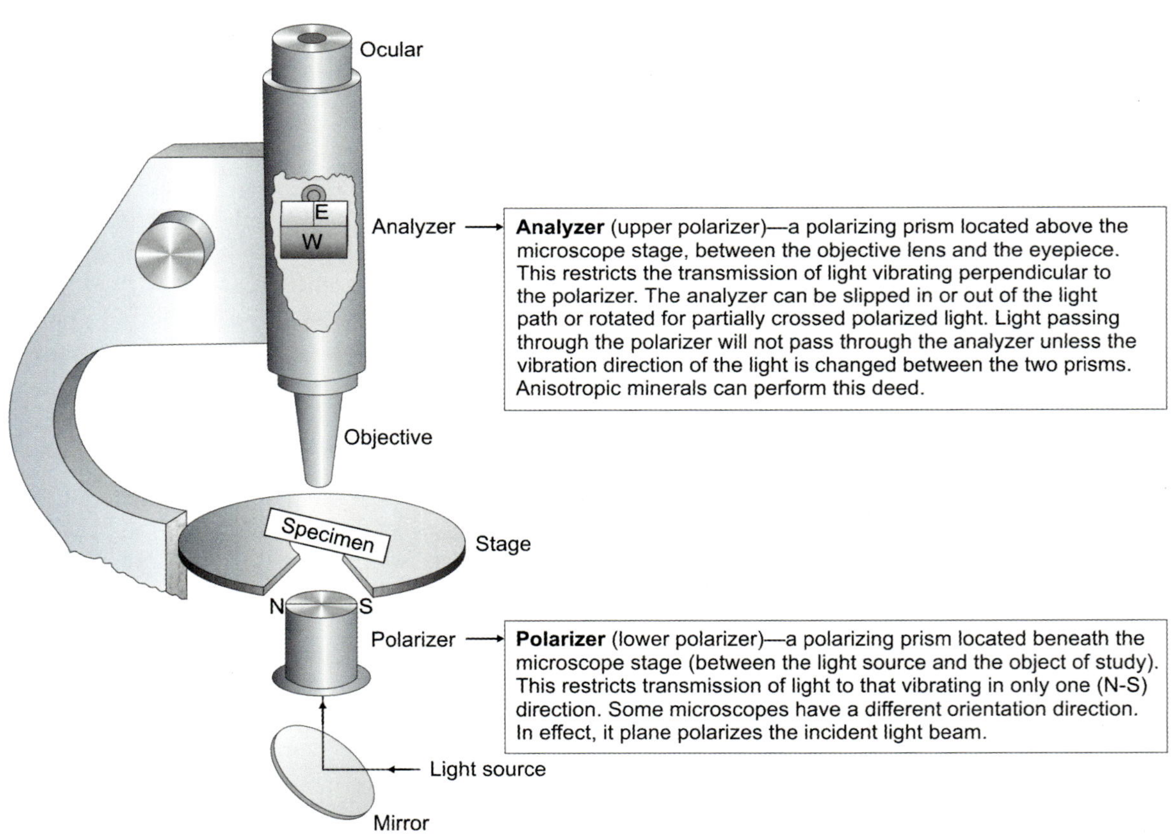

Fig. 2 Polarized light microscope

an extruded first PB, which is considered to be arrested in metaphase II, have aligned chromosomes in the metaphase plate? When can one expect to observe chromosomal alignment in the metaphase plate? The lack of adequate checkpoints during fertilization of the oocyte may cause chromosomal aberrations.[9] Spindle imaging using PLM could identify oocytes that are at risk for developing nondisjunction, thereby avoiding injection of oocytes that have failed to organize their meiotic spindles and have not reached their meiotic maturity. Wang et al. (2001) reported that spindle imaging with the PLM could predict embryo developmental competence and fertilization rate by better preinjection assessment of

oocyte quality **(Figs 3A and B)**.[10] They also concluded that oocytes that showed a meiotic spindle had a higher rate of blastulation.

Rienzi et al. (2003) studied the angle between the spindle and first PB. They observed a 74% fertilization rate if spindle and PB were more or less aligned and a reduced fertilization (50%) if the angle between them was less than 90°.[11] A meta-analysis performed by Peterson et al. (2009) compared the visualization of meiotic spindles with the intracytoplasmic sperm injection (ICSI) outcome. All parameters, such as fertilization rate (P < 0.0001), zygote morphology (P < 0.003), cleavage rate (P < 0.0001), embryo quality (P < 0.003), as well as rate of blastocyst

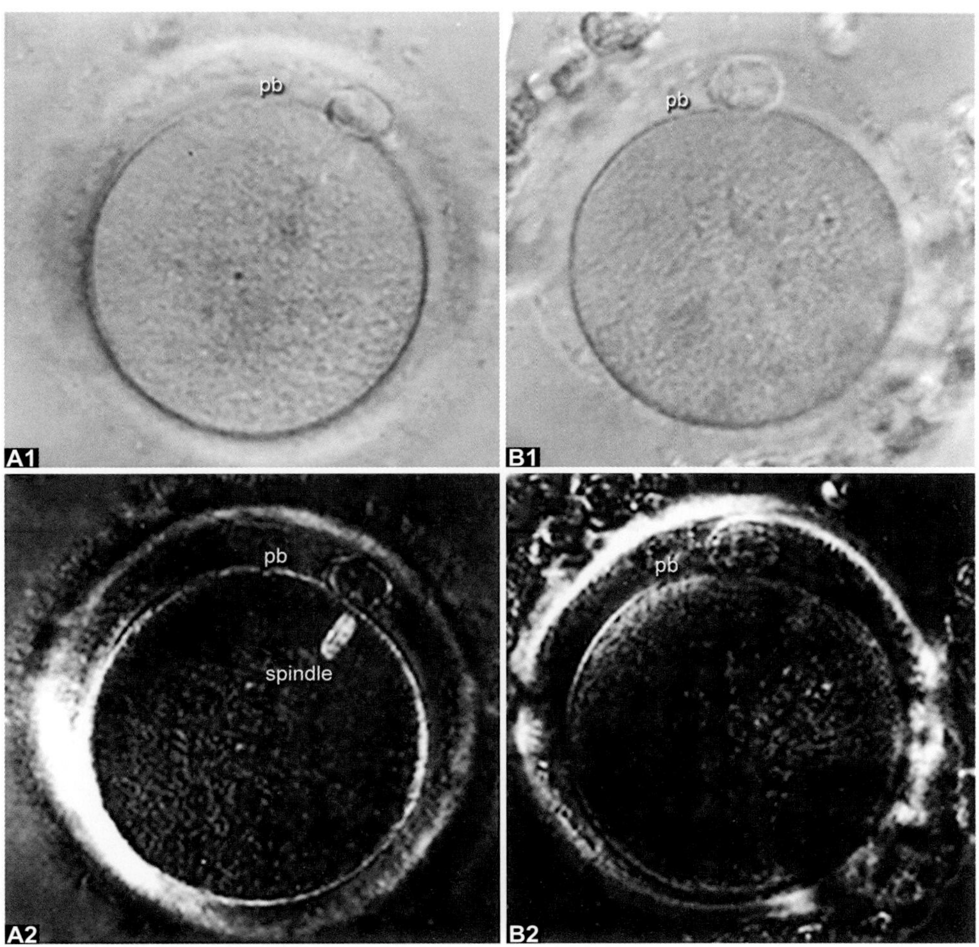

Figs 3A and B (A1 and B1) Human oocytes imaged with contrast microscopy (CM) and (A2 and B2) with the polarized light microscopy (PLM). Figures A1 and A2 show an oocyte with birefringent spindle, which was not visible with CM optics (as in Figure A1), but was imaged with the PLM (as in Figure A2). The spindle is located just under the plasma membrane where the polar body was situated. Figures B1 and B2 show an oocyte without spindle birefringence imaged with both CM (as in Figure B1) and the PLM (as in Figure B2)

formation (P < 0.0001) were higher than in the spindle negative counterparts.[12] However, Montag et al. (2008) recorded video sequences that showed the disappearance of the spindle apparatus during the transition from metaphase I to metaphase II for approximately 1 hour.[6] This supports the idea that in some oocytes the absence of the spindle is more likely an indicator of physiological progression through an important developmental stage of meiosis rather than a cellular disturbance.[6]

Table 1 shows the different studies that evaluated the presence of meiotic spindles and its association with the fertilization rate.

Spindle Quality and Retardance

The microtubules present within the spindle are responsible for the birefringence and signals detected by PLM and the retardance signals are directly proportional to the microtubule density.[16] Single and bundled microtubules can be measured adequately and the spindles composed of numerous highly ordered microtubules have a higher retardance than spindles with poor organization.

Montag and Van der Ven (2008) showed that good quality zygotes with good pronuclear morphology were derived from oocytes with a significantly (P < 0.05) higher spindle retardance (1.72 nm) than those zygotes stemming from intermediate (1.53 nm) and bad patterns (1.52 nm).[6] The retardance of oocytes that led to the formation of abnormal zygotes or bad quality pronuclei had a low retardance of approximately 1.39 nm.[6] Shen et al. (2005) studied the pole to pole distance (long axis) between the meiotic spindles along with the retardance of the same to determine the quality of the embryo.[15] They concluded that spindle length was not related to pronuclear pattern; however, in the case of shortened spindles, the risk of pronuclear misalignment was significantly higher (P < 0.001).[15]

Some studies have shown a positive correlation between the numbers of blastomeres on day 3 compared to the magnitude of spindle retardance.[17] Spindle retardance of more than 3 nm showed improved progression (P < 0.05) to blastocyst stage (61%) compared to oocytes with a retardance of 2–3 nm (25%) or less than 2 nm (14%). Additionally, a correlation was found between spindle length and blastocyst formation. If the spindle was longer than 12 nm, survival to day 5 was significantly (P < 0.05) better (45%) than in the groups with shorter spindles, e.g. 10–12 nm (34%) and 10 nm (20%).

However, more studies and multicentric trials are required to prove the reliability of spindle birefringence as a tool for evaluating oocyte competence. This is more so, as spindle arrangement is highly dynamic and is also dependent on physiologic and environmental conditions.[6]

Table 1 Presence of the meiotic spindle and its association with fertilization rate. Adapted from Ebner et al (2009)

Author	Spindle positive	Fertilization rate	
		Spindle	None
Wang et al.[10]	327/533 (61.4)	202 (61.8)*	91 (44.2)*
Rienzi et al.[11]	484/532 (91.0)	362 (74.8)†	16 (33.3)†
Moon et al.[12]	523/626 (83.6)	444 (84.9)*	78 (75.7)*
Cooke et al.[13]	115/124 (92.7)	81 (72.4)	nda
Cohen et al.[8]	585/770 (76.0)	413 (76.0)*	115 (62.2)*
Shen et al.[14]	739/897 (82.4)	676 (91.5)†	116 (73.4)†
Rama Raju et al.[15]	160/205 (78.1)	132 (82.5)*	14 (31.1)*

Note: Values in parentheses are percentages

Keys:

*P < 0.05

†P < 0.001

Abbreviation: nda, no data available

Source: Ebner T, Omar S, Yaman C, et al. A review of possible applications of polarization microscopy in IVF. J Turk Ger Gynecol Assoc. 2009;10:104-8.

ICSI after Spindle Assessment by PLM

Performing ICSI using PLM to determine the location of the spindle can be useful as in many cases the spindle is not located directly below the PB. Some authors used PLM to derive the location of the meiotic spindle and perform ICSI thereafter so as to prevent damage to the spindle.[14] This technique was compared with the usual PB aligned ICSI. Interestingly, the number of blastomeres on day 2 (P < 0.05) and morphology of the embryos were superior in the spindle-aligned group versus the PB aligned cohort (P < 0.01). However, the fertilization rate remained unaffected.

Polarized light microscopy was also used to time the performance of ICSI depending on the appearance of the meiotic spindle as it was observed that many oocytes were not in metaphase II at the time of ICSI.[8] Using PLM, Cohen et al. discovered that after 38 hours post human chorionic gonadotropin administration most of the oocytes obtained were in metaphase II. Therefore, the use of PLM prior to ICSI may be beneficial in patients that have a limited number of oocytes.

Imaging of the Zona Pellucida

The ZP has a multilaminar structure that exhibits birefringence on PLM. It is the inner layer of the ZP that is important in this respect which is evaluated using PLM.[14] It has been reported that the birefringence of the inner zona is directly proportional to its thickness.[14,15] Shen et al. found a 30% higher retardance of ZP in conception cycles compared to non-conception cycles.[14]

Montag et al. noted better embryo quality (day 3) in zonae with higher retardance.[6] Similarly, an Indian group observed that if the zona inner layer retardance was less than 3 nm, the blastulation rate was 60.9% as compared to 14.1%, if retardance was lower than 2 nm.[16] Since all data dealing with zona imaging were of a retrospective character, a prospective study was set up in order to determine the potential of PLM in the study of ZP retardance.[18] It was shown that the only if the retardance of the inner zona layer **(Fig. 4)**, the blastulation rate was better.[18]

To summarize, ZP retardation on PLM can be a valuable marker in determining oocyte competence, which is directly related to folliculogenesis and oocyte maturation.

Spindle Assessment Related to Positive Pregnancy Rate

Kilani et al. assessed the spindle morphology using PLM in oocytes by two separate researchers. They studied a total

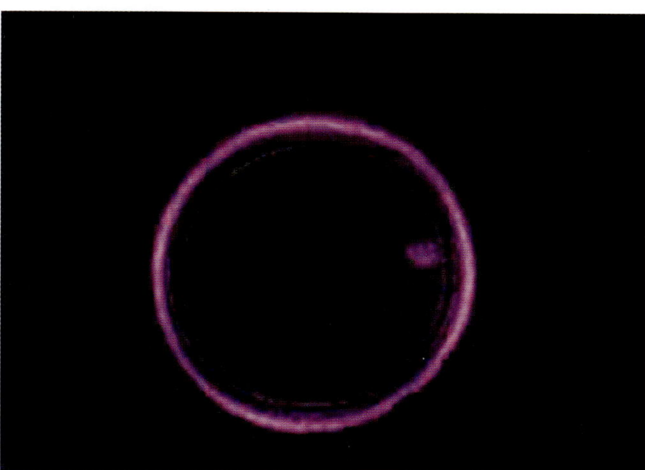

Fig. 4 Automatic user-independent zona pellucida imaging of mature oocyte

of 808/920 oocytes in metaphase II. Of those, 711 (88%) had a visible spindle wherein 205 (29%) were normal spindles (NS) and 506 (71%) abnormal spindles (AS). Fertilization rates were significantly higher in NS oocytes. Although NS and AS oocytes both formed morphologically good quality blastocysts, implantation and live birth rates were higher from NS oocytes. All ongoing pregnancies resulted from NS oocytes.[19]

Sperm Birefringence

In a mature sperm nucleus, there is a strong intrinsic birefringence associated with nucleoprotein filaments. Additionally, the subacrosomal protein filaments cause a similar type of birefringence. Even the tail is in part birefringent due to the microtubular organization.[20] Gianoroli et al. used sperm birefringence to compare the embryo development and implantation potential. Their criterion for sperm selection was the presence of birefringence in the sperm head, regardless of whether it was associated with the nucleus or the acrosome.[21] They concluded that the quality of embryos obtained were better with sperms demonstrating a higher retardance of the nucleus (33% vs 20%, P < 0.05). Additionally, the implantation rate was also higher in birefringent sperms compared to the conventional treatment group.[21]

■ CONCLUSION

To summarize, PLM can be a useful tool in evaluating oocyte competence by the study of the birefringence of the meiotic spindle, its position and retardation, as well as the thickness of the ZP. The study of sperm birefringence can also be done to evaluate the fertilization potential of an individual sperm and may aid in selection prior to ICSI. The use of PLM can prove to be invaluable if selection of gametes is required, i.e. in countries where the production of surplus embryos and their cryopreservation is legally not permissible. In conclusion, more studies and randomized trials are needed to evaluate the use of this technology and to determine its standing in recent ART practice.

■ REFERENCES

1. Molinari E, Evangelista F, Racca C, et al. Polarized light microscopy-detectable structures of human oocytes and embryos are related to the likelihood of conception in IVF. J Assist Reprod Genet. 2012;29(10):1117-22.
2. Balaban B, Urman B. Effect of oocyte morphology on embryo development and implantation. Reprod Biomed Online. 2006;12(5):608-15.
3. Rienzi L, Vajta G, Ubaldi F. Predictive value of oocyte morphology in human IVF: a systematic review of the literature. Hum Reprod Update. 2011;17(1):34-45.
4. Keefe D, Liu L, Wang W, et al. Imaging meiotic spindles by polarization light microscopy: principles and applications to IVF. Reprod Biomed Online. 2003;7(1):24-9.
5. Ebner T, Omar S, Yaman C, et al. A review of possible applications of polarization microscopy in IVF. J Turk Ger Gynecol Assoc. 2009;10:104-8.
6. Montag M, van der Ven H. Symposium: innovative techniques in human embryo viability assessment. Oocyte assessment and embryo viability prediction: birefringence imaging. Reprod Biomed Online. 2008;17(4):454-60.
7. Oldenbourg R. A new view on polarization microscopy. Nature. 1996;381(6585):811-2.
8. Cohen Y, Malcov M, Schwartz T, et al. Spindle imaging: a new marker for optimal timing of ICSI? Hum Reprod. 2004;19(3):649-54.
9. Champion MD, Hawley RS. Playing for half the deck: the molecular biology of meiosis. Nat Cell Biol. 2002;4(Suppl):s50-6.
10. Wang WH, Meng L, Hackett RJ, et al. Developmental ability of human oocytes with or without birefringent spindles imaged by Polscope before insemination. Hum Reprod. 2001;16(7):1464-8.
11. Rienzi L, Ubaldi F, Martinez F, et al. Relationship between meiotic spindle location with regard to the polar body position and oocyte developmental potential after ICSI. Hum Reprod. 2003;18(6):1289-93.
12. Moon JH, Hyun CS, Lee SW, et al. Visualization of the metaphase II meiotic spindle in living human oocytes using the Polscope enables the prediction of embryonic developmental competence after ICSI. Hum Reprod. 2003;18(4):817-20.
13. Cooke S, Tyler JP, Driscoll GL. Meiotic spindle location and identification and its effect on embryonic cleavage plane and early development. Hum Reprod. 2003;18(11):2397-405.
14. Shen Y, Stalf T, Mehnert C, et al. High magnitude of light retardation by the zona pellucida is associated with conception cycles. Hum Reprod. 2005;20(6):1596-606.
15. Rama Raju GA, Prakash GJ, Krishna KM, et al. Meiotic spindle and zona pellucida characteristics as predictors of embryonic development: a preliminary study using PolScope imaging. Reprod Biomed Online. 2007;14(2):166-74.
16. Sato H, Ellis GW, Inoue S. Microtubular origin of mitotic spindle form birefringence. Demonstration of the applicability of Wiener's equation. J Cell Biol. 1975;67(3):501-17.
17. Trimarchi JR, Karin RA, Keefe DL. Average spindle retardance observed using the PolScope predicts cell number in day 3 embryos. Fertil Steril. 2004;82:S268.
18. Ebner T, Balaban B, Moser M, et al. Automatic user-independent zona pellucida imaging at the oocyte stage allows for the prediction of preimplantation development. Fertil Steril. 2010;94(3):913-20.
19. Kilani S, Cooke S, Tilia L, et al. Does meiotic spindle normality predict improved blastocyst development, implantation and live birth rates? Fertil Steril. 2011;96(2):389-93.
20. Baccetti B. Microscopical advances in assisted reproduction. J Submicrosc Cytol Pathol. 2004;36(3-4):333-9.
21. Gianaroli L, Magli MC, Collodel G, et al. Sperm head's birefringence: a new criterion for sperm selection. Fertil Steril. 2008;90(1):104-12.

26

IMSI in Daily Laboratory Practice: Lights and Shadows

Fabien Murisier, Françoise Urner, Alain Chanson, Marc Germond, Alfred Senn

■ INTRODUCTION

When in vitro fertilization (IVF) started several decades ago, numerous studies have tried to correlate the morphology of the spermatozoa and the male fertility potential.[1,2] The morphology classification described by the World Health Organization Laboratory Handbook (1980–2010) has been adopted by many laboratories in the world. The World Health Organization (WHO) reference limits for sperm morphology were based on the evaluation of a thousand or more ejaculates from men who had conceived less than a year before and were set as the 5th percentile. Interestingly, during the subsequent editions, the morphology reference limit dropped from 30% in 1984 to 14% in 1999, and finally 4% in the last edition. This decline can be mainly attributed to the progressive introduction of strict criteria for the evaluation of sperm morphology,[3] as these were leading to better correlations with the fertility outcome both in intrauterine insemination[4] and classical IVF.[5-7]

The power of intracytoplasmic sperm injection (ICSI) as a tool to overcome fertilization failures in IVF procedures has led to a first common acceptance by embryologists that morphology of the selected sperm for injection was of secondary importance.[8] Every IVF laboratory has experienced that even sperm samples with quite low percentages of normal forms were able to fertilize and to produce viable embryos both in normal IVF and ICSI. In a large retrospective analysis, De Vos et al. (2003) showed that the injection of morphologically abnormal spermatozoa affected fertilization, implantation and pregnancy rates.[9] Several other authors suspected a possible negative influence of the paternal heritage on embryo development.[10-12]

In 2001, a series of ICSI procedures in which sperm was selected on the basis of a high magnification morphology evaluation was published.[13] The new technique was named IMSI (Intracytoplasmic Morphologically selected Sperm Injection), and the evaluation procedure MSOME (Motile Sperm Organelle Morphology Evaluation).[14] The results showed a significant benefit of the selection procedure on the ongoing pregnancies rates, but less so on the fertilization rates.[13,15-19] A link between the presence of large vacuoles in the head, an increased DNA fragmentation[20-22] and a decreased blastocyst formation rates was drawn.[23]

The demands for the use of IMSI became more outspoken, mainly among patients who were informed about this new technique through Internet chats, but also among IVF clinicians who were confronted to a lack of alternatives in cases of repeated treatment failures.

The aim of this paper is to summarize our experience using IMSI and to elaborate a strategy for the identification of the patients who would benefit from IMSI.

■ MATERIAL AND METHODS

Intracytoplasmic Morphologically Selected Sperm Injection Procedure

Intracytoplasmic morphologically selected sperm injection and pre-IMSI tests were performed using the OCTAX cytoScreen™ system (Medical Technology Vertriebs-GmbH, Bruckberg, Germany) installed on an Olympus IX71 microscope. A 60x air objective is used in combination with Hoffman's contrast and an OCTAX high resolution camera. Using a 1.6x magnification enhancer a total magnification of 960x can be achieved **(Fig. 1)**. Associated with the real-time digital image enhancement, the setup provides an excellent image quality with a total on-screen magnification of about 5,400x. Observation and selection of the spermatozoa are performed on the same microscope as the one used for oocyte injection.

The spermatozoa selection (IMSI) and oocyte injection (ICSI) are performed in two separated dishes. First 2–5 µL of a suspension of spermatozoa prepared by discontinuous density gradient centrifugation (Isolate, Irvine Scientific, USA) are deposited in a 20 µL PVP

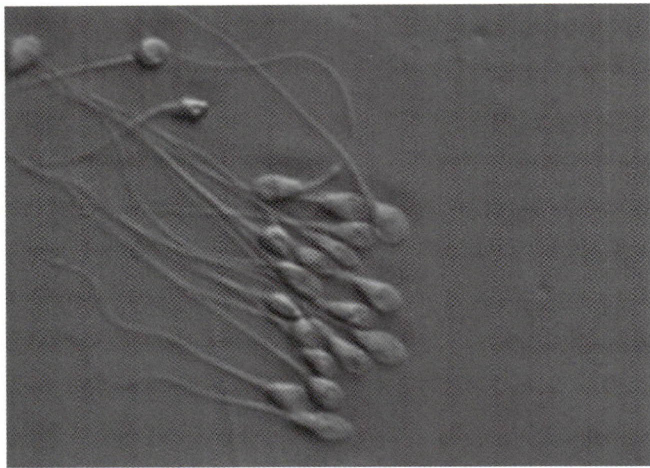

Fig. 1 Live spermatozoa observed under 960x magnification. Shape and presence of vacuoles can be clearly examined

Table 1 Grading and classification of spermatozoa observed under motile sperm organelle morphology evaluation

Grade	Description
I	Normal or borderline shapes, no vacuoles
II	Normal or borderline shapes with ≥ 1 vacuole(s)
III	Abnormal shape $\pm$ vacuoles(s)

microdroplet (ICSI medium, Vitrolife, Sweden) in a glass bottom Petri dish (Willco Wells, The Netherlands). Motile spermatozoa are observed using the CytoScreen setup and those that are judged as morphologically normal are aspirated in an ICSI injection pipette and transferred in a 5 µL microdroplet of G-MOPS medium (Vitrolife, Sweden) in a plastic Petri dish that will be used to perform the ICSI procedure.

Selecting motile sperm with normal morphology (normal head lacking vacuoles, normal midpiece without cytoplasmic droplets and aligned with the head main axis, normal tail clearly constituted of a single axoneme) is a critical step which needs some practice and may take several minutes per spermatozoon depending on sperm characteristics.

Pre-Intracytoplasmic Morphologically Selected Sperm Injection Tests

In pre-IMSI tests, sperm of patients with poor prognosis for successful ICSI cycle were tested to determine whether an IMSI would be indicated and technically feasible. For this test, the sperm preparation and observation were performed as described above. One hundred motile spermatozoa were submitted to MSOME evaluation and categorized according to the classification given in **Table 1**. The proportion of vacuolated sperm (PVS) heads among normal shapes was calculated as PVS = [grade II/ (grade I + grade II)] in percent.

In ICSI cycles, normal looking spermatozoa corresponding to grade I or II were used. In IMSI cycles, all collected mature oocytes were injected with spermatozoa that had been selected as morphologically normal (grade I). In a few cases, no normal spermatozoa could be identified and the selection was based on the second best (grade II or III) criteria.[18]

Patient Selection

Patient selection for IMSI was performed by the medical doctors in charge of the couple using either one of the following indications:
1. Repeated implantation failures,
2. Repeated early abortions,
3. Rnhanced sperm DNA fragmentation or
4. Severe teratozoospermia. For technical reasons, cryptozoospermia and/or severe asthenozoospermia (<0.05 million motile spermatozoa after preparation) were exclusion criteria.

A historical control group was constructed using regular ICSI cycles performed during the same period of time without any exclusion. This group does not necessarily represent an equivalent set of patients (male, female) to that of the IMSI group. The main purpose of this control group is to illustrate overall ICSI results obtained in our center during this period.

End Points

As supernumerary fertilized oocytes have to be cryo-preserved at the pronucleate stage in Switzerland,[24] the treatment outcome was expressed as the cumulated pregnancies obtained after fresh and frozen-thawed embryo transfers.[25]

Statistical Analysis

All data were extracted from our in-house IVF database (FileMaker Pro, USA) and exported in Microsoft Excel files. A statistical package (SPSS v18, Zürich, Switzerland) was used to perform the statistical analysis. Comparisons between the intracytoplasmic morphologically selected sperm injection and ICSI groups were performed using Student's t-test.

■ RESULTS

Pre-Intracytoplasmic Morphologically Selected Sperm Injection Tests

The pre-IMSI results of 30 patients are presented in **Table 2**. All patients were candidates for IMSI according to either sperm characteristics or clinical indications.

The mean grade values show that only 10.5% of spermatozoa were of grade I. The majority of spermatozoa were considered as abnormal or containing too many vacuoles (89.5%). When looking at the PVS values, the mean was 66.4%, indicating that only one out of three spermatozoa with a normal shape is vacuole free and suitable for injection. A threshold of 30% has been used to discriminate between sperm that can be used in regular ICSI (PVS <30%) or sperm that need an IMSI selection (PVS >30%). The percentages of grade I spermatozoa vary greatly among patients.

Intracytoplasmic Morphologically Selected Sperm Injection Results

Results obtained with the IMSI procedure are presented in **Table 3** and are compared to a group of 358 regular ICSI cycles performed over the same period. Most female parameters were comparable between the two groups, except for age (p = 0.048) and attempt number (p = 0.004). In the 62 IMSI cycles, a mean additional time of 40.0 minutes was needed for the sperm selection procedure. The fertilization rates were comparable in the two groups (76.4 versus 75.9%). The number of frozen zygotes and the number of embryos transferred were also the same. The day of transfer was significantly higher in the IMSI group, as more cultures up to the blastocyst stage were performed in this group; however, only a maximum of three zygotes were cultured in these cases. This explains why the number of frozen zygotes was slightly lower in the IMSI group.

Intracytoplasmic Morphologically Selected Sperm Injection Outcome in Young and Older Patients

The cumulative pregnancy rates were calculated among the two groups (IMSI and ICSI), in relation to the age of the patients at the time of oocytes pickup (OPU). Pregnancies obtained after fresh and frozen-thawed cycles were cumulated and expressed as the rate of pregnancies per OPU. Results are graphically presented in **Figure 2**.

Table 2 Distribution of sperm quality in pre-intracytoplasmic morphologically selected sperm injection tests

	Grade I (%)	Grade II (%)	Grade III (%)	Proportion of vacuolated sperm (%)
Mean	10.5	18.1	71.4	66.4
Minimum	0	1	40	30.0
Maximum	42	32	99	100.0

Table 3 Summary of the intracytoplasmic morphologically selected sperm injection and ICSI cycles

	IMSI	ICSI	P
Number of cycles	62	358	
Age (female)	36.6 ± 3.7	35.9 ± 4.6	0.048
Attempt number	1.8 ± 0.9	1.4 ± 0.7	0.004
Collected oocytes	11.2 ± 5.5	10.8 ± 5.8	0.351
Injected oocytes	9.4 ± 4.6	8.9 ± 5.1	0.269
Additional time for sperm selection (min)	40.0 ± 19.3	–	
Additional time for sperm selection per oocyte (min)	3.8 ± 2.6	–	
Fertilization rates (%)	76.4 ± 21.1	75.9 ± 22.0	0.636
Zygotes (2PN)	7.1 ± 3.7	6.8 ± 4.3	0.123
Frozen zygotes	4.7 ± 3.4	4.9 ± 4.2	0.047
Transferred embryos	1.9 ± 0.4	1.9 ± 0.4	0.291
Day of transfer	3.3 ± 1.4	2.6 ± 0.9	0.001

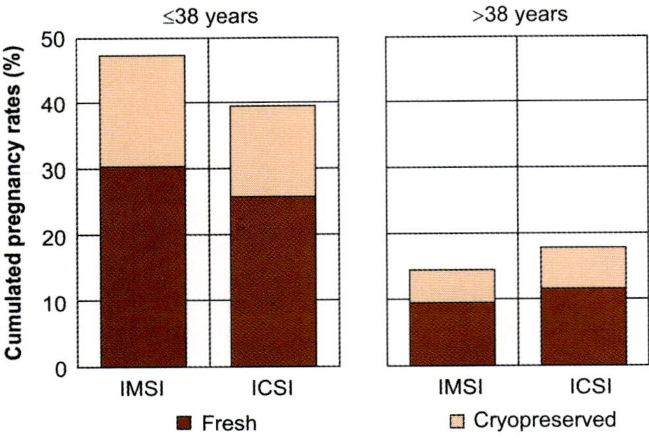
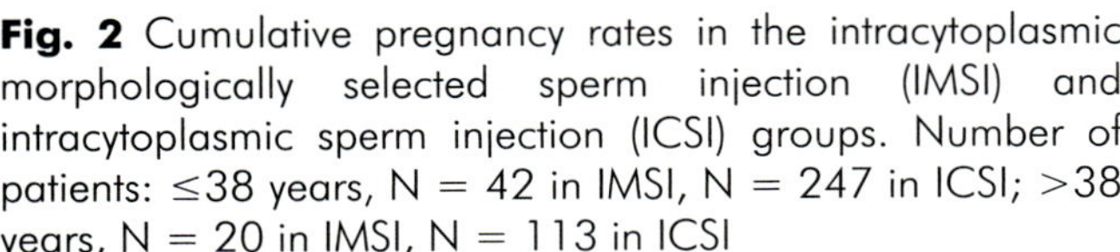

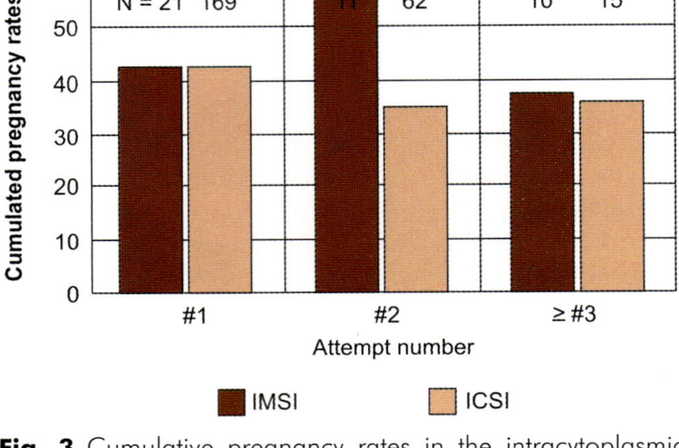

Fig. 2 Cumulative pregnancy rates in the intracytoplasmic morphologically selected sperm injection (IMSI) and intracytoplasmic sperm injection (ICSI) groups. Number of patients: ≤38 years, N = 42 in IMSI, N = 247 in ICSI; >38 years, N = 20 in IMSI, N = 113 in ICSI

Fig. 3 Cumulative pregnancy rates in the intracytoplasmic morphologically selected sperm injection (IMSI) and intracytoplasmic sperm injection (ICSI) groups in younger patients according to the attempt number

In younger patients (≤38 years old) cumulative pregnancy rates of 47.6% versus 40.2% (p > 0.1) were obtained in the IMSI versus ICSI groups. In older patients, these rates were 15.0% versus 18.0% (p > 0.1) respectively.

The abortion rate in less than or equal to 38-year-old patients was 10.0% in the IMSI group, and 18% in the ICSI group. In the older patient group, these values were 66.6% and 38% respectively. Due to the small number of cases, all rates shown in **Figure 2** were not statistically different.

Intracytoplasmic Morphologically Selected Sperm Injection Outcome According to the Attempt Number in Less than or Equal to 38-Year-Old Patients

The cumulative pregnancy rates were calculated among the two groups (IMSI and ICSI), in relation to the attempt number in the younger patients group. Pregnancies obtained after fresh and frozen-thawed cycles were cumulated and expressed as the rate of pregnancies per oocyte collection. Results are presented in **Figure 3**. The beneficial effect of IMSI is particularly visible during the second attempt, but the number of cases is too small to reach statistical significance.

■ DISCUSSION

In our hands, the IMSI procedure performed with CytoScreen was on average 40 minutes longer than a conventional ICSI procedure. When considering the number of injected oocytes, this figure was about 3.8 minutes per oocyte. The overall IMSI procedure is thus roughly twice as long as a regular ICSI. It is thus important to reserve sufficient amount of time within the routine schedule of the laboratory. The CytoScreen system has the advantage over oil based objectives to allow an easy and fast change of dishes between the sperm selection glass dish and the regular plastic dish used for sperm storage and ICSI injection.

The duration of oocyte exposure to external conditions can be reduced to lengths similar to those of ICSI, provided that the oocytes are kept inside the incubator during the sperm selection procedure.

We have observed repeatedly in the IMSI group of patients, that the presence of vacuoles in the sperm head is quite common and that the number of sperm suitable for injection is low (10.5%, minimum-maximum: 0-42). The role of the pre-IMSI test is thus crucial as it may help the laboratory staff to reserve sufficient time to complete the IMSI procedure. It is not disputed in the literature that gross head malformations can easily be detected with 20x–40x conventional Hoffman objectives, but this may not be the case for the detection of vacuoles. The advantage of the IMSI procedure is to achieve both a selection of morphologically normal and vacuole-free spermatozoa.

As shown in **Table 3**, the fertilization rates observed in the IMSI and ICSI groups are comparable, as already mentioned by various studies.[16,21]

There is an intrinsic difficulty when comparing IMSI with ICSI, as our IMSI group is composed of bad prognosis patients. As shown in **Figure 2**, IMSI does not appear to be beneficial in terms of pregnancy rates per oocyte collection both for younger (≤38 years old) and older (>38 years) patients. The recorded abortion rate was lower in the IMSI group (10%) than in the ICSI group (18%). This observation is in accordance with other studies,[18] however, our IMSI group is too small to allow valid statistical comparisons. In older patients, the abortion rates were much higher and did not seem to differ whether IMSI or ICSI was applied. This observation highlights the fact that in older patients the improvement brought by IMSI cannot compensate for the oocyte genetic defects associated with age.

Most published studies on IMSI rely on retrospective analysis, involving a comparison with previous cycles for the same patients or with a matched control group.[13,16-19,21] There is only one published prospective study, which clearly shows a beneficial effect of IMSI in term of pregnancy rates.[15] However, more prospective randomized studies are needed to confirm the advantage of IMSI in certain groups of patients. The ideal prospective randomized study should be blinded both to the clinician, the patient and the ICSI operator. Assembling all these conditions is difficult as it requires proper counseling of the patients and avoidance of ethical pitfalls associated with experimentation with human gametes. In addition, a deliberate injection of spermatozoa presenting defects, such as vacuolated or dysmorphic heads, is likely to be unacceptable both for the patients and the embryologists.

The indications for IMSI found in the literature are essentially indirect ones, such as recurrent implantation failures or repeated early abortions.[15,16,21] At the level of the spermatozoa, the indications are not well defined except for enhanced DNA fragmentation.[21,20] In our center, we have retained three major indications for IMSI:

1. Repeated unexplained implantation failures or recurrent abortions.
2. A severe teratozoospermia or enhanced sperm DNA fragmentation.
3. A pre-IMSI test indicating that IMSI might improve sperm selection before ICSI (PVS >30%).

In conclusion, the IMSI procedure has changed our perception of what a normal spermatozoon suitable for injection looks like. There appears to be classes of patients which benefit from this technique, but the clinical indications are scarce and derived mainly from the history of the patients and careful pretest analysis of the sperm suspension.

■ REFERENCES

1. Bostofte E, Serup J, Rebbe H. Relation between morphologically abnormal spermatozoa and pregnancies obtained during a twenty-year follow-up period. Int J Androl. 1982;5:379-86.
2. Coetzee K, Kruge TF, Lombard CJ. Predictive value of normal sperm morphology: a structured literature review. Hum Reprod Update. 1998;4:73-82.
3. Kruger TF, Acosta AA, Simmons KF, et al. New method of evaluating sperm morphology with predictive value for human in vitro fertilization. Urology. 1987;30:248-51.
4. Van Waart J, Kruger TF, Lombard CJ, et al. Predictive value of normal sperm morphology in intrauterine insemination (IUI): a structured literature review. Hum Reprod Update. 2001;7:495-500.
5. Acosta AA, van der Merwe JP, Doncel G, et al. Fertilization efficiency of morphologically abnormal spermatozoa in assisted reproduction is further impaired by antisperm antibodies on the male partner's sperm. Fertil Steril. 1994;62:826-33.
6. Grow DR, Oehninger S, Seltman HJ, et al. Sperm morphology as diagnosed by strict criteria: probing the impact of teratozoospermia on fertilization rate and pregnancy outcome in a large in vitro fertilization population. Fertil Steril. 1994;62:559-67.
7. Kruger TF, Acosta AA, Simmons KF, et al. Predictive value of abnormal sperm morphology in in vitro fertilization. Fertil Steril. 1988;49:112-7.
8. Lundin K, Soderlund B, Hamberger L. The relationship between sperm morphology and rates of fertilization, pregnancy and spontaneous abortion in an in vitro fertilization/intracytoplasmic sperm injection programme. Hum Reprod. 1997;12:2676-81.
9. De Vos A, Van De Velde H, Joris H, et al. Influence of individual sperm morphology on fertilization, embryo morphology, and pregnancy outcome of intracytoplasmic sperm injection. Fertil Steril. 2003;79:42-8.
10. Shoukir Y, Chardonnens D, Campana A, et al. Blastocyst development from supernumerary embryos after intracytoplasmic sperm injection: a paternal influence? Hum Reprod. 1998;13:1632-7.
11. Spano M, Seli E, Bizzaro D, et al. The significance of sperm nuclear DNA strand breaks on reproductive outcome. Curr Opin Obstet Gynecol. 2005;17:255-60.
12. Tesarik J, Mendoza C, Greco E. Paternal effects acting during the first cell cycle of human preimplantation development after ICSI. Hum Reprod. 2002;17:184-9.
13. Bartoov B, Berkovitz A, Eltes F. Selection of spermatozoa with normal nuclei to improve the pregnancy rate with intra-cytoplasmic sperm injection. N Engl J Med. 2001;345:1067-8.
14. Bartoov B, Berkovitz A, Eltes F, et al. Real-time fine morphology of motile human sperm cells is associated with IVF-ICSI outcome. J Androl. 2002;23:1-8.
15. Antinori M, Licata E, Dani G, et al. Intracytoplasmic morphologically selected sperm injection: a prospective randomized trial. Reprod Biomed Online. 2008;16:835-41.

16. Bartoov B, Berkovitz A, Eltes F, et al. Pregnancy rates are higher with intracytoplasmic morphologically selected sperm injection than with conventional intracytoplasmic injection. Fertil Steril. 2003;80:1413-9.

17. Berkovitz A, Eltes F, Ellenbogen A, et al. Does the presence of nuclear vacuoles in human sperm selected for ICSI affect pregnancy outcome? Hum Reprod. 2006;21:1787-90.

18. Berkovitz A, Eltes F, Lederman H, et al. How to improve IVF-ICSI outcome by sperm selection. Reprod Biomed Online. 2006;12:634-8.

19. Berkovitz A, Eltes F, Yaari S, et al. The morphological normalcy of the sperm nucleus and pregnancy rate of intracytoplasmic injection with morphologically selected sperm. Hum Reprod. 2005;20:185-90.

20. Franco JG Jr, Baruffi RL, Mauri AL, et al. Significance of large nuclear vacuoles in human spermatozoa: implications for ICSI. Reprod Biomed Online. 2008;17:42-5.

21. Hazout A, Dumont-Hassan M, Junca AM, et al. High-magnification ICSI overcomes paternal effect resistant to conventional ICSI. Reprod Biomed Online. 2006;12:19-25.

22. Oliveira JB, Massaro FC, Baruffi RL, et al. Correlation between semen analysis by motile sperm organelle morphology examination and sperm DNA damage. Fertil Steril. 2010;94(5):1937-40.

23. Vanderzwalmen P, Hiemer A, Rubner P, et al. Blastocyst development after sperm selection at high magnification is associated with size and number of nuclear vacuoles. Reprod Biomed Online. 2008;17:617-27.

24. Germond M, Senn A. A law affecting medically assisted procreation is on the way in Switzerland. J Assist Reprod Genet. 1999;16:341-3.

25. Germond M, Urner F, Chanson A, et al. What is the most relevant standard of success in assisted reproduction?: The cumulated singleton/twin delivery rates per oocyte pick-up: the CUSIDERA and CUTWIDERA. Hum Reprod. 2004;19:2442-4.

27

Role of Preimplantation Genetic Diagnosis in ART

Sunita R Tandulwadkar, Sejal Naik

INTRODUCTION

In current practice of IVF the embryos are selected and transferred on the basis of morphological characteristics. PGD helps in detection of genetically abnormal embryos and thus avoids transferring them. It is becoming an established approach especially in patients with advanced age, X-linked disorders, autosomal recessive conditions, specific gene diagnosis, etc. At present, PGD may be performed by three major approaches:

1. *First and second polar body biopsy*: Removal following maturation and fertilization of oocytes (day 0 and/or day 1) **(Fig. 1)**
2. *Blastomere biopsy*: At the cleavage stage (6–10 cells stage) (day 3) **(Fig. 2)**.
3. *Blastocyst biopsy*: (day 5/6) **(Figs 3A and B)**

Each PGD methods has advantages and disadvantages, and their choice depends on circumstances; however, in some cases the combination of two or three methods may be required. All these methods require breaching the ZP in order to facilitate the removal of cellular material. The biopsied material is tested for single gene disorders using PCR analysis, or for chromosomal abnormalities using FISH analysis. Thus, the abnormal embryos are removed and only normal embryos are transferred to improve implantation rate and overall pregnancy outcome.

METHODS OF BREACHING THE ZONA

Three methods are used primarily to breach the ZP to facilitate the removal of cells for testing.

Partial Zona Dissection

This mechanical technique was first used successfully by Cohen et al. to facilitate sperm penetration.

Technique: The fine needle is penetrated into and under the ZP, the skewered section of zona is then cut by gentle

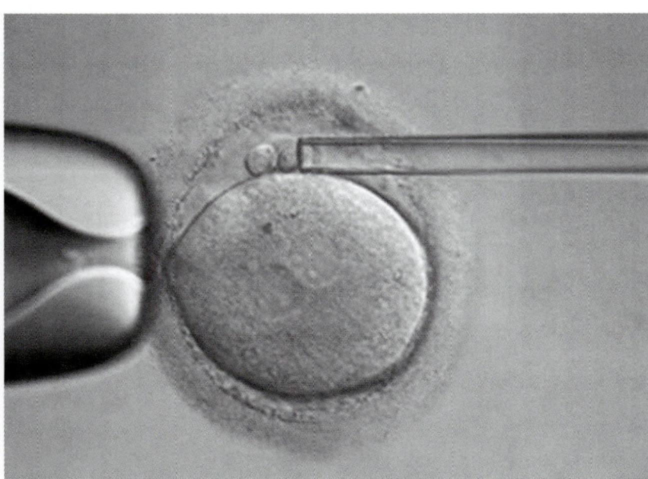

Fig. 1 Polar body biopsy

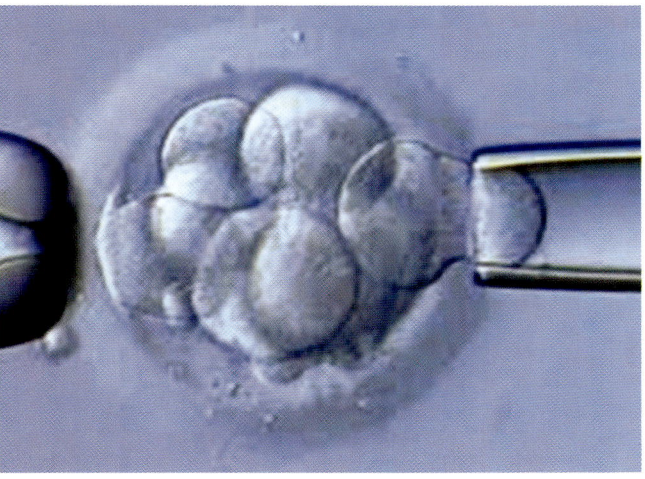

Fig. 2 Blastomere biopsy on day 3

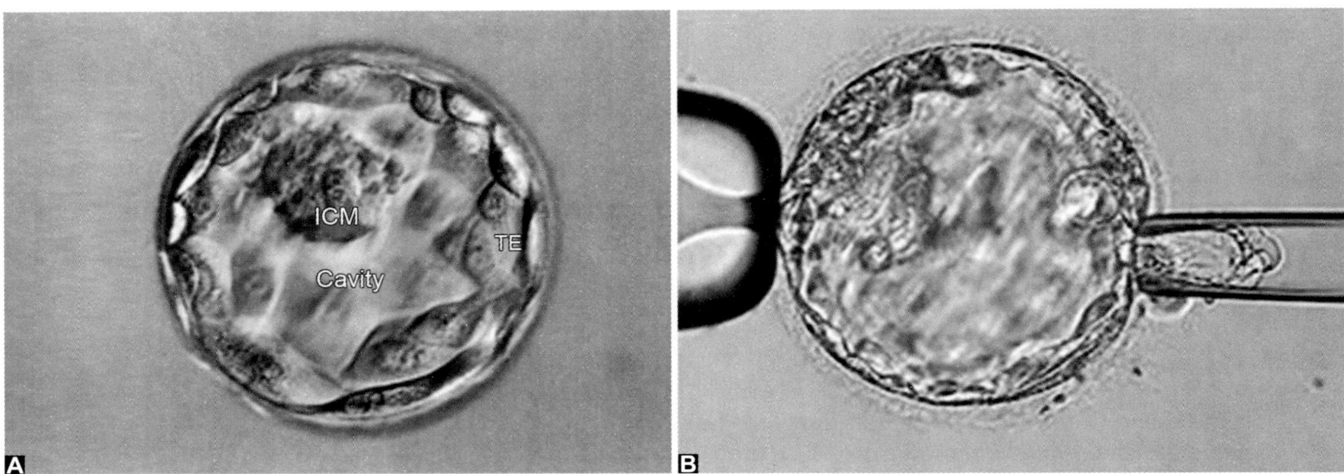

Figs 3A and B Blastocyst and blastocyst biopsy on day 5

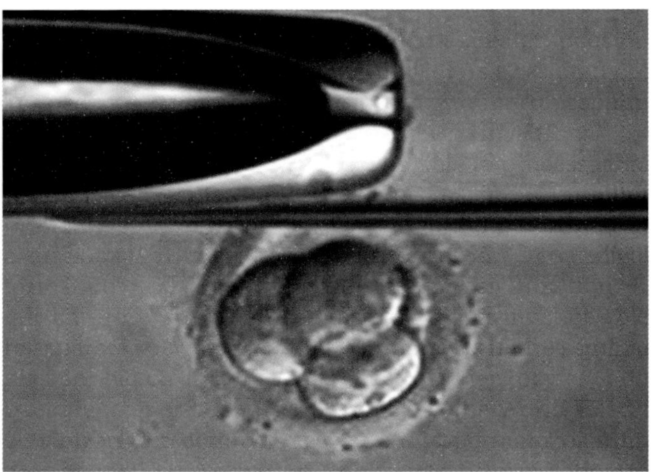

Fig. 4 Mechanical opening (partial zona dissection) by glass microneedle

rubbing against the holding pipette creating a slit-type opening. A modification of "three-dimensional partial zona dissection" was developed, in which a second intersecting slit is made at a right angle to the first, creating a flap opening in the ZP. Through this flap, the biopsy pipette can be introduced to remove polar bodies or blastomeres **(Fig. 4)**.

Advantage: No change in pH, or temperature.

Disadvantage: Requires a double tool holder for PZD needle and biopsy pipette. It also requires practice to quickly rotate the oocyte or embryo so that the slit is in focus and in the right position, therefore longer learning curve.

Zona Drilling

Chemical digestion of ZP with acidified Tyrode's solution (pH 2.2–2.4) was first applied to enhance fertilization in the presence of oligospermia.

Technique: The embryo is held in fixed position with holding pipette, and a small micropipette is used to apply acid to the outer surface of the ZP. The embryo is then thoroughly rinsed to remove any residual acidic solution. This procedure allows for a rapid creation of a 20–30 μm opening in the ZP.

Advantage: Does not require expensive equipment.

Disadvantage: Requires considerable skill to create the correct hole size while not exposing the embryo to excessive acid.

Studies have shown considerable intracellular pH changes in oocyte following procedure is unable to compensate acidosis, causing developmental arrest after fertilization. Therefore, zona drilling with acid has never been the method of choice prior to PB biopsy. However, this technique has been widely used for assisted hatching at the cleavage stage. Quick and careful application of the acidic solution followed by thorough rinsing does not seem to have a negative effect on embryo development and has been shown to enhance implantation with selective application for poor-prognosis patients.

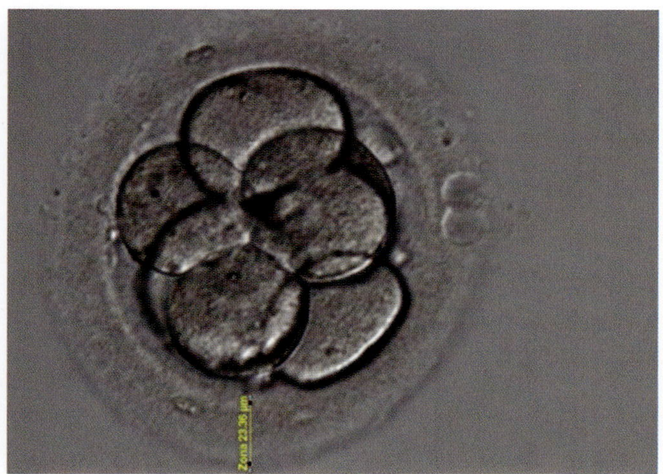

Fig. 5 Laser-assisted breach in zona on day 3 embryo

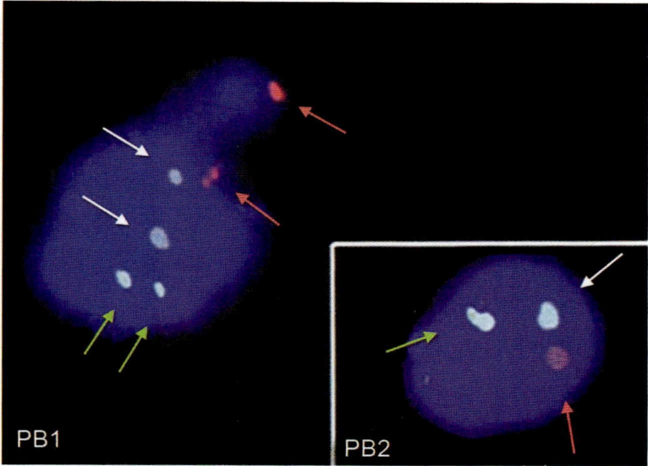

Fig. 6 Fluorescence in situ hybridization pattern in polar body 1 and 2

Laser

The most recently applied method involves the use of a computer-controlled noncontact 1,480 nm infrared diode laser beam. The use of lower laser intensity and more than one pulse could safely generate a sufficiently sized hole for complete hatching. This method is found more accurate and effective and resulted in a greater number of intact blastomeres obtained compared to zona drilling **(Fig. 5)**.

Advantage: The uniformity of the opening with each embryo, reducing operator variability. It requires less time and reducing the time the embryos are outside the incubator.

Disadvantage: Concerns regarding the proper use to avoid heat damage by keeping the firing position of the laser away from the nearest blastomere as well as firing in a row, moving across the ZP from outside to inside in a location adjacent to the largest perivitelline space.

■ POLAR BODY BIOPSY

Polar body biopsy involves the removal of both the PB1 and PB2 in order to make an accurate diagnosis of the oocyte. They can be removed together for aneuploidy testing after fertilization or separately for single gene disorder. In latter, the PB1 is removed shortly after retrieval and PB2 on day 1 after intracytoplasmic sperm injection (ICSI).

Polar body 1 is the by-product of the first meiotic division and normally contains a double signal for each chromosome, each representing a single chromatid on FISH **(Fig. 6)**.

In contrast to PB1, the normal FISH pattern of PB2 is represented by one signal for each chromosome (chromatid).

Advantages

- Use to determine chromosomal aneuploidy related to maternal meiosis.
- Detect maternally derived unbalanced translocation chromosomes.
- Detect single-gene defects in the maternal genome.
- Allow day 3 embryo transfer.
- Polar body is naturally extruded from oocytes as a result of maturation and fertilization; removal of PB1 and PB2, on the other hand, should not have any effect on embryo viability.

Disadvantages

- They provide no information on paternally derived anomalies, even if this constitutes less than 10% of chromosomal errors in preimplantation embryos.
- Due to legislation in some countries, PGD can only be performed prior to syngamy, creating a small window of time in which to complete PB analysis. Because of this constraint, the removal of only first PB, termed "preconception genetic diagnosis" is performed, providing information on the first meiotic division only.
- Moreover, FISH can be difficult and technically demanding to perform on polar bodies due to limitations in the number of chromosomes which can be investigated, requiring several rounds of hybridization.

CLEAVAGE-STAGE EMBRYO BIOPSY

The day 3 embryo biopsy has been the most common method utilized in past two decades. The embryo is totipotent at this stage; each blastomere is capable of developing into an entire organism. Traditionally, blastomeres have been removed using gentle suction from a biopsy pipette with a diameter of 30 μm but more recently by displacement caused by positive pressure generated from the expulsion of medium under the ZP. The optimum number of cells (6–10) required at the time of biopsy so as not to remove a considerable portion of embryonic cell mass with detriment to further development and implantation. For the same reason, the removal of a single blastomere has been found to be less detrimental to blastocyst formation and implantation when compared to the removal of two cells to ensure a more accurate diagnosis.

Cleavage-stage biopsy can be performed with the use of Ca^{2+} or Mg^{2+} free medium, which has been found to ease the removal of a single blastomere with less chance of embryo damage since it allows for the dissociation of blastomeres by loosening the membrane adhesions.

The FISH pattern of blastomeres is represented by two signals for each chromosome tested, so any deviation from this pattern suggests the chromosomal abnormality **(Fig. 7)**.

Advantages

- Blastomere biopsy allows the detection of maternal and paternal genetic contributions for single gene mutations, human leukocyte antigen compatibility, chromosomal rearrangements, and aneuploidy. Paternally derived abnormalities constitute less than 10% of chromosomal errors in preimplantation embryos.
- Single blastomere biopsy is found nondetrimental to further development.

Disadvantages

- Possible embryo cell number reduction, which might have a potential influence on embryo viability. Studies on polarity of the embryo, however, have challenged this dogma, suggesting the removal of even a single cell can be detrimental due to the uneven distribution of mitochondria and regulatory proteins within the cells of the preimplantation embryo. Embryo biopsy has been shown to reduce pyruvate and glucose uptake in biopsied embryos compared to control and results in fewer cells in the embryo at the blastocyst stage. Moreover, it also leaves the embryo fragile and less likely to survive slow freezing methods.
- Its limitation due to a high mosaicism rate in cleaving embryos, particularly when single blastomere is tested. It is the major cause attributed to misdiagnosis. In such cases, normal or viable embryos may be discarded due to false misdiagnosis of aneuploidy.
- In order to allow time for genetic testing and embryo transfer within the same cycle, day 3 embryo biopsy requires subsequent culture to the blastocyst stage, and therefore an excellent blastocyst culture system.
- Some studies reported poor benefit or risk ration, specifically regarding aneuploidy testing and lower rate of implantation and pregnancy rates. This may be due to over-exposure to Ca^{2+} or Mg^{2+} free medium, or due to the removal of more than one blastomere.

BLASTOCYST BIOPSY

Trophectoderm biopsy was explored early in 1990 by Dokras et al. It was not universally applied due to poor pregnancy rates with few embryos reaching the blastocyst stage. Also, extreme tight time constraints do not allow for fresh transfer, requiring cryopreservation and transfer in a future cycle. With the introduction of several key technologies, blastocyst biopsy is now a reality.

- The advancements in embryo culture, low-oxygen and sequential culture systems using chemically defined media formulated to meet the needs of the embryo's metabolism at particular stages has enabled the culture to the blastocyst stage become common practice for many laboratories.

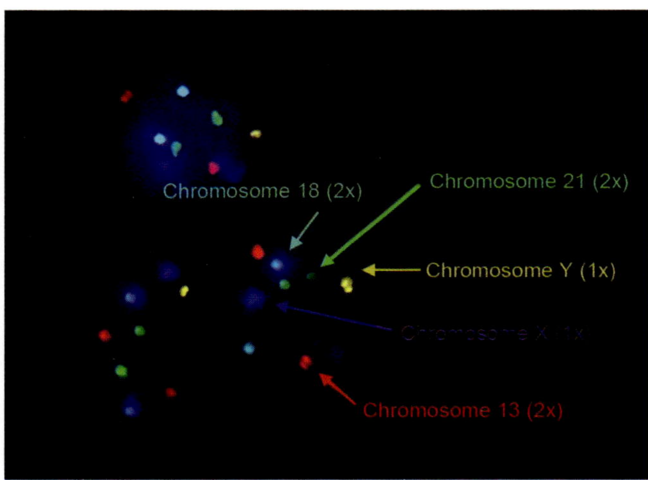

Fig. 7 Fluorescence in situ hybridization pattern of blastomere

- The development of noncontact infrared laser as an effective means of biopsying trophectoderm cells with ease and without negative impacting the viability of human blastocysts.
- The improved method of cryopreservation using vitrification, which allows for biopsied human embryos to be cryopreserved with a high rate of efficiency.
- The appearance of comprehensive chromosomal screening techniques and advanced understanding in genetics, real-time PCR, etc. have all recently been developed to assess all 23 pairs of chromosomes simultaneously from trophectoderm biopsies.

Technique

On day 3 prior to transferring cleavage-stage embryos to extended culture medium, the ZP is breached using a noncontact laser. Trophectoderm cells will herniate through the opening upon further development, formation and expansion of the blastocoel cavity. A small breach in ZP is made in an area of considerable perivitelline space. This is accomplished with 100% power and a 200-µs pulse, creating a hole approximately 5 µm in diameter. This size opening allows for sufficient herniation of the trophectoderm so that approximately four to eight cells can safely be removed on day 5 and 6 without disturbing the inner cell mass.

On the day 5, blastocyst development is assessed and the expanding blastocyst undergoes trophectoderm biopsy. After biopsy is complete, each blastocyst is individually rinsed in equilibrated blastocyst medium and placed in separate appropriately labeled organ culture dishes for further culture until vitrification is performed. The FISH pattern applies to blastocyst analysis is the same as blastomere pattern.

Advantages

- The negative impact on embryonic cell mass is greatly reduced as a smaller fraction of cells is removed from the developing embryo.
- It has an advantage of analyzing not one, but a group of cells for aneuploidy testing, obviating the problem of mosaicism, at least to some extent.
- It can also be utilized for single gene mutation analysis. Removal of several cells for single gene disorders may alleviate the problem of failed amplification and allele dropout in PCR-based protocols due to increased amount of deoxyribonucleic acid (DNA) template and therefore may reduce the potential for misdiagnosis and uninformative outcome.
- This can also be applied to embryos previously frozen at the blastocyst stage; the ZP is breached immediately after thawing, before the embryo has a chance to fully re-expand.
- Fewer embryos progress to the blastocyst stage, even in the best culture systems, and as a result there are fewer embryos requiring biopsy.
- Unlike PB biopsy, assessment of the trophectoderm allows for an assessment of both the maternal and paternal contribution to the embryo's chromosomal status.
- Unlike cleavage-stage biopsy, the presence of several cells in the biopsied material allows for a larger DNA template to work with and therefore a better chance to get an accurate result and fewer embryos with "no result" outcome with the trophectoderm biopsy.
- Trophectoderm cells have shown similar genetic pattern as developing embryo and can give accurate diagnosis.

Disadvantages

- Excellent blastocyst culture system is required. High-quality sequential culture media with oil overlay and 5% oxygen gas phase is a critical component of success. The use of modified neonatal isolette to maintain temperature and pH. A Ca^{2+}/Mg^{2+} free medium is not required.
- Blastocyst cryopreservation facilities such as blastocyst vitrification are required because chromosomal analysis (i.e. full embryonic karyotype) can take 2 to 4 weeks.
- Noncontact laser is required to breach zona.

■ CHROMOSOMAL ANEUPLOIDIES

The majority of chromosomal abnormalities originate from female meiosis, and according to DNA polymorphism studies, derives mainly from meiosis I. Common trisomies were shown to increase with maternal age, which may be due to the age-related reduction of meiotic recombination. In a large study 52% of oocytes were found aneuploid for chromosomes 13, 16, 18, 21 and 22 in women of 35 years or older. Overall 41.8% oocytes had meiosis I errors and 37.3% had meiosis II errors. The peri-implantation embryos show 60% aneuploidy rate. More than 40% of abnormal oocytes from women of advanced reproductive age were found to have complex errors, including an error of the same chromosome in both meiotic divisions (meiosis I and II) (21.5%), or an error of different chromosomes (78.5%), which may also be due to spindle formation errors.

As PB1 and PB2 have no biological significance in development of embryo, their removal and testing may become useful tool in ART to identify the aneuploidy-free oocytes with the highest potential for establishing viable pregnancies and thus improving IVF efficiency.

To perform PGD for chromosomal aneuploidies both PB1 and PB2 are removed simultaneously the next day after insemination of the matured oocytes or ICSI, and analyzed by FISH. PB1 contains a double signal, each representing single chromatid. Accordingly, in case of meiosis I error, instead of a double signal, four different patterns may be observed:

1. *No signal*: Chromosome non-disjunction
2. *One signal*: Chromatid mis-segregation
3. *Three signals*: Chromatid mis-segregation
4. *Four signals*: Chromosome non-disjunction.

The genotype of the oocytes will, accordingly be opposite to the PB1 genotype, i.e. missing signals will suggest extra chromosome material in the corresponding oocyte, while an extra signal (or signals) will indicate monosomy or nullisomy status of the tested chromosome.

The normal FISH pattern of PB2 is one signal for each chromatid, so any deviation from this, such as no signal or two signals suggest meiosis II error.

Testing of one and even more blastomeres at the cleavage stage might not represent the actual chromosome number in the embryo with the possibility of misdiagnosis due to mosaicism. The diagnostic accuracy may be improved by combination of PB and blastomere testing.

CHROMOSOMAL TRANSLOCATIONS

Because carriers of translocations have an extremely poor pregnancy outcome, translocations have been one of the most important indications for PGD, which was first performed by PB1 analysis. However, because without PB2 the meiotic outcome of translocations cannot be accurately established, interphase blastomere analysis was used in most cases. The available data after PGD for translocation show normal/balanced embryos were available for transfer in 69% of the clinical cycles with 35% clinical pregnancy rate. The clinical outcome is poorer in reciprocal than in Robertsonian translocations, with pregnancy rates of 23% and 33% respectively. The presence of high frequency of mosaicism in cleavage stage still presents problems for diagnosis even with application of combination of commercially available probes. Therefore, for maternally derived translocations the PGD strategy may still be based on PB1 and PB2 testing, applying the blastomere technique only if further testing is required. It is also observed that embryos with unbalanced chromosome complements have the potential to reach the blastocyst stage in extended culture, suggesting some of the detected chromosomal rearrangements may not be lethal, explaining an extremely high spontaneous abortion rate in couples carrying translocations.

Because PGD is practically the only hope for couples with translocations to have an unaffected child without fear of repeated spontaneous abortions, increasing numbers of PGD cycles for this indication have been performed. PGD will permit these couples to establish pregnancies which are unaffected from the onset and offer them the opportunity to have children of their own, instead of multiple unsuccessful attempts of prenatal diagnosis and subsequent termination of pregnancy.

BLASTOCYST TRANSFER FOLLOWING BIOPSY

The pituitary is downregulated with gonadotropin-releasing hormone agonist in previous cycle with oral contraceptive pills. The estrogen tablet or transdermal patches can be used on 3rd day of bleeding. When the adequate endometrial thickness is achieved and serum estradiol levels are appropriate, progesterone is started either intramuscularly or vaginally to make the endometrium "in phase" with embryo stage. On the 6th day of progesterone administration, the blastocyst-stage embryos, which have been deemed chromosomally normal after genetic testing, are warmed and transferred. Generally, no more than two blastocysts are transferred at any one time due to their high implantation rates.

Embryo survival after biopsy, vitrification, and warming was found excellent (97%). To date, 100 live births and many more ongoing pregnancies are under way. Of all embryos biopsied, about half were diagnosed as aneuploid, and in 10% diagnosis was not obtained.

IMPACT OF PGD ON IVF OUTCOME

Although more data has to be collected to exclude short-term and/or long-term side effects completely, the data currently available show no evidence of any detrimental effect of PB, blastomere or blastocyst biopsy. Overall PGD for aneuploidy has been applied in more than 5,000 clinical cycles, and resulted in the birth of at least 1,000 unaffected children, showing a comparable prevalence of congenital abnormalities to that in the general population, which suggests that there is no detrimental effect of any of the biopsy procedures mentioned above.

Preimplantation genetic diagnosis for chromosomal aneuploidy contribute to an improvement of the pregnancy outcome of IVF patients of advanced reproductive age, poor-prognosis patients, including those with repeated IVF failures and repeated spontaneous abortions. However, an improvement of the outcome of PGD may be expected only when the number of embryos biopsied is equal to or higher than the number of embryos expected to be replaced without PGD.

In one study, implantation, spontaneous abortions and take-home baby rates were analyzed before and after PGD in different cycles of same patients; implantation rates appeared to be significantly improved, 7.2% without PGD in contrast to 34.8% after PGD. Six-fold reductions in spontaneous abortion rate in patients with translocation, take-home baby rate was 11.5% before PGD and 79.4% after PGD application.

■ CONCLUSION

- There are many factors which play a role in the success of performing biopsy procedures for PGD
  - A high quality culture system capable of development to the blastocyst stage
  - The developmental stage of the sampled material which will provide the information
  - The manner in which the ZP is breached
  - The amount of material to be removed in order to obtain sufficient information without detriment to the embryo
  - A successful cryopreservation method allowing for embryo transfer in subsequent nonstimulated cycle.
- Fewer embryos progress to the blastocyst stage, even in the best culture systems, and as a result there are fewer embryos requiring blastocyst-stage biopsy. The fact that an embryo has developed to the blastocyst stage reflects its quality and hardiness and perhaps a higher tolerance for biopsy when compare to biopsy on day 1 or 3 of embryo development.
- Unlike PB biopsy, assessment of the trophectoderm allows for an assessment of both the maternal and paternal contribution to the embryo's chromosomal status.

- Unlike cleavage-stage biopsy, the presence of several cells in the biopsied material allows for a larger DNA template to work with and therefore a better chance to get an accurate result and fewer embryos with "no result" outcome with the trophectoderm biopsy.
- Mosaicism is thought to be less of problem at the blastocyst stage as compared to the cleavage stage since several cells are analyzed, reducing the chance of missing mosaicism.
- Couples with previous IVF failures can be effectively assessed with blastocyst culture and trophectoderm aneuploidy screening. If these patients fail to achieve blastocyst development in an excellent sequential culture system in addition to previously failed day 3 embryo transfers, their cause of IVF failure is self-evident. If blastocyst formation does occur, aneuploidy screening will determine whether any of the embryos developing are in fact chromosomally normal. If chromosomally normal blastocysts are obtained and implantation continues to fail, a uterine factor must be considered. The diagnostic potential allows patients to move onto appropriate therapies such as egg donation or the use of a gestational carrier.
- The continuous emphasis on single-embryo transfer to avoid multiple pregnancies, low birth weight babies and congenital malformations demands clinicians and embryologists to determine which single embryo has the greatest developmental potential. Blastocyst culture, trophectoderm biopsy and chromosomal screening guide to this goal.
- It may be predicted that PGD will soon become standard practice for IVF patients of advanced reproductive age. It cannot be excluded that preselection of aneuploidy-free embryos may appear of even higher value for younger IVF patients, because of the higher number of oocytes available for testing. This may contribute to improving overall standards of ART, by substituting the present practice of selection of embryos for transfer using morphological parameters with the preselection of chromosomally normal embryos with a higher potential of resulting in a normal pregnancy.

28 Assisted Hatching of Human Embryos

Sunita R Tandulwadkar, Devika Chopra

■ INTRODUCTION

According to the World Health Organization (WHO), one in six couples experience delay in conception and an increasing number of patients require assisted conception procedures of in vitro fertilization (IVF) and/or intracytoplasmic sperm injection (ICSI).[1] However, despite many developments in the field of assisted reproduction, the implantation rate per embryo transfer is 10–15% for day 2 or day 3 transfers and 23–25% for blastocyst transfers.[1] The success of embryo implantation depends upon the intricate relationship between the transferred embryo and endometrium. The implantation potential of an embryo depends upon the quality of the originating gametes, intrinsic chromosomal composition and the quality of its cytoplasm and cytoskeletal elements.[2] Implantation failure following IVF/ICSI may have many causative factors including poor embryo quality, poor uterine receptivity or lower rate of hatching of the zona pellucida (ZP) following embryo culture.[3]

More recently, the failure of ZP to rupture following blastocyst formation has emerged as an important cause of lowered implantation rates observed following IVF or ICSI. Elasticity and thinning of the ZP are essential for embryo hatching process and its implantation, both of which can be adversely influenced by advancing maternal age, in vitro culture conditions or the freezing-thawing process.[4] An emerging technique known as assisted hatching (AH) has been proposed as a method for improving the implantation potential of embryos.[1] The AH involves the artificial disruption of the ZP and various techniques such as zona thinning, zona drilling and complete removal of the zona (using chemicals, lasers and mechanical techniques) have been developed.[5] This chapter will focus on the different techniques that are in use currently for AH and their importance in recent assisted reproductive technology (ART) practice.

■ STRUCTURE AND FUNCTION OF ZONA PELLUCIDA

The ZP is an extracellular matrix glycoprotein layer that surrounds the oocyte and has multiple functions.[6] The ZP is mainly composed of three major proteins namely, ZP1, ZP2, ZP3 **(Fig. 1)**.[3] ZP1 provides structural integrity to the embryo whereas ZP2 is species-specific and prevents polyspermy.[3] ZP3 initiates the acrosomal reaction of the bound spermatozoa.[3] Prior to fertilization, the ZP permits only acrosome intact sperm to fertilize the oocyte and prevents polyspermy.[7] After the embryo formation, the zona maintains the integrity of the same and facilitates the free passage of the embryo through the Fallopian tube. The ZP acts as a protective barrier and prevents infection of the embryo by bacterial and fungal agents in the reproductive tract.[6] Additionally, it prevents the separation of dividing blastomeres in cleaving embryos.[6]

Following sperm fusion with the oocyte, cortical granules within the oocyte release their contents into the perivitelline space in an event termed "cortical reaction".[8] This reaction alters the properties of the ZP and cause the ZP to become refractory to sperm binding and penetration.[8] This "zona hardening" process after fertilization involves inactivation of sperm receptors and an increased ZP resistance to dissolution by a variety of agents including heat, proteases, reducing agents and low pH.[8] The hardening of the ZP that occurs in IVF cycles is due to suboptimal culture media, advancing age in vivo, increased hormonal stimulation and smoking. At the ultrastructure level, this occurs due to the cross-linking of its component glycoproteins. In the absence of any other qualitative definition to label a "hardened" ZP, a thickness of more than 15 μm is considered as a thick zona and may require intervention to "assist" implantation. About 15% of cases have ZP thickness of more than 15 μm.[9]

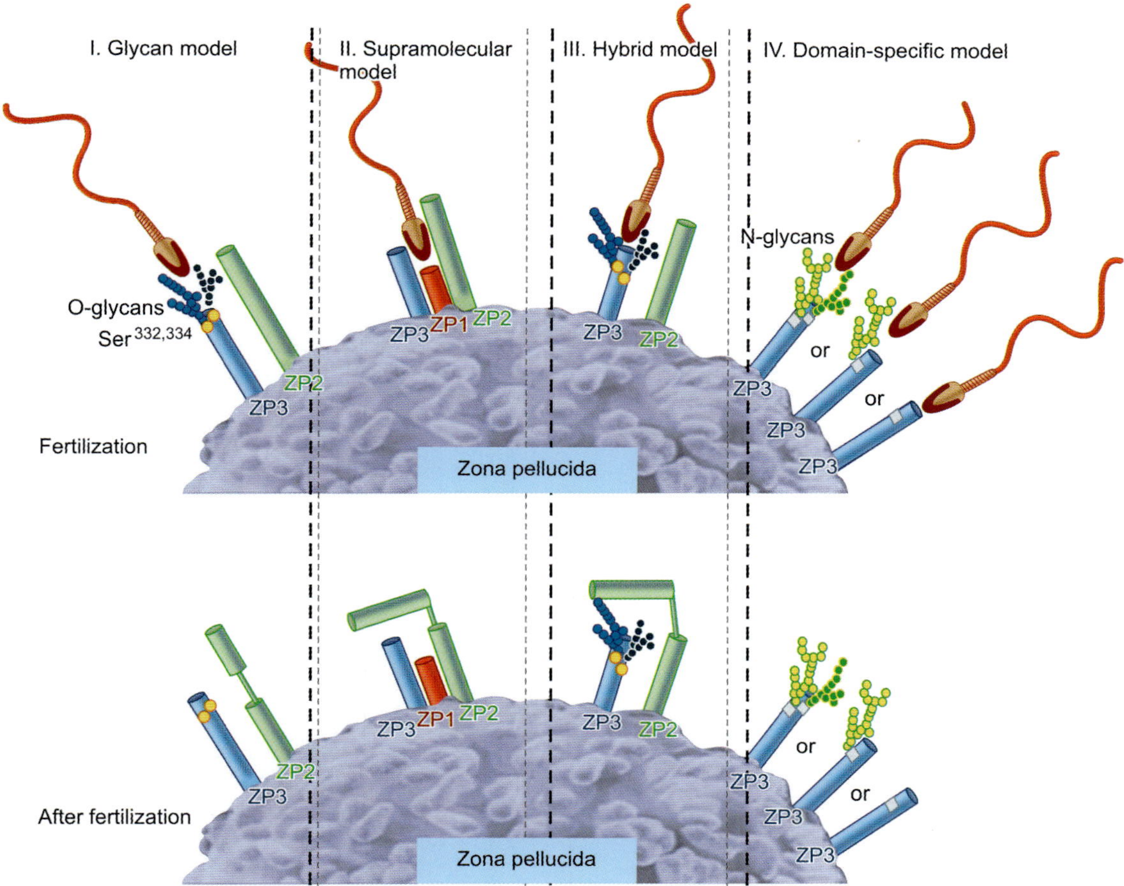

Fig. 1 Putative models of sperm-zona pellucida binding. (I) The glycan model proposes that sperm binding is initiated via O-linked glycans that are attached at residues Ser^{332} and Ser^{334} of ZP3. After fertilization, these residues are deglycosylated thereby preventing further sperm adhesion; (II) The supramolecular structure model is based on the premise that the physical structure of the matrix formed by the three ZP glycoproteins is critical for the binding of sperm. Following fertilization, ZP2 is processed in such a way that it prevents further sperm adhesion; (III) The hybrid model incorporates aspects of both the glycan model and the supramolecular model and proposes that O-linked glycosylation is a critical determinant of sperm recognition. However, the key O-glycans reside on residues other than Ser^{332} and Ser^{334}. Furthermore, the modification of ZP2 that accompanies fertilization renders these O-glycans inaccessible to sperm; (IV) In contrast, the domain-specific model proposes that sperm bind with a variety of N-linked glycans attached to ZP3 and/or the peptide backbone of the glycoprotein depending upon its glycosylation status

■ INDICATIONS FOR ASSISTED HATCHING

The localized thinning of the ZP is an important step in cleaving embryos that helps in the implantation process. Embryos that have uniform ZP without any localized thinning are less likely to implant.[9,10] It is also proposed that this inability to implant is usually associated with zona resilience rather than its actual thickness. Zona manipulation in order to decrease its resilience or drilling a hole into the ZP in order to facilitate its implantation is the rationale behind AH. Additionally, AH may overcome a deficiency in the production of an embryonic lysin/hatching factor that promotes hatching following blastocyst expansion.[11] Zona manipulation/AH in some form can be offered in the following cases:[9]

- Elderly women (age >35 years)[12]
- Women with high follicle-stimulating hormone (FSH) levels
- Oocytes undergoing in vitro maturation
- Prior to embryo transfer in frozen thaw cycles
- Following recurrent implantation failure.

MECHANISM OF ASSISTED HATCHING

There are many explanations which postulate the mechanism by which AH promotes embryo implantation; although, the exact mechanism remains unclear. The implantation window is a critical period wherein the precise synchronization between embryos and endometrium is essential. Most embryos hatch during this implantation window.

Embryos with artificial gaps in their ZP initiate hatching earlier than zonae intact embryos.[13] Therefore, AH may facilitate implantation by increasing embryo-endometrium contact. A two-way transport of metabolites and growth factors across the ZP is facilitated by the artificial gap. These nutrients enhance embryo development and blastocyst formation.[1]

TECHNIQUES OF ASSISTED HATCHING

Since the first AH technique introduced in 1980s, several approaches have been proposed to assist zona thinning. These techniques are:

- Mechanical incision of the ZP[13]
- Chemical zona drilling with acidic medium[14]
- Chemical zona thinning[15]
- Laser-assisted hatching (LAH)[16]
- Piezo micromanipulation.[17]

The mechanical and the chemical methods of AH are extremely tedious and require skilled precision to produce uniform, well controlled and standardized micro holes.[1] AH is usually performed on after day 2 once the adherence between the blastomeres has increased.

Mechanical Techniques

The first mechanical technique of AH was described by Cohen et al. and it was named as partial zona dissection (PZD).[14] The process involves holding the embryo gently by suction using the holding pipette. The microneedle first pierces the embryo and is then advanced tangentially at the largest perivitelline space in the ZP until it pierces the ZP again **(Figs 2A to H)**. The embryo is then released from the holding pipette and held by the microneedle. The small part of the ZP trapped against the microneedle is rubbed against the holding pipette, thus opening the area between the two sides pierced by the microneedle. The mechanism of PZD is quick to perform but there is variability in the holes produced by this method which is not always optimal.[18]

Another technique known as "three-dimensional PZD" has been described wherein a second cut is made in the ZP under the first at a right angle leaving a cross shaped hole on the ZP.[19] This technique allows the protection of ZP by flaps of the cruciate incision and at the same time creating a hole in the ZP. Nijs et al. described a technique of rubbing the ZP with the microneedle and reducing the ZP matrix thickness. There is no gap in the ZP thereby preventing loss of blastomeres.[20] However, care should be taken at the time of multiple embryo transfers as AH can result in multiple pregnancies.[20]

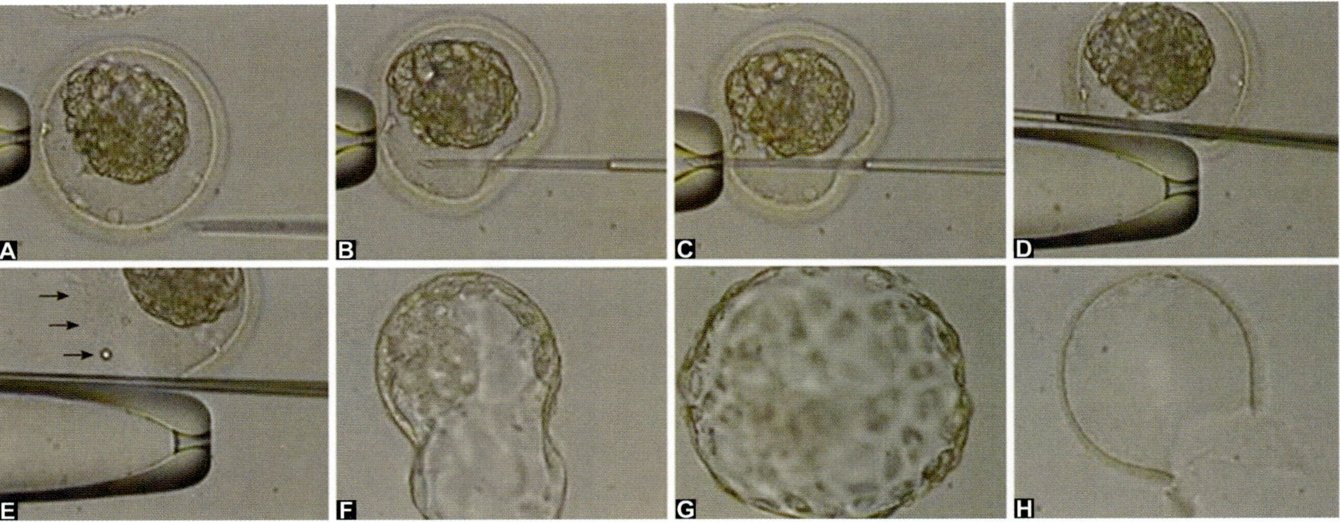

Figs 2A to H The process of partial zona dissection (PZD)

Mechanically Expanding the ZP

In a study by Cong et al. (2010), a technique of mechanically expanding the ZP using hydrostatic pressure was described. This type of AH neither thins nor breached the ZP rather it expands the embryo and stretches the ZP via injected hydrostatic pressure. It was observed that a higher clinical pregnancy rate was obtained by this technique compared to controls.[21]

Chemical Techniques

Assisted hatching using acid Tyrode's was described by Cohen et al.[14] The embryo is held by the holding pipette and acid Tyrode's solution is preloaded in the microneedle. The suction is controlled by mouth suction and acidic solution is expelled slowly over a small area (blastomere free) until the ZP is breached **(Fig. 3)**. Suction is immediately applied after breaching the ZP in order to prevent excess acid entering the perivitelline space. This technique requires very quick handling and precision in order to avoid exposure of the embryos to the acidic solution.

Cruciate thinning of the ZP with acid Tyrode's is also described by Tucker et al.[22] This involves biaxial application of the acid to make a cruciate thinning over one-third of the circumference of the ZP. However, Tucker et al. did not find this technique to be effective in human embryos.

Piezo Micromanipulation

Piezo technology involves the use of vibratory movements produced by a piezoelectric pulse for zona drilling **(Fig. 4)**.[17] The vibratory pulses are generated by a controller and are used to carve a conical area in the ZP. Five to eight applications in adjacent areas are required to produce a large hole, which facilitates hatching of the embryo.[17]

■ LASER-ASSISTED HATCHING

In 1991, two groups Tadir and Palanker separately described the procedure of LAH.[23,24] The laser hole may be drilled in a contact mode or in a noncontact mode using an optical lens tangential to the embryo. The laser presents an ideal tool for zona hatching as the energy is focused directly on a targeted area producing a precise constant hole without interoperator variation. The contact mode of LAH uses ultraviolet (UV) laser delivered by a glass pipette or infrared (IR) laser delivered with a quartz fiber. However, the advantage of a noncontact mode and the potential of UV radiation to cause damage to the embryo have made the noncontact IR 1.48 µm diode laser the preferred method of LAH **(Fig. 5)**.[25]

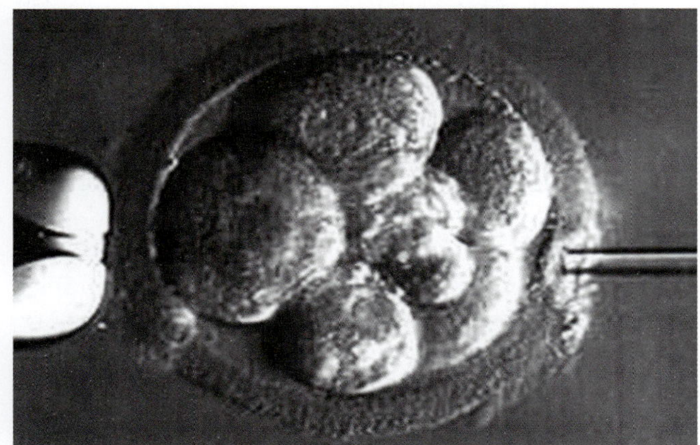

Fig. 3 Assisted hatching using acid Tyrode's solution

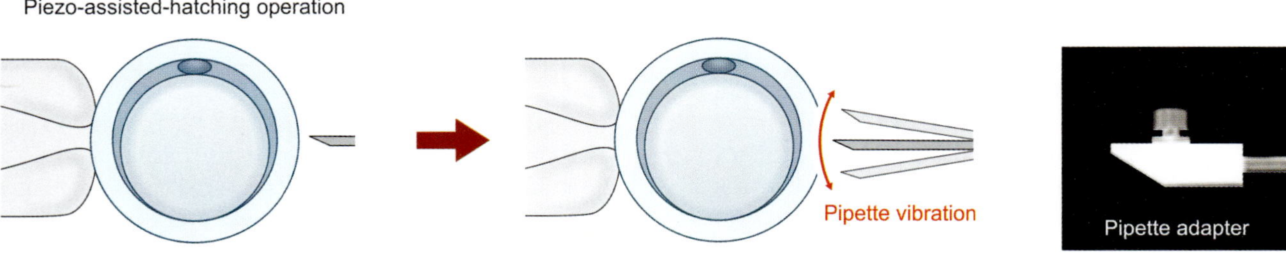

Fig. 4 Piezo-assisted hatching

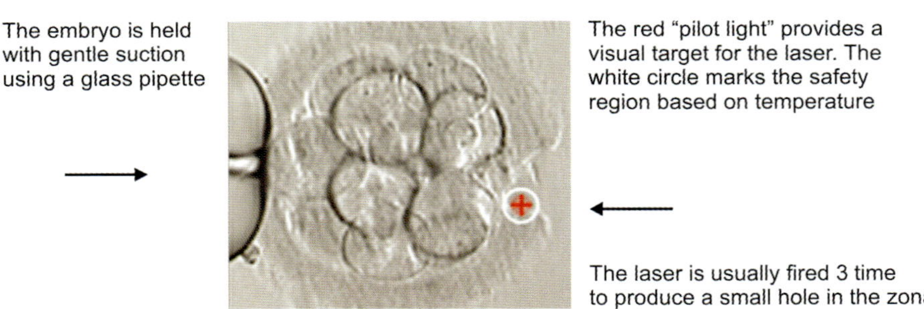

Fig. 5 Laser-assisted hatching

Initially, a full thickness hole was made using LAH. Recently, however, zona thinning without creating a hole in the ZP has shown to demonstrate a significant increase in hatching in vitro.[26,27] LAH of the ZP can be done with high precision and repeatability with no negative impact on embryo development. Both light and scanning electron microscopy revealed no ultrastructural degenerative alterations of the ZP.[1]

REVIEW OF LITERATURE

A meta-analysis performed by Martins et al. (2011) revealed that AH was related to an increased clinical pregnancy and multiple pregnancy rates in women with repeated implantation failure or in frozen thaw cycles (RR: 1.1, 95% CI: 1.00–1.24).[7] Additionally, they also concluded that AH was unlikely to improve clinical pregnancy rates when performed in fresh embryos or in unselected/poor prognosis women or in women with advanced age (RR: 1.03, 95% CI: 0.91–1.16).[7] Their study, however, could not provide a firm conclusion with regards to miscarriage or live birth rates due to the small sample evaluated by their pool of included studies.[7] In a retrospective cohort study of 22,949 cycles from 2004 to 2011 in USA, Butts et al. reported that AH was associated with a lower live birth rate in women with diminished ovarian reserve when compared to non-AH cycles.[28]

A 2009 Cochrane reviewing 28 trials that were described in 25 publications concluded that there was no difference in live birth rate following AH (7 trials; OR: 1.1, 95% CI: 0.83–1.55). Only the clinical pregnancy rate was higher after AH versus no AH (28 trials, OR: 1.3, 95% CI: 1.12–1.49).[29]

In 2008, the practice committee of the American Society for Reproductive Medicine (ASRM) recommended that individual ART programs needed to evaluate their own patient populations in order to improve their ART success rates and that the routine performance of AH in the treatment of all IVF patients was unwarranted.[30] In 2014, a Level C recommendation by the ASRM was that AH should not be practiced in all patients undergoing IVF.[31]

RISKS ASSOCIATED WITH ASSISTED HATCHING

A hole in the ZP deprives the embryo of its protective coat and may expose the embryo to microorganisms within the reproductive tract. Blastomeres may get trapped in the hole in the ZP, which may cause a failure of the hatching process.[4] LAH and acid Tyrode's used in chemical hatching may cause lethal damage to the growing embryo and reduce embryo viability. Additionally, handling of the ZP may increase the risk of monozygotic twinning.[20] Embryonic death, vesiculization and loss of blastomeres are other complications of AH.[14]

Monozygotic twinning after AH may occur due to two reasons. Trapping of the blastomeres after AH may cause a figure 8 shape of the hatching embryo. Subsequent subdivision of the embryo may result in monozygotic twins. The second reason is premature hatching of the blastomeres which may result in the development of an identical embryo. Thus, AH involves techniques that require highly skilled operators and precision.

CONCLUSION

There are several techniques that are currently in use to assist hatching, which differ both in efficacy and risks. LAH has the lowest procedural risk and is relatively easier to perform with consistency between operators. However, the routine use of AH is inappropriate in view of the lack of evidence suggesting universal benefit of its use. Multicentric trials are required to confirm the safest technique to use and the patients which may benefit before they have several unsuccessful treatment cycles. In conclusion, AH proves a promising intervention that helps ART specialists in treating recurrent implantation failure and can improve clinical pregnancy rates in frozen thaw cycles.

■ REFERENCES

1. Hammadeh ME, Fischer-Hammadeh C, Ali KR. Assisted hatching in assisted reproduction: a state of the art. J Assist Reprod Genet. 2011;28(2):119-28.
2. Huisman GJ, Fauser BC, Eijkemans MJ, et al. Implantation rates after in vitro fertilization and transfer of a maximum of two embryos that have undergone three to five days of culture. Fertil Steril. 2000;73(1):117-22.
3. Nikander E. Assisted hatching. In: Kovacs G, editor. How to Improve Your ART Success Rates: An Evidence based Review of Adjuncts to IVF. Austrailia: Cambridge University press; 2012. p. 1242.
4. Cohen J. Assisted hatching: indications and techniques. Acta Eur Fertil. 1993;24(5):215-9.
5. Balaban B, Urman B, Alatas C, et al. A comparison of four different techniques of assisted hatching. Hum Reprod. 2002;17(5):1239-43.
6. Sifer C, Sellami A, Poncelet C, et al. A prospective randomized study to assess the benefit of partial zona pellucida digestion before frozen-thawed embryo transfers. Hum Reprod. 2006;21(9):2384-9.
7. Martins WP, Rocha IA, Ferriani RA, et al. Assisted hatching of human embryos: a systematic review and meta-analysis of randomized controlled trials. Hum Reprod Update. 2011;17(4):438-53.
8. Boccaccio A, Frassanito MC, Lamberti L, et al. Nanoscale characterization of the biomechanical hardening of bovine zona pellucida. J R Soc Interface. 2012;9(76):2871-82.
9. Das S, Seif MW. Assisted hatching. In: Kovacs G, editor. How to Improve Your ART Success Rates: An Evidence based Review of Adjuncts to IVF: Cambridge University Press; 2011. pp. 156-60.
10. Wright G, Wiker S, Elsner C, et al. Observations on the morphology of pronuclei and nucleoli in human zygotes and implications for cryopreservation. Hum Reprod. 1990;5(1):109-15.
11. Schiewe MC, Hazeleger NL, Sclimenti C, et al. Physiological characterization of blastocyst hatching mechanisms by use of a mouse antihatching model. Fertil Steril. 1995;63(2):288-94.
12. Loret De Mola JR, Garside WT, Bucci J, et al. Analysis of the human zona pellucida during culture: correlation with diagnosis and the preovulatory hormonal environment. J Assist Reprod Genet. 1997;14(6):332-6.
13. Malter HE, Cohen J. Blastocyst formation and hatching in vitro following zona drilling of mouse and human embryos. Gamete Res. 1989;24(1):67-80.
14. Cohen J, Elsner C, Kort H, et al. Impairment of the hatching process following IVF in the human and improvement of implantation by assisting hatching using micromanipulation. Hum Reprod. 1990;5(1):7-13.
15. Khalifa EA, Tucker MJ, Hunt P. Cruciate thinning of the zona pellucida for more successful enhancement of blastocyst hatching in the mouse. Hum Reprod. 1992;7(4):532-6.
16. Miyata H, Matsubayashi H, Fukutomi N, et al. Relevance of the site of assisted hatching in thawed human blastocysts: a preliminary report. Fertil Steril. 2010;94(6):2444-7.
17. Nakayama T, Fujiwara H, Yamada S, et al. Clinical application of a new assisted hatching method using a piezo-micro-manipulator for morphologically low-quality embryos in poor-prognosis infertile patients. Fertil Steril. 1999;71(6):1014-8.
18. Cohen J, Feldberg D. Effects of the size and number of zona pellucida openings on hatching and trophoblast outgrowth in the mouse embryo. Mol Reprod Dev. 1991;30(1):70-8.
19. Cieslak J, Ivakhnenko V, Wolf G, et al. Three-dimensional partial zona dissection for preimplantation genetic diagnosis and assisted hatching. Fertil Steril. 1999;71(2):308-13.
20. Nijs M, Vanderzwalmen P, Segal-Bertin G, et al. A monozygotic twin pregnancy after application of zona rubbing on a frozen-thawed blastocyst. Hum Reprod. 1993;8(1):127-9.
21. Fang C, Li T, Miao BY, et al. Mechanically expanding the zona pellucida of human frozen thawed embryos: a new method of assisted hatching. Fertil Steril. 2010;94(4):1302-7.
22. Tucker M, Luecke N, Wiker S, et al. Chemical removal of the outside of the zona pellucida of day 3 human embryos has no impact on implantation rate. J Assist Reprod and Genet. 1993;10(3):187-91.
23. Tadir Y. Ten years of laser assisted gametes and embryo manipulation. Contemp Ob/Gyn. 1998;9:2-10.
24. Palanker D, Ohad S, Lewis A, et al. Technique for cellular microsurgery using the 193-nm excimer laser. Lasers Surg Med. 1991;11(6):580-6.
25. Rink K, Delacretaz G, Salathe RP, et al. Non-contact microdrilling of mouse zona pellucida with an objective-delivered 1.48-microns diode laser. Lasers Surg Med. 1996;18(1):52-62.
26. Moser M, Ebner T, Sommergruber M, et al. Laser-assisted zona pellucida thinning prior to routine ICSI. Hum Reprod. 2004;19(3):573-8.
27. Blake DA, Forsberg AS, Johansson BR, et al. Laser zona pellucida thinning—an alternative approach to assisted hatching. Hum Reprod. 2001;16(9):1959-64.
28. Butts SF, Owen C, Mainigi M, et al. Assisted hatching and intracytoplasmic sperm injection are not associated with improved outcomes in assisted reproduction cycles for diminished ovarian reserve: an analysis of cycles in the United States from 2004 to 2011. Fertil Steril. 2014;102(4):1041-7.e1.
29. Das S, Blake D, Farquhar C, et al. Assisted hatching on assisted conception (IVF and ICSI). Cochrane Database Syst Rev. 2009(2):Cd001894.
30. The role of assisted hatching in in vitro fertilization: a review of the literature. A Committee opinion. Fertil Steril. 2008; 90(5 Suppl):S196-8.
31. Role of assisted hatching in in vitro fertilization: a guideline. Fertil Steril. 2014;102(2):348-51.

Culture of Embryos and Transfer

29 Culture and Evaluation of Embryos: From Fertilization to Transfer

Rajvi H Mehta

INTRODUCTION

Assisted reproductive technologies (ARTs) have now become a routine modality of treating infertility. The success of any ART programs depends upon multiple factors ranging from the *intrinsic factors* like the age of the couple, the cause of infertility, response to ovarian stimulation and the quality of the gametes; to the *extrinsic factors* like the skills of the ART specialists and embryologists; the culture laboratory and culture conditions which in term determine the quality of the embryos that are available for transfer.

To a great extent, the ART laboratory aims at mimicking the endogenous environment of the Fallopian tube as well as the uterus. This is achieved by creating an optimal laboratory environment in terms of the culture media and culture conditions. Good healthy gametes in good culture media under good laboratory conditions can give good healthy embryos. However, even the best gametes cannot lead to good embryos if the media and culture conditions are compromised.

CULTURE MEDIA FOR ART

In the early days of ART, embryos were cultured in a variety of culture media such as simple salt solutions like Earle's Balanced Salt Solution (EBSS) or the complex Ham's F-10—media that were conventionally used for tissue culture. However, it was soon realized that the nutritional requirements of gametes differed from cell lines and attempts were made to formulate culture media based on the composition of human tubal fluid.[1]

Another approach that led to the evolution of human ART culture media was to understand the metabolism of human embryos and then specifically formulate media as per the nutritional requirements of the embryos. The evidence that the nutritional requirements of human embryos varies with the stage of development led to the concept of using different types of media for cleavage stage embryos and blastocysts.[2,3] This is now commonly termed as sequential culture. Biggers put forth the concept of "let the embryo choose" wherein a single culture medium is provided and the embryo "chooses" the nutrients that it requires.[4]

In the early days of ART, most laboratories prepared their own culture media either from dehydrated formulations or by individually adding the different components which constituted the medium. However, this led to a lot of batch-to-batch variation with the biggest "culprit" being the quality of water that was used. This batch-to-batch variation often led to the differences in the outcome of IVF.

Now, almost all ART laboratories depend on ready-to-use culture media which are commercially available. These media have their own quality control assessments which reduce the batch-to-batch variations. However, the limitation of these media would be the transit time from the manufacturing unit, the source, to the ART laboratory. The cold chain maintenance is crucial during the transportation from the manufacturing unit to the laboratory lest the components degrade in transit! It is not merely the transportation time from country to country but also the time taken to clear local import and customs regulations!

BASIC COMPOSITION OF CULTURE MEDIA FOR ART

The basic formulation of any ART culture media would be carbohydrates such as glucose, lactate any pyruvate; amino acids and proteins and buffering systems. Some media contain additional growth factors and vitamins. Antibiotics like gentamycin are added for prophylactic purposes along with pH indicators like phenol red to "alert" the embryologist of any drastic changes to the pH.

Carbohydrates

A vascular perfused preparation of the Fallopian tube was developed as a model to study the formation and composition of human tubal fluid. These studies revealed that the concentration of glucose and pyruvate were very low (approximately between 0.17 mM and 0.53 mM) while that of lactate were 8 mM.[5] When the concentration of these metabolites were measured in the Fallopian tube and the uterus in naturally cycling women, it was observed that pyruvate in the oviduct did not vary with the day of cycle, the mean value was 0.24 mM. Lactate and glucose concentrations varied with the day of cycle; lactate increasing from 4.87 mM in the follicular phase to 10.50 mM at the time of ovulation, whereas glucose decreased from 3.11 mM in the follicular phase to 0.50 mM midcycle and subsequently increased to 2.32 mM in the luteal phase. The concentrations of pyruvate, lactate and glucose in uterine fluid remained constant throughout the cycle (0.10, 5.87 and 3.15 mM, respectively).[6]

Site	Cycle phase	Pyruvate (mM)	Lactate (mM)	Glucose (mM)
Fallopian tube	Mid cycle	0.32	10.5	0.5
Uterus	Other phases	0.1	5.9	3.2

Glucose is the major energy substrate in the oviduct and is utilized by the tube for events such as secretory activity, muscular and ciliary movement of the tube. These studies suggested that an optimal culture media formulation for human IVF especially those supporting the development of zygotes to cleavage stage embryos should have low glucose and higher concentration of lactate which is in sync with the environment in the Fallopian tube where zygotes develop into cleavage stage embryos.

Proteins and Amino Acids

Both essential and non-essential amino acids are added to culture media. The amino acids that are added vary from formulation to formulation. The amino acids serve as a substrate during protein synthesis especially when the embryonic genome takes over. Some amino acids also act as a source of energy while they also act as buffers.

Glutamine is found to be an absolutely essential component for media. A higher proportion of embryos reached the morula (89% vs 68%, respectively) and blastocyst (71% vs 54%, respectively) stages when cultured with glutamine compared with embryos cultured

without glutamine.[7] Glutamine plays multiple roles. It acts as a source of energy by entering the tricarboxylic acid (TCA) cycle generating several molecules of adenosine triphosphate in the process; it also works as an osmolyte which protects the embryos from the high salt concentrations; it is a carrier of the amine group, which is necessary for the synthesis of ADP, RNA, DNA, amino acids as well as proteins. Deamination of glutamine results in the generation of glutamic acid which serves as a precursor for the other amino acids.

Despite the "benefits" of using amino acids, one has to be cautious as many amino acids break down to ammonia which can be toxic to embryos.[8] To minimize ammonium generation in the culture media, these should not be preincubated for more than 72 hours.

Glutamine and alanine are some of the most labile of the amino acids. It is advisable to use media containing glutamine in its more stable form as alanyl glutamine. And, instead of adding alanine to the media, one can optimize by using pyruvate which breaks down to alanine.

Proteins such as human serum albumin, recombinant albumin or synthetic serum substitute which consists of albumin and macroglobulins are also added to culture media.

Antibiotics

As the culture media are in rich in nutrients—they can also "nourish" contaminating microorganisms either from the environment or in some instances from semen. Therefore, the culture medium is supplemented with antibiotics as a prophylactic measure. The most preferred antibiotic is gentamycin as it is a broad spectrum antibiotic; acts on the mycoplasma which can contaminate semen and does not lead to allergic reactions as compared with antibiotic like penicillin.

Buffers

As the embryos are very sensitive to changes in pH, excellent buffering systems are required to maintain the pH in the culture media. The two most commonly used buffering systems are the sodium bicarbonate and HEPES (2-hydroxyethyl piperazine-N-2-ethanesulfonic acid) buffering system. The former is used for embryo culture while the latter is more common in the media used for sperm preparation. Media containing sodium bicarbonate buffering system should always be pre-equilibrated in a CO_2 incubator so that the medium achieves the desired pH.

pH Indicators

As the medium is very susceptible to pH changes, a pH indicator aids in detecting any major changes in pH. For example, if there is any contamination of the medium then the color of the medium would turn yellow. On the other hand, if there is a drop in the CO_2 levels then the color of the medium would change to dark pink. These pH indicators are not indicative of minor pH changes which are crucial for optimal embryonic development.

■ SEQUENTIAL VERSUS SINGLE STEP CULTURE MEDIUM

Sequential Media

In vivo, cleavage stage embryos develop in the Fallopian tube while it is only the blastocyst that enters the uterus. Therefore it appeared to be "logical" to culture blastocysts and then transfer them to the uterus. Very few embryos managed to develop to blastocyst with the conventional media used in the earlier days of ART.

An improved understanding of the embryo metabolism and realization that the nutrient requirements of cleavage stage embryos differed from those of morula and blastocyst—two different culture media were formulated, viz. cleavage and blastocyst media. Early cleavage stage human embryos are cultured in relatively simple media with minimal glucose which is in sync with the low glucose concentrations detected in the human Fallopian tubes and minimal amino acids. These embryos are then transferred to the blastocyst culture medium which is rich in glucose and also contains growth factors and complex nutrients.

Research on sequential media was independently carried out in various laboratories worldwide and these are now available commercially.[2,3,9] The concentration of the various components remains unknown in these commercial brands but the manufacturers do provide information on the constituents used.

Single Step Media

The concept that embryos can "choose what they want" from the culture media led to the refinement of the sequential media into single step media for culture of embryos from the zygote to the blastocyst stage. As long as the "additional" constituents are in a tolerable range would not be detrimental for the embryos. The reader can refer to a detailed review on this topic by Summers and Biggers.[4]

The pH and osmolality of the culture media have to be tested and adjusted to the optimal values (as described later) and tested for endotoxin and sterility. The efficacy of medium would depend not merely on its composition but how it is handled. A good culture media has to be handled well for it to give us the desired results.

■ IN VITRO CULTURE CONDITIONS

The three main variables that need to be controlled to make the medium optimally support embryonic development are: (1) temperature, (2) pH and (3) osmolality.

Temperature

Human zygotes and embryos have to be maintained at 37°C under all times. The culture media used for human zygotes and embryos need to be pre-equilibrated at 37°C by incubating the medium into the CO_2 incubator for a minimum of 6 hours prior to its actual use for the gametes. For the sake of convenience, one can even incubate them the evening before.

It has been shown that if the temperature of the medium drops below 33°C for even 5 minutes then the spindle gets damaged.[10] Therefore, maintaining the temperature of the medium is crucial because spindle damage would result in abnormal development of the embryos. It is not only the incubation temperature but also even the ambient temperature during embryo handling that influences them.

pH

The intracellular pH determines the intracellular activities. The mean pH of cleavage stage embryos is 7.0–7.3 (mean 7.12±0.01) and therefore the optimal pH of the culture medium should be similar to the intracellular pH. There are two mechanisms to relieve the pH changes. The HCO_3^-/Cl^- exchanger to relieve alkalosis and the Na^+/H^+ antiporter to relieve acidosis which in turn is maintained by the buffering system such as sodium bicarbonate which in turn is regulated by the circulating CO_2. The pH of the culture medium is primarily regulated by a balance of CO_2 concentration, supplied by the incubator, and by the concentration of bicarbonate in the media. Because bicarbonate concentrations are set by commericial suppliers of media, it is easiest to adjust CO_2 concentration in the incubator to adjust the pH. Raising CO_2 lowers media pH while lowering CO_2 raises the pH of the medium.[11]

Relationship between pH and Embryonic Development

Quinn studied the relationship between the pH of the culture medium and the embryonic and blastocyst development potential (unpublished observations). Sixty to eighty percent of the zygotes developed into 8-celled embryos in the pH range of 7.1–7.25 but when the pH of culture medium increased to 7.3 then the percentage of embryos that developed dropped to nearly 40%. This data had been obtained from the observation of 96,000 embryos. This clearly indicates the importance of maintaining the pH of the culture medium and even a slight variation could be detrimental to their development.

Maintenance of pH

The pH of the medium is maintained by the CO_2 concentration in the incubator and the sodium bicarbonate concentration in the medium. Higher the CO_2 lowers the pH while lowering the CO_2 raises the pH. As the ambient CO_2 levels are very low, the medium needs to be pre-equilibrated for a minimum of 6 hours and the minimal exposure of the medium to the outside environment as that would immediately lead to the rise in pH. CO_2 out-gassing has to be prevented by keeping culture dishes and medium under the CO_2 atmosphere as much as possible and renewing the desired CO_2 concentration as quickly as possible after culture dishes are returned to the incubator. The CO_2 levels in the incubator drops when the doors are opened and the sensors of the incubators need to be such that they are capable of immediately detecting the drop and allow the CO_2 to be readjusted.

Epigenetic Effects of pH Fluctuation

Koustas et al. (2011) have demonstrated the epigenetic effects of pH stress on mouse embryos. Such embryos have a reduced blastocyst formation; lower cell numbers in the blastocyst, reduced hatching, increased apoptosis and even the fetal weight was reduced.[12]

Although such studies cannot be replicated in humans for obvious ethical reasons, it clearly shows that maintaining of the pH of the culture medium is crucial. This can be achieved by using more incubators, minimal opening of the doors, minimal exposure of the embryos to the external environment and very efficient handling to minimize trauma due to pH fluctuation.

Osmolality

Osmolality is the "concentration" of a solution. It is defined as the number of osmoles of solute per kilogram of solvent. It is expressed in terms of osmol/kg. The osmolality of the medium is adjusted at the time of manufacturing but exposure to the environment can alter its osmolality.

Factors That Influence the Osmolality

The osmolality of the medium would increase with the decrease in the size of the drop. Smaller the drop, the greater it is prone to "evaporation" which is further enhanced at higher temperatures. Culture of embryos in larger volumes reduces osmolality changes during culture and incubation; and covering of the culture droplet with oil.[13]

When embryos are to be cultured in droplets, care should be taken that these drops are not prepared on a heated surface as this could affect the osmolality of the medium. Unlike the pH which can be adjusted on pre-equilibration, the osmolality once increased cannot decrease on equilibration! This change in osmolality is evident within 5 minutes of exposure of the drop to a heated surface and this affects mice embryonic development.[13]

Oil

When embryos are cultured in small droplets ranging 20–100 uL; it becomes mandatory to cover these droplets with oil to reduce changes in pH and osmolality. The mineral oil that is used is obtained after an extensive refinement process from crude oil and is comprised of a mixture of various hydrocarbons. Those with unsaturated hydrocarbons are more susceptible to peroxidation which is embryotoxic.

Otsuki et al. (2012) have demonstrated that oil can also lead to embryotoxicity.[14,15] This could be due to presence of embryo toxins, including zinc and peroxides. The degree of peroxidation depends on the exposure to heat, UV light and extended storage. The peroxidation of oils increases with light and heat. Therefore oils should be stored in dark and lower temperatures. Prewashing the oil with culture medium reduces peroxides and embryotoxicty.[16] Nowadays, commercially available oils for ART are generally prewashed with culture medium. Any new batch of oil should be tested for toxicity before utilizing it for ART.

Thus, an ideal culture medium utilized under optimal culture conditions would create an environment which is possibly as close to the in vivo environment to facilitate embryonic development.

■ EVALUATION OF ZYGOTES AND EMBRYOS

One of the greatest dilemmas faced by clinical embryologists is selecting the right embryo for transfer.

After all the time and efforts taken to stimulate, monitor and recover the oocytes; assist fertilization either by coincubation of the oocytes and sperms as in conventional IVF or through intracytoplasmic sperm injection (ICSI) and providing the ideal environment for embryonic development—it is very crucial to assess the quality and the developmental potential of these embryos—so that the couple has the highest chance of achieving a pregnancy following the transfer of the embryo.

Like the fetal milestones reflect the health of the new born; like the milestones during infant development reflect the development potential of the child—the milestones of embryonic development could be indicative of their future development.

Timeline of Embryonic Development

Presence of two pronuclei and the release of the second polar body are indicative of fertilization. This can be observed about 18–20 hours post-insemination or ICSI. Fertilization check is an important step in any ART procedure. Zygotes with more than two pronuclei also develop into morphologically normal appearing embryos. However, such aneuploid embryos would not develop further and even if they do, they would result in the first trimester loss. Therefore, one should always do a "fertilization check on Day 1 post-insemination or ICSI.

Fertilized oocytes, zygotes, develop into 2–4 cells on Day 1 (with Day 0 being the day of insemination or ICSI); approximately 8 cells on Day 3, morula on Day 4 and a blastocyst on Day 5. Apart from the number of blastomeres in each embryo which is indicative of their development, they need to assessed for their "quality" **(Figs 1A to H)**.

Morphological assessment of the embryos still remains the hall mark of assessing embryo quality and recently morphokinetic assessment is also being used to determine the developmental and implantation potential of embryos.

Criteria for Grading Embryos

The following criteria are commonly used for the grading of embryos:
- The number of cells (blastomeres)
- The size and uniformity of blastomeres
- The level and type of fragmentation
- Presence of multinucleation in the blastomeres
- Rate of development of the embryos.

The Number of Cells

As mentioned earlier, about 2–4 cells should be presented in the embryos of Day 2; 6–8 on Day 3 and blastocysts on Day 5. If the number of cells is lower in number then that it is indicative of poor development status.

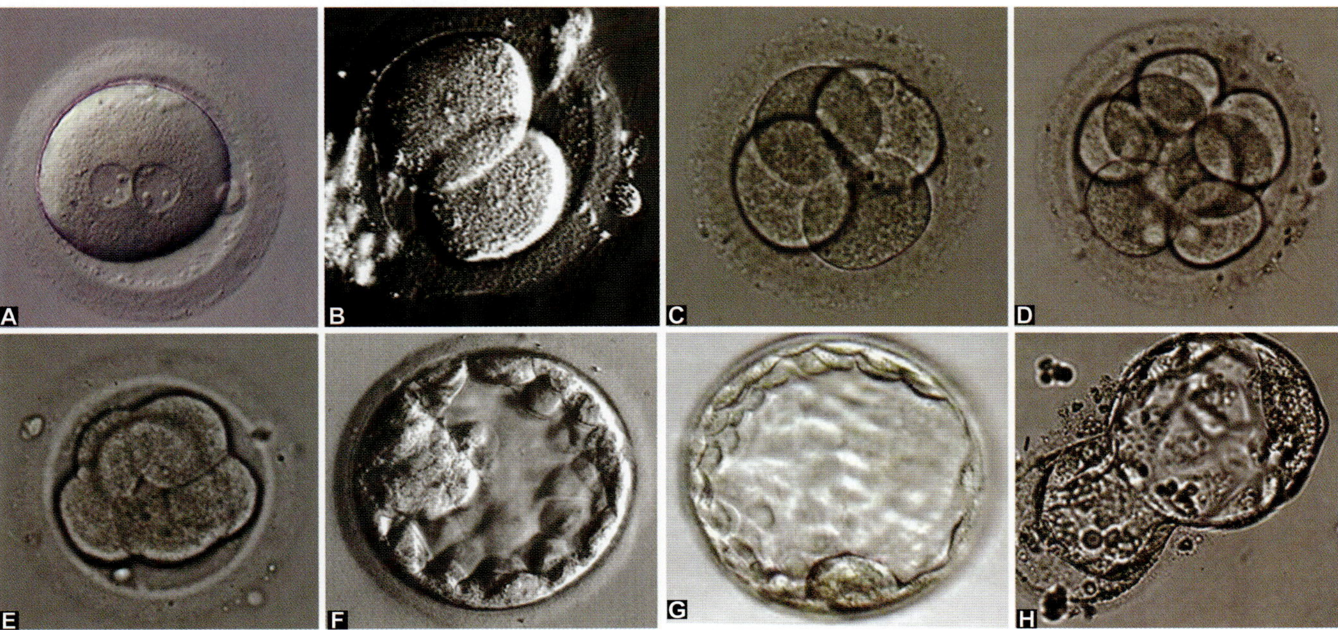

Figs 1A to H Timeline of embryonic development (from Day 1—fertilization to Day 6 hatched blastocyst)

(*Source: Sunita Tandulwadkar*)

Size and Uniformity of Blastomeres

A "good" embryo is considered to be the one where all the blastomeres are of identical size. However, if there are an odd number of blastomeres then it could be possible that one of the blastomeres has still not completed cell division and therefore is larger in size.

Fragmentation

The percentage and location of fragmentation is reflective of the quality of the embryo. Minor fragmentation is often detected in embryos and this has not been found to be detrimental to the implantation of the embryos. Recent studies with time lapse imaging systems show that fragments do get resolved with time in some cases. Twelve percent of the embryos show moderate fragmentation and in 89% of the embryos, the fragments do get resorbed within 9 hours[17] **(Fig. 2)**.

Secondly, the location or the dispersion of fragments is also reflective of their quality. Concentrated fragments are better than fragments which are scattered across the embryo.[19] Each of the blastomere of the embryo is totipotent and is capable of developing into a blastocyst. Therefore, localized concentrated fragmentation may be reflective of a single damaged blastomere. However, when the fragmentation is scattered then it is indicative of damage to many blastomeres; such embryos are associated with increased incidence of chromosomal abnormalities and such embryos have a poor developmental potential **(Figs 3 and 4)**.

So, if one has to select between a good 2-cell embryo without any fragmentation and equal blastomeres and a 4-cell embryo with minor localized fragmentation then the latter would be preferable.

What are these fragments? These fragments are of blastomere origin. But their "purpose" is unclear. These could be normal occurrences facilitating "reorganization" of the dividing cells. Or, fragmentation could be a result of suboptimal culture conditions which could lead to a deficiency of the cytoplasmic organelles compromising the quality of the embryo. Embryos do have nuclear and chromosomal abnormalities, and mosaicism has been detected even in in vivo generated embryos. These fragments could also be apoptotic bodies which removing cellular abnormalities.

Some of the iatrogenic causes of fragmentation could be the improper culture conditions, or presence of toxins or absence of growth factors.

The impact of fragmentation depends upon the amount of fragmentation, day of observation and localization of the fragments. A total lack of fragmentation is not essentially good.

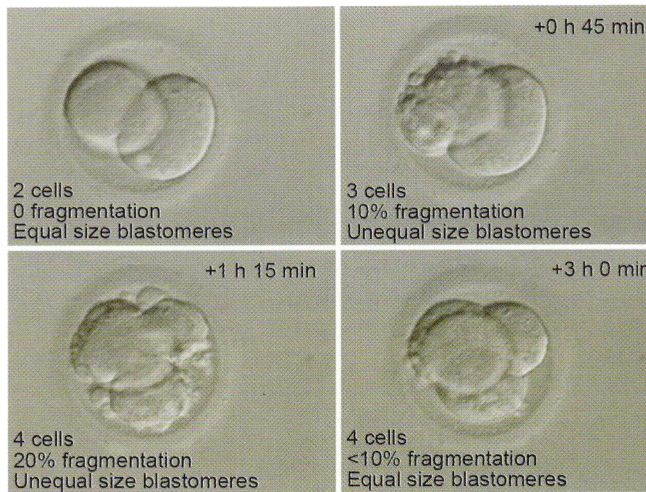

Fig. 2 Fragmentation of the embryos
(*Source:* Lemmen et al[18])

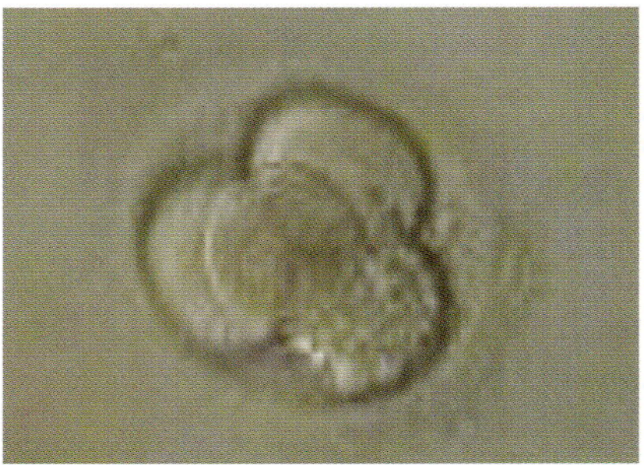

Fig. 3 Concentrated fragmentation

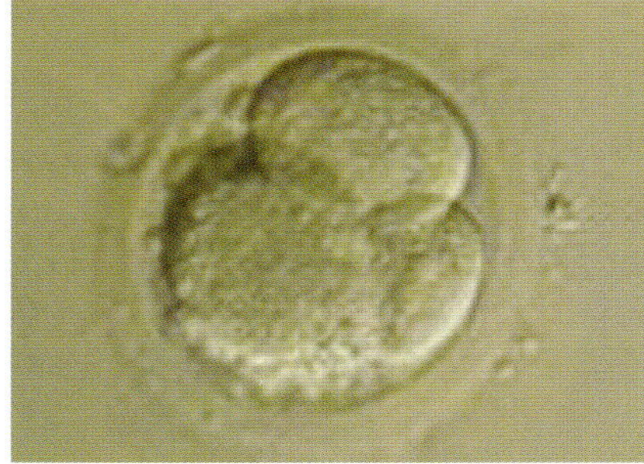

Fig. 4 Scattered fragmentation

Multinucleation

The number of nuclei in the blastomere reflects embryo quality. Multinucleated blastomeres are indicative of poor embryo quality. However, nuclei are not easily visible in the blastomere. Bar-Yoseph et al. (2011) have demonstrated

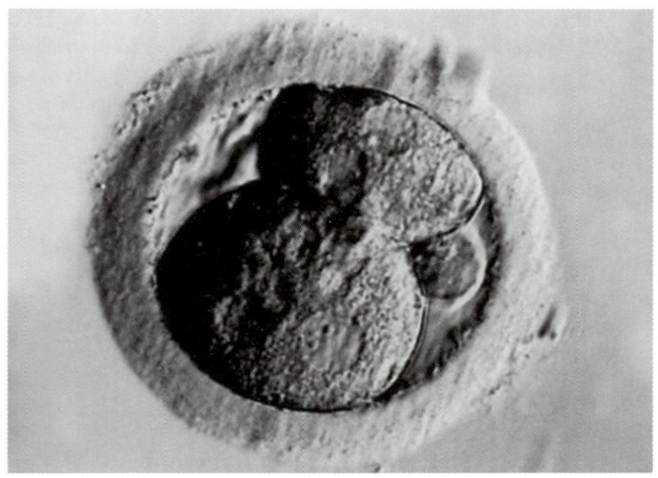

Fig. 5 Multinucleated embryo

that observation of single nucleus in all blastomeres leads to a higher implantation rate as compared with those with multinucleation.[20] Assessment of embryo morphology on Day 2 is associated with implantation rate. The nuclear scoring including: 1 nucleus in all blastomeres, 1 nucleus in part of the blastomeres, no visualization, and multinucleation showed high association with IR = 32.7%, 22.9%, 14.8% and 9.1%, respectively[20] **(Fig. 5)**.

Grading of Embryos

Different grading systems have been evolved by different professional bodies giving different weightage to the morphological parameters. This makes the assessment more objective and facilitates the decision in selecting the embryos for transfer.

Some grading systems assess embryos based on the number of blastomeres and percentage of fragmentation.

Grading of Blastocysts

Blastocysts are graded on the basis of the blastocoel, the inner cell mass (ICM) and the trophectoderm. For a long time, it was believed that the ICM was more important than the trophectoderm. This belief was based on the fact that the ICM would develop into the fetus. However, recent studies have clearly shown that trophectoderm morphology is an independent predictor of clinical pregnancy and livebirth.[21,22] A blastocyst with a complete trophectoderm without breaks and a lesser number of cells in the ICM is considered to be better than the one with a better ICM but an "incomplete" trophectoderm.

Gardner et al. had created a simple scoring system for the assessment of blastocysts.[23] The blastocysts are graded

Table 1 Simple scoring system for the assessment of blastocysts (Gardner et al)

Degree of expansion	1 = not expanded	4 = well expanded
Inner cell mass	A = many cells	C = few cells
Trophectoderm	A = many cells	C = few cells

on the extent of expansion, the number of cells in the ICM and the number of cells in the trophectoderm **(Table 1)**.

Thus, the best blastocyst would be graded 4AA while the worst would be 1CC.

Time Lapse Imaging

Conventionally, one can "observe" the embryos once or twice a day as too much exposure of the environment would be detrimental to their development. On the other hand, multiple observations give a better picture on the overall development as compared with a single observation. Most laboratories managed to grade and select embryos based on single point observations per day rather than expose embryos frequently to the external environment to assess their development.

This limitation is now overcome with the time lapse imaging systems which make it possible to make hundreds of observation of the embryos without disturbing incubating conditions. With time lapse systems, it is now possible to have morphokinetic data on embryo development. Such data include disappearance of pronuclei; exact timing of first and subsequent cleavages; synchrony of divisions; fragmentation history; appearance of nuclei after division.[23] These data have been used to evolve models that can predict the implantation potential of embryos and thereby aid in selecting the right embryo for transfer.[24]

Attempts are being made to have better assessment of embryos by quantifying the level of metabolites in the spent culture media. But, these are still not in the state of clinical application.

■ CONCLUSION

The ART laboratory and the embryologists are the one of the key players in an ART program. These personnel not only need the skills to perform the various ART procedures but also should pay critical attention to the selection and maintenance of culture media and culture conditions to facilitate the growth of human embryos. The grading and selection of the embryos is one of the last but important steps in ART—not only to select the embryo for transfer and cryopreservation but also for the overall assessment of the ART laboratory and culture conditions.

■ REFERENCES

1. Quinn P, Kerin J, Warnes G. Improved pregnancy rates in human in vitro fertilization with the use of medium based on the composition of human tubal fluid. Fertil Steril. 1985;44:493-8.
2. Gardner DK, Lane M. Culture of viable human blastocysts in defined sequential serum free media. Hum Reprod. 1998;13 (Suppl 3):148-59.
3. Menezo Y, Veiga A, Benkhalifa M. Improved methods for blastocyst formation and culture. Hum Reprod. 1998;13(Suppl 4): 256-65.
4. Summers MC, Biggers JD. Chemically defined media and the culture of mammalian preimplantation embryos: historical perspectives and current issues. Hum Reprod Update. 2003;9:557-82.
5. Dickens CJ, Maguiness SD, Corner MT, et al. Human tubal fluid: formation and composition during vascular perfusion of the Fallopian tube. Hum Reprod. 1995;10:505-8.
6. Gardner DK, Lane M, Calderon I, et al. Environment of the pre-implantation human embryo in vivo: metabolite analysis of oviduct and uterine fluids and metabolism of cumulus cells. Fertil Steril. 1996;65:349-53.
7. Devreker F, Winston RM, Hardy K. Glutamine improves human preimplantation development in vitro. Fertil Steril. 1998;69:293-9.
8. Lane M, Gardner DK. Ammonium induces aberrant blastocyst differentiation, metabolism, pH regulation, gene expression and subsequently alters fetal development in the mouse. Biol Reprod. 2003;69:1109-17.
9. Behr B, Pool TB, Milki AA, et al. Preliminary clinical experience with human blastocyst development in vitro without co-culture. Hum Reprod. 1999;14:454-7.
10. Wang WH, Meng L, Hackett RJ, et al. Limited recovery of meiotic spindles in living human oocytes after cooling-rewarming observed using polarized light microscopy. Hum Reprod. 2001;16:2374-8.
11. Swain JE. Optimizing the culture environment in the IVF laboratory: impact of pH and buffer capacity on gamete and embryo quality. Reprod Biomed Online. 2010;21:6-16.
12. Zander-Fox DL, et al. Alterations in mouse embryo intracellular pH by DMO during culture impair implantation and fetal growth. Reprod Biomed Online. 2010;21(2):219-29.
13. Swain JE, Cabrera L, Xu X, et al. Microdrop preparation factors influence culture-media osmolality, which can impair mouse embryo preimplantation development. Reprod Bio Med Online. 2011;24:142-7.
14. Otsuki J, Nagai Y, Chiba K. Peroxidation of mineral oil used in droplet culture is detrimental to fertilization and embryo development. Fertil Steril. 2007;88:741-3.
15. Otsuki J, Nagai Y, Chiba K. Damage of embryo development caused by peroxidized mineral oil and its association with albumin in culture. Fertil Steril. 2009;91:1745-9.
16. Morbeck DE, Khan Z, Barnidge DR, et al. Washing mineral oil reduces contaminants and embryotoxicity. Fertil Steril. 2010;94:2747-52.
17. Pribenszky C, Losonczi E, Molnár M, et al. Prediction of in-vitro developmental competence of early cleavage-stage mouse embryos with compact time-lapse equipment. Reprod Biomed Online. 2010;20(3):371-9.
18. Lemmen JG, Agerholm I, Ziebe S. Kinetic markers of human embryo quality using time-lapse recordings of IVF/ICSI-fertilized oocytes. Reprod Biomed Online. 2008;17:385-91.
19. Magli MC, Gianaroli L, Ferraretti AP, et al. Embryo morphology and development are dependent on the chromosomal complement. Fertil Steril. 2006;87:534-41.
20. Bar-Yoseph H, Levy A, Sonin Y, et al. Morphological embryo assessment: reevaluation. Fertil Steril. 2011;95:1624-8.
21. Thompson SM, Onwubalili N, Brown K, et al. Blastocyst expansion score and trophectoderm morphology strongly predict successful clinical pregnancy and livebirth following elective single embryo blastocyst transfer (eSET): a national study. J Assist Reprod Genet. 2013;30(12):1577-81.
22. Hill MJ, Richter KS, Heitmann RJ, et al. Trophectoderm grade predicts outcomes of single-blastocyst transfers. Fertil Steril. 2013;99:1283-9.
23. Meseguer M, Herrero J, Tejera A, et al. The use of morphokinetics as a predictor of embryo implantation. Hum Reprod. 2011;26:2658-71.
24. Rubio I, Galán A, Larreategui Z, et al. Clinical validation of embryo culture and selection by morphokinetic analysis: a randomized, controlled trial of the EmbryoScope. Fertil Steril. 2011;102:1287-94.

Proteomics and Metabolomics in ART

Devika Chopra

■ INTRODUCTION

Infertility inflicts 15% of the population and irrespective of whether the male or female is infertile, the couple is affected.[1] With significant advances in molecular biology research, large-scale analysis of male and female reproductive functions have gained an impetus thereby deepening our insight into pathological causes of infertility; however, much still remains to be known. Genomics, proteomics and metabolomics are rapidly evolving sciences in recent times that have potential applications in molecular and cellular biology. Application of proteomic tools have contributed toward identification of relevant protein biomarkers that can potentially change the strategies for early diagnosis and treatment of several disease conditions.[1] Proteomics and metabolomics enable scientists to map proteins and secretomes at the cellular levels and decipher their function. The absence or presence of a protein/metabolite, and its association to a certain disease condition has enabled scientists to elucidate the mechanism of disease processes at the cellular level.

Reproductive biologists have also made sincere attempts to exploit proteomic and metabolomic tools for studying infertility related pathologies. Profiling and mapping various tissues (e.g. testes, ovary, placenta, epididymis and endometrium) and concurrent mapping of gametes and embryos have enabled researchers to scrutinize a variety of events in normal reproduction. In this chapter, we have focused on proteomics and metabolomics, and their use in assisted reproductive technology (ART).

■ WHAT ARE GENOMICS, PROTEOMICS AND METABOLOMICS?

Genomics is a discipline in genetics concerned with the study of the genomes of organisms. The field includes efforts to determine the entire DNA sequence of organisms and fine-scale genetic mapping. The investigation of the roles and functions of single genes is a primary focus of molecular biology or genetics and is a common topic of modern medical and biological research.

Proteomics is the large-scale study of proteins, particularly their structures and functions. The term "proteomics" was first coined in 1997 to make an analogy with genomics, the study of the genes. The word "proteome" is a blend of "protein" and "genome", and was coined by Marc Wilkins in 1994 while working on the concept as a PhD student. The proteome is the entire complement of proteins, including the modifications made to a particular set of proteins, produced by an organism or system. This will vary with time and distinct requirements, or stresses and illness, that a cell or organism faces during its lifespan.

Finally, metabolomics is the scientific study of chemical processes involving metabolites. Specifically, metabolomics is the "systematic study of the unique chemical fingerprints that specific cellular processes leave behind", the study of their small-molecule metabolite profiles. The metabolome represents the collection of all metabolites in a biological cell, tissue, organ or organism, which are the end products of cellular processes. Thus, while mRNA gene expression data and proteomic analyses do not tell the whole story of what might be happening in a cell, metabolic profiling can give an instantaneous snapshot of the physiology of that cell **(Fig. 1)**.

■ PROTEOMICS IN ART

In recent times, proteomic mapping of reproductive tissues such as oocyte, sperm, endometrium, ovary, epididymis and testis have been made, and these have enriched our knowledge on proteins expressed in these tissues. Efforts are also being made in identifying the proteins, which contribute to the pathology in various reproductive health disorders, such as azoospermia, oligozoospermia in men and endometriosis (EOS) and polycystic ovarian syndrome (PCOS), etc. Gel-based approaches like two-dimensional electrophoresis (2DE), differential in gel electrophoresis (DIGE), etc. and gel-free approaches, like liquid chromatography-based workflows, mass spectrometry (MS) are being used to identify the proteins significant in endowing male or female gametes with their specific functions [e.g. spermatogenesis, sperm maturations, folliculogenesis, oogenesis, endometrial receptivity and implantation **(Figs 1 and 2)**].[1]

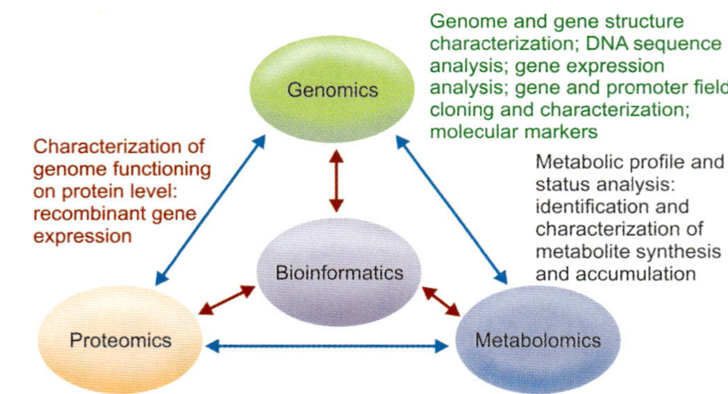

Fig. 1 Workflow representing genomics, proteomics and metabolomics

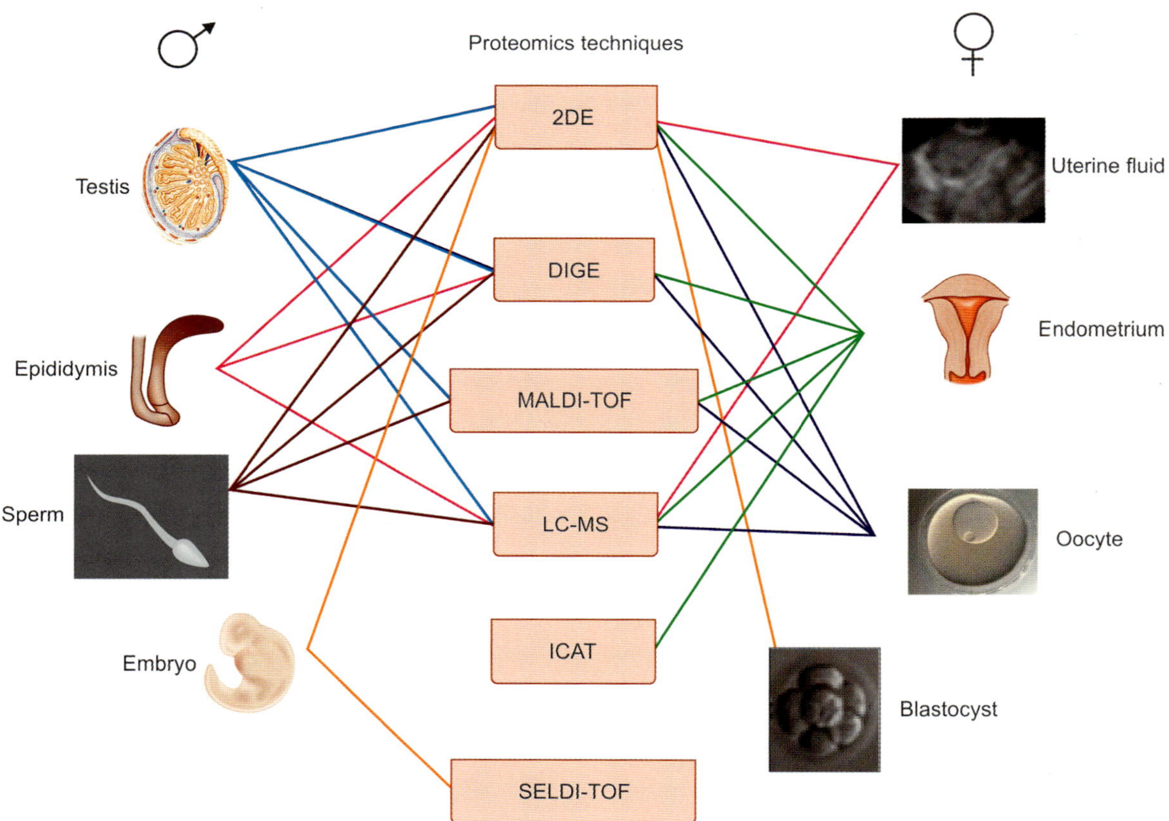

Fig. 2 A diagrammatic representation of proteomic techniques and the various tissues that can be mapped using proteomics

Abbreviations: 2DE, two-dimensional electrophoresis; DIGE, differential in gel electrophoresis; MALDI-TOF, matrix-assisted laser desorption ionization time-of-flight; LC–MS, liquid chromatography–mass spectrometry; ICAT, isotope-coded affinity tag; SELDI-TOF, surface-enhanced laser desorption/ionization

■ PROTEOMIC STUDIES ON THE MALE REPRODUCTIVE SYSTEM

Recently, 1908 proteins that are testis specific have been identified by 2DE techniques.[2] Such a 2DE database will be useful for comparative proteomics analyses of normal and diseased human testis thereby paving the way for the discovery of novel biomarkers.[2] Studies done on testicular tissue samples with normal and pathological testes have shown 10 differentially expressed spermatogenesis related proteins. Of them, four proteins viz phospholipid hydroperoxide glutathione peroxidase, peroxiredoxin 4, heat shock protein beta-1 (HSP 27) and cathepsin D are found to play important roles in various spermatogenic processes including germ cell movement and spermiation.[3]

Studies on proteins specific to sperm-milieu, which are secretions of testis and epididymis, have also been done. Li et al. have carried out testicular mapping of the sperm-located proteins by 2DE and matrix-assisted laser desorption ionization time-of-flight (MALDI-TOF) MS. This has revealed 725 unique proteins, of which the presence of 240 proteins in the sperm-milieu was confirmed by Western blotting and localization of 167 proteins in the mature spermatozoa by immunocytochemistry **(Fig. 3)**.[4]

Using 2DE and MALDI-TOF-MS, Heredia et al. have identified 98 proteins from human spermatozoa. Of these, 10% have been attributed to have an important functional role in cytoskeleton, flagella and cell movement.[5] Several researchers have investigated proteins differentially expressed in asthenozoospermatozoa in order to identify diagnostic and prognostic markers for poor sperm motility.[6-8] Thirty-five proteins that are differentially expressed in globozoospermia have been identified by MS and DIGE.[5] Out of these 35, 9 proteins were upregulated and 26 were downregulated on proteomic analyses.[5]

Although preliminary, the use of proteomics in male infertility needs more research and may prove to be a useful tool in the future to identify disease processes leading to infertility.

Proteomics Studies on the Female Reproductive System

Several studies have now been focused on proteomic studies of the ovary, fallopian tubes, uterus and the endometrium. Proteins secreted by these tissues during normal reproductive cycles have revealed several thousand proteins that may be altered leading to infertility.

The molecular composition of endometrium during the receptive phase is expected to unearth the reasons underlying the low success rate of in vitro fertilization–embryo transfer (IVF-ET) and infertility in women. Parmar et al. used 2DE to identify alterations in the proteome of mid-secretory phase endometrium as compared to that in late proliferative phase of menstrual cycle in women with normal menstrual cycles. Proteins found downregulated were identified to be calreticulin, fibrinogen adenylate kinase isoenzyme-5 and transferrin, and upregulated were annexin-5, alpha-1-antitrypsin, peroxidin-6 and creatine kinase in the mid-secretory phase or receptive phase.[1] Proteomic analysis of human endometrium by DIGE identified 41 different gene products as differentially regulated between the mid-proliferative (non-receptive) and mid-secretory (receptive) phases of the menstrual cycle.[9]

In addition to endometrial tissues, uterine fluid samples in different phases of the menstrual cycle have been analyzed using proteomic tools. Casado-Vela et al. identified 803 different proteins in uterine fluid samples. The use of high-performance liquid chromatography (HPLC), sodium dodecyl sulfate–polyacrylamide gel electrophoresis. (SDS–PAGE) and liquid chromatography–

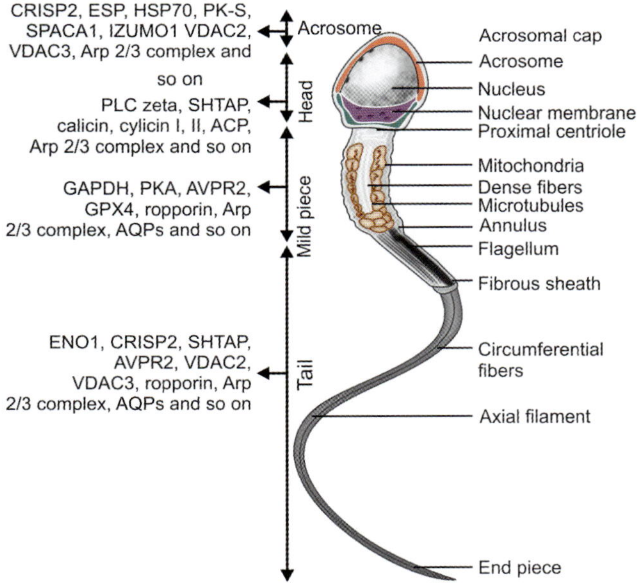

Fig. 3 Diagram showing a mature human spermatozoon with proteins localized in acrosome, head, mid-piece, and tail that are mainly involved in capacitation and acrosomal reaction, spermatozoa-oocyte interaction (zona binding), energy production and metabolism and motility and metabolism, respectively

mass spectrometry (LC–MS) led to identification of interleukin-18, matrix metalloproteinase-9 (MMP-9), mucins-1 and -16, vitamin D-binding protein and glycodelin.[10] While this study provided a list of proteins present in uterine fluid, it did not identify the proteins, which show differential abundance in the mid-secretory phase as compared to that in other phases of menstrual phase.

Endometriosis afflicts 2–48% of infertile women.[11] Investigation of endometrial tissue using 2DE techniques identified secretory proteins, i.e. apolipoprotein A2, peroxiredoxin-2, chaperonins, proteins associated with DNA metabolism and catabolism in women with and without EOS.[12] Zhang et al. compared the protein expression of endometria and sera in women with or without EOS using 2DE.[11] In their study, they identified 13 and 11 differentially expressed proteins in sera and endometrium between the two study groups, respectively.[11] HSP 90-alpha and beta were found downregulated in the women with EOS.[13] A 20 kDa fragment of HSP 70 was found to be increased in the endometrium of EOS patients.[14]

Polycystic ovary syndrome is known to affect approximately 5–10% of women of reproductive age.[15] Proteomic technologies can identify the markers and therapeutic targets for PCOS. However, a major hindrance in identification of the proteins associated with the pathogenesis of PCOS has been the non-availability of ovaries from healthy women. Ma et al., using 2DE coupled to MALDI-TOF-MS, identified 69 out of 110 proteins to be differentially expressed between PCOS and normal ovaries.[16] Majority of the differentially expressed proteins were known to be associated with the regulation of cellular physiological processes such as proliferation and metabolism.[16]

The oocyte proteome directly affects the oocyte function and ultimately affects fertilization and pregnancy outcome. A pioneering study by Meng et al., profiling mouse mature cumulus–oocyte complexes using 2DE and MS identified 156 individual proteins that were involved in cell signaling/communication, cell division, gene/protein expression, cell metabolism, cell structure and motility.[17] A more recent study reported that the proteome of metaphase II mouse oocyte contains 3,699 proteins, of which 28 proteins were also present in the proteome of undifferentiated mouse embryonic stem cells, majority of which were associated to nuclear reprograming of proteins, RNAs, lipids and small molecules.[18] Thus, oocyte proteomics will reveal invaluable information regarding mechanisms of oocyte maturation, fertilization and embryo development contributing significantly to the field of human and animal reproduction.

Proteomics of Embryos

The transcriptome and proteome of the embryo reflects its developmental potential. Using surface-enhanced laser desorption ionization time-of-flight mass spectrometry (SELDI-TOF/MS), Katz-Jaffe et al. have delineated proteomes of early, expanded and degenerating blastocysts.[19,20] Comparison of early blastocysts with expanded blastocysts revealed two negatively charged proteins of approximately 5 kDa and 6.3 kDa as being significantly upregulated in expanded blastocysts and one negatively charged protein/biomarker of approximately 3.8 kDa significantly downregulated in early and expanded blastocysts. This study emphasized that two blastomeres at same stages can differ in their proteomes. Preliminary database searching highlighted that the potential candidates for 6.3 kDa protein was parathyroid hormone-related peptide. Parathyroid hormone-related peptide is abundant in human syncytiotrophoblast and plays an important role in maternal–fetal calcium homeostasis. In addition, degenerating embryos exhibit a different protein expression profile than developing blastocysts with significant upregulation of numerous proteins/biomarkers. Preliminary database searching has identified potential candidates involved in apoptotic and growth-inhibiting pathways, which are directly linked to embryogenesis.[19,21]

Use of proteomics tools has indeed broadened the knowledge of proteins, which make up the reproductive tissue/organs. Yet, we know that reproductive biology proteomics is still in its infancy and major challenges include obtaining reproductive tissue samples, ethical issues of blastocyst and embryo proteomics are obstacles that need to be overcome. However, availability of the reference proteome maps of the reproductive tissues will definitely open up the avenues for the discovery of biomarkers for reproductive diseases such as PCOS, EOS, endometrial cancer, reduced sperm count and also in turn male and female infertility.[1]

■ METABOLOMICS IN ART

Metabolomics is the identification and quantification of all the metabolites in the metabolome,[22,23] where metabolites are the low molecular weight end-products which are essential for cellular reactions, and the metabolome is the complete collection of all the metabolites in an organism.[24] Metabolomics can be applied to ART by obtaining and examining the metabolic profiles of oocytes follicular fluid (FF) and embryos (culture media or blastocoel fluid) for biomarkers of oocyte/embryo quality. One of the most common analytical platforms for metabolomics is nuclear magnetic resonance (NMR) spectroscopy, which measures the presence of certain nuclei (most commonly, 1H) in a sample, where the positions of the signals on the *x*-axis (chemical shift in ppm) reflect the chemical environments of the corresponding nuclei (and hence enable identification of the metabolites), and the intensities of the signals indicate the number of nuclei in the given chemical environment (so the area under the signal gives a measure of the concentration of the metabolite).[25] The second most commonly used platform is MS, which offers a much greater sensitivity than NMR.[25]

This section has focused on the potential use of metabolomics in improving outcomes in assisted conception.

Selecting the Best Embryo

While morphokinetics is becoming the new "gold standard" for determining embryo developmental potential, the methods are still in their infancy.[26] Clinical markers for embryo quality may overcome some of the limitations of morphological assessments and could be complementary to morphokinetic assessments. Studies have analyzed the uptake and secretion of various metabolites by the embryo into the surrounding culture medium. Good-quality early human embryos have shown an increased uptake of glucose compared to poor-quality embryos.[27]

Houghton et al. measured the turnover of amino acids by human embryos during culture, and observed that a low amino acid turnover was associated with better development.[28] This finding was reinforced in a later study by the same group, along with the observation that decreased culture medium levels of glycine and leucine and increased levels of asparagine correlated with clinical pregnancy and livebirth.[29] Differences in amino acid turnover between genetically normal and abnormal embryos have also been observed during different stages of culture. Most recently, it has been suggested that monitoring patterns of oxygen consumption in human embryos in culture for up to 72 hours may be informative of embryo viability.[30]

In recent years, studies of embryo metabolism have moved away from targeted metabolite analysis and toward metabolomics. The first metabolomics study of embryo culture medium to assess oocyte potential was carried out using near infrared and Raman spectroscopy by Seli et al. in 2007.[31] Higher values of viability scores (higher metabolomic profile) were associated with live birth. Marhuenda-Egea et al. have used HPLC–MS and 1H-NMR-based metabolomics to identify differences in culture media from embryos with and without

pregnancy.[32,33] The authors postulated that all embryo culture medium amino acids played a crucial role in the embryo metabolism.[33]

Selecting the Best Oocyte

Cellular predictors of good oocyte quality include a high content of oocyte mitochondrial DNA,[34] adequate redistribution, differentiation and transcription of mitochondria;[35] varying levels of adenosine triphosphate in the cytoplasm produced by the oocyte;[36] and low glucose-6-phosphate dehydrogenase activity in oocytes.[37] This method however is invasive and does not preserve the oocyte for future use. Noninvasive metabolite analysis involving the measurement of energy substrate levels in culture media has been performed. Preis et al. quantified glucose and lactate consumption and release into culture media from mouse oocytes.[38] They found the oocytes that consumed larger amounts of glucose and produced more lactate had the highest potential for fertilization.[38]

In another study, oocytes from patients with PCOS exhibited greater rates of glucose and pyruvate consumption compared to controls.[39] Additionally, higher pyruvate consumption was also associated with abnormal oocyte karyotypes.[39] Some have investigated the respiration rate of oocytes as a marker for oocyte viability; Scott et al. found that human oocytes with respiration rates between 0.48 nanoliter and 0.55 nanoliter O_2/ hour were viable, whereas those with lower rates did not mature or became atretic in vitro.[40]

While all of these investigations are exhaustive, they have not yet led to the discovery of suitable methods for selecting oocytes with good potential in clinical practice. A non-invasive, reproducible, and high-output metabolomic method for predicting oocyte quality remains to be discovered.[25]

Metabolomic Assessment of Follicular Fluid

Follicular fluid provides the microenvironment for the oocyte in the follicle and is therefore important for studying the metabolites available to the oocyte during its maturation and during ovulation. Additionally, it also contains the metabolites excreted by the oocyte and the follicular cells. FF would be an ideal medium in which to test oocyte quality since it is obtained along with the oocyte during follicular aspiration as part of the standard IVF procedure and is usually discarded.

In 2012, Wallace et al. published the first metabolomics study of human FF to assess oocyte viability.[41] Lower FF levels of lactate and choline/phosphocholine and higher levels of glucose and high-density lipoproteins were associated with oocytes, which failed to cleave. In terms of pregnancy test outcome, patients who tested positive were associated with a lower FF level of glucose and higher levels of proline, lactate, leucine, and isoleucine.[41]

Thus, metabolomics although in its infancy can provide us with useful biomarkers for embryo, oocytes and FF, that may help improve the outcome in ART.

■ CONCLUSION

Research into biomarkers of IVF outcome is essential if we are to improve clinical pregnancy rates and live birth rates, increase the numbers of elective single embryo transfer (eSET) performed, to reduce the incidence of chromosomal abnormalities and without compromising the overall success rate in assisted conception. A large amount of knowledge has been gained over the years from targeted studies of embryo culture medium, oocytes, semen, FF and plasma, but still no biomarker is in routine clinical use.[25] The move from proteomics to metabolomics in recent years has offered a much greater potential for unraveling the mechanisms of infertility and for identify groups of diagnostic markers or models from which disease processes can be predicted. Ultimately, if a biomarker can distinguish between two groups of samples then it is a legitimate biomarker. With such improvements over the coming years, the possibility of identifying biomarkers of IVF outcome using proteomics and metabolomics could become a reality, which is a very exciting prospect.[25]

■ REFERENCES

1. Upadhyay RD, Balasinor NH, Kumar AV, et al. Proteomics in reproductive biology: beacon for unraveling the molecular complexities. Biochim Biophys Acta. 2013;1834(1):8-15.
2. Guo X, Zhao C, Wang F, et al. Investigation of human testis protein heterogeneity using two dimensional electrophoresis. J Androl. 2010;31(4):419-29.
3. Huo R, He Y, Zhao C, et al. Identification of human spermatogenesis-related proteins by comparative proteomic analysis: a preliminary study. Fertil Steril. 2008;90(4):1109-18.
4. Li J, Liu F, Liu X, et al. Mapping of the human testicular proteome and its relationship with that of the epididymis and spermatozoa. Mol Cell Proteomics. 2011;10(3):M110.004630.
5. Martinez-Heredia J, Estanyol JM, Ballesca JL, et al. Proteomic identification of human sperm proteins. Proteomics. 2006;6(15):4356-69.
6. Zhao C, Huo R, Wang FQ, et al. Identification of several proteins involved in regulation of sperm motility by proteomic analysis. Fertil Steril. 2007;87(2):436-8.
7. Martinez-Heredia J, de Mateo S, Vidal-Taboada JM, et al. Identification of proteomic differences in asthenozoospermic sperm samples. Hum Reprod. 2008;23(4):783-91.
8. Siva AB, Kameshwari DB, Singh V, et al. Proteomics-based study on asthenozoospermia: differential expression of proteasome alpha complex. Mol Hum Reprod. 2010;16(7):452-62.
9. Chen JI, Hannan NJ, Mak Y, et al. Proteomic characterization of midproliferative and midsecretory human endometrium. J Proteome Res. 2009;8(4):2032-44.
10. Casado-Vela J, Rodriguez-Suarez E, Iloro I, et al. Comprehensive proteomic analysis of human endometrial fluid aspirate. J Proteome Res. 2009;8(10):4622-32.
11. Zhang H, Niu Y, Feng J, et al. Use of proteomic analysis of endometriosis to identify different protein expression in patients with endometriosis versus normal controls. Fertil Steril. 2006;86(2):274-82.
12. Scotchie JG, Fritz MA, Mocanu M, et al. Proteomic analysis of the luteal endometrial secretome. Reprod Sci. 2009;16(9):883-93.
13. Fowler PA, Tattum J, Bhattacharya S, et al. An investigation of the effects of endometriosis on the proteome of human eutopic endometrium: a heterogeneous tissue with a complex disease. Proteomics. 2007;7(1):130-42.
14. Chehna-Patel N, Warty N, Sachdeva G, et al. Proteolytic tailoring of the heat shock protein 70 and its implications in the pathogenesis of endometriosis. Fertil Steril. 2011;95(5):1560-7.e1-3.
15. Dunaif A. Insulin resistance and the polycystic ovary syndrome: mechanism and implications for pathogenesis. Endocr Rev. 1997;18(6):774-800.
16. Ma X, Fan L, Meng Y, et al. Proteomic analysis of human ovaries from normal and polycystic ovarian syndrome. Mol Hum Reprod. 2007;13(8):527-35.
17. Meng Y, Liu XH, Ma X, et al. The protein profile of mouse mature cumulus-oocyte complex. Biochim Biophys Acta. 2007;1774(11):1477-90.
18. Pfeiffer MJ, Siatkowski M, Paudel Y, et al. Proteomic analysis of mouse oocytes reveals 28 candidate factors of the "reprogrammome". J Proteome Res. 2011;10(5):2140-53.
19. Katz-Jaffe MG, Linck DW, Schoolcraft WB, et al. A proteomic analysis of mammalian preimplantation embryonic development. Reproduction. 2005;130(6):899-905.
20. Katz-Jaffe MG, Schoolcraft WB, Gardner DK. Analysis of protein expression (secretome) by human and mouse preimplantation embryos. Fertil Steril. 2006;86(3):678-85.
21. Katz-Jaffe MG, Gardner DK, Schoolcraft WB. Proteomic analysis of individual human embryos to identify novel biomarkers of development and viability. Fertil Steril. 2006;85(1):101-7.
22. Fiehn O. Combining genomics, metabolome analysis, and biochemical modelling to understand metabolic networks. Comp Func Genomics. 2001;2(3):155-68.
23. Wishart DS. Metabolomics: the principles and potential applications to transplantation. Am J Transplant. 2005;5(12):2814-20.
24. Wishart DS. Proteomics and the human metabolome project. Expert Rev Proteomics. 2007;4(3):333-5.
25. McRae C, Sharma V, Fisher J. Metabolite profiling in the pursuit of biomarkers for IVF outcome: the case for metabolomics studies. Int J Reprod Med. 2013;2013:16.

26. Meseguer M, Herrero J, Tejera A, et al. The use of morphokinetics as a predictor of embryo implantation. Hum Reprod. 2011;26(10):2658-71.

27. Gardner DK, Lane M, Stevens J, et al. Noninvasive assessment of human embryo nutrient consumption as a measure of developmental potential. Fertil Steril. 2001;76(6):1175-80.

28. Houghton FD, Hawkhead JA, Humpherson PG, et al. Non-invasive amino acid turnover predicts human embryo developmental capacity. Hum Reprod. 2002;17(4):999-1005.

29. Brison DR, Houghton FD, Falconer D, et al. Identification of viable embryos in IVF by non-invasive measurement of amino acid turnover. Hum Reprod. 2004;19(10):2319-24.

30. Tejera A, Herrero J, Viloria T, et al. Time-dependent O_2 consumption patterns determined optimal time ranges for selecting viable human embryos. Fertil Steril. 2012;98(4):849-57.e1-3.

31. Seli E, Sakkas D, Scott R, et al. Noninvasive metabolomic profiling of embryo culture media using Raman and near-infrared spectroscopy correlates with reproductive potential of embryos in women undergoing in vitro fertilization. Fertil Steril. 2007;88(5):1350-7.

32. Marhuenda-Egea FC, Martinez-Sabater E, Gonsalvez-Alvarez R, et al. A crucial step in assisted reproduction technology: human embryo selection using metabolomic evaluation. Fertil Steril. 2010;94(2):772-4.

33. Marhuenda-Egea F, Gonsálvez-Álvarez R, Martínez-Sabater E, et al. Improving human embryos selection in IVF: non-invasive metabolomic and chemometric approach. Metabolomics. 2011;7(2):247-56.

34. Santos TA, El Shourbagy S, St John JC. Mitochondrial content reflects oocyte variability and fertilization outcome. Fertil Steril. 2006;85(3):584-91.

35. Au HK, Yeh TS, Kao SH, et al. Abnormal mitochondrial structure in human unfertilized oocytes and arrested embryos. Ann N Y Acad Sci. 2005;1042:177-85.

36. Van Blerkom J, Runner MN. Mitochondrial reorganization during resumption of arrested meiosis in the mouse oocyte. Am J Anat. 1984;171(3):335-55.

37. Alm H, Torner H, Lohrke B, et al. Bovine blastocyst development rate in vitro is influenced by selection of oocytes by brillant cresyl blue staining before IVM as indicator for glucose-6-phosphate dehydrogenase activity. Theriogenology. 2005;63(8):2194-205.

38. Preis KA, Seidel G Jr, Gardner DK. Metabolic markers of developmental competence for in vitro-matured mouse oocytes. Reproduction. 2005;130(4):475-83.

39. Harris SE, Maruthini D, Tang T, et al. Metabolism and karyotype analysis of oocytes from patients with polycystic ovary syndrome. Hum Reprod. 2010;25(9):2305-15.

40. Scott L, Berntsen J, Davies D, et al. Human oocyte respiration-rate measurement–potential to improve oocyte and embryo selection? Reprod BioMedicine Online. 2008;17(4):461-9.

41. Wallace M, Cottell E, Gibney MJ, et al. An investigation into the relationship between the metabolic profile of follicular fluid, oocyte developmental potential, and implantation outcome. Fertil Steril. 2012;97(5):1078-84.e1-8.

31. Time-lapse Microscopy

Sunita R Tandulwadkar, Devika Chopra

INTRODUCTION

Over the past 37 years, success rates with in vitro fertilization (IVF) have improved remarkably. However, the ability to identify the most viable embryo remains a challenge as many assisted reproductive technology (ART) centers still depend on morphological assessment using light microscopy as the first-line approach for embryo selection.[1] To date, determining why some embryos develop normally while others fail to do so is a vital question that remains unanswered. Until recently, we knew little about the exact timing and sequence of events involved in embryo development. In recent times, one particularly promising development is the use of "time-lapse microscopy" (TLM) or/and computer-assisted technologies to visualize the early development of embryos in vitro. These new developments are ideal tools to monitor the early stages of embryo development that generate morphological, quantitative and dynamic data in a noninvasive manner.[2] In addition to external factors like temperature, light and culture media; morphological characteristics such as cleavage rate, fragmentation, size and distribution of blastomeres have been shown determine the development of embryos in vitro and subsequent pregnancy rates.[3] By using TLM, the best embryo based on morphology and developmental grade can be selected subsequently improving the ART outcome.

STAGES OF EMBRYO DEVELOPMENT

Viewing biological processes as they occur can provide invaluable insight into cell behavior. TLM is a tool that enables scientists to explore various dynamics of cell morphology and development, which would remain unidentified with routine light microscopy assessment.

In mammals, preimplantation embryo development involves molecular mechanisms encompassing various morphological and biological processes. Embryo development begins with the fusion of a sperm to an egg to create a zygote, which undergoes rapid mitotic divisions and cellular differentiations to form an embryo. During early cleavage stages (4–8 cells), the zygote also undergoes epigenetic reprogramming. The early cleaving embryo relies upon the mRNA and protein reserves of the egg for a series of divisions until the point of embryonic genome activation. After serial mitotic divisions, a morula (16-cell stage) is formed which subsequently undergoes division to form a blastocyst consisting of an inner cell mass and trophectoderm. **Figure 1** gives a pictorial representation of various stages of embryo development prior to implantation. These preimplantation processes need to be precisely executed for successful embryo development. Hence, monitoring these processes is crucial during not only for a successful ART cycle but also for a healthy pregnancy.

TIME-LAPSE MICROSCOPY

Time-lapse microscopy is a breakthrough technology that has transformed the dynamics of ART. It comprises of a multi-gas incubator, a microscope attached to a camera that takes images of dividing embryos at preset time intervals. The incubator allows detailed observation of the embryo in every stage of in vitro fertilization. The monitoring system is noninvasive and minimizes the need to remove the embryo from the incubator. As a result, embryo survival rates are much higher. The images that are captured are recorded and evaluated using a computer program at the very same ART clinic **(Figs 2A and B)**.

Advantages of Time-lapse Microscopy

Morphological Assessment of Embryos in a Continuous Time Period

Time-lapse chromatography or its more popular name "embryoscope" makes embryo selection from a cohort of embryos easier by capturing images at defined intervals over a specific period of time. Images of developing

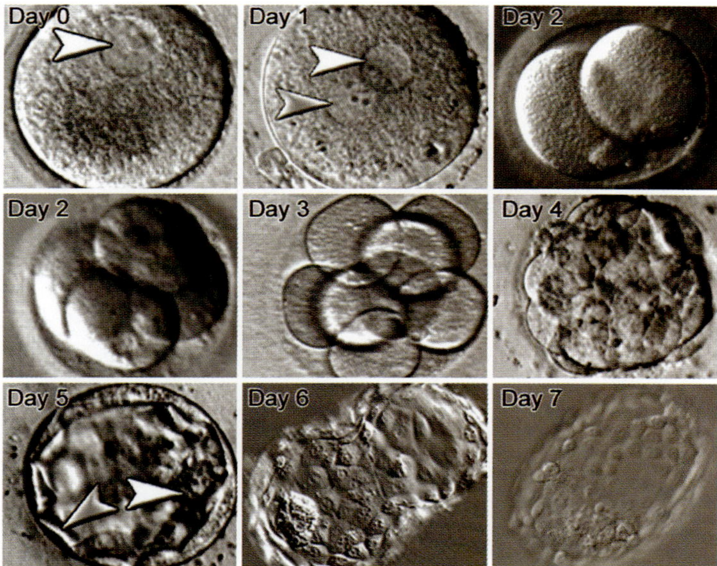

Fig. 1 Stages of human preimplantation embryo development. Phase-contrast images of human embryo development from day 0 to day 7. Arrowheads in day 0 and day 1 indicate pronuclei. On or around day 4, the embryo compacts, resulting in the formation of a morula that consists of 16 cells (or blastomeres). The blastocyst, which forms on day 5, is a fluid-filled structure composed of an inner cell mass (white arrowhead) and trophectoderm (gray arrowhead). On day 6, the blastocyst "hatches" and it is ready to implant into the uterine wall on day 7[4]

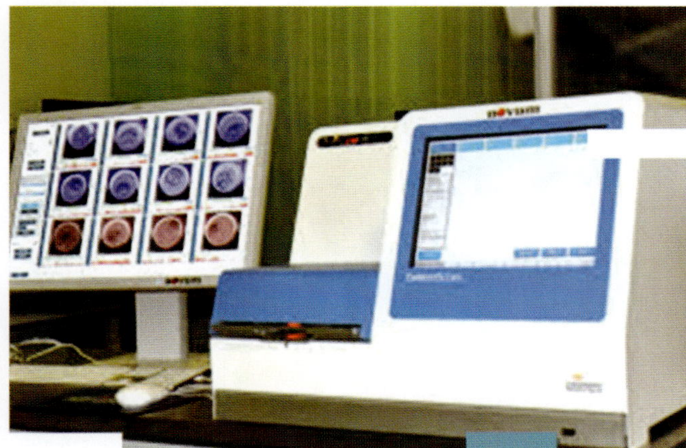

Fig. 2A An embryoscope with a computer screen taking live time-lapse images

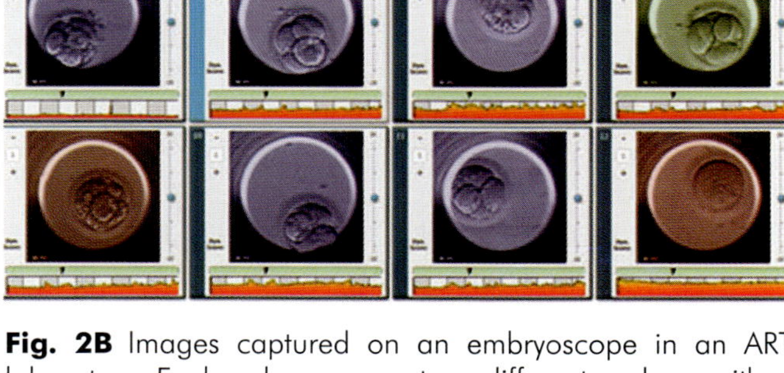

Fig. 2B Images captured on an embryoscope in an ART laboratory. Each cube represents a different embryo with a different stage of development

embryos can be captured at varied intervals ranging from 20 minutes, 10 minutes to even 10 seconds.[5] Embryo morphology can undergo a change within a short-time interval and thus may be misleading if assessment is done at a static time point. Monitoring over specific time scales can aid better embryo selection criteria. For example, two morphologically similar embryos that may appear similar at one specific time point could have arisen from two varied developmental stages. One could be normal whereas the other could have suffered from fragmentation followed by fragment reabsorption or one may have undergone abnormal divisions with disturbance of the cell cycle.[2] Azarello et al. (2012) noted that the timing of pronuclear formation and pronuclear breakdown (PNB) was a vital parameter which determined embryo implantation and live birth rate. In their study, they found that PNB occurred significantly later in embryos resulting in live birth and PNB in live birth embryos never occurred before 20 hours and 45 minutes.[6] **Figures 3A to D** shows morphological parameters of good quality and poor quality embryos.[7] Uneven cleavage, multinucleated blastomeres and several degrees of fragmentation are markers of poor quality embryos. **Table 1** depicts studies that have used morphological markers used to evaluate embryo quality and competence. These studies show that certain embryonic morphological markers can predict whether an embryo will form a blastomere or result in a healthy pregnancy.

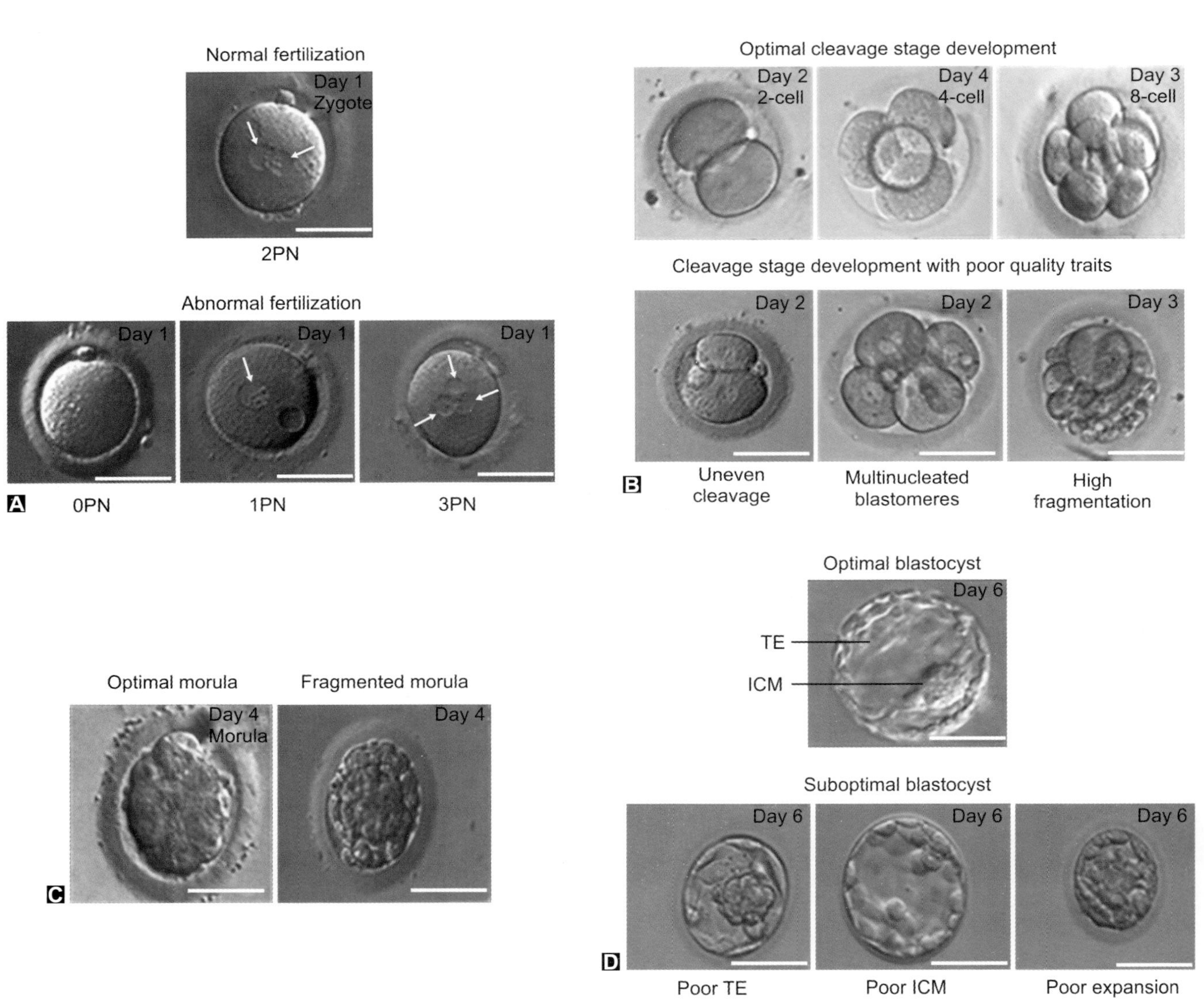

Figs 3A to D (A) The assessment of normal fertilization on day 1 of embryonic development shows two pronuclei (PN), 2PN (top panel). Abnormally fertilized day 1 embryos (bottom) containing 0PN, 1PN or 3PN are of poor quality; (B) A comparison of cleavage-stage embryos (day 2, two-cell stage; day 2, four-cell stage and day 3, eight-cell stage) with optimal development and embryos exhibiting traits that depict poor quality, including uneven cleavage, multinucleated blastomeres and several degrees of fragmentation; (C) An optimal morula-stage embryo (day 4) and a fragmented morula; (D) Human blastocysts (day 6) can be assessed for optimal or suboptimal blastocoel expansion[7]

Abbreviations: TE, trophectoderm; ICM, inner cell mass

Table 1 Morphological markers of human embryo competence evaluated using embryoscope[8]

Event	Author	Endpoint	No. of embryos analyzed	Statistically associated
Fast PB extrusion	Payne et al. (1997)	Day 3 quality	30	Yes
Synchrony in male and female PN formation	Payne et al. (1997)	Day 3 quality	30	Yes
Fast PN abuttal	Payne et al. (1997)	Day 3 quality	30	Yes
Early disappearance of pronuclei	Lemmen et al. (2008)	Day 2 blastomere number	102	Yes
Duration of first cytokinesis	Wong et al. (2010)	Development to blastocyst	100	Yes
First cleavage/time point of 2-cell stage	Meseguer et al. (2011)	Pregnancy	102	Yes
	Lemmen et al. (2008)	Day 2 blastomere Numbers	102	Yes
Fast reappearance of nuclei after first cleavage	Lemmen et al. (2008)	Day 2 blastomere Numbers	29	Yes
		Pregnancy	19	Yes
Synchrony of reappearance of nuclei after first division	Lemmen et al. (2008)	Day 2 blastomere Numbers	102	No
		Pregnancy	10	Yes
Early second division/time point of 3-cell stage	Meseguer et al. (2011)	Pregnancy	246	Yes
	Wong et al (2010)	Development to blastocyst	100	Yes
Duration of the 2-cell stage	Meseguer et al. (2011)	Pregnancy	246	Yes
Interval between second and third division/synchrony in second cell cycle (duration of 3-cell stage)	Meseguer et al. (2011)	Pregnancy	243	Yes
	Wong et al. (2010)	Development to blastocyst	100	Yes
Time point of the 4-cell stage	Meseguer et al. (2011)	Pregnancy	243	Yes
Time point of the 5-cell stage	Meseguer et al. (2011)	Pregnancy	228	Yes

Abbreviations: PB, polar bodies; PN, pronuclei

Morphokinetics: The time-bound "Milestones" embryos must comply with:

"Morphokinetics" is a term coined to define embryonic developmental milestones that need to be crossed by healthy embryos at specified time periods. Kinetic parameters of an embryo are shown to have an impact on its implantation and subsequent developmental potential.[9] Ziebe et al. (1998) noted that embryos showing 10% or lesser cellular fragmentation at the 4-cell cleavage stage had a higher implantation rate.[10] Zhan et al. (2013) noted that the time to blastomere alignment (tBR) and time to morula (tM) formation was significantly shorter in good quality embryos and that tBR is positively correlated with tM (r = 0.34; P = 0.03) in the implanted group. However, no correlation was found in nonimplanted embryos.[11] In their study, Kumtepe et al. (2013) concluded that embryos that maintain even cell stages synchronous to each other exemplify a high implantation potential.[12] Additionally, predictive morphokinetic parameters include direct cleavage from the 1- to 3-cell stage or the 2- to 5-cell stage within less than 5 hours. **Table 2** summarizes time estimates to achieve certain developmental milestones observed in two different studies. **Table 3** enlists the proposed morphokinetic parameters that can be used to assess embryo quality using an embryoscope.

Table 2 Comparison of estimates in time (in hours) from fertilization and reaching specified stages of development[1,13]

Expected stage of development	Edwards et al. (1981)	Istanbul consensus workshop (2011)[a]
2-cell stage	33.2 ± 1.3	26 ± ICSI 28 ± 1 post IVF
4-cell stage	49.0 ± 1.3	44 ± 1
8-cell stage	64.8 ± 1.8	68 ± 1
Morula	96.8 ± 1.9	92 ± 2
Blastocyst	112.7 ± 2.9	116 ± 2

Values are mean hours ± SD
ICSI = intracytoplasmic sperm injection
[a]Alpha Scientists in Reproductive Medicine and ESHRE Special interest Group of Embryology (2011)

Table 3 Proposed morphokinetic parameters for time-lapse analysis[8]

Proposed parameter	Description
First cytokinesis	Time point and duration of the first cytokinesis
Cleavage pattern	Time point for each cell division until compaction stage
Synchronicity	Time from beginning of one cleavage cycle till the beginning of the next
Embryo kinetics	Time points and duration of compaction, morula and blastocyst stages
Blastocoel pattern	Time points, duration and number of collapses of the blastocoel. Extent of collapses
Nuclei	Time points for appearance and disappearance of nuclei

Maintenance of External Environment Homeostasis

Embryos that are placed in an embryoscope are subjected to less frequent handling and lesser environmental disturbances. As embryos are placed in a closed incubator, there is less fluctuation in its pH and temperature. Additionally, embryos are very susceptible to light, humidity and CO_2 changes. Thus, any disturbance in the external environment homeostasis of the embryos can prove to be detrimental. **Figure 4** shows the comparison between standard embryo evaluation and time-lapse based embryo evaluation.

Molecular Level Assessment of Embryos

Time-lapse chromatography can also be used to visualize and quantify embryo behavior using molecular tools. The cloning of green fluorescent protein (GFP) 15 years ago revolutionized visualization of molecular mechanisms within living cells and dividing embryos.[15] In 1995, Stricker SA used time-lapse confocal microscopy to observe calcium fluctuations in zebrafish embryos and

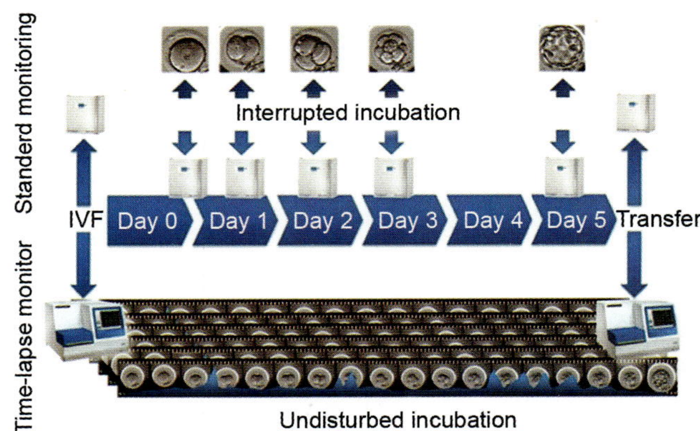

Fig. 4 Comparison between standard embryo monitoring and time-lapse based monitoring. Time-lapse based embryo evaluation allows continuous automated embryo images with a continuous culture and external environment; thus avoiding fluctuations in embryo external homeostasis. The Figure also shows recommended time intervals at which embryo assessment is required according to the Alpha-ESHRE consensus workshop[14]

subsequent calcium oscillations postfertilization using calcium-sensitive fluorochrome calcium green (CG) and the calcium-insensitive dye rhodamine (Rh) for dual-channel confocal ratioing.[16] More recently, the use of time-lapse confocal microscopy has been used by scientists to study neutrophil migration in zebrafish embryos. Similar setups can also be applied to image other motile cell types and signaling processes in translucent embryos or tissues.[17,18] Similarly, Fasulo and Sullivan (2014) used live time-lapse confocal analysis to distinguish between mutant and drug treated *Drosophila* embryos.[18] This research however, is limited only to animal models. The use of human embryos for confocal time-lapse microscopy research is confounded by ethical and moral issues, and is yet to be initiated.

Eliminating the Need for PGD

The current morphologically-based selection of human embryos fails to detect most chromosome aneuploidies. So far, preimplantation genetic diagnosis (PGD) or screening (PGS) is used to diagnose chromosomal anomalies in selected high-risk cases. PGD/PGS involves the biopsy of polar bodies or blastomeres and the use of microarray technology for aneuploidy screening. The routine preimplantation and prenatal genetic diagnosis requires testing in an aggressive manner. These procedures may be invasive to the growing embryo and potentially may compromise the clinical outcome. The use of time-lapse imaging to detect morphokinetic parameters like delayed initiation of compaction, increased time to reach full blastocyst stage and delayed initiation of blastulation have been shown to be associated with aneuploidy in embryos.[19] This noninvasive method of time-lapse imaging may be used to avoid selecting embryos with high risk of aneuploidy and aid in selecting those with reduced risk. With continued effort, the refinement of morphokinetic risk classification and modeling systems may improve the predictive ability to determine embryonic aneuploidy. However, embryo biopsy, followed by PGD/PGS still remains the most reliable method to assess chromosomal complement of preimplantation embryos.[20]

Noninvasive TLM Markers

One of the most popular techniques to improve ART success rates is to transfer embryos at the blastocyst stage which has shown to have a significant improvement in pregnancy rate.[21] However, not many embryos survive to this stage and there are concerns that prolonged exposure to artificial culture may cause epigenetic disorders. The identification of markers that demonstrate the potential of embryos to develop into blastocysts while they are still at an early developmental stage, thereby allowing culture times to be shortened, would be highly advantageous. Interestingly, all embryo parameters studied at present occur before day 3 of development suggesting that the fate of the embryo is determined before embryonic gene activation.[2] **Table 4** shows a few studies that have studied noninvasive TLM markers as a predictor of embryo competence.

Critical Evaluation of TLM

Phototoxicity is a major concern whilst using TLM. Light, especially ultraviolet (UV) radiation has been implicated to cause DNA damage in growing embryos. It has been reported that visible light is less harmful in comparison to UV light. Thus, bright field imaging (the use of simple light absorbance to create contrast) and dark field imaging (the use of simple light scattering to create a contrast) with filters are used in TLM to reduce phototoxicity.[22] The exposure to light is only for a few minutes for image acquisition. Moreover, this exposure to light is far lower in comparison to routine IVF laboratory practice for morphological analysis.[3]

Embryos do not always remain static in their culture media. Space constraints as well as the inability of a camera to move along with the embryos can be a setback. However, this issue can be resolved by using moving optics, motorized plates or multi-well culture plate dishes.[5,23] Multi-well plates can be tracked easily throughout TLM imaging as they are separately loaded. Not only can many embryos of a single patient be kept in it, the exchange of growth factors between embryos has been shown to be beneficial.[24,25]

Some studies have shown that TLM does not significantly improve the selection of high quality

Table 4 Noninvasive TLM markers used by scientists for embryo selection[8]

Research group	Marker adopted
Payne et al.	Time between fertilization and PN abuttal
Lemmen et al.	Appearance of nuclei after first cleavage
Wong et al.	Duration of first cytokinesis; time between first and second mitosis; synchronicity of second and third mitosis
Meseguer et al.	Time between first and second mitosis; synchronicity of second and third mitosis; time to reach 5-cell stage; computer-assisted technologies

embryos, predict blastocyst formation or improve pregnancy outcome.[22,26] These studies however, cannot refute the fact that TLM can reduce the number of embryos transferred and therefore the overall multiple pregnancy rate in ART. Additionally, TLM can improve cycle efficiency by improving implantation rates.[3]

Computer-assisted Analysis: Alternative to TLM

Based on digital image sequences, blastomere size and nuclear structures can be analyzed using a computer software **(Fig. 5)**.[27] Additionally, CAA can store multi-level images of embryos in a rapid manner thereby limiting the time of exposure to external, less favorable environment.[28] Calculations of embryo characteristics using mathematical equations, such as the degree of fragmentation and the size of blastomeres, are possible using CAA software. This reduces the inter- and intraobserver variability in morphological assessment of embryos. CAA however has the disadvantage of being time consuming, as every blastomere has to be measured manually. This can be counteracted by an automatic blastomere counting and measuring software. More research is needed however for evaluating the cost-effectiveness versus the predictive value of CAA with regards to ART success rates.

■ FUTURE PROSPECTS

In the current research and clinical scenario, events occurring after embryonic genome activation such as compaction, blastulation, length of the 5- to 8-cell interval, and timing of fourth cleavage are assessed manually.

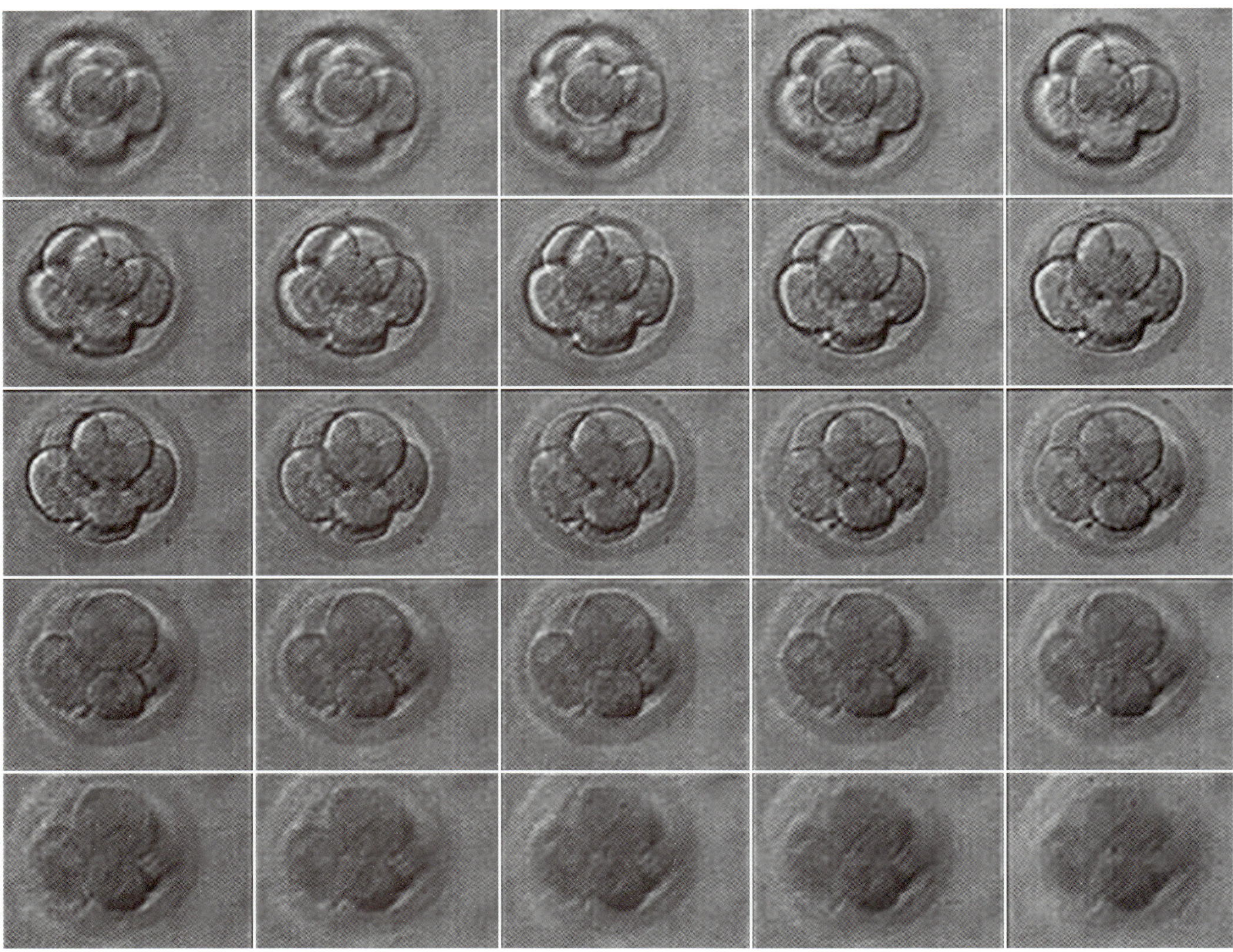

Fig. 5 Digital image sequence of a 7-cell embryo using CAA at 5 micron intervals[27]

Additional research may be required to develop accurate scoring systems that can be performed in real time and scalable enough to accommodate many embryos at one time. This requires the development of sophisticated computer algorithms, appropriate illumination techniques and additional focal planes that capture embryonic events.[22] Development of automated software that utilizes more time points for embryo assessment and measurements could be another arena where research should be directed. Multiple scoring scales (cumulative mean of individual scores at different time points) could be the best guide for embryo scoring in the future.[29]

Events occurring prior to pronuclear formation, such as calcium oscillations and cytoskeletal movements can be evaluated using confocal time-lapse imaging. Oocyte activation is an important event that may be responsible for the developmental potential of an embryo.[30] Assessment of these earlier molecular events occurring early on during embryo formation may therefore be an area of interest in future research.

■ CONCLUSION

In ART practice, embryo selection criteria should be standardized, objective, easy to assess, should cause minimal harm to the embryo and must have a high correlation with pregnancy rates.[1] These requirements are fulfilled by TLM. Although some studies have shown no benefit of TLM over standard light microscopy, the use of TLM allows better selection of embryos, which are less probable to have an euploidy. CAA scoring systems allow assessment of embryos at multiple levels and the development of new algorithms to assess embryos via multiple scoring systems is the need of the hour. However, there are some disadvantages associated with TLM and CAA such as maintenance cost, user subjectivity and slight phototoxicity. These limitations need to be corrected for the more widespread use of these technologies. In conclusion, although TLM is not being used in every ART center, a significant body of both scientific and clinical research is being undertaken to evaluate, test and improve this revolutionary technology.

■ REFERENCES

1. Machtinger R, Racowsky C. Morphological systems of human embryo assessment and clinical evidence. Reproductive Biomed Online. 2013;26:210-21.
2. Wong CC, Loewke K, Bossert NL, et al. Non-invasive imaging of human embryos before embryonic genome activation predicts development to the blastocyst stage. Nature Biotechnology. 2010;28:1115-21.
3. Meseguer M, Rubio I, Cruz M, et al. Embryo incubation and selection in a time-lapse monitoring system improves pregnancy outcome compared with a standard incubator: a retrospective cohort study. Fertil Steril. 2012;98(6):1481-9.e10.
4. Niakan KK, Han J, Pedersen RA, et al. Human pre-implantation embryo development. Development. 2012;139(5):829-41.
5. Meseguer M, Herrero J, Tejera A, et al. The use of morphokinetics as a predictor of embryo implantation. Hum Reprod. 2011;26(10):2658-71.
6. Azzarello A, Hoest T, Mikkelsen AL. The impact of pronuclei morphology and dynamicity on live birth outcome after time-lapse culture. Hum Reprod. 2012;27(9):2649-57.
7. O'Leary T, Heindryckx B, Lierman S, et al. Derivation of human embryonic stem cells using a post-inner cell mass intermediate. Nat Protoc. 2013;8(2):254-64.
8. Kirkegaard K, Agerholm IE, Ingerslev HJ. Time-lapse monitoring as a tool for clinical embryo assessment. Hum Reprod. 2012;27(5):1277-85.
9. Wittemer C, Bettahar-Lebugle K, Ohl J, et al. Zygote evaluation: an efficient tool for embryo selection. Hum Reprod. 2000;15(12):2591-7.
10. Ziebe S, Petersen K, Lindenberg S, et al. Embryo morphology or cleavage stage: how to select the best embryos for transfer after in-vitro fertilization. Hum Reprod. 1997;12(7):1545-9.
11. Zhan Q, Zaninovic N, Malmsten J, et al. Is time of blastomere realignment related to embryo quality and implantation: time-lapse study. Fertil Steril. 2013;100(3):S241.
12. Centinkaya M, Pirkevi C, Kumtepe Y, et al. Synchronicity of cleavage cycles predicts blastocyst formation and quality. Fertil Steril. 2013;100(3):S238.
13. The Istanbul consensus workshop on embryo assessment: proceedings of an expert meeting. Hum Reprod. 2011;26(6):1270-83.
14. Quinn P. Culture Media, Solutions, and Systems in Human ART. Cambridge University Press; 2014. p. 296.
15. Muzzey D, van Oudenaarden A. Quantitative time-lapse fluorescence microscopy in single cells. Annu Rev Cell Dev Biol. 2009;25:301-27.
16. Stricker SA. Time-lapse confocal imaging of calcium dynamics in starfish embryos. Dev Biol. 1995;170(2):496-518.
17. Lam PY, Fischer RS, Shin WD, et al. Spinning disk confocal imaging of neutrophil migration in zebrafish. Methods Mol Biol. 2014;1124:219-33.
18. Fasulo B, Sullivan W. Live confocal analysis of mutant- and drug-treated Drosophila embryos. Methods Mol Biol. 2014;1075:243-55.
19. Campbell A, Fishel S, Bowman N, et al. Modelling a risk classification of aneuploidy in human embryos using non-invasive morphokinetics. Reprod Biomed Online. 2013;26(5):477-85.
20. Swain JE. Could time-lapse embryo imaging reduce the need for biopsy and PGS? J Assist Reprod Genet. 2013;30(8):1081-90.

21. Papanikolaou EG, Camus M, Kolibianakis EM, et al. In vitro fertilization with single blastocyst-stage versus single cleavage-stage embryos. N Engl J Med. 2006;354(11):1139-46.

22. Wong C, Chen AA, Behr B, et al. Time-lapse microscopy and image analysis in basic and clinical embryo development research. Reprod Biomed Online. 2013;26(2):120-9.

23. Pribenszky C, Losonczi E, Molnar M, et al. Prediction of in-vitro developmental competence of early cleavage-stage mouse embryos with compact time-lapse equipment. Reprod Biomed Online. 2010;20(3):371-9.

24. Glujovsky D, Blake D, Farquhar C, et al. Cleavage stage versus blastocyst stage embryo transfer in assisted reproductive technology. Cochrane Database Syst Rev. 2012;7:CD002118.

25. Ciray HN, Aksoy T, Goktas C, et al. Time-lapse evaluation of human embryo development in single versus sequential culture media—a sibling oocyte study. J Assist Reprod Genet. 2012;29(9):891-900.

26. Chen AA, Tan L, Suraj V, et al. Biomarkers identified with time-lapse imaging: discovery, validation, and practical application. Fertil Steril. 2013;99(4):1035-43.

27. Hnida C, Engenheiro E, Ziebe S. Computer-controlled, multilevel, morphometric analysis of blastomere size as biomarker of fragmentation and multinuclearity in human embryos. Hum Reprod. 2004;19(2):288-93.

28. Paternot G, Debrock S, D'Hooghe T, et al. Computer-assisted embryo selection: a benefit in the evaluation of embryo quality? Reprod Biomed Online. 2011;23(3):347-54.

29. Santos Filho E, Noble JA, Poli M, et al. A method for semi-automatic grading of human blastocyst microscope images. Hum Reprod. 2012;27(9):2641-8.

30. Ramadan WM, Kashir J, Jones C, et al. Oocyte activation and phospholipase C zeta (PLCzeta): diagnostic and therapeutic implications for assisted reproductive technology. Cell Commun Signal. 2012;10(1):12.

32 Embryo Transfer: Catheters and Techniques

Hrishikesh Pai

INTRODUCTION

The success rate of treatment with in vitro fertilization (IVF) depends on the characteristics of the couple being treated and the performance of the clinic. The former factor cannot be changed hence a continuous effort has been put toward optimizing the embryological procedures.

The procedure of embryo transfer (ET), apart from embryo quality and endometrial receptivity, happens to be a crucial determinant of the success of any IVF cycle.[1]

Recent studies have identified the relationship between IVF outcome and transfer techniques and have noted a pregnancy rate of 33.3% for *excellent transfers* and 10.5% for *poor transfers*.[2,3] The cardinal tenet of a good ET is gentle and atraumatic placement of good quality embryos into the uterine cavity.

HISTORICAL ASPECTS

The history of IVF and ET dates back as early as the 1890s when Walter Heape a professor and physician at the University of Cambridge, England, who had been conducting research on reproduction in a number of animal species, reported the first known case of embryo transplantation in rabbits, long before the applications to human fertility were even suggested.[4]

However, it was not until 1959 that indisputable evidence of IVF was obtained by Chang[5] who was the first to achieve births in a mammal (a rabbit) by IVF. The newly ovulated eggs were fertilized, in vitro by incubation with capacitated sperm in a small Carrel flask for 4 hours, thus opening the way to assisted procreation.

Patrick Steptoe and Robert Edwards conducted the first successful ET in humans in 1978. In 1985, Strickler et al. reported first transabdominal ET done under ultrasound guidance.

PREPARATORY TECHNIQUES

Role of Hysteroscopy Prior to Embryo Transfer

Hysteroscopy is the gold standard to visualize the uterine cavity. It has an advantage of simultaneously treating intrauterine abnormalities. A pre-IVF endometrial cavity evaluation is mandatory prior to treatment. The preferred method is hysteroscopy especially in patients with previous history of implantation failures, and those with high suspicion of uterine or cervical anomalies.

Jyotsna Pundir and Omanwa, in 2014, conducted a meta-analysis of 23 studies that included a total of 3,179 participants and they concluded that performing hysteroscopy before IVF treatment significantly increases the chance of pregnancy and livebirth rate (RR 1.44, P = 0.01) in the subsequent IVF cycle especially in women who had one or more failed IVF cycles.[6]

Balmaceda et al. have shown that up to 45% of patients, undergoing IVF had a detectable uterine abnormality. Shamma et al. showed that about 43% patients with normal hysterosalpingography had abnormal findings on hysteroscopy such as small uterine septa **(Fig. 1)**, small submucous fibroids, uterine hypoplasia and cervical ridges.

The author routinely performs hysteroscopy prior to IVF in all patients. However, there is no definitive evidence that all infertile patients, will greatly benefit from a hysteroscopy done in previous cycles.

Medication Prior to Embryo Transfer

Uterine Relaxants

A variety of substances, such as prostaglandins, play a role in the delicate process of embryo apposition, attachment and invasion into the endometrium. β-sympatho-

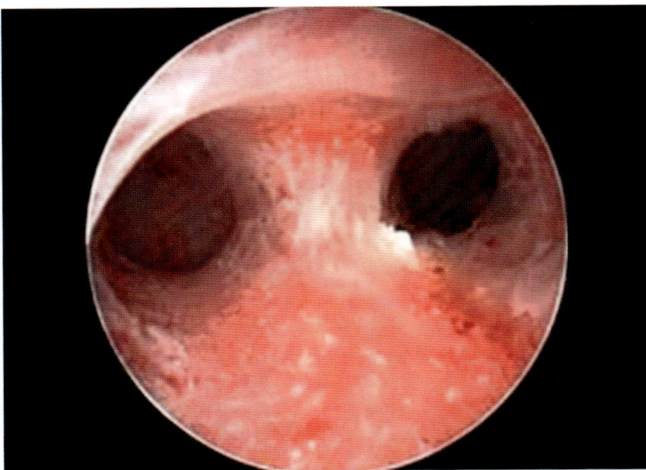

Fig. 1 Hysteroscopy: intrauterine septum

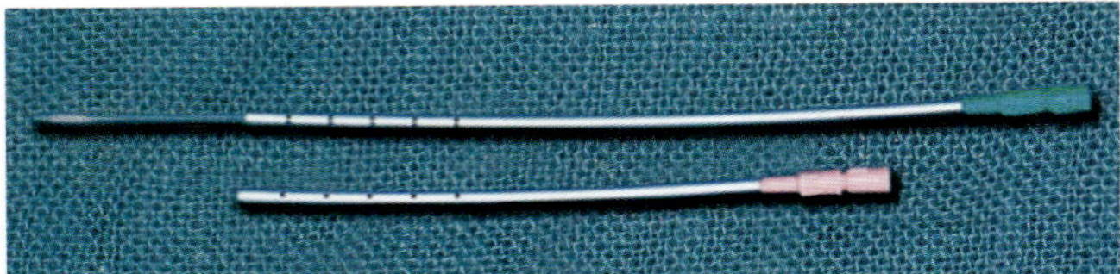

Fig. 2 Wallace embryo transfer catheter

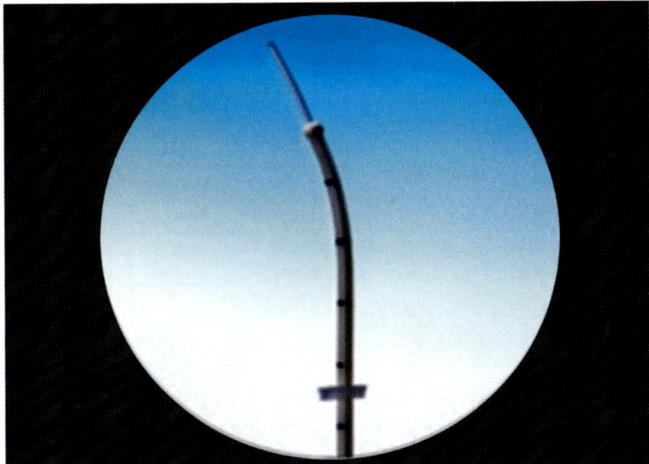

Fig. 3 Labotect embryo transfer catheter

mimetics as well as prostaglandin synthetase inhibitors have been proposed and used to achieve uterine quiescence at the time of transfer and to improve the pregnancy rates. In addition, it has been published that the pregnancy rate was higher in patients that exhibited endometrial waves (45%/ET, 20/44) in comparison to those that showed a quiescent uterus (16%/ET, 12/77, P < 0.001).[7]

Prophylactic Antibiotic Administration

It has been demonstrated that a significant reduction of pregnancy and implantation rates occurs in patients with positive microbial catheter tip cultures. In light of this information, Egbase et al. have presented data to show that the use of antibiotics at the time of oocyte aspiration significantly reduced the incidence of positive cultures of catheter tips 48 hours later.[8]

Choice of Catheter

Though the procedure of ET itself has undergone little change over the years, the technicalities of the procedure have been an issue of constant study. Embryo transfer catheters may be classified according to:
- Tip characteristics
- Flexibility
- Presence of fixed or detached outer sheath
- Malleability
- Shape memory of the material
- Gauge and length.

The commercially available catheters may be broadly divided into soft and firm catheters. The common catheters used in clinical practice are:

- Edward Wallace coaxial catheter (**Fig. 2**)
- Labotect coaxial catheter (**Fig. 3**)
- Cooks trans-soft coaxial catheter
- Frydman catheter
- Tomcat catheter.

Soft vs Rigid

Soft catheters such as Wallace allow the catheter to gently follow the curvatures of the uterocervical canal thus minimizing trauma to the endometrium. However, their extreme flexibility makes them liability in difficult transfers. On the other hand, catheters with rigid outer sheath make catheter placement much easier.[9,10] However, their rigid nature may cause bleeding, mucous plugging, retention of embryos and uterine contractions—factors which may compromise pregnancy rates.[11,12] Various studies have demonstrated better results with the use of a soft catheter.[1,13,14] The author too prefers to use a soft catheter and reserves the use of a firm catheter in cases where negotiating the cervical canal with a soft catheter is deemed *impossible*.

The ultimate decision of the catheter to be used is based on the skill, experience and catheter familiarity of the clinician performing ET.

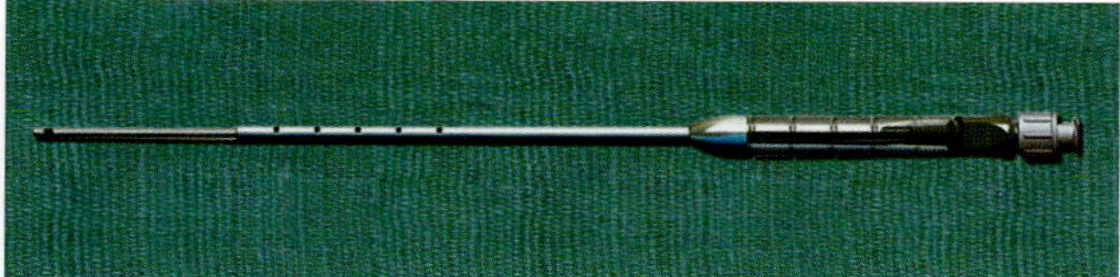

Fig. 4 Echo-Cath

Newer Catheters

Echo-Cath: It consists of a high reflection echo band proximal to the tip to provide immediate identification of catheter tip position **(Fig. 4)**.

Timing of Embryo Transfer

Historically, most ETs were carried out on day 2 which is 48 hours after oocyte retrieval. However, it has been noted that delaying the transfer till day 3 has no detrimental effects on pregnancy rates. In fact, a day 3 transfer may allow selection of embryos with better prognosis for development **(Fig. 5)**.

Patients with three or more good quality embryos on day 3 may be subjected to a blastocyst transfer on day 5. The success rate of blastocyst transfer is in the range of 50–60%.[15] However, a caveat remains. Only about 60% of good embryos may grow to blastocysts **(Fig. 6)**, hence in the absence of rigorous selection criteria, the transfer procedure may need cancelation due to absence of blastocyst formation.

However, a meta-analysis conducted by Glujovski and Blake in 2013 showed that cumulative pregnancy rates (after both fresh and frozen thaw ETs) are more in those women who had cleavage stage transfers compared with blastocyst stage transfer.[16]

Sequential Embryo Transfer

Some clinicians have tried to perform a second transfer in the same cycle after replacement on day 2 or day 3. The second transfer was then performed on day 5. One philosophy is to have the benefits of blastocyst transfer without the drawbacks of culture to day 5, i.e. arrest of all embryos after day 2 or 3, and hence having no transfer at all. It is still unclear whether the patient benefits from this approach, however this seems unlikely.

Role of Ultrasound in Embryo Transfer

- To exclude any newly developed contraindications to ET (hydrometra).

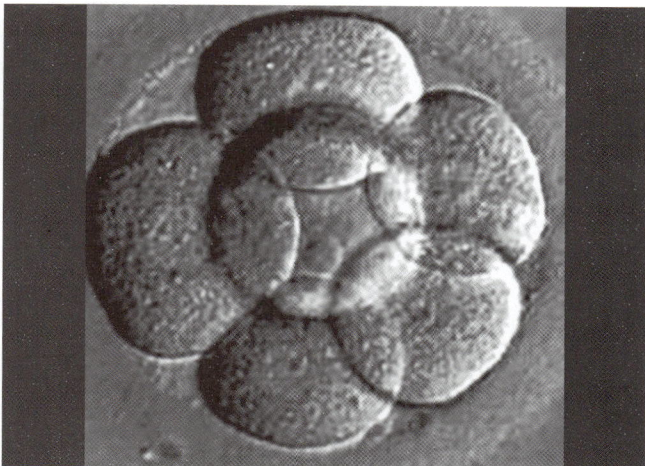

Fig. 5 Six-cell, grade 1 embryo

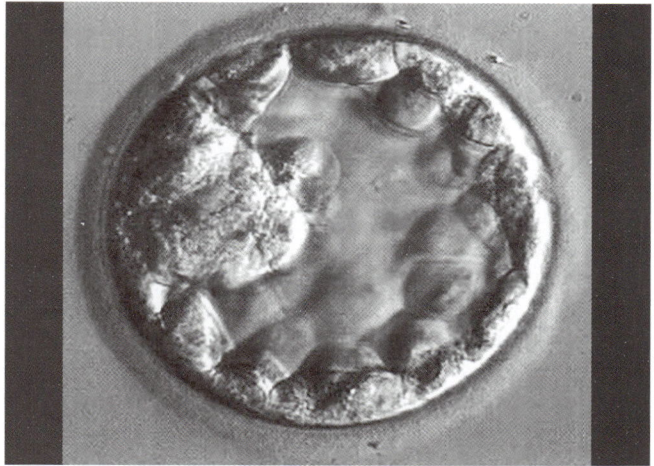

Fig. 6 A blastocyst

- To measure the endometrial thickness and the uterocervical length.
- To assess ovarian size to confirm that risk of ovarian hyperstimulation syndrome (OHSS) is not great.
- To measure the uterocervical angle and bend the tip of the catheter accordingly.
- To confirm that the embryos are deposited in the uterine cavity in the area of maximum implantation potential.[17,18]
- To confirm that the embryos are not displaced from the uterine cavity.[19]

Brown and Buckingham confirmed in 2010 that the ultrasound-guided method of ET **(Fig. 7)** improves the rate of clinical pregnancies compared to the clinical touch method.[20]

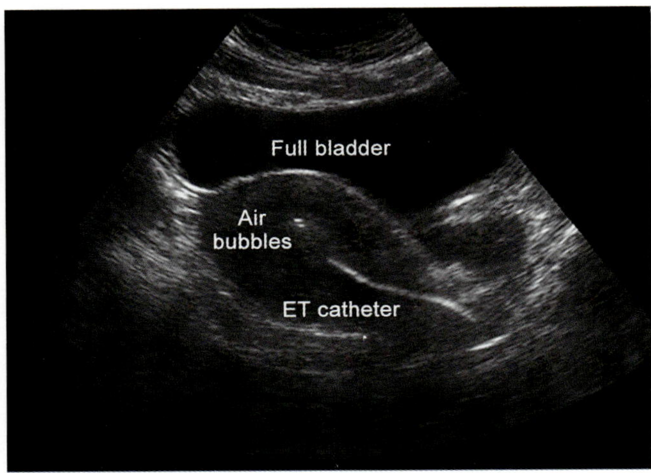

Fig. 7 Ultrasound-guided embryo transfer

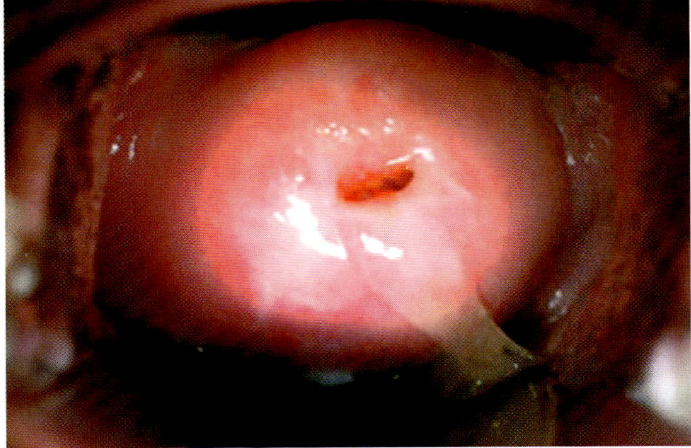

Fig. 8 Removing cervical mucous: an important step in embryo transfer

Procedure of ET

An embryo transfer procedure consists essentially of the following important steps:

1. *Confirmation of patient identity:*
   - Confirm the name and identity of the patient who is made ready for transfer.
   - Check that relevant consents forms are filled and duly signed.
   - Tally the embryo dishes with the patient's identity. This is a crucial step to avoid mismatched transfer and further medicolegal litigation.

2. *Patient preparation*
   - A brief check is made to confirm an adequately full bladder. Normal saline is used as the coupling medium for transabdominal ultrasound.
   - The patient is placed in lithotomy position. An abdominal ultrasound is performed to confirm proper visualization of the endometrial cavity and straightening of the cervicouterine axis.
   - The person aiding performing the abdominal scan as well as the clinician doing the transfer wear plastic gloves that have been pre-rinsed with saline and dried with a sterile towel.
   - The private parts are painted with normal saline.
   - The cervix is visualized with the help of Cusco's speculum or two sims speculums. The cervix is cleaned and the cervical mucus is gently removed. Buffered culture medium is finally used to rinse the cervix.

3. *Removal of cervical mucous:*
   - Cervical mucous **(Fig. 8)** can cause plugging of the catheter tip leading to retention of embryos and embryo damage. It may also lead to bacterial contamination of the endometrial cavity.[8,21,22]

4. *Loading of catheter:*
   - Embryos may be loaded into the transfer catheter in a pre-loading or after-loading fashion.
   - The after-loading technique carries a higher risk of temperature and pH changes in the embryo-carrying medium through the delicate inner sheath of the catheter. The author hence prefers to pre-load the embryos.

5. *Actual transfer:*
   - The catheter is passed under ultrasound control, 1.5 cm below the fundus or 5 cm from the external os.
   - Midcavity deposit of the embryos is made by depressing the piston of the syringe, slowly. After deposition, there should be gentle pressure maintained on the syringe piston. One can withdraw the ET catheter immediately or after 30 seconds of expulsion of embryos. A real-time ultrasound is done to confirm the proper placement of embryos.
   - During removal of the catheter, the pressure on the piston is maintained to avoid sucking in of embryos.
   - The catheter is checked for presence of blood, mucus or retained embryos.

6. *Immediate post-transfer:*
   - The patient is rested on the ET table for 20 minutes. After that, the patient is discharged with proper instructions.
   - Proper documentation is done.

Post-transfer Instructions

- To take antibiotics for 2 days.
- Adequate luteal support in form of vaginal or injectable progesterone.
- To report in case of pain in abdomen, nausea, giddiness or bleeding.
- Follow-up for an ultrasound 5–7 days after transfer, in patients at high-risk of OHSS.
- To undergo a human chorionic gonadotropin test 14 days after transfer and to repeat the test after 2 days.
- Not to stop luteal support unless told by the doctor.
- Avoid physical exertion.

Number of Embryos Transferred

The number of embryos transferred depends on the age of the patient, associated infertility factors and the stage at which the transfer is being carried out. Most countries have their own laws or rules that regulate the maximum number of embryos that may be transferred per attempt.

In India, the regulations allow no more than three embryos to be transferred in women less than 37 years of age.[7]

When a blastocyst transfer is planned, only two blastocysts may be transferred into a woman during each transfer attempt.

However, a maximum of four embryos may be transferred in exceptional cases such as in women who are more than 37 years of age or have adenomyosis or have had more than two previous implantation failures.

Single Embryo Transfer

A meta-analysis of eight clinical trials performed by Mc Lernon et al. in 2010 showed that elective single ET results in a higher chance of delivering a term singleton livebirth compared with double ET. Although this strategy yields a lower pregnancy rate than a double ET in a fresh IVF cycle, this difference is almost completely overcome by an additional frozen single ET cycle.[23]

The American society of Reproductive Medicine advocates considering single ET in good prognosis patients who are less than 35 years of age.

Difficult Embryo Transfer

Difficult ET was associated with very poor pregnancy rates (4%) as compared to easy transfers (20%). A difficult transfer may provoke subendometrial-myometrial contractions.[24,25] If there are more than four uterine contractions per minute, on ultrasound, there is a lowering of pregnancy rate (Fanchin et al.).[26]

Normally, the author follows the following sequence in case of difficult transfer:

1. All ETs are done under ultrasound guidance as a rule. Manipulation of cervix with speculum and or guiding of the catheter tip with long artery forceps or ring forces is done to negotiate the internal os, wherever necessary.
2. In case of previous history of difficult ET or difficult mock transfer, one can use an outer catheter sheath with a malleable stylet or mandril. Once this catheter is negotiated under ultrasound guidance into the ideal spot, the inner ET catheter is loaded with the embryos, the mandril is removed and the inner catheter is threaded in, and transfer is performed.
3. In case the catheter cannot pass through the canal, one can hold the anterior lip with a tenaculum or ellis and gently give traction on the cervix. This helps in straightening out of the uterocervical canal. One should not clamp the tenaculum, as the pressure will create immense pain and muscular contractions.
4. A constant watch is kept on time, once the embryos are loaded into the ET catheter. In case, the embryos are not replaced into the uterine cavity 2 minutes from the time of loading, they are returned to the laboratory and replaced in the Petri dish to prevent cooling effect and pH damage to the embryos (Brinsden et al.).[3]
5. If everything else fails, one may have to resort to cervical dilatation. This may be done without anesthesia or under sedation. In case the patient is not starving, one can wait for a few hours and then do the dilatation and the transfer. The dilatation is done with 1 or 2 mm diameter steel dilators. Alternately, one can do it with rigid catheters such as TDT or soft catheters such as Wallace with malleable mandarin (stylet).
6. In extreme cases, where the cervix cannot be negotiated, one can go for transmyometrial ET.
7. In case, there is difficulty in passing the cervix and the tubes are normal, one can do a laparoscopic transfer of the embryos into the Fallopian tube (Tubal embryo transfer or TET).
8. In worst case scenarios, where cervical dilatation has led to excessive bleeding, one can reposit the embryos into culture and transfer them the next day.

Rest After Embryo Transfer

The embryo carrying fluid in a transfer catheter is generally less than 30 µL. This small volume, coupled with the sticky secretions of the endometrial lining and the contractile peristaltic forces of the apposing endomyometrial surfaces result in proper retention of embryos. A standing patient coupled with gravity is not adequate enough to expel the embryos out of the uterus. Multiple studies support that standing immediately after transfer does not influence the position of embryos and does not affect the result. Hence, a patient can easily walk home following 15–30 minutes of rest, following ET (Sheriff et al.).[26]

OTHER TECHNIQUES

Frozen Thaw Embryo Transfer

There is growing interest in a "freeze-all" embryo policy in IVF. Such an approach, which cryopreserves all embryos generated in a stimulated IVF cycle for later transfer in a nonstimulated natural cycle, would avoid any of the adverse effects which ovarian stimulation might have on endometrial receptivity during the treatment cycle. Ovarian stimulation has been shown to have adverse effects on endometrial receptivity and the risk of OHSS is also increased when ET is performed in the stimulated cycle.

The first meta-analysis on this subject indicates that the chance of a clinical pregnancy is around 30% higher when all embryos are frozen for later transfer than with fresh ET. The results were presented by Professor Miguel Angel Checa from the Hospital Universitari del Mar in Barcelona, Spain.[27]

The study was a systematic review of the entire literature, which provided a pool of 64 relevant studies-with three randomized trials-performed before December 2011. The current review was based on information from 633 IVF/ICSI cycles in which 316 were randomized to fresh ET and 317 to frozen embryo transfer (FET). Results showed (based on a relative risk calculation) that the probability of a clinical pregnancy is significantly higher from freeze-all cycles (50%) than in fresh ETs (38%), a relative risk of 1.31, which was statistically significant. The miscarriage rates did not show significant differences between the two groups.

Role of Granulocyte Colony-stimulating Factor

A few early studies have shown intrauterine instillation of granulocyte colony-stimulating factor to be beneficial in patients with thin endometrium and recurrent implantation failures (Kunicki et al. 2014).[28]

However, due to absence of randomized controlled trials the use of granulocyte colony-stimulating factor is still considered experimental.

CONCLUSION

Thirty percent of failure in assisted reproductive technology (ART) is due to a poorly performed ET. The transfer procedure has largely remained unchanged over time. However, the importance of a skillfully performed ET cannot be highlighted enough. Due to insufficient evidence from clinical trials, it is not clear which variables are crucial to optimising the success of ET in IVF. But studies remain unanimous in one conclusion that the clinician behind the procedure happens to be the most important determinant of a successful ART program.

REFERENCES

1. Diedrich K, Van der ven H, Al-Hasani S, et al. Establishment of pregnancy related to embryo transfer techniques after in vitro fertilization. Hum Reprod. 1989;4(Suppl. 8):111–4.
2. Cohen J. Embryo replacement technology. San Francisco 31st Annual Post Graduate Course. ASRM; 1998.
3. Brinsden P. Oocyte recovery and Embryo transfer technique. A textbook of IVF and ART, 2nd edition. The Parthenon Publishing Group; 1999.
4. Dorn C, Reinsberg J, Schlebusch H, et al. Serum oxytocin concentration during embryo transfer procedure. Eur J Obstet Gynecol Reprod Biol. 1999;87(1):77–80.
5. Chang MC. Fertilization of rabbit ova *in vitro*. Nature. 1959; 8:184. (suppl 7) 466.
6. Pundir J, Pundir V, Omanwa K, et al. Hysteroscopy prior to the first IVF cycle: A systematic review and meta-analysis. Reprod BioMedicine Online. 2014;28(2):151-61.
7. ICMR ART Regulations. Ministry of Health and Family Welfare, Government of India, New Delhi; 2010.
8. Egbase PE, al-Sharhan M, al-Othman S, et al. Incidence of microbial growth from the tip of the embryo transfer catheter after embryo transfer in relation to clinical pregnancy rate following in-vitro fertilization and embryo transfer. Hum Reprod. 1996;11(8):1687–9.
9. Meriano J, Weissman A, Greenblatt EM, et al. The choice of embryo transfer catheter affects embryo implantation after IVF. Fertil Steril. 2000;74(4):678–82.
10. Mortimer S, Fluker M, Yuzpe A. Effect of embryo transfer catheter on implantation rates [abstract]. 58th Annual meeting of the American Society for Reproductive Medicine. Fertil Steril. 2002;78(3): S17–8.
11. Curfs MHJM, Cleine JH, van Kamp AA, et al. Comparison of the Wallace versus TDT embryo-transfer catheter: a prospective, randomized study. Third Biennial Alpha Conference, September 8–11, 2001, New York, USA. Reprod Biomed Online. 2001;3(Suppl. 1).
12. Foutouh IA, Youssef M, Tolba M, et al. Does embryo transfer catheter type affect pregnancy rate? Middle East Fertil Soc J. 2003;8:154–8.
13. Mcllveen M, Lok D, Pritchard J, et al. A randomised controlled trial comparing two embryo transfer catheters. Hum Reprod. 2004;19:127S.
14. Boone WR, Johnson JE, Blackhurst DM, et al. Cook versus Edwards–Wallace: are there differences in flexible catheters? J Assist Reprod Genet. 2001;18(1):15–7.
15. Gardner DK, Lane M, Stevens J, et al. Blastocyst score affects implantation and pregnancy outcome: towards a single blastocyst transfer. Fertil Steril. 2000;73(6):1155-8.

16. Glujovsky D, Blake D, Farquhar C, et al. Cleavage stage versus blastocyst stage embryo transfer in assisted reproductive technology. Cochrane Database Syst Rev. 2012;7.
17. Birnholz JC. Ultrasound visualization of endometrial movements. Fertil Steril. 1984;41(1):157–8.
18. Amorcho B, Gomez E, Pontes L, et al. Does the selection of catheter for embryo transfer affect the success rate of an ART unit? [abstract] 15th Annual Meeting of the ESHRE (Tours, France), 1999. Hum Reprod. 1999;14(Suppl. 1):205.
19. Coroleu B, Carreras O, Veiga A, et al. Embryo transfer under ultrasound guidance improves pregnancy rates in in vitro fertilization. Hum Reprod. 2000;15(3):616–20.
20. Brown JA, Buckingham K, Abou-Setta A, et al. Ultrasound versus 'clinical touch' for catheter guidance during embryo transfer in women. Cochrane Database Syst Rev. 2007;24(1):1469-93.
21. Moore DE, Soules MR, Klein NA, et al. Bacteria in the transfer catheter tip influence the live-birth rate after in vitro fertilization. Fertil Steril. 2000;74(6):1118–24.
22. Al-Shawaf T, Dave R, Harper J, et al. Transfer of embryos into the uterus: how much do technical factors affect pregnancy rates? J Assist Reprod Genet. 1993;10:31–6.
23. Kunicki M, Łukaszuk K, Woclawek-Potocka I, et al. Evaluation of granulocyte colony-stimulating factor effects on treatment-resistant thin endometrium in women undergoing in vitro fertilization. BioMed Res Int. 2014. p. 5.
24. McDonald JA, Norman RJ. A randomized controlled trial of a soft double lumen embryo transfer catheter versus a firm single lumen catheter: significant improvements in pregnancy rates. Hum Reprod. 2002;17(6):1502-6.
25. Fanchin R, Righini C, Olivennes F, et al. Uterine contractions at the time of embryo transfer alter pregnancy rates after in vitro fertilization. Hum Reprod. 1998;13(7):1968–74.
26. Ghazzawi IM, Al-Hasani S, Karaki R, et al. Transfer technique and catheter choice influence the incidence of transcervical embryo expulsion and the outcome of IVF. Hum Reprod. 1999;14(3):677–82.
27. Roque M, Lattes K, Serra S, et al. Fresh embryo transfer versus frozen embryo transfer in *in vitro* fertilization cycles: a systematic review and meta-analysis. Fertil Steril. 2013;99(1):156-62.
28. McLernon DJ, Harrild K, Bergh C, et al. Clinical effectiveness of elective single versus double embryo transfer: meta-analysis of individual patient data from randomised trials BMJ. 2010;341:c6945.

Implantation

33 Endometrial Receptivity

Jure Knez, Christophe Blockeel

INTRODUCTION

The process of embryo implantation involves the attachment of the nascent embryo at the blastocyst stage to the endometrium, invasion into the stroma and formation of the placenta. This requires a careful synchronization between blastocyst development and the endometrium. The soluble growth factors, hormones, adhesion molecules, extracellular matrix (ECM) and prostaglandins establish a complex dialogue between the endometrium and the embryo.[1] Thus, the coordination of the steps by which the embryo attaches to the epithelium, breaches the basement membrane and invades into the stroma is enabled.[2] Subsequently, decidualization, the process of extensive stromal transformation and angiogenesis to provide the embryo with its needs is initiated. These early events are crucial for the successful establishment of eventual pregnancy.

However, the implantation rates in human are estimated to be around 25–35% per menstrual cycle, which is low compared to some of the other animal species.[3,4] While the embryo with its characteristic high rates of aneuploidy can be responsible for the failure of implantation, the lack of uterine receptivity on the other hand is also of importance.[5,6] The priming of endometrium to optimize the window of implantation (WOI) phase has been a subject of interest for decades, and much research has been devoted to understanding the preparation and capability of the endometrial wall to create a hospitable environment for the interaction with the blastocyst. This chapter gives a concise description of the physiologic aspects of implantation, the current evidence about the endometrial receptivity markers and the reasons for failure of implantation in humans and animal models.

THE PROCESS OF IMPLANTATION

The implantation process involves three stages: apposition, adhesion and penetration of the embryo. Apposition is an unstable adhesion of the blastocyst to the endometrial surface. During this stage, the trophoblast becomes closely apposed to the luminal epithelium.[2] In the following adhesion stage, the association of the trophoblast and the luminal epithelium becomes sufficiently intimate to resist dislocation of the blastocyst by flushing the uterine lumen. This is mediated by adhesion molecules, immune cells, and cytokines.[7] The first sign of attachment reaction occurs on day 20–21 of the menstrual cycle in humans, and coincides with the localized increase in the stromal vascular permeability at the site of blastocyst attachment.[1] Following adhesion, the embryo invades through the luminal epithelium into the stroma to establish a relationship with the maternal vasculature; although this activity is mainly controlled by the trophoblast, the decidua also limits the extent of invasion.[1] In response to this invasion and the presence of progesterone stimulation, the endometrial stromal cells and endometrial ECM undergo decidualization that is essential for the viability of the pregnancy. If the endometrium is not competent to participate in all of these stages, the implantation of the embryo will fail. Actual implantation of the blastocyst into the endometrium occurs 6–7 days after fertilization and after 10 days, the blastocyst is completely embedded in the uterine wall.[8] In most pregnancies, human chorionic gonadotropin (hCG) secreted by the embryo is detectable in maternal serum within 8–10 days of ovulation. Several benign gynecological disorders have been correlated with decreased cycle fecundity and endometrial receptivity, including: endometriosis, hydrosalpinx, leiomyoma and polycystic ovarian syndrome (PCOS).[9]

ENDOMETRIAL RECEPTIVITY

The term "endometrial receptivity" refers to the ability of the uterine lining to accept and accommodate a nascent embryo, resulting in a successful pregnancy. The human endometrium undergoes a complex series of organized proliferative and secretory changes in each menstrual cycle, and exhibits only a short period of receptivity, known as the "window of implantation".[10] Endometrial development resulting in endometrial receptivity during the WOI requires the subtle collaboration of an extremely large number of different factors.[6]

Embryo transfer studies in rodents have shown that the endometrium becomes receptive to implantation for a very limited period of approximately 24 hours.[11] In rats and mice, this receptive phase occurs between day 4 and day 5 after mating. Embryos, entering the uterine cavity outside this "WOI" do not implant. The timing of the WOI in humans was first described by the early work of Herting et al. (1956),[12] in a unique study of uterine samples in women attempting pregnancy before hysterectomy. By looking at the early embryos in the process of attachment and invasion, the group defined for the first time, the earliest events in embryo implantation in the human, finding that early attachment and invasion occurred 5–6 days after ovulation. They observed free floating embryos within the uterine lumen before days 19–20 of the menstrual cycle, whereas from day 21 onwards, blastocysts were found already implanted. These data have been corroborated in oocyte donation cycles in which fertilized oocytes were transferred to the uterus of recipient women during spontaneous and induced cycles with exogenous steroids.[12] The findings led to the conclusion that the human WOI occupies a 4–5 days interval during the secretory phase of the cycle, coinciding with the peak plasma progesterone levels. When implantation does not occur, a timely destruction of the fully developed endometrium leads to menstruation. On the other side, if implantation does occur, the endometrium continues to grow and undergoes further morphological and molecular changes to provide sufficient support for the growing embryo.[10]

The existence of the "WOI" has triggered several studies to investigate how the endometrium is brought to this receptive state and to define the morphological and molecular markers that identify this state. By knowing the answers to these questions, possible diagnostic criteria for predicting poor implantation could be developed and the appropriate treatments could be designed.

■ THE ROLE OF STEROID HORMONES

Ovarian hormones, estrogen and progesterone, which modulate uterine events in a spatiotemporal manner, are primarily responsible for the endometrial transition and establishment of a receptive endometrium.[13] The importance of these steroid hormones cannot be understated as pregnancy cannot occur without them. They act primarily through the nuclear receptors estrogen receptor alpha (ERα), ERβ, progesterone receptor α (PRα) and PRβ, respectively, which act to alter gene expression.[14]

Each of the mentioned receptor subtypes is present in the epithelial as well as stromal cells of the endometrium. Thus, the levels of these receptors and concentrations of hormones are equally important for successful implantation.[14] Both receptors decline in the epithelium at the opening of the WOI due to the influence of progesterone.[15] At the same time, epithelial cells express several secretory proteins and cell surface markers that are important for the receptivity. Some of these effects are mediated by the epithelial cells through the progesterone receptors on the stromal cells. This is exemplified in humans by the expression of integrin $\alpha v \beta 3$ in epithelial cells, which is mediated by heparin binding epidermal growth factor (HB-EGF) secreted from stromal cells under progesterone induction. The effect of steroid hormones is to organize endometrium appropriately so that local cytokines and chemokines can direct activities in implantation.

Studies in laboratory animals, primates and women undergoing oocyte donation in hormone replacement cycles indicate that the development of receptive endometrium requires only adequate priming with estradiol and then exposure to progesterone for a period matching the developmental stage of the embryo.[11] In humans and primates, exogenous estrogen in the luteal phase is not essential for receptivity, although this does not exclude local estrogen production by the endometrium or the embryo by itself, both of which can synthesize estradiol through the action of the enzyme aromatase.[16-18]

■ MORPHOLOGIC AND MOLECULAR MARKERS OF RECEPTIVITY IN HUMAN ENDOMETRIUM

The endometrium undergoes precisely defined morphological changes that lead toward the WOI. As described in the early studies of human endometrium by Noyes et al.[19] histological examination of the midluteal phase endometrial biopsy provides the evidence of progesterone-induced secretory changes of the estradiol-primed endometrium. However, it has become clear that normal "in phase" endometrial biopsy does not necessarily reflect normal endometrial function or receptivity. Hence, in addition to morphological changes, researchers have tried to find reliable genetically based molecular markers of implantation.

The molecules secreted by or expressed on the surface of endometrium are today known to represent a complex matrix that includes a number of mediators that modulate endometrial receptivity, and that may be involved in the maintenance and nurturing of ascending spermatozoa and the preimplantation embryo. A number of normal endometrial development markers, expressed at different stages of the luteal phase have been described in the last decade. Subtle differences in the molecular repertoire expressed by the endometrium of fertile women compared with patients who show subfertility have been revealed. It is still questionable though, to what extent these apparent differences in molecular markers reflect a functionally compromised endometrium that is not receptive. Today, none of the known markers has a sufficient discriminatory value to serve as a test for endometrial receptivity in routine clinical practice. As opposed to a single marker, it is more likely that a complex profile of markers will provide the most sensitive and specific means of assessing endometrial receptivity in the future.[20]

However, before the introduction of high-density oligonucleotide microarray technology, a one-by-one approach to identify candidate markers of uterine receptivity expressed during the putative WOI was used. Today, the whole genetic signature of the endometrium at a certain time point can be determined. Hence, several markers and their possible interactions can be studied simultaneously.[21,23]

Histological Evidence

The Noyes criteria have remained the gold standard for endometrial evaluation since the introduction over half a century ago.[19] However, the usefulness of endometrial dating has been questioned since the histological delay in endometrial maturation fails to discriminate between fertile and infertile couples.[23] A few studies have shown that endometrial histological features fail to reliably distinguish specific menstrual cycle days or narrow intervals of days of endometrial receptivity, leading to the conclusion that histological dating has neither the accuracy nor the precision to be useful in the clinical management of patients.[24,25] However, in contrary to these findings, it has recently been shown that by using microarray technology, genetic profile can discriminate between women with and without endometrial advancement after ovarian stimulation cycles.[26]

Pinopodes

Electronic microscopic scanning has allowed visualizing further aspects of the endometrium. Thus, cytoplasmic protrusions on the apical surface of the luminal epithelium, termed pinopodes or uterodomes have been visualized. Their appearance has been shown to coincide with the period of receptivity in rodents. In humans, they appear around day 19 of the cycle and are reported to persist for no more than 48 hours, although there is some disagreement about this duration.[27,28] Human blastocysts are reported to attach preferentially to cultured endometrial epithelial cells expressing pinopodes rather than to the areas of microvilli.[29] This has led to suggestion that they are involved in the initial attachment of the blastocyst to the endometrium in vivo. Their appearance is induced by progesterone and the timing of this is modified by treatments such as controlled ovarian hyperstimulation or hormone replacement cycles for oocyte recipients.[29,30] However, even in the fertile women, there is a considerable variation in the time they form, appearing between 5 and 8 days after ovulation. Moreover, the quantitation of pinopodes proved highly subjective. Thus, most of the recent studies have failed to show a reliable pattern for their expression.[28,31,32] Hence, their significance as markers of endometrial receptivity remains unproven. Furthermore, morphological features seldom provide the information regarding the molecular mechanisms taking place in the tissue throughout the menstrual cycle, which may allow a better understanding of the physiological status of the endometrium. Some of the most researched receptivity biomarkers will be briefly discussed in the following sections.

Genetic Factors: Role of Homeobox Genes

Homeobox or *HOX* genes are essential for endometrial growth. Both *HOXA10* and *HOXA11* are expressed in human endometrial epithelial and stromal cells, and their expression is significantly higher in the mid- and late-secretory phases, coinciding with the time of embryo implantation.[33-35] In the case of successful implantation, the decidua of the early pregnancy continues to express high levels of *HOXA10* and *HOXA11* mRNA.[34,36] Both estrogen and progesterone act independently and in concert to upregulate *HOXA10* and *HOXA11* expression in the endometrium.

As transcription factors, *HOX* genes regulate other downstream target genes leading to the proper development of the endometrium and receptivity to implantation. Both of these genes are necessary for fertility in mice. Although, *HOXA10* and *HOXA11* knockout mice produce normal embryos and these embryos can survive in the wild-type surrogate, wild-type embryos from surrogate mice cannot implant in *HOXA10* and *HOXA11* knockout mice. This suggests uterine factor infertility due to an implantation defect.[37-39] The importance of *HOXA10* in implantation is also supported by experiments using antisense oligonucleotides to *HOXA10* that were injected into the mouse uterus, resulting in decrement of implantation rates.[40]

A number of other molecular and morphological markers specific to implantation window are regulated by *HOX* genes, including pinopodes and insulin-like growth factor-binding-protein-I (IGFBP-I). *HOXA10* antisense treatment diminishes pinopode number, whereas an increase is observed when uterine *HOXA10* expression is upregulated.[41] There are no documented mutations in *HOXA10* or *HOXA11* likely due to widespread function of these genes in development and their necessity for reproduction. However, women with decreased expression of either of these two genes during the secretory phase have lower implantation rates as seen in endometriosis, PCOS, hydrosalpinx and fibroids.[42,43] Thus, the *HOX* genes clearly play a role in endometrial function but their involvement in endometrial receptivity also remains unproven.

Cellular Adhesion Molecules Family

The cellular adhesion molecule (CAM) family is composed of four members, known as integrins, cadherins, selectins, and immunoglobulins. These surface ligands mediate cell-to-cell adhesion. Their classical functions include maintenance of tissue integration, wound healing, morphogenic movements, cellular migrations and tumor metastasis.

Integrins

Integrins are a class of cell transmembrane heterodimeric glycoproteins that are anchored to the plasma membrane and serve multiple functions within cells,[44] including functions within the endometrium.[6,45] Heterodimers of α and β integrins serve as receptors for ECM ligands such as collagen, laminin and fibronectin, as well as transducing signals from soluble ligands such as osteopontin.[46] To date, 18α and 8β chains have been identified in mammals that can form 24 distinct heterodimers.[47]

A large variety of integrins have been described within the luminal and glandular endometrial epithelium.[48,49] Whereas the majority of the integrins are constitutively expressed throughout the entire menstrual cycle, others exhibit an interesting regulating pattern within the menstrual cycle.[48] Integrins whose expression is increased in the mid-luteal phase were proposed as the markers for the WOI. Three cycle-specific integrins are expressed by the human endometrium defined histologically on days 20–24 of the menstrual cycle: α1β1, α4β1 and αvβ3. However, only the integrins with β3 mRNA subunit expression were shown to increase after day 19 and were not detected beforehand. Thus, one of the most investigated endometrial biomarkers related to infertility is the αvβ3 integrin.[50] The appearance of αvβ3 integrin on the apical surface is due to its presence in the subnuclear secretory granules that typically complete their transit by cycle day 19–20. Expression of the molecule is rate-limited by the production of β3 unit that is regulated directly by the transcription factor HOXA10. A failure to upregulate β3 integrin at the appropriate time has been observed in patients with poor reproductive performance. Although, this has been reported to occur also in normal fertile women, it is much more common in women with endometriosis, PCOS, hydrosalpinges or unexplained infertility.[50-52] It is clear that the expression of β3 coincides with the WOI and can provide a marker of endometrial receptivity, but the evidence supporting its diagnostic reliability as a marker is inconclusive. In mice, β3 is expressed on the surface of blastocyst and epithelium at the time of implantation. When injected with neutralizing antibodies, significantly reduced implantation rates were observed.[53] However, the β3 knockout mice can be fertile and β3 deficient humans can also be fertile.[54] This shows that it is difficult to identify a single responsible gene for implantation deficiency, because of the redundancy inherent in the system. β3 is upregulated in the normal epithelium at the time of implantation, and this could be disturbed in subfertile women. Still, these subtle alterations in gene expression can occur in the absence of any histological signs of maturation delay and may indicate an altered response to progesterone. Moreover, the endometrium can often subsequently "catch up" and integrin expression is normal later in the menstrual cycle. Thus, the β3 expression is not a reliable marker of endometrial receptivity.

Selectins

Selectins are glycoproteins which also belong to the CAM family. They include P-selectin, L-selectin and E-selectin. The human L-selectin, which is important for implantation process, consists of a large, highly glycosylated extracellular domain, a single spanning transmembrane domain and a small cytoplasmic tail.[55] Selectins play an important role in leukocyte transendothelial trafficking. They are expressed on leukocytes and interact with their carbohydrate-based ligands on the endothelium.[56] Selectins are responsible for the tether and roll mechanism on endothelial surface. A parallel can be made between the leukocytes' "rolling" phenomenon and blastocyst apposition to the endometrial epithelium.[7,57] Namely, hatched blastocysts also express L-selectin and use this molecule to mediate its attachment to the luminal epithelial surface. The lack of L-selectin ligand MECA-79 in mid-luteal biopsies has been shown to be indicative of low chance of pregnancy.[56]

Cytokines

Cytokines are multifunctional glycoproteins that are involved in numerous physiological processes, including implantation and immune function. Both pleiotropy and redundancy characterize the cytokine family and the molecules often exert overlapping or even opposing roles. Several cytokines have been suggested to participate in the process of human embryo implantation.[58]

Interleukins

Interleukin-1 (IL-1) is a known product of monocytes and macrophages and modulates cell proliferation and differentiation in a number of cell types, and is also present in both the endometrium and the embryo.[59,60] IL-1 was shown to regulate the expression of several molecules in the endometrium, including IL-6, IL-8, leukemia-inhibiting factor (LIF), tumor necrosis factor-α (TNF-α), cyclooxygenase-2 (COX-2) and several prostaglandins.[61] Animal models have shown that blocking of IL-1 system in mice results in significant loss in the number of implanted blastocysts.[59,62,63] Decreased levels of IL-1β mRNA in human endometrium were also correlated to recurrent pregnancy loss.[64]

Interleukin-11 in normal uterus is involved in the process of decidualization. A number of IL-11 regulated ECM component genes, which might participate in the decidualization process, were identified using microarray analysis of pseudopregnant type α IL-11 receptor-deficient mice.[65] *In vitro* studies have also shown that it promotes progesterone-induced decidualization of human stromal cells.[66] In women with recurrent miscarriage, decreased synthesis of IL-11 in epithelial endometrium has been reported.[67] However, the current knowledge about IL-11 role in the implantation process is still insufficient and should be validated in future studies. Other ILs, such as IL-6, IL-10, IL-15 and IL-18 have also been associated with different aspects of the implantation process,[58,68] but again, there is insufficient data to identify these molecules as reliable biomarkers of endometrial receptivity.

Leukemia Inhibiting Factor

Leukemia-inhibiting factor (LIF) is a pleiomorphic glycoprotein that can act on a variety of tissues and cell types, including those of embryonic, hematopoietic and endothelial origin to exert proliferative and differentiating effects.[69] In humans and several animals, it is expressed from the endometrium at the time of blastocyst implantation, and is associated with normal implantation.[70,71] LIF knock-out mice are unable to initiate decidualization and support blastocyst implantation.[70,72] If mice are injected with LIF, the implantation is rescued. In humans; however, the association between endometrial LIF production and infertility is controversial, as studies have provided inconclusive results.[64] To date, there is little evidence regarding the mechanisms of LIF in the process of embryo implantation. It is mainly present in the uterine epithelial cells and lumen and may exert an important role in implantation process by stimulating trophoblast outgrowth, invasion through the epithelium and decidualization.

Tumor Growth Factor β (TGFβ)

Tumor growth factor β family (-1 to -3) was shown to modulate maternal immunotolerance during implantation and regulate several implantation related molecules. TGFβ-3 is also cycle dependent, increasing during the secretory phase, with the maximal expression in the early pregnancy decidua.[10] Because TGFβ-binding sites are also present on trophoblast cells, they could act as autocrine or paracrine factors to regulate placental development and function. TGFβ may play a role in human implantation by promotion of adhesion of trophoblast cells to the ECM via their stimulation of fibronectin or vascular endothelial growth factor (VEGF). In vitro, TGFβ can regulate proteins such as insulin-like growth factor binding protein-1 (IGFBP-1) and LIF. Trophoblast invasive capacity can also be inhibited by treatment with TGFβ1, probably by the inhibition of matrix metalloproteinase-9 (MMP-9) and plasmin. There are several more functions of TGFβ demonstrated in 'in vitro' conditions, but it is of question how many of these functions are actually active 'in vivo', where the full repertoire of modulators is present.[58]

■ NON-INVASIVE ASSESSMENT OF ENDOMETRIAL RECEPTIVITY

Although in many ways promising, the discussed markers currently do not have adequate diagnostic capacity for endometrial receptivity, are expensive and not applicable to routine clinical practice. However, there are aspects of endometrium that indicate receptivity and can be assessed by non-invasive methods.

Transvaginal ultrasonography can provide some insight to the state and development of the endometrium and the capability to be receptive for embryos. Endometrial thickness is one of the most investigated ultrasonic markers of receptivity. When measured on the day before oocyte retrieval, it may be indicative about the possibility of implantation,[73-75] but this is controversial as some studies did not show any correlation between endometrial thickness and implantation rates.[76] Even a very thin endometrium (<6 mm) is not a reliable predictor for lower embryo implantation potential.[77] When considering morphologic characteristics of the endometrium, namely the multilayered echogenic pattern (triple line appearance), it has been shown that they can be predictive of pregnancy.[76,78] With regard to ultrasonic markers, blood flow through the endometrium has also been proposed as a sign of endometrial receptivity; however, it did not prove to be of reliable clinical significance.[79,80] It does also not appear that different pattern of endometrial contractility on the day of embryo transfer is predictive for possibility of pregnancy.[74]

CONCLUSION

Normal implantation is crucial for the establishment of pregnancy. For the couples facing subfertility and their treating physician, a better understanding of the process of implantation will enable better diagnosis and treatment planning. Today, endometrial receptivity appears to be a major limiting factor in increasing the success rates of medically assisted reproduction. It is clear that the frequency of abnormal expression of some endometrial receptivity markers such as integrin $\alpha vb3$ is increased in subfertile patients. However, there is a substantial overlap with regard to receptivity markers between the group of patients suffering from subfertility and healthy controls. Furthermore, it does not appear that any independent factor plays a determining role in the establishment of endometrial receptivity. To completely understand the implantation process it is still necessary to investigate the mechanisms of action and the interactions between different regulators determining endometrial receptivity. This can lead to new strategies in treating implantation failure and improve pregnancy rates in medically assisted reproduction.

MESSAGE BOX

The process of embryo implantation requires a careful synchronization between blastocyst development and the endometrium. By the collaboration of a large number of different factors, only a short period of endometrial receptivity is achieved in humans. It is clear that abnormal expression of several receptivity markers is increased in subfertile women. The mechanisms of action and interactions between different receptivity regulators have yet to be studied in order to elucidate new strategies to treat implantation failure and improve pregnancy rates in medically assisted reproduction.

REFERENCES

1. Sharkey AM, Smith SK. The endometrium as a cause of implantation failure. Best Pract Res Clin Obstet Gynaecol. 2003;17:289-307.
2. Tabibzadeh S, Babaknia A. The signals and molecular pathways involved in implantation, a symbiotic interaction between blastocyst and endometrium involving adhesion and tissue invasion. Human Reprod. 1995;10:1579-602.
3. Wilcox AJ, Weinberg CR, O'Connor JF, et al. Incidence of early loss of pregnancy. N Engl J Med. 1988;319:189-94.
4. Boomsma CM, Macklon NS. What can we do to improve implantation? Reprod Biomed Online. 2006;13:845-55.
5. Macklon NS, Geraedts JP, Fauser BC. Conception to ongoing pregnancy: the 'black box' of pregnancy loss. Hum Reprod Update. 2002;8:333-43.
6. Achache H, Revel A. Endometrial receptivity markers, the journey to successful embryo implantation. Hum Reprod Update. 2006;12:731-46.
7. Dominguez, F. Yanez-Mo M, Sanchez-Madrid F, et al. Embryonic implantation and leukocyte transendothelial migration: different processes with similar players? FASEB J. 2005;19:1056-60.
8. Van Mourik MS, Macklon NS, Heijnen CJ. Embryonic implantation: cytokines, adhesion molecules, and immune cells in establishing an implantation environment. J Leukoc Biol. 2009;85:4-19.
9. Donaghay M, Lessey BA. Uterine receptivity: alterations associated with benign gynecological disease. Semin Reprod Med. 2007;25:461-75.
10. Strowitzki T, Germeyer A, Popovici R, et al. The human endometrium as a fertility-determining factor. Hum Reprod Update. 2006;12:617-30.
11. Navot D, Bergh PA, Williams M, et al. An insight into early reproductive processes through the in vivo model of ovum donation. J Clin Endocrinol Metabol. 1991;72:408-14.
12. Hertig AT, Rock J, Adams EC. A description of 34 human ova within the first 17 days of development. Am J Anat. 1956;98:435-93.

13. Paulson RJ. Hormonal induction of endometrial receptivity. Fertil Steril. 2011;96:530-5.

14. Lessey BA. Two pathways of progesterone action in the human endometrium: implications for implantation and contraception. Steroids. 2003;68:809-15.

15. Slayden OD, Zelinski-Wooten MB, Chwalisz K, et al. Chronic treatment of cycling rhesus monkeys with low doses of the antiprogestin ZK 137 316: morphometric assessment of the uterus and oviduct. Human Reprod. 1998;13:269-77.

16. Edgar DH, James GB, Mills JA. Steroid synthesis by early human embryos in culture. Hum Reprod. 1993;8:277-8.

17. Ghosh D, Sengupta J. Another look at the issue of peri-implantation oestrogen. Hum Reprod. 1995;10:1-2.

18. Bulun SE, Yang S, Fang Z, et al. Role of aromatase in endometrial disease. J Steroid Biochem Mol Biol. 2001;79:19-25.

19. Noyes RW, Hertig AI, Rock J. Dating the endometrial biopsy. Fertil Steril. 1950;1:3-25.

20. Cheong Y, Boomsma C, Heijnen C, et al. Uterine secretomics: a window on the maternal-embryo interface. Fertil Steril. 2013;99:1093-9.

21. Critchley HO, Robertson KA, Forster T, et al. Gene expression profiling of mid to late secretory phase endometrial biopsies from women with menstrual complaint. Am J Obstet Gynecol. 2006;195:406.e1-16.

22. Ponnampalam AP, Weston GC, Susil B, et al. Molecular profiling of human endometrium during the menstrual cycle. Aust NZ J Obstet Gynaecol. 2006;46:154-8.

23. Coutifaris C, Myers ER, Guzick DS, et al. Histological dating of timed endometrial biopsy tissue is not related to fertility status. Fertil Steril. 2004;82:1264-72.

24. Murray MJ, Meyer WR, Zaino RJ, et al. A critical analysis of the accuracy, reproducibility, and clinical utility of histologic endometrial dating in fertile women. Fertil Steril. 2004;81;1333-43.

25. Diedrich K, Fauser BC, Devroey P, et al. The role of the endometrium and embryo in human implantation. Hum Reprod Update. 2007;13:365-77.

26. Van Vaerenbergh I, Van Lommel L, Ghislain V, et al. In GnRH antagonist/rec-FSH stimulated cycles, advanced endometrial maturation on the day of oocyte retrieval correlates with altered gene expression. Hum Reprod. 2009;24:1085-91.

27. Nikas G, Psychoyos A. Uterine pinopodes in peri-implantation human endometrium. Clinical relevance. Ann N Y Acad Sci. 1997;816:129-42.

28. Acosta AA, Elberger L, Borghi M, et al. Endometrial dating and determination of the window of implantation in healthy fertile women. Fertil Steril. 2000;73:788-98.

29. Bentin-Ley U, Horn T, Sjorgen A, et al. Ultrastructure of human blastocyst-endometrial interactions in vitro. J Reprod Fertil. 2000;120:337-50.

30. Martel D, Monier MN, Roche D, et al. Hormonal dependence of pinopode formation at the uterine luminal surface. Hum Reprod. 1991;6:597-603.

31. Usadi RS, Murray MJ, Bagnell RC, et al. Temporal and morphologic characteristics of pinopod expression across the secretory phase of the endometrial cycle in normally cycling women with proven fertility. Fertil Steril. 2003;79:970-4.

32. Quinn C, Ryan E, Claessens EA, et al. The presence of pinopodes in the human endometrium does not delineate the implantation window. Fertil Steril. 2007;87:1015-21.

33. Gendron RL, Paradis H, Hsieh-Li HM, et al. Abnormal uterine stromal and glandular function associated with maternal reproductive defects in Hoxa11 null mice. Biol Reprod. 1997;56:1097-105.

34. Taylor H, Arici A, Olive D, et al. HOXA10 is expressed in response to sex steroids at the time of implantation in the human endometrium. J Clin Invest. 1998;101:1379-84.

35. Sarno JL, Kliman HJ, Taylor HS. HOXA10, Pbx2, and Meis1 protein expression in the human endometrium: formation of multimeric complexes on HOXA10 target genes. J Clin Endocrinol Metab. 2005;90:522-8.

36. Taylor HS, Bagot C, Kardana A. HOX gene expression is altered in the endometrium of women with endometriosis. Hum Reprod. 1999;14:1328-31.

37. Hsieh-Li HM, Witte DP, Weinstein M, et al. HOXA 11 structure, extensive antisense transcription, and function in male and female fertility. Development. 1995;121:1373-85.

38. Satokata I, Benson G, Maas R. Sexually dimorphic sterility phenotypes in HOXA 10 deficient mice. Nature. 1995;374:460-63.

39. Benson GV, Lim H, Paria BC, et al. Mechanisms of reduced fertility in HOXA10 mutant mice: uterine homeosis and loss of maternal HOXA10 expression. Development. 1996;122:2687-96.

40. Bagot CN, Troy PJ, Taylor HS. Alteration of maternal HOXA10 expression by uterine gene transfection affects implantation. Gene Ther. 2000;7:1378-84.

41. Bagot CN, Kliman HJ, Taylor HS. Maternal HOXA10 is required for pinopod formation in the development of mouse uterine receptivity to embryo implantation. Dev Dyn. 2001;222:538-44.

42. Daftary GS, Taylor HS. Hydrosalpinx fluid diminishes endometrial cell HOXA10 expression. Fertil Steril. 2002;78:577-80.

43. Cermik D, Selam B, Taylor HS. Regulation of HOXA-10 expression by testosterone in vitro and in the endometrium of patients with polycystic ovary syndrome. J Clin Endocrinol Metab. 2003;88:238-24.

44. Albelda SM, Buck CA. Integrins and other cell adhesion molecules. FASEB J. 1990;4:2868-80.

45. Singh H, Aplin JD. Adhesion molecules in endometrial epithelium: tissue integrity and embryo implantation. J Anat. 2009;215:3-13.

46. Humphries MJ. Integrin structure. Biochemical Soc Trans. 2000;28:311-39.

47. Hynes RO. Integrins: bidirectional, allosteric signalling machines. Cell. 2002;110:673-87.

48. Lessey BA, Damjanovich L, Coutifaris C, et al. Integrin adhesion molecules in the human endometrium. Correlation with the normal and abnormal menstrual cycle. J Clin Invest. 1992;90:188-95.

49. Lessey BA, Castelbaum AJ, Buck CA, et al. Further characterization of endometrial integrins during the menstrual cycle and in pregnancy. Fertil Steril. 1994;62:497-506.

50. Lessey BA, Gui Y, Apparao KB, et al. Regulated expression of HB-EGF in the human endometrium: a potential paracrine role during implantation. Mol Reprod Devel. 2002;62:446-55.

51. Meyer WR, Castelbaum AJ, Somkuti S, et al. Hydrosalpinges adversely affects markers of endometrial receptivity. Hum Reprod. 1997;12:1393-8.

52. Ota H, Tanaka T. Integrin adhesion molecules in the endometrial glandular epithelium of patients with endometriosis and adenomyosis. J Obstet Gynaecol Res. 1997;23:485-91.

53. Illera MJ, Cullinan E, Gui Y, et al. Blockade of the alpha(v) beta(3) integrin adversely affects implantation in the mouse. Biol Reprod. 2000;62:1285-90.

54. Hodivala-Dilke KM, McHugh KP, Tsakiris DA, et al. β3 integrin deficient mice are a model for Glanzmann thrombasthenia showing placental defects and reduced survival. J Clin Invest. 1999;103:229-38.

55. Smalley DM, Ley K. L-selectin: mechanisms and physiological significance of ectodomain cleavage. J Cell Mol Med. 2005;9:255-66.

56. Foulk RA, Zdravkovic T, Genbavec O, et al. Expression of L-selectin ligand MECA-79 as a predictive marker of human uterine receptivity. J Assist Reprod Genet. 2007;24:316-21.

57. Genbancev OD, Prakobphol A, Foulk RA, et al. Trophoblast L-selectin- mediated adhesion at the maternal–fetal interface. Science. 2003;299:405-8.

58. Dimitriadis E, White CA, Jones RL, et al. Cytokines, chemokines and growth factors in endometrium related to implantation. Hum Reprod Update. 2005;11:613-30.

59. Simón C, Frances A, Piquette G, et al. Interleukin-1 system in the materno-trophoblast unit in human implantation: immunohistochemical evidence for autocrine/paracrine function. J Clin Endocrinol Metabol. 1994;78:847-54.

60. de los Santos MJ, Mercader A, Frances A, et al. Role of endometrial factors in regulating secretion of components of the immunoreactive human embryonic interleukin-1 system during embryonic development. Biol Reprod. 1996;54:563-74.

61. Minas V, Loutradis D, Makrigiannakis A. Factors controlling blastocyst implantation. Reprod BioMed Online. 2005;10:205-16.

62. Zheng H, Fletcher D, Kozak W, et al. Resistance to fever induction and impaired acute-phase response in interleukin-1 beta-deficient mice. Immunity. 1995;3:9-19.

63. Abbondanzo SJ, Cullinan EB, McIntyre K, et al. Reproduction in mice lacking a functional type 1 IL-1 receptor. Endocrinology. 1996;137:3598-601.

64. Laird SM, Tuckerman EM, Li TC. Cytokine expression in the endometrium of women with implantation failure and recurrent miscarriage. Reprod Biomed Online. 2006;13:13-23.

65. White CA, Robb L, Salamonsen LA. Uterine extracellular matrix components are altered during defective decidualization in interleukin-11 receptor alpha deficient mice. Reprod Biol Endocrinol. 2004;2:76.

66. Dimitriadis E, Robb L, Liu YX, et al. IL-11 and IL-11Ralpha immunolocalisation at primate implantation sites supports a role for IL-11 in placentation and fetal development. Reprod Biol Endocrinol. 2003;1:34.

67. Linjawi S, Li TC, Tuckerman EM, et al. Expression of interleukin-11 receptor alpha and interleukin-11 protein in the endometrium of normal fertile women and women with recurrent miscarriage. J Reprod Immunol. 2004;64:145-55.

68. Makrigiannakis A. Mechanisms of implantation. Reprod Biomed Online. 2007;14:102-9.

69. Hilton DJ, Gough NM. Leukemia inhibitory factor: a biological perspective. J Cell Biochem. 1991;46:21-6.

70. Stewart CL, Kaspar P, Brunet LJ, et al. Blastocyst implantation depends on maternal expression of leukaemia inhibitory factor. Nature. 1992;359:76-9.

71. Yue ZP, Yang ZM, Wei P, et al. Leukemia inhibitory factor, leukemia inhibitory factor receptor, and glycoprotein 130 in rhesus monkey uterus during menstrual cycle and early pregnancy. Biol Reprod. 2000;63:508-12.

72. Chen JR, Cheng JG, Shatzer T, et al. Leukemia inhibitory factor can substitute for nidatory estrogen and is essential to inducing a receptive uterus for implantation but is not essential for subsequent embryogenesis. Endocrinology. 2000;141:4365-72.

73. Lenz S, Lindenberg S. Ultrasonic evaluation of endometrial growth in women with normal cycles during spontaneous and stimulated cycles. Hum Reprod. 1990;5:377-81.

74. Vlaisavljević V, Reljič M, Gavrić-Lovrec V, et al. Subendometrial contractility is not predictive for in vitro fertilization (IVF) outcome. Ultrasound Obstet Gynecol. 2001;17:239-44.

75. Fanchin R. Assessing uterine receptivity in 2001: ultrasonographic glances at the new millennium. Ann N Y Acad Sci. 2001;943:185-202.

76. Leibovitz Z, Grinin V, Rabia R, et al. Assessment of endometrial receptivity for gestation in patients undergoing in vitro fertilization, using endometrial thickness and the endometrium-myometrium relative echogenicity coefficient. Ultrasound Obstet Gynecol. 1999;143:194-9.

77. Dain L, Bider D, Levron J, et al. Thin endometrium in donor oocyte recipients: enigma or obstacle for implantation? Fertil Steril. 2013;100(5):1289-95.

78. Fanchin R, de Ziegler D, Taieb J, et al. Human chorionic gonadotropin administration does not increase plasma androgen levels in patients undergoing controlled ovarian hyperstimulation. Fertil Steril. 2000;73:275-9.

79. Bloechle M, Schreiner T, Küchler I, et al. Colour Doppler assessment of ascendent uterine artery perfusion in an in-vitro fertilization-embryo transfer programme after pituitary desensitization and ovarian stimulation with human recombinant follicle stimulating hormone. Hum Reprod. 1997;12(8):1772-7.

80. Ng EH, Chan CC, Tang OS, et al. Changes in endometrial and subendometrial blood flow in IVF. Reprod Biomed Online. 2009;18(2):269-75.

34 Embryo Endometrial Dialogue

Sunita R Tandulwadkar, Kamala Selvaraj, Devika Chopra

■ SYNOPSIS

Implantation

Successful implantation needs a healthy viable embryo (blastocyst stage) and an endometrial window of maximum receptivity.

Successful Implantation

Immediately after fertilization the embryo needs to have a dialogue along the rest of its path by way of signals to the ovary, endometrium and myometrium.

Embryo: Uterine Interaction During Implantation

The embryo and endometrium interact with each other via several mediators.
- Vasoactive mediators
- Growth factors (GFs) and cytokines
- Endometrial integrins and specific proteins
- Hormonal and immunological factors.

The final outcome is a healthy viable embryo and a successful pregnancy.

■ INTRODUCTION

Pregnancy is a complex interaction of the male immunological system with the female immunological system. This is made possible by maternal immunological adjustments at the chemical and ultimately at the molecular level. Surely this has to involve a great dialogue not only between the embryo and the implantation site, but also to the rest of the body. The attraction and attachment of human embryo to the receptive endometrium is a cascade of events studied basically from animal models like mice, rodents, rabbits and so on.

The implantation sequence involving three stages has to occur in coordinated fashion for successful implantation and growth of the fetus. This involves many biochemical, immunological and endocrinological events at autocrine, paracrine and molecular levels. For no known reasons, the floating blastocyst is attracted to a portion of endometrium, anterior, posterior or fundus and decides to grow or gets rejected to be washed out in the form of biochemical pregnancy (14%).

Implantation is a complex developmental process that involves an intimate "crosstalk" between the embryo and uterus. Synchronized development of the embryo to the blastocyst stage and differentiation of the uterus to the receptive state are essential in this process. Successful execution of the events of implantation involves participation of steroid hormones, locally derived growth factors (GFs), cytokines, transcription factors and lipid mediators.[1]

A successful implantation depends on a coordinated sequence of events before, at, and immediately after nidation of the conceptus in the wall of the uterus. In human, the conceptus makes contact with the endometrium about 5–8 days before the onset of next menstrual flow. It is at this fixed-framed window that many things such as occult abortion by way of damage to the conceptus before touching the endometrium and nidation can occur. It is during this broad window of implantation that delicate changes can occur that affect the pre, peri- and postimplantation stages of an embryo.

Molecular interactions at the embryo-maternal interface at the time of implantation is an exciting field demanding a wide effort in order to understand the crucial process of embryonic implantation. This pathway of molecular interactions is apparently initiated by the endometrium in the presence of an implanting blastocyst. It is mediated through the embryonic interleukin (IL)-la + IL-lp, and the target is the endometrial epithelial β3 integrin subunit. Communication between them, and the reciprocal effect on each other is an exciting and as yet unsolved paradigm in reproductive medicine.[2]

PREIMPLANTATION EMBRYO DEVELOPMENT

The endometrium is an active, versatile and hormonally regulated "organ" which plays a major role in the process of implantation and in maintaining a viable pregnancy. It has traditionally been perceived as a passive counterpart. Recent evidence, however, suggests that the maternal endometrium has to be prepared, in that it is "receptive" to an implanting blastocyst only within a "window of implantation", which is temporally and spatially restricted.

The crucial role of steroid hormones to prepare and drive the endometrium for successful embryonic implantation is beyond any doubt. However, it is clear that steroid hormones are not the final effectors, rather they may initiate a "downstream" cascade of molecular events through local paracrine or autocrine molecules which account for the intimate mechanisms of receptivity. We are just beginning to understand the expression, regulation, and mode of action of several cytokines, GFs, and adhesion molecules during the implantation window.[3]

These effector molecules include members of the epidermal growth factor (EGF) family, leukemia-inhibitory factor (LIF) and IL-1. A newly discovered member of the EGF family, heparin-binding EGF (HPEGF) is expressed in uterine luminal epithelium at the site of implantation before any other sign of blastocyst attachment and disappears when implantation is delayed by administration of progesterone.[4]

There is no evidence that estrogen and/or progesterone act directly on the preimplantation embryo. Embryonic development is considered to depend on growth-promoting factors originating from the reproductive tract under the influence of these hormones. However, normal development in defined media cultures suggests that preimplantation embryos themselves produce the growth-promoting factors (reviewed in Paria and Dey, 1990). This is consistent with the expression of several GFs, cytokines and their receptors in the embryo and uterus, as well as beneficial effects of these factors on embryonic development and functions.[5]

UTERINE RECEPTIVITY AND IMPLANTATION

Stage I: Fertilization at the lateral end of the Fallopian tube.

Stage II: Initiation of cell division.

Stage III: The morula enters the uterine cavity and further divides to form the blastocyst.

Stage IV: Corresponds to the time of adhesion/apposition, penetration and invasion.

Stage V: Development of placenta approximately 11–12 days of the implantation.

The first conspicuous sign that the implantation process has been initiated is an increased uterine vascular permeability at the sites of blastocyst apposition. These processes are accompanied by remodeling of the extracellular matrix and angiogenesis in the stromal bed. Estrogen stimulates proliferation of uterine epithelial cells, and progesterone stimulates stromal cell proliferation. These two steroids together further potentiate stromal cell proliferation.[6] Similar hormonal stimulation of cell-specific proliferation occurs in the preimplantation uterus. Preovulatory ovarian estrogen secretion induces proliferation of the luminal and glandular epithelial cells during the first 2 days of pregnancy.

Development of the endometrium depends on the programmed secretion of ovarian steroids, i.e. estradiol (E2) and progesterone. Peak of serum progesterone coincides with implantation which is about 7–10 days after ovulation. The endometrium under the influence of estrogen proliferates and the epithelial cells forms the thickness of the endometrium with an increase in the estrogen and progesterone receptors. The secretory phase represents a period of conversion from epithelial to stromal dominance and starts protein synthesis and secretion. This is the time when there is expression of specific gene that may facilitate and/or limit the ability of the blastocyst and trophoblast to invade. Embryo invasion causes endometrial decidualization and progesterone level rises in response to the embryo with rapid changes in stromal protein expression. These changes represent decidualization of the endometrial stroma with expression of extracellular mass (ECM) components, cell surface receptors and cellular proteins. The time of endometrial receptivity corresponds to the entry of the blastocyst in the uterine cavity (72–96 hours) after fertilization. When the embryo hatches out of the zona pellucida, its exposed elements on the outer trophoblast, of epithelial surface which are probably involved in embryo endometrial inter-reactions. Embryo attachment, however, has to wait until the endometrium recognizes the trophoblast. Hatching of the embryo occurs on day 5 about 110–120 hours after ovulation.

IMPLANTATION WINDOW

This is a specified period of days of receptivity when the primed endometrium allows the conceptus to implant. This specified period assists implantation by further enhancing factors like:

- Immune cells
- Cytokines
- Growth factors

- Chemokines
- Adhesion molecules.

Pinopods may serve as a pseudo-basal surface that allows the embryo to attach and intrude. This shows how two epithelial apical surfaces might interact. The function of pinopods is still unclear and helps in endocytosis and pinocytosis. Pinocytosis is involved in implantation by the uptake of macromolecules, withdrawal of uterine fluid and facilitating adhesion of blastocyst. Pinopods are strictly progesterone dependent and it is a marker of uterine receptivity and should appear on day 6.

The embryo once gets attached starts invasion to access the vascularized maternal endometrium. As it increases in size and grows, its metabolism also increases requiring more quantities of nutrition, oxygen and better management of cellular waste for survival. Once the embryo has burrowed and well below the luminal surface, it is surrounded by layer of cytotrophoblast which will soon bud to form the placental villi.

During pregnancy, the placenta and extra-placental membranes interface directly with maternal blood and tissue. Among the many functions of the placenta, one of which is avoidance of immune rejection of paternally inherited antigens.

SUSCEPTIBILITY TO IMMUNITY

- The embryo floats free for few days during preimplantation and contains very few cells to stimulate maternal immune mechanism.
- Spermatozoa are taken up by the endometrial macrophages and may initiate little maternal sensitization.
- Pre-existing cytotoxic maternal immunity may at times affect preimplantation embryo.
- Zona pellucida forms a protective covering for the preimplantation embryo.
- Defense mechanisms.
- Before hatching the zona pellucida may serve as a barrier to natural killer cells and cytotoxic T lymphocytes (CTL) effector cells.

RELEVANCE OF THE LEPTIN SYSTEM IN THE EMBRYO: ENDOMETRIAL DIALOGUE

Obesity has always been correlated with infertility and is on the increase in many countries. High body mass index (BMI) has been associated with low in vitro fertilization (IVF) and pregnancy rates suggesting a link between adipose tissue and reproductive system and also endometrial receptivity and implantation.

Leptin is a 16 kDa non-glycosylated polypeptide of 146 amino acids discovered in 1994 by Zhang.[7] It is thought to be secreted by adipose tissue and related to food consumption, energy balance and body weight. Recently, leptin has been linked to the regulation of reproductive function.

Obesity is not characterized by leptin deficiency, possibly it causes leptin resistance. It is yet to be known whether leptin exerts its effect as endocrine or paracrine mediator but has a direct effect on the brain especially the pituitary. Leptin production may be influenced by ovarian function and is secreted by blastocyst and endometrial epithelial cells (EEC). Leptin expression is detected specifically at the blastocyst stage and there is leptin signaling system in the endometrium and regulation of leptin secretion by EEC due to the presence of the human embryo implicating the leptin system in the embryo endometrial dialogue.

In another study, endometrial fluid obtained transcervically by aspiration immediately prior to embryo transfer was analyzed and the protein profile in each sample was determined. Recently, Van der Gaast et al. investigated the effect of ovarian stimulation in IVF on endometrial secretion and markers of receptivity in the midluteal phase.[8]

The endometrium is hormonally regulated tissue that responds to paracrine pathways to the presence of the blastocyst. Transcriptomic and other biochemical changes are thought to be crucial for acquiring receptivity.

Chemokines produced locally by epithelium may act to recruit leukocytes and further induce second wave of cytokines which by binding to specific receptors regulate the expression of adhesion molecules essential for the adhesion of the blastocyst. Other genes products are involved in the complex phenomena.

The endometrium represents a barrier to implantation except under appropriate and defined hormonal conditions. Synchrony between the corpus luteum, endometrium and embryo appears to be crucial element of normal implantation.

The events during implantation are the result of regulated changes in gene transcriptions that ultimately control the expression of embryonic and endometrial proteomes. Proteomics together with genomics and metabolomics are complementary approaches which will improve our understanding of the complexity of the implantation process. All these approaches and information needs to be integrated into a system biology approach to understand endometrial receptivity and the embryo-endometrial dialogue in a holistic way.[9]

POTENTIAL MOLECULAR SIGNALING DURING IMPLANTATION

Recent progress in genetics and molecular biology has remarkably increased our knowledge regarding the roles of locally derived GFs, cytokines, homeobox gene products and lipid mediators during implantation and decidualization. These factors are produced by the uterus or embryo independently or cooperatively under the influence of steroid hormones. For successful implantation, the blastocyst on hatching, signals to the mother for early pregnancy factor (EPF), platelet-activating factor (PAF), placental protein [pregnancy-associated plasma protein A (PAPP-A)] and endometrial proteins (placental proteins 12 and 14).

Autocrine Secretion

Autocrine signaling refers to signals secreted by a cell that may bind to that cell or to a neighboring cell of similar phenotype.

Paracrine Secretion

Paracrine signaling refers to signals produced by a cell to which that cell type cannot respond but other cell types can.

Juxtacrine Signals

Contact-mediated signals require two adjacent cells to be in contact, as these types of signals are not secreted extracellularly from the producing cell. Such signals can be transmitted through transmembrane receptors or through membrane channels.

Locally produced signaling molecules includes:
- Cytokines
- Growth factors
- Homeobox transcription factors
- Lipid mediators and
- Morphogen genes.

IMMUNOMODULATION

Hormonal and Immunological Factors: Progesterone as an Immunomodulatory Molecule (Flow chart 1)

The actions of progesterone on uterus and endometrium are to modify the distribution of estrogen receptors, stimulate secretary activity/stromal edema, increase the volume of blood vessels/angiogenesis, prime decidual cells/stabilize lysosomes, inhibit activation of phospholipase C, might be an immunosuppressant, reduce uterine irritability and contractility, activate 17-hydroxy dehydrogenase, stimulate the formation of PINOPODS, facilitate decidual prolactin synthesis, may stimulate GFs and binding protein, stimulate the formation of fibronectin and may regulate the formation of reactive oxygen species.

Progesterone-induced blocking factor (PIBF) is allogenic stimulation occurring during pregnancy allows the binding of progesterone to specific lymphocyte expressed receptors resulting in the synthesis of mediator protein named PIBF. It inhibits arachidonic acid release by direct action on the phospholipase A2 enzyme, induces T helper 2 (Th2) immune response, controls natural killer (NK) cell activity, produces asymmetrical antibodies and exerts antiabortive effect.

Role of human chorionic gonadotropin (hCG) in immunomodulation is luteotrophic and binds to ovarian receptors. Half-life of hCG is 30 hours and stepwise increment of hCG prolonged the luteal phase and raises progesterone levels. It also binds to receptors in the endometrium and plays a role in endometrial physiology by paracrine secretion, binds to trophoblast via receptor and this binding mediates the effect on the differentiation of syncytiotrophoblast from cytoblast. hCG also causes cytoplasmic maturation of the developing preovulatory oocyte. Progesterone and hCG are effective immunosuppressant and facilitates acceptance of fetal allograft.

Growth factors are chemical and are like cellular dance which prelude to implantation. Both the trophoblast and the decidua produce GFs, inducers, cytokines, proteinases, glycoproteins, hormones and other paracrine factors. GFs are implantation-promoting GF (IMGF), platelet-derived GF (PDGF), fibroblast GF (FGF), insulin GF (IGF), transforming GF (TGF), EGF, colony-stimulating factor (CSF) and interleukins (ILs) are IL-3, 4, 6, 7, 8, 11 and 12, cytokines and interferons.

CYTOKINES

These are small multifunctional glycoproteins whose biological actions are mediated by specific cell-surface receptors and act as potent intercellular signals regulating functions of the endometrial cells and embryo maternal interactions.

Entry of blastocyst into the uterine cavity is important to initiate the production of cytokines by trophoblast cells and uterine epithelium which can modulate the uterine receptivity.

Cytokines such as leukemia inhibitory factor (LIF) and IL-1 and their specific receptors, properly

Flow chart 1 The role of immunomodulation in implantation and subsequent pregnancy

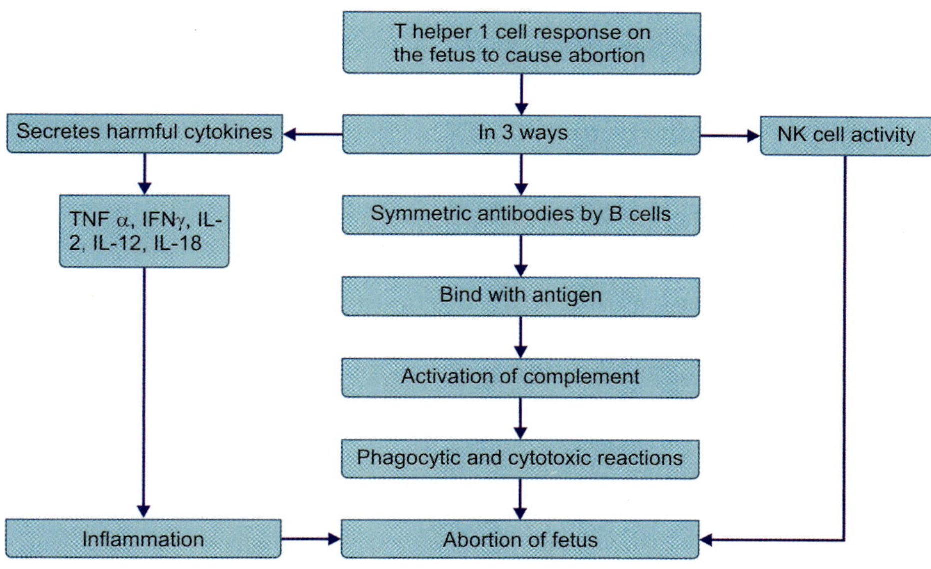

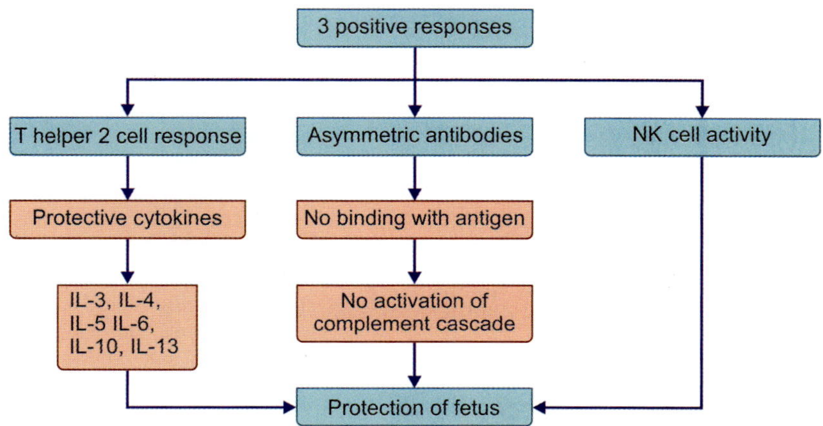

distributed throughout endometrium and embryo and adequately controlled at the endocrine and paracrine or autocrine (cytokine and GF) levels, may start the mutual recognition of implanting blastocyst and endometrium. Cytokines and GFs may also serve as the link in the regulation of molecules that provide the physical contact between embryo and uterus, referred to as adhesion molecules. Since redundancy is one premise to assure the effectiveness of crucial biological processes, many communication possibilities between embryo and endometrium must exist, but unique systems could also be at play.[10]

Cytokines are the products of Th cells which are relevant to pregnancy and may be generally divided into two categories **(Fig. 1)**.
1. *Th1 type cytokines*: Potentially deleterious for pregnancy by increasing cell-mediated immunity.
2. *Th2 type cytokines*: Potentially beneficial effect by inhibiting cellular responses.

Endometrial integrins, Cadherins and other specific proteins helps in adhesion and communicating molecules. These are transmembrane glycoproteins and heterodimeric complexes of α and β subunits (α4 β1 and α5 β1). Integrins like α4 and β3 (produced by secretory

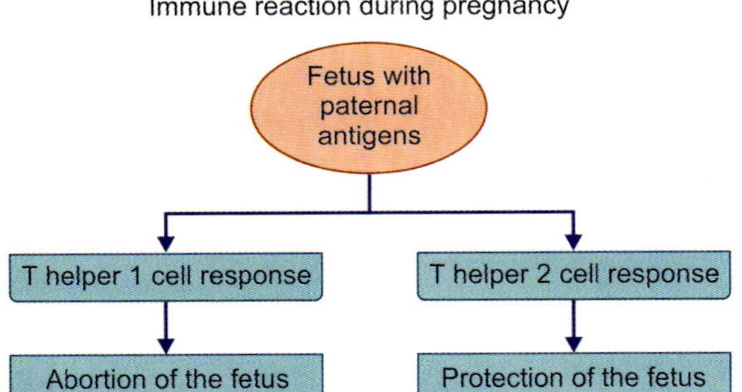

Fig. 1 Pregnancy is associated in altered Th1 and Th2 balance. Protection of the fetus from a harmful maternal immune response is based on a complex mechanisms and cascade of events via cytokines. Immunoglobulin synthesis in pregnant woman is increased and cell-mediated responses are decreased

Abbreviation: Th, T helper

endometrium) are found to rise at the time of maximum uterine receptivity. Fibronectin, vitronectin and receptor integrin αv β3 is of current interest as a marker for uterine receptivity.

Carbohydrate Chains of Glycoproteins Expression

The first structure the blastocyst opposes is the apical surface of the uterine luminal epithelium. The luminal epithelium undergoes a change in the expression of a number of surface glycoproteins. Relocation of adhesion factors on the apical uterine surface resulting in a sticky surface that fixes the slowly moving blastocyst. Large glycoprotein type 1 cell—the mucin MUC1 inhibits both cell-cell and cell-matrix adhesion, high peri-implantation levels could play a role in shielding the impending blastocyst from other inhibitory factors on the epithelial surface and variable number of tandem repeats (VNTR). Infertile women were found to have reduced number of *VNTR* and *MUC1* gene.

CONCLUSION

The first step in implantation is a dialog between free-floating blastocyst and the receptive endometrium, which is mediated by hormones and GFs is followed by apposition, where the trophoblast cells adhere to the receptive luminal epithelium. Microprotrusions present on the surface of uterine epithelium known as pinopodes may have a role in this process. Consequently, blastocyst adheres to the endometrial basal lamina and stromal extracellular matrix through local paracrine signaling between the embryo and endometrium.

Finally the invasion process, which involves penetration of the embryo through the luminal epithelium into the stroma thereby establishing a vascular relationship with the mother.

Thus, success of implantation depends on a receptive endometrium, a functionally normal blastocyst and a synchronized cross-talk between embryonic and maternal tissues.

■ REFERENCES

1. Bibhash CP, Haengseok S, Sudhansu KD. Implantation: molecular basis of embryo-uterine dialogue. Int J Dev Biol. 2001;45:597-605.
2. Carlos S, Carlos M, Jose R, et al. Molecular interactions between embryo and uterus in the adhesion phase of human implantation. Hum Reprod. 1998;13(supplement 3):219-32.
3. Giudice LC. Growth factors and growth hormone modulators in human uterine endometrium: their potential relevance to reproductive medicine. Fertil Steril. 1994;61:1-17.
4. Das SK, Wang X-N, Paria BC, et al. Heparin binding EGF-like growth factor gene is induced in the mouse uterus temporally by the blastocyst solely at the site of its apposition: a possible ligand for interaction with blastocyst EGF receptor in implantation. Development. 1994;120:1071-83.
5. Carson DD, Bagchi I, Dey SK, et al. Embryo implantation. Dev Biol. 2000;223:217-37.
6. Huet-Hudson YM, Andrews GK, Dey SK. Cell type-specific localization of c-myc protein in the mouse uterus: modulation by steroid hormones and analysis of the periimplantation period. Endocrinol. 1989;125:1683-90.
7. Zhang Y, Proenca R, Maffei M, et al. Positional cloning of the mouse obese gene and its human homologue. Nature. 1994;372:425-32.
8. Van der Gaast MH, Classen-Linke I, Krusche CA, et al. Impact of ovarian stimulation on mid-luteal endometrial tissue and secretion markers of receptivity. Reprod Biomed Online. 2008;4:553-63.
9. Najwa AR, Sujata L, Parameswaran GL, et al. Endometrial receptivity and human embryo implantation. Am J Reprod Immunol. 2011;66(Suppl 1):23-30.
10. Simon C, Gimeno MJ, Mercader, A. et al. Cytokines-adhesion molecules-invasive proteinases. The missing paracrine/autocrine link in embryonic implantation? Mol Hum Reprod. 1996;2(6):405-24.

35 Physiology of Implantation in Natural Cycle Versus Stimulated Cycle

Jana AlShalati, Togas Tulandi

INTRODUCTION

Implantation requires an interaction between the human embryos and the endometrium. This process is mediated by cytokines, growth factors, and adhesion molecules, which are secreted by the endometrium and blastocyst.[1] Implantation consists of three stages: apposition of the embryos to the endometrium, attachment and invasion, and culminates when placenta starts to form. The main purpose of implantation is to provide an appropriate environment for embryo growth and development, in order to achieve a successful pregnancy.[2,3] The two main factors that determine the success of implantation are embryo quality and endometrial receptivity.

CHANGES IN ENDOMETRIUM DURING MENSTRUAL CYCLE

Endometrium undergoes cyclical changes in response to the ovarian hormones. The endometrium consists of two layers, the functional layer at the upper two-thirds and the basal layer at the lower one-third of endometrium.[4,5] In the follicular or proliferative phase, the endometrium responds to increasing estrogen concentration produced by the growing follicles. Endothelial cells proliferate and the stroma becomes hyperplastic and edematous, leading to an increasing surface of the mucosal layer. Angiogenesis takes place throughout the menstrual cycle, but becomes prominent in the proliferative phase.[6] Angiogenesis where the blood vessels elongate[7] is dependent on many factors including nitric oxide, matrix metalloproteinase, and a few growth factors such as fibroblast growth factor, epidermal growth factor, and vascular endothelial growth factor.[8]

Estrogen also induces the expression of steroid receptors, such as progesterone receptors, estrogen receptors (ERa, ERb), and androgen receptors.[9] After ovulation, corpus luteum forms and secretes progesterone. The secretory phase is characterized by marked coiling of

Table 1 Physiological changes of the menstrual cycles

Proliferative phase	Secretory phase
↑ estrogen	↑ progesterone
Growing follicles	Corpus luteum formation
Glands → long and straight	Coiling of the glands
Angiogenesis → blood vessel elongation	↑ vascularity (by intussusceptions)
Endothelial cells proliferate	↓ cellular activity and proliferation
Stroma → hyperplastic and edematous	↑ vacuolization of the cytoplasm + glycogen content
Nuclei of the epithelial cells → midway between basal and luminal borders	Nuclei → more basal location

Abbreviations: ↑, increase; ↓, decrease

the glands and increased vascularity of the stromal layer. The secretory activity of the glands peaks at the mid-secretory phase, when implantation is expected to occur. At the mid to late-secretory phase, the endometrium is infiltrated by bone marrow derived immune cells including large granulated lymphocytes [decidual natural killer (NK) cells], T cells and macrophages.[7] Failure of implantation leads to degeneration of the corpus luteum resulting in a sudden decrease of progesterone and estrogen levels, followed by menstruation. A summary of physiological changes during menstrual cycles is demonstrated in **Table 1**.

EARLY EMBRYO DEVELOPMENT AND IMPLANTATION

In a normal condition, fertilization takes place in the Fallopian tube, 24–48 hours after ovulation.[2,10] The fertilized oocyte or zygote is then transported into the uterine cavity and enters the uterus at the morula stage, 2–3 days after fertilization or around day 18 of the cycle. A blastocyst forms and sheds its zona pellucida (non-adhesive protective coating) and apposes superficially to the endometrium. At this point, the interaction between the embryo and the endometrium is unstable. Increasing interaction between the blastocyst and endometrium leads to a more stable adhesion. The trophoblasts then invade the endometrium, the underlying stroma, the inner-third of the myometrium and the uterine vasculature resulting in placentation.[10]

For successful implantation, the endometrium undergoes morphological and physiological changes to host the conceptus. This period of time is called *window of implantation* that corresponds to day 7–10 after ovulation or day 19–24 of a cycle.[11] This is the time when the uterine receptivity is optimal for a competent embryo to implant. During this period of time, the endometrium produces proteins and other molecules in a cycle-dependent manner which may help to identify uterine receptivity.[11,12] For example, on a cellular level, pinopodes are prominently displayed on apical surface of luminal endometrial epithelium. They are progesterone-dependent[13] and become visible between days 20–21 of a natural cycle.[14] By assessment of pinopode as receptivity marker, the window of implantation appears only open for 48 hours[15] and it is 1–2 days earlier in a stimulated cycle.[16]

Mucin-1 is one of the mucin-like proteins that increases during implantation period.[17] In addition, the embryo needs to cleave MUC-1 layer on the epithelium to facilitate implantation.[18] Integrins alpha and beta subunits, the cell adhesion molecules play a role in the implantation process.[19] Absent or low expression of integrin is associated with infertility such as in unexplained or endometriosis-related infertility,[20] and in women with hydrosalpinx.[21]

Another substance that is found abundantly at the secretory endometrium during the implantation window is glycodelin, one of the glycoproteins. Its main function is to suppress the activity of NK cells,[22] Similarly, HOXA10 and 11 show maximal upregulation during the window of implantation. HOXA10 expression is diminished in hydrosalpinx and endometriosis-related infertility.[9] There are many other factors including cytokines and growth factors that play an important role in implantation and might act as potential prognostic markers for implantation.[2,19] Factors involved in implantation are shown in **Box 1**.

◼ STIMULATED CYCLE

During ovarian stimulation, estradiol (E2) production increases tremendously. This high level of E2 seems to

Box 1 Factors involved in implantation

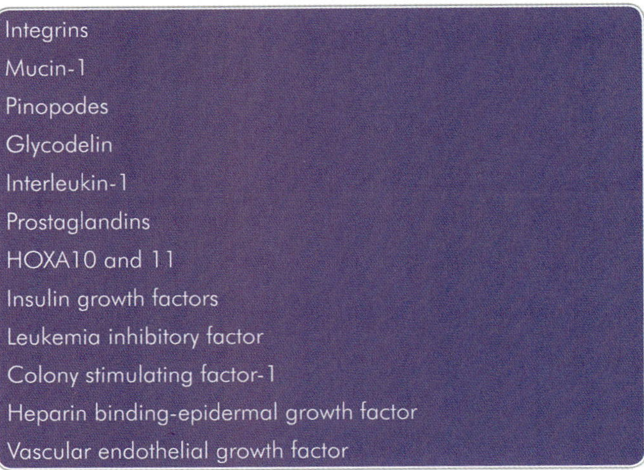

impair endometrial maturation and diminishes uterine receptivity for implantation compared to a natural cycle.[23] It has been shown that E2 levels of over 2500 pg/mL leads to a significant reduction in implantation rate.[24] On the other hand, when a step-down protocol was used, ensuring lower E2 levels, implantation and pregnancy rates were significantly better in comparison with a standard stimulation protocol.[25] However, in a large retrospective comparative study between in vitro fertilization-embryo transfer (IVF-ET) patients and recipients of donated oocytes, Levi et al., 2001,[26] reported that embryo implantation and pregnancy and delivery rates were similar.

Implantation window is affected by the use of GnRH agonist or antagonist. For example, ovarian stimulation with a standard GnRH analog and gonadotropin advances endometrial maturation around the time of ovulation by 2–4 days[9] and the ratio between progesterone and estrogen and their receptors is reduced.[27] With GnRH antagonist stimulation protocols, supraphysiological steroid levels seem to impair the luteal phase.[28,29] Here, luteal support to improve the endometrial development could be considered.[30] Yet, there was no significant difference in advanced endometrial maturation on the day of oocytes retrieval and the mid-luteal phase between agonist and antagonist cycle.[31]

Clomiphene stimulated cycles are also associated with a reduction in pinopode formation at the mid-luteal phase, and negatively impacts the implantation process.[9]

◼ CONCLUSION

Implantation is a complex process mediated by cytokines, growth factors, adhesion molecules and other substances. It is crucial for a successful pregnancy. For a successful implantation, the endometrium undergoes morphological and physiological changes to host the conceptus. This period of time is called *window of implantation* that corresponds to day 7–10 after ovulation. Compared to a natural cycle, this window is opened 1–2 days earlier in the stimulated cycle. In fact, the use of medications including GnRH agonist, GnRH antagonist, and clomiphene citrate might impair implantation.

■ REFERENCES

1. Lindhard A, Bentin-Ley U, Ravn V, et al. Biochemical evaluation of endometrial function at the time of implantation. Fertil Steril. 2002;78(2):221-33.
2. Guzeloglu-Kayisli O, Basar M, Arici A. Basic aspects of implantation. Reprod Biomed Online. 2007;15(6):728-39.
3. Krüssel JS, Bielfeld P, Polan ML, et al. Regulation of embryonic implantation. Eur J Obstet Gynecol Reprod Biol. 2003;110 (Suppl 1):S2-9.
4. Owen JA. Physiology of the menstrual cycle. Am J Clin Nutr. 1975;28(4):333-8.
5. Sherman BM, Korenman SG. Hormonal characteristics of the human menstrual cycle throughout reproductive life. J Clin Invest. 1975;55(4):699-706.
6. King AE, Critchley HO. Oestrogen and progesterone regulation of inflammatory processes in the human endometrium. J Steroid Biochem Mol Biol. 2010;120(2-3):116-26.
7. Gambino LS, Wreford NG, Bertram JF, et al. Angiogenesis occurs by vessel elongation in proliferative phase human endometrium. Hum Reprod. 2002;17(5):1199-206.
8. Print C, Valtola R, Evans A, et al. Soluble factors from human endometrium promote angiogenesis and regulate the endothelial cell transcriptome. Hum Reprod. 2004;19(10):2356-66.
9. Strowitzki T, Germeyer A, Popovici R, et al. The human endometrium as a fertility-determining factor. Hum Reprod Update. 2006;12(5):617-30.
10. Norwitz ER, DJ Schust, SJ Fisher. Implantation and the survival of early pregnancy. N Engl J Med. 2001;345(19):1400-8.
11. Wilcox AJ, Baird DD, Weinberg CR. Time of implantation of the conceptus and loss of pregnancy. N Engl J Med. 1999;340(23):1796-9.
12. Lessey BA. Endometrial receptivity and the window of implantation. Baillieres Best Pract Res Clin Obstet Gynaecol. 2000;14(5):775-88.
13. Martel D, Monier MN, Roche D, et al. Hormonal dependence of pinopode formation at the uterine luminal surface. Hum Reprod. 1991;6(4):597-603.
14. Nikas G, Drakakis P, Loutradis D, et al. Uterine pinopodes as markers of the 'nidation window' in cycling women receiving exogenous oestradiol and progesterone. Hum Reprod. 1995;10(5):1208-13.
15. Nikas G, Psychoyos A. Uterine pinopodes in peri-implantation human endometrium. Clinical relevance. Ann NY Acad Sci. 1997;816:129-42.
16. Nikas G. Pinopodes as markers of endometrial receptivity in clinical practice. Hum Reprod. 1999;14 (Suppl 2):99-106.
17. Hey NA, Graham RA, Seif MW, et al. The polymorphic epithelial mucin MUC1 in human endometrium is regulated with maximal expression in the implantation phase. J Clin Endocrinol Metab. 1994;78(2):337-42.
18. Meseguer M, Aplin JD, Caballero-Campo P, et al. Human endometrial mucin MUC1 is up-regulated by progesterone and down-regulated in vitro by the human blastocyst. Biol Reprod. 2001;64(2):590-601.
19. Hoozemans DA, Schats R, Lambalk CB, et al. Human embryo implantation: current knowledge and clinical implications in assisted reproductive technology. Reprod Biomed Online. 2004;9(6):692-715.
20. Lessey BA, Castelbaum AJ, Sawin SW, et al. Integrins as markers of uterine receptivity in women with primary unexplained infertility. Fertil Steril. 1995;63(3):535-42.
21. Meyer WR, Castelbaum AJ, Somkuti S, et al. Hydrosalpinges adversely affect markers of endometrial receptivity. Hum Reprod. 1997;12(7):1393-8.
22. Okamoto N, Uchida A, Takakura K, et al. Suppression by human placental protein 14 of natural killer cell activity. Am J Reprod Immunol. 1991;26(4):137-42.
23. Martínez-Conejero JA, Simón C, Pellicer A, et al. Is ovarian stimulation detrimental to the endometrium? Reprod Biomed Online. 2007;15(1):45-50.
24. Simón C, Cano F, Valbuena D, et al. Clinical evidence for a detrimental effect on uterine receptivity of high serum oestradiol concentrations in high and normal responder patients. Hum Reprod. 1995;10(9):2432-7.
25. Simón C, Garcia Velasco JJ, Valbuena D, et al. Increasing uterine receptivity by decreasing estradiol levels during the preimplantation period in high responders with the use of a follicle-stimulating hormone step-down regimen. Fertil Steril. 1998;70(2):234-9.
26. Levi AJ, Drews MR, Bergh PA, et al. Controlled ovarian hyperstimulation does not adversely affect endometrial receptivity in in vitro fertilization cycles. Fertil Steril. 2001;76(4):670-4.
27. Bourgain C, Ubaldi F, Tavaniotou A, et al. Endometrial hormone receptors and proliferation index in the periovulatory phase of stimulated embryo transfer cycles in comparison with natural cycles and relation to clinical pregnancy outcome. Fertil Steril. 2002;78(2):237-44.
28. Kolibianakis E, Bourgain C, Albano C, et al. Effect of ovarian stimulation with recombinant follicle-stimulating hormone, gonadotropin releasing hormone antagonists, and human chorionic gonadotropin on endometrial maturation on the day of oocyte pick-up. Fertil Steril. 2002;78(5):1025-9.
29. Ubaldi F, Bourgain C, Tournaye H, et al. Endometrial evaluation by aspiration biopsy on the day of oocyte retrieval in the embryo transfer cycles in patients with serum progesterone rise during the follicular phase. Fertil Steril. 1997;67(3):521-6.
30. Diedrich K, Fauser BC, Devroey P, et al. The role of the endometrium and embryo in human implantation. Hum Reprod Update. 2007;13(4):365-77.
31. Saadat P, Boostanfar R, Slater CC, et al. Accelerated endometrial maturation in the luteal phase of cycles utilizing controlled ovarian hyperstimulation: impact of gonadotropin-releasing hormone agonists versus antagonists. Fertil Steril. 2004;82(1):167-71.

Recurrent Implantation Failure: Strategies and Intervention

Sadhana K Desai, Partha Guha Roy

INTRODUCTION

Many infertile couples fail to achieve a pregnancy after repeated transfers of morphologically good quality embryos produced by in vitro fertilization (IVF) treatment. These patients who have had three or more consecutive IVF cycles without clinical pregnancy are regarded as having recurrent implantation failure (RIF).

Recurrent implantation failure is today the major reason for women completing several IVF/intra-cytoplasmic sperm injection (ICSI) attempts without having achieved a child and is probably also the explanation for many cases of unexplained infertility. Implantation is a complicated process that requires the orchestration of a series of events involving both the embryo and the endometrium.

The success of assisted reproduction, although gradually increasing over the years, is still less than satisfactory. Even when embryos are of high quality, implantation rates remain around 25–35%.[1] Faced with the frustratingly low success rates following embryo transfer, IVF providers are therefore searching for strategies and interventions designed to increase the chance of successful implantation.

Of late, IVF clinicians have watched their laboratory colleagues make progress in improving embryo quality and selection for transfer. However, in the same period only marginal improvement of the implantation and pregnancy rate per transfer has been achieved. So, the clinicians have sought to develop clinical interventions aimed at enhancing implantation rates from IVF. The fierce competitive scenario of IVF practice has often led to the early adoption of promising new interventions before clear evidence for their efficacy and safety has been established.

In this chapter, the various clinical strategies employed by the clinicians to increase the chance of implantation are reviewed.

There are two basic causes for RIF: (1) problem in embryo quality and (2) problem in endometrial receptivity.

EMBRYO AS A POSSIBLE CAUSE OF RIF: STRATEGIES AND INTERVENTION

Suspect if age more than 38 years
Poor responder
Polycystic ovary syndrome

Ovarian Stimulation Regimen

Ovarian stimulation and the supraphysiological estradiol concentration have been shown to impact negatively on endometrial receptivity. This may be due to advanced postovulatory endometrial maturation and defective induction of progesterone receptors.[2] The stimulation of large number of follicles may result in the generation of poor quality of oocytes, and hence lower quality of embryos. Increasing knowledge of the physiology of ovarian follicle development, together with availability of gonadotropin-releasing hormone (GnRH) antagonists, has presented the opportunity to develop novel, milder approaches to ovarian stimulation for IVF.[3,4]

Although more oocytes are retrieved in conventional ovarian stimulation, the oocytes from milder stimulation group showed an increased percentage of euploid embryos per number of oocytes retrieved.[5] Employing mild stimulation regimens may aid embryo selection by increasing the chance that the transferred embryo is euploid.

Adjusting the dose of ovarian stimulation to the individual patient with the aim of inducing a mild ovarian stimulation can be challenging because ovarian response varies substantially between patients. Pharmacogenetics has emerged as an attractive tool to individualize follicle-stimulating hormone (FSH) dosing. Number of antral follicles, ovarian volume, age and smoking habits are the initial screening parameters to determine the response dose of FSH. Using this screening model, a randomized controlled trial (RCT) has showed a higher pregnancy rate in the individual dose group.[6]

> *Milder stimulation*
> ↓Estradiol level
> Endometrium in phase
> ↑Euploid embryos

Blastocyst Transfer

In women who do not conceive with repeated day 3 transfer, blastocyst transfer may be attempted. Blastocyst stage transfer is more physiological as the endometrium is synchronized with the developmental stage of embryos. Similar to cleavage stage embryos, not all blastocysts are equally implantation competent.[7] Transfer of expanded blastocysts with a normal inner cell mass yielded higher implantation rate.[8]

The value of blastocyst transfer has been questioned and a recent meta-analysis concluded that blastocyst stage transfer does not confer any advantage over cleavage stage embryo transfer.[9] Another recent prospective randomized study that compared embryo transfer on day 2, 3 and day 6, however failed to show any difference in implantation and pregnancy rates.[10,11]

> *Higher implantation rate*
> With expanded blastocyst with normal inner cell mass

Sequential Embryo Transfer

Loutradis et al.[12] evaluated the outcome of sequential embryo transfers on days 2 and 4 or 5 in patients who repeatedly fail to conceive despite the transfer of good quality embryos. A 38–60% clinical pregnancy rate was achieved in women who had day 2 and day 4 and day 2 and day 5 sequential embryo transfer respectively. Whether sequential embryo transfer can serve as a viable option in women with RIF, however remains to be determined in prospective randomized trials.

Assisted Hatching

Assisted hatching is based on the presumption that creating artificial openings in the zona pellucida might assist the in vivo hatching process of embryos that are kept in culture. Some centers use assisted hatching for poor prognosis patients such as women with advanced age, poor quality embryos, embryos with thick zona pellucida and previous implantation failures.

It is current policy to perform assisted hatching using the laser in the subgroup of patients with advanced age (>37 years), one or more previous implantation failures and with poor embryo characteristics such as suboptimal embryo quality and thick zona pellucida.

Cocultures

Coculture has been proposed as a salvage treatment option in couples with RIF.[13] Different human and non-human cells and cell lines have been used for cocultures. Since the advent of complex sequential media those yield very high blastocyst formation and blastocyst implantation rates, the need for cocultures has been questioned. Simon et al. were the first to report the results of autologous endometrial coculture in couples with RIF following IVF-embryo transfer or oocyte donation.[14]

In the era of complex sequential media, cocultures should no longer be offered to patients undergoing assisted reproduction and whether cocultures are beneficial in patients with repeated implantation failures should be investigated in randomized trials.

Preimplantation Genetic Diagnosis for Aneuploidy Screening

Choosing chromosomally normal embryos among a cohort may also improve embryo selection and increase pregnancy rates. Many couples have benefited from this technique particularly women of advanced age, couples with RIF and recurrent aborters.[15-17] When all other factors leading to RIF have been eliminated embryonic aneuploidy is usually blamed for non-implantation.

The data of the European Society of Human Reproduction and Embryology (ESHRE) preimplantation genetic diagnosis (PGD) consortium, which include PGD cycles from 25 centers, reported that implantation rate in RIF was only 11% compared with 32–36% in aneuploidy screening for other indications.[18] PGD does not seem to increase the success of assisted reproduction in couples with RIF. However, it provides additional information for counseling the couple regarding the etiology of previous failed treatment cycles.

Evaluating Embryonic Potential

The complications of multiple gestations following IVF have introduced strict IVF transfer policies involving elective transfer of single embryo. It is also known that only 5–7% of the oocytes retrieved during IVF will lead to pregnancy, and only 10–15% of the embryos will result in the birth of a child.[19] So search is on to identify the embryo with maximum potential to implant from the cohort of developing embryos.

In everyday practice, the embryologist checks the embryos for progress once every 24 hours and thus is aware of the daily progress but does not know how the embryos advance from one developmental stage to the next. Time-lapse monitoring allows continuous observation of the embryos without removing them from the incubators to maintain ideal culturing conditions. A camera is built into the incubator that takes a picture of the embryo every 5–10 minutes and a short film is created thereby allowing precise observation of the dynamics of the embryo's development.

The timing and duration of cellular division are very important. Embryos those start to divide late or slow to complete the divisions are less likely to reach the blastocyst stage and are therefore less likely to be eligible for implantation. It is also important to observe the synchronization of these early events. Embryos those spend minimal time at stages with uneven blastomeres (3-, 5- and 7-cell stages) have better implantation potential.[20] Fragmentation typically is considered a poor morphological sign. Time-lapse monitoring has shown that the appearance and disappearance of fragments also are a dynamic process, and by observing the embryo only once daily, one may miss some of these fragments.

Many techniques have been explored in recent years. It is well-known, there is significant proportion of the embryos are aneuploid, and therefore do not implant. Genetic screening to identify the euploid embryos is expected to raise pregnancy and delivery rates. Available information suggests an increase of approximately 50% in implantation rates, but randomized trial data are limited, and the associated expenses must also be considered.[21,22]

Analysis of metabolic products, protein secretory products and oxygen consumption of the embryo has provided mixed results, and is not ready for routine clinical use. Gene expression profiling of the cumulus cells is another area of interest but also is not available for clinical use.

Until better tools for embryo selection become routinely available, we have to use the tools we have. Time-lapse monitoring already is available for embryo selection. With the increase in the number of continuously observed cycles, new embryo developmental signs are identified; those could aid the selection for transfer. It is hoped that the benefits of this observation will soon be confirmed by randomized studies and a widespread applications of this technique can be recommended.

■ ENDOMETRIUM AS POSSIBLE CAUSE OF RIF: STRATEGIES AND INTERVENTION

Embryo Transfer Technique

Significant improvements in clinical pregnancy rates can be achieved by giving due attention to embryo transfer technique. Stiff catheters as compared to soft ones make catheter placement easier, but may cause more trauma and bleeding. In a recent meta-analysis of seven RCTs comparing soft and stiff embryo catheters, significantly increased pregnancy rates were observed with the former.[23]

Controversy exists concerning the depth from fundus and embryo replacement. Traditionally, the embryo transfer was aimed at placing the embryos 1 cm below the fundus of the uterus.[24] However, it has been suggested that transferring embryos lower in the uterine cavity may improve implantation rates. Significantly better results were obtained when the catheter tip was positioned close to the middle of the uterine cavity.[25] Another randomized study revealed significantly higher implantation rates when embryos were deposited 1.5 cm or 2 cm from the fundus as compared with 1 cm.[26] As a result of these studies, many centers have adjusted their embryo transfer procedure.

The blind nature of traditional "Clinical Touch" embryo transfer had led to the suggestion of a role for ultrasound in improving IVF outcome. A meta-analysis of four RCT comparing ultrasound-guided embryo transfer versus clinical touch showed a higher pregnancy rate and implantation rate after ultrasound-guided transfer.[27]

Screening Hysteroscopy

As implantation failure after embryo transfer is one of the main problems of the IVF, and intrauterine pathology can lead to higher abortion rates, it appears necessary to exclude all factors that could negatively influence IVF outcome.[28-30] Different opinions exist on the importance of hysteroscopy as part of the routine basic diagnostic of infertility, especially in patients plan for IVF.

In a study on 375 patients with primary infertility in normal basic sonography, every tenth patient suffers from intrauterine pathology (mainly adhesions), which could influence the outcome of later sterility treatment.[31] Screening hysteroscopy is therefore suggested to minimize any negative anatomical intrauterine influence on IVF outcome before including patients in a IVF program or better before any infertility treatment.

Endometrial Injury

Endometrial receptivity is one of the key factors regulating blastocysts implantation, and it has been shown that mechanical trauma to the endometrium alters gene expressions, enhances secretion of growth factors and makes it more receptive for implantation.[32] Interestingly, this effect has been shown to last in the subsequent cycle possibly because the monocytes recruited to the injured sites are long lived and reside in tissues for a long time.[33]

Pooling of seven control studies (four randomized and three non-randomized), with 2,062 participants showed that local endometrial injury induced in the cycle preceding ovarian stimulation is 70% more likely to results in a clinical pregnancy as opposed to no intervention.[34] The mechanical manipulation and local injury to the endometrium can be induced by endometrial biopsy or hysteroscopy.

Thin Endometrium

Different thresholds of endometrial thickness were suggested as essential for successful implantation and most demonstrated that no pregnancy was established with the thickness of the preovulatory endometrium was less than 6 mm. The incidence of thin endometrium in natural cycles has been reported 5% in women less than 40 years of age and 25% in women 41–45 years of age.[35] Thin endometrium may be after effect of tuberculous endometritis, multiple curettage following induced abortion or miscarriage and other pelvic inflammatory diseases.

Various empirical treatments with combination of steroid hormones with sildenafil and aspirin with low dose of heparin have been tried in an effort to improve the endometrial thickness with an adequate endometrial response being defined as an ultrasonographic thickness more than and equal to 7 mm. No treatment was found to be better than the other, and these patients had a poor reproductive prognosis even if some endometrial thickening or implantation did occur. Proper counseling regarding the very low live birth rate achieved by IVF and alternatives such as surrogacy and adoption should be discussed with these patients.

> Tuberculous endometritis
> Multiple curettage
> Other pelvic inflammatory disease

■ IMMUNOLOGICAL FACTORS

Allogeneic Lymphocyte Therapy

There is strong evidence that locally secreted cytokines control the implantation process and can cause implantation failure.[36,37] Normal pregnancy is proposed to be a T helper (Th)2 immune response. Th2 cells induce antibody-mediated immunity and secrete cytokines such as IL-4, 5 and 10 which favor successful pregnancy. Women with recurrent spontaneous abortion and multiple implantation failures after IVF-embryo transfer have significantly higher Th1/Th2 ratio as compared with normal fertile woman.[38] Other cytokines, particularly, leukemia inhibitory factor (LIF) have gained widespread attention. LIF expression is increased during the luteal phase and implantation is severely impaired in the absence of LIF in animal models. Third party or husband-derived lymphocyte isoimmunization has been proposed to induce the Th1 to Th2 shift and enhance the implantation process. Some immunotherapy specialists postulate that excess Th1 cytokines cause all implantation failure and should be corrected by allogeneic leukocyte isoimmunization.[38,39] However, implantation is a very complex process involving many steps, and thus failure of implantation is not likely to be treated with a single universal approach. Although no randomized trials exist or implantation failure, a large randomized trial in women with recurrent spontaneous abortion failed to show any beneficial effect of allogeneic leukocyte immunization.[40]

Thrombophilia

Presence of thrombophilia may also lead to implantation failure. Women with RIF should be evaluated for thrombophilia and if found to be positive then should be treated with low-dose heparin and ecosprin.

Transfer in Hormone Replacement Therapy Cycles

In fresh cycle of IVF due to hyperstimulation and increased estradiol level, the endometrium remains out of phase and thereby implantation failure is high. With the hormone replacement therapy cycle the frozen embryos when replaced have a better implantation rate as the endometrium is in phase.

Concept of Personalized Embryo Transfer and Endometrial Receptivity Assay

Endometrial receptivity refers to a hormone limited period in which the endometrial tissue acquires a functional and transient ovarian steroid dependent status allowing blastocyst adhesion. Functional genomic studies of the human endometrium in natural cycles have demonstrated that endometrial receptivity is an active process involving upregulation and downregulation of hundreds of genes.[41]

The IVI group from Spain led by Carlos Simon has developed the endometrial receptivity assay (ERA) tool, a customized array of 238 genes coupled to a computational predictor capable of diagnosing a functionally receptive endometrium regardless of its histological appearance.[42] The accuracy of the diagnostic ERA tool has been demonstrated to be superior to endometrial histology and results are completely reproducible 29–40 months later.[43] This concept of personalized embryo transfer in patients with implantation failure guided by ERA has been developed to identify the window of implantation successfully regardless of histological appearance of the endometrium. This has shown promising results and is currently being validated in an ongoing RCT.

Some implantation failure patients should not be categorized as having a pathological condition but as patients in whom embryo transfer timing should be personalized as their endometrial timing is different.

■ ADJUVANT PHARMACEUTICAL THERAPIES

Aspirin

Low-dose aspirin is very often used as an adjuvant drug in IVF with the aim of enhancing blood flow to the uterus and ovaries. There are several studies in the literature that have evaluated the effectiveness of aspirin cotreatment in unselected patients undergoing IVF or ICSI.[44-46] The results are conflicting, but a recent meta-analysis concluded that there was no statistically significant benefit of aspirin use in infertile women undergoing ART.[47] An RCT was performed comparing aspirin and heparin treatment from the time of embryo transfer with placebo in 143 antiphospholipid or antinuclear antibody-seropositive women with a previous history of IVF implantation failure.[48] No significant differences in

implantation or pregnancy rates were observed. Current evidence suggests that the use of aspirin at present is at best equivocal and may be associated with side effects.

Nitric Oxide Donors

Nitric oxide has been shown to be an important modulator of folliculogenesis, fertilization, decidualization and implantation.[49,50] It acts as a relaxant of arterial and smooth muscle, and inhibits platelet aggregation. Uterine vasodilatation induced by a nitric oxide donor during IVF might improve endometrial receptivity. More recent studies suggested a detrimental effect of nitric oxide on implantation.[51,52] Although subgroups of women may be identified who benefited from nitric oxide donor therapy, at present the available data demand caution in its use.

Aromatase Inhibitors

By preventing excessive estradiol synthesis, it has been postulated that the adjuvant treatment with aromatase inhibitors during gonadotropin ovarian stimulation may result in less disruption of endometrial receptivity. Three non-randomized trials showed comparable pregnancy rate with aromatase inhibitors as an adjunct treatment in normal responders.[53-55] While of considerable potential value, further studies are required to confirm the value and safety of aromatase inhibitors in IVF.

Ascorbic Acid

Transient high plasma concentrations can be achieved by high-dose intake of ascorbic acid, which can exert anti-inflammatory and immunostimulant effects. These effects might benefit embryo implantation. However, an RCT investigating the effect of high dose of ascorbic acid versus placebo during the luteal phase in 620 women undergoing IVF showed no difference in implantation rates.[56]

Prolonged Progesterone

Following ovarian stimulation and IVF, the luteal phase is abnormal compared with natural cycle, the characteristic features being elevated progesterone level in early luteal phase followed by a dramatic and premature fall in the unsupported mid-luteal phase. The luteal phase can be restored by stimulating the corpora lutea with human chorionic gonadotropin or supplementation with progesterone.

The optimal duration of progesterone administration remains to be clarified. Many centers continue it till first trimester of pregnancy citing the uterine relaxing properties of progesterone. Uterine contractions were significantly decreased on the day of embryo transfer when vaginal progesterone was started on the day of oocyte retrieval.[57] In addition, progesterone has potentially beneficial immunomodulatory properties.

Extended progesterone supplementation needs to be viewed within the context of the endocrinology of early pregnancy after IVF. Studies of luteal function in the early pregnancy among pregnant women following IVF reported markedly raised progesterone concentration for up to 9 weeks of gestation compared with spontaneous pregnancies.[58] RCT comparing 5 weeks versus 2 weeks of progesterone therapy from oocyte retrieval onward showed no difference in outcome.[59] Since the multiple corpora lutea resulting after IVF produce high concentrations of progesterone in early pregnancy, extending therapy beyond the luteal phase is probably superfluous.

Estradiol Supplementation

The application of luteal estradiol supplementation remains controversial. A meta-analysis of three RCTs, using a long GnRH agonist protocol reported no difference in pregnancy rates when estrogen was added to progesterone in luteal phase.[60] In contrast, a recent RCT of 166 women undergoing ICSI, reported significantly higher pregnancy and implantation rates after estradiol supplementation.[61]

Glucocorticoids Use

The uterine receptivity is controlled by locally acting growth factors, cytokines and uterine natural killer cells. It has been shown that uterine natural killer cells may have an important role in early implantation, since they accumulate around arteries supplying the implantation site.[62] A defect in the integrity of the number of uterine natural killer cells has also been implicated in implantation failure. A higher number of natural killer cells were reported in endometrial biopsies from women with implantation failure versus fertile controls.[63] In women with recurrent miscarriage, prednisolone has been shown to reduce the expression of uterine natural killer cells in the endometrium.[64] There is therefore evidence to support a possible role for glucocorticoids in improving the intrauterine environment by acting as immunomodulators.

The Cochrane Systematic Review data on glucocorticoids on embryo implantation show insufficient evidence to support the empirical use of glucocorticoids to improve implantation in IVF. In certain group of patients with antiphospholipid antibody syndrome, there may be specific role for this therapy. Women with positive antinuclear antibody, anticardiolipin antibody, antidouble-stranded DNA and lupus anticoagulant reported significantly higher pregnancy rates after glucocorticoid administration. However, further research is necessary to clarify its role in an aid to implantation.

Insulin Sensitizing Agents

No effect on implantation rate has been reported when metformin has been used in women with polycystic ovary syndrome (PCOS). A meta-analysis of eight RCT investigating metformin in women with PCOS demonstrated no significant differences in pregnancy rates.[65] Caution should be applied before insulin sensitizing drugs are prescribed as adjuvant treatment for IVF, since there is no evidence supporting their use in non-selected IVF population.

■ ALTERNATIVE MEDICINES TO IMPROVE IMPLANTATION

Stress is part of infertility, especially in assisted reproduction patients due to personal, social, familiar, ethical, cultural, financial and even religious issues. Abnormal stress or inadequate coping strategies reduce uterine flow and induce uterine contraction that decreases embryo implantation rates. Measures to reduce stress before, during or after embryo transfer embrace good medical care with pharmacologic, psychological or different types of relaxation techniques. This type of complementary and alternative medicine is gaining popularity throughout the world. The mostly used of them are acupuncture, hypnosis, transcendental meditation, yoga and spirituality. There are few serious studies with enough scientific evidence of their real efficacy and safety in infertility patients.

There is lack of enough randomized, controlled prospective studies to know for sure the real value and safety of these measures in infertility, especially in assisted reproduction patients during specific steps of treatment like oocyte retrieval or embryo transfer. Simple measures are beneficial as also the pharmacological, psychological or alternative medicine approaches. All of them are able to decrease uterine contraction, increase blood flow and make the procedure more tolerable. More studies are needed to evaluate the safety and efficacy of these measures in embryo transfer. It is recommended to offer them because they are based in sound scientific principles and make the procedure more tolerable. Alternative medicine is a compliment not an opposite of traditional medicine.[66]

SURROGACY AND GAMETE DONATION

With repeated implantation failure due to thin endometrium, intrauterine adhesions with grade III and IV, one may opt for surrogacy. When embryos are in doubt, one may opt for gamete donation which may produce a good embryo leading to implantation. Nowadays, the surrogacy and gamete donation programs are well-known and easily accepted by the patient.

CONCLUSION

Multiple factors result in embryo implantations failure. Hence, no single additional treatment is likely to provide the key solution. Until an understanding of the factor that determine the ability of an embryo to successfully implant increases, it is unlikely that additional medical interventions such as those reviewed in this chapter will be shown to have anything but a marginal effect on IVF outcomes.

REFERENCES

1. Andersen AN, Gianaroli L, Felberbaum R, et al. European IVF–monitoring programme. Assisted Reproductive Technology in Europe 2001. Results generated from European registers by ESHRE. Hum Reprod. 2005;20:1158-76.
2. Devroey P, Bourgain C, Macklon NS, et al. Reproductive biology and IVF: ovarian stimulation and endometrial receptivity. Trends Endocrinol Metab. 2004;15:84-90.
3. Fauser BC, Macklon NS. Medical approaches to ovarian stimulation for infertility. In: Strauss JF, Barbieri R (eds) Yen and Yaffe's Reproductive Endocrinology. Philadelphia: Elsevier Saunders; 2004.
4. Macklon NS, Stouffer RL, Giudice LC, et al. The science behind 25 years of ovarian stimulation for in vitro fertilization. Endocr Rev. 2006;27:170-207.
5. Baart Eb et al. Does the magnitude of ovarian stimulation for IVF affect chromosomal competence of embryos as assessed by PGS? 21st Annual meeting of the ESHRE. Hum Reprod. 2005;20:191-2 [Abstract O-246].
6. Popovic-Todorovic B, Loft A, Bredkjaeer HE, et al. A prospective randomized clinical trial comparing an individual dose of recombinant FSH based on predictive factors versus a standard dose of 150 IU/day in 'standard' patients undergoing IVF/ICSI treatment. Hum Reprod. 2003;18:2275-82.
7. Balaban B, Urman B. Embryo culture as a diagnostic tool. Reprod Biomed Online. 2003;7:671-82.
8. Kovacic B, Vlaisavljevic V, Reljic M, et al. Development capacity of different morphological types of day 5 human morulae and blastocysts. Reprod Biomed Online. 2004;8:687-94.
9. Blake D, Proctor M, Johnson N, et al. Cleavage stage versus blastocyst stage transfer in assisted conception. Cochrane Database Syst Rev. 2002;(2):CD002118.
10. Pantos K, Makrakis E, Karantzis P, et al. A blastocyst versus early cleavage embryo transfer: a retrospective analysis of 4165 transfers. Clin Exp Obstet Gynecol. 2004;31:42-4.
11. Pantos K, Makrakis E, Stavrou D, et al. Comparison of embryo transfer on day 2 and 3 and day 6: a prospective randomized study. Ferti Steril. 2004;81:454-5.
12. Loutradis D, Drakakis P, Dallianidis K, et al. A double embryo transfer on day 2 and 4 or 5 improves pregnancy outcome in patients with good embryos but repeated failures in IVF/ICSI. Clin Exp Obstet Gynecol. 2004;31:63-6.
13. Spandorfer D, Clark R, Park J, et al. Autologus endometrial on co-culture (AECC): an effective tool for patients with multiple failed IVF attempts. Fertil Steril. 2003;80(Suppl 3):S6.
14. Simon C, Mercader A, Garcia-Velasco J, et al. Co-culture of human embryo with autologous human endometrial epithelial cells in patients with implantation failure. J Clin Endocrinol Metab. 1999;84:2638-46.
15. Pehlivan T, Rubio C, Rodrigo L, et al. Impact of preimplantation of genetic diagnosis on IVF outcome in implantation failure patients. Reprod Biomed Online. 2003;6:232-7.
16. Caglar G, Asimakopoulos B, Nikolettos N, et al. Preimplantation genetic diagnosis for aneuploidy screening in case of repeated implantation failure. Reprod Biomed Online. 2005;10:381-8.
17. Kuliev A, Verlinsky Y. Thirteen years' experience of preimplantation diagnosis: report of the Fifth International Symposium on preimplantation Genetics. Reprod Biomed Online. 2004;8:229-35.
18. ESHRE PGD Consortium Steering Committee. ESHRE preimplantation genetic diagnosis consortium data collection III (May 2001). Hum Reprod. 2002;17:233-46.
19. Kovalevsky G, Patrizio P. High rates of embryo wastage with use of assisted reproductive technology: a look at the trends between 1995 and 2001 in the United States. Fertil Steril. 2005;84:325-30.
20. Kirkegaard K, Agerholm IE, Ingerslev HJ. Time lapse monitoring as a tool for clinical embryo assessment. Hum Reprod. 2012;27:1277-85.
21. Kovacs P. Multiple pregnancies after ART and how to minimize their occurrence. Curr Womens Health Rev. 2012;8:289-96.
22. Herrero J, Meseguer M. Selection of high potential embryos using time lapse imaging. The era of morphokinetics. Fertil Steril. 2013;99:1030-34.
23. Buckett WM. A review and meta-analysis of prospective trials comparing different catheters used for embryo transfer. Fertil Steril. 2006;85:728-34.
24. Schoolcraft W. Embryo transfer. Textbook of Assisted Reproductive Techniques; Laboratory and Clinical Perspectives, 2nd edition. London: Taylor and Francis; 2001. p. 751.

25. Oliveira JB, Martins AM, Baruffi RL, et al. Increased implantation in pregnancy rate obtained by placing the tip of the transfer catheter in the central area of the endometrial cavity. Reprod Biomed Online. 2004;9(4):435-41.
26. Coroleu B, Barri PN, Carreras O, et al. The influence of the depth of embryo replacement into uterine cavity on implantation rates after IVF: a controlled ultrasound guided study. Hum Reprod. 2002;17:341-6.
27. Buckett WM. A meta-analysis of ultrasound guided versus clinical touch embryo transfer. Fertil Steril. 2003;80:1037-41.
28. Grijmbizis GF, Camus M, Tarlatzis BC, et al. Clinical implications of uterine malformations and hysteroscopic treatment results. Hum Reprod Update. 2001;7:161-74.
29. Nawroth F, Schmidt T, Freise C, et al. Uterus septus with primary infertility—an operating indication? Zentralbl Gynakol. 2001;123:644-47.
30. Nawroth F, Schmidt T, Freise C, et al. Is it possible to recommend an 'optimal' postoperative management after hysteroscopic metroplasty? A retrospective study with 52 patients showing a septate uterus. Acta Obstet Gynecol Scand. 2002;81:55-7.
31. Nawroth F, Foth D, Schmidt T. Mini-hysteroscopy as in essential part of routine basic diagnostics in patients with primary infertility. J Am Assoc Gynecol Laparosc. 2003;10:396-8.
32. Klma Y, Granot I, Gnainsky Y, et al. Endometrial biopsy induced gene modulation: first evidence for the expression of bladder-transmembranal uroplack lb in human endometrium. Fertil Steril. 2009;91:1042-49.
33. Gnainsky Y, Granot I, Aldo PB, et al. Local injury of the endometrium induces an inflammatory response that promotes successful implantation. Fertil Steril. 2010;94: 2030-36.
34. Potdar N, Gelbaya T, Nardo LG. Endometrial injury to overcome recurrent embryo implantation failure: a systematic review and meta-analysis. Reprod Biomed Online. 2012;25(6):561-71.
35. Shufaro Y, Simon A, Laufer N, et al. Thin unresponsive endometrium—a possible complication of surgical curettage compromising ART outcome. J Assist Reprod Genet. 2008;25(8):421-25.
36. Ledee-Bataille N, Laprée-Delage G, Taupin JL, et al. Concentration of leukemia inhibitory factor (LIF) in uterine flushing fluid is highly predictive of embryo implantation. Hum Reprod. 2002;17:213-8.
37. Kwak Kim JY, Chung-Bang HS, Ng SC, et al. Increased T helper I cytokine responses by circulating T cells are present in women with recurrent pregnancy losses and in fertile women with multiple implantation failure after IVF. Hum Reprod. 2003;18:767-73.
38. Ng SC, Gilman-Sachs A, Thaker P, et al. Expression of intracellular TH1 and TH2 cytokines in women with recurrent spontaneous abortion, implantation failures after IVF ET or women with normal pregnancy. Am J Reprod Immunol. 2002;48:77-81.
39. Ntrivalas El, Kwak-Kim JY, Gilman-Sachs A, et al. Status of peripheral blood natural killer cells in women with recurrent spontaneous abortions and infertility of unknown etiology. Hum Reprod. 2001;16:855-61.
40. Ober C, Karrison T, Odem RR, et al. Mononuclear cell immunization in prevention of recurrent miscarriages: a randomized trial. Lancet. 1999;354:365-69.
41. Riesewijk A, Martin J, van Os R, et al. Gene expression profiling of human endometrial receptivity on days LH+2 versus LH+7 by micro array technology. Mol Hum Reprod. 2003;9:253-64.
42. Simon C, Ruiz-Alonso M, Blesa D, et al. Endometrial receptivity array for diagnosis and personalized embryo transfer as a treatment for patients with repeated implantation failure. Fertil Steril. 2013;100(3):818-24.
43. Dias-Gimeno P, Horcajadas JA, Martínez-Conejero JA, et al. A genomic diagnostic tool for human endometrial receptivity based on the transcriptomic signature. Fertil Steril. 2011;95: 50-60.
44. Unnan B, Mercan R, Alatas C, et al. Low dose aspirin does not increase implantation rate in patients undergoing ICSI: a prospective randomized study. J Assist Reprod Genet. 2000; 17:586-90.
45. Lok IH, Yip SK, Cheung LP, et al. Adjuvant dose of aspirin therapy in poor responder undergoing IVF: a prospective randomized double blind placebo controlled trial. Fertil Steril. 2004;81:556-61.
46. WaldenStrom U, Hellberg D, Nilsson S, et al. Low dose aspirin in a short regimen a standard treatment in IVF: a randomized prospective study. Fertil Steril. 2004;81:1560-64.
47. Daya Salim et al. Aspirin and other adjuvant in assisted reproduction proceedings of 7th World congress in controversies in obstetrics and gynecology and infertility. E Oren. 2005;272-83.
48. Stern C, Chamley L, Norris H, et al. A randomized double blind placebo controlled trial of heparin and aspirin for women with IVF implantation failure and antiphospholipid or antinuclear antibodies. Fertil Steril. 2003;80:376-83.
49. Hefler LA, Greg AR. Inducible and endothelial nitric oxide synthase genetic background affects ovulation in mice. Fertil Steril. 2002;77:147-51.
50. Chwalisz K, Garfield RE. Role of nitric oxide in implantation and menstruation. Hum Reprod. 2000;15(Suppl 3):96-111.
51. Battagalia C, Regnani G, Marsella T, et al. Adjuvant L-arginine treatment in controlled ovarian hyperstimulation: a double-blind, randomized study. Hum Reprod. 2002;17:659-65.
52. Ohi J, Lefebvre-Maunnoury C, Writtemer C, et al. Nitric oxide donors for patients undergoing IVF. A prospective, double-blind, randomized, placebo-controlled trial. Hum Reprod. 2002;17:2615-20.
53. Healey S, Tan SL, Tulandi T, et al. Effects of letrozole on superovulation with gonadotropins in women undergoing intrauterine insemination. Fertil Steril. 2003;80:1325-9.
54. Mitwally MF, Casper RF. Aromatase inhibition reduces the dose of gonadotropin required for controlled ovarian hyperstimulation. J Soc Gynecol Investig. 2004;11:406-15.
55. Mitwally MF, Casper RF. Aromatase inhibition reduces the dose of gonadotropin required for controlled ovarian stimulation in women with unexplained infertility. Hum Reprod. 2003;18:1588-97.
56. Gresinger G, Franke K, Kinast C, et al. Ascorbic acid supplement during luteal phase in IVF. J Assist Reprod Genet. 2002;19:164-8.

57. Fanchin R, Righini C, de Ziegler D, et al. Effects of vaginal progesterone administration on uterine contractility at the time of embryo transfer. Fertil Steril. 2001;75:1136-40.
58. Costea DM, Gunn LK, Hargreaves C, et al. Delayed luteoplacental shift of progesterone production in IVF pregnancy. Int J Gynaecol Obstet. 2000;68:123-29.
59. Nyboe AA, Popovic-Todorovic B, Schmidt KT, et al. Progesterone supplement during early gestations after IVF or ICSI has no effects on the delivery rates. A randomized controlled trial. Hum Reprod. 2002;17:357-61.
60. Prits EA, Atwood AK. Luteal phase support in infertility treatment: a meta-analysis of the randomized trials. Hum Reprod. 2002;17:2287-99.
61. Lukaszuk K, Liss J, Lukaszuk M, et al. Optimization of estradiol supplementation during the luteal phase improves the pregnancy rate in women undergoing in vitro fertilization embryo transfer cycles. Fertil Steril. 2005;83:1372-76.
62. Croy BA, Chantakru S, Esadeg S, et al. Decidual natural killer cells: key regulators of placental of development (a review). J Reprod Immunol. 2002;57:151-68.
63. Ledee-Bataille N, Bonnet-Chea K, Hosny G, et al. Role of the endometrial tripod interleukin-18, -15, and -12 in adequate uterine receptivity in patients with a history of repeated IVF–embryo transfer failure. Fertil Steril. 2005;83:598-605.
64. Quenby S, Kalumbi C, Bates M, et al. Prednisolene reduces preconceptual endometrial natural killer cells in women with recurrent miscarriage. Fertil Steril. 2005;84:980-4.
65. Costello MF, Chapman M, Conway U. A systematic review and meta analysis of randomized controlled trials on metformin co-administration during gonadotrophin ovulation induction or IVF in women with polycystic ovary syndrome. Hum Reprod. 2006;21:1387-99.
66. Perez- Pena E, alternative medicine and embryo transfer, WARM: In-vitro embryology: new trends and reproductive medicine.

37 Implantation and the Endometrium in Uterine Fibroid

Sesh Kamal Sunkara

INTRODUCTION

Uterine fibroids are the most common pelvic tumors, occurring in 30% of women over the age of 30 years.[1] Their incidence increases with age, and they are more common in Afro-Caribbean women. Although most women affected with fibroids are fertile, fibroids may interfere with fertility with the effect being dictated largely by the location and size of the fibroid.[2,3] Fibroids are traditionally classified according to their anatomical location and are divided into submucous, intramural (the most common site) or subserous fibroids. Submucous fibroids are those that distort the uterine cavity, intramural fibroids are contained within the uterine wall with less than 50% of the tumor protruding into the serosal surface of the uterus, and fibroids protruding greater or equal to 50% out of the serosal surface are subserosal fibroids. Fibroids are multiple in around two-thirds of cases.

FIBROIDS AND FERTILITY

Whilst fibroids are associated with infertility in 5–10% of cases, they are estimated to be the sole cause of infertility in 1–2.4% of cases.[4] The mechanism by which fibroids have a detrimental effect on fertility remains controversial with various theories being postulated. It has been suggested that the mechanism by which fibroids cause infertility are mechanical in nature. The fibroids, if subendometrial or tubal in position, may directly block the passage of spermatozoa. Any fibroid that distorts the shape or elongates the endometrial cavity may affect the establishment and maintenance of early pregnancy. Subendometrial fibroids are capable of causing endometrial erosion with subsequent inflammation. This state alters the biochemical nature of intrauterine fluid, and thus results in hostile environment for the spermatozoa. Alternatively, the subendometrial fibroids may disrupt the endometrial blood supply, thus affecting nidation and sustenance of the early embryo. It has also been suggested that the hyperestrogenic environment associated with fibroids may impair fertility.

A decreased risk of fibroids in parous women when compared with nulliparous women has been repeatedly reported. The observation that parity is associated with a reduction in the risk of fibroids could be interpreted in two ways. Parity may be a protective factor or, alternatively, fertility may be partly compromised in women with fibroids. Studies investigating the association between fibroids and history of infertility may be of help in clarifying this issue, but unfortunately evidence on this regard is scarce. Overall, the question therefore remains about causality of the association. Does pregnancy protect from fibroid development or, conversely, do fibroids affect fertility.

FIBROIDS AND IN VITRO FERTILIZATION TREATMENT OUTCOME

The advent of assisted reproductive techniques (ART) and, in particular, of in vitro fertilization (IVF) treatment has offered a useful tool to elucidate the relationship between fibroids and fertility. Results from IVF treatment provide precious information on the impact of uterine fibroids on embryo implantation.

There have been meta-analyses that have aimed to assess the impact of fibroids in IVF cycles. Somigliana et al. published a meta-analysis of studies investigating the influence of fibroids located at different sites in IVF cycles.[5] Overall, their results showed that myomas negatively affect pregnancy rates. Although based on a small number of studies, submucous fibroids appeared to strongly interfere with the chance of pregnancy: odds ratio (OR) (95% CI) for conception and delivery being 0.3 (0.1–0.7) and 0.3 (0.1–0.8) respectively. The impact of intramural fibroids was less dramatic although still statistically significant: OR (95% CI) for conception and delivery being 0.8 (0.6–0.9) and 0.7 (0.5–0.8) respectively. In general, these effects appeared to be more relevant when considering the delivery rate compared to the clinical pregnancy rate. Conversely, subserosal fibroids did not seem to affect pregnancy rates.

A recent updated systematic review by Pritts et al. evaluated the effects on fertility by location of fibroids.[6] Their results were consistent in showing that women actively attempting to conceive and with submucous fibroids, compared to women without fibroids, demonstrated a significantly lower clinical pregnancy rate (RR 0.36; 95% CI 0.17–0.73), implantation rate (RR 0.28; 95% CI 0.12–0.64), and ongoing pregnancy/live birth rate (RR 0.31; 95% CI 0.11–0.85) and a significantly higher spontaneous abortion rate (RR 1.67; 95% CI 1.37–2.05). Women with intramural fibroids also produced significantly lower implantation rate (RR 0.79; 95% CI 0.69–0.90) and ongoing pregnancy/live birth rate (RR 0.78; 95% CI 0.69–0.88), and a significantly higher spontaneous abortion rate (RR 1.89; 95% CI 1.47–2.42). When women with subserous fibroids were compared with women without fibroids, no difference was observed for any outcome measure.

There is controversy on the impact of intramural fibroids that do not distort the uterine cavity on IVF treatment outcome. This was addressed in a recent systematic review Sunkara et al. that looked at 19 observational studies comprising a total of 6,087 IVF cycles.[7] Meta-analysis of these studies showed a significant decrease in clinical pregnancy (RR 0.85; 95% CI 0.77–0.94) live birth and rates (RR 0.79; 95% CI 0.70–0.88) in women with non-cavity distorting intramural fibroids compared to those without fibroids, following IVF treatment.

The inverse relationship between IVF outcome and the presence of submucous and intramural fibroids may be explained by altered uterine vascular perfusion, myometrial contractility, endometrial function or myometrial/endometrial gene expression.

FERTILITY AFTER MYOMECTOMY

Myomectomy is the surgical treatment option for women with fibroids wishing to conceive. The procedure may be performed abdominally, laparoscopically or hysteroscopically. Several reviews of literature on pregnancy rates following myomectomy have been published. One of the early reviews focusing on studies published between 1933 and 1980 by Buttram and Reiter reported a 40% pregnancy rate following abdominal myomectomy (480 out of 1202 cases).[8] This rate was 54% when patients with other causes of infertility were excluded. Another review by Vercellini et al. confirmed this rate of success following myomectomy.[9] They reported a postsurgical pregnancy rate of 57% across prospective studies. When including women with unexplained infertility, this rate was 61%. The advent of endoscopic surgery did not seem to modify this result. In a review by Donnez and Jadoul the pregnancy rate among women undergoing hysteroscopic and laparoscopic myomectomy was reported as 45% and 49% respectively.[4] These findings have further been confirmed by more recent and larger studies.

IN VITRO FERTILIZATION OUTCOME AFTER MYOMECTOMY

Whilst there is a consistent body of literature on the adverse influence of fibroids on pregnancy outcome following IVF treatment, the impact of myomectomy has been less extensively investigated. Narayan and Goswamy investigated the effect of myomectomy on a small group of women with submucosal fibroids (n = 27).[10] They found that the delivery rate was not significantly different in women who underwent myomectomy compared to women without fibroids (37% and 22% respectively, p = 0.13). Surrey et al. reported a pregnancy rate of 62% and 68% respectively in women operated for submucous fibroids and controls without fibroids following IVF treatment.[11] From these studies, we can infer that although the overall evidence is scarce, myomectomy for submucous fibroids did not seem to negatively affect the pregnancy rate following IVF treatment.

A comparative study by Bulletti et al. looked at the effectiveness of myomectomy prior to IVF treatment in women with intramural and/or subserosal fibroids with at least one lesion greater than 5 cm.[12] Women were allocated to myomectomy (n = 84) or no surgery (n = 84) based on their decision. They reported a live birth rate of 25% and 12% respectively in women who did and did not undergo surgery prior to IVF treatment. It is worthy of note that this study involved small numbers and this evidence therefore does not justify advocating routine myomectomy for these women; a favorable risk benefit analysis of this surgical intervention or any other interventions, in this clinical context, is currently lacking.

From this evidence, it can be concluded that fertility outcomes are decreased in women with submucosal fibroids, and removal seems to confer benefit. Subserosal fibroids do not affect fertility outcomes, and removal does not confer benefit. Intramural fibroids appear to decrease fertility, but the results of therapy are unclear.

ALTERNATIVE TREATMENTS FOR FIBROIDS

Several non-surgical approaches for the treatment of fibroid associated symptoms have emerged over the last several years with medical therapies as well as radiological interventions being proposed. Gonadotropin-releasing hormone (GnRH) agonists, the mainstay of medical therapy for fibroids, work by creating a hypogonadotropic hypogonadal state, and produce a significant reduction in fibroid size. Their use in the context of infertility treatment remains questionable since ovulation is generally inhibited during treatment, and the fibroids usually resume their pretreatment dimension within a few months after stopping treatment. Other medical options that may reduce the size of fibroids include androgenic steroid, danazol; antiprogestogen, mifepristone; selective estrogen receptor modulator, raloxifene; and aromatase inhibitor, fadrozole. Again, because of reasons mentioned above, their use in the context of infertility treatment remains questionable.

Nonmedical alternative treatment options for fibroids that have been developed over the recent past include fibroid embolization, laparoscopic myolysis and magnetic resonance imaging (MRI) guided focused ultrasound. Data regarding pregnancy outcome with these interventions is scanty as most women who wish to conserve fertility have been excluded from these treatments due to safety concerns. Particularly, information on laparoscopic myolysis and MRI-guided focused ultrasound are absolutely insufficient, and the effect of these techniques on pregnancy therefore unknown. Recently, more evidence has been emerging on the effects of fibroid embolization on pregnancy outcome. In a large survey of 1,200 women, Walker and McDowell recorded 108 women who attempted to become pregnant of whom 31% were successful.[13] This rate appears to be lower than surgery, but it is difficult to draw definite conclusions as there was no control group. Data regarding pregnancy outcome following uterine artery embolization tends to support a detrimental effect. An increased risk of miscarriage, preterm delivery, IUGR, abnormal placentation and postpartum hemorrhage has been reported. However, these results are controversial, as studies are underpowered. Based on present evidence fibroid embolization cannot be recommended in daily clinical practice to women wishing to conserve their fertility.

Given the current evidence, clinicians should pursue a comprehensive and personalized approach taking into account the pros and cons of myomectomy, including the impact of fibroids on fertility, the risks associated with fibroids during pregnancy on one hand, and the risks associated with surgery on the other hand.

■ REFERENCES

1. Verkauf BS. Myomectomy for fertility enhancement and preservation. Fertil Steril. 1992;58:1-15.
2. Ubaldi F, Tournaye H, Camus M, et al. Fertility after hysteroscopic myomectomy. Hum Reprod Update. 1995;1: 81-90.
3. Rackow BW, Arici A. Fibroids and in-vitro fertilisation: which comes first? Curr Opin Obstet Gynecol. 2005;17:225-31.
4. Donnez J, Jadoul P. What are the implications of myomas on fertility? A need for a debate? Hum Reprod. 2002;17:1424-30.
5. Somigliana E, Vercellini P, Dagauti R, et al. Fibroids and female reproduction: a critical analysis of evidence. Hum Repro Update. 2007;13:465-76.
6. Pritts EA, Parker WH, Olive DL. Fibroids and Infertility: an updated systematic review of evidence. Fertil Steril. 2009;91:1215-23.
7. Sunkara SK, Khairy M, El-Toukhy T, et al. The effect of intramural fibroids without uterine cavity involvement on the outcome of IVF treatment: a systematic review and meta-analysis. Hum Repro. 2010;25:418-29.
8. Buttram VC Jr, Reiter RC. Uterine leiomyomata: etiology, symptomatology, and management. Fertil Steril. 1981;36: 433-45.
9. Vercellini P, Maddalena S, De Giorgi O, et al. Abdominal myomectomy for infertility: a comprehensive review. Hum Reprod. 1998;13:873-9.
10. Narayan R, Goswamy RK. Treatment of submucous fibroids and outcome of assisted conception. J Am Assoc Gynecol Laparosc. 1994;1:307-11.
11. Surrey ES, Minjarez D, Stevens J, et al. Effects of myomectomy on the outcome of assisted reproductive technologies. Fertil Steril. 2005;83:1473-9.
12. Bulletti C, DE Ziegler D, Levi Setti P, et al. Myomas, pregnancy outcome, and in vitro fertilisation. Ann N Y Acad Sci. 2004;1034:84-92.
13. Walker WJ, McDowell SJ. Pregnancy after uterine artery embolization for leiomyomata: a series of 56 completed pregnancies. Am J Obstet Gynecol. 2006;195:1266-71.

38 Implantation in Endometriosis

Sunita R Tandulwadkar, Anupama Singh

INTRODUCTION

Implantation is the final step in successful establishment of pregnancy. It is a secret shared by the embryo and the endometrium, the subject of widespread speculations tried by many but still an enigma for all. Despite rapid advances in the field of in vitro fertilization (IVF) since the first success in 1978,[1] the success rate of IVF has stagnated around 25–30%,[2] mainly limited due to our failure to improve implantation rates.

Human embryo implantation is a three-stage process (apposition, adhesion and invasion) involving synchronized crosstalk between a receptive endometrium and a functional blastocyst.[3] This ovarian steroid-dependent phenomenon can only take place during the window of implantation,[4] a self-limited period of endometrial receptivity spanning between day 20 and day 24 of the menstrual cycle. Implantation involves a complex sequence of signaling events, consisting of the acquisition of adhesion ligands together with the loss of inhibitory components, which are crucial to the establishment of pregnancy.

PHYSIOLOGY OF IMPLANTATION

The process by which a foreign blastocyst is accepted by the maternal endometrium is complex and requires an interplay of many systems. The process of apposition, adhesion, and invasion is orchestrated by sequential appearance and disappearance of molecules in the endometrial epithelium and stroma brought about by steroid hormonal signaling and manifested histologically by changes in the appearance of epithelium and stroma in various stages. The key to the process is the establishment of controlled aggression orchestrated by a family of chemokines, adhesion molecules and T cells, uterine natural killer (NK) cells and T regulatory (T_{reg}) cells.

The rising estrogen levels during the first part of menstrual cycle enhance endometrial proliferation. Following ovulation progesterone secreted by luteinized follicles leads to differentiation of these cells. The fine-tuning of window of implantation timing is crucial and is under the control of prostaglandins[5] that in turn induce a variety of molecules playing a pivotal role in implantation. These mediators include a large variety of inter-related molecules including adhesion molecules, growth factors cytokines and lipids.[5]

Endometrial receptivity involves acquisition of adhesion ligands together with the loss of inhibitory molecules that may act as a barrier to the attaching embryo.[6] Inadequate uterine receptivity is responsible for approximately two-thirds of implantation failures, whereas the embryo itself is responsible for only one-third of these failures.[7] A major process in implantation is decidualization, in which the endometrium undergoes extensive changes in morphology and expression and secretion pattern to help the implanting blastocyst to gain access to the maternal system that is brought about by the sequential interplay of steroid hormones. Initial studies into the implantation process involving histological features[8] revealed characteristic microvillar protrusions on the luminal surface of the endometrium—pinopods, during the window of implantation,[8,9] which are the hallmark of endometrial receptivity. Blastocyst attachment occurs at the site of pinopod expression.[10]

The key to successful implantation is the establishment of a two-way dialogue between the embryo and the endometrium through a host of molecules, which is an area of active research. Molecular studies reveal that there is a chemokine gradient in the uterus, which guides the implanting blastocyst to the most appropriate site.[11] The major players in the process of implantation are:

Cytokines

An important class of molecules involved in the process is interleukin-6 (IL-6) family, which includes leukemia inhibitory factor (LIF), IL-11 and IL-6 all of which have intracellular signaling through gp130. LIF and IL-6 are proinflammatory cytokines, which act on the stromal cells and control the migration of macrophages and T cells into the endometrium[12] while IL-11 is an anti-inflammatory one, which controls trophoblast invasion.[13] LIF and IL-6 receptors are also present on the embryo, which indicate a role in the cross talk.[14]

Another important group is the IL-1 family, which consists of two agonists IL-1a and IL-1b, two receptors IL-1R1 and IL-1R2, an accessory protein IL-1RAcP and a naturally occurring antagonist IL-1RA and IL-18. IL-1 stimulates LIF production, upregulates integrin β3 and aids in decidualization. IL-1 is also produced by the blastocyst, and it also expresses its receptors.[15,16] IL-18 is a proinflammatory cytokine produced by the stromal as well as epithelial cells which has an important role in decidualization. IL-18 induces Th1 response but in the absence of IL-12, it affects type 2 helper T cell (Th2) response.[17]

Leptin is another molecule playing a crucial role by modulating the action of cytokines, upregulating integrin β3[18] and regulating the action of molecules involved in tissue remodeling like matrix metalloproteases (MMPs).[19] Leptin receptors are also found in early blastocyst.[20]

The insulin-like growth factor (IGF)/IGF binding protein (IGFBP) system also has an important role in implantation. IGF-2 is secreted by trophoblast, which helps in invasion while IGFBP-1 expressed by endometrium controls the invasion. An imbalance between two may impair implantation.[21,22]

Glycodelin is upregulated in the peri-implantation period, which has a suppressive effect on the maternal immune system to the fetal allograft.[23] Osteopontin is also upregulated in the secretory phase under the influence of IL-1, TNFα, TGFβ and IFNγ, which helps in cell–cell attachment and communication.[24]

Adhesion Molecules

Selectins are a group of molecules involved in apposition and adhesion. L-selectins are expressed on both endometrium and blastocyst indicating a role in communication.[25] Integrins, especially integrin αvβ3, are another class of molecules proposed to play an important role in adhesion being expressed on both endometrium and blastocyst.[26] MUC-1 is another class of molecules, which aids in implantation by global upregulation and selective downregulation at most suitable implantation site during the implantation window.[27] Cadherins are a class of molecules, which have a role in adhesion junction formation. E-cadherin is especially implicated in guiding the invasion of implanting embryo by forming

a permeability barrier in the endometrium. Both endometrium and embryo express this molecule.[28]

Immune Cells, Complement Factors and Major Histocompatibility Complex

Uterine NK cells, which are phenotypically similar to peripheral CD56+ T cells, play an important role in decidualization by elaboration of IFNγ and TNFα. They also aid in implantation through their interaction with blastocyst HLA-G molecules preventing immune rejection and at the same time controlling trophoblastic invasion by a complex interplay of pro- and anti-inflammatory cytokines.[29,30] They also play an important role in vascularization of the endometrium by elaboration of VEGF.[31]

T cells also play an important role in implantation. The shift of balance of Th1–Th2 in pregnancy as previously postulated is now known to be not as clear-cut. Th1 response is required in peri-implantation period. In fact Th1 by elaboration of cytokines helps to shift the balance toward Th2. Elaboration of IL-11 to IL-18 is so complex that their classification into Th1/Th2 seems to be an over simplification.[32] T_{reg} cells are an important mediator in the implantation. They are derived from peripheral CD4+ cells and help in controlling maternal immune response to embryo by modulating T cell activity.[33]

Macrophages are present in high density in the peri-implantation endometrium. Many roles of these macrophages has been proposed, e.g. elaboration of cytokines to maintain a proper cytokine environment, clearing up apoptotic material resulting from apoptosis of trophoblast throughout pregnancy.[34,35]

Besides uterine NK cells and macrophages, dendritic cells (DCs) also form an important population of cells in endometrium. They are the sentinels of the immune system activating it as and when provoked. However, they can also induce immune tolerance. Immature DCs differentiate into CD83+ DCs around the time of implantation mediated by cytokines and facilitate Th2 response.[36,37] NK and DCs are in close relation in the endometrium and help in each other's differentiation and maturation and also regulate each other's action through negative feedback loop.[38]

The embryo which enters the endometrial cavity in search of a suitable site for implantation also responds by expressing receptors for the cytokines, adhesion molecules, e.g. LIF, α5 integrin, etc. and secretes certain factors like human chorionic gonadotropin, corticotropin-releasing hormone (CRH), carcinoembryonic antigen 1, etc., which in turn modulate the uterine environment further facilitating implantation. The expression of

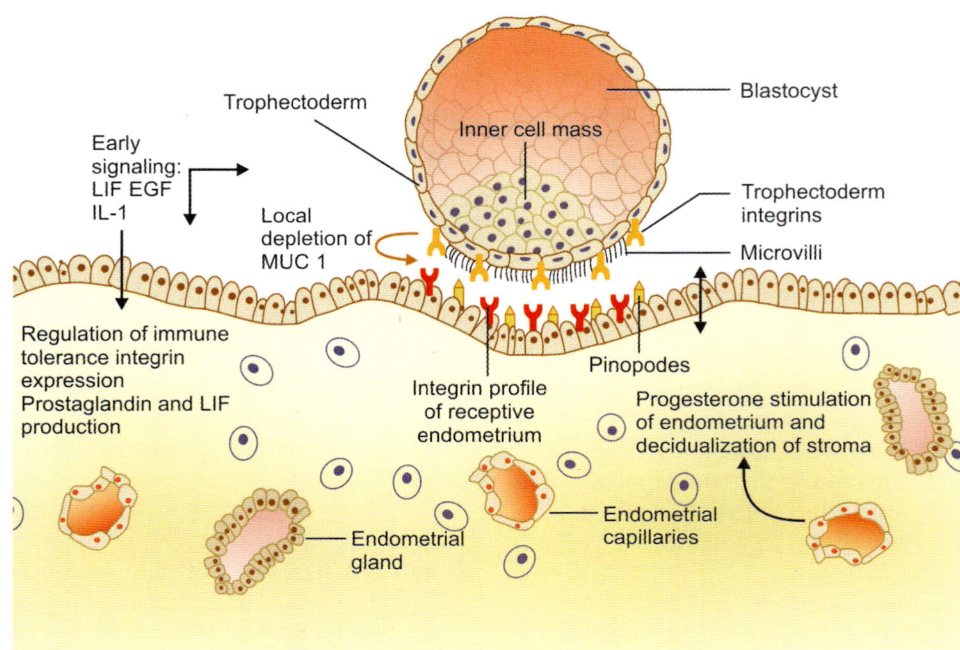

Fig. 1 Embryo-endometrium dialogue

complementary molecules and their receptors on the blastocyst and endometrium provides insights into the ways by which both participate in the two-way dialogue **(Fig. 1)**.

In more simplistic terms, implantation can be viewed as an act of aggression on the part of the embryo or an act of invitation on the part of endometrium or more precisely a combination or balance of the two, disturbance of which leads to either complete failure of implantation or recurrent miscarriages.

PATHOGENESIS OF DEFECTIVE IMPLANTATION

Endometriosis has been associated with infertility; however, the exact mechanism by which it causes is unknown and is a matter of intense research. Endometriosis is encountered in 35–50% couples seeking infertility treatment.[39] The fecundity rate in women with endometriosis is reduced to 2–10%[40,41] compared to 15–20% in normal couples. With the advent of IVF, we have had an opportunity to investigate the effects of endometriosis at specific stages of the reproductive process including folliculogenesis, fertilization, embryo development and implantation. Even with assisted reproductive techniques, the success rates in cases with endometriosis are lower than other causes of infertility.[42] Despite well-known association between endometriosis and infertility, there is difficulty in proving any causal association due to the multiple mechanisms that might be involved. Major pelvic adhesions, including those that result from endometriosis can impair oocyte release from the ovary or inhibit ovum capture or transport.[43] IVF studies have revealed poor ovarian response, lower oocyte quality and yield poorer embryo quality and defective implantation[44,45] as the cause of infertility.

The inflammatory effects of the disease process affects both oocyte production and ovulation in the ovary,[46] and in advanced cases, there may be impaired gamete transport due to distortion of the pelvic anatomy. Earlier studies emphasized on the adverse effects of hostile peritoneal environment prevailing in endometriosis, which proves toxic to the growing oocyte and impairs its developmental potential to varying extent reflected in impaired fertilization and cleavage rates. Then there have been theories about the inflammatory environment affecting the sperm quality reflected in poor fertilization rates.[47] Controversies abound, but the recent studies have refuted any effect of the disease on oocyte quality per se.[48] Poorer ovarian response may be due to reduced ovarian reserve due to repeated surgeries leading to loss of cortex[49] or impaired blood supply, and hence impaired delivery of gonadotropins to the growing follicles.[50]

Despite speculations about quality of gametes, and hence embryos persisting in endometriosis focus has now shifted to the endometrial quality which leads to decreased implantation as being one of the major contributors to subfertility.

The exact mechanism is unknown but many hypotheses have been proposed. There is common consensus that the histological appearance of the eutopic endometrium is unaltered[51] leading to earlier conclusions about non-involvement of endometrium. There is higher prevalence of endometrial polyps in women with endometriosis.[52] This may be an incidental finding or may be due to imbalance between cellular proliferation and apoptosis.[53]

However, recent studies focusing on the molecular defects have unraveled newer secrets. Cells migrate from ectopic endometrial implants to the eutopic endometrium.[54] Wnt7a expression is essential to estrogen mediated uterine growth and implantation by signaling between epithelium and stroma.[55-57] Aberrant activation of Wnt pathway disturbs endometrial development during implantation window.[58] The increased expression of Wnt7a outside of the gland in endometriosis likely disrupts the normal epithelial and stromal polarity required for normal fertility **(Table 1)**.

Failure of downregulation of progesterone receptors during the window of implantation[59] is associated with reduced *HOXA-10* and -11 genes expression[60,61] that lead to decreased $\alpha v \beta 3$ integrin expression,[62] which is critical to attachment of the blastocyst. Concurrent with this endometrial CRH and urocortin peptides involved in endometrial decidualization is downregulated in endometriosis. There is also an altered expression of activin A, which increases MMP activity helping in neovascularization and trophoblastic invasion.[63] Membrane bound IL-1RAcP expression is unaltered in endometriosis while soluble IL-1RAcP is decreased in patients of endometriosis which is critical in binding to IL-1 to reduce its activity[64] critical to implantation.

The action of steroid hormones especially progesterone is basically mediated by methylation and demethylation of specific promoter regions of the genes for proteins and cytokines, which mark endometrial receptivity. Endometriosis is associated with the aberrant expression of these genes, which in turn may be due to relative progesterone resistance state. Thus, many authors have postulated that the defects seen in this disease is basically an epigenetic phenomenon.[65]

Earlier it was believed that there is a shift in Th1 to Th2 type immunity during window of implantation leading to successful establishment of pregnancy, which now seems to be oversimplification of the mechanisms involved. Uterine NK cells play a pivotal role in implantation by controlling maternal immune response to fetal allograft as

Table 1 Summary of changes in the implantation window

Normal endometrium (Upregulated)	Eutopic endometrium in endometriosis
1. $\alpha v \beta 3$ integrin	*Upregulated*
2. Selectins	1. Uterine NK cells (CD16)
3. Soluble ICAM	2. Cadherins
5. MUC-1	3. MUC-1
6. LIF	4. Glycodelin
7. IL-6	5. Osteopontin
8. Soluble IL-1RAcP	6. LIF
9. Uterine NK (CD56) cells	
10. Osteopontin	*Downregulated*
11. Glycodelin	1. $\alpha v \beta 3$ integrin
12. Leptin	2. Soluble ICAM
13. IGFBP-1	3. Soluble IL-1RAcP
14. E-cadherin	4. T_{reg} cells
15. Dendritic cells CD83+	5. Dendritic cells CD83+
16. Macrophages	6. Macrophages

Abbreviations: ICAM, intercellular cell adhesion molecule; LIF, leukemia inhibitory factor; MUC-1, mucin 1, cell surface associated

well as trophoblast invasion and modulating endometrial neovascularization.[66] T_{reg} cells is another population of T cells, which appear around window of implantation essential for establishment of allotolerance by controlling autoreactive T cells.[66] DCs facilitate Th2 response. Close association of DCs and uterine NK cells stimulate each other maturation and maintain a negative feedback loop on each other activity.[38]

There is a significant decrease in the DC population in the basal as well as the functional layer of the endometrium in cases of endometriosis.[67] In addition to this, there is no increase in the macrophage population in the endometrium of endometriosis normally seen during the window of implantation, which may be associated with altered immune cell environment.[68]

T_{reg} population is decreased in eutopic endometrium while it is increased in ectopic sites which leads to recruitment of NK cells crucial in the implantation process from eutopic to ectopic sites and hence the disruption of the entire process.[69]

■ TREATMENT OF ENDOMETRIOSIS

Patients with endometriosis-associated infertility have a reduced or similar pregnancy rates compared to other causes of infertility is a matter of debate.[70,71] IVF success rates are diminished compared to other causes of infertility but IVF likely maximizes cycle fecundity for those with endometriosis.[44] However Society for Assisted Reproductive Technology emphasizes similar outcomes compared to other infertile population in its latest review.[72]

However, there are a few therapies, which have been well established in management of endometriosis patients.

Medical therapy: Medical therapy as such is discouraged in patients with endometriosis who are trying to conceive as all therapies revolve around suppression of ovulation.[73]

However, in the setting of IVF, gonadotropin-releasing hormone (GnRH) agonist therapy prior to IVF has proven to improve success rates.[74,75] Proposed mechanisms are by means of increased oocyte retrieval, higher implantation rates and reduced preclinical abortions[76] by suppressing the vicious cycle of inflammatory and immune processes.

Similar to the GnRH agonist therapy, 4–6 weeks of continuous oral contraceptive pill therapy results in improved outcomes.[77]

Surgical therapy: Surgery has a definite role to play in this disease at all stages. Possible effects may be due to correction of anatomical distortion, removal of implants and endometrioma and resulting decreased inflammation, which has an effect on all aspects of fertility. Even in earlier stages of the disease, surgery has significant benefit over no intervention in terms of pregnancy rates.[78]

■ FUTURE RESEARCH AREAS

A number of novel medical therapies are being currently examined for benefits in endometriosis related infertility. As research is throwing light on the various molecular mechanisms, the focus of treatment is gradually shifting from ablation or suppression of the disease foci to complete eradication of the disease by attacking the underlying process leading to persistence of the disease. Some of areas of focus are:

Immunoconjugates (ICON): They are meant to specifically target aberrantly expressed tissue factors on endometriotic endothelium and prompt regression of the disease probably by devascularization.[78] It has the potential to destroy pre-existing implants in a non-toxic, non-hormonal manner, which could potentially improve fertility rates.

Aromatase inhibitors: Aromatase is found in eutopic endometrium, where it is normally absent, which may impact estradiol levels and implantation. In fact, use of aromatase inhibitors has been shown to improve implantation in preliminary trials.[79]

Genetic engineering: The underlying cause of all defects in endometriosis is gradually being traced to aberrant expression of genes due to abnormal hyper/hypomethylation of promoter or repressor regions without causing any change in the actual genetic makeup. Some of the genes involved are *HOXA-10*, progesterone receptor, E-cadherins, estrogen receptor and steroidogenic factor-1.[62,80] Potential future treatments could involve targeting these altered molecular pathways and correcting abnormal methylation.

Stem cell therapy: Bone-derived stem cells can give rise to endometrial cells. Damaged endometrium can be replaced with stem cells. This is especially appealing given the epigenetic damage to the endometrium in women with endometriosis; epigenetic alterations are persistent, and at present, there are no known therapy to reverse this damage. Replacement of endometrium with a stem cell based therapy may be optimal way to restore normal endometrial function and implantation in women with endometriosis.[81]

■ REFERENCES

1. Steptoe PC, Edwards RG. Birth after the reimplantation of a human embryo. Lancet. 1978;2(8085):366.
2. des los Santos MJ, Mercader A, Galan A, et al. Implantation rates after two, three, or five days of culture. Placenta. 2003;24 (Suppl B):S13-9.
3. Enders AC, Schlafke S. A morphological analysis of early implantation stages in the rat. Am J Anat. 1967;120:185-229.
4. Paria BC, Reese J, Das SK, et al. Deciphering the cross-talk of implantation: advances and challenges. Science. 2002;296(5576):2185-8.
5. Ye X, Hama K, Contos JJ, et al. LPA3-mediated lysophosphatidic acid signaling in embryo implantation and spacing. Nature. 2005;435(7038):104-8.
6. Alpin JD. The cell biological basis of human implantation. Baillieres Best Prect Res Clin Obstet Gynaecol. 2000;14(5):757-64.
7. Ledee-Bataille N, Taupin JL, Dubanchet S, et al. Concentration of leukemia inhibitory factor (LIF) in uterine flushing fluid is highly predictive of embryo implantation. Hum Reprod. 2002;17(1):213-8.
8. Usadi RS, Murray MJ, Bagnell C, et al. Temporal & morphological characteristics of pinopod expression across the secretory phase of the endometrial cycle in normally cycling women with proven fertility. Fertil Steril. 2003;79: 970-4.
9. Staverus EA, Nikas G, Landgren BM, et al. Formation of pinopods in human endometrium is associated with the concentration of progesterone & progesterone receptors. Fertil Steril. 2001;76:782-91.
10. Bertin-Ley U, Sjogren A, Nilsson L, et al. Presence of uterine pinopods at the embryo endometrial interface during human implantation in vitro. Human Repro. 1999;14:575-80.
11. Dominguez F, Yanez-Mo M, Sanchez-Madrid F, et al. Embryonic implantation and leukocyte transendothelial migration: different processes with similar players? FASEB J. 2005;19(9):1056-60.
12. Kimber SJ. Leukemia inhibitory factor in implantation and uterine biology. Reproduction. 2005;130:131-45.
13. Cork BA, Tuckerman EM, Li TC, et al. Expression of interleukin (IL)-11 receptor by the human endometrium in vivo and effects of IL-11, IL-6 and LIF on the production of MMP and cytokines by human endometrial cells in vitro. Mol Hum Reprod. 2002;8(9):841-8.
14. Sharkey AM, Dellow K, Blayney M, et al. Stage-specific expression of cytokine and receptor messenger ribonucleic acids in human preimplantation embryos. Biol Reprod. 1995;53(4):974-81.
15. Krussel JS, Bielfeld P, Polan ML, et al. Regulation of embryonic implantation. Eur J Obstet Gynecol Reprod Biol. 2003;110 (Suppl 1):S2-9.
16. Fazleabas AT, Kim JJ, Strakova Z. Implantation: embryonic signals and the modulation of the uterine environment—a review. Placenta. 2004;25 (Suppl A):S26-31.
17. Croy BA, Esadeg S, Chantakru S, et al. Update on pathways regulating the activation of uterine natural killer cells, their interactions with decidual spiral arteries and homing of their precursors to the uterus. J Reprod Immunol. 2003;59(2): 175-91.
18. Gonzalez RR, Rueda BR, Ramos MP, et al. Leptin-induced increase in leukemia inhibitory factor and its receptor by human endometrium is partially mediated by interleukin 1 receptor signaling. Endocrinology. 2004;145(8):3850-7.
19. Gonzalez RR, Simon C, Caballero-Campo P, et al. Leptin and reproduction. Hum Reprod Update. 2000;6(3):290-300.
20. Antczak M, Van Blerkom J. Oocyte influences on early development: the regulatory proteins leptin and STAT3 are polarized in mouse and human oocytes and differentially distributed within the cells of the preimplantation stage embryo. Mol Hum Reprod. 1997;3(12):1067-86.
21. Fowler DJ, Nicolaides KH, Miell JP. Insulin-like growth factor binding protein-1 (IGFBP-1): a multifunctional role in the human female reproductive tract. Hum Reprod Update. 2000;6(5):495-504.
22. Lathi RB, Hess AP, Tulac S, et al. Dose-dependent insulin regulation of insulin-like growth factor binding protein-1 in human endometrial stromal cells is mediated by distinct signaling pathways. J Clin Endocrinol Metab. 2005;90(3):1599-606.
23. Vigne JL, Hornung D, Mueller MD, et al. Purification and characterization of an immunomodulatory endometrial protein, glycodelin. J Biol Chem. 2001;276(20):17101-5.
24. Kimber SJ. Molecular interactions at the maternal-embryonic interface during the early phase of implantation. Semin Reprod Med. 2000;18(3):237-53.
25. Genbacev OD, Prakobphol A, Foul RA, et al. Trophoblast L-selectin-mediated adhesion at the maternal-fetal interface. Science. 2003;299(5605):405-8.
26. Aplin JD. Adhesion molecules in implantation. Rev Reprod. 1997;2(2):84-93.
27. Meseguer M, Aplin JD, Caballero-Campo P, et al. Human endometrial mucin MUC1 is up-regulated by progesterone and down-regulated in vitro by the human blastocyst. Biol Reprod. 2001;64:590-601.
28. Paria BC, Zhao X, Das SK, et al. Zonula occludens-1 and E-cadherin are coordinately expressed in the mouse uterus with the initiation of implantation and decidualization. Dev Biol. 1999;208(2):488-501.
29. Kimber SJ. Leukemia inhibitory factor in implantation and uterine biology. Reproduction. 2005;130(2):131-45.
30. Croy BA, van den Heuvel MJ, Borzychowski AM, et al. Uterine natural killer cells: a specialized differentiation regulated by ovarian hormones. Immunol Rev. 2006;214:161-85.
31. Dosiou C, Giudice LC. Natural killer cells in pregnancy and recurrent pregnancy loss: endocrine and immunologic perspectives. Endocr Rev. 2005;26(1):44-62.
32. Chaouat G, Zourbas S, Ostojic S, et al. A brief review of recent data on some cytokine expressions at the materno-foetal interface which might challenge the classical Th1/Th2 dichotomy. J Reprod Immunol. 2002;53(1-2):241-56.
33. Aluvihare VR, Kallikourdis M, Betz AG. Regulatory T cells mediate maternal tolerance to the fetus. Nat Immunol. 2004;5(3):266-71.

34. Abrahams VM, Kim YM, Straszewski SL, et al. Macrophages and apoptotic cell clearance during pregnancy. Am J Reprod Immunol. 2004;51(4):275-82.

35. Dietl J, Honig A, Kämmerer U, et al. Natural killer cells and dendritic cells at the human feto-maternal interface: an effective cooperation? Placenta. 2006;27(4-5):341-7.

36. Kämmerer U, Schoppet M, McLellan AD, et al. Human decidua contains potent immunostimulatory CD83(+) dendritic cells. Am J Pathol. 2000;157(1):159-69.

37. Miyazaki S, Tsuda H, Sakai M, et al. Predominance of Th2-promoting dendritic cells in early human pregnancy decidua. J Leukoc Biol. 2003;74:514-22.

38. Rose-John S. Coordination of IL-6 by membrane bound and soluble receptors. Adv Exp Med Biol. 2001;495:145-51.

39. Von Wolff M, Stieger S, Lumpp K, et al. Endometrial IL-6 in vitro is not regulated directly by female steroid hormone but by pro-inflammatory cytokines and hypoxia. Mol Hum Reprod. 2002;8(12):1096-102.

40. Gonzalez RR, Leavis P. Leptin upregulates beta3-integrin expression and interleukin-1beta, upregulates leptin and leptin receptor expression in human endometrial cell cultures. Endocrine. 2001;16(1):21-8.

41. Comijn J, Berx G, Vermassen P, et al. The two-handed E box binding zinc finger protein SIP1 downregulates E-cadherin and induces invasion. Mol Cell. 2001;7(6):1267-78.

42. Somkriti SG, Yuan L, Fritz MA, et al. Epidermal growth factors and sex steroids dynamically regulate a marker of endometrial receptivity in Ishikawa cells. J Clin Endocrinol Metab. 1997;82(7):2192-7.

43. Donnez J. Endometriosis: enigmatic in pathogenesis and controversial in therapy. Fertil Steril. 2012;98(3):509-10.

44. Practice Committee of the American Society for Reproductive Medicine. Endometriosis and infertility: a committee opinion. Fertil Steril. 2012;98(3):591-8.

45. Hughes EG, Fedorkow DM, Collins JA. A quantitative overview of controlled trials in endometriosis associated infertility. Fertil Steril. 1993;59(5):963-70.

46. Brosens I. Endometriosis and the outcome of in vitro fertilization. Fertil Steril. 2004;81(5):1198-200.

47. Olivennes F. Results of IVF in women with endometriosis. J Gynecol Obstet Biol Reprod (Paris). 2003;32(8 Pt 2):S45-7.

48. Holoch KJ, Lessey BA. Endometriosis and infertility. Clin Obstet Gynecol. 2010;53(2):429-38.

49. Benaglia L, Bermejo A, Somigliana E, et al. In vitro fertilization outcome in women with unoperated bilateral endometriomas. Fertil Steril. 2013;99(6):1714-9.

50. Arici A, Olive DL, Huzsar G, et al. Peritoneal fluid from women with moderate or severe endometriosis inhibits sperm motility: the role of seminal fluid. Fertil Steril. 1996;66(5):787-92.

51. Filippi F, Benaglia L, Paffoni A, et al. Ovarian endometriomas and oocyte quality: insights from in vitro fertilization cycles. Fertil Steril. 2014;101(4):988-93.

52. Somigliana E, Benaglia L, Vigano P, et al. Surgical excision of endometriomas and ovarian reserve: a systematic review on serum antimüllerian hormone level modifications. Fertil Steril. 2012;98(6):1531-8.

53. Velasco G, Nikas G, Pellices A, et al. Endometrial receptivity in terms of pinopod expression is not impaired in women with endometriosis. 54th Annual Meeting ASRM. 1998.

54. Shen L, Wang Q, Huang W, et al. High prevalence of endometrial polyps in endometriosis related infertility. Fertil Steril. 2011;95(8):2722-4.

55. Park JS, Lee JH, Kim M, et al. Endometrium from women with endometriosis shows increased proliferation activity. Fertil Steril. 2009;92(4):1246-9.

56. Santamaria X, Massasa EE, Taylor HS. Migration of cells from experimental endometriosis to the uterine endometrium. Endocrinology. 2012;153(11):5566-74.

57. Hou X, Tan Y, Li M, et al. Canonical Wnt signaling is critical to estrogen-mediated uterine growth. Mol Endocrinol. 2004;18(12):3035-49.

58. Kao LC, Germeyer, Tulac S, Lobo S, et al. Expression profiling of endometrium from women with endometriosis reveals candidate genes for disease-based implantation failure and infertility. Endocrinology. 2003;144(7):2870-81.

59. Mohamed OA, Jonnaert M, Kuroda K, et al. Uterine Wnt/β-catenin signaling is required for implantation. Proceedings of the National Academy of Sciences of the United States of America. 2005;102(24):8579-84.

60. Liu Y, Kodithuwakku SP, Ng PY, et al. Excessive ovarian stimulation up-regulates the Wnt-signaling molecule DKK1 in human endometrium and may affect implantation: an in vitro co-culture study. Hum Reprod. 2010;25(2):479-90.

61. Mote PA, Balleine RL, McGowan EM, et al. Colocalization of progesterone receptors A and B by dual immunofluorescent histochemistry in human endometriosis during menstrual cycle. J Clin Endocrin Metabol. 1999;84(8):2963-71.

62. Bagot C, Kardana A, Olive D, et al. HOX gene expression is altered in the endometrium of women with endometriosis. Hum Reprod. 1999;14(5):1328-31.

63. Rocha AM, Cavalho FM, Pereira RMA, et al. The role of the *Hoxa10/HOXA10* gene in the etiology of endometriosis and its related infertility: a review. J Assist Reprod Genet. 2010;27(12):701-10.

64. Castelbaum AJ, Sawin SW, Buck CA, et al. Aberrant integrin expression in the endometrium of women with endometriosis. Clin Endocrin Metabol. 1994;79(2):643-9.

65. Novembri R, Rocha AL, Carraelli P, et al. Altered expression of activin, cripto, and follistatin in the endometrium of women with endometrioma. Fertil Steril. 2011;95(7):2241-6.

66. Guay S, Michaud N, Bourcier N, et al. Distinct expression of the soluble and the membrane-bound forms of interleukin-1 receptor accessory protein in the endometrium of women with endometriosis. Fertil Steril. 2011;95(4):1284-90.

67. Guo SW. Epigenetics of endometriosis. Mole Hum Reprod. 2009;15(10):587-607.

68. van Mourik MSM, Macklon NS, Heijnenet CJ, et al. Embryonic implantation: cytokines, adhesion molecules and immune cells in establishing implantation environment. J Leucocyte Biol. 2009;85;14-9.

69. Schulke L, Berbic M, Marconi F, et al. Dendritic cell population in ectopic and eutopic endometrium of women with endometriosis. Hum Reprod. 2009;24(7):1695-703.

70. Berbic M, Schulke L, Markhan R, et al. Macrophage expression in endometrium of women with or without endometriosis. Hum Reprod. 2008;24(2):325-32.

71. Brandmeier A, Jackson K, Hastings J, et al. Induction of endometriosis alters the peripheral and endometrial T cell population in non-human primate. Hum Reprod. 2012;27(6):1712-22.

72. Reproductive technology in United States, 2010 Results generated from the American Society for Reproductive Medicine/Society for Assisted Reproduction. 2012.

73. Ozkan S, Murk W, Arici A. Endometriosis and infertility: epidemiology and evidence-based treatments. Ann N Y Acad Sci. 2008;1127:92-100.

74. Guo YH, Lu N, Zhang Y, et al. Comparative study on the pregnancy outcomes of in vitro fertilization-embryo transfer between long-acting gonadotropin-releasing hormone agonist combined with transvaginal ultrasound-guided cyst aspiration and long-acting gonadotropin-releasing hormone agonist alone. Contemp Clin Trials. 2012;33(6):1206-10.

75. Ozkan S, Arici A. Advances in treatment options of endometriosis. Gynaec and Obstet Invest. 2009;67(2):81-91.

76. Benschop L, Farquhar C, Heineman MJ, et al. Interventions for women with endometrioma prior to assisted reproductive technology. Cochrane Database Sys Rev. 2010;(11):CD008571.

77. de Ziegler, Gayet V, Wolf JP, et al. Use of oral contraceptives in women with endometriosis before assisted reproduction treatment improves outcomes. Fertil Steril. 2010;94(7): 2796-9.

78. Jacobson TZ, Duffy JM, Barlow D, et al. Laparoscopic surgery for subfertility associated with endometriosis. Cochrane Database Sys Rev. 2010;(1):CD001398.

79. Taylor HS, Osteen KG, Bruner Tran KL, et al. Novel therapies targeting endometriosis. Reprod Sci. 2011;18(9):814-23.

80. Patel BG, Bushnell G, Higdon HL, et al. Letrozole use in frozen-thawed embryo transfer cycles: clinical pregnancy outcomes in patients with and without endometriosis. Fertil Steril. 2011;96(3):276.

81. Senapati S, Barnhart K. Managing endometriosis associated infertility. Clin Obstet Gynecol. 2011;54(4):720-6.

Cryopreservation

39   # Oocyte Cryopreservation

Dominic Stoop

■ INTRODUCTION

The first human pregnancy after oocyte cryopreservation was reported by Chen in 1986.[1] The success rate with this slow-freezing technique was relatively low but the introduction of the vitrification technique has significantly improved the outcome of oocyte cryopreservation.[2] During vitrification, cryoprotectants are added at a high concentration while the oocyte is at room temperature. To further protect against ice crystal formation, an extremely rapid rate of cooling is achieved by exposing the oocytes directly to the liquid nitrogen (LN_2).

The introduction of successful oocyte vitrification had a great impact on several clinical aspects of artificial reproductive technology (ART). Vitrification has revolutionized oocyte donation and allows women without a partner to independently preserve their fertility. The aim of this chapter is to provide current knowledge on oocyte cryopreservation and its clinical applications.

■ EFFICIENCY OF OOCYTE CRYOPRESERVATION

Clinical Outcome

Most of the peer reviewed literature report successful oocyte cryopreservation with the use of "open" vitrification systems. These systems allow direct contact between the oocyte and the LN_2, however allowing the hypothetical risk of disease transmission through the unsterile LN_2. Therefore, "open" vitrification is now commonly performed with the use of sterilized LN_2[3] through ultraviolet radiation. Sterile storage of the oocytes can then be performed by capping the carriers or by storing the oocytes in the vapor phase of LN_2.[4] Alternatively, oocytes can be vitrified in a hermetically sealed carrier which avoids the need for LN_2 sterilization.[5] A recent prospective randomized trial has compared open versus closed oocyte vitrification.[6] The authors found that the replacement of the open vitrification system by a closed system had no impact on clinical pregnancy and implantation rates.

Reportedly, oocytes preserved using vitrification have consistently good outcome with survival rates of about 85% and a fertilization rate of 75%.[7] Rienzi et al., have found that vitrified oocytes in comparison to sibling fresh oocytes are not inferior in terms of fertilization and embryo development.[8] A large randomized trial did confirm that vitrified oocytes are not inferior as compared to fresh oocytes in terms of ongoing pregnancies in a oocyte donation setting.[9] Clinical pregnancy rate (CPR) per cycle (50.2 versus 49.8%; P = 0.933) or per embryo-transfer (55.4 versus 55.6%; P = 0.974), and implantation rate (39.9 versus 40.9%; P = 0.745) were similar for patients receiving either vitrified of fresh oocytes.[9] Excellent results with oocyte cryopreservation were also achieved in the non-donor population and in women of a more advanced age. Chang et al. performed a controlled study to evaluate laboratory and clinical outcomes of oocytes vitrification obtained in in vitro fertilization (IVF) patients aged 30–39 years.[10] The authors concluded that the impact of vitrification was reduced to a minimal level, making it possible to achieve high pregnancy rates and implantation rates in this age group of IVF patients. The same authors were the first to report a successful pregnancy obtained following oocyte vitrification and embryo re-vitrification.[11]

These reports of efficient cryopreservation in peer reviewed literature has led to the removal of oocyte cryopreservation's experimental label by the American Society for Reproductive Medicine (ASRM) in 2012.[12]

Neonatal Outcome

A systematic review collected 22 papers presenting information on neonatal health of children born after oocyte freezing.[13] The authors found limited information on birth weight or karyotype examinations and in most studies the only information given about children was "healthy". A large study has been published on the neonatal outcome of 200 children born after oocyte vitrification.[14] As the vitrification technique is fairly recent, there is no data available on the long-term child follow-up.

■ CLINICAL APPLICATIONS

Infertile Patients

The aspiration and cryopreservation of excess oocytes in stimulated intrauterine insemination cycles lowers the risk of multiple pregnancy and offers additional pregnancy chances through later use of the cryopreserved oocytes.[15] IVF with these oocytes, accumulated over several intrauterine insemination cycles, avoids the need of ovarian stimulation in these patients often a risk for ovarian hyperstimulation syndrome (OHSS).

An obvious use of oocyte vitrification is for rescuing oocytes in case of an unexpected absence of sperm on the day of oocyte retrieval.

Furthermore, In IVF treatments, a clinician can also decide to opt for a freeze-all oocyte policy in case of a threatening OHSS,[16] especially in a gonadotropin-releasing hormone (GnRH) agonist protocol.

This freeze-all approach is advocated by some as a method for performing IVF for all patients in order to completely eradicate OHSS.[17] Although human chorionic gonadotropin is the gold standard for ovulation triggering, due to its long half-life, it is responsible for an increased incidence of OHSS. The utilization of GnRH agonist for triggering in GnRH antagonist cycles is a breakthrough as it eliminates early OHSS. A freeze-all approach, or segmentation, further eliminates the late OHSS in case of a pregnancy. Moreover, it no longer exposes the embryo to the suboptimal endometrium caused by the hyperphysiological steroid concentrations associated with ovarian stimulation.[16]

Some authors advocate the accumulation of oocytes from several ovarian stimulation protocols in low-responder patients.[18] A study by Cobo et al., published in 2012, found a statistically higher live birth rate per patients with this approach as compared to the poor responder group treated with fresh oocytes.[18]

Oocyte Donation

Oocyte donation is nowadays widespread within ART clinic as it allows many women without or with defective oocytes to achieve a pregnancy. The first successful oocyte vitrification was performed in an oocyte donation program.[2] Reports of highly efficient vitrification following the protocol by Kuwayama, triggered a large scale use of oocyte vitrification worldwide.[19,20] Since then, Egg bank donation has revolutionized the way oocyte donation is done. The banking of oocytes has many advantages as compared to fresh oocyte donation. The synchronization of donor and recipient is no longer needed and the matching between donor and recipient for phenotype and blood groups has become easier to organize. In many countries with a scarcity of oocyte donors, the freezing of oocytes makes it much more practical to share the oocytes of one oocyte donor over several recipients, allowing a much more efficient use of the available oocytes. Moreover, several studies have indicated that the outcomes obtained with vitrified oocytes are as good as with fresh oocytes.[9,21] Last but not least, the egg bank donation strategy makes the procedure safer by permitting a more accurate screening of infectious diseases among donors as with cryopreserved semen in sperm donation.

Fertility Preservation

The advent of vitrification enables many young and single women to preserve their fertility in the absent of a partner. Although fertility preservation may initially be performed in cancer patients, there are many other non-oncological conditions and treatments that may compromise fertility.[22] Recent publications have indicated that even young girls can undergo ovarian stimulation and oocyte vitrification at a pre-pubertal age.[23]

An alternative is the cryopreservation of ovarian cortex, which can be combined with the maturation of immature follicles found during cortex dissection. Vitrification of these immature follicles is performed preferably after in vitro maturation as this offers a better outcome.[24,25]

Banking for AGE (Anticipated Gamete Exhaustion)

An innovative application of oocyte cryopreservation is its use for the expansion of the reproductive lifespan. Unlike men, women just recently gained the opportunity to independently preserve their fertility without the need to create embryos.[26] In 2010, Knopman et al., reported a pregnancy in a 41-year-old woman who has preventively cryopreserved oocytes at the age of 39. As intrauterine inseminations and IVF failed, the use of the oocytes consequently resulted in a live birth.[27]

The use of this technique has caused controversy as it is considered by some as an unnatural tool for selfish women who want to delay motherhood in favor of their careers. Clinical experience does however learn that most of these women turn to such treatments because they are single. The Taskforce on Law and Ethics of the European Society Human Reproduction and Embryology (ESHRE) advises to refrain from passing judgments.

As for other forms of fertility preservation, it remains impossible to predict the number of oocytes that need to be cryopreserved in order to guarantee a future pregnancy. It has been calculated that the chance for one oocyte, retrieved after ovarian stimulation, to become a live birth before the age of 38 years is about 4–5%.[28] Cryopreservation at a later age appears to be less successful as the changes for a live birth at the age of 40 years drop to 2.5%. Cil et al., performed a meta-analysis based on original data from 10 studies including 2,265 cycles from 1,805 patients.[29] The authors calculated the probabilities of live birth at different ages of cryopreservation enabling more accurate counseling and informed decisions for women considering oocyte cryopreservation.[29]

It remains unclear whether it is cost efficient to cryopreservation of oocytes in anticipation of future age-related fertility loss.[30] A Dutch cost-effectiveness study concluded that oocyte freezing is more cost effective compared to IVF at an advanced age, if at least 61% of the women return to collect their oocytes.[31] An American study on the other hand that analyzed both oocyte as ovarian cortex cryopreservation, concluded that it was not cost effective.[32] The authors attribute their opposing conclusions to different clinical situations, expected outcomes and assumed costs of the treatments.[30]

■ CONCLUSION

Oocyte cryopreservation has become a simple, safe and efficient procedure. The clinical applications are often related to the fact that it allows preservation of female gametes without the need of prior fertilization. Oocyte cryopreservation is therefore an important tool in fertility preservation prior to gonadotoxic therapy or to prevent age-related fertility decline. Fertility centers worldwide are turning to egg bank donation to replace fresh oocyte donation for reasons of practicality and serological safety.

■ REFERENCES

1. Chen C. Pregnancy after human oocyte cryopreservation. Lancet. 1986;1(8486):884-6.
2. Kuleshova L, Gianaroli L, Magli C, et al. Birth following vitrification of a small number of human oocytes: case report. Hum Reprod. 1999;14(12):3077-9.
3. Parmegiani L, Accorsi A, Cognigni GE, et al. Sterilization of liquid nitrogen with ultraviolet irradiation for safe vitrification of human oocytes or embryos. Fertil Steril. 2010;94(4):1525-8.
4. Cobo A, Romero JL, Pérez S, et al. Storage of human oocytes in the vapor phase of nitrogen. Fertil Steril. 2010;94(5):1903-7.
5. Stoop D, De Munck N, Jansen E, et al. Clinical validation of a closed vitrification system in an oocyte-donation programme. Reprod Biomed Online. 2012;24(2):180-5.
6. Papatheodorou A, Vanderzwalmen P, Panagiotidis Y, et al. Open versus closed oocyte vitrification system: a prospective randomized sibling-oocyte study. Reprod Biomed Online. 2013;26(6):595-602.
7. Rienzi L, Cobo A, Paffoni A, et al. Consistent and predictable delivery rates after oocyte vitrification: an observational longitudinal cohort multicentric study. Hum Reprod. 2012;27(6):1606-12.
8. Rienzi L, Romano S, Albricci L, et al. Embryo development of fresh "versus" vitrified metaphase II oocytes after ICSI: a prospective randomized sibling-oocyte study. Hum Reprod. 2010;25(1):66-73.
9. Cobo A, Meseguer M, Remohí J, et al. Use of cryo-banked oocytes in an ovum donation programme: a prospective, randomized, controlled, clinical trial. Hum Reprod. 2010;25(9):2239-46.
10. Chang CC, Elliott TA, Wright G, et al. Prospective controlled study to evaluate laboratory and clinical outcomes of oocyte vitrification obtained in in vitro fertilization patients aged 30 to 39 years. Fertil Steril. 2013;99(7):1891-7.
11. Chang CC, Shapiro DB, Bernal DP, et al. Two successful pregnancies obtained following oocyte vitrification and embryo re-vitrification. Reprod Biomed Online. 2008;16(3):346-9.
12. Practice Committees of American Society for Reproductive Medicine, Society for Assisted Reproductive Technology. Mature oocyte cryopreservation: a guideline. Fertil Steril. 2013;99(1):37-43.
13. Wennerholm UB, Söderström-Anttila V, Bergh C, et al. Children born after cryopreservation of embryos or oocytes: a systematic review of outcome data. Hum Reprod. 2009;24(9):2158-72.
14. Chian RC, Huang JYJ, Tan SL, et al. Obstetric and perinatal outcome in 200 infants conceived from vitrified oocytes. Reprod Biomed Online. 2008;16(5):608-10.
15. Stoop D, Van Landuyt L, Paquay R, et al. Offering excess oocyte aspiration and vitrification to patients undergoing stimulated artificial insemination cycles can reduce the multiple pregnancy risk and accumulate oocytes for later use. Hum Reprod. 2010;25(5):1213-8.
16. Garcia-Velasco JA. Agonist trigger: what is the best approach? Agonist trigger with vitrification of oocytes or embryos. Fertil Steril. 2012;97(3):527-8.
17. Devroey P, Polyzos NP, Blockeel C. An OHSS-Free Clinic by segmentation of IVF treatment. Hum Reprod. 2011;26(10):2593-7.
18. Cobo A, Garrido N, Crespo J, et al. Accumulation of oocytes: a new strategy for managing low-responder patients. Reprod Biomed Online. 2012;24(4):424-32.
19. Katayama KP, Stehlik J, Kuwayama M, et al. High survival rate of vitrified human oocytes results in clinical pregnancy. Fertil Steril. 2003;80(1):223-4.
20. Kuwayama M, Vajta G, Kato O, et al. Highly efficient vitrification method for cryopreservation of human oocytes. Reprod Biomed Online. 2005;11(3):300-8.
21. Solé M, Santaló J, Boada M, et al. How does vitrification affect oocyte viability in oocyte donation cycles? A prospective study

to compare outcomes achieved with fresh versus vitrified sibling oocytes. Hum Reprod. 2013;28(8):2087-92.

22. Garcia-Velasco JA, Domingo J, Cobo A, et al. Five years' experience using oocyte vitrification to preserve fertility for medical and nonmedical indications. Fertil Steril. 2013;99(7):1994-9.

23. Stoop D, De Vos M, Tournaye H, et al. Fertility preservation utilizing controlled ovarian hyperstimulation and oocyte cryopreservation in a premenarcheal female with myelodysplastic syndrome. Fertil Steril. 2012;98(5):1121-2.

24. Fasano G, Demeestere I, Englert Y. In-vitro maturation of human oocytes: before or after vitrification? J Assist Reprod Genet. 2012;29(6):507-12.

25. Fasano G, Moffa F, Dechène J, et al. Vitrification of in vitro matured oocytes collected from antral follicles at the time of ovarian tissue cryopreservation. Reprod Biol Endocrinol. 2011;9:150.

26. Polge C, Smith AU, Parkes AS. Revival of spermatozoa after vitrification and dehydration at low temperatures. Nature. 1949;164(4172):666.

27. Knopman JM, Noyes N, Grifo JA. Cryopreserved oocytes can serve as the treatment for secondary infertility: a novel model for egg donation. Fertil Steril. 2010;93(7):2413.e7-9.

28. Stoop D, Ermini B, Polyzos NP, et al. Reproductive potential of a metaphase II oocyte retrieved after ovarian stimulation: an analysis of 23 354 ICSI cycles. Hum Reprod. 2012;27(7):2030-5. Erratum in: Hum Reprod. 2013;28(1):286.

29. Cil AP, Bang H, Oktay K. Age-specific probability of live birth with oocyte cryopreservation: an individual patient data meta-analysis. Fertil Steril. 2013;100(2):492-9.e3.

30. Hirshfeld-Cytron J, van Loendersloot LL, Mol BW, et al. Cost-effective analysis of oocyte cryopreservation: stunning similarities but differences remain. Hum Reprod. 2012;27(12):3639.

31. van Loendersloot LL, Moolenaar LM, Mol BWJ, et al. Expanding reproductive lifespan: a cost-effectiveness study on oocyte freezing. Hum Reprod. 2011;26(11):3054-60.

32. Hirshfeld-Cytron J, Grobman WA, Milad MP. Fertility preservation for social indications: a cost-based decision analysis. Fertil Steril. 2012;97(3):665-70.

Embryo Cryopreservation

Yasser Orief, Engie Al Salman

INTRODUCTION

It is essential in every assisted reproductive technology (ART) unit to have a well-established frozen/thawed embryo transfer program. Freezing and storing of surplus embryos allows the number of replaced embryos in both fresh and frozen/thawed embryo transfers to be reduced. This diminishes the risk of multiple pregnancies, in addition to increasing the cumulative pregnancy rates of in vitro fertilization (IVF) and intracytoplasmic sperm injection (ICSI) procedures.

Nowadays, there is a continuous debate about which cryopreservation method should be used and whether we should stick to the conventional cryopreservation techniques or to move towards the new method of vitrification. In conventional cryopreservation, the cells are suspended in a suitable solution, cooled, stored in liquid nitrogen (LN_2), warmed to room temperature, and returned to a physiological solution. During each step of this process, cells are at risk for various types of injuries. The primary injury is that caused by the formation of intracellular ice during cooling and warming. To prevent this injury, inclusion of a cryoprotectant is essential for large cells like mammalian embryos. However, the cryoprotectant introduces other kinds of injuries, i.e. chemical toxicity of the agent and osmotic over-swelling of the cells during removal of the permeated cryoprotectant.

During their removal, embryos are usually exposed to a hypertonic solution with sucrose, and embryos can be injured by osmotic over-shrinkage in some cases. In addition, embryos can be dissected physically by a fracture plane during passage through the glass transition temperature.

Furthermore, certain types of embryos are injured just by chilling at –20° to 0°C. In order for embryos to survive cryopreservation, the effect of each of these injuries must be minimized. Slow cooling procedures have also the disadvantage in that they are time consuming and require accurately controlled expensive freezing units, making them unsuitable for use where cost and time is a consideration. On the other hand, vitrification, in which not only the cells but also the whole solution is solidified without ice crystallization, is relatively simple. It includes two major benefits: (1) the process can be completed in only few minutes and (2) it does not require specialized equipment in contrast to conventional slow freezing techniques. Vitrification is a reasonable and effective strategy for preventing the primary cause of injury, the intracellular ice formation. Fracture damage and chilling injury may also be minimized in vitrification. In addition, the survival of embryos is more likely if the embryo treatment is optimized.

However, the procedure still might have some disadvantages; solutions for vitrification must include a high concentration of permeating cryoprotectants, which may cause injury through the toxicity of the agents. This could be overcome by applying the ultra-rapid vitrification technique using minute tools, such as electron microscopic grids, thin capillaries, minute loops, minute sticks, or as micro-drops instead of the conventional vitrification using insemination straws.

This way, a lower concentration of the permeating cryoprotectants is used, thus having a lower toxicity. In addition, the ultra-rapid cooling/warming helps to prevent ice formation. There was also a report of possible embryo infection after exposure to LN_2 artificially mixed with high concentrations of virus. Nevertheless, because it is highly unlikely such an adverse environment exists and actual cases of contamination have not occurred in previous surveys, there is hardly any concern in real terms. However, in some countries like USA, legal provisions are beginning to be considered for the future to avoid such a risk.

Viral infection mediated by LN_2 can be prevented by completely sealing the cryopreservation container prior to immersing the sample in LN_2. Kuwayama et al.[1] developed a vitrification method for this purpose, the vitritip method, which is able to realize complete sealing of the container along with ultra-rapid cooling and warming rates comparable to the Cryotop method.

We still have other causes minimizing the practical impact of vitrification, the presence of a wide variety of different carriers and vessels in addition to the many different vitrification solutions that have been formulated, which has not helped to focus efforts on perfecting a single approach **(Table 1)**.

Table 1 Comparison of vitrification with slow cooling

	Vitrification	Slow freezing
Duration of procedure	Few minutes (3–15 mins)	Prolonged (1–3 hours)
Costs	No expensive equipment required	Expensive slow freezers
Ice crystal formation	Less likely	More likely
Toxicity	More likely	Less likely
Osmotic shock	More likely	Less likely
Fractures	More likely	Less likely
Operator	More operator sensitive	Less operator sensitive

■ CRYOPRESERVATION OF TWO PRONUCLEAR STAGE ZYGOTES

Several protocols of freezing have been formulated for cryopreservation of human pronuclear (PN) zygotes among which the conventional (slow) freezing has been the most widely used method of storage. Other methods for freezing of the PN zygotes have been postulated like ultra-rapid freezing technique and vitrification.

Slow Freezing Technique

Preparation of Oocytes

Following oocyte retrieval, the cumulus and corona radiata are removed mechanically under a stereomicroscope, after exposure to 0.5% hyaluronidase solution for 30 seconds. IVF or ICSI are performed as usual. Pronucleate zygotes must have an intact zona pellucida and healthy cytoplasm with two distinct pronuclei clearly visible. When pronuclei start to migrate before syngamy the mitochondrial system is highly vulnerable to temperature fluctuation leading to possible scattering of the chromosomes. Ludwig et al.[2] recently published a new scoring system for zygotes at the PN stage. This score is based on the fact that a faster developmental process after fertilization demonstrates a better quality of the zygotes and resulting embryos. Their score included not only the morphological appearance of the pronuclei, but also the further development up to the PN membrane breakdown and first cleavage

division. This last item (PN membrane breakdown and first cleavage division within 24–26 hours post oocyte retrieval) constituted two fifths of the maximum score. Scoring was done at 16–18 hours post-ICSI according to: (1) the position of the pronuclei; (2) the alignment of nucleoli at the junction of the two pronuclei, and (3) the appearance of the cytoplasm. In Germany, for example, this item cannot be included, since only selection at the PN stage is allowed and supernumerary PN zygotes must be cryopreserved at the PN stage or discarded.

Freezing and Thawing Procedures

The supernumerary zygotes of the collecting cycles are cryopreserved 18 hours after the IVF or ICSI procedure. Ham's F-10 supplemented with 20% human umbilical cord serum is used as freezing solution. The cryoprotectants 1,2-propanediol (PROH) and sucrose are used at concentrations of 1.5 mol/L and 0.1 mol/L, respectively. PN stage embryos are then equilibrated in two steps (first step: 1.5 mol/L PROH, second step: 1.5 mol/L PROH and 0.1 mol/L sucrose) at room temperature, each for 10 minutes. A biological freezer working with an open freezing system and self-seeding is used for cryopreservation. Up to three, two pronuclei zygotes are transferred with medium to each ministraw. The ministraws are cooled slowly from room temperature to –33°C. They should be kept at –33°C for 30 minutes and then they are plunged directly into LN_2 for storage. The thawing procedure begins with the direct transfer of ministraws to a 30°C water bath, for 30 seconds. After this, the cryoprotectants are diluted in four steps, using different solutions: first, with 1 mol/L PROH and 0.2 mol/L sucrose; second, with 0.5 mol/L PROH and 0.2 mol/L sucrose; third, with 0.2 mol/L sucrose; and finally with Ham's F-10 medium alone. Each step should last 5 min. PN stage zygotes are then cultured in Ham's F-10 for 2–3 hours and then inspected for survival under both a stereomicroscope (magnification 50) and an inverted microscope (magnification 200–400).

Ultra-Rapid Freezing Technique

The zygotes are again first exposed to a cryoprotectant, equilibration prior to freezing is carried out as described in the slow freezing method. Zygotes are then drawn up into plastic straws, also electron microgrids can be used as a physical support, before they are plunged directly into LN_2 after 2–4 minutes. For thawing, the straw is gently expulsed into a phosphate buffered solution containing 20% fetal calf serum and 0.25 mol/L sucrose for 10 minutes at room temperature. The zygotes are then placed in culture and incubated for 2-4 hours before transfer into the recipient uterus. A freezing solution is often used consisting of 30% ethylene glycol (EG), 18% Ficoll, 0.5 mol/L sucrose, 10% fetal bovine serum with added modified Dulbecco's phosphate buffered saline, supplemented with sodium pyruvate (0.33 mmol/L), glucose (5.6 mmol/L), penicillin G (0.0375 g/L) and streptomycin (0.025 g/L).

Vitrification

The physical definition of vitrification is the solidification of a solution (water is rapidly cooled and formed into a glassy, vitrified state from the liquid phase) at low temperature, not by ice crystallization but by extreme elevation in viscosity during cooling. This method combines the use of concentrated solutions with rapid cooling in order to avoid ice formation. The samples reach low temperature in a glassy state which has the molecular structure of a viscous liquid and is not crystalline. Today, human PN zygotes can be cryopreserved successfully by vitrification. The efficacy of a rapid freezing method using the electron microscope copper grid or the Flexipet denuding pipette (FDP) for human PN embryos has already been reported. With respect to survival, cleavage on day 2, and blastocyst formation, a high survival and cleavage rate of multi-PN zygotes was also documented. Liebermann and Tucker,[3] using 5.5 M EG, 1.0 M sucrose, and an FDP as a carrier for the vitrification, observed 90% of two pronuclei survival after warming and 82% of two pronuclei cleavage on day 2. On day 3 in the vitrified two pronuclei group, approximately 80% of embryos cleaved to become an embryo with four or more blastomeres, and 30% of two pronuclei embryos eventually became blastocysts. More recently, successful pregnancies after vitrification of human zygotes have been reported.[4]

It is stated that the PN stage is well able to withstand the vitrification and warming conditions. Probably, this might be due to the processes during and after the fertilization, such as the cortical reaction and subsequent zona hardening that may give the ooplasmic membrane more stability to cope with the low temperature and osmotic changes. Finally, the low toxicity of EG, together with the good survival, cleavage, blastocyst formation and pregnancy rates obtained after vitrification of PN zygotes, may satisfy the real need in countries where cryopreservation of later-stage human embryos is not allowed by law or for ethical reasons.

■ COMPARISON OF THE DIFFERENT CRYOPRESERVATION TECHNIQUES

Because of the low water permeability and a low surface to volume ratio of the two pronucleate zygotes, a slow cooling rate may be advantageous. At slow cooling rates the compositional changes in the intracellular solution can follow those in the extracellular solution. Intracellular freezing is avoided because the water content of the zygote has approached the equilibrium water content before reaching the homogeneous nucleation temperature. On the other hand, the slow freezing method requires expensive equipment and is time consuming.

With the ultra-rapid freezing method the need for a computer controlled freezing apparatus is avoided and the time required for freezing and thawing is greatly reduced. However, the extreme toxicity of the high concentration of the cryoprotectant solution is the main disadvantage of this method. Van den Abbeel et al.[5] compared a slow controlled rate freezing procedure with a rapid cooling procedure using one-cell human embryo. They showed that slow controlled rate freezing is more efficient than rapid cooling.

Vitrification can be an alternative to the conventional slow freezing protocol with advantages of the lack of the ice crystal formation and ease of operation. The method also has the advantage of taking only a few seconds to cool embryos. Furthermore, it does not require a controlled rate cooling apparatus. However, Uechi et al.,[6] by comparing the conventional slow controlled rate freezing and vitrification on two-cell mouse embryos, showed that the implantation rate of blastocysts developed in vitro from vitrified two-cell embryos was significantly lower than that from slow controlled rate frozen embryos (10.2% versus 22.1%).

Vitrification may, therefore, exert a more harmful effect than the slow controlled rate freezing in two-cell embryos.

Cryopreservation of Cleavage Embryos

There is much debate as to the developmental stage at which human embryos are best cryopreserved. The disadvantage of two-pronucleate stage embryos is that nothing is known regarding their developmental competence. A major complication of cleavage-stage embryos on the other hand is that after thawing, damaged blastomeres often coexist with intact ones and it has been demonstrated convincingly that the implantation potential of such embryos is much lower than that of fully intact ones. Selection of fresh embryos for transfer on the basis of observations, such as growth rate, morphology and early cleavage, can enhance the outcome of embryo transfer, but usually relies on multiple embryos from which the "best" can be selected. Similarly, selection on the basis of survival and resumption of mitosis can enhance the outcome from cryopreserved embryo transfer. Clinical success with cryopreservation depends on many factors, including patient age and stimulation protocol, quality of embryos selected for freezing, developmental stage at freezing, media formulation (including type of cryoprotectants used) and parameters of cooling and warming. Vitrification has improved viability and survival rates of cells owing to the prevention of intracellular ice crystallization. Nevertheless, this procedure requires much higher concentrations of cryoprotectants that may also cause possible toxic and osmotic effects when compared with slow freezing. More recently, it has been addressed as the future of cryopreservation of human gametes and embryos due to the highest survival and pregnancy rates.

Is Vitrification More Favorable than Slow Freezing of Cleaved Stage Embryos?

The primary disadvantages to slow human embryo cryopreservation are the requirement for an expensive programmable freezing machine and the time-consuming nature of the procedure. The introduction of a technique that could be performed without the use of costly equipment and could be completed by one cryopreservation specialist within minutes would provide significant benefits for any busy IVF program. Vitrification of embryos and oocytes may offer a solution to this problem.

The considerable advantages of vitrification include elimination of ice crystal formation, which may increase their chances for survival, it is a simple technique involving direct plunging into LN_2 and the time required for equilibration and cooling is considerably reduced. On the other hand, disadvantages of vitrification are the required high cryoprotectant concentration and, consequently, the increased risk of toxic and osmotic damage, and the need to use special tools permitting high cooling rate by reducing radically the volume of solutions containing the embryos.

The effectiveness of zygote and cleavage-stage embryo cryopreservation in terms of embryo survival has been the subject of several studies. However, few studies have directly compared the results of different freezing strategies utilizing either zygote or cleavage-stage embryo cryopreservation, and these studies have yielded highly controversial results, either similar results for zygotes (74.4%) and day 2 embryos (77.4%)[7] or better results for day 2 embryos (73.9%) than for zygotes (64.4%).[8]

A retrospective study, conducted by Salumets et al., was devised to evaluate the impact of developmental stage of embryos on the pregnancy outcome of frozen embryo transfer.[9] A total of 4,006 embryos were analyzed, the highest survival rate was observed for zygotes (86.5%),

followed by day 2 (61.7%) and day 3 (43.1%) embryos, with overall clinical pregnancy and implantation rates of 20.7 and 14.2% respectively.

There were no significant differences in clinical pregnancy, implantation, delivery and birth rates between frozen zygote, day 2 and 3 embryo transfers. The findings of this study support the conclusions of a group that reported a better survival rate for zygotes (80.4%) than for day 2 embryos.[10]

The majority of studies of vitrification of human embryos reported high survival rates (>85%) and pregnancy rates of approximately 22–30%, which were completely in acceptable ranges and much higher than the rates of slow freezing.[11] El-Danasouri and Selman reported that survival rates following vitrification are positively correlated with the number of blastomeres in the cleavage-stage embryos.[12] In addition, higher pregnancy and slightly higher survival rates were commonly attributed to the further stages of human embryos, such as eight cells and blastocyst stage. More notable is the observation that vitrification either at blastocyst stage or at cleavage and PN stage, along with subsequent embryo transfer either at day 3 or 5, was shown to result in almost similar pregnancy rates as fresh cycles. Furthermore, the rate of blastocyst formation after vitrification, either at PN or cleavage stage, was similar to fresh cycles and commonly above 40–50%. These findings suggest the advantage of early-stage vitrification based on the similar survival rates of vitrification at different stages and high blastulation rates, comparable to fresh cycles **(Table 2)**.[11,13-18]

Cryopreservation of Blastocyst Stage Embryos

Culture and transfer of human embryos at the blastocyst stage has gained widespread popularity during the last decade. The low implantation rates, in the range of 10–20%, commonly observed following transfer of cleavage-stage (day 2 or 3) embryos indicate that the efficiency of this conventional approach is rather low, since more than 80% of embryos never implant. In order to overcome the implantation barrier, it has been common in the past to transfer a high number of embryos, resulting in an unacceptably high rate of multiple pregnancies, the major complication of assisted reproduction treatment. Advances in understanding the different metabolic needs of cleavage and blastocyst-stage embryos have resulted in the development of sequential media systems, which have improved the capability of in vitro blastocyst formation. By using sequential media, the reported rate of blastocyst formation varies between 33% and 93%. Transfer at the blastocyst stage has been reported to improve success

Table 2 Outcome of recent studies on vitrification of human zygote and early stage embryos

Study	Embryo stage	Cryoprotectants	Cryocarrier	Vitrified embryos (N)	SR (%)	PR (%)	Notes
Al-Hasani et al.[13]	Zygote	EG/DMSO/S	Cryotop	339	89	36.8	Abortion rate: 17.42%
Kuwayama et al.[14]	PN stage	EG/DMSO	Cryotip	1300	100		Delivery rate: 48–51%
	Cleavage stage		Cryotop		98	27	
					90	53	
Zhu et al.[15]	Embryos	EG-based	Open-pulled straws	957	72.2	19–22	
Rama Raju et al.[16]	Embryos (8 cells)	EG-based	Open-pulled straws	40	95	35	
Hredzák et al.[11]	Cleavage stage	EG/S	100 µL pipetting tip	215	69	27	
Isachenko et al.[17]	PN stage	EG-based	Open-pulled straws	59	71		
Liebermann et al.[3,23]	Embryos (8 cells)	EG-based	FDP	266	83.8		

Abbreviations: PN, pronuclear; EG, ethylene glycol; DMSO, dimethyl sulfoxide; S, sucrose; FDP, Flexipet denuding pipette; SR, survival rate; PR, pregnancy rate.

rates by identifying potentially superior quality embryos. The blastocyst transfer allowed the transfer of a single embryo, while maintaining a high implantation potential. This achieves greater significance with the regulations limiting the number of transferred embryos. It also becomes helpful for patients who have suffered multiple previous implantation failures.

The possible advantages of extended culture and transfer at the blastocyst stage can be summarized in the following points:

- Selection of embryos with increased implantation potential after the initiation of embryonic genome activation
- Improved endometrial-embryonic synchrony (physiologic)
- Transfer of fewer embryos leading to reduced probability of high-order multiple pregnancies
- Transfer of embryos with a greater likelihood of being chromosomally competent
- Ample time and possibilities to perform preimplantation genetic diagnosis.

However, adopting blastocyst transfer would require achieving an adequate rate of blastocyst development in culture. This requires precise control of laboratory conditions, in addition to mastering the extended culture systems with possible incorporation of co-culture from endometrial epithelial cells. A low blastulation rate may be one limitation to the adoption of blastocyst transfer which may leave many labs preferring to transfer available embryos on day 3. It has also been shown that poor responders are not good candidates for blastocyst

transfer. This may be related to the original oocyte quality. The number of eight-cell embryos at day 3 may be a good predictor of blastocyst development rate. In order to transfer two blastocysts, the woman must produce seven or eight viable oocytes, each with a fertilization rate of 80%, cleavage rate of 90% and blastocyst formation rate of 50%. The cryopreservation of surplus blastocysts would be mandatory. There are two main categories of cryopreservation, slow freezing and vitrification. Slow freezing of blastocysts has been successfully reported as early as 1992.[19]

The sudden increase in demand for blastocyst surplus storage in the late 90s coincided with major developments in vitrification techniques. After its success in oocyte preservation which was a highly challenging task for slow freezing, vitrification seemed to be a better approach for the other challenging specimens in the ART lab such as the blastocyst.

Key Points of Blastocysts Vitrification Improvement

Studies have shown that blastocyst vitrification has evolved through time, with improving results and reproducibility. This evolution can be attributed to many developments in the vitrification procedures. Improvements in vitrification techniques, along with a better understanding of vitrification and of specific blastocysts requirements have allowed for such improvements. We are trying to analyze this evolution by relating it to its essential components as a guide for future improvements.

Blastocyst Selection for Vitrification

Some improvement in blastocyst vitrification can be controlled by blastocyst selection. The selection can be in terms of the quality of the originating embryo and/or the timing in which the blastocyst is vitrified.

Influence of Early Embryonic Quality

The quality of the development of the early embryo determines the quality of the blastocyst and the final result. In their study, Vanderzwalmen et al.[20] observed as a side finding in their experiment that vitrified blastocysts which originated from a cohort of early embryos of optimal quality had survival rates, implantation rates and ongoing pregnancy rates of 73%, 32% and 19% respectively. In contrast, when the blastocysts came from embryos of suboptimal quality, the rates of survival, implantation and ongoing pregnancy were only 38%, 9% and 6%. These findings underline the importance of following the day-by-day development of each embryo to select the blastocyst with the best potential for vitrification.

Day 5 Versus Day 6 Vitrification

Expanded blastocysts are blastocysts that have exhibited more resilience and development competence by further in vitro development. Blastulation of human embryo usually occurs on day 5 or may be delayed till day 6. Blastocelic cavity continues to expand till the zona hatches and the blastocyst escapes. The blastocyst is considered nonexpanded if blastocele/total volume is less than 50%. It is considered expanded if blastocele/total volume is more than 50%. The transfer of fresh day 5 blastocysts seems to result in higher pregnancy rates than the transfer of fresh day 6 blastocysts. This may be related to the slower blastocyst development that mandated a day 6 blastocyst transfer. Interestingly, the transfer of cryopreserved day 6 blastocysts results in similar or superior results compared to day 5 cryopreserved blastocysts. This may be related to better endometrial synchrony in cryopreserved blastocyst transfer cycles while endometrial receptivity window may be missed in day 6 fresh transfer. From a cryopreservation perspective, the extension of culture of blastocysts may make them more vulnerable to cryopreservation. The blastocelic volume increases, the number of blastomeres increases and they become more metabolically demanding and sensitive to suboptimal conditions. **Table 3** summarizes the different studies that compared day 5 to day 6 blastocyst cryopreservation.[21-24]

We may conclude from the previous studies that day 5 blastocysts have in general shown more resilience to cryopreservation specifically to vitrification and better clinical results than day 6 blastocysts. This may be related to a lower quality day 6 blastocysts that were retarded in development, which was the case in most clinical trials. However, given this explanation, the results of vitrification of day 6 retarded blastocysts should then be well appreciated. Another possible explanation is that the degree of expansion of the blastocyst may increase the chances of ice crystal formation or decrease the chances of vitrification, thereby causing more damage to the blastocyst. This effect may be the sole effector in case of embryos that are not retarded in development and therefore should be then highly considered. In other words, a well-progressing embryo may be better vitrified when it is still nonexpanded on day 5, whereas, delayed embryos may still be vitrified on day 6. The rate of development and the degree of expansion at time of vitrification are better parameters to affect the outcome than the day of vitrification. Afterall, transferred vitrified embryos will benefit from a better endometrial synchrony which will dampen a negative effect of the blastocyst cryostorage.

Table 3 Different studies comparing the slow preservation and/or vitrification of day 5 and day 6 blastocysts in terms of survival after warming, implantation and pregnancy rates

	Slowly frozen day 5 blastocysts	Slowly frozen day 6 blastocysts	Vitrified day 5 blastocysts	Vitrified day 6 blastocysts
Mukaida et al.[21]			Survival: 87%	Survival: 55%
Stehlik et al.[22]	Survival: 83.1%;	Survival: 89.5%;	Survival: 100%;	Survival: 100%;
	Pregnancy rate: 16.7%	Pregnancy rate: 18.5%	Pregnancy rate: 50%	Pregnancy rate: 33%
Liebermann et al.[23]	Survival: 91.4%;	Survival: 94.8%;	Survival: 95.9%;	Survival: 97.5%;
	Implantation: 29.6%;	Implantation: 28.2%;	Implantation: 33.4%;	Implantation: 25.9%;
	Pregnancy rate: 42.8%	Pregnancy rate: 43.1%	Pregnancy rate: 48.7%	Pregnancy rate: 42.8%
Kader et al.[24]	DNA integrity index: 94.76 ± 4.70	DNA integrity index: 90.87 ± 6.16	DNA integrity index: 84.36 ± 8.76	DNA integrity index: 77.61 ± 16.65

Post-thawing Selection

Post-warming, viable blastocysts re-expand and are usually allowed 4–6 hours of incubation to regain their vitality before being transferred. An important marker of post-warming blastocyst performance is blastocyst re-expansion timing. The earlier the blastocyst expands, the better it is expected to perform after transfer.

Interventions

Previtrification Interventions

The blastocyst represents a particularly challenging developmental stage to cryopreserve due to several intrinsic factors. Both the presence of the zona pellucida and the multicellular shape of the blastocyst are physical barriers to the permeation of cryoprotectant. Furthermore, the fluid-filled cavity called the blastocele can be difficult to dehydrate or deliver high concentration of cryoprotectants into, which may result in ice crystal formation that can impair the post-thaw survival of the cryopreserved blastocysts.

Zonal hatching: Assisted hatching can be performed prior to vitrification to introduce a small point of structural weakness in the zona pellucida. This intervention is thought to facilitate embryo escape from the zona pellucida, thus avoiding degeneration of the blastocyst upon failure to hatch and improving implantation and pregnancy rates. In addition, this point of weakness would allow better access of the cryoprotectants to reach the blastocysts when being prepared for vitrification.

Blastocele evacuation: Apart from zonal effects, much attention has been paid to the volume of the blastocele prior to vitrification and its effect on the overall success of vitrification. A negative correlation between blastocelic volume and outcome measures has been attributed to intracellular ice formation in an inadequately dehydrated blastocele. Consequently, assisted shrinkage was developed as an effective method of reducing blastocelic volume prior to vitrification. Assisted shrinkage can be performed in a variety of ways, including microneedle puncture of the zona pellucida, laser-pulse opening of the zona pellucida, repeated micropipetting of the blastocele, and microsuction of the blastocelic contents **(Figs 1A to E)**. Another variation on artificial shrinkage is microsuction of blastocelic fluid. **Table 4** summarizes the results of different previtrification interventions on blastocyst vitrification outcome.[25-32]

Post-warming Intervention

This is mainly done by assisted hatching in the zona pellucida after warming. Vanderzwalmen et al.[20] achieved significantly better implantation and pregnancy rates after transferring warmed than zona hatched blastocysts. Ongoing pregnancy rates were 38% and 19% respectively for assisted hatched and nonhatched blastocysts. Implantation rate was 22% in the hatched group compared to 13% in the nonhatched group. They also demonstrated that zona pellucida is hardened by vitrification which may limit the success of transferring nonhatched vitrified blastocysts.

Improvements in Vitrification Methods

All improvements in vitrification techniques should be relevant to the equation:

Probability of vitrification

$$= \frac{\text{Cooling and warming rates} \times \text{Viscosity}}{\text{Volume}}$$

Improving Media Protocols

Increasing the concentrations of permeable cryoprotectants to increase the viscosity and thereby increase the probability of vitrification was the earliest approach tested to achieve vitrification. Since the inception of vitrification as a technique, many different media protocols have been tested to achieve high intracellular cryoprotectant delivery.

Searching for ways to attain improvements in outcome measures, experimenters aimed to elucidate the best protocol in terms of the composition of the cryoprotectants, the concentration of cryoprotectants, and the number of steps before vitrification or after warming.

The goal of immersing the blastocysts in cryoprotectant solutions is to allow for permeation of these cryoprotectants into the blastocele, replacing the water in the cavity with cryoprotectant to minimize the propensity of blastocelic fluid to form ice crystals.

The use of two cryoprotectants in the vitrification solution has a synergistic effect. It allows better cryoprotection through different mechanisms while reducing the toxicity to the blastocysts by using less concentration of any given cryoprotectant. In addition to using two cryoprotectant solutions to deliver high intracellular cryoprotectant concentrations, extracellular disaccharides and macromolecules are commonly added to the solutions in current practice. The extracellular presence of a disaccharide, usually sucrose, helps draw water out of the blastocele to attain better dehydration, as well as reduce osmotic shock. By using macromolecules, such as Ficoll and synthetic serum substitute, we can reduce the mechanical shock blastocysts endure during the freezing process and again reduce toxicity

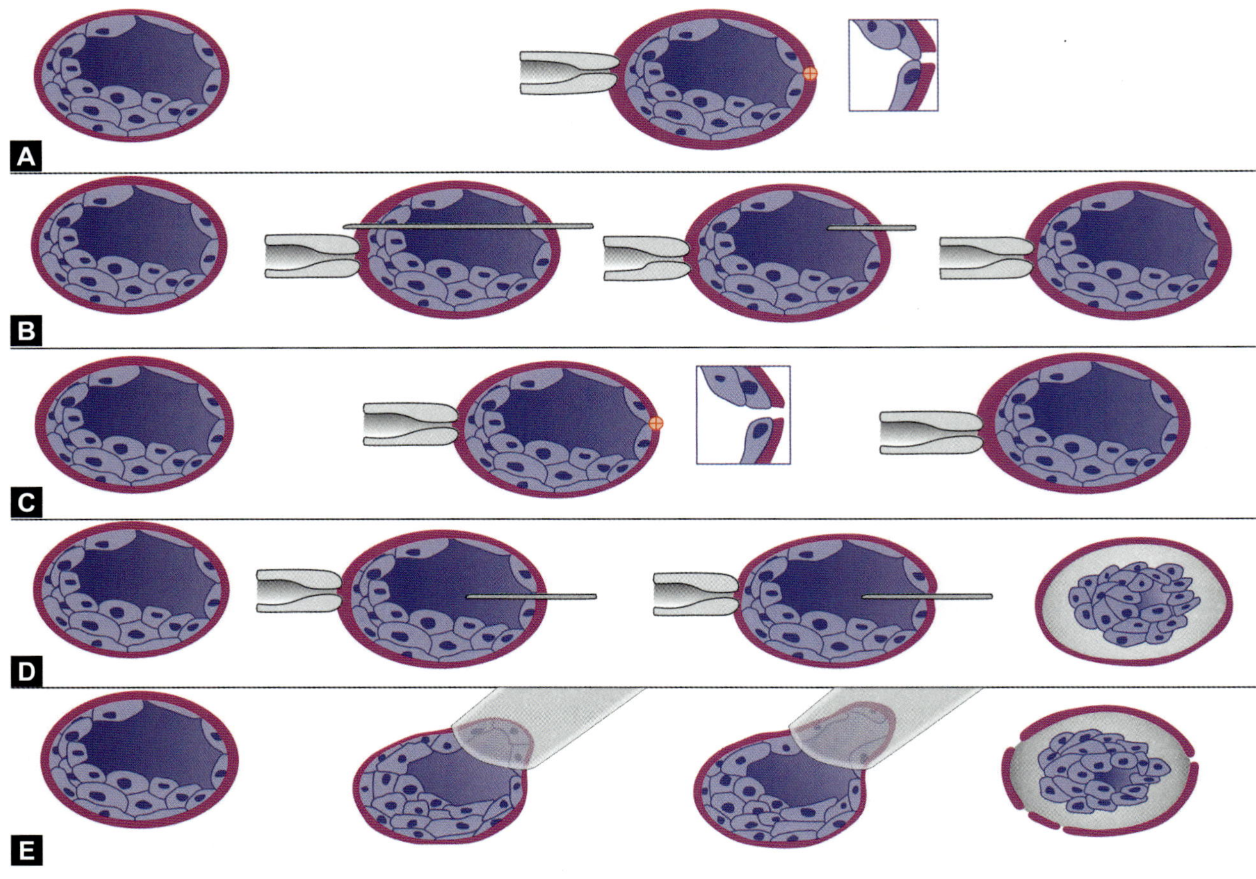

Figs 1A to E (A) Assisted hatching; (B) Needle blastocele puncture; (C) Laser blastocele puncture; (D) Blastocele aspiration; (E) Micropipetting

of the cryoprotectants by permitting the use of lower concentrations.

A single cryoprotectant exposure subjects the blastocyst to an increased risk of osmotic shock, particularly when the cryoprotectant used is highly concentrated compared to the blastocelic fluid. Depending on the duration of exposure, a single immersion may not allow enough time for adequate cryoprotectant permeation into the blastocele. Survival rates began to improve in subsequent years, partly due to the evolution of two-step protocols that would replace the one-step method. The two-step protocols called for an equilibration step of a few minutes at lower cryoprotectant concentration before a shorter exposure to the vitrification solution of higher concentration. Immersion of the blastocysts at lower cryoprotectant concentration for a few minutes allowed more time for cryoprotectant permeation while reducing osmotic shock and toxicity. Survival and hatching rates tend to decline when the concentrations of cryoprotectants used become too high, especially in the blastocyst stage, which requires a delicate balance between high cryoprotectant delivery and ensuing cellular toxicity. One of the most commonly used current protocols consists of an equilibrium solution of 7.5% EG and 7.5% dimethyl sulfoxide (DMSO) mixture, to be followed by a vitrification solution of 15% EG and 15% DMSO. Currently, most commonly applied warming protocol is performed in a 3-step procedure, beginning with 0.3 mol/L sucrose in base medium, followed by transfer to 0.2 mol/L sucrose in base medium, and finally to a solution only containing base medium.

Minimal Volume Vitrification

A small volume of media allows minimal delay in the cooling/heat transfer by minimizing the propagation time across an ultra-short distance. It also minimizes the effect of insulating nitrogen bubble formation surrounding the specimen or the loading device that may hamper the cooling/heat transfer.

Theoretically, a very small drop (~5 nL) of pure water should vitrify, if cooled very rapidly (107°C/s), the

Table 4 Studies showing different methods of blastocysts' previtrification interventions and their outcome parameters

Blastocele evacuation						
Authors	Species	Method	Intervention sample size	Outcome parameter	Intervention	Control
Vanderzwalmen et al.[25]	Human	Microneedle puncture	75	Survival rate	70.6%	20.3%
				Pregnancy rate	20.5%	4.5%
				Implantation rate	18.4%	7.1%
Son et al.[26]	Human	Microneedle puncture	90	Survival rate	90.0%	---
				Pregnancy rate	48.0%	---
				Implantation rate	29.0%	---
Hiraoka et al.[27]	Human	Micropipetting	48	Survival rate	98.0%	---
				Pregnancy rate	50.0%	---
				Implantation rate	33.0%	---
Chen et al.[28]	Mice	Microsuction	108	Survival rate	92.0%	80.0%
Mukaida et al.[29]	Human	Microneedle puncture	462	Survival rate	97.2%	85.0%
				Pregnancy rate	60.2%	34.1%
				Implantation rate	46.5%	---
Mukaida et al.[29]	Human	Laser pulse	40	Survival rate	97.5%	85.0%
				Pregnancy rate	61.5%	34.1%
				Implantation rate	48.6%	---
Kader et al.[30]	Mice	Microsuction	22	DNA integrity index	90.1%	77.6%
Zonal hatching						
Zech et al.[31]	Human	Spontaneous and Assisted (Mechanically)	38	Survival rate	82%	64%
				Pregnancy rate	35%	21%
				Implantation rate	26%	12%
Isachenko et al.[32]	Human	Assisted (Laser drilling)	73 (Open system)	Re-expansion rate	80.9%	–
			73 (Closed system)	Re-expansion rate	80.4%	–
Kader et al.[30]	Mice	Assisted (Acidified Tyrod's)	16	DNA integrity index	94.6%	84.4%
		Spontaneous	12	DNA integrity index	88.5%	77.6%

glass transition temperature (Tg) would then be around –140°C. In case drops are larger, cooling rates are slower, presence of impurities or a temperature above the (Tg), ice nucleation is likely to occur. Ice nucleation is a critical event and must be avoided. A single nucleation event in the liquid material will trigger immediate crystallizations of the entire specimen.

In order to achieve the maximal cooling rates, different improvements have been introduced to the vitrification systems and devices in order to minimize the vitrifying volume. In its infancy, vitrification was tried out using the available tools for slow freezing such as regular straws. These represent a great challenge to the heat transfer rate and contain a large volume that will be an extra challenge for vitrification.

A major shift in the development concepts was by encouraging minimal volumes of vitrification solution to surround the specimen. Different innovations to achieve vitrification in minimal volumes led to the development of different loading devices. Devices that provide minimal volume are electron microscopy grid, cryoloop™, cryotip™, cryoleaf™ high security straws™. The currently most acceptable target in designing vitrification loading devices for oocytes or embryos is to use a small volume (< 1 μL) of high-concentration cryoprotectant (~ 30%), and very rapid cooling rates of 15,000–30,000°C/min.

It is of no doubt that the development and standardization of current devices as well as determining the requirements for further device developments all led to a dramatic improvement in reports on blastocysts vitrification.

Increasing Cooling and Warming Rates

High cooling and warming rates are crucial to achieve proper vitrification and survival after warming. Cooling rate is specially challenging as it would entail either the direct contact of the sample with the LN_2 or indirectly if contained in a closed carrier. Improvements in cooling rates are more challenging due to the difficulty of having the specimen directly contact the LN_2 with the subsequent LN_2 evaporation and insulating gas bubble formation. This bubbling effect can be minimized by either stirring the sample going into LN_2, not allowing the evaporating nitrogen to accumulate and form gas bubbles or by decreasing the temperature of nitrogen below the evaporation temperature.

Direct contact vitrification: In this method, a high cooling rate is achieved by totally avoiding any delay that may be caused by the carrier walls. In combination with minimal volume, this method was considered the gold standard for vitrification, until the LN_2 contamination concerns required more protection of the specimen in a closed system. Examples of old open methods are the electron microscopy grid. Examples of open systems are the cryoloop™, cryotop™, cryoleaf™ and cut standard straw.

Closed system vitrification: In a closed system, the specimen is not allowed to directly come in contact with the LN_2. Therefore, a carrier will be required to deliver maximum cooling/heat transfer rate to the contained specimen which is usually in a minimal volume of cryoprotectant. Closed containers try to achieve this minimal impedance of heat transfer by design (being ultra-thin, containing microvolumes) and by material selection. The most recent developments in the closed systems are the (CryoTip)™ and the high security straws (HSS)™.

Cut standard straw is a system that can be used as open (by direct contact with LN_2) and closed if placed inside a sealed standard straw (straw within straw). It holds the embryos in a 0.75 μL with a cooling rate of 15,000°C/min if open and 600°C/min if closed.

Decreasing the temperature of LN_2: An alternative way to increase the cooling rate is to decrease the temperature

of the LN_2. This increases the cooling through two mechanisms: (1) wider difference in temperature leads to more rapid transfer, (2) delays the evaporation of LN_2 around the specimen, allowing the specimen or the device to come in contact with cooler LN_2 without intervening evaporating LN_2.

Two mechanisms have been described to achieve this phenomenon:
1. Vacuum application over the LN_2 would decrease the LN_2 temperature to (–200°C up to –210°C) away from its original boiling temperature of –196°C.
2. *Liquid nitrogen slush:* LN_2 slush is at -210°C which is 16°C less than the boiling temperature for LN_2.

Warming: Proper warming is as important as rapid cooling to avoid ice crystals from forming during warming and avoid fractures. This is usually handled by immediate transfer of the sample to a physiologically warm (37°C) environment while making sure this temperature is immediately available to the sample. This can be done in open methods by mixing the sample in ample amount of pre-warmed media or in closed methods by plunging in a warm water bath. In a closed system, heating rate will be controlled by the same factors that control the cooling rate.

Operator Training

The late interest in the technique could primarily be explained by the apprehension of many researchers to expose embryos to high concentrations of cryoprotectants (30–50%) necessary to obtain a vitrified state. In addition, with the early reports of vitrification being erratic, most ART centers elected to maintain slow freezing as their method of cryopreservation. This led to a delay in the acquisition of training required to perform vitrification among qualified embryologists. The early erratic results were mostly related to the technique being under development, in protocols and devices. This was followed by another era of embryologists being gradually introduced to the technique, with preservation in applying it. As with the current vitrification standards, the procedure remains operator-dependent, requiring a totally different training than with slow freezing. The performing embryologist should be able to adapt to an ultra-rapid handling and propagation of embryos in microvolumes. The high viscosity of media makes this handling an uneasy task. Any delay in handling may result in severe damage to the embryos. Also, with different loading devices available, some training and standardization will be required for each one of them. The lab should also be set to meet the specific requirements for vitrification in general and for the elected loading device. Failure may simply happen because of misplacement of instruments, like far away tanks, a lot of traveling of the straws in the air, badly calibrated sealers or using the media at undesired temperatures. The embryologist needs to have a good deal of understanding of the fundamentals of vitrification as well as become familiar with the tools he/she chooses to work with to achieve reliable results. He/she should be aware of the different variables that can affect the effectiveness vitrification, which can be summarized as follows:

- The type and concentration of cryoprotectant used and their toxicity threshold (almost every kind of cryoprotectant is toxic)
- The temperature of the vitrification solution at exposure
- Avoidance of media mixing in multiple steps protocols
- The duration of exposure to the final cryoprotectants (high concentration) before plunging into LN_2
- The rapid loading and sealing in a sealed system
- System validation (loading, sealing)
- The type of device that is used for vitrification (which influences the size of the vapor coat and cooling rate) and required movement to minimize the vapor effect.

With recently accumulating results pointing toward the superiority of the technique in cryopreservation of oocytes, embryos and blastocysts, it became more appealing for most ART centers to consider gradual partial or total shift of their practice with slow freezing to vitrification with less worries. Once the technique has become established in a wide range of ART clinics and the proper experience with it has been acquired, we would expect dramatic qualitative and quantitative changes in reports.

■ FUTURE PERSPECTIVES

From the technological development side, different companies are working on providing additional loading devices, which are a cornerstone of vitrification rather than being just a vessel. A great focus is toward development of closed systems with added ease of use. Technological developments are also extended to involve certain auxiliary devices aiming at easing the handling of embryos or adding safety to the devices such as sealers.

From the clinical embryologist perspective, we believe that it is almost time to narrow the gaps and come closer to a consensus or algorithm that can be a guide to blastocysts vitrification. It may also advise experienced and inexperienced embryologists on ways to improve their results and may be inspiring for additional methods of improvement of this technology and its specific application.

■ KEY POINTS

- Freezing and storing of surplus embryos allow the number of replaced embryos in both fresh and frozen embryo transfers to be reduced, thereby diminishing the risk of multiple pregnancies
- All embryos could be cryopreserved if the woman has a risk of developing ovarian hyperstimulation syndrome
- The pregnancy rates obtained from vitrification of the human embryos are at least equal to, or significantly better than, those obtained with traditional slow cooling
- Vitrification appears to be a rapid and simple technique that favors the biological integrity of both human oocytes and embryos, resulting in higher survival and pregnancy rates
- Vitrification of blastocysts can be successfully carried out using many loading devices. It could eventually replace slow freezing of blastocysts
- Though effect on perinatal outcome has not been fully investigated due to the novelty of the technique in clinical practice, however, the available data supports its potential safety
- Other than the patient clinical parameters, the clinical success of transferring vitrified blastocysts would rely on a multitude of factors:
  - The selection of a good quality embryo on preferably day 5 postfertilization is the first step
  - The selection of blastocysts that show earlier re-expansion post-thaw for transfer could improve the outcome from transferring vitrified blastocysts
  - The assisted hatching and induction of blastocele collapse prior to vitrification have also shown to improve the blastocyst vitrification outcome
  - Current media protocols and loading devices are capable of achieving proper vitrification attaining high level of viscosity and dehydration of the blastocysts and delivering high freezing and warming rates
  - Finally, the embryologist training would have a major bearing on the vitrification.

■ REFERENCES

1. Kuwayama M, Kato O. All round vitrification of human oocytes and embryos. J Assist Repro Genetic. 2000;17(8):477.
2. Ludwig M, Schöpper B, Al-Hasani S, et al. Clinical use of a pronuclear stage score following intracytoplasmic sperm injection: impact on pregnancy rates under the conditions of the German embryo protection law. Hum Reprod. 2000;15(2):325-9.
3. Liebermann J, Tucker MJ. Effect of carrier system on the yield of human oocytes and embryos as assessed by survival and

developmental potential after vitrification. Reproduction. 2002;124:483-9.

4. Jelinkova L, Selman HA, Arav A, et al. Twin pregnancy after vitrification of 2-pronuclei human embryos. Fertil Steril. 2002; 77:412-4.

5. Van den Abbeel E, Camus M, Van Waesberghe L, et al. Viability of partially damaged human embryos after cryopreservation. Hum Reprod. 1997;12:2006-10.

6. Uechi H, Tsutsumi O, Morita Y, et al. Comparison of the effects of controlled-rate cryopreservation and vitrification on 2-cell mouse embryos and their subsequent development. Hum Reprod. 1999;14:2827-32.

7. Horne G, Critchlow JD, Newman MC, et al. A prospective evaluation of cryopreservation strategies in a two-embryo transfer programme. Hum Reprod. 1997;12:542-7.

8. Kattera S, Shrivastav P, Craft I. Comparison of pregnancy outcome of pronuclear- and multicellular-stage frozen-thawed embryo transfers. J Assist Reprod Genet. 1999;16:358-62.

9. Salumets A, Tuuri T, Mäkinen S, et al. Effect of developmental stage of embryo at freezing on pregnancy outcome of frozen-thawed embryo transfer. Hum Reprod. 2003;18:1890-5.

10. Sean A, Vozzi C, Chanson A, et al. Prospective randomized study of two cryopreservation policies avoiding embryo selection: the pronucleate stage leads to a higher cumulative delivery rate than the early cleavage stage. Fertil Steril. 2000; 74:946-52.

11. Hredzák R, Ostró A, Zdilová V, et al. Clinical experience with a modified method of human embryo vitrification. Ceska Gynekol. 2005;70:99-103.

12. El-Danasouri I, Selman H. Successful pregnancies and deliveries after a simple vitrification protocol for day 3 human embryos. Fertil Steril. 2001;76:400-2.

13. AI-Hasani S, Ozmen B, Koutlaki N, et al. Three years of routine vitrification of human zygotes: is it still fair to advocate slow-rate freezing? Reprod Biomed Online. 2007;14:288-93.

14. Kuwayama K, Vajta G, Ieda S, et al. Comparison of open and closed methods for vitrification of human embryos and the elimination of potential contamination. Reprod Biomed Online. 2005;11:608-14.

15. Zhu GJ, Jin L, Zhang HW, et al. Vitrification of human cleaved embryos in vitro fertilization-embryo transfer. Zhonghua Fu Chan Ke Za Zhi. 2005;40:682-4.

16. Rama Raju GA, Haranath GB, Krishna KM, et al. Vitrification of human 8-cell embryos a modified protocol for better pregnancy rates. Reprod Biomed Online. 2005;11:434-7.

17. Isachenko V, Selman H, Isachenko E, et al. Modified vitrification of human pronuclear oocytes: efficacy and effect on ultrastructure. Reprod Biomed Online. 2003;7:211-6.

18. Vajta G, Nagy ZP. Are programmable freezers still needed in the embryo laboratory? Review on vitrification. Reprod Biomed Online. 2006;12:779-96.

19. Ménézo Y, Nicollet B, Herbaut N, et al. Freezing cocultured human blastocysts. Fertil Steril. 1992;58(5):977-80.

20. Vanderzwalmen P, Bertin G, Debauche Ch, et al. Vitrification of human blastocysts with the Hemi-Straw carrier: application of assisted hatching after thawing. Hum Reprod. 2003;18(7): 1504-11.

21. Mukaida T, Nakamura S, Tomiyama T, et al. Vitrification of human blastocysts using cryoloops: clinical outcome of 223 cycles. Hum Reprod. 2003;18:384-91.

22. Stehlik E, Stehlik J, Katayama KP, et al. Vitrification demonstrates significant improvement versus slow freezing of human blastocysts. Reprod Biomed Online. 2005;11:53-7.

23. Liebermann J, Tucker MJ. Comparison of vitrification and conventional cryopreservation of day 5 and day 6 blastocysts during clinical application. Fertil Steril. 2006;86:20-6.

24. Kader A, Agarwal A, Abdelrazik H, et al. Evaluation of post-thaw DNA integrity of mouse blastocysts after ultrarapid and slow freezing. Fertil Steril. 2009;91(5 suppl);2087-94.

25. Vanderzwalmen P, Bertin G, Debauche CH, et al. Births after vitrification at morula and blastocyst stages: effect of artificial reduction of the blastocoelic cavity before vitrification. Hum Reprod. 2002;17:744-51.

26. Son WY, Yoon SH, Yoon HJ, et al. Pregnancy outcome following transfer of human blastocysts vitrified on electron microscopy grids after induced collapse of the blastocoele. Hum Reprod. 2003;18:137-9.

27. Hiraoka K, Kinutani M, Kinutani K. Blastocoele collapse by micropipetting prior to vitrification gives excellent survival and pregnancy outcomes for human day 5 and 6 expanded blastocysts. Hum Reprod. 2004;19(12):2884-8.

28. Chen SU, Lee TH, Lien YR, et al. Microsuction of blastocoelic fluid before vitrification increased survival and pregnancy of mouse expanded blastocysts, but pretreatment with the cytoskeletal stabilizer did not increase blastocyst survival. Fertil Steril. 2005;84 (Suppl 2):1156-62.

29. Mukaida T, Oka C, Goto T, et al. Artificial shrinkage of blastocoeles using either a micro-needle or a laser pulse prior to the cooling steps of vitrification improves survival rate and pregnancy outcome of vitrified human blastocysts. Hum Reprod. 2006;21:3246-52.

30. Kader A, Sharma RK, Falcone T, et al. Mouse blastocyst previtrification interventions and DNA integrity. Fertil Steril. 2010;93(5):1518-25.

31. Zech NH, Lejeune B, Zech H, et al. Vitrification of hatching and hatched human blastocysts: effect of an opening in the zona pellucida before vitrification. Reprod Biomed Online. 2005;11:355-61.

32. Isachenko V, Katkov II, Yakovenko S, et al. Vitrification of human laser treated blastocysts within cut standard straws (CSS): novel aseptic packaging and reduced concentrations of cryoprotectants. Cryobiology. 2007;54(3):305-9.

41. Cryopreservation of Ovarian Tissue

Sunita R Tandulwadkar, Sejal Naik

INTRODUCTION

History

First ovarian transplant with cryopreserved ovarian tissue was performed by Dr Kutluk Oktay in 1999. In September 2004, Professor Donnez of Louvain in Belgium reported the first successful birth from slow or controlled rate, frozen ovarian tissue. In 1997, samples of ovarian cortex were taken from a woman with Hodgkin's lymphoma and cryopreserved in a rate freezer (Planer, UK) and stored in liquid nitrogen. Chemotherapy was initiated and after the patient had premature ovarian failure. In 2003, after freeze-thawing, orthotopic autotransplantation of ovarian cortical tissue was done by laparoscopy and 5 months after reimplantation signs indicated recovery of regular ovulatory cycles. Eleven months after reimplantation a viable intrauterine pregnancy was confirmed, which resulted in a livebirth of Tamara. There has, however, been a great deal of controversy surrounding the Louvain claim. Colleagues refute the claims by Donnez, stating that it is not sure whether the mother was indeed infertile.[1]

The first birth following transplantation of ovarian tissue, which has been stored at a central cryo bank after overnight transport, has been achieved by centers of the FertiProtekt network in Germany 2011. This demonstrated that ovarian tissue can be stored centrally in specialized centers.[2,3]

Indications

Ovarian tissue cryopreservation is currently considered to be experimental techniques of fertility preservation. This procedure is an option to patients who require immediate gonadotoxic treatment for aggressive malignancies, when there is insufficient time to allow the woman to undergo ovulation induction, oocytes retrieval and cryopreservation of embryos and/or oocytes.[4] It is the only option for prepubertal girls as they are at risk for premature ovarian failure, and this procedure is as feasible and safe as comparable operative procedures in children:[5]

- Patients who are planning surgery for another reason may be good candidates for OTC. Specifically, this may include women planning an oophorectomy as part of their treatment for endometrial cancer, etc.
- Patients undergoing urgent aggressive chemotherapy and/or radiotherapy for example in hematologic malignancies or breast cancer.[6]
- Prepubertal girls and women having hormone-sensitive malignancies.
- Women anticipating hematopoietic stem cells transplantation for the benign hematological conditions, e.g. sickle cell anemia, thalassemia major, aplastic anemia.
- Women with autoimmune diseases who have failed to immunosuppressive therapy as a prophylactic procedure for preservation of fertility.
- For fertility preservation in women with genetic mutations that poses a high-risk for premature ovarian failure, who are unable to pursue nonexperimental fertility preservation approaches.

Ovarian tissue cryopreservation is generally not recommended in women who:

1. Are more than 41 years old.
2. Have a large ovarian cyst on the ovary to be cryopreserved.
3. Have received prior chemotherapy that has significantly impaired ovarian function.
4. Ovarian tissue cryopreservation should not be offered to women who wish to delay childbearing or to women with benign conditions that are best managed by fertility enhancing minimally invasive surgeries.

Procedure

The procedure is to take a part of the ovary and carry out slow freezing before storing it in liquid nitrogen whilst therapy is undertaken. Tissue can then be thawed and implanted near the Fallopian, either orthotopic (on the natural location) or heterotopic (on the abdominal wall),[7] where it starts to produce new eggs, allowing normal conception to take place.[8] A study of 60 procedures concluded that ovarian tissue harvesting appears to be safe.[7] The ovarian tissue may also be transplanted into mice that are immunocompromised (severe combined immunodeficiency mice) to avoid graft rejection, and tissue can be harvested later when mature follicles have developed.[8]

OVARIAN CORTICAL TISSUE

Most oocytes are located into the primodial follicles in the ovarian cortex; therefore, obtaining small volume from cortical tissue potentially enables cryopreservation of large number of oocytes **(Flow chart 1)**. Whenever possible, OTC should be obtained prior to initiate treatment. However, for leukemic patients, who harbors cancer cells within ovarian blood vessels, obtaining ovarian tissue after first remission and before bone marrow transplant may decrease the risk of transmission from reimplanted thawed tissue.

The most common method to obtain tissue is by laparoscopy, although, the tissue may also be obtained by minilaparotomy, or while doing ovarian transposition surgery. Once tissue is obtained, it is cut into small slivers of tissue that are typically 0.3–2 mm in thick and then cryopreserved.

Limitations: Ovarian tissue is fragile under hard freezing conditions and putting it back into the body carries the risk of reintroducing cancerous cells.

WHOLE OVARY CRYOPRESERVATION

In patients in whom complete ovarian failure is anticipated, this can be another option. In this method, whole ovary is removed by laparoscopy (sometimes by laparotomy) with a large part of vascular pedicle left attached. Inclusion of large vascular pedicle enables use of special perfusion equipment to introduce cryoprotectant to all cells within the ovary and remove cryoprotectant from all cells at the time of thawing via vascular pedicle. It also facilitate organ transplant. The advantage of whole ovary cryopreservation is, it provides immediate blood supply to the graft, possibly limiting ischemia of the ovary and compromised long-term ovarian function.

Limitations: Challenging procedure, longer surgical time, risk of thromboembolism and ischemia of ovarian tissue and possibility of reintroducing malignant cells.

Flow chart 1 Different methods of cryopreservation: advantages

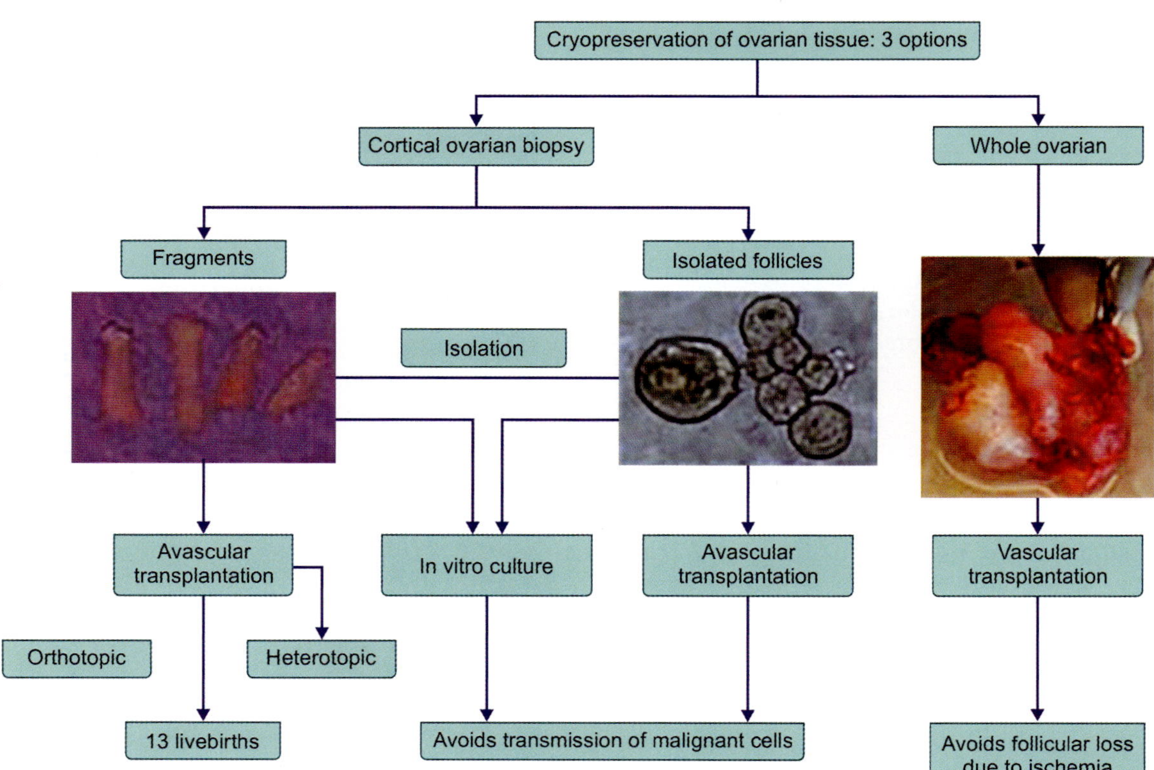

METHODS OF FREEZING

Slow Freezing

It is a classical method of OTC. It refers to exposure of tissue to cryoprotectant and cooling the tissue slowly in programmable fashion approximately –140°C, after which time tissue is put into liquid nitrogen at –196°C for storage.

Vitrification

It is a rapid method of OTC developed to eliminate the risk of ice-crystal formation in ovarian tissue. In vitrification, high concentration of cryoprotectants are used in fast cooling fashion (within minutes).

In systematic comparison of these two methods of slow freezing and vitrification for OTC demonstrated that outcome is similar for preservation of morphologic integrity of ovarian tissue. Although, oocyte survival was similar, granulosa cells survival and integrity of stroma were improved by vitrification. Although initial data suggests vitrification may be favored approach, outcome studies are needed before vitrification replaces slow freezing as a standard method for OTC.[9,10]

PREGNANCY AFTER OVARIAN TISSUE CRYOPRESERVATION

It is important to emphasize that OTC is experimental, and that a very limited number of pregnancies have resulted from this technology **(Figs 1A and B)**. **Table 1** gives a summary of live-births after autologous transplantation of cryopreserved-thawed ovarian tissue **(Flow chart 2)**.[11-20]

TRANSPLANTATION

Orthotropic Transplantation of Ovarian Cortex

Transplantation of very thin (<1.0–1.5 mm) strips of ovarian tissue that have been successfully thawed into either medullary portion of the remaining ovary or the peritoneum of the ovarian fossa. Resumption of normal menstruation has been reported within 4–9 months after transplantation. Tissue ischemia with loss of primodial follicles is the concern because these grafts require neovascularization.

Advantage: Possibility of natural conception as ovarian tissue is in close proximity to Fallopian tube.

Disadvantage: Requires invasive surgical procedure for transplant, limitation of number of fragments transplanted owing to ovarian size.

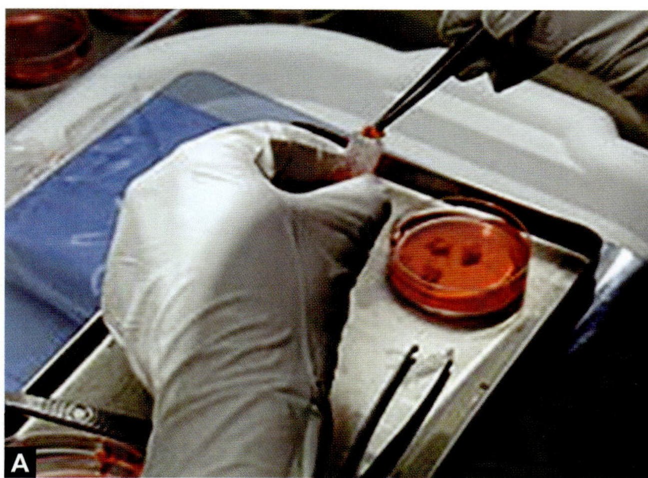
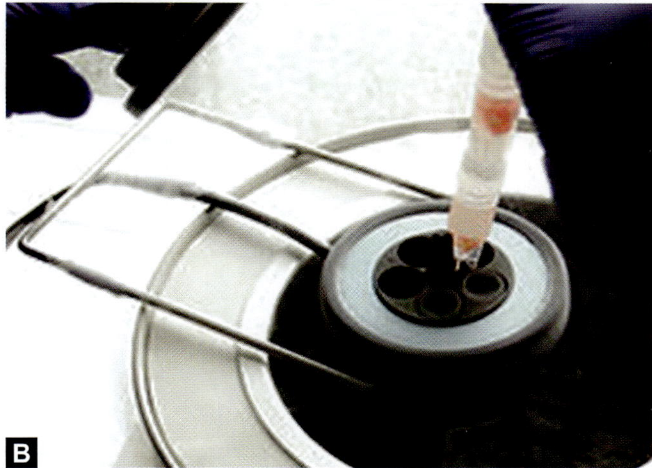

Figs 1A and B Ovarian tissue cryopreservation

Heterotropic Transplantation of Ovarian Cortical Tissue

It is the transplantation of ovarian cortical tissues in the forearm, chest wall and abdominal wall. In this case, pregnancy can be achieved only by oocyte retrieval and in vitro fertilization. However, there is no pregnancy reported after heterotropic transplant.

Advantages: Monitoring of follicular growth, oocytes retrieval for in vitro fertilization and monitoring of recurrence of cancer is easy because easy access location of transplant.

Disadvantages: Compromised viability of graft because heterotropic sites are less likely to undergo neovascularization, assisted reproductive technology requires for pregnancy to achieve, less cosmetically

Table 1 Overview of success after ovarian tissue cryopreservation

Diagnosis	Age at Cryo (years)	Prior chemo-therapy	Surgical method	Reimplantation site	Conception
Hodgkin's lymphoma	25	No	Ovarian biopsies	Orthotopic	Spontaneous singleton
Non-Hodgkin's lymphoma	28	Yes	Ovarian biopsies	Orthotopic	IVF singleton
Hodgkin's lymphoma	24	Yes	Unilateral oophorectomy	Orthotopic and heterotopic (abdominal wall)	Spontaneous singleton Spontaneous singleton
Hodgkin's lymphoma	26	Yes	Unilateral oophorectomy	Orthotopic	IVF singleton
Ewing's sarcoma	27	No	Ovarian biopsies	Orthotopic	IVF singleton Spontaneous singleton
Sickle cell anemia	20	No	Unilateral oophorectomy	Orthotopic	Spontaneous singleton
Breast cancer	36	No	Ovarian biopsies	Orthotopic	IVF twins
Metastatic neuroectodermic tumor	17	No	Ovarian biopsies	Orthotopic	Spontaneous singleton
Hodgkin's lymphoma	20	No	Ovarian biopsies	Orthotopic	Spontaneous singleton
Microscopic polyangitis	27	Yes	Unilateral oophorectomy	Orthotopic	IVF singleton

Source: Adapted from Kondapalli. LA. Ovarian tissue cryopreservation and transplantation. Cancer Treat Res. 2012.
Abbreviation: IVF, in vitro fertilization

Flow chart 2 Outcomes of ovarian tissue cryopreservation

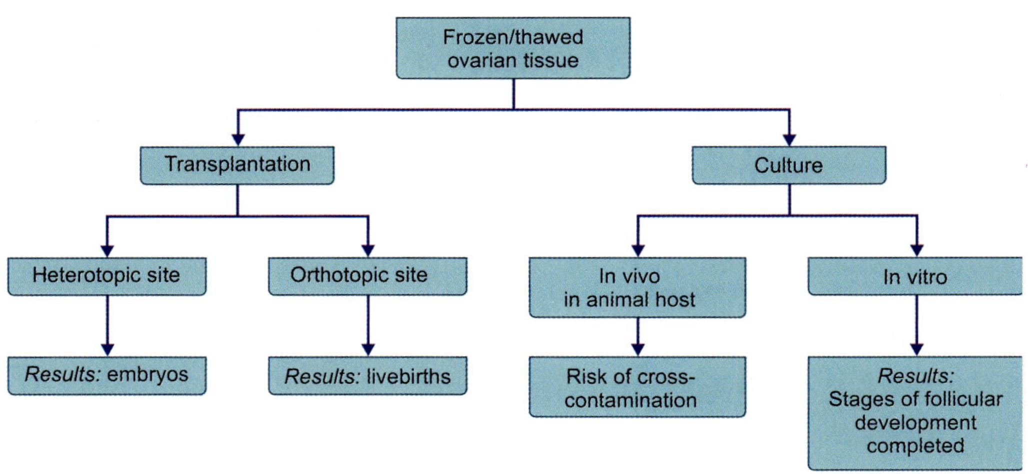

appealing site for ovary especially while follicular development.

While there have been some pregnancies and livebirths after allografting ovarian tissue between identical and nonidentical sisters,[20] transplantation is generally not regarded as a safe option for women with cancer. One study, looking at autopsy files, ovarian metastasis was found in 8.4–55.5% of women younger than 40 years old.[21] Certain types of cancers had higher rates of metastasis than others (gastric cancer – 55%, leukemia – 8.4%). Given that there are no reliable methods to detect minimal residual disease in the cryopreserved tissue, the safety of transplantation is in question.

■ RISK OF CANCER RECURRENCE

For autotransplantation of cryopreserved ovarian tissue in cancer survivors, metastasis have been repeatedly detected in ovarian tissue obtained from patients with leukemia, as well as in one patient with Ewing's sarcoma.[22] Ovarian tissue autotransplantation may pose a risk of cancer recurrence in patients with colorectal, gastric and endometrial cancer.[22] However, no metastasis have been detected in ovarian tissue from lymphoma and breast cancer patients who have been undergoing ovarian tissue cryopreservation.[22] It is not recommended in patients with blood-borne malignancies such as leukemia or with inherited risk of ovarian cancers.

ALTERNATIVES TO OVARIAN TISSUE CRYOPRESERVATION

In Vitro Maturation

For cancer patients, the general recommendation is to avoid transplantation of ovarian tissue in cases where there is concern about reseeding cancer cells, and instead, to consider in vitro maturation of oocytes. Researchers are working on in vitro maturation of oocytes, using follicle culture with alginate hydrogels. They are working with cell cultures, animal models, and translation research with human tissue, with the hope of developing a protocol to allow quiescent oocytes to grow in vitro to the point of fertilization. To date, in humans, there have not been successful fertilizations or pregnancies from this technique.

CONCLUSION

- Ovarian tissue cryopreservation and transplantation is experimental.
- Ovarian tissue cryopreservation is the option for patients who require immediate gonadotoxic treatment and is the only option available for prepubertal girls.
- Ovarian tissue cryopreservation should not be offered to patients with benign condition or for the purpose of delaying childbearing.
- Ovarian tissue cryopreservation in human has been cryopreserved as a cortical biopsies or strips or as a whole ovary.
- Ovarian tissue can be transplanted into the pelvis (orthotropic transplantation) or extrapelvic (heterotropic) site.
- Pregnancies and livebirths have been achieved only with orthotropic transplantation of cortical strips; however, data are confounded by the fact that the pregnancy could have been resulted from ovulation from native ovary.
- No pregnancies have been reported to date either from thawed ovarian tissue transplanted to heretotropic site or as a result of thawed whole ovary transplantation.
- Ovarian tissue transplantation carries a potential risk of reimplantation of malignancies.

REFERENCES

1. http://retractionwatch.wordpress.com/2012/07/26/ovarian-transplant-update-authors-of-2004-live-birth-follow-up-letter-ask-lancet-to-retract-it/
2. Dittrich R, Lotz L, Keck G, et al. Live birth after ovarian tissue autotransplantation following overnight transportation before cryopreservation. Fertil Steril. 2012;97:387-90.
3. Andreas Müller, Katja Keller, Jennifer Wacker, et al. Retransplantation of Cryopreserved Ovarian Tissue: the First Live Birth in Germany. Dtsch Arztebl Int. 2012;109:8-13.
4. Isachenko V, Lapidus I, Isachenko E, et al. Human ovarian tissue vitrification versus conventional freezing: morphological, endocrinological, and molecular biological evaluation. Reproduction. 2009;138(2):319-27.
5. Oktay K, Oktem O. Ovarian cryopreservation and transplantation for fertility preservation for medical indications: report of an ongoing experience. Fertil Steril. 2008;93(3):762–8.
6. Jadoul P, Dolmans M, Donnez J. Fertility preservation in girls during childhood: is it feasible, efficient and safe and to whom should it be proposed? Human Reproduction Update. 2010;16(6):617.
7. Livebirth after orthotopic transplantation of cryopreserved ovarian tissue. The Lancet. Sep 24, 2004.
8. Lan C, Xiao W, Xiao-Hui D, et al. Tissue culture before transplantation of frozen-thawed human fetal ovarian tissue into immunodeficient mice. Fertil Steril. 2008;93(3):913–9.
9. Keros V, Xella S, Hultenby K, et al. Vetrification versus controlled-rate freezing in cryopreservation of human ovarian tissue. Hum Reprod. 2009;24:1670-83.
10. Silber S, Kagawa N, Kuwayama M, et al. Duration of fertility after fresh and frozen transplantation. Fertil Steril. 2010;94:2191-6.
11. Donnez J, Dolmans M, Demylle D, et al. Livebirth after orthotopic transplantation of cryopreserved ovarian tissue. Lancet. 2004;364:1405-10.
12. Meirow D, Levron J, Eldar-Geva T, et al. Pregnancy after transplantation of cryopreserved ovarian tissue in a patient with ovarian failure after chemotherapy. N Eng J Med. 2005;353:58-63.
13. Demeestere I, Simon P, Emiliani S, et al. Fertility preservation: successful transplantation of cryopreserved ovarian tissue in a young patient previously treated for Hodgkin's disease. Oncologist. 2007;12:1437-42.
14. Demeestere I, Simon P, Moffa F, et al. Birth of a second healthy girl more than 3 years after cryopreserved ovarian graft. Human Reproduction. 2010;25:1590-1.
15. Andersen CY, Rosendahl M, Byskov AG, et al. Two successful pregnancies following autotransplantation of frozen/thawed ovarian tissue. Human Reproduction. 2008;23:2266-72.
16. Ernst E, Bergholdt S, Jorgensen JS, et al. The first woman to give birth to two children following transplantation of frozen/thawed ovarian tissue. Human Reproduction. 2010;25:1280-81.

17. Roux C, Amiot C, Agnani G, et al. Live birth after ovarian tissue autograft in a patient with sickle cell disease treated by allogeneic bone marrow transplantation. Fertil Steril. 2008;93:e15-2413.e19.

18. Sánchez-Serrano M, Crespo J, Mirabet V, et al. Twins born after transplantation of ovarian cortical tissue and oocyte vitrification. Human Reproduction. 2010;93:e11–3.

19. Donnez J, Squifflet J, Jadoul P, et al. Pregnancy and live birth after autotransplantation of frozen-thawed ovarian tissue in a patient with metastatic disease undergoing chemotherapy and hematopoietic stem cell transplantation. Fertil Steril. 2011;95:e1-4.

20. Donnez J, Silber S, Anderson CY, et al. Children born after autotransplantation of cryopreserved ovarian tissue. A review of 13 live births. Ann Med. 2011;43(6):437-50.

21. Kyono K, Doshida M, Toya M, et al. Potential indications for ovarian autotransplantation based on the analysis of 5,571 autopsy findings of females under the age of 40 in Japan. Fertil Steril. 93:2429-30.

22. Bastings L, Beerendonk CCM, Westphal JR, et al. Autotransplantation of cryopreserved ovarian tissue in cancer survivors and the risk of reintroducing malignancy: A systematic review. Human Reproduction Update. 2013;19(5): 483-506.

42 In Vitro Maturation of Oocytes

Sunita R Tandulwadkar, Devika Chopra

INTRODUCTION

Controlled ovarian hyperstimulation (COH) or superovulation is commonly used in assisted reproductive technology (ART) with the aid of exogenous drugs or hormones to facilitate multiple follicle ovulations. This superovulation is needed for obtaining multiple oocytes at the time of oocyte retrieval for the purpose of in vitro fertilization (IVF) or intracytoplasmic sperm injection (ICSI). Many times, these superovulation protocols result in ovarian hyperstimulation syndrome (OHSS), a multisystem disorder whose underlying etiology is that of increased vascular permeability. The clinical entity of OHSS can range from a mild abdominal discomfort to a fatal thromboembolism. OHSS can occur during the stimulation cycle, at the time of embryo transfer or during early pregnancy. Severe OHSS is reported in 0.5–5% of all cases undergoing COH necessitating an intensive care management for these cases. The diagnosis of OHSS results in the cancelation of the stimulation protocol, cancelation of embryo transfer in addition to the physical and psychological trauma to the patient.

Patients with polycystic ovarian syndrome (PCOS) are at a high risk of developing OHSS. This is attributed to the fact that these women have the highest number of antral follicles **(Figs 1A and B)** that are sensitive to exogenous gonadotropins. OHSS in PCOS patients can be avoided by regular follicular monitoring during stimulation, regular

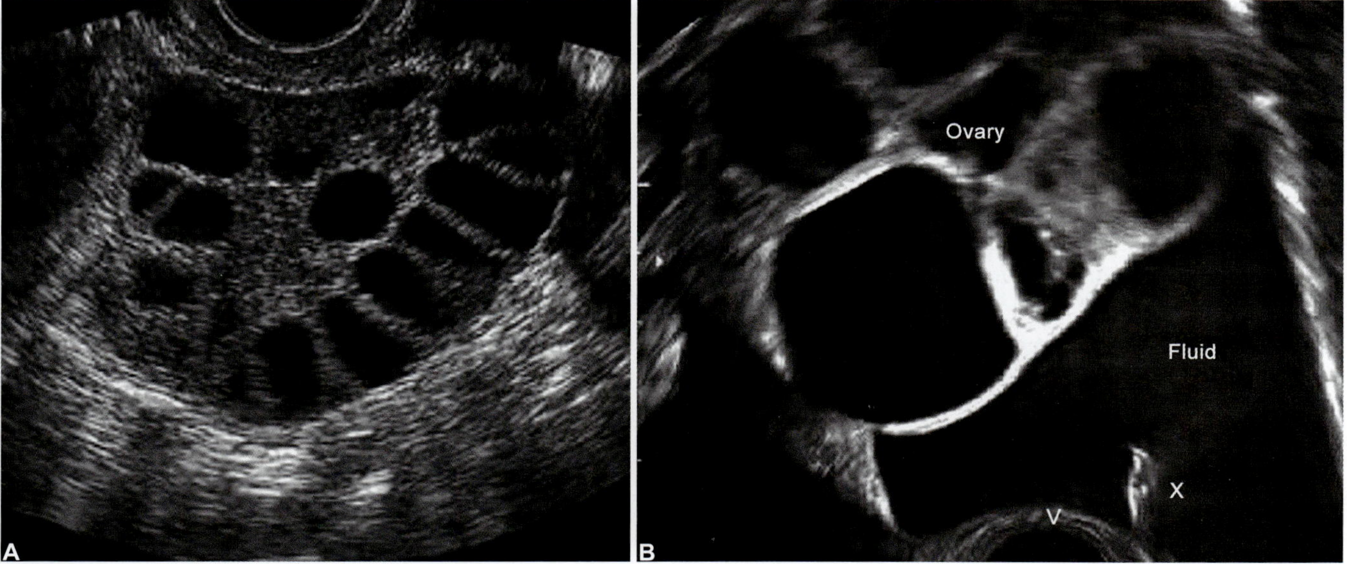

Figs 1A and B (A) An unstimulated polycystic ovary. This ovary has many antral follicles that are receptive to exogenous gonadotropins; (B) The same polycystic ovary after gonadotropin stimulation. The patient has developed OHSS, with free fluid seen in the pouch of Douglas

blood estrogen level tests, by using low-dose gonadotropin regimes and using antagonist protocols. However, despite these precautions some PCOS patients, yet develop OHSS and need an alternative management to achieve ovulation and a successful pregnancy following ART.

■ HISTORY OF IN VITRO MATURATION OF OOCYTES

The occurrence of OHSS in PCOS patients emphasized the need of developing alternative methods to COH to retrieve oocytes that were developmentally competent. Developmental competence is the ability of an oocyte to resume meiosis, undergo fertilization, form a blastocyst, and develop into a normal fetus that grows uneventfully to term.[1] The development of in vitro maturation (IVM) is reported to date back as early as the mid-1930s **(Fig. 2)**. Initially, the process of IVM was far from being as efficient as IVF. The first IVM baby was reported by Veeck. The first baby born by a PCOS patient following IVM was reported by Trounson et al. in 1994.[2] The first IVM babies in the United Kingdom were a pair of twins delivered on October 18, 2007, by the efforts of scientists and clinicians in the oxford fertility unit (OFU). Since then there have been several IVM pregnancies worldwide that have resulted in live births.[3]

■ IN VITRO MATURATION OF OOCYTES

In vitro maturation entails ultrasonography aided aspiration of antral follicles before the emergence of a dominant follicle from an unstimulated or minimally stimulated ovary.[4] These oocytes are then cultured in the laboratory under controlled conditions for 24–48 hours till the extrusion of the first polar body is completed. The oocyte then can be used for IVF or ICSI.

1878: First attempt to fertilize mammalian eggs in vitro
1935: Pincus and Enzmann IVM in rabbit
1959: First report of animal (rabbit) produced through IVF
1965: Edwards IVM of human oocytes
1968: Edwards and Bavister fertilized the first human egg
1983: Veeck first IVM baby (GV rescue)
1989: Cha et al. First IVM babies (triplets)
1993: Cha et al. Further 4 IVM babies
1994: Trounson et al. First IVM baby from PCOS
1995: Barnes et al. PCOS
1996: Mikkelsen, Schmidt, Lindenberg
2008: More than 3000 pregnancies from IVM

Fig. 2 History of in vitro maturation (IVM). The first attempt at IVM was performed in 1878. In 1935, Pincus and Enzmann performed IVM in rabbit oocytes. The first IVM baby was reported by Veeck. Since then several IVM babies have been born throughout the world

■ APPLICATIONS OF IN VITRO MATURATION

The applications of IVM are manifold. PCOS patients are greatly benefited by IVM as this procedure can be done with little or no gonadotropin stimulation. This negates the risk of OHSS in these patients. IVM can also be used in cancer patients where preservation of fertility is important prior to chemotherapy or radiotherapy. Oocytes are retrieved and cryopreserved in young cancer patients. At a later date, when the patient is desirous of bearing a child, IVM followed by IVF or ICSI is performed. Porcu et al. (2008) reported the birth of twins following oocyte cryopreservation and IVM in a cancer patient who had undergone bilateral oophorectomy.[5]

Another proposed application of IVM is inpatients who face repeated failures by conventional IVF or who have poor embryo quality and recurrent miscarriages following IVF. IVM is also useful in patients who choose less drug administration. There is a growing interest in "natural cycle IVF" and minimal ovarian stimulation protocols in order to reduce the long-term risk of gynecological cancers associated with COH.[4] Another potential advantage of IVM is substantial reduction in the cost of an IVF cycle. As the drugs that are used for COH are costly, IVM can provide a good alternative to COH in order to reduce the cost of IVF cycles. IVM also provides a source of oocytes for research into cloning, stem cells and fertilization.

■ DISADVANTAGES OF IN VITRO MATURATION

Till date, the use of IVM has not become mainstream in ART with COH being the favored approach. This can be due to the reduced fertilization, pregnancy and implantation rates observed after IVM of oocytes. In a study by Khashavi and Karimzadeh in 2004, higher oocyte maturation rate, fertilization rate and blastocyst formation rate were seen in conventional IVF compared to IVM.[6] More recently however, a study conducted by Junk and Yeap (2012) showed that in women with polcystic ovaries (PCO) or PCOS, improved implantation, higher clinical pregnancy, and higher live birth rates could be achieved after the use of IVM.[7]

There is very little data on the health of children that have been conceived via IVM. This is in contrast to a significant volume of high quality studies that have followed up children conceived following standard IVF and ICSI. Laboratory studies have reported high rates of chromosomal abnormalities in embryos fertilized following IVM, with a higher rate of abnormalities linked to longer period of maturation in vitro.[8] This may in part explain the higher rate of miscarriage observed in IVM pregnancies.[9] In cattle, IVM is a standard protocol for assisted reproduction but is associated with a risk of "large offspring syndrome". It has been proposed that the mechanism by which IVM causes this effect may be through inducing permanent epigenetic changes in the expression of imprinted genes.[8]

ANIMAL MODELS FOR IN VITRO MATURATION

The study of animal oocyte development and maturation in vitro has aided in strengthening the knowledge on IVM protocols. Since 1992, a lot of experiments on IVM using slaughterhouse ovaries have been performed to establish the best medium at different stages of development.[10] Ultimately, the maturation media used for IVM of human oocytes comes from research on animal models of IVM. In 2008, Prada and Vandevoort studied the effect of growth hormone on the IVM of rhesus monkey oocytes. They observed an increased maturation of oocytes in culture media containing recombinant human growth hormone,

thereby emphasizing the role of growth hormone and other growth factors in IVM culture media.[11] Fukui et al. 2000 studied the effect of different culture media on the growth of bovine oocytes.[12] These studies emphasize the role of animal models in the understanding of the process of IVM and the research applications of IVM.

DISCUSSION

In vitro maturation of oocytes was developed in cows in the mid-1980s, not as a clinical requirement but as a research tool.[13] The maturation medium used for the IVM of bovine oocytes has undergone a lot of research and improvement over the last 25 years. Animal models, therefore can provide useful information on the process of IVM and can be used for research into the improvement of maturation media for the same.

Growth factors are produced by the cumulus cells, granulosa cells and theca cells within the ovary. There is a cross talk among these cells during folliculogenesis **(Fig. 3)**. This cross talk plays an important role in the in vivo development and maturation of oocytes. In a study

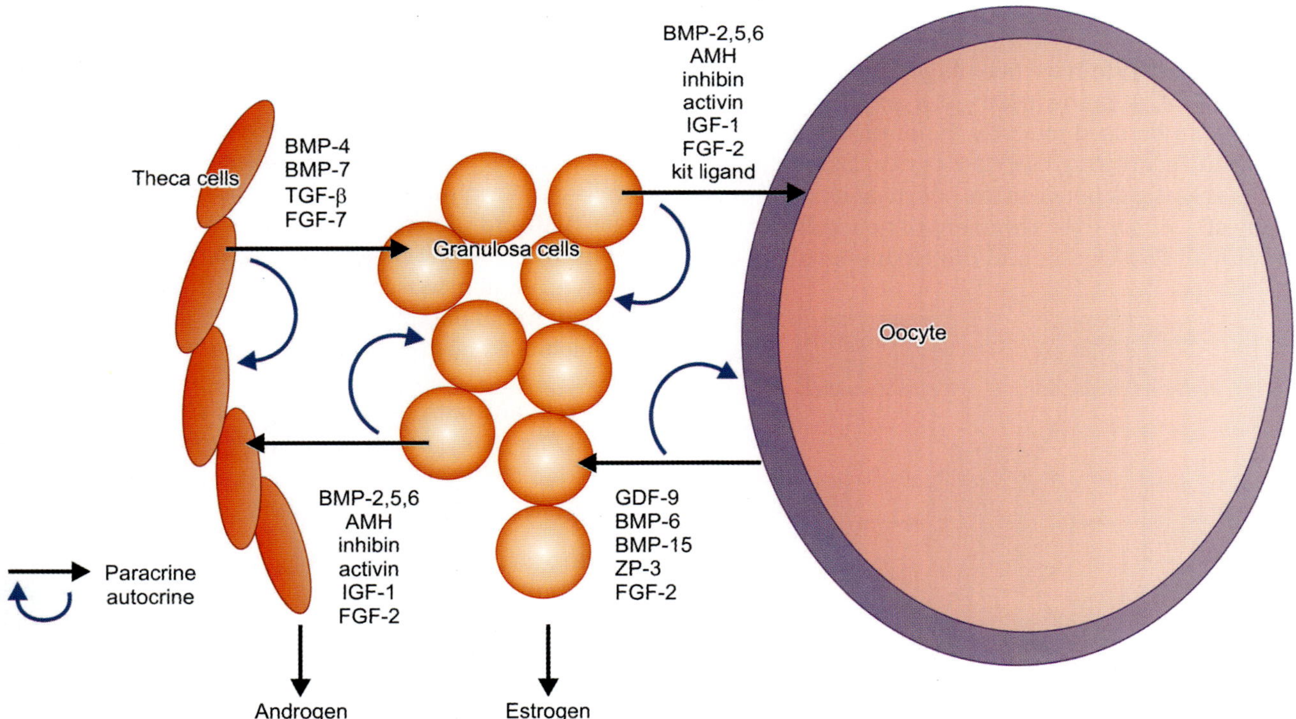

Fig. 3 Growth factors involved during folliculogenesis in mouse oocytes. Hypothetical factors and related interactions are indicated. Ovarian folliculogenesis requires the coordinated actions of an array of autocrine and paracrine growth factors, their corresponding receptors and signaling pathways

conducted by Illera et al. in 1998, it was concluded that growth factors such as epidermal growth factor (EGF) and insulin-like growth factor 1 (IGF1) has a stimulatory effect on the maturation and fertilization of pig oocytes. Another study conducted by Hasegawa et al. in 2009 emphasized the role of growth factors in the maturation of mouse oocytes.[14] Somatic cells (cumulus cells) and germ cells (oocytes) form a functional unit consisting of physical contacts between the cells, mediated by a dense web of gap junctions, and a paracrine signaling system. While, traditionally, communication was believed to occur only between the granulosa cells and the oocytes, an increasing amount of evidence has clearly demonstrated that the communication is actually bidirectional.[15] In particular, growth differentiation factor-9 and bone morphogenetic protein-15 (also called GDP-8) play a key role in the communication process.[16] Thus, oocytes lacking healthy cumulus complexes failed to show any development. On the other hand, deleterious effects of compact cumulus complexes have been shown in studies.[17]

The maturation medium must contain the right balance of antioxidants, growth factors and antibiotics to favor the maturation of the oocyte. **Figure 4** highlights the factors that influence the oxidative stress status of the oocyte and the importance of a good maturation medium in IVM.[17]

The uses of IVM have been highlighted earlier. More recently, IVM is being used as a promising research tool that can be used to study the maturation and gene expression in growing oocytes. It can also be used to study the cross talk between the oocyte and cumulus cells thereby allowing the development of new culture media. The study of fertilization and the factors involved in the

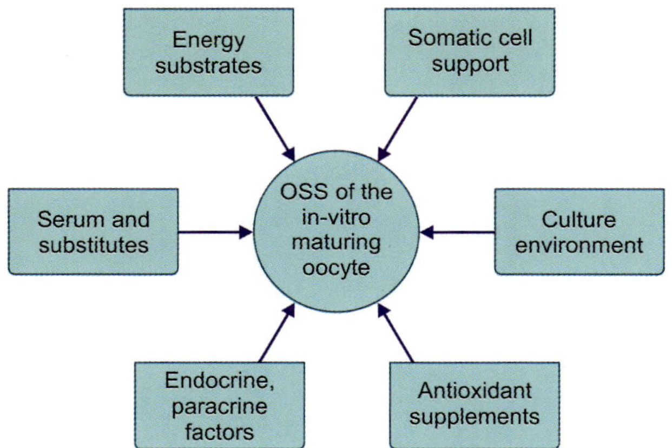

Fig. 4 Factors that may influence the oxidative stress status of oocytes (Combelles et al. 2009). The availability of antioxidants, energy substrates, growth factors and cumulus cell support are vital for the maturation of the IVM oocyte

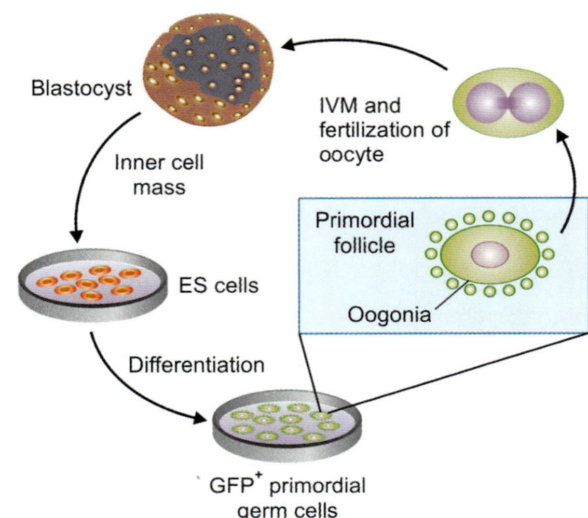

Fig. 5 In vitro differentiation of mouse embryonic stem cells yields oocytes, which undergo IVM followed by fertilization to form blastocysts

activation of the oocyte can be studied by using IVM of immature oocytes obtained during COH protocols. The more distant future offers the exciting prospect of an unlimited source of oocytes from any given female obtained through the generation of oocytes from embryonic stem cells (ESCs). While the capacity of these cells to differentiate into most types of adult tissues is well established, recently it has been observed that these cells can form mature egg-like cells that can be cultured via IVM and are capable of developing into blastocysts **(Fig. 5)**. This would alter the current dogma that the oocyte population is finite. It may be possible to stimulate this germinal population and amplify the oocyte number available at birth via IVM.[18] There are several ethical issues with respect to the use of ESCs for developing germ line cells and currently the culture of ESCs to form human germ line cells is not permitted by certain ethical bodies.

■ CONCLUSION

In vitro maturation is a novel reproductive technology that is currently being underused due to the lower maturation, fertilization, pregnancy and implantation rates obtained after its use. Despite the disadvantages of IVM, its lower costs and prevention of OHSS has made IVM is a clinically valuable technology in human assisted reproduction, with clear application for young PCO and PCOS patients. The use of IVM for research into the gene expression of immature oocytes and the study of fertilization has piqued the interests of scientists worldwide. To conclude,

IVM is an invaluable technology that can have future uses coupled with ESC culture to obtain an unlimited source of oocytes, provided ethical approval is obtained.

■ REFERENCES

1. Sirard MA, Richard F, Blondin P, et al. Contribution of the oocyte to embryo quality. Theriogenol. 2006;65(1):126-36.
2. Trounson A, Wood C, Kausche A, et al. In vitro maturation and the fertilization and developmental competence of oocytes recovered from untreated polycystic ovarian patients. Fertil Steril. 1994;62(2):353-62.
3. Son WY, Lee SY, Yoon SH, et al. Pregnancies and deliveries after transfer of human blastocysts derived from in vitro matured oocytes in in vitro maturation cycles. Fertil Steril. 2007;87(6):1491-3.
4. Chian R, Buckett W, Tan S, et al. In-vitro maturation of human oocytes. Reprod Biomed Online. 2004;8(2):148-66.
5. Porcu E, Venturoli S, Damiano G, et al. Healthy twins delivered after oocyte cryopreservation and bilateral ovariectomy for ovarian cancer. Reprod Biomed Online. 2008;17(2):265-7.
6. Khashavi M, Karimzadeh M. Comparison of unstimulated in vitro maturation and stimulated in vitro fertilization in women with poly cystic ovarian syndrome. J Res Med Sci. 2004;(6):260-3.
7. Junk S, Yeap D. Improved implantation and ongoing pregnancy rates after single-embryo transfer with an optimized protocol for in vitro oocyte maturation in women with polycystic ovaries and polycystic ovary syndrome. Fertil Steril. 2012;98(4): 888-92.
8. Basatemur E, Sutcliffe A. Health of IVM children. J Assist Reprod Genet. 2011;28(6):489-93.
9. Lindenberg S. History and Role of IVM in ART. Copenhagen: Copenhagen Fertility Centre; 2009.
10. Talukder M, Iqbal A, Khandoker M, et al. Collection grading and evaluation of cumulus-oocyte complexes for in vitro maturation in sheep. The Bangladesh Veterinarian. 2011;28(1):31-8.
11. Prada J, VandeVoort C. Growth hormone and in vitro maturation of rhesus macaque oocytes and subsequent embryo development. J Assist Reprod Genet. 2008;25(4):145-58.
12. Fukui Y, Kikuchi Y, Kondo H, et al. Fertilizability and developmental capacity of individually cultured bovine oocytes. Theriogenol. 2000;53(8):1553-65.
13. Sirarad M, Parrish JJ, Ware CB, et al. The culture of bovine oocytes to obtain developmentally competent embryos. Biol Reprod. 1988;(39):546-52.
14. Hasegawa A, Kumamoto K, Mochida N, et al. Gene expression profile during ovarian folliculogenesis. J Reprod Immunol. 2009;83(1-2):40-4.
15. Albertini D, Combelles C, Benecchi E, et al. Cellular basis for paracrine regulation of ovarian follicle development. Reproduction. 2001;121(5):647-53.
16. Eppig JJ. Oocyte control of ovarian follicular development and function in mammals. Reproduction. 2011;122(6):829-38.
17. Sirard MA. Follicle environment and quality of in-vitro matured oocytes. J Assist Reprod Genet. 2011;28:483-8.
18. Gandolfi F, Brevini TA, Cillo F, et al. Cellular and molecular mechanisms regulating oocyte quality and the relevance for farm animal reproductive efficiency. Rev Sci Tech. 2005;24(1):413-23.

43

Semen Banking

Natachandra Chimote, Bindu Chimote, Nishad Chimote

GENERAL ASPECTS OF SEMEN BANKING

The advent of low-temperature banking has rendered reproductive medicine unimaginable without the benefit of preserving and shipping germplasm. Cryopreservation of semen and spare embryos has become a mainstay of the assisted reproduction technology (ART) laboratory. Fertility preservation is so dependent on cryopreservation that most of the chapters in books are increasingly being dedicated to this topic.[1]

BJ Luyet[2] formulated the first theory of cryopreservation in the 1930s, moving this endeavor from the realms of speculation toward a scientific course. There is double trouble for cells cooled below freezing temperatures; water crystallizes to form ice and salt concentrations rise. Thus, the key to successful cryopreservation of cells of every type and species is to avoid ice inside cells and the side effects of freezing outside.

Cryoprotective agents (CPAs) like glycerol are small, water-soluble molecules that serve as colligative antifreeze agents by disrupting hydrogen bonds between water. They must be "nontoxic": glycerol has a robust claim as a natural metabolite of the body, and it accumulates at concentrations that protect some insects from freezing. Other species, including a few vertebrate species, derive protection from nonpermeating sugars and/or proteins, although the mechanisms of action are different. The so-called primary CPAs, such as glycerol, must diffuse inside cells to provide any benefit, and only a few other compounds with the necessary qualities have been adopted in practice. Polge et al.[3] noted that propanediol and ethylene glycol prevented damage to human sperm and both compounds are now used for a wide range of cell types. In every case, a compelling requirement is low toxicity, although none is completely safe.

Cryopreservation is widely used in many assisted conception units to preserve male fertility, for example, before cytotoxic chemotherapy,[4] radiotherapy or certain surgical treatments that may lead to testicular failure or ejaculatory dysfunction. Freezing of sperm before initiation of treatment provides patients with "fertility insurance" and may allow them to father their own children through the use of in vitro fertilization (IVF) or intracytoplasmic sperm injection (ICSI). Cryopreservation of sperm is mandatory in donor-insemination programs. The use of frozen semen allows screening of donors for infections such as human immunodeficiency virus and hepatitis B before release for insemination.[5] Cryopreservation is also widely used for storage of sperm retrieved from azoospermic patients who have undergone testicular sperm extraction (TESE) or percutaneous epididymal sperm aspiration (PESA), avoiding the need for repeat biopsies or aspiration.

Despite many refinements in cryopreservation methodology, the salvage of post-thaw sperm remains poor.[6] The most commonly reported detrimental effect of cryopreservation on human sperm is a marked reduction in motility.[7] This decrease is in both percentage of motile sperm and the velocity of their movement[8] and may be associated with the extensive damage caused.

THE PRINCIPAL VARIABLES OF CRYOPRESERVATION: SOLUTIONS, TEMPERATURES AND RATE CHANGES

Three major factors serve as principal determinants of survival of all types of mammalian cells, including spermatozoa, oocytes and embryos, when they are subjected to cryopreservation.

1. *Temperature:* Mammalian cells have evolved to function within a rather narrow temperature range from approximately 35°C to 40°C. Although they may tolerate brief exposure to lower temperatures, mammalian cells die if cooled and held at temperatures near 0°C for extended times. The specific limits of time and temperature depend on the cell type. Oocytes and spermatozoa, for example, seem to be especially

susceptible to damage when cooled to 0°C; this commonly is referred to as "chilling injury".

2. *Rate of temperature change:* The rate at which cells are cooled from physiological temperatures to low subzero temperatures is critical to their survival. Equally important, if not more important, is the rate at which cryopreserved cells are warmed from subzero temperatures to physiological ones. Again, depending on the cell type, the rate of cooling and/or the rate of warming may damage or kill cells.

3. *Medium used:* Finally, there is the role of the medium in which the cells are suspended when cooled or frozen to low temperatures.

SPERM CRYOPRESERVATION

Freezing and thawing methods expose spermatozoa to much physical and chemical damage, and thus several improvements have been made to the process of cryopreservation and thawing.[9]

Cryoprotectants are low molecular weight and highly permeable chemicals that serve to protect spermatozoa from freeze damage by ice crystallization. There are four main known cryoprotectants: (1) Glycerol (2) ethylene glycol (3) dimethyl sulfoxide and (4) 1,2-propanediol. Cryoprotectants act by decreasing the freezing point of a substance, reducing the amount of salts and solutes present in the liquid phase of the sample and by decreasing ice formation within the spermatozoa.[10]

There are two main freezing techniques used in sperm cryopreservation—(1) slow freezing and (2) rapid freezing (vitrification). The slow freezing method may be manual or automated involving a semi-programmable freezer. It is performed by simultaneously decreasing the temperature of the semen while adding cryoprotectant in a stepwise manner and eventually plunging the samples into liquid nitrogen. This method can cause ice crystallization to form if the cooling rate is too fast or too slow. The rapid freezing method, vitrification, is a process by which the samples are exposed to nitrogen vapor, equilibrated for some time and are then directly plunged into liquid nitrogen. This method does not allow ice crystallization to occur[9] (Nawroth et al. 2005). Cryoinjury is not limited to the freezing process but may also occur during thawing. Ice crystals melt during thawing and could result in damage of the sperm organelles. Therefore, the thawing phase and cryoprotectant removal must be conducted in a stepwise manner, similar to freezing[11] Normozoospermic semen samples appear to be more tolerant to damage induced by freezing and thawing compared with oligozoospermic samples. It was reported that motile spermatozoa could be recovered after five refreeze–thaw cycles in normozoospermic samples and after two refreeze–thaw cycles in oligozoospermic specimens samples.[12]

APOPTOSIS IN EJACULATED HUMAN SPERMATOZOA

Apoptosis, a programmed cell death mechanism, is vital to many eukaryotes as it regulates cell count and removes unnecessary cells that compromise survival. It involves a series of biochemical events that trigger cellular morphological alterations eventually leading to cellular termination. Apoptotic changes are typified by nuclear fragmentation, chromatin condensation, mitochondrial enlargement and irregular changes to the plasma membrane.[13]

The removal of dead cells by neighboring phagocytic cells has been termed efferocytosis. Dying cells that undergo the final stages of apoptosis display phagocytotic molecules, such as phosphatidylserine, on their cell surface. Elevated apoptosis markers have also been found to negatively correlate with oocyte penetration capacity. It has been reported that semen samples with lowered penetrative ability contain spermatozoa with higher concentrations of apoptotic markers (phosphatidylserine externalization, disrupted mitochondrial membrane potential, activated caspase-3) as compared to semen samples with normal penetrative ability.[14]

MECHANISMS AND MANIFESTATIONS OF CRYOINJURY IN SPERMATOZOA

There are many risks associated with cryopreservation. Freezing to subzero temperatures cause irreversible injury in spermatozoa, which gets aggravated during the thawing procedure, thereby reducing the sperm cryosurvival rate. Cryoprotectants themselves can be toxic if used in high concentrations since spermatozoa are vulnerable to osmotic changes induced by cryoprotectants.[15] Spermatozoa can also undergo intracellular and extracellular ice formation, excessive dehydration (due to increased solute concentration) and denaturation of proteins due to shifts in pH as well as membrane damage caused by close proximity freezing of cells **(Flow chart 1)**.

The cooling rate plays an important role in determining the extent of cryoinjury to the spermatozoa. During freezing, ice nucleates in the extracellular matrix, eliciting an osmotic gradient. During freezing, water will move across the membrane from the intracellular to the extracellular space and intracellular ice formation will occur with rapid cooling rates. If the cooling rate is too slow, water can join the ice phase of the extracellular space and the cells become osmotically inactive due to

Flow chart 1 Schematic diagram of the detrimental effects of cryopreservation on sperm integrity and associated events leading to apoptosis and to the decline in sperm function. Appropriate use of sperm selection techniques and cryoprotectants should be used to minimize these detrimental effects

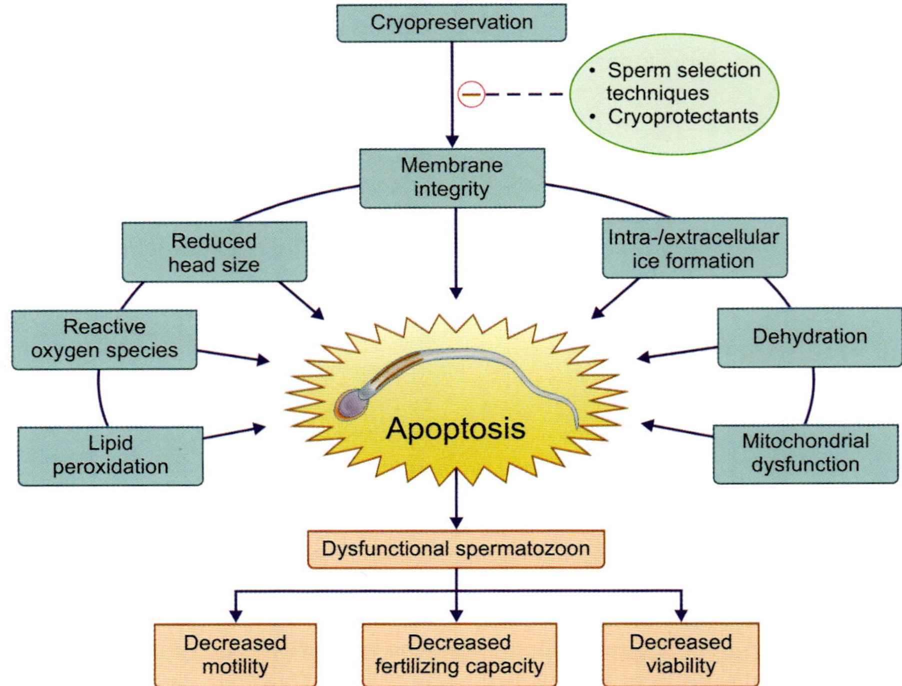

intracellular ice formation and loss of cell membrane integrity.[16] Thus, the cooling rate is very critical—too rapid will cause severe intracellular ice formation but too slow can expose the cells to toxicity damage by high solute concentrations. Sperm motility, plasma membrane integrity and mitochondrial function are inversely correlated with cooling rates, which indicates that too fast or too slow cooling rates can cause these parameters to be compromised.[17]

Osmotic changes during the cryopreservation process expose spermatozoa to changes in osmotic conditions resulting in cellular damage. According to few studies, survival of human cryopreserved spermatozoa is decreased at hypo-osmotic conditions due to cellular swelling leading to lysis and that spermatozoa are initially resistant to hyperosmotic conditions; however, significant cell damage occurs when returned to isosmotic conditions.[18,19]

The membrane integrity is an important factor for the sperm motility and viability. Membrane fluidity has been positively correlated with the recovery of motile, viable spermatozoa from a cryopreserved sample.[20] The integrity of the sperm membrane is affected during cryopreservation and thawing processes. Alterations in sperm membrane integrity have been well observed in

ultrastructural studies.[21] The stability of the membrane is affected by changes in temperature, volume changes associated with the movement of water, cryoprotectants and osmotic stress due to increased salt concentration. During cryopreservation, the initial cooling process causes phase transitions of the membrane lipids and impairs the function of membrane proteins, which are responsible for ion transport and metabolism.[22] These changes compromise the membrane integrity and cause loss of function. Glycerol has been found to have a direct effect on the membrane by altering its fluidity via increasing the order of the fatty acids.[23] Cryopreservation of human spermatozoa is also known to have negative effects on sperm motility and velocity due to membrane swelling and acrosomal leakage and degeneration. It has been reported that irregular interaction between deoxyribonucleic acid (DNA) and nuclear proteins can lead to impaired motion parameters in spermatozoa.[10]

Implication of Apoptosis in Sperm Cryoinjury/ Increased Apoptosis in Cryopreserved Spermatozoa

Studies have revealed that apoptosis markers tend to increase in spermatozoa following cryopreservation and thawing. In an animal model, cryopreservation increased apoptosis manifestations including mitochondrial membrane potential, caspase activation, membrane permeability and phosphatidylserine externalization.[24]

In general, the occurrence of sperm DNA fragmentation during cryopreservation remains to be elucidated. The current body of evidence suggests that sperm DNA fragmentation is associated with an increase in oxidative stress during cryopreservation, rather than the activation of caspases and apoptosis.[25] The alteration in the mitochondrial membrane fluidity that occurs during cryopreservation will lead to a rise in mitochondrial membrane potential and the release of reactive oxygen species (ROS). Subsequently, released ROS cause DNA damage in spermatozoa that present with high frequencies of single- and double-strand DNA breaks. The process of ROS generation during cryopreservation and thawing of spermatozoa has been well documented. It has been reported that ROS production by both human spermatozoa and seminal leukocytes increases on cooling to 4°C.[26] Thus, cryopreserved semen samples containing leukocytes may be more prone to DNA fragmentation. In addition, the cryopreservation process has been shown to diminish the antioxidant activity of the spermatozoa making them more susceptible to ROS-induced damage.[27] In a recent study, the improvement in the post-thaw integrity of cryopreserved human spermatozoa was tested, specifically from men with abnormal semen parameters. The addition of an antioxidant, e.g. vitamin E to cryopreservation medium, has been found to be significantly associated with post-thaw motility, but neither sperm viability nor DNA fragmentation is affected.[28] Similarly, it has been recently reported that increased ROS concentrations in post-thaw spermatozoa were significantly reduced by both ascorbate and catalase.[29]

The occurrence of the sperm DNA fragmentation may not be the result of cryopreservation but may be more associated with the thawing. A rapid increase in sperm DNA fragmentation over time was shown with the highest rate of fragmentation occurring during the first 4 hours after thawing. Therefore, thawed sperm samples should be used in the clinical setting as quickly as possible.[30] The DNA integrity during cryopreservation also appears to be independent of the method used (slow versus vitrification) or presence of cryoprotectants.[31]

Comparison of fresh versus cryopreserved spermatozoa has shown that cryopreservation significantly increases the percentage of spermatozoa with activated pan-caspases from 21% to 47%. Interestingly, the concentration of activated caspases positively correlated with increasing glycerol concentration from 7% to 14%.[32]

In support, a significant increase of activated caspase-1 in healthy donors, caspase-8 in unselected infertility patients and caspase-9 in both patient and donor groups were reported after cryopreservation.[33]

The extent of apoptosis in spermatozoa appears to be related to the type of cryoprotectant used and the protocols for cryopreservation. The application of 14% glycerol resulted in higher amounts of activated caspase than 7% glycerol. Therefore it is postulated that glycerol may also contribute to activation of caspases directly via toxic effects to mitochondria during sperm cryopreservation.[33]

APOPTOSIS IN CRYOPRESERVED SUBFERTILE SEMEN SAMPLES

Spermatozoa from infertile men seem to be more prone to cryoinjury, DNA damage and cell death after cryopreservation than normal semen sample. It was noted that the severity of cryoinjury in human spermatozoa was greater in subfertile males and the extent of damage was correlated to the degree of oligoasthenoteratozoospermia.[22] Increased concentrations of ROS cause peroxidative damage to the sperm plasma membrane, leading to reduced membrane integrity. This can deleteriously affect sperm motility by damaging the axonemal structure of the spermatozoa.[34] Most importantly, more recent findings documented that spermatozoa with lower motility are more susceptible to cryodamage and, consequently, have lower fertilizing capacity.[35]

Sperm DNA in infertile men was found to be less resistant to damage during cryopreservation compared with spermatozoa from fertile men.[36] Cryopreserved semen samples from cancer patients were also found to have higher DNA fragmentation compared with healthy donors.[37] It has been reported that men with oligozoospermia present with higher rates of sperm DNA fragmentation both pre- and postcryopreservation compared with fertile men.[38]

METHODS TO DECREASE APOPTOSIS DURING SPERM CRYOPRESERVATION

Optimization of the sperm preparation techniques, concentrations of cryoprotectant and freezing and thawing protocols should minimize the induction of apoptosis during sperm cryopreservation, which in turn should translate into higher success rates during assisted reproductive techniques **(Fig. 1)**. Before freezing, semen samples should be processed in a way to enhance the postfreeze sperm quality. The swim-up method

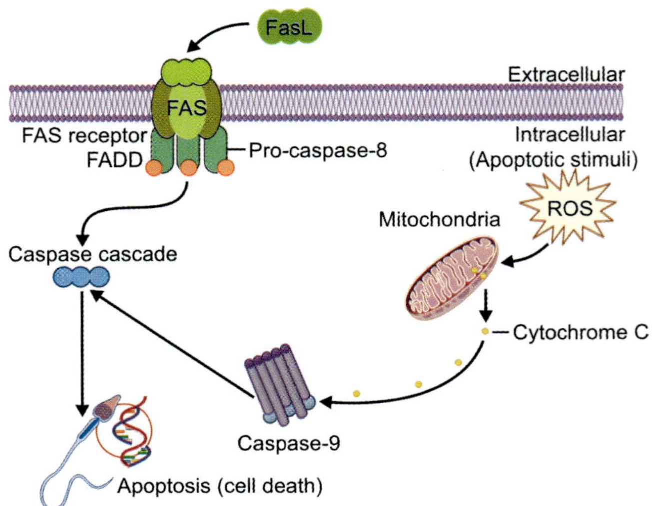

Fig. 1 Apoptosis during sperm cryopreservation

Abbreviation: ROS, reactive oxygen species

to separate motile spermatozoa and the two density-gradient centrifugation techniques are both used to ensure the isolation of functionally and morphologically normal spermatozoa.[39] In a comparative study, it was found that semen samples from infertile patients prepared by a double density-gradient technique yielded higher recovery of motile spermatozoa following cryopreservation–thaw compared with those samples prepared by swim-up.[40] On the other hand, both density-gradient centrifugation and swim-up techniques were demonstrated to significantly reduce the extent of apoptotic spermatozoa compared with raw semen.[41]

The exclusion of apoptotic spermatozoa before cryopreservation may lead to recovery of higher quality spermatozoa that are functionally normal following thawing. Magnetic cell sorting (MACS) using annexin V-conjugated microbeads is a technique that has the ability to separate non-apoptotic from apoptotic spermatozoa based on phosphatidylserine externalization. It has been well documented that the separation of a distinctive population of non-apoptotic spermatozoa with intact membranes using annexin V-MACS may optimize cryopreservation–thaw outcome. The technique, if performed prior to the freezing, was found to enhance the percentage of spermatozoa with higher motility, intact membrane mitochondrial potential and survival rates following cryopreservation.[42,43] The use of MACS can also improve motility and enhance oocyte penetration potential.[44-46]

It is also important to consider the protective capacity of the seminal fluid when performing cryopreservation.

The seminal plasma contains protective agents that can increase the resistance to freezing damage; however, it remains a controversy whether freezing raw or prepared samples yield better results. Sperm preparation methods are commonly used to select mature and functional spermatozoa but these procedures eliminate the presence of the antioxidant supply from the seminal plasma. Supplements can always be included in vitro to compensate for this deficiency. Multiple studies show the advantage of using TEST-yolk buffer as a cryoprotectant with glycerol to prevent damage in spermatozoa.[47,48] Using TEST-yolk buffer in combination with glycerol is preferred compared with using glycerol alone. This combined approach was shown to preserve higher motility, morphology and sperm membrane integrity.[47] It also decreases the number of spermatozoa with phosphatidylserine externalization[49] and prevents excess chromatin structure damage and morphology changes.[50]

▪ PROCESSING OF SEMEN CAN RESULT IN INCREASED SPERM DEOXYRIBONUCLEIC ACID FRAGMENTATION

Processing of semen for ART entails a number of procedures. Sometimes, semen samples are not processed immediately after semen collection, remaining in the laboratory for several hours before they are processed for ART. Previous studies have shown that incubation of semen is associated with oxygen radical-mediated attack of membrane phospholipids, which results in lipid peroxidation, leading to loss of motility and of sperm fertilizing ability.[51,52] It has been previously reported that the production of oxygen radicals and of superoxide anion, in particular, increases during thawing of cryopreserved ejaculated sperm.[53] Motility loss during thawing of cryopreserved sperm appears to be related, atleast in part, to oxidation of reduced glutathione.[54] Processing of semen for ART, including incubation and cryopreservation of semen, may result in increased sperm DNA fragmentation. Therefore, unnecessary incubation of semen in the laboratory should be avoided.

EFFECTS OF CRYOPRESERVATION ON HUMAN SPERM DEOXYRIBONUCLEIC ACID INTEGRITY

Cryopreservation is known also as a cell damaging procedure and may lead, due to temperature variations, to deleterious changes in sperm structure (e.g. membrane, mitochondria and DNA).[49,55-57] Evaluating the impact on sperm chromatin after cryopreservation is of extreme importance as DNA integrity is essential in achieving fertilization and embryo development; it is crucial to guarantee the success of ART.[58,59]

Oxidative stress was studied as a possible mechanism for the origin of sperm DNA damage. It was widely reported that ROS are associated with poor semen quality and defective functional competence of human spermatozoa.[60,61] ROS are also known to play an important role in the pathophysiology of damage to human spermatozoa.[62,63] Therefore, it is thought that sperm DNA damages including DNA fragmentation, base modifications, chromatin cross-linking, and other alterations, are linked to oxidative stress.[62-64]

Among all of these alterations, DNA fragmentation was the most studied and associated with male infertility and sperm parameters defects but its origin is still unclear. It could be attributed to oxidative stress but also to apoptosis and defective chromatin packaging.[60,62,65] Terminal deoxynucleotidyl transferase (Tdt) mediated deoxyuridine triphosphate (dUTP) nick end labeling is one of the most used tests to detect DNA fragmentation either with fluorescence microscopy or by flow cytometry.[66] The oxidative DNA biomarker 8-oxoguanine commonly used to evaluate oxidative DNA alterations due to its high specificity and sensitivity, relative abundance in DNA and potent mutagenicity.[22]

Actually there is clinical evidence to show that sperm DNA damage is detrimental to reproductive outcomes and extensive data exist on the relationship between DNA damage and ART outcomes, particularly on pregnancy rates.[67,68]

CANCER AND FERTILITY: STRATEGIES TO PRESERVE FERTILITY

As a result of treatment innovations, the survival rates of young people with cancer have improved markedly. The most commonly occurring cancers among young people aged 15–24 years include Hodgkin's lymphoma, testicular cancer and malignant melanoma.[69,70] 5-year survival rates of over 90% for these malignancies are now reported in young people.[70]

However, the management of many common malignancies involves aggressive radiotherapy or chemotherapy, which may permanently impair reproductive function.[71] Iatrogenic infertility is a distressing consequence for many cancer survivors and their families. Accordingly, there is increasing interest among oncologists and reproductive specialists alike to consider fertility preservation as an essential component of a comprehensive approach to cancer treatment. This demand has driven the recent development of a number of novel strategies to preserve fertility.

EFFECTS OF CANCER AND ITS TREATMENT ON FERTILITY

Male Reproductive System

Almost 30% of men with testicular cancer have semen abnormalities at the time of diagnosis. Interestingly, semen abnormalities are also common among young men at the time of diagnosis with other cancers.[72]

Spermatogenesis is a highly prolific process.[73] Therefore, the germinal epithelium is extremely sensitive to the effects of chemotherapy and radiotherapy, which target rapidly dividing cells. Subfertility is observed in the majority of men who receive alkylating agents plus radiotherapy (above or below the diaphragm) for the treatment of cancer. Radiation doses of only 0.1–1.2 Gray (Gy) can impair spermatogenesis and doses of more than 4 Gy may cause permanent damage.[74] The mechanism of disruption of spermatogenesis is uncertain, but is believed to involve depletion of both stem cells and differentiating spermatogonia.[74,75]

Spermatogenesis declines 3–6 months following chemotherapy or radiotherapy for testicular cancer, but steadily recovers thereafter,[76] 2 years after treatment, 97% and 94% of men treated with chemotherapy or radiotherapy (with shielding of the contralateral testicle), respectively, show good recovery of spermatogenesis. In contrast, the prevalence of azoospermia among men treated for lymphoma is reported to be as high as 59%

and a long recovery period (45 months) is needed to achieve the highest sperm concentration.[77] The impact of chemotherapy regimens on spermatogenesis depends on the type of chemotherapeutic agents used and the cumulative dose given.[78]

PRESERVATION OF FERTILITY FOR YOUNG ADULTS WITH CANCER

Preservation of fertility should be offered to all young people who receive potentially curative gonadotoxic cancer therapies. Experts agree that fertility preservation should be considered as early as possible in the course of cancer treatment. However, evidence suggests that cancer treatment often commences without adequate consideration of fertility preservation[79] and those current services could be much improved.[80]

Infertility is a major concern for young people with cancer.[81] Oncologists are, therefore, encouraged to provide information on the risk of infertility conferred by their cancer treatment and offer a specialist referral to discuss options for fertility preservation.[82] Storage of gametes, embryos, blastocysts or gonadal tissue prior to cancer treatment should also be considered for young people who require aggressive chemotherapy or radiotherapy.

CRYOPRESERVATION TECHNIQUES

Cryopreservation of gametes and embryos is being offered with increasing frequency following guidelines to limit the number of fresh embryos transferred per cycle of ART and improvements in laboratory techniques and clinical outcomes. Cryostorage is now a valuable component of standard IVF and ICSI regimens.

All cryopreservation protocols involve equilibration of cells in cryoprotectant followed by chilling, freezing and storage in liquid nitrogen at −196°C.[72] Cryoprotectants, such as ethylene glycol and dimethylsulfoxide, partially replace intracellular fluid and prevent the formation of intracellular ice crystals during the freezing process. The samples are subsequently thawed and the cryoprotectant is removed. The type, concentration and volume of cryoprotectant used in the solution have an impact on the outcome of cryopreservation.[83]

Both open and closed cryopreservation systems are commercially available. In closed systems, specimens are sealed inside carriers before being plunged into liquid nitrogen. Open systems involve direct contact of the specimen with liquid nitrogen and carry a theoretical risk of contamination and cross-infection.

MALE FERTILITY PRESERVATION

Cryopreservation of Sperm

Sperm banking is a simple and low-cost intervention for men who require fertility preservation. If men are unable to ejaculate semen for storage, sperm can be obtained by epididymal aspiration or testicular biopsy. The use of ICSI largely circumvents the issues of low sperm counts or poor sperm motility that are common in patients with cancer.[74] Therefore, cryopreservation of sperm is recommended for all men prior to potentially gonadotoxic cancer treatment.

Despite the advantages of sperm banking, evidence suggests that it is not universally offered prior to cancer treatment. Although utilization rates vary, it seems that few cancer survivors (2–27%) proceed to use cryopreserved sperm to attempt a pregnancy.[84] The reasons for the low rates of utilization are unknown, but it has been suggested that patients either do not have access to ART or fear transmitting the disease to their children.[85] Despite the low utilization rates of cryopreserved sperm, discussion of fertility preservation provides reassurance of the curative intent of cancer treatment and is, therefore, beneficial for many patients and their families.

SPERM VACUOLES ARE NOT MODIFIED BY FREEZING–THAWING PROCEDURES

Nomarski interference contrast microscopy at high magnification (X 6,000 to X 10,000) revealed a new morphological criterion in human spermatozoa: the presence of nuclear vacuoles. Real-time observation of motile spermatozoa by this technique, motile sperm organelle morphology examination (MSOME), was first used by Bartoov et al.[86] to select spermatozoa with as few vacuoles as possible before microinjection into the oocyte by intracytoplasmic morphologically selected sperm injection (IMSI). IMSI may improve the pregnancy rate compared with conventional ICSI, mainly after several failures of ICSI, as confirmed by a prospective randomized controlled trial.[87]

Despite the success of cryopreservation of spermatozoa in ART, the freezing–thawing process is undoubtedly associated with alterations of sperm quality. The primary cause of cell injury during cryopreservation is the formation of intracellular ice crystals. In addition, during cooling, crystallization of the extracellular medium increases the concentration of solutes in suspension in the liquid phase and therefore the osmolarity of the extracellular medium, which may lead to excessive intracellular dehydration. These different physical events are associated with mechanical damage during cold shock and so may result in rupture of the plasma membrane and disturbance of cellular organelles.

As far as it is known, 10 years after the development of a new concept called MSOME for observing the sperm head vacuoles by high magnification with Nomarski contrast before IMSI, there is no data on the use of this detailed morphological analysis after sperm cryopreservation in liquid nitrogen.

No difference in the vacuole criteria before and after freezing–thawing in terms of relative vacuole area, total vacuole area or vacuole area in the anterior, median and basal parts of the head, nor in terms of distribution of the subpopulations of spermatozoa with small or large vacuoles.[88] The freezing process (dehydration and rehydration of the cell, formation of intracellular crystals and cooling shock) thus has no impact on the sperm cephalic vacuoles.

Furthermore, DNA integrity is more affected by freezing in teratospermic when compared with normospermic men.[89] It is therefore postulated that the impact of freezing and thawing on fine sperm head morphology could be less detectable in this population of fertile men. Further studies are therefore needed in infertile population. However, it must be highlighted that, although less susceptible, all sperm parameters affected by the freeze–thawing procedure in infertile men are also affected in fertile men while the vacuolar criteria are remarkably stable.[90]

SIMPLE VITRIFICATION FOR SMALL NUMBERS OF HUMAN SPERMATOZOA

In cases of azoospermia, cryopreservation of testicular spermatozoa can avoid repeated testicular biopsy and it is useful for effective treatment and management. However, traditional freezing techniques are not suitable for spermatozoa from the testis because of their low number and poor in situ motility.[91] The lack of an easily implemented technology has remained a major bottleneck for the cryopreservation of small numbers of spermatozoa.

A previous publication[92] reported a successful vitrification method for a single spermatozoon using the Cryotop (Kitazato Biopharma, Japan), which consists of non-biological material and is available commercially. However, the samples are in direct contact with liquid nitrogen (LN_2) because the Cryotop is an open system, and this may result in microbial contamination.[93]

Some authors have reported successful pregnancies using a few spermatozoa stored in empty zona pellucida.[94,95] However, use of zona pellucida generates many ethical problems and is only available on a limited basis, because the procedure depends on biological material from human or animal sources and there is the potential for disease transmission. Furthermore, it is difficult to obtain the zona pellucida from a partner unless she decides to undergo oocyte retrieval specifically for uncertain sperm cryopreservation. Therefore, other authors have attempted to cryopreserve small numbers of spermatozoa using various types of containers such as droplets on plastic dishes.[96] Further, Gimenez et al.[97] have presented the negative evidence of cross-contamination mediated by LN_2 between human pathogens and oocytes/embryos that were clinically vitrified using an open device. Taken together, these results may suggest that the risk of the cross-contamination between gametes and LN_2 is vanishingly small.

It is possible to cryopreserve small numbers of spermatozoa using the cell sleeper.[98] Using this method, spermatozoa could be vitrified easily and recovered efficiently and quickly. It is arguable whether the spermatozoa would be infected with bacteria or pathogens mediated by LN_2, which have leaked into the cell sleeper during storage in a cryobank. No case of transmission of infectious disease has ever been reported and no report mentions LN_2 as a probable vehicle for disease transmission in assisted reproduction treatment.

Cell sleeper is a useful container for the cryopreservation of small numbers of spermatozoa and the method is a quick, easy and simple. The cell sleeper is commercially available and easy to prepare for use. Clinical application of this procedure to extremely poor sperm specimens will be necessary in order to confirm these findings.

PROTOCOLS FOR LABORATORY PROCEDURES

Equipment and Reagents

- Microwell counting chambers from conception technologies
- 5 mL eppendorf® pipette
- Aliquot mixer
- Vortex
- −20°C freezer
- LN_2 container with racks
- Sterile specimen container
- Sterile 15 mL centrifuge tubes with caps
- Sterile serological pipettes (1 mL, 2 mL and 5 mL capacity)
- Sterile Nunc cryovials (1 mL and 2 mL capacity)
- Colored cryomarkers

- Test tube racks (for 15 mL test tubes)
- Cryovial racks
- Stainless steel canes for cryovials
- Plastic cryosleeves
- Cryogloves
- Latex gloves
- 37°C incubators
- LN_2 from suppliers
- Eosin-Nigrosin stain
- Microslide
- Coverslip
- Sperm washing media
- Makler chamber
- Freezing medium (TEST-yolk buffer with glycerol: with TYB–G)
- Sperm washing media [Human tubal fluid (HTF)].

■ PROCEDURES (ASPIRATION FROM SURGERY)

Technical Note

Sterile techniques should be used throughout specimen processing. Gloves are mandatory for all procedures dealing with body fluids. Latex, however, may be toxic to sperm. Therefore, care should be taken to prevent contamination of the specimen with latex or talc. Vinyl gloves are available alternative.

- Cryopreservation worksheet labeled with the patient's name, diagnosis, and LN_2 container and rack. If there is more than one specimen, then have a worksheet for each specimen.
- Every time a laboratory receives the notice that an aspiration is ready, take one bottle of frozen TEST-yolk media and put into the 37°C incubator to thaw.
- A technologist will go to the surgery room to retrieve the specimen(s). Keep the vials warm in your hands.
- Normally, two to three specimen will arrive from surgery. Make sure the name of patient as well as the specimen number.
- Using sterile technique, measure the volume of each specimen and record on the appropriate cryopreservation sheet.
- Centrifuge the specimen in the original container for 5 minutes at 1,600 rpm.
- Label three sterile 15 mL conical centrifuge tubes with the patient's name and specimen number.
- Transfer the supernatant of specimen one and specimen two, and if there is specimen three also in the supernatant tube.
- Add 0.5 mL HTF (sperm washing media) to each pellet to resuspend. Mix gently.

- Transfer a drop of each specimen into a prelabeled conical cap for semen analysis.
- Perform the following on each specimen aspirate: regular manual semen analysis. Endtz test (leuko-cytospermia test) eosin-nigrosin stain procedure, Tygerberg's strict criteria from morphology evaluation.
- Always notify the surgeon if no motile sperm on the wet prep.
- Warm within 1 hour of specimen collection; add an aliquot of freezing medium equal to 25% of the resuspended aspirate volume to the centrifuge tube with a sterile pipette.
  Note: Since the resuspended volume for each aspirate is 0.5 mL, then divide 0.5 by 4 to obtain 0.13. Therefore add 0.13 of freeze media four times to the specimen.
- Gently, rock the specimen(s) with the freezing media for 5 minutes on an aliquote mixer.
- Repeat steps 13 and 14 three times or until the volume of freezing media equal to the specimen volume in step 9.
- Centrifuge the tube labeled "supernatant" for 5 minutes at 1,600 rpm.
- Remove the supernatant from the "supernatant" tube. Resuspend the pellet with 0.5 mL of HTF. Mix gently. Remove one drop for a semen analysis.

Note: If no motile sperm is found in the "supernatant" tube, then do not start freezing. If motile sperm is found, then freeze as in steps.[13-15]

During the mixing step above, use appropriate colored cryomarkers to label 2 mL cryovials and canes. The volume added to the vial should not exceed 1.8 mL/vial.[99]

- Label an additional 1.0 mL cryovial as in for each specimen. This will contain a left over aliquot of the cryodiluted specimen to be assessed of cryovial 24 hours after freezing in LN_2.
- A visual inspection should therefore be made of cryodiluted specimen for motility. A manual motility can be done using a microcell chamber or Makler chamber and a Nikon 2 phase microscope. The percent motility should be documented on the cryopreservation worksheet under cryodilution motility.
- Distribute the well-mixed, cryodiluted semen into prelabeled vials using a 1 mL or 2 mL sterile serological pipette. Add atleast 0.2 mL to the smaller 1.0 mL cryovial.
- Place labeled vials into a plastic freezing rack along with canes and cryosleeves and put into a –20°C freezer for 8 minutes. Do not open the freezer in any circumstance during this incubation.

Note: Exposure to freezing conditions should occur within 1.5 hours of specimen collection.

- After the 8 minutes incubation, remove the rack and canes from the –20°C freezer. Place a maximum of two cryovials into bottom slots of canes upside down. Put into cryosleeves.
- After minimum 2 hours incubation in LN_2 vapors, turn cases upside down, immerging them into LN_2.
- After a minimum of 24 hours in LN_2, thaw the aliquot in the 1.0 mL cryovial.
- Using cryogloves, remove cane containing the vial and snap it out. Loosen the cap and place in the 37°C incubation for 20 minutes.
- Mix the vial well and analyze manually.
- Record the cryovial area of the cryopreservation worksheet.
- Assess cryosurvival in the formula:

$$\frac{\%\ \text{motility of post-thaw specimen}}{\%\ \text{motility of prefreeze specimen}}$$

■ PROCEDURE (SEMEN FROM EJACULATE)

Technical Note

Sterile techniques should be used throughout specimen processing. Gloves are mandatory for all procedures dealing with body fluids. Latex, however, may be toxic to sperm. Therefore, care should be taken to prevent contamination of the specimen with latex or talc. Vinyl gloves are available as alternative.

- Cryopreservation worksheet labeled with the patient's name, diagnosis, and LN_2 container and rack. If there is more than one specimen, then have a worksheet for each specimen.
- Using sterile technique, measure the volume of each specimen and record on the appropriate cryopreservation worksheet.
- Perform the following on the semen sample: regular manual semen analysis, Endtz test, eosin-nigrosin stain procedure, Tygerberg's strict criteria for morphology evaluation.
- Within 1 hour of specimen collection, add an aliquot of freezing medium equal to 25% of the resuspended aspirate volume to the centrifuge tube with a sterile pipette.

Note: Since the resuspended volume for each aspirate is 0.5 mL, then divide 0.5 by 4 to obtain 0.13. Therefore add 0.13 of freeze media four times to the specimen.

- Gently, rock the specimen(s) with the freezing media for 5 minutes on an aliquot mixer.
- Repeat step 4 three times or until the volume for freezing media added is equal to the specimen volume in step 2.

- During the mixing steps above, use appropriately colored cryomarkers to label 2 mL cryovials and canes. The volume added to the vial should not exceed 1.8 mL/vial.
- Label an additional 1.0 mL cryovial as in for each specimen. This will contain a leftover aliquot of the cryodiluted specimen to be assessed for cryosurvival 24 hours after freezing in LN_2.
- A visual inspection should therefore be made of cryodiluted specimen for motility. A manual motility can be done using a microcell chamber or Makler chamber and a Nikon 2 phase microscope. The percent motility should be documented on the cryopreservation worksheet under cryodilution motility.
- Distribute the well-mixed, cryodiluted semen into prelabeled vials using a 1 mL or 2 mL sterile serological pipette. Add atleast 0.2 mL to the smaller 1.0 mL cryovial.
- Place lebeled vials into a plastic freezing rack along with canes and cryosleeves and put into a –20°C freezer for 8 minutes. Do not open the freezer in any circumstance during this incubation.

Note: Exposure to freezing conditions should occur within 1.5 hours of specimen collection.

- After 8 min incubation, remove the rack and canes from the –20°C freezer. Place a maximum of two cryovials into bottom slots of canes upside down. Put into cryosleeves.
- After minimum 2 hours incubation in LN_2 vapors, turn cases upside down, immerging them into LN_2.
- After a minimum of 24 hours in LN_2, thaw the aliquot in 1.0 mL cryovial.
- Using cryogloves, remove cane containing the vial and snap it out. Loosen the cap and place in the 37°C incubation for 20 minutes.
- Mix the vial well and analyze manually.
- Record the cryovial area of the cryopreservation worksheet.
- Assess cryosurvival in the formula:

$$\frac{\%\ \text{motility of post-thaw specimen}}{\%\ \text{motility of prefreeze specimen}}$$

■ SUMMARY

Cryopreservation is an integral component of fertility management and much of its successful application will affect success rates of assisted reproduction treatments. Whether sperm cryopreservation is applied as a fertility preservation measure or for a backup for assisted reproduction, the recovery rate of functionally competent spermatozoa is critical. Apoptosis has been correlated with decreased fertilizing capacity of spermatozoa and male infertility. Increased apoptosis markers have been documented in response to cryopreservation and thawing in human spermatozoa. This poses a serious threat to success rates following the use of cryopreserved spermatozoa for assisted reproduction. Thus, different aspects associated with apoptosis deserve attention during sperm cryopreservation in order to conserve vital sperm functions after thawing. Technical measures should be applied to provide maximal protection to the spermatozoa during cryopreservation and thawing to prevent induction of apoptosis. Appropriate use of cryoprotectants and sperm selection technologies appears to have the most impact on preventing apoptosis and thereby improving sperm cryosurvival rates.

Although the origin of cryopreservation-induced DNA damages is not well elucidated, we can presume that DNA fragmentation would be attributed to an ROS assault but also to an apoptotic mechanism, whereas DNA oxidation is mainly a consequence of oxidative stress. Further investigations of the apoptotic process and oxidative stress should be conducted to elucidate the mechanisms by which cryopreservation/thawing affect sperm DNA integrity.

The possible future effects of chemotherapy or radiotherapy on fertility should be discussed with all cancer patients who have reproductive potential. Moreover, fertility preservation should be considered for all young people undergoing potentially gonadotoxic treatment. The age and relationship status of the patient, the type of cancer and stage at diagnosis, the type and dose of chemotherapy and radiotherapy required and the time available before initiation of cancer treatment will influence individual patient management. Therefore, a variety of safe and effective options for fertility preservation are required. Early referral of patients to a fertility specialist will allow consideration and discussion of the full range of fertility preservation options.

Sperm banking is a simple and low-cost intervention that should be recommended to all men prior to gonadotoxic cancer treatment.

■ REFERENCES

1. Donnez J, Kim SS. Principles and practice of fertility preservation. Cambridge, UK: Cambridge University Press; 2011.
2. Luyet BJ. The vitrification of organic colloids and of protoplasm. Biodynamica. 1937;1:1-14.
3. Polge C, Smith AU, Parkes AS. Revival of spermatozoa after vitrification and dehydration at low temperatures. Nature. 1949;164:666.
4. Sanger WG, Olson JH, Sherman JK. Semen cryobanking for men with cancer—criteria change. Fertil Steril. 1992;58:1024-7.
5. Sherman JK. Current status of clinical cryobanking of human semen. In: Paulson JD, Negro-Vlar A, Lucena E, Martini L (Eds). Andrology: Male Fertility and Sterility. Orlando, FL: Academic Press; 1986. pp. 517-47.
6. Agrawal A, Tolentine MV, Sidhu RS, et al. Effect of cryopreservation on semen quality in patients with testicular cancer. Urology. 1995;46:382-9.
7. Englert Y, Delvigne A, Vekemans M, et al. Is fresh or frozen semen to be used in in vitro fertilization with donor sperm. Fertil Steril. 1989;51:661-4.
8. Graczykowski JW, Siegel MS. Motile sperm recovery from fresh and frozen-thawed ejaculates using a swim-up procedure. Fertil Steril. 1991;55:841-3.
9. Nawroth F, Rahimi G, Isachenko E, et al. Cryopreservation in assisted reproductive technology: new trends. Semin Reprod Med. 2005;23:325-35.
10. Royere D, Barthelemy C, Hamamah S, et al. Cryopreservation of spermatozoa: a 1996 review. Hum Reprod Update. 1996;2:553-9.
11. Verheyen G, Pletincx I, Van Steirteghem A. Effect of freezing method, thawing temperature and post-thaw dilution/washing on motility (CASA) and morphology characteristics of high-quality human sperm. Hum Reprod. 1993;8:1678-84.
12. Verza S, Feijo CM, Esteves SC. Resistance of human spermatozoa to cryoinjury in repeated cycles of thaw-refreezing. Int Braz J Urol. 2009;35:581-90.
13. Kerr JF, Wyllie AH, Currie AR. Apoptosis: a basic biological phenomenon with wide-ranging implications in tissue kinetics. Br J Cancer. 1972;26:239-57.
14. Grunewald S, Said TM, Paasch U, et al. Relationship between sperm apoptosis signalling and oocyte penetration capacity. Int J Androl. 2008;31:325-30.
15. Gao DY, Ashworth E, Watson PF, et al. Hyperosmotic tolerance of human spermatozoa: separate effects of glycerol, sodium chloride, and sucrose on spermolysis. Biol Reprod. 1993;49:112-23.
16. Frim J, Mazur P. Interactions of cooling rate, warming rate, glycerol concentration, and dilution procedure on the viability of frozen-thawed human granulocytes. Cryobiology. 1983;20:657-76.
17. Henry MA, Noiles EE, Gao D, et al. Cryopreservation of human spermatozoa. IV. The effects of cooling rate and warming rate on the maintenance of motility, plasma membrane integrity, and mitochondrial function. Fertil Steril. 1993;60:911-8.
18. Curry MR, Watson PF. Osmotic effects on ram and human sperm membranes in relation to thawing injury. Cryobiology. 1994;31:39-46.
19. Meyers SA. Spermatozoal response to osmotic stress. Anim Reprod Sci. 2005;89:57-64.
20. Giraud MN, Motta C, Boucher D, et al. Membrane fluidity predicts the outcome of cryopreservation of human spermatozoa. Hum Reprod. 2000;15:2160-4.
21. Barthelemy C, Royere D, Hammahah S, et al. Ultrastructural changes in membranes and acrosome of human sperm during cryopreservation. Arch Androl. 1990;25:29-40.

22. Oehninger S, Duru NK, Srisombut C, et al. Assessment of sperm cryodamage and strategies to improve outcome. Mol Cell Endocrinol. 2000;169:3-10.
23. Hammerstedt RH, Graham JK, Nolan JP. Cryopreservation of mammalian sperm: what we ask them to survive. J Androl. 1990;11:73-88.
24. Martin G, Sabido O, Durand P, et al. Cryopreservation induces an apoptosis-like mechanism in bull sperm. Biol Reprod. 2004;71:28-37.
25. Thomson LK, Fleming SD, Aitken RJ, et al. Cryopreservation-induced human sperm DNA damage is predominantly mediated by oxidative stress rather than apoptosis. Hum Reprod. 2009;24:2061-70.
26. Wang AW, Zhang H, Ikemoto I, et al. Reactive oxygen species generation by seminal cells during cryopreservation. Urology. 1997;49:921-5.
27. Lasso JL, Noiles EE, Alvarez JG, et al. Mechanism of superoxide dismutase loss from human sperm cells during cryopreservation. J Androl. 1994;15:255-65.
28. Taylor K, Roberts P, Sanders K, et al. Effect of antioxidant supplementation of cryopreservation medium on post-thaw integrity of human spermatozoa. Reprod Biomed Online. 2009;18:184-9.
29. Li Z, Lin Q, Liu R, et al. Protective effects of ascorbate and catalase on human spermatozoa during cryopreservation. J Androl. 2009.
30. Gosalvez J, Cortes-Gutierez E, Lopez-Fernandez C, et al. Sperm deoxyribonucleic acid fragmentation dynamics in fertile donors. Fertil Steril. 2009;92:170-3.
31. Isachenko V, Isachenko E, Katkov II, et al. Cryoprotectant-free cryopreservation of human spermatozoa by vitrification and freezing in vapor: effect on motility, DNA integrity, and fertilization ability. Biol Reprod. 2004;71:1167-73.
32. Grunewald S, Paasch U, Wuendrich K, et al. Sperm caspases become more activated in infertility patients than in healthy donors during cryopreservation. Arch Androl. 2005;51:449-60.
33. Wundrich K, Paasch U, Leicht M, et al. Activation of caspases in human spermatozoa during cryopreservation—an immuno-blot study. Cell Tissue Bank. 2006;7:81-90.
34. Saleh RA, Agarwal A. Oxidative stress and male infertility: from research bench to clinical practice. J Androl. 2002;23:737-52.
35. Borges Jr E, Rossi LM, Locambo de Freitas CV, et al. Fertilization and pregnancy outcome after intracytoplasmic injection with fresh or cryopreserved ejaculated spermatozoa. Fertil Steril. 2007;87:316-20.
36. Donnelly ET, Steele EK, McClure N, et al. Assessment of DNA integrity and morphology of ejaculated spermatozoa from fertile and infertile men before and after cryopreservation. Hum Reprod. 2001;16:1191-9.
37. Said TM, Tellez S, Evenson DP, et al. Assessment of sperm quality, DNA integrity and cryopreservation protocols in men diagnosed with testicular and systemic malignancies. Andrologia. 2009;41:377-82.
38. de Paula TS, Bertolla RP, Spaine DM, et al. Effect of cryopreservation on sperm apoptotic deoxyribonucleic acid fragmentation in patients with oligozoospermia. Fertil Steril. 2006;86:597-600.
39. Sakkas D, Manicardi GC, Tomlinson M, et al. The use of two density gradient centrifugation techniques and the swim-up method to separate spermatozoa with chromatin and nuclear DNA anomalies. Hum Reprod. 2000;15:1112-6.
40. Allamaneni SS, Agarwal A, Rama S, et al. Comparative study on density gradients and swim-up preparation techniques utilizing neat and cryopreserved spermatozoa. Asian J Androl. 2005;7:86-92.
41. Ricci G, Perticarar S, Boscolo R, et al. Semen preparation methods and sperm apoptosis: swim-up versus gradient-density centrifugation technique. Fertil Steril. 2009;91:632-8.
42. Grunewald S, Paasch U, Said TM, et al. Magnetic-activated cell sorting before cryopreservation preserves mitochondrial integrity in human spermatozoa. Cell Tissue Bank. 2006;7:99-104.
43. Said TM, Grunewald S, Paasch U, et al. Effects of magnetic-activated cell sorting on sperm motility and cryosurvival rates. Fertil Steril. 2005;83:1442-6.
44. Said T, Agarwal A, Grunewald S, et al. Selection of nonapoptotic spermatozoa as a new tool for enhancing assisted reproduction outcomes: an in vitro model. Biol Reprod. 2006;74:530-7.
45. Said TM, Agarwal A, Grunewald S, et al. Evaluation of sperm recovery following annexin V magnetic-activated cell sorting separation. Reprod Biomed Online. 2006;13:336-9.
46. Said TM, Agarwal A, Zborowski M, et al. Utility of magnetic cell separation as a molecular sperm preparation technique. J Androl. 2008;29:134-42.
47. Hallak J, Sharma RK, Wellstead C, et al. Cryopreservation of human spermatozoa: comparison of TEST-yolk buffer and glycerol. Int J Fertil Womens Med. 2000;45:38-2.
48. Nallella KP, Sharma RK, Allamanen SS, et al. Cryopreservation of human spermatozoa: comparison of two cryopreservation methods and three cryoprotectants. Fertil Steril. 2004;82:913-8.
49. Duru NK, Morshedi MS, Schuffner A, et al. Cryopreservation-thawing of fractionated human spermatozoa is associated with membrane phosphatidylserine externalization and not DNA fragmentation. J Androl. 2001;22:646-51.
50. Hammadeh ME, Greiner S, Rosenbaum P, et al. Comparison between human sperm preservation medium and TEST-yolk buffer on protecting chromatin and morphology integrity of human spermatozoa in fertile and subfertile men after freeze-thawing procedure. J Androl. 2001;22:1012-8.
51. Alvarez JG, Storey BT. Evidence for increased lipid peroxidative damage resulting from freeze/thaw-induced loss of superoxide dismutase activity as a mode of sublethal cryodamage to human sperm during cryopreservation. J Androl. 1992;13:232-41.
52. Muratori M, Maggi M, Spinelli S, et al. Spontaneous DNA fragmentation in swim-up-selected human spermatozoa during long-term incubation. J Androl. 2003;24:253-62.
53. Chatterjee S, Gagnon C. Production of reactive oxygen species by spermatozoa undergoing cooling, freezing and thawing. Mol Reprod Dev. 2001;59:451-8.
54. Chatterjee S, de Lamirande E, Gagnon C. Cryopreservation alters sulphydryl status of bull spermatozoa: protection by oxidized glutathione. Mol Reprod Dev. 2001;60:498-506.

55. Gandini L, Lombardo F, Lenzi A, et al. Cryopreservation and sperm DNA integrity. Cell Tissue Bank. 2006;7:91-8.

56. Schuffner A, Morshedi M, Oehninger S. Cryopreservation of fractionated, highly motile human spermatozoa: effect on membrane phosphatidylserine externalization and lipid peroxidation. Hum Reprod. 2001;16:2148-53.

57. Watson PF. The causes of reduced fertility with cryopreserved semen. Anim Reprod Sci. 2000;2:481-92.

58. Lopes S, Sun J, Jurisicova A, et al. Sperm deoxyribonucleic acid fragmentation is increased in poor-quality semen samples and correlates with failed fertilization in intracytoplasmic sperm injection. Fertil Steril. 1998;69:528-32.

59. Meseguer M, Martinez-Conejero JA, O'Connor JE, et al. The significance of sperm DNA oxidation in embryo development and reproductive outcome in an oocyte donation program: a new model to study a male infertility prognostic factor. Fertil Steril. 2008;89:1191-9.

60. Moustafa MH, Sharma RK, Thornton J, et al. Relationship between ROS production, apoptosis and DNA denaturation in spermatozoa from patients examined for infertility. Hum Reprod. 2004;19:129-38.

61. Pasqualotto FF, Sharma RK, Nelson DR, et al. Relationship between oxidative stress, semen characteristics, and clinical diagnosis in men undergoing infertility investigation. Fertil Steril. 2000;73:459-64.

62. Cocuzza M, Sikka SC, Athayde KS, et al. Clinical relevance of oxidative stress and sperm chromatin damage in male infertility: an evidence based analysis. Int Braz J Urol. 2007;33:603-21.

63. Aitken RJ, Gordon E, Harkiss D, et al. Relative impact of oxidative stress on the functional competence and genomic integrity of human spermatozoa. Biol Reprod. 1998;59:1037-46.

64. Kodama H, Yamaguchi R, Fukuda J, et al. Increased oxidative deoxyribonucleic acid damage in the spermatozoa of infertile male patients. Fertil Steril. 1997;68:519-24.

65. Henkel R, Kierspel E, Hajimohammad M, et al. DNA fragmentation of spermatozoa and assisted reproduction technology. Repro Biomed Online. 2003;7:477-84.

66. Dominguez-Fandos D, Camejo MI, Ballesca JL, et al. Human sperm DNA fragmentation: correlation of TUNEL results as assessed by flow cytometry and optical microscopy. Cytometry A. 2007;71:1011-8.

67. Zini A, Libman J. Sperm DNA damage: clinical significance in the era of assisted reproduction. CMAJ. 2006;175:495-500.

68. Shamsi MB, Kumar R, Dada R. Evaluation of nuclear DNA damage in human spermatozoa in men opting for assisted reproduction. Indian J Med Res. 2008;127:115-23.

69. Cancer Research UK (2009). CancerStats. [online] Available from http://info.cancerresearchuk.org/cancerstats/ [Accessed February, 2015].

70. Gatta G, Zigon G, Capocaccia R, et al. Survival of European children and young adults with cancer diagnosed. Eur J Cancer. 2009;45:992-1005.

71. Donnez J, Martinez-Madrid B, Jadoul, et al. Ovarian tissue cryopreservation and transplantation: a review. Hum Reprod Update. 2006;12:519-35.

72. Rueffer U, Breuer K, Josting A, et al. Male gonadal dysfunction in patients with Hodgkin's disease prior to treatment. Ann Oncol. 2001;12:1307-11.

73. Orwig KE, Schlatt S. Cryopreservation and transplantation of spermatogonia and testicular tissue for preservation of male fertility. J Natl Cancer Inst Monogr. 2005;34:51-6.

74. Wallace WH, Anderson RA, Irvine DS. Fertility preservation for young patients with cancer: who is at risk and what can be offered? Lancet Oncol. 2005;6:209-18.

75. Meistrich ML, Finch M, da Cunha MF, et al. Damaging effects of fourteen chemotherapeutic drugs on mouse testis cells. Cancer Res. 1982;42:122-31.

76. Gandini L, Sgro P, Lombardo F, et al. Effect of chemo or radiotherapy on sperm parameters of testicular cancer patients. Hum Reprod. 2006;21:2882-9.

77. Bahadur G, Ozturk O, Muneer A, et al. Semen quality before and after gonadotoxic treatment. Hum Reprod. 2005;20:774-81.

78. Dohle GR. Male infertility in cancer patients: review of the literature. Int J Urol. 2010;17:327-31.

79. Chian RC, Huang JY, Gilbert L, et al. Obstetric outcomes following vitrification of in vitro and in vivo matured oocytes. Fertil Steril. 2009;91:2391-8.

80. Andersen CY, Rosendahl M, Byskov AG, et al. Two successful pregnancies following autotransplantation of frozen/thawed ovarian tissue. Hum Reprod. 2008;23:2266-72.

81. Partridge AH, Gelber S, Peppercorn J, et al. Web-based survey of fertility issues in young women with breast cancer. J Clin Oncol. 2004;22:4174-83.

82. Ethics Committee of the American Society for Reproductive Medicine. Fertility preservation and reproduction in cancer patients. Fertil Steril. 2005;83:1622-8.

83. Fernandez-Santos MR, Esteso MC, Montoro V, et al. Influence of various permeating cryoprotectants on freezability of Iberian red deer (Cervus elaphus hispanicus) epididymal spermatozoa: effects of concentration and temperature of addition. J Androl. 2006;27:734-45.

84. Menon S, Rives N, Mousset-Simeon N, et al. Fertility preservation in adolescent males: experience over 22 years at Rouen University Hospital. Hum Reprod. 2009;24:37-44.

85. Blackhall FH, Atkinson AD, Maaya MB, et al. Semen cryopreservation, utilisation and reproductive outcome in men treated for Hodgkin's disease. Br J Cancer. 2002;87:381-4.

86. Bartoov B, Berkovitz A, Eltes F. Selection of spermatozoa with normal nuclei to improve the pregnancy rate with intra cytoplasmic sperm injection. N Engl J Med. 2001;345:1067-8.

87. Antinori M, Licata E, Dani G, et al. Intracytoplasmic morphologically selected sperm injection: a prospective randomized trial. Reprod Biomed Online. 2008;16:835-41.

88. Gatimel N, Leandri R, Parinaud J. Sperm vacuoles are not modified by freezing–thawing procedures. Reprod Biomed Online. 2013;26:240-6.

89. Kalthur G, Adiga SK, Upadhya D, et al. 2008. Effect of cryopreservation on sperm DNA integrity in patients with teratospermia. Fertil Steril. 2008;89:1723-7.

90. Hammadeh ME, Greiner S, Rosenbaum P, et al. Comparison between human sperm preservation medium and TEST-yolk buffer on protecting chromatin and morphology integrity of human spermatozoa in fertile and subfertile men after freeze–thawing procedure. J Androl. 2001;22:1012-8.

91. AbdelHafez F, Bedaiwy M, El-Nashar SA, et al. Techniques for cryopreservation of individual or small numbers of human spermatozoa: a systematic review. Hum Reprod Update. 2009;15:153-64.

92. Endo Y, Fujii Y, Shintani K, et al. Single spermatozoon freezing using Cryotop. J Mamm Ova Res. 2011;28:47-52.

93. Bielanski A, Vajta G. Risk of contamination of germplasm during cryopreservation and cryobanking in IVF units. Hum Reprod. 2009;24;2457-67.

94. Cohen J, Garrisi GJ, Congedo-Ferrara TA, et al. Cryopreservation of single human spermatozoa. Hum Reprod. 1997;12:994-1001.

95. Walmsley R, Cohen J, Ferrara-Congedo T, et al. The first births and ongoing pregnancies associated with sperm cryopreservation within evacuated egg zonae. Hum Reprod. 1998;13(Suppl 4):61-70.

96. Vajta G, Reichart A. Risk of contamination of germplasm during cryopreservation and cryobanking in IVF units. Hum Reprod. 2011;26:i42-3.

97. Gimenez JR, Cabal AC, Santos MJ, et al. Viral screening of spent culture media and liquid nitrogen samples of oocytes or embryos coming from HIV, HCV, and HBV chronically infected women undergoing IVF cycles. Hum Reprod. 2011;26:i45.

98. Endo Y, Fujii Y, Shintani K, et al. Simple vitrification for small numbers of human spermatozoa. RBM Online. 2012;24:301-7.

99. Cayli S, Jakab A, Ovari L, et al. Biochemical markers of sperm function: male fertility and sperm selection for ICSI. Reprod Biomed Online. 2003;7:462-8.

44 Fertility Preservation in Cancer (Male and Female)

Bina Vasan

INTRODUCTION

For many people, cancer is the most feared health diagnosis imaginable and brings about immediate thoughts of death. Even cancer healthcare providers have been shown to exhibit a sense of hopelessness and negative attitudes toward a cancer diagnosis.[1] Yet, overall cancer survival rates have been increasing over the past 30 years, suggesting that a diagnosis of cancer should not necessarily be associated with impending death or giving up hope of survival.[2] Five-year cancer survival rates over the past 30 years have increased from 56% to 64% for adults and 56% to 75% for pediatric and adolescent cancers.[3] As a result, there are approximately 450,000 cancer survivors between the ages of 19 and 39 in the current population. The exact risk of infertility from chemotherapy or radiation depends mostly on the age of the patient, the type of therapy, the site of the cancer, and the stage of the disease.[4] Studies suggest that between 40% and 80% of female cancer patients are at risk of becoming infertile, and between one-third and three-quarters of male cancer patients may become sterile following treatment for cancer.[5]

EFFECTS OF CANCER AND ITS TREATMENT ON FERTILITY

Early detection and improvements in screening have increased the number of premenopausal women diagnosed with cancer. As a result, it is estimated that a malignancy will be diagnosed in one among 46 women under the age of 40 years. Based on the cancer diagnosis, it is estimated that approximately half of these women will receive some form of gonadotoxic treatment; hence approximately 1% of females with reproductive potential are at risk. With recent advances in cancer therapy, many of these patients will be cured by combination treatment with chemotherapy, radiotherapy and/or surgery.[6] The ovary is particularly sensitive to the adverse effects of cancer treatments because of the set number of follicles present in the postnatal ovary. Reproductive lifespan is determined by the follicle pool, and therefore, cancer treatments that cause follicular depletion accelerate the onset of menopause.[7] Medical interventions including chemotherapy, radiotherapy and surgery act as insults to ovarian reserve, and may result in premature ovarian failure and infertility. However, of all the patients at risk for premature ovarian failure, very few are advised to go for fertility preservation **(Fig. 1)**.

The extent of ovarian damage is drug and dose dependent and correlates to age at the time of treatment. There is an increased potential for ovarian failure with advancing age of the patient.[8] Total body, abdominal or pelvic irradiation can cause ovarian and uterine damage depending on radiation dose, fractionation schedule and age at the time of treatment. Multiple strategies have emerged aiming to preserve fertility in women with different types of malignancies.[9] These include embryo and oocyte cryopreservation, cortical and whole ovary cryopreservation, ovarian transplantation, ovarian transposition and gonadotropin-releasing hormone (GnRH) agonist protection. Currently, embryo and mature oocyte cryopreservation following in vitro fertilization (IVF) are the only techniques endorsed by the American Society of Reproductive Medicine, and the other methods are still considered to be investigational. In males, cryopreservation of sperms is a well-standardized treatment. Other methods of fertility preservation in men include cryopreservation of testicular tissue and radiation shielding of the testes during radiation therapy.

Male Reproductive System

Almost 30% of men with testicular cancer have semen abnormalities at the time of diagnosis. Interestingly, semen abnormalities are also common among young men at the time of diagnosis with other cancers. For example, in a study of 158 untreated men (aged 16–52

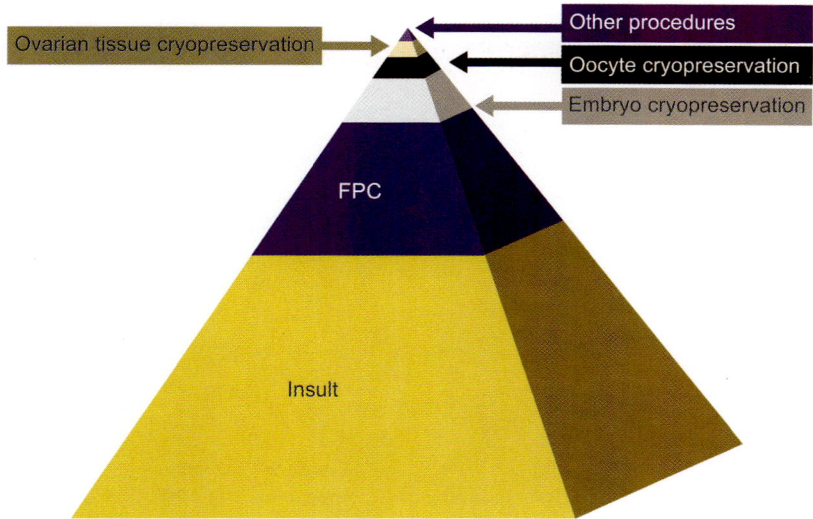

Fig. 1 Pyramid of cancer risk and fertility preservation

years) recently diagnosed with Hodgkin's lymphoma, 111 (70%) had semen abnormalities prior to treatment.[10]

Spermatogenesis is a highly prolific process. Therefore, the germinal epithelium is extremely sensitive to the effects of chemotherapy and radiotherapy, which target rapidly dividing cells.[11] Subfertility is observed in a majority of men who receive alkylating agents plus radiotherapy (above or below the diaphragm) for the treatment of cancer. Radiation doses of only 0.1–1.2 Gray (Gy) can impair spermatogenesis and doses of more than 4 Gy may cause permanent damage. The mechanism of disruption of spermatogenesis is uncertain, but is believed to involve depletion of both stem cells and differentiating spermatogonia.[12,13] Spermatogenesis declines during the 3–6 months following chemotherapy or radiotherapy for testicular cancer, but steadily recovers thereafter.[14] Following 2 years after treatment, 97% and 94% of men treated with chemotherapy or radiotherapy (with shielding of the contralateral testicle), respectively, show good recovery of spermatogenesis.[14] In contrast, the prevalence of azoospermia among men treated for lymphoma is reported to be as high as 59% and a long recovery period (up to 45 months) is needed to achieve the highest sperm concentration.[15]

Figure 2 represents the types of damage occurring to the sperm from various cancer treatments. Chemotherapeutic agents have deleterious effects on spermatogenesis. Similar to radiation therapy, Leydig cells may incur damage following chemotherapy resulting in subsequent hypogonadism.[16] However, with advances in chemotherapy delivery, side effects have been minimized using synergistic agents at lower toxic doses but a risk of

infertility is still present. The extent of gonadal damage is largely dependent on the type, the age of the patient, and the extent of the chemotherapeutic agent administered. **Table 1** highlights some common chemotherapeutic agents and their effect on spermatogenesis.

There is compelling evidence of short-term deoxyribonucleic acid (DNA) damage to sperm following cancer treatment,[17,18] but a reduction in DNA integrity among long-term survivors has yet to be proven.[19] The impact of chemotherapy regimens on spermatogenesis depends on the type of chemotherapeutic agents used and the cumulative dose given.[20] Chemotherapeutic agents may disrupt spermatogenesis by targeting various testicular cell types (Leydig cells, Sertoli cells and germ cells) and by activating numerous molecular pathways involved in germ-cell metabolism. In particular, p53 and the Fas system have been shown to have roles as modulators of proapoptotic activity in the testis.[16] Alkylating agents,

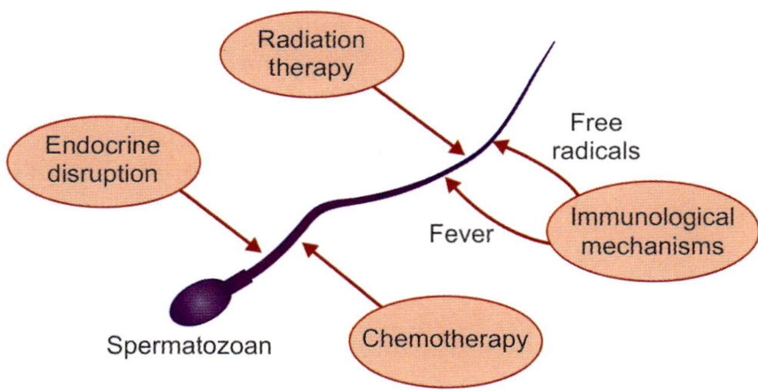

Fig. 2 Etiology of sperm damage during cancer treatment

Table 1 Effect of chemotherapeutic agents on spermatogenesis

Agent	Mechanism of action	Example(s)	Some diseases utilizing drugs	Effect on spermatogenesis
Platinum-based agents	Cross-linking DNA, impair DNA synthesis/ transcription and function	Cisplatin, carboplatin	Bladder cancer, germ cell tumor, HL, NHL	Spermatogensis affected, possible chromosomal aberrations[19] Less impact with carboplatin
Antimetabolites	Interferes with DNA transcription	Fluorouracil, 6-mercaptopurine, methotrexate, gemcitabine	Colorectal cancer, HL, NHL, bladder cancer, leukemia	Spermatogenesis affected[21], possible chromosomal aberrations
Vinca alkyloids	Inhibit microtubule polymerization	Vincristine, vinblastine	HL, NHL, leukemia	Arrest in spermatogesis and affects spermatozoa motility[23] Vinblastine is cytotoxic to primary spermatocytes[24]
Alkylating agents	DNA base pair alkylation, formation of abnormal DNA cross-bridges, and mis-pairing of nucleotides	Busulfan, cyclophosphamide, chlorambucil, procarbazine, ifosdamide	Germ cell tumors, sarcomas, HL, NHL	Most toxic class; Induces azoospermia withing 90 days[25] Irreversible effect[7,26] mutagenic in all stages of spermatogenesis; but does not cause aneuploidy[27]
Topoisomerase inhibitors	Prevents DNA supercoiling and interfere with DNA transcription/replication	Etoposide, doxorubicine	Sarcomas, germ cell tumors, HL, NHL	Cytotoxic with possible chromosomal anomalies[28]

Abbreviations: HL, Hodgkin's lymphoma; NHL, Non-Hodgkin's lymphoma; DNA, Deoxyribonucleic acid

such as procarbazine, cyclophosphamide and cisplatin, carry the greatest risks of infertility.[21] A high incidence of aneuploidy in sperm has been reported following some chemotherapy regimens.[22] Animal studies suggest that combination treatment with bleomycin, etoposide and cis-platinum, a chemotherapy cocktail used to treat testicular cancer, alters sperm chromatin quality which may have adverse effects on progeny outcome.[23] However, there is no evidence to date on the increased incidence of congenital abnormalities among the children of male cancer survivors.[24,25]

The somatic (Sertoli and Leydig) cells of the testis are more resistant to the effects of cancer treatments than germ cells. Doses of 30 Gy are required to cause Leydig cell dysfunction in adults.[26] Therefore, steroidogenesis in males is usually maintained after radiotherapy treatment, albeit by compensatory elevation of luteinizing hormone (LH) concentrations.[15] Nonetheless, men should be informed of the potential gonadotoxicity of cancer treatment **(Table 2)**.

Female Reproductive System

There is no evidence of a direct effect of cancer on the female reproductive system; however, its treatment may adversely affect various sites in the reproductive tract. Doses of radiation of 14–30 Gy administered in childhood to the whole body or abdomen compromise growth and development of the uterus.[27-31] Uterine radiotherapy in childhood or adolescence is associated with an increased incidence of spontaneous miscarriage and intrauterine growth retardation in subsequent pregnancies. These effects are believed to be secondary to vascular damage and reduced elasticity of the myometrium. Data from the Childhood Cancer Survivor Study showed that women treated with pelvic irradiation and/or increasing alkylating agent doses were at risk for acute ovarian failure, premature menopause and having offspring born small for gestational age.[30] Small ovarian volume in female survivors of childhood cancer has also been reported.[31] Exposure to chemotherapy or radiotherapy profoundly depletes the number of follicles present in the ovary. Follicular damage

Table 2 Cytotoxic agents according to degree of gonadotoxicity

Level of risk	Cytotoxic agent
High-risk	Cyclophosphamide, chlorambucil, melphalan, busulfan, nitrogen mustard, procarbazine
Intermediate risk	Cisplatin, adriamycin
Low/no risk	Methotrexate, 5-fluorouracil, vincristine, bleomycin, actinomycin D

in females affects both endocrine and reproductive functions. As the size of the ovarian follicular pool is predefined, follicular destruction may cause premature ovarian failure or advanced menopause. The lethal dose of radiation required to kill half of the primordial follicles in the ovaries is estimated to be less than 2 Gy. Treatment with alkylating agents such as, cyclophosphamide during adolescence increases the risk of premature ovarian failure.[32] Cyclophosphamide treatment appears to exert its ovarian toxicity by significantly reducing primordial follicle count; this has been demonstrated in animals[33] and a real-time quantitative evidence of such an effect has been described in a human ovarian xenograft model.[34] Premature ovarian failure following chemotherapy occurs more frequently in older than younger women.[35] It is suggested that exposure to gonadotoxic treatment at a younger age leads to the loss of more follicles than at an older age.[36] Thus, younger women treated for cancer lose more years of normal ovarian function than do their older counterparts.[36] However, as noted above, older patients have lower ovarian reserve than younger women, and therefore, have a higher risk of ovarian failure during or after chemotherapy or radiation therapy. Markers of ovarian age, such as the antral follicle count and anti-Müllerian hormone (AMH), before, during and after chemotherapy may help to evaluate the extent of ovarian damage due to cancer treatment.[37,38] A recent study of 17 women undergoing chemotherapy showed that AMH and inhibin B concentrations immediately declined in response to chemotherapy and that the follicular target of chemotherapy appeared to be growing follicles.[39] High pretreatment AMH concentrations were predictive of a higher post-treatment AMH concentration. The extent of damage induced by radiotherapy depends on the field of treatment, total dose and fractionation schedule. Low-dose cranial irradiation for central nervous system tumors may impair fertility by disruption of the hypothalamic-pituitary-ovarian axis,[40-42] although this effect may become apparent only after many years cancer treatment. Radiation causes a dose-related reduction in the primordial follicle pool.[43] The human oocyte is extremely sensitive to radiation, and irradiation at ovarian dose more than 6 Gy usually causes irreversible ovarian failure and demonstrated that less than 4 Gy is enough to destroy half of the oocyte population (LDL_{50} <4 Gy). However, very recently, Meirow et al. used a revised mathematical model to suggest that the LDL_{50} of the oocytes was <2 Gy. Age at the time of exposure to radiotherapy, extent and type of radiation therapy (e.g. abdominal, pelvic external beam irradiation and intracavitary brachytherapy) and fractionation schedule are important prognostic indicators for development of ovarian failure.[44]

PATIENTS' DILEMMA: COPING WITH CANCER AND DECISION ON FERTILITY PRESERVATION

Diagnosis of any malignancy has a major impact on the life of any person. The extent of impact can vary with the type of cancer, treatment prospects, emotional support available, financial resources and loss of career due to physical debility. In a young individual there may be additional burden due to potential loss of reproductive function.[45] After the acute phase of diagnosis and treatment, patients must adjust to living their lives as cancer survivors. A survey of cancer patients has found that many of them expressed a strong desire to be informed about the available options for fertility preservation. The same survey also revealed their desire to have children if there was remission or cure. If cancer survivors are not able to reproduce by normal sexual activity, they have the option of assisted reproduction or storage of gametes and tissues.[46] Donor gametes and gestational surrogacy are also the other options available. However, fertility preservation in children is more complicated as there are ethical considerations.

MALIGNANT CONDITIONS NECESSITATING FERTILITY PRESERVATION

Childhood Cancers

Cancer is the second leading cause of death in children between the ages of 1 year and 14 years.[47] The cure rates from childhood cancers have improved markedly over the last three decades, thanks to cancer treatment that includes combined chemotherapy and/or radiotherapy, and hematopoietic stem cell transplantation. Five-year survival is now more than 80% for all cancers combined, which is between 80% and 86% for childhood acute lymphoblastic leukemia (ALL), and more than 90% for Hodgkin's disease.[48-50] Around 2,000 patients are estimated to become long-term survivors of ALL each year, the most common childhood malignancy.[51] In addition to leukemias, patients who face the risk of ovarian failure due to cytotoxic treatment are those with Hodgkin's lymphoma, neuroblastoma, non-Hodgkin's lymphoma, Wilms' tumor, Ewing's sarcoma and osteosarcoma of the pelvis and genital rhabdomyosarcoma.[52-55]

Breast Cancer

Breast cancer is the most common malignant disease in women of reproductive age. In the USA, an estimated 200,000 new cases of invasive breast cancer were expected to be diagnosed each year (Flow chart 1). The incidence of female breast cancer has increased since 1986, but the death rates decreased in the early 1990s; 2.5% per year in white women, and 1.0% per year in black women.[56] One out of every 228 women will develop breast cancer before the age of 40 years, and about 15% of all breast cancer cases are estimated to occur at less than 40 years.[57] Many of these patients will be subjected to multi-agent, mainly cyclophosphamide-based, cytotoxic chemotherapy.[58] In breast cancer, because chemotherapy is usually initiated 6 weeks after the surgery, there is adequate time for controlled ovarian stimulation (COS) to preserve fertility by oocyte or embryo cryopreservation. Because conventional ovulation induction regimens are deemed risky for breast cancer patients due to resultant surge in estradiol levels, potentially safer regimens including tamoxifen or aromatase inhibitors have been introduced.[59] Embryo cryopreservation using letrozole is a novel stimulation protocol in breast cancer patients; however, long-term follow-up data are awaited. Cryopreservation of ovarian tissue and oocyte are experimental technologies.[60]

Cancer of the Cervix

Cancer of the cervix is a serious health problem affecting 500,000 women each year worldwide. In the year 2002, 13,000 new cervical cancer cases were diagnosed in North America and roughly half of them occurred before the age of 35 years.[60] Over the past three decades, while the incidence of squamous cell carcinoma of the cervix decreased by 42%, the incidence of adenocarcinoma of the cervix has increased by 29%.[61] Ovarian involvement is extremely rare in squamous cell cervical carcinoma, but it is encountered in up to 12% of the cases with adenocarcinoma and adenosquamous carcinoma of the cervix.[62,63]

Patients Receiving Pelvic Radiation

Radiotherapy is utilized to improve prognosis or to achieve local tumor control in some solid tumors presenting in the pelvis, such as, Ewing sarcoma, osteosarcoma, retroperitoneal sarcoma, and in some benign bone tumors.[64-69] Radiation therapy also plays an important part in the management of rectal cancer.[70] These patients can resort to ovarian, oocyte or embryo cryopreservation, and alternatively oophoropexy may also be considered, especially if an abdominal surgery is necessary for the treatment of the primary disease.

Endometrial Cancer

Endometrial cancer is an estrogen-sensitive malignancy which is encountered in women of reproductive age. The accepted treatment of endometrial cancer in young women requires total abdominal hysterectomy and bilateral salpingo-oophorectomy. However, many of these patients have not initiated or completed child bearing and

Flow chart 1 A proposed algorithmic approach to decision-making for fertility preservation in breast cancer patients

Abbreviations: TMX, tamoxifen; FP, fertility preservation; cryo, cryopreservation

progestin treatment has been used to preserve fertility in women with stage 1, grade 1–2 endometrial carcinoma. In earlier studies where assisted reproductive technologies were used in cases with existing endometrial cancer, typically a high-dose progestin treatment was performed prior to attempts for IVF with conventional stimulation protocols. Those stimulation regimens generally expose patients to high estrogen levels, and no attempt was made to protect the endometrium against the effects of estrogen. As the elevation of estradiol levels is undesirable, the use of aromatase inhibitors has been developed for ovarian stimulation in patients with endometrial cancer. As tamoxifen is stimulatory on the endometrium, it cannot be used for ovarian stimulation in cases of endometrial cancer. Embryo cryopreservation is a good option for patients who cannot have conservative management or, who do not respond to progestins and need surgical treatment.

Cancers in Males

Male survivors of childhood cancer have an estimated 46% overall reduction in the likelihood of eventually siring a pregnancy.[71] Thomson et al. have reported that only 33% of male survivors of childhood cancers have normal semen quality.[72] The germinal epithelium is very sensitive to chemotherapy, especially to the alkylating agents which exert their effects via direct damage to DNA and ribonucleic acid (RNA) as well as the induction of apoptosis.[73,74] Sixty-three percent of adolescent patients treated with mechlorethamine, vincristine, procarbazine and prednisone for Hodgkin disease were azoospermic after a median duration of 10 years of treatment.[75] Leydig cells appear to be much less sensitive to most chemotherapeutic regimens; however, elevated stimulated LH levels were demonstrated in 87.8% of boys who underwent treatment for Hodgkin disease, likely secondary to procarbazine administration.[76] The germinal epithelium is also sensitive to the effects of irradiation.

The largest cohort study to date, with greater power than previous studies, examined all singleton births in Denmark and Sweden between 1994 and 2004, to show that a 17% increased risk of major congenital abnormalities exists in the offspring of male cancer survivors.[77] This risk was independent of whether natural conception or assisted reproductive technology was employed. Whether this increased risk can be attributed to the effects of cancer treatment, a systemic genetic instability leading to both the development of cancer and conception of a child with a birth defect, or an effect of the cancer itself on the integrity of sperm DNA remains to be fully investigated.[78]

The process of fertility preservation in male cancer patients may be taken according to the **Flow chart 2**.

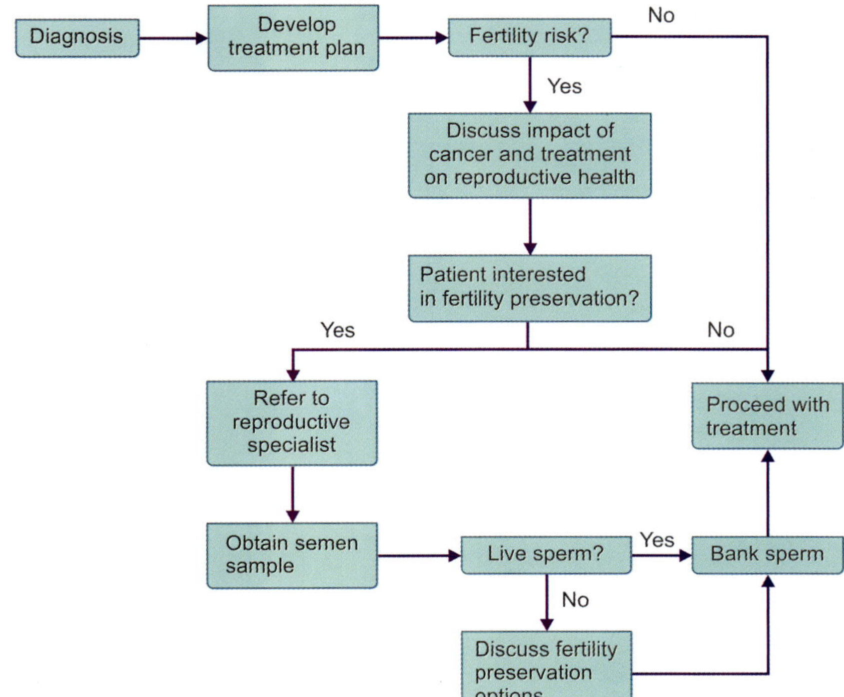

Flow chart 2 Process of fertility preservation in male cancer patients

■ METHODS OF FERTILITY PRESERVATION IN MALES

Fertility Preservation Options for the Adult Male

There are two standard options for men diagnosed with cancer who wish to preserve their fertility:
1. Sperm banking prior to cancer therapy
2. Radiation shielding of the testes during radiation therapy.

The American Society of Clinical Oncology (ASCO) and the American Society for Reproductive Medicine (ASRM) recommend that, when possible, at-risk patients should be referred to a fertility preservation specialist prior to starting cancer treatment. Men who are interested in fertility preservation prior to starting cancer therapy will provide a semen sample for analysis. The following chart illustrates fertility preservation options based on the results of the semen sample analysis **(Flow chart 3)**.

Semen Cryopreservation

Cryopreservation of sperm from semen samples is the most reliable option for fertility preservation in adult male patients. If time before cancer treatment allows, three samples of semen, produced at least 48 hours apart, may be preserved to maximize yield. Well-established, successful methods for the cryopreservation of human spermatozoa include the use of Tris-TES egg yolk-citrate medium with a slow cooling to 5°C followed by a faster freezing to -80°C, and then a rapid freeze to -196°C in about 30 seconds.[79] Glycerol is added as a cryoprotectant to help prevent ice crystal formation which can be damaging to cell membranes. However, glycerol may be toxic to human spermatozoa and thus they should be removed as quickly as possible after thawing.[79] Freezing spermatozoa with the seminal plasma appears to offer protection from cryoinjury.[80] One large study of male survivors of cancer with a mean follow-up of 57 months showed a rate of 9.6% for the use of cryopreserved semen.[81]

Flow chart 3 Fertility preservation options in males

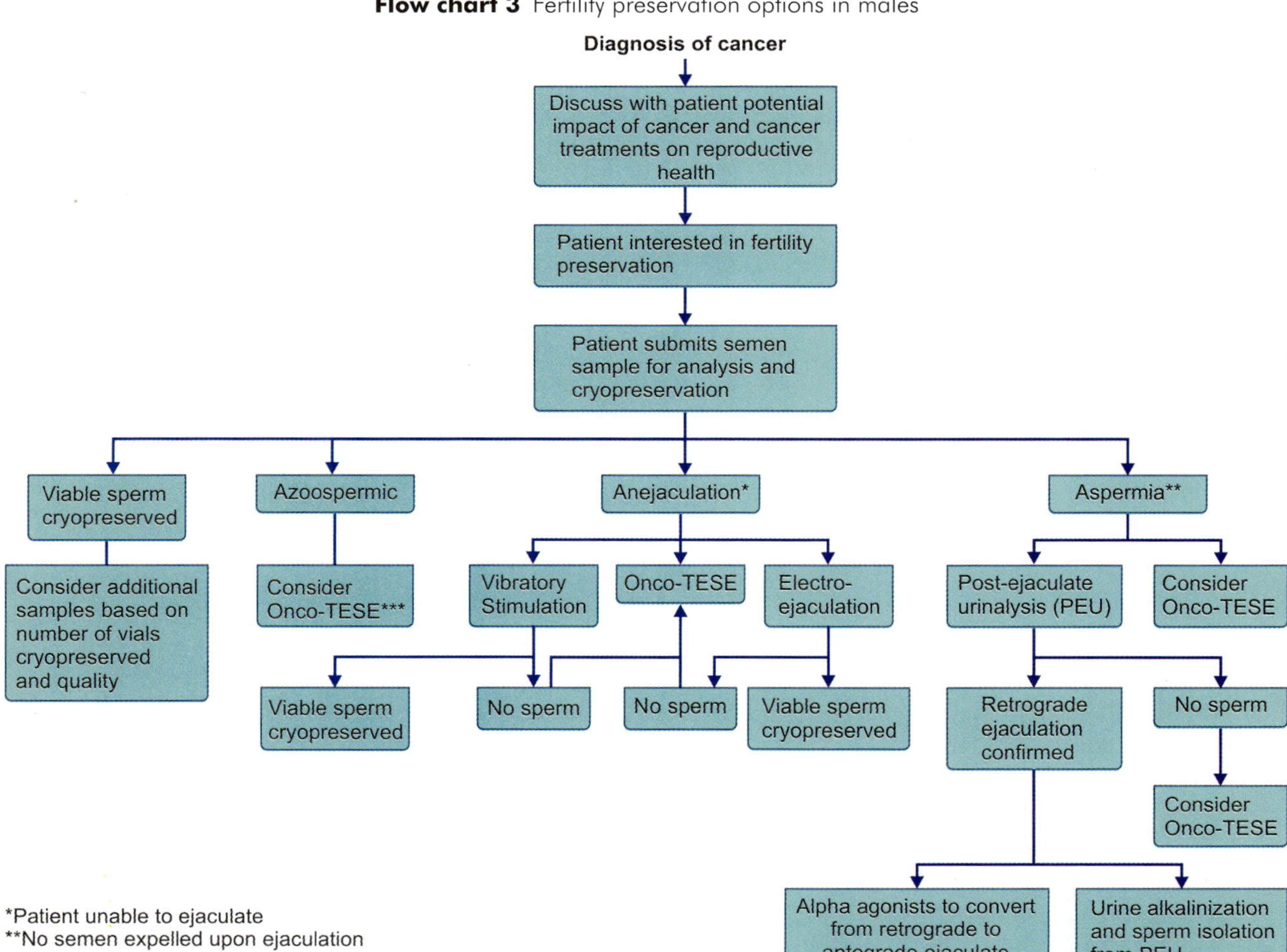

*Patient unable to ejaculate
**No semen expelled upon ejaculation
***Oncological testicular sperm extraction (Onco-TESE)

Many men with testicular and hematologic malignancies may present initially with subfertility. In one series, 49.8% of patients referred for semen banking were found to have fewer than 10,106 motile sperm per ejaculate, 13.8% were azoospermic, and 2.6% were unable to produce a sample.[82] Males with testicular cancer (the most common malignancy in men aged 15–35 years) are most likely to present with poor semen parameters before initiation of gonadotoxic therapies.[83] This may be related to a common risk factor for infertility and the development of testis cancer: cryptorchidism, immune mediated infertility, or the stress effects on spermatogenesis. In fact, sometimes the diagnosis of infertility precedes the cancer diagnosis.[84] Treatment may include orchiectomy, chemotherapy, retroperitoneal lymph node dissection with possible injury to the sympathetic nerves responsible for ejaculation, and in the case of seminoma, radiation therapy. With the advent of intracytoplasmic sperm injection (ICSI), conception is now possible for men with severe oligospermia or even azoospermic men with spermatozoa extracted from testicular tissue. In cases of nonobstructive azoospermia, sperm can be retrieved by microsurgical testicular sperm extraction (TESE) with a focus on identifying seminiferous tubules that appear wider in caliber and more opaque, which, therefore, may be more likely to harbor active spermatogenesis. Testicular spermatozoa should be cryopreserved to allow for future availability without the need for another surgical intervention. Baukloh et al. showed that the quality of isolated sperm from fresh testicular tissue was equivalent to that of thawed cryopreserved testicular sperm and yielded identical pregnancy rates.[85]

Cryopreservation of Testicular Tissue

Cryopreservation of intact testicular tissue has been more challenging because of loss of cell-cell adhesions, water trapped in tubules leading to ice crystal formation, and the different cryobiological properties of various cell types.[86] Vitrification—involving rapid freezing after dehydration and permeation of the cryoprotectant—has been the subject of recent investigations.[87] In mouse models, Gouk et al. have shown that the preservation of post-warming cell viability is superior with vitrification of testicular tissue compared to conventional slow freezing.[88]

Fertility Preservation Options in Prepubertal Males

For prepubertal patients who have not initiated spermatogenesis, investigators are examining cryopreservation of testicular tissue through either cell suspension or whole tissue as a possible option for fertility preservation. Tissue can be obtained through the techniques previously described, including TESE, microscopic epididymal sperm aspiration and testicular biopsy.

Cryopreservation of sperm in adolescent oncology patients as young as 13.5 years can be performed with success rates similar to adults, provided a semen sample can be produced.[89] Penile vibratory stimulation and electroejaculation under general anesthesia have been used to obtain sperm in pubertal boys who are not psychologically ready to produce a semen sample.[90]

Investigators from the Children's Hospital of Philadelphia recently published reports of 24 prepubertal boys who underwent testicular biopsy with tissue cryopreservation for fertility preservation at the time of surgical central line placement.[91] Despite this and other similar experimental protocols reporting preservation of prepubertal testicular tissue, no study to date has demonstrated a technique to transform this immature, cryopreserved testicular tissue into functional gametes either in vivo or in vitro.

Cryopreserved testicular tissue from prepubertal boys cannot currently be used in a clinical setting, because the post-meiotic sperm required for fertilization has not yet been developed. Although there is potential for the future development of technology allowing the use of immature testicular tissue for fertilization, current uses of such tissue are considered strictly experimental; therefore, the ethical issues involved in its procurement, including obtaining informed consent, are complicated. Three potential strategies are under active investigation for the use of harvested spermatogonial stem cells from prepubertal boys:[92]

1. Germ cells could be transplanted using a cryopreserved single-cell suspension infused back into the testis after gonadotoxic therapy. This was achieved in a mouse model in 1994 by Brinster and Zimmermann by injection of spermatogonia into seminiferous tubules.[93,94] Human spermatogonial stem cells have been successfully cultured and propagated in vitro. An experimental protocol for cryopreserving a human germ cell suspension has been developed with 66% post-thaw viability regardless of the cryopreservative used.[95]

2. Spermatozoa could be generated from spermatogonial stem cells via in vitro differentiation. Alternatively, germ cells could potentially be derived from embryonic stem cells, as they have been in a murine model.[96] Adult human germ line stem cells have been successfully derived from testicular spermatogonial cells.[97,98]

3. Immature cryopreserved testicular tissue could be grafted into another organism when the infertile cancer patient desires to father children. After differentiation occurs, sperm could be retrieved from the tissue for ICSI.

Beyond the current technical limitations in being able to transform cryopreserved spermatogonia into mature, functional sperm, there are hypothetical risks associated with tissue preservation. Given the underlying malignancy in patients undergoing testicular tissue extraction, there is concern regarding the potential for reseeding the cancer when the cryopreserved tissue is reintroduced into the native host.[99] Studies in rat have demonstrated leukemic relapse in previously treated animals when as few as 20 leukemic cells were reintroduced.[100] This is further supported by the observation of increased risk of CNS relapse in leukemic patients undergoing traumatic lumbar punctures.[101] This concern, combined with technological factors, limits the current utility of testicular tissue preservation.

Currently, the options for fertility preservation in the prepubertal male are limited and are investigatory.[102] Patients and families must be counseled and any procedure adopted should be considered highly investigational at this time.

■ METHODS OF FERTILITY PRESERVATION IN FEMALES

Embryo Cryopreservation

In cancer patients, IVF can be performed to store embryos for future use, if the patient has a partner and enough time prior to treatment. Survival rates per thawed embryo range between 35% and 90%, implantation rates between 8% and 30%, and cumulative pregnancy rates can be more than 60%.[78-81] In breast cancer, there is typically a 6-week hiatus between surgery and chemotherapy which would be adequate to perform ovarian stimulation and IVF. Nevertheless, since conventional controlled hyperstimulation regimens in IVF cycles typically result in estradiol levels that may be 10-fold higher than peak levels seen in a natural cycle, they are not recommended in breast cancer patients.[82-85] After its discovery in 1963, tamoxifen became an important part in the treatment of breast cancer, and has been tested for the chemoprevention of this disease.[86,87] While tamoxifen was originally used as a contraceptive agent in the UK, it was later found to be a useful ovulation induction agent.[88] It can be safely used for ovarian stimulation and IVF in breast cancer patients. Even though tamoxifen results in an increase in peak estradiol levels, it is well known to block the effects of supraphysiological levels of estrogen on breast tissue, and inhibits the growth of breast tumors by competitive antagonism of estrogen at its receptor site. In fact, mean estradiol levels are chronically elevated in breast cancer patients who are on long-term tamoxifen treatment, and can be higher than the levels seen in patients undergoing ovarian stimulation with tamoxifen.[89,90]

Mature Oocyte Cryopreservation

Embryo cryopreservation may not be an option for single women unless they choose to use sperm donation. In these patients, if they have time to complete ovarian stimulation prior to cancer therapy, freezing mature or immature oocytes can be considered as an alternative. Over 1,000 live births have been reported as a result of oocyte cryopreservation[91-93] with some centers reporting pregnancy rates similar to those of standard fresh IVF treatments. Although still considered experimental by the ASRM (Practice Committee Bulletin, 2008), a recently published survey, reporting that more than 50% of US infertility clinics currently offer oocyte cryopreservation for cancer patients, implies that the technology is becoming a mainstream technique. In addition, ovarian stimulation parameters and oocyte yield (both the total number and the percentage of mature oocytes) in cancer patients have been shown to be comparable to those of healthy women undergoing fertility treatment.

Ovarian Tissue Cryopreservation

Cryopreservation of ovarian tissue has several potential advantages over that of oocytes and embryos. Firstly, the human ovarian cortex contains many primordial follicles with oocytes arrested in the diplotene stage of prophase of first meiotic division. Secondly, ovarian tissue cryopreservation can preserve the endocrine functions of the ovary. Third, ovarian tissue can be harvested by laparoscopy or laparotomy at any time, independent of the stage of the menstrual cycle. Fourth, primordial follicles are theoretically less cryosensitive than mature oocytes. It has been suggested that relatively high surface/volume ratio, low metabolic rate and the absence of zona pellucida make primordial follicles less susceptible to cryodamage. However, it also has disadvantages since it involves two surgical procedures, for harvesting and for transplantation.

Ovarian tissue cryopreservation and transplantation studies date back to the 1950s. Initial studies were disappointing until the discovery of effective modern cryoprotectants and the availability of automated cryopreservation machines. Glycerol was the only available cryoprotectant in 1960s, but was found ineffective for cryopreservation of human oocytes and ovarian tissue. With the advent of more effective cryoprotectants such as ethylene glycol, Dimethyl Sulfoxiab (DMSO) and propanediol, animal studies were repeated and successful deliveries were reported in a number of species. In humans, resumption of ovarian endocrine function could also be demonstrated.

Development of Human Ovarian Transplantation Techniques

There have been two main approaches in auto-transplantation of ovarian cortical pieces in humans. Orthotopic transplants involve grafting these strips near the infundibulopelvic ligaments or possibly on a post-menopausal ovary. In the heterotopic transplant, tissues can be grafted subcutaneously at various locations including forearm and abdominal wall.

Orthotopic Ovarian Transplantation

While transplantation may allow a natural pregnancy to occur, it requires abdominal surgery and general anesthesia.[98] A laparoscopic approach makes this surgery less invasive but technically more challenging. In the first case of laparoscopic orthotopic transplantation procedure with frozen ovarian tissue in a 27-year-old woman, ovarian cortical pieces had been cryopreserved in 1.5 mol/L propanediol using a slow-freeze protocol. After tissues had been thawed, they were sutured to two triangular frames made from an absorbable cellulose membrane. Then we laparoscopically transplanted them beneath the left pelvic peritoneum of the ovarian fossa. With the expectation of improving vascularization, aspirin 80 mg/day p.o. and FSH 150 IU/day IM were given for a week after the operation. Fifteen weeks after grafting, the patient was stimulated with daily menopausal gonadotropins which were gradually increased from 150 IU/day to 675 IU/day, and ovulation was confirmed by elevated progesterone levels, ultrasonographic demonstration of a corpus luteum, free fluid in the cul-de-sac, and change in endometrial pattern on ultrasound. Ovarian function could not be demonstrated beyond 9 months of follow-up.

Heterotopic Ovarian Transplantation

Auto-transplanting tissue to a heterotopic site is a well-known concept, and it has long been utilized for implanting fresh or frozen-thawed parathyroid tissue following total parathyroidectomy. Heterotopic transplantation has significant advantages like non-requirement of general anesthesia or abdominal surgery. In addition, it is easy to monitor follicle development and to remove the transplanted tissue from a subcutaneous site when necessary. One of the potential limitations of ovarian tissue cryopreservation and transplantation is loss of a large fraction of follicles during the initial ischemia after transplantation. Previous work has indicated that while the loss due to freezing is relatively small, up to two-thirds of follicles are lost after transplantation. Consequently, it is not recommended to freeze ovarian tissue in patients aged above 40 years.

Risk of Metastatic Disease

Ovarian tissue can be grafted once the patient survives malignancy or is considered cured. It is naturally of concern that the frozen-thawed tissue might harbor malignant cells, and the cancer could be reseeded by ovarian transplantation. Fortunately, most of the malignant tumors of reproductive age women do not metastasize to ovaries, with the exception of some hematological malignancies such as leukemia's, Burkitt's lymphoma and some advanced stage solid tumors such as, breast and colon cancers. In children, ovarian metastasis has been demonstrated in 25 ± 50% of neuroblastoma cases in postmortem examinations. Breast cancer has a low-to-intermediate risk of ovarian involvement in early stages. In the absence of clinical and radiological evidence of distant metastasis, ovarian involvement is extremely rare, and most cases could be detected by a thorough clinical and radiological evaluation **(Table 3)**.

Table 3 Cancers with risk of ovarian involvement

Low-risk	Wilms' tumor Ewing's sarcoma Breast cancer—Stage I–III (Infiltrative ductal histological subtype) Non-Hodgkin's lymphoma Hodgkin's lymphoma Non-genital rhabdomyosarcoma Osteogenic sarcoma Squamous cell carcinoma of the cervix
Moderate risk	Adenocarcinoma Adenosquamous carcinoma of the cervix Colon cancer Breast cancer Stage IV (Infiltrative lobular histological subtype)
High risk	Leukemia Neuroblastoma Burkitt's lymphoma Ovarian transposition (oophoropexy)

Shielding of Ovaries

Ovaries can be moved out of the radiation field so that direct effects of ionizing radiation may be avoided. If the patient is to undergo an abdominal surgery, ovaries can be transposed simultaneously, or if she is to be treated non-surgically, laparoscopic transposition can be performed before the scheduled radiotherapy. The success with fertility preservation by ovarian transposition prior to radiotherapy varies between 16% and 90%. This variation in success rates is due to variations in the degree of scatter radiation, vascular compromise, the age of the patient, dose of radiation, whether the ovaries were shielded, whether concomitant chemotherapy is used, and whether vaginal brachytherapy or pelvic external beam irradiation plus brachytherapy was used. Even though ovarian transposition may decrease the risk of ovarian failure, ovaries are still subjected to a significant amount of radiation despite proper shielding. This is mainly due to scatter radiation and transmission through the shield, which may amount to as much as 8 ± 15% of the total pelvic radiation dose. In addition, this surgical procedure is not without complications; Fallopian tube infarction, chronic ovarian pain, ovarian cyst formation and migration of ovaries back to their original position before radiotherapy have been reported, some of which may require additional gynecological surgeries.

GnRH Analog Co-treatment

There are several possible mechanisms through which GnRH agonists may protect the ovary during chemotherapy. Proposed mechanisms include protection via reduced levels of gonadotropins, a direct influence of GnRH on the ovary and reduced blood flow to the ovary. In the adult ovary, a cohort of primordial follicles is recruited every month where the majority will undergo atresia and one will become a dominant follicle. The basal follicular growth is independent of gonadotropins. It is possible that suppressing the gonadotropin level with GnRH analogs preserves these follicles that have initiated growth and reached the gonadotropin-dependent stage. However, growing follicles constitute 10% of all follicles and once growth has been initiated, they are destined either to become atretic or to ovulate. Therefore, this explanation for a protectant mechanism for GnRH agonists could not explain a long-term effect. Another possibility is that there is a decline in ovarian blood flow during GnRH therapy, reducing the dose of chemotherapy reaching the ovary and therefore limiting the damage to the ovarian reserve. Other additional models which may explain a GnRH agonist effect include up-regulation of an intragonadal

anti-apoptotic molecule such as, sphingosine-1-phosphate, and protection of the undifferentiated germ line stem cells. It has been demonstrated that there are no prospective, randomized, controlled trials showing a significant effect of GnRH agonist in protecting the ovary from the damage of chemotherapy. At this time a conclusion cannot be drawn regarding the efficiency of GnRH agonists for fertility preservation in young female patients receiving chemotherapy.

In Vitro Maturation of Oocytes

In vitro maturation (IVM), for oocyte or embryo cryopreservation, involves the retrieval of immature oocytes after minimal or no gonadotropin stimulation, followed by IVM and subsequent cryopreservation of matured oocytes (or embryos, if a male partner is involved). Advantages of this approach are that it is minimally invasive and can be accomplished rapidly in the absence of gonadotropin stimulation, even in the luteal phase, in order to start cancer treatment without delay. The recently reported outcomes of two oocyte IVM vitrification trials involving 58 patients without cancer have resulted in a total of 19 live births and 26 healthy newborns. This group has also demonstrated the feasibility of IVM followed by oocyte and embryo vitrification in a group of breast cancer patients. The technology of IVM holds promise but further studies are necessary to assess the widespread utility as a fertility preservation measure in patients newly diagnosed with malignancy. IVM is a useful strategy to improve the mature oocyte yield of fertility preservation cycles. Immature oocytes retrieved during oocyte/embryo cryopreservation cycles should not be discarded to improve the future potential of fertility.

In Vitro Grown Human Ovarian Follicles

Human follicle development can be achieved in vitro in a bioengineered culture system. The in vitro growth of immature follicles derived from ovaries collected prior to the commencement of cancer treatment is an important direction for research. The purpose of the in vitro human follicle growth system is to mimic the in vivo process by providing follicles with appropriate growth factors and hormones, in correct amounts at the right time, which allows growth of the follicle and oocyte while maintaining the essential connections between somatic cells and the oocyte called transzonal projections **(Figs 3A to D)**. In vitro follicle growth provides the opportunity to expand research initiatives in follicle development as well as to potentially provide expanded options to young cancer patients.

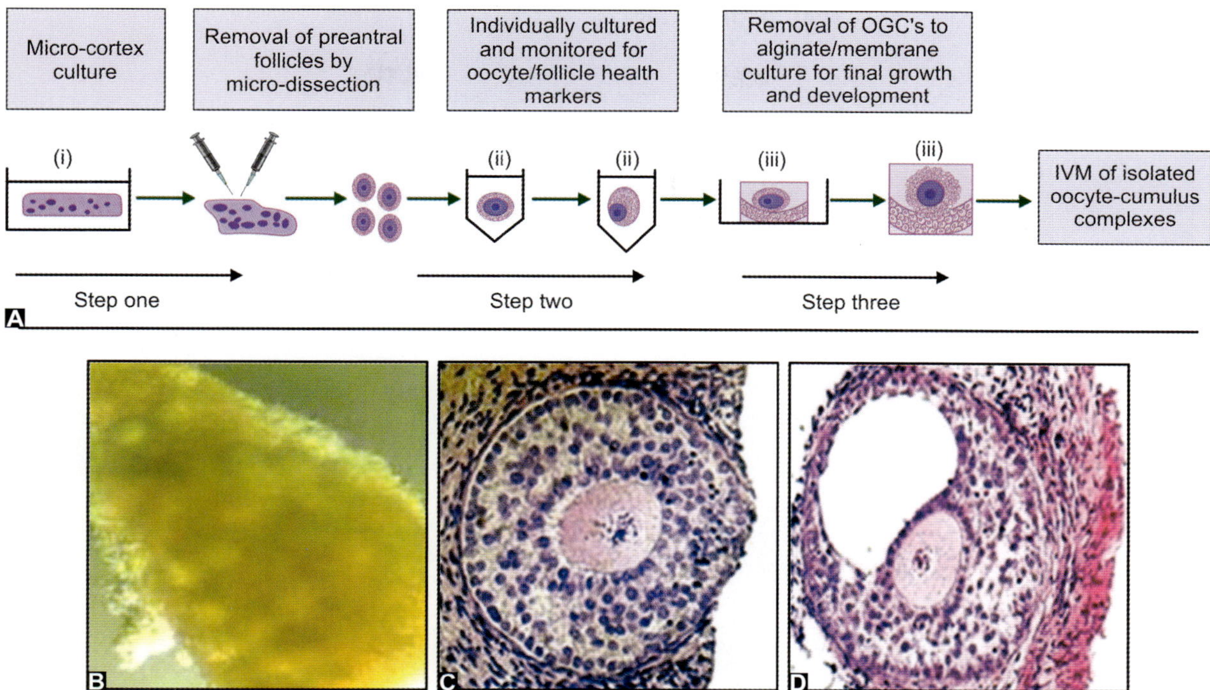

Figs 3A to D *Multistep culture system to support human follicle development in vitro* (A) Steps involved in the culture of human primordial follicles to antral stages (i–ii) and removal of oocyte granulosa cell complexes (OGCs) for placement in alginate bead/membrane (iii) for further growth and development, and subsequent in vitro maturation (IVM). Human follicles can be developed from primordial (B) to preantral (C) and antral stages (D) in serum free medium

Donor Oocytes and Surrogacy

In vitro fertilization with donor oocytes is another alternative in patients who suffer from premature menopause or low ovarian reserve due to cancer treatment. The success rates with appropriate oocyte donors are now more than 60% per embryo transfer. Gestational surrogacy can also be employed in patients who had undergone hysterectomy or received pelvic radiation for cervical cancer. Patients with breast cancer who are considered high risk for recurrence, or who have to be on lifelong therapy with aromatase inhibitors, may also resort to gestational surrogacy. However, laws and regulations regarding this procedure vary significantly between countries.

■ SPECIAL CONSIDERATIONS FOR OVARIAN STIMULATION IN CANCER PATIENTS

The patients referred for fertility preservation due to malignancy are different from subfertile patients coming for IVF (Flow chart 4). Cancer may affect multiple tissues throughout the body and can result in variety of complications during COS. Therefore, the goals during COS in cancer patients are to prevent these serious life-threatening complications with prophylaxis, and to recognize and manage them effectively when they occur.[57] Ovarian stimulation protocols using GnRH antagonists should be preferred, as they are associated with a lower risk of ovarian hyperstimulation syndrome (OHSS). The risk of OHSS can further be decreased by triggering final oocyte maturation by GnRH agonists. The use of GnRH agonists can also speed the interval from oocyte retrieval to next menses as well as reducing the likelihood and extent of residual ovarian cyst formation. This in turn improves the chances of multiple back-to-back cycles before initiating cancer treatment.[58,59] During stimulation, there is a potential risk that the supraphysiologic estradiol levels resulting from ovarian stimulation with gonadotropins may promote the growth of estrogen-sensitive tumors, such as endometrial and estrogen receptor-positive breast cancers. The rise in estradiol is directly proportional to the number of follicles recruited to grow. Alternative safer protocols, like natural cycle IVFs or stimulation protocols

Flow chart 4 Fertility preservation strategies

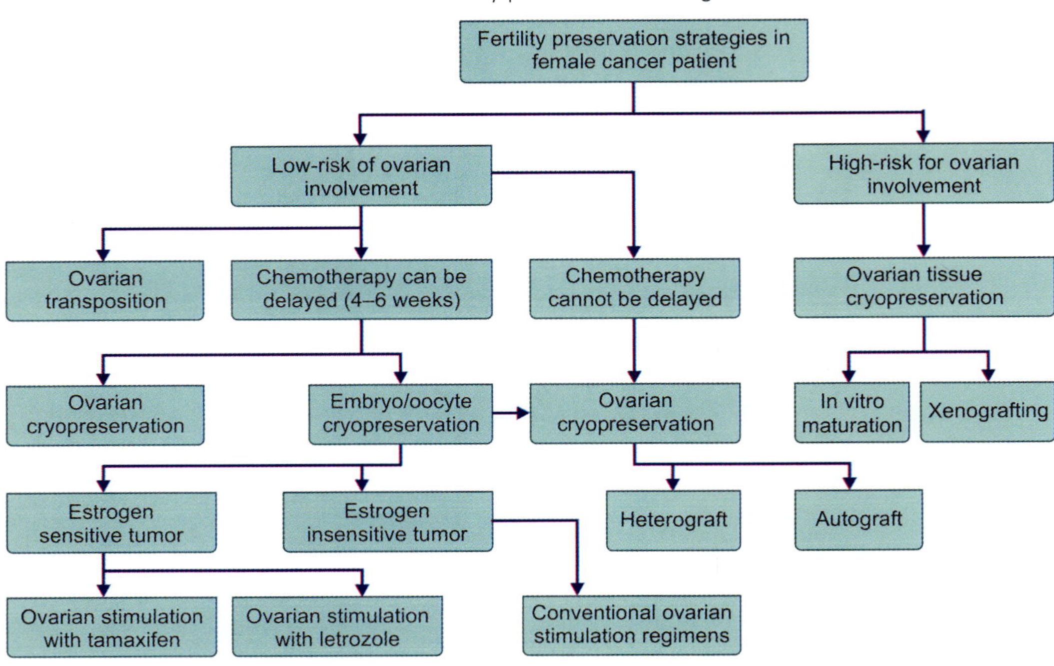

Source: Reprinted from M. Sonmezer and K. Oktay. Hum Reprod Update. 2004.

with tamoxifen or aromatase inhibitors, are advocated to reduce estrogen production.

OBSTACLES TO FERTILITY PRESERVATION

The patient's own lack of awareness of the option for fertility preservation is the first challenge to ensure fertility preservation for all those who may desire it. For patients who have been told about fertility preservation at the time of diagnosis, looking beyond their own survival can be difficult.

The physician's own lack of knowledge relating to fertility preservation options constitutes another hurdle. An oncologist may not refer a patient to a fertility specialist to avoid the risk of delaying treatment, the patient's limited resources or feeling that a discussion of fertility preservation is inappropriate in the midst of fighting the disease. A recent study has determined that with supportive resources available, the time required for stimulation of mature oocytes for cryopreservation does not significantly extend the duration between diagnosis and the start of chemotherapy. Discussion and management of preserving reproductive potential are the most challenging aspects of care and inadequate counseling results from lack of multidisciplinary approach to providing fertility preservation.

ETHICAL DILEMMA

For young girls and females without a partner at the time of preservation, embryo cryopreservation may not be an acceptable modality. In the case of children, it may be difficult to accurately gain informed consent, or even for a parent to make an informed decision. The use of oocyte cryopreservation is an alternative choice but procedure is still experimental and not offered routinely. Ovarian tissue cryopreservation also avoids the dilemma of using donor sperm, yet it is also experimental and has the faint risk of reintroducing malignant cells.

CURRENT GUIDELINES FOR FERTILITY PRESERVATION

There is possibility that cancer patients might be faced with impaired fertility or sterility in the future, and options they have for future childbirth and or parenting need to be considered. The ASCO and the ASRM recommend that physicians should discuss the risks of infertility with all cancer patients of reproductive age. They further suggest that interested patients should be provided with information to answer their questions about possible fertility preservation, and should be referred to reproductive specialists and psychosocial providers as needed.

ASCO Guidelines for Fertility Preservation

Key recommendations of the ASCO include:

- Discuss fertility preservation with all patients of reproductive age (and with parents or guardians of children and adolescents) if infertility is a potential risk of therapy.
- Refer patients who express an interest infertility preservation (and patients who are ambivalent) to reproductive specialists.
- Address fertility preservation as early as possible, before the start of treatment.
- Document fertility preservation discussions in the medical record.
- Answer basic questions about whether fertility preservation may have an impact on successful cancer treatment.
- Refer patients to psychosocial providers, if they experience distress about potential infertility.
- Encourage patients to participate in registries and clinical studies.

Adult Males

- Present sperm cryopreservation (sperm banking) as the only established fertility preservation method.
- Do not recommend hormonal therapy in men; it is not successful in preserving fertility.
- Inform patients that other methods (e.g. testicular tissue cryopreservation, which does not require sexual maturity, for the purpose of future reimplantation or grafting of human testicular tissue) are experimental.
- Advise men of a potentially higher risk of genetic damage in sperm collected after initiation of chemotherapy.

Adult Females

- Present both embryo and oocyte cryopreservation as established fertility preservation methods.
- Discuss the option of ovarian transposition (oophoropexy) when pelvic radiation therapy is performed as cancer treatment.
- Inform patients of conservative gynecologic surgery and radiation therapy options.
- Inform patients that there is insufficient evidence regarding the effectiveness of ovarian suppression (GnRH analogs) as a fertility preservation method, and these agents should not be relied on to preserve fertility.
- Inform patients that other methods (e.g. ovarian tissue cryopreservation, which does not require sexual maturity, for the purpose of future transplantation) are still experimental.

Children

- Use established methods of fertility preservation (semen cryopreservation and oocyte cryopreservation) for postpubertal minor children, with patient assent, if appropriate, and parent or guardian consent.
- Present information on additional methods that are available for children but are still investigational.
- Refer for experimental protocols, when available.

Although addressing potential fertility loss may be overwhelming for newly diagnosed patients and their families, multiple studies suggest that failure to confront the possibility can cause regret and distress to cancer survivors, and significantly impact their quality of life. Multiple studies with survivors, particularly adult survivors of pediatric or young adult cancer, suggest patients do not recall having a discussion about loss of fertility. It is not known if these discussions did in fact occur for the majority of patients but resulted in patients not remembering them or if the conversations did not take place at all. What is known is that the ability to parent a biological child is of great importance to cancer survivors. Several studies suggest that as many as 75% of childless patients who are diagnosed with cancer wish to have a child in the future. Studies conducted among survivors of pediatric cancer indicate a strong fear that they will be rejected by future partners due to their inability to have a child.

Current guidelines attribute the onus of these multifaceted conversations to oncologists. However, patient-provider interactions are complex and providing an optimal exchange of information along the continuum of care for cancer patients is challenging. The current ASCO guidelines, perhaps, fail to account for the fact that discussions about fertility preservation need to be ongoing and must be modified to meet the specific needs of each patient. For example, at the point of diagnosis, information on fertility preservation may not take precedence over information about survival. Healthcare providers should insist that patients and families hear and consider fertility preservation information regardless of patients being overwhelmed or distraught. During treatment, patients should be given information on how that particular treatment regime may affect their future fertility. Finally, after patients are cancer-free or have completed treatment, they may have questions about childbearing in regard to their health and the health of their potential offspring. Thus, discussing fertility preservation should not be viewed as a one-time task to be checked off on a care plan, but as an evolution of health information exchanges between healthcare providers, patients and their families. Providing this information in a comprehensive, honest and consistent manner may improve the patient's long-term health related to their quality of life.

Role of Oncologists

Physicians treating younger patients for cancer and non-cancerous conditions should be aware of the adverse effects of treatment on fertility and ways to minimize those effects. Issues to be considered in choosing a treatment plan include the risk of gonadal failure and/or uterine damage with the proposed treatment program, the overall prognosis for the patient, the potential risks of delaying treatment, the impact of any future pregnancy upon the risk of tumor recurrence, and the impact of any required hormonal manipulation on the cancer itself. If gonadal toxicity is unavoidable, physicians also should be knowledgeable about options for fertility preservation, and offer patients a referral to a fertility specialist. With the growing number of cancer survivors, much attention is now focused on their quality of life and the physical, psychological, social and spiritual issues that they confront.[22] There is some evidence that not all oncologists are as attentive to issues of fertility as patients might wish them to be.[23] A recent study showed that although 60% of oncologists reported an awareness of the ASCO guidelines for fertility preservation, less than 25% of the respondents said they follow them on a regular basis, distribute any type of educational materials, or refer patients for fertility preservation discussions.[24] Unless patients are informed or properly referred before treatment, options for later reproduction may be lost. Fertility specialists and patient organizations should work with cancer specialists and cancer organizations to make certain that information is appropriately conveyed and options explained.

◼ CONCLUSION

Patients facing gonadotoxic treatments have important needs in preserving fertility and cancer, and fertility specialists should try to protect patients' needs. When damage to reproductive organs due to gonadotoxic treatment is unavoidable, healthcare providers should inform patients of options for storing gametes, embryos, or gonadal tissue and refer them to fertility specialists who can provide or counsel them about those services. Counseling by a qualified mental health professional and genetic counselor, when appropriate, should also be offered.

Fertility programs should counsel patients and survivors on the risks of gonadotoxic treatment on fertility, and the options for and the risks of preserving fertility and reproducing after cure or remission. Fertility preservation

procedures that have not been shown to be safe and effective could be offered to patients only in an experimental setting under Institution Review Board (IRB) oversight. Parents may act to preserve reproductive options of minor children undergoing gonadotoxic treatment as long as the minor assents, the intervention does not pose undue risk, and the intervention offers a reasonable chance of net benefit to the child. Programs storing gametes, embryos or gonadal tissue for cancer patients should request clear instructions about what should be done with stored materials in the event of the patient's death, unavailability, non-payment of storage fees or other contingency.

◼ REFERENCES

1. Schover LR, Brey K, Lichtin A, et al. Oncologists' attitudes and practices regarding banking sperm before cancer treatment. J Clin Oncol. 2002;20(7):1890-7.
2. Quinn GP, Vadaparampil ST, Gwede CK, et al. Discussion of fertility preservation with newly diagnosed patients: oncologists' views. J Cancer Surviv. 2007;1(2):146-55.
3. Quinn GP, Vadaparampil ST, Fertility Preservation Research Group. Fertility preservation and adolescent/young adult cancer patients: physician communication challenges. J Adolesc Health. 2009;44(4):394-400.
4. Jemal A, Murray T, Samuels A, et al. Cancer statistics, 2003. CA Cancer J Clin. 2003;53(1):5-26.
5. Adashi EY. Ovulation induction. In: Adashi EY, Rock JA, Rosenwaks Z (Eds). Reproductive Endocrinology, Surgery and Technology, 1st edition. Philadelphia, PA: Lippincott-Raven Publishers; 1996.
6. Al-Hasani S, Diedrich K, Ven H van der, et al. Cryopreservation of human oocytes. Hum Reprod. 1987;2(8):695-700.
7. Rodriguez-Wallberg KA, Oktay K. Options on fertility preservation in female cancer patients. Cancer Treat Rev. 2012;38(5):354-61.
8. Sklar CA, Mertens AC, Mitby P, et al. Premature menopause in survivors of childhood cancer: a report from the childhood cancer survivor study. J Natl Cancer Inst. 2006;98(13):890-6.
9. Anderson RA, Wallace WHB. Fertility preservation in girls and young women. Clin Endocrinol (Oxf). 2011;75(4):409-19.
10. Hovatta O. Cryopreservation of testicular tissue in young cancer patients. Hum Reprod Update. 2001;7:378-83.
11. Ginsberg JP, Carlson CA, Lin K, et al. An experimental protocol for fertility preservation in prepubertal boys recently diagnosed with cancer: a report of acceptability and safety. Hum Reprod. 2010;25(1):37-41.
12. Franck P, Duffner U, Schulze-Seemann W, et al. Testicular relapse after 13 years of complete remission of acute lymphoblastic leukemia. Urol Int. 1998;60(4):239-41.
13. Jahnukainen K, Hou M, Petersen C, et al. Intratesticular transplantation of testicular cells from leukemic rats causes transmission of leukemia. Cancer Res. 2001;61(2):706-10.
14. Rech A, de Carvalho GP, Meneses CF, et al. The influence of traumatic lumbar puncture and timing of intrathecal therapy on outcome of pediatric acute lymphoblastic leukemia. Pediatr Hematol Oncol. 2005;22(6):483-8.

15. Stensvold E, Magelssen H, Oskam IC. Fertility-preserving measures for boys and young men with cancer. Tidsskr Nor Laegeforen. 2011;131:1433-5.

16. Dohle GR. Male infertility in cancer patients: review of the literature. Int J Urol. 2010;17:327-31.

17. Holoch P, Wald M. Current options for preservation of fertility in the male. Fertil Steril. 2011;96:286-90.

18. Brannigan RE. Fertility preservation in adult male cancer patients. Cancer Treat Res. 2007;138:28-49.

19. Lee SJ, Schover LR, Partridge AH, et al. American Society of Clinical Oncology recommendations on fertility preservation in cancer patients. J Clin Oncol. 2006;24:2917-31.

20. Fertile Hope. Cancer and Fertility: Fast Facts for Reproductive Professionals. 2008. www.fertilehope.org/uploads/pdf/FH_RP_FastFacts_08.pdf. Accessed February 11, 2011.

21. Ethics Committee of the American Society for Reproductive Medicine. Fertility preservation and reproduction in cancer patients. Fertil Steril. 2005;83:1622-28.

22. Jeruss JS, Woodruff TK. Preservation of fertility in patients with cancer. N Engl J Med. 2009;360:902-11.

23. Tschudin S, Bitzer J. Psychological aspects of fertility preservation in men and women affected by cancer and other life-threatening diseases. Hum Reprod Update. 2009;15:587-97.

24. Schover LR, Brey K, Lichtin A, et al. Knowledge and experience regarding cancer, infertility, and sperm banking in younger male survivors. J Clin Oncol. 2002;20(7):1880-9.

25. CDC—The National Action Plan for Cancer Survivorship [Internet]. [cited 2015 Feb 11]. http://www.cdc.gov/cancer/survivorship/what_cdc_is_doing/action_plan.htm

26. Rueffer U, Breuer K, Josting A, et al. Male gonadal dysfunction in patients with Hodgkin's disease prior to treatment. Ann Oncol. 2001;12(9):1307-11.

27. Bath LE, Critchley HO, Chambers SE, et al. Ovarian and uterine characteristics after total body irradiation in childhood and adolescence: response to sex steroid replacement. Br J Obstet Gynaecol. 1999;106(12):1265-72.

28. Critchley HOD, Wallace WH. Impact of cancer treatment on uterine function. J Natl Cancer Inst Monogr. 2005;(34):64-8.

29. Critchley HO, Wallace WH, Shalet SM, et al. Abdominal irradiation in childhood; the potential for pregnancy. Br J Obstet Gynaecol. 1992;99(5):392-4.

30. Green DM, Sklar CA, Boice JD, et al. Ovarian failure and reproductive outcomes after childhood cancer treatment: results from the Childhood Cancer Survivor Study. J Clin Oncol. 2009;27(14):2374-81.

31. Larsen EC, Müller J, Schmiegelow K, et al. Reduced ovarian function in long-term survivors of radiation- and chemotherapy-treated childhood cancer. J Clin Endocrinol Metab. 2003;88(11):5307-14.

32. Byrne J, Fears TR, Gail MH, et al. Early menopause in long-term survivors of cancer during adolescence. Am J Obstet Gynecol. 1992;166(3):788-93.

33. Plowchalk DR, Mattison DR. Phosphoramide mustard is responsible for the ovarian toxicity of cyclophosphamide. Toxicol Appl Pharmacol. 1991;107(3):472-81.

34. Oktem O, Oktay K. A novel ovarian xenografting model to characterize the impact of chemotherapy agents on human primordial follicle reserve. Cancer Res. 2007;67(21):10159-62.

35. Petrek JA, Naughton MJ, Case LD, et al. Incidence, time course, and determinants of menstrual bleeding after breast cancer treatment: a prospective study. J Clin Oncol. 2006;24(7):1045-51.

36. Wallace WHB, Thomson AB, Kelsey TW. The radiosensitivity of the human oocyte. Hum Reprod. 2003;18(1):117-21.

37. Anderson RA, Themmen APN, Al-Qahtani A, et al. The effects of chemotherapy and long-term gonadotrophin suppression on the ovarian reserve in premenopausal women with breast cancer. Hum Reprod. 2006;21(10):2583-92.

38. Broekmans FJ, Soules MR, Fauser BC. Ovarian aging: mechanisms and clinical consequences. Endocr Rev. 2009;30(5):465-93.

39. Rosendahl M, Andersen CY, la Cour Freiesleben N, et al. Dynamics and mechanisms of chemotherapy-induced ovarian follicular depletion in women of fertile age. Fertil Steril. 2010;94(1):156-66.

40. Bath LE, Anderson RA, Critchley HO, et al. Hypothalamic-pituitary-ovarian dysfunction after prepubertal chemotherapy and cranial irradiation for acute leukaemia. Hum Reprod. 2001;16(9):1838-44.

41. Littley MD, Shalet SM, Beardwell CG, et al. Radiation-induced hypopituitarism is dose-dependent. Clin Endocrinol (Oxf). 1989;31(3):363-73.

42. Hall JE, Martin KA, Whitney HA, et al. Potential for fertility with replacement of hypothalamic gonadotropin-releasing hormone in long term female survivors of cranial tumors. J Clin Endocrinol Metab. 1994;79(4):1166-72.

43. Gosden RG, Mullan J, Picton HM, et al. Current perspective on primordial follicle cryopreservation and culture for reproductive medicine. Hum Reprod Update. 2002;8(2):105-10.

44. Meirow D, Nugent D. The effects of radiotherapy and chemotherapy on female reproduction. Hum Reprod Update. 2001;7(6):535-43.

45. Brenner H, Kaatsch P, Burkhardt-Hammer T, et al. Long-term survival of children with leukemia achieved by the end of the second millennium. Cancer. 2001;92(7):1977-83.

46. Pui C-H, Cheng C, Leung W, et al. Extended follow-up of long-term survivors of childhood acute lymphoblastic leukemia. N Engl J Med. 2003;349(7):640-9.

47. Robison LL, Bhatia S. Late-effects among survivors of leukaemia and lymphoma during childhood and adolescence. Br J Haematol. 2003;122(3):345-59.

48. Gurney JG, Severson RK, Davis S, et al. Incidence of cancer in children in the United States. Sex-, race-, and 1-year age-specific rates by histologic type. Cancer. 1995;75(8):2186-95.

49. Arndt CA, Donaldson SS, Anderson JR, et al. What constitutes optimal therapy for patients with rhabdomyosarcoma of the female genital tract? Cancer. 2001;91(12):2454-68.

50. Franchi-Rezgui P, Rousselot P, Espié M, et al. Fertility in young women after chemotherapy with alkylating agents for Hodgkin and non-Hodgkin lymphomas. Hematol J. 2003;4(2):116-20.

51. Ozaki T, Flege S, Kevric M, et al. Osteosarcoma of the pelvis: experience of the Cooperative Osteosarcoma Study Group. J Clin Oncol. 2003;21(2):334-41.

52. Rödl RW, Hoffmann C, Gosheger G, et al. Ewing's sarcoma of the pelvis: combined surgery and radiotherapy treatment. J Surg Oncol. 2003;83(3):154-60.

53. Weir HK, Thun MJ, Hankey BF, et al. Annual report to the nation on the status of cancer, 1975-2000, featuring the uses of surveillance data for cancer prevention and control. J Natl Cancer Inst. 2003;95(17):1276-99.

54. Oktay KH, Yih M. Preliminary experience with orthotopic and heterotopic transplantation of ovarian cortical strips. Semin Reprod Med. 2002;20(1):63-74.

55. Kaufmann M, von Minckwitz G, Smith R, et al. International expert panel on the use of primary (preoperative) systemic treatment of operable breast cancer: review and recommendations. J Clin Oncol. 2003;21(13):2600-8.

56. Oktay KH, Buyuk E, Rosenwaks Z. Novel use of an aromatase inhibitor for fertility preservation via embryo cryopreservation in endometrial cancer: a case report. Fertil Steril. 2003;80:144.

57. Waggoner SE. Cervical cancer. Lancet. 2003;361(9376):2217-25.

58. Smith HO, Tiffany MF, Qualls CR, et al. The rising incidence of adenocarcinoma relative to squamous cell carcinoma of the uterine cervix in the United States—a 24-year population-based study. Gynecol Oncol. 2000;78(2):97-105.

59. Nakanishi T, Wakai K, Ishikawa H, et al. A comparison of ovarian metastasis between squamous cell carcinoma and adenocarcinoma of the uterine cervix. Gynecol Oncol. 2001;82(3):504-9.

60. Yamamoto R, Okamoto K, Yukiharu T, et al. A study of risk factors for ovarian metastases in stage Ib-IIIb cervical carcinoma and analysis of ovarian function after a transposition. Gynecol Oncol. 2001;82(2):312-6.

61. Feigenberg SJ, Marcus RB, Zlotecki RA, et al. Megavoltage radiotherapy for aneurysmal bone cysts. Int J Radiat Oncol Biol Phys. 2001;49(5):1243-7.

62. Ferguson WS, Goorin AM. Current treatment of osteosarcoma. Cancer Invest. 2001;19(3):292-315.

63. Bacci G, Ferrari S, Mercuri M, et al. Multimodal therapy for the treatment of nonmetastatic Ewing sarcoma of pelvis. J Pediatr Hematol Oncol. 2003;25(2):118-24.

64. Ozaki T, Flege S, Kevric M, et al. Osteosarcoma of the pelvis: experience of the Cooperative Osteosarcoma Study Group. J Clin Oncol. 2003;21(2):334-41.

65. Pisters PWT, Ballo MT, Fenstermacher MJ, et al. Phase I trial of preoperative concurrent doxorubicin and radiation therapy, surgical resection, and intraoperative electron-beam radiation therapy for patients with localized retroperitoneal sarcoma. J Clin Oncol. 2003;21(16):3092-7.

66. Kapiteijn E, Marijnen CA, Nagtegaal ID, et al. Preoperative radiotherapy combined with total mesorectal excision for resectable rectal cancer. N Engl J Med. 2001;345(9):638-46.

67. Green DM, Kawashima T, Stovall M, et al. Fertility of male survivors of childhood cancer: a report from the Childhood Cancer Survivor Study. J Clin Oncol. 2010;28(2):332-9.

68. Thomson AB, Campbell AJ, Irvine DC, et al. Semen quality and spermatozoal DNA integrity in survivors of childhood cancer: a case-control study. Lancet. 2002;360(9330):361-7.

69. Hsiao W, Stahl PJ, Osterberg EC, et al. Successful treatment of postchemotherapy azoospermia with microsurgical testicular sperm extraction: the Weill Cornell experience. J Clin Oncol. 2011;29(12):1607-11.

70. Jahnukainen K, Ehmcke J, Hou M, et al. Testicular function and fertility preservation in male cancer patients. Best Pract Res Clin Endocrinol Metab. 2011;25(2):287-302.

71. Heikens J, Behrendt H, Adriaanse R, et al. Irreversible gonadal damage in male survivors of pediatric Hodgkin's disease. Cancer. 1996;78(9):2020-4.

72. Brämswig JH, Heimes U, Heiermann E, et al. The effects of different cumulative doses of chemotherapy on testicular function. Results in 75 patients treated for Hodgkin's disease during childhood or adolescence. Cancer. 1990;65(6):1298-302.

73. Ståhl O, Boyd HA, Giwercman A, et al. Risk of birth abnormalities in the offspring of men with a history of cancer: a cohort study using Danish and Swedish national registries. J Natl Cancer Inst. 2011;103(5):398-406.

74. al-Shawaf T, Yang D, al-Magid Y, et al. Ultrasonic monitoring during replacement of frozen/thawed embryos in natural and hormone replacement cycles. Hum Reprod. 1993;8(12):2068-74.

75. Senn A, Vozzi C, Chanson A, et al. Prospective randomized study of two cryopreservation policies avoiding embryo selection: the pronucleate stage leads to a higher cumulative delivery rate than the early cleavage stage. Fertil Steril. 2000;74(5):946-52.

76. Son W-Y, Yoon S-H, Yoon H-J, et al. Pregnancy outcome following transfer of human blastocysts vitrified on electron microscopy grids after induced collapse of the blastocoele. Hum Reprod. 2003;18(1):137-9.

77. Wang JX, Yap YY, Matthews CD. Frozen-thawed embryo transfer: influence of clinical factors on implantation rate and risk of multiple conception. Hum Reprod. 2001;16(11):2316-9.

78. Pittaway DE, Wentz AC. Evaluation of the exponential rise of serum estradiol concentrations in human menopausal gonadotropin-induced cycles. Fertil Steril. 1983;40(6):763-7.

79. Chen C-H, Zhang X, Barnes R, et al. Relationship between peak serum estradiol levels and treatment outcome in in vitro fertilization cycles after embryo transfer on day 3 or day 5. Fertil Steril. 2003;80(1):75-9.

80. Peña JE, Chang PL, Chan LK, et al. Supraphysiological estradiol levels do not affect oocyte and embryo quality in oocyte donation cycles. Hum Reprod. 2002;17(1):83-7.

81. Harper MJ, Walpole AL. A new derivative of triphenylethylene: effect on implantation and mode of action in rats. J Reprod Fertil. 1967;13(1):101-19.

82. Veronesi U, Maisonneuve P, Rotmensz N, et al. Italian randomized trial among women with hysterectomy: tamoxifen and hormone-dependent breast cancer in high-risk women. J Natl Cancer Inst. 2003;95(2):160-5.

83. Klopper A, Hall M. New synthetic agent for the induction of ovulation: preliminary trials in women. Br Med J. 1971;1(5741):152-4.

84. M Klijn JG, Beex LV, Mauriac L, et al. Combined treatment with buserelin and tamoxifen in premenopausal metastatic breast cancer: a randomized study. J Natl Cancer Inst. 2000;92(11):903-11.

85. Shushan A, Peretz T, Mor-Yosef S. Therapeutic approach to ovarian cysts in tamoxifen-treated women with breast cancer. Int J Gynaecol Obstet. 1996;52(3):249-53.

86. Noyes N, Knopman J, Labella P, et al. Oocyte cryopreservation outcomes including pre-cryopreservation and post-thaw meiotic spindle evaluation following slow cooling and vitrification of human oocytes. Fertil Steril. 2010;94(6):2078-82.

87. Noyes N, Labella PA, Grifo J, et al. Oocyte cryopreservation: a feasible fertility preservation option for reproductive age cancer survivors. J Assist Reprod Genet. 2010;27(8):495-9.

88. Rudick B, Opper N, Paulson R, et al. The status of oocyte cryopreservation in the United States. Fertil Steril. 2010;94(7):2642-6.

89. Nagy ZP, Chang CC, Shapiro DB, et al. Clinical evaluation of the efficiency of an oocyte donation program using egg cryo-banking. Fertil Steril. 2009;92(2):520-6.

90. Cobo A, Meseguer M, Remohí J, et al. Use of cryo-banked oocytes in an ovum donation programme: a prospective, randomized, controlled, clinical trial. Hum Reprod. 2010;25(9):2239-46.

91. Oktay K, Economos K, Kan M, et al. Endocrine function and oocyte retrieval after autologous transplantation of ovarian cortical strips to the forearm. JAMA. 2001;286(12):1490-3.

92. Oktay K, Nugent D, Newton H, et al. Isolation and characterization of primordial follicles from fresh and cryopreserved human ovarian tissue. Fertil Steril. 1997;67(3):481-6.

93. Gosden RG, Baird DT, Wade JC, et al. Restoration of fertility to oophorectomized sheep by ovarian autografts stored at -196 degrees C. Hum Reprod. 1994;9(4):597-603.

Luteal Phase in ART

45. **Luteal Phase Support in ART**
Sunita R Tandulwadkar, Sejal Naik, Chaithra SK

45 Luteal Phase Support in ART

Sunita R Tandulwadkar, Sejal Naik, Chaithra SK

INTRODUCTION

The luteal phase starts after ovulation and is relatively fixed at 12–14 days of menstrual cycle. The corpus luteum with highest blood flow per mass transforms into highly active temporary glands producing progesterone up to 40 mg/day. Progesterone along with estrogen and other hormones produced by the corpus luteum brings various changes in the endometrium making it receptive for implantation. In absence of pregnancy, corpus luteum degenerates 9–11 days after ovulation and luteal phase ends with the onset of menstruation. Once the pregnancy is established, human chorionic gonadotropin (hCG), not luteinizing hormone (LH), drives the corpus luteum until luteo-placental shift at 7–10 weeks of pregnancy.

LUTEAL PHASE IN NATURAL CYCLES

Granulosa theca cells luteinization is triggered by pituitary derived LH. Estradiol synthesis increases progressively from the dominant follicle and initiates the LH surge, which reflects the increasing LH pulse amplitude and frequency leading up to the LH surge. A surge lasting for 24–36 hours is sufficient to induce resumption of oocyte meiosis, luteinization of granulosa cells and initial support of corpus luteum (CL).[1] After the LH surge, there is rapid production of progesterone from the luteinized theca cells. During conception cycle, the regression of CL is prevented by the hCG produced by the trophoblastic cells. Maintenance of CL is essentially by LH, however its regression is caused by reduction in the responsiveness of aging CL to LH, which can be overcome in the fertile cycle by elevated hCG.[2]

Progesterone is synthesized in two enzymatic steps: conversion of cholesterol to P5 by P450ssc (rate limiting step) and its subsequent conversion to progesterone by 3 beta-hydroxysteroid dehydrogenase (HSD). The expression of StAR protein is very essential for the synthesis of progesterone which is expressed in greater levels during luteal phase.[3] CL is also the site of estrogen biosynthesis under the influence of LH and insulin-like growth factor-1 (IGF-1) and not follicle-stimulating hormone (FSH).[4] In a non-fertile cycle, decline in StAR protein expression leads to decline in other steroidogenic enzymes leading to luteolysis. In a conception cycle, CL is rescued by the hCG from trophoblastic cells in the developing embryo around the time of implantation (day 8 after ovulation). There is increase in the size of CL due to proliferation of nonsteroidogenic cells without a parallel increase in progesterone levels. There exists a positive correlation between CL volume, relaxin and beta hCG levels.

Role of Progesterone in Luteal Phase

- Progesterone acts on the endometrium to bring about secretory changes for implantation.
- It promotes local vasodilatation by inducing nitric oxide synthesis in decidua which improves endometrial growth and secretory changes.
- It causes decidualization, pinopode formation,[5] downregulation of estrogen receptors (ERs), leukemia inhibiting factor (LIF) and beta 3 integrin.
- It causes upregulation of vascular endothelial growth factor (VEGF), mucin 1, integrins, selectins, cathedrins, immunoglobulins, IGF-1, interleukin (IL), HOXA genes, endometrial cytokines and growth factors like epidermal growth factor (EGF), transforming growth factor (TGF), VEGF, platelet-derived growth factor (PDGF).[6-8]
- It promotes uterine quiescence by relaxing uterine musculature.

LUTEAL PHASE DEFECT

Luteal phase defect (LPD) is defined as a condition where endogenous progesterone production is insufficient to support a functional endometrium resulting in infertility

effective for LPS in stimulated cycles with respect to clinical pregnancy rates.[36]

DURATION OF LUTEAL SUPPORT

Optimum Timing of the LPS Initiation

While progesterone supplementation is essential, it is very important not to advance the endometrial maturation out of phase with embryo development. If starting progesterone too early in the cycle has a negative effect on the outcome, starting too late could be equally detrimental. Starting progesterone on the day of oocyte retrieval is documented to decrease uterine contractility on the day of embryo transfer. A randomized prospective study with patients on a GnRH suppression protocol reported no significant differences in pregnancy rate when LPS was started on the day after hCG administration, on the day of ovum pick up or the day of embryo transfer.[37] Referring to published data, one can conclude that most IVF clinicians start LPS after oocyte retrieval and before embryo transfer, but the optimal time is still unknown.

Discontinuation of Luteal Phase Support

The timing of discontinuation of LPS is still a matter of debate. A randomized controlled study by Schmidt et al. concluded that there is no benefit of continuing the LPS beyond the positive pregnancy test.[38] Another school of thought suggests discontinuation after the first ultrasound, 4–6 weeks after the embryo transfer. Since the luteo-placental shift takes place around 7–10 weeks, most clinicians still continue LPS till 8–10 weeks. The primary reason for this practice is the lack of courage to discontinue earlier although there seems to be no strong evidence of benefit from continuation till 7–10 weeks.

ADJUNCT THERAPY FOR LUTEAL PHASE SUPPORT

Esradiol

The endometrial quality is dependent on both estrogen and progesterone though the role of estrogen in the luteal phase is not clear. However, in IVF cycles, the levels of estrogen and progesterone drop in mid to late luteal phase. It is not clearly established whether this fall in mid luteal phase has any effect on clinical pregnancy rates. In a meta-analysis, Fatemi et al. found no differences between the groups supplemented with estrogen and progesterone as compared to progesterone alone.[39] This is true with both agonist and antagonist suppressed cycles.

However, two recent randomized controlled trials (RCTs) by Lukaszuk et al. reported positive outcomes in the form of higher pregnancy rates when supplemented with 4 mg oral E2 valerate and progesterone combination starting on the day of oocyte retrieval than progesterone alone.[40]

GnRH Agonist

Gonadotropin-releasing hormone is hypothesized to support CL by stimulating the release of LH from the pituitary. Peripheral GnRH receptor systems may serve as regulators of hCG synthesis and implantation, and may play a crucial role in antiproliferation and apoptosis.[41] GnRH is always used in combination with progesterone for the luteal phase support, its efficacy as a single agent has not been established. GnRH is usually administered as a single dose 6 days after oocyte retrieval or 3 days after embryo transfer. A recent study in 2013 concluded that administration of GnRH may increase implantation and pregnancy rates in IVF and intracytoplasmic sperm injection (ICSI) cycles.[42]

Human Chorionic Gonadotropin

With the introduction of GnRH antagonists protocols for the prevention of premature LH surge, triggering the final oocyte maturation and ovulation with a single bolus of GnRH agonist which prevented ovarian hyperstimulation syndrome (OHSS) became a popular option. However, due to shorter duration and smaller amplitude, total gonadotropin released is significantly reduced. To overcome this luteal deficiency, administration of a bolus of 1,500 IU of hCG was suggested. This secured the luteal phase and improved implantation and pregnancy rates.[43] The implantation and pregnancy rates when hCG is used as luteal phase are comparable with that of progesterone[44] although some trials have shown superiority of hCG over progesterone. Several studies have compared combined use of progesterone and hCG as luteal phase support with progesterone alone, yielding mixed results. The only disadvantage of hCG is the potential risk of OHSS. Studies have shown a statistically significant higher rates of moderate and severe OHSS.[45] Hence hCG should be used cautiously in patients at risk of OHSS.

LUTEAL PHASE IN SPECIAL CASES

- *Frozen embryo transfer and donor recipient*: These cycles are very different from stimulated cycles as there is no endogenous production of progesterone. Hence, luteal phase should be created in these patients. Combination of oral estradiol and IM/vaginal progesterone seems to be the best luteal phase support as it provides physiologic replacement by providing adequate serum progesterone levels while maintaining high local concentrations in the uterine cavity.[46]

- *Endometriosis*: In these cases there will be progesterone resistance due to alterations in the progesterone receptors in the endometrium.[47] To overcome this and to improve ART outcomes, ovarian suppression for short period of 6–8 weeks with oral contraceptive pills (OCPs) or long-term suppression of 3–6 months using GnRH agonists are recommended.[48,49]
- *Polycystic ovarian syndrome (PCOS)*: PCOS is another condition known to have progesterone resistance due to endometrial alterations due to persistent elevation in androgen levels. It is not proven yet whether this hyperandrogenic state could be overcome by ovarian suppression with pretreatment with OCPs.[50] Further studies are warranted to understand the progesterone resistance in these patients.

■ CONCLUSION

In conclusion, an overwhelming evidence suggests LPD in ART cycles and LPS is mandatory to optimize ART outcome. LPS is a well-established practice that will continue in the future. LPS is best initiated on the day of oocyte retrieval and continued up to 7–10 weeks of gestation. Pregnancy rates were similar for different forms of progesterone, with vaginal route being the preferred choice. In most randomized studies, there are no significant differences in pregnancy rates with progesterone supplementation alone or in combination with estradiol, hCG or hCG alone. The use of GnRH agonist as LPS is a novel approach and appears to be very promising. LPS in progesterone resistance cases like PCOS and endometriosis are worth further investigation.

■ REFERENCES

1. Devoto L, Fuenten A, Kohen P, et al. The human corpus luteum: life cycle and function in natural cycles. Fertil Steril. 2009;92(3):1067-79.
2. Zeleznik AJ. In vivo responses of the primate corpus luteum to the luteinizing hormone and chorionic gonadotrophin. Proc Natl Acad Sci USA. 1998;95:11002-7.
3. Kiriakidou M, McAllister JM, Sugawara T, et al. Expression of steroidogenic acute regulatory protein (StAR) in the human ovary. J Clin Endocrinol Metab. 1996;81:4122-8.
4. Deveto L, Kohen P, Vega M, et al. Control of human luteal steroidogensis. Mol Cell Endocrinol. 2002;186:137-41.
5. Nikas G, Aghajanova L. Endometrial pinopodes: Some more understanding on human implantation? Reprod Biomed Online. 2002;4(Suppl 3):18-23.
6. Cavagna M, Mantese JC. Biomarkers of endometrial receptivity: a review. Placenta. 2003;24:39-47.
7. Strowitzki T, Germeyer A, Popovici R, et al. The human endometrium as fertility-determining factor. Hum Reprod Update. 2006;12:617-30.
8. Dimitriadis E, White CA, Jones RL, et al. Cytokines, chemokines, and growth factors in endometrium related to implantation. Hum Reprod Update. 2005;11:613-30.
9. Jones GE. Some newer aspects of management of infertility. JAMA. 1949;141:1123-29.
10. Davis OK, Berkeley AS, Naus GJ, et al. The incidence of luteal phase defect in normal fertile women determined by serial endometrial biopsies. Fertil Steril. 1989;51(4):582-6.
11. Jordan J, Craig K, Clifton DK, et al. Luteal phase deficiency: the sensitivity and specificity of diagnostic methods in common clinical use. Fertil Steril. 1994;62:54-62.
12. Steele PA, Braund W, Judd SJ. Regulation of pulsatile secretion of progesterone during the human luteal phase. Clin Repro Fertil. 1986;2:117-24.
13. Practice Committee of the American Society for Reproductive Medicine. The clinical relevance of luteal phase deficiency: a committee opinion. Fertil Steril. 2012;98(5):1112-7.
14. Fatemi HM, Popovic-Todorovic B, Papanikolaou E, et al. An update of luteal phase support in stimulated IVF cycles. Hum Reprod Update. 2007;13(6):581-90.
15. Shaarawy M, Shabaan HA, Eid MM, et al. Plasma beta-endorphin levels in case of luteal phase deficiency. Fertil Steril. 1991;56:248-53.
16. Basi GS, O WS, Ng EH, et al. Morphometric analysis of peri-implantation endometrium in patients having excessively high oestradiol concentrations after ovarian stimulation. Hum Reprod. 2001;16:435-40.
17. Smitz J, Erard P, Camus M, et al. Pituitary gonadotrophin secretory capacity during the luteal phase in super ovulation using GnRH agonists and HMG in a desensitization or flare up protocol. Hum Reprod. 1992;7:1225-9.
18. Macklon NS, Fauser BC. Impact of ovarian hyperstimulation on the luteal phase. L Reprod Fertil Suppl. 2000;55:101-8.
19. Miyake A, Aono T, Kinugasa T, et al. Suppression of serum levels of luteinizing hormone by short and long loop negative feedback in ovariectomized women. J Endocrinol. 1979;80:353-6.
20. de Ziegler D, Franchin R, de Moustier B, et al. The hormone control of endometrial receptivity: estrogen and progesterone. J Reprod Immunol. 1998;39:149-66.
21. Smitz EM, Anthony FW, Gadd SC, et al. Trial of support treatment with hCG in the luteal phase after treatment with buserelin and hMG in women taking part in an IVF programme. Br Med J. 1989;298:1483-6.
22. Smith J, Devroey P, Camus M, et al. The luteal phase and early pregnancy after combined GnRH-agonist/HMG treatment for superovulation in IVR or GIFT. Hum Reprod. 1988;3:585-90.
23. Belaisch-Allart J, De Mouzon J, Lapousterle C, et al. The effect of HCG supplementation after combined GnRH agonist/HMG treatment in an IVF programme. Hum Reprod. 1990;5:163-6.
24. Albano C, Grimbizis G, Smitz J, et al. The luteal phase of non supplemental cycles after ovarian super ovulation with hMG and the GnRH antagonist Cetrorelix. Fertil Steril. 1998;70:357-9.

25. de Jong D, Macklon NS, Fauser BC. A pilot study involving minimal ovarian stimulation for IVF: extending the follicle stimulating hormone window combined with GnRH antagonist Cetrorelix. Fertil Steril. 2000;73:1051-4.

26. Kolibianalis EM, Bourgain C, Platteau P, et al. Abnormal endometrial development occurs during the luteal phase of non supplemental donor cycles treated with r-FSH ad GnRH antagonists. Fertil Steril. 2003;80:464-6.

27. Al-Inany H, Aboulghar M. GnRH antagonist in assisted reproduction: a Cochrane review. Hum Reprod. 2002;17:874-85.

28. Ziad R, Suheil J. Luteal supplementation in in vitro fertilization: more questions than answers. Fertil Steril. 2008;89(4):749-58.

29. Miles RA, Paulson RJ, Lobo RA, et al. Pharmacokinetics and endometrial tissue levels of progesterone after administration by IM and vaginal routes: a comparative study. Fertil Steril. 1994;62:485-90.

30. de Ziegler D. Hormonal control of endometrial receptivity. Hum Reprod. 1995;10:4-7.

31. Cicinelli E, de Ziegler D, Morgese S, et al. 'First pass uterine effect' is observed when estradiol is placed in the upper but not lower third of vagina. Fertil Steril. 2001;75:1136-40.

32. Chakravarty BN, Shirazee HH, Dam P, et al. Oral dydrogesterone versus intravaginal micronized progesterone as LPS in ART cycles: results of a randomized study. J Steroid Biochem Mol Biol. 2005;97:416-20.

33. Friedler S, Raziel A, Schachter M, et al. Luteal support with micronized progesterone following IVF using a down regulation protocol with GnRH agonist: a comparison study between vaginal and oral administration. Hum Reprod. 1999;14:1944-8.

34. Licciardi FL, Kwiatkowski A, Noyes NL, et al. Oral versus intramuscular progesterone for IVF: a prospective study. Fertil Steril. 1999;71:614-8.

35. Smith J, Devroey P, Camus M, et al. A randomized prospective study comparing supplementation of the luteal phase and early pregnancy by natural progesterone administered by IM or vaginal route. Rev Fr Gynecol Obstet. 1992;87:507-16.

36. Polyzos NP, Messini C, Papanikolau E, et al. Vaginal progesterone gel for the luteal phase support on IVF/ICSI cycles: a meta-analysis. Fertil Steril. 2010;94:2083-7.

37. Mochtar MH, Van Wely M, Van der Veen F. Timing luteal phase support in GnRH agonist down regulated cycles. Hum Reprod. 2006;21:905-8.

38. Schmidt KL, Ziebe S, Popovic B, et al. Progesterone supplementation during early gestation after IVF has no effect on delivery rate. Fertil Steril. 2001;75:337-41.

39. Fatemi HM, Kolibianakis EM, Camus M, et al. Addition of estradiol to progesterone for luteal supplementation in patients stimulated with GnRH antagonists/rFSH for IVF: a randomized controlled trial. Hum Reprod. 2006;21:2628-32.

40. Lukaszuk K, Liss J, Lukaszuk M, et al. Optimization of estradiol supplementation during the luteal phase improves the pregnancy rate in women undergoing IVF-ET cycles. Fetil Steril. 2005;83:1372-6.

41. Yu B, Ruman J, Christman G. The role of peripheral gonadotrophin releasing hormone receptors in female reproduction. Fertil Steril. 2011;95(2):465-73.

42. Brigante C.M.M, Mignini Renzini, Dal Canto, et al. Efficacy of luteal phase support with GnRH agonist: a preliminary comparative study. Fertil Steril. 2013;100(3):299.

43. Humaidan P, Ejdrup Bredkjaer H, Westergaard LG, et al. 1,500 IU of HCG at oocyte retrieval rescues the luteal phase when GnRH agonist is used for ovulation induction: a prospective, randomized controlled study. Fertil Steril. 2010;93(3):847-54.

44. Pritts EA, Atwood AK. Luteal phase support in infertility treatment: a meta-analysis of the randomized trials. Hum Reprod. 2002;17:2287-99.

45. Daya S, Gunby J. Luteal phase support in assisted reproductive cycles. Cochrane Database Syst Rev. 2004;(3):(CD004830).

46. Leonard PH, Hokenstad AN, Khan Z, et al. Luteal phase support for frozen embryo transfers: Does route of progesterone administration make a difference? Fertil Steril. 2013;99(3):S33-S34.

47. Engemise SL, Willets JM, Taylor AH, et al. Changes in glandular and stromal ER and PR isoform expression in eutopic endometrium following treatment with LNG- IUS. Eur J Obstet Gynecol Reprod Biol. 2011;157:101-6.

48. de Ziegler D, Gayet V, Aubriot FX, et al. Use of OCPs in women with endometriosis before ART improves outcomes. Fertil Steril. 2010;94:2796-9.

49. Surrey ES, Silverberg KM, Surrey MW, et al. Effect of prolonged GnRH agonist therapy on the outcome of IVF-ET in patients with endometriosis. Fertil Steril. 2002;78:699-704.

50. Daftary GS, Taylor HS. Endometrial regulation of HOX genes. Endocr Rev. 2006;27:331-55.

ART in Special Conditions

46

Endometriosis and ART

Israel Ortega, Juan A García-Velasco

■ INTRODUCTION

Endometriosis is an estrogen-dependent inflammatory disease that is characterized by the presence of viable endometrial tissue, including glandular epithelia and stromal cells, outside the uterine cavity. It represents one of the most common causes of chronic pelvic pain, dysmenorrhea and infertility, affecting several tissues, such as ovaries, pelvic organs (ureter, bladder, bowel and intestines), pelvic peritoneum and rectovaginal septum.[1]

Endometriosis is a common gynecological condition that affects approximately 10–15% of the female population during their reproductive years of any ethnic or social group and 10–25% of patients requiring assisted reproduction treatment (ART). Endometriotic ovarian cysts may be present in up to 20–40% of women with endometriosis scheduled for in vitro fertilization (IVF), whereas bilateral endometriomas may represent 19–28% of cases.[2,3]

The best medical approach to treat endometriotic ovarian cysts is controversial, and whether there is any benefit or not of removing endometriomas prior to IVF is still a matter of debate. The old notion of a systematic removal of all ovarian endometriotic cysts has recently been replaced with a more evidence-based approach, assessing the advantages as well as the complications of cyst removal prior to ART in each individual case.

In the present review, we have discussed in detail the impact of both conservative and surgical approaches for ovarian endometriosis on ovarian reserve. Furthermore, we will address the limitations and risks of both, to finally provide some guidelines for the management of ovarian endometriosis prior to IVF.

■ MEDICAL TREATMENT PRIOR TO IN VITRO FERTILIZATION

Endometriosis is a challenging condition associated with substantial morbidity and clinical sequelae, such as pain and infertility, which may have devastating impacts on the physical, mental and social well-being of afflicted women, and their overall quality of life.

Medical management of endometriosis must be individualized and aimed at alleviating pain and other symptoms, reducing the size of the endometriotic lesions and improving the quality of life of affected individuals. To date, medical treatment for alleviation of endometriosis-related pain is generally successful, with no medical agent being more efficacious than the other in spite of significantly differing side-effect profiles. However, the present evidence that supports preoperative medication prior to IVF treatment is too poor to make a recommendation on such regimens.

It has been suggested that pituitary suppression with the administration of gonadotropin-releasing hormone (GnRH) analogs for a few months prior to IVF may increase the success rate in patients diagnosed with endometriomas. The potential beneficial effects of this medication may be due to the induced amenorrhea, a similar endocrine environment to hypogonadotropic hypogonadism, to the effects of GnRH analogs on aromatase expression or on uterine natural killer (NK) cells. In a recent meta-analysis, the administration of GnRH agonists for a period of 3–6 months prior to IVF or intracytoplasmic sperm injection (ICSI) cycles in women with endometriosis increased the odds of clinical pregnancy by fourfold. However, these results should be interpreted with caution since they were extracted just from 165 patients and 78 pregnancies. In addition, none of the three trials included in the meta-analysis were specifically focused on ovarian endometriomas.[4] Thus, further clinical trials are needed to determine the benefit of this approach in patients with endometriosis before undergoing IVF treatment.

Ultrasound-guided aspiration of ovarian endometriomas represents an alternative to surgery in those patients who decline it, or in whom surgical removal is contraindicated. Furthermore, this procedure allows the concomitant use of in situ irrigation or injection with a sclerosing agent, such as tetracycline, interleukin-2, ethanol and methotrexate.[5,6] This combined approach is aimed to reduce recurrence rate and size of ovarian endometriomas, leading to a better access to follicles during oocyte retrieval as well as to a better response to ovarian stimulation after loss of ovarian tissue compression. However, the current experience is not convincing, and further studies are needed to clarify the impact of this combined approach on reproductive outcomes before its clinical use in routine IVF practice.

■ MANAGEMENT OF OVARIAN ENDOMETRIOMAS

Expectant Approach: Impact on Reproduction

The current evidence suggests that ovarian reserve is damaged after excision of ovarian endometriomas. However, the gonadal damage due to the presence of an endometrioma per se cannot be ruled out. Indeed, Benaglia et al.[7] evaluated the ovulation rate in 70 women with monolateral endometriomas, who had not undergone previous adnexal surgery. Ovulation was observed in the affected ovary in 31% of the cases, indicating that physiological mechanisms leading to ovulation are deranged in ovaries with endometriomas.

Ovarian response has been shown to be decreased in infertile patients diagnosed with ovarian endometriosis. Anti-Müllerian hormone (AMH) is a reliable marker of ovarian response with high sensitivity and the advantage of being independent of the cycle day. Garcia-Velasco et al.[8] evaluated 28 women undergoing IVF/ICSI cycle in whom an endometrioma more than 2 cm was clearly visible in ultrasound in one of the ovaries and not in the other. A group of 28 egg donors were included as a control group. Follicular fluid from the largest follicle of each ovary (with or without endometrioma) was individually collected prior to the rest of the follicular aspiration, and similarly in the control group. In this study, AMH levels in the ovaries with a large endometrioma were significantly lower (4.1 ± 2.7 ng/mL) than in the contralateral ovary (4.9 ± 2.6 ng/mL) and the control group (6.2 ± 3.0 ng/mL). Thus, AMH concentration in follicular fluid is diminished in women with endometriosis and may also decrease AMH levels in surrounding follicles. These findings may be of clinical relevance when counseling patients about their reproductive options.

Growing evidence indicates that women with endometriosis undergoing IVF treatment present poor reproductive outcomes. Gupta et al.[9] conducted a meta-analysis aimed to evaluate the ovarian reserve and ovarian responsiveness to stimulation, and assisted reproduction outcomes in patients with ovarian endometrioma. A decreased ovarian responsiveness to stimulation in patients with ovarian endometrioma was found compared with controls, probably due to deleterious effects of endometriosis on folliculogenesis, impaired follicular environment and reduced rates of follicular growth resulting in poor quality oocytes. Similarly, the odds of spontaneous abortion in those with ovarian endometrioma were significantly increased in comparison with those without. In contrast, the odds for fertilization and clinical pregnancy were not significantly affected in patients with endometrioma compared with controls.

Even though, some groups question whether the negative impact of ovarian endometriosis on reproductive outcome is due to the space-occupying effect of an ovarian endometrioma, rather than endometriosis itself. To this end, Kumbak et al.[10] evaluated the reproductive outcomes during IVF treatment in 85 women with unilateral ovarian endometriomas and 83 women with basal ovarian cysts. Gonadotropin consumption was higher and significantly fewer numbers of oocytes were retrieved in the endometrioma group. Moreover, embryo quality was found to be better in the cyst group compared to endometrioma group (79.7 versus 70.7%). Implantation rate was shown to be higher in the cyst group (28 versus 19%), whereas pregnancy and ongoing pregnancy rates were similar. Therefore, the negative impact of endometriosis on reproductive outcomes in women undergoing IVF treatment is due to the disease itself, and not to the presence of a cystic mass.

However, whether embryo implantation may play a role in the infertility associated with endometriosis is still a matter of debate. To address this issue, Diaz et al.[11] carried out a matched case-control study in which 25 recipients with stage III-IV endometriosis (group I) and 33 without the disease (group II) were included. On the day of retrieval, oocytes from a single donor were donated to recipients from both groups. Reproductive outcome comparison between patients with severe endometriosis who receive donor oocytes and patients without endometriosis provides an appropriate setup to address how this disease may affect fertility. Pregnancy, implantation and miscarriage rates were not affected by stage III-IV endometriosis when compared with control group. The livebirth rate was 28.0% in the group with endometriosis and 27.2% in the control group. The authors concluded that implantation is not affected by stage III-IV endometriosis and, thus, poor reproductive outcomes observed in these patients must be due to other factors.

Surgical Approach: Impact on Reproduction

Over the past decade, there is a general consensus that endometriomas require surgical treatment due to ineffectiveness of medical therapies. Indeed, laparoscopic management of endometrioma has been the gold standard for women with endometriosis-related pain and infertility until recently. Laparoscopic minimally invasive approach has the advantage of combining diagnostic and therapeutic procedures in a single operation is a better approach than laparotomy for the management of endometriosis. Furthermore, laparoscopy is associated with reduced blood loss, shortened hospital stay and costs, less complications and reduced need for analgesia compared to laparotomy.

However, surgical management for endometriosis increases time to achieve a pregnancy, costs and is related to a potential risk of significant damage to ovarian reserve. Cystectomy has been associated with concomitant excision of normal ovarian tissue resulting in significant follicle loss with possible subsequent reduction in ovarian reserve. Of note, it has been reported that surgical treatment of ovarian cysts that have well-defined ovarian capsules (dermoids, serous and mucinous cysts) resulted in some ovarian tissue being removed in 6% of cases. Conversely, a small portion of tissue containing primordial follicles is removed in more than 50% of endometriomas.[12] This difference is probably due to the difficulty in removing an endometrioma attached to the normal ovarian tissue.

A recent meta-analysis published by Raffi et al.[13] evaluated the impact of surgery for endometriomas on ovarian reserve as determined by serum AMH. It was conducted for eight studies that included a total of 237 patients who underwent cystectomy for unilateral or bilateral endometriomas. The overall average preoperative AMH was 3.0 ng/mL, and this fell by a statistically significant amount (38%) postoperatively, suggesting a negative impact of excision of endometriomas on ovarian reserve.

Adverse effects of surgical approach on ovarian reserve have been confirmed by assessing a change of the frequency of ovulation from affected ovaries during the natural cycle of patients with unilateral endometriomas before and after surgery. Horikawa et al.[14] retrospectively evaluated twenty-eight infertile women with unilateral ovarian endometriomas who underwent laparoscopic cystectomy. In this study, laparoscopic cystectomy caused a reduction of the ovarian reserve, as evidenced by the reduced ovulation rate of the affected ovary after surgery compared to before cystectomy (16.9 ± 4.5% versus 34.4 ± 6.6%, p = 0.013).

There are significant concerns regarding the potential negative impact of surgical treatment of endometrioma on ovarian reserve. A retrospective, case-control study demonstrated significantly fewer mature follicles recruited and fewer oocytes retrieved in women who underwent surgical treatment of endometrioma compared with those who had surgical removal of a non-endometriotic benign cyst.[15] Indeed, women who have undergone surgical removal of endometriomas before an ICSI cycle present a significantly longer stimulation, a significantly higher total recombinant follicle-stimulating hormone (FSH) dose and a lower number of mature oocytes compared to untreated women. In contrast, there was no statistically significant difference in terms of fertilization, implantation or pregnancy rates.[16] Thus, the negative effects of surgical removal of endometriomas on IVF outcome seem to be quantitative rather than qualitative.

In addition, surgeon's experience may play a role in surgery-induced negative effect on ovarian response and reproductive outcome. Yu et al.[17] evaluated 149 IVF-ICSI cycles with infertile patients who previously underwent laparoscopic conservative surgery for ovarian endometriomas; there were 76 cycles with an inexperienced surgeon and 73 cycles with an experienced surgeon. In this study, the number of antral follicle count (7.5 ± 3.8 versus 9.6 ± 6.6; p = 0.011), and live-born rate per cycle (9.3% versus 32.9%; p <0.001) were significantly lower in the inexperienced group comparing with the experienced group. Thus, the experience of the laparoscopist may affect ovarian reserve and live-born rate after treating ovarian endometrioma in infertile women with IVF-ICSI.

To date, there is growing evidence indicating that surgical treatment of endometrioma may exert deleterious effects on reproductive outcomes in women undergoing IVF. In addition, the negative impact of surgical removal of endometriomas on IVF outcome is closely related to the severity of endometriosis. Kuivasaari et al.[18] carried out an observational study evaluating 98 women who underwent IVF or ICSI treatment and had endometriosis diagnosed by laparoscopy or laparotomy and classified as minimal to mild endometriosis (American Society for Reproductive Medicine I/II) (n = 31) or moderate to severe endometriosis (American Society for Reproductive Medicine III/IV) (n = 67). In this study, 87 women with tubal infertility were included as a control group. A significantly lower pregnancy rate per fresh embryo transfer was found among women with stage III/IV endometriosis (22.6%) compared to stage I/II group (40.0%) or tubal infertility (36.6%). These findings indicate that stage III/IV endometriosis have a worse prognosis for IVF/ICSI treatments compared to milder stages or tubal factors.

Tsoumpou et al.[19] recently published a meta-analysis that compared surgery versus no treatment of endometrioma in women undergoing IVF. No significance difference was found between the two groups with regard to the outcome measures used to evaluate the response to controlled ovarian hyperstimulation with gonadotropins. Similarly, there was no significant difference regarding clinical pregnancy rate between the treated and the untreated groups. Therefore, surgical removal of endometriomas in order to improve reproductive outcome is not justified in those asymptomatic patients waiting for IVF treatment.

■ RISKS OF EXPECTANT MANAGEMENT AND SURGERY

Expectant Management

Missing an Occult Early Stage Malignancy

Histological examination after ovarian cyst removal must be performed not only for setting the diagnosis but also to rule out the presence of a potential occult early stage malignancy. Malignant transformation of endometriosis is rare, but may occur in up to 1% of women, with the most common site being the ovary.[20] Therefore, careful sonographic evaluation of ovarian endometriomas prior to IVF treatment is mandatory.

Development of a Pelvic Abscess

It should be noted that the bloody content of the cyst may serve as an excellent culture medium and may facilitate the spread of infection. The development of pelvic abscess after oocyte retrieval has been previously reported, but its incidence is really low. Benaglia et al.[21] evaluated the frequency of pelvic abscess in 214 patients with endometriomas undergoing oocyte retrieval, reporting that none of the women develop this complication. As a result, the potential risk of development of pelvic abscess should not determine the decision-making process regarding the ovarian cyst removal prior to IVF cycle.

Impairment of Endometriosis

Endometriosis is an estrogen-dependent disease and the number of ovulatory events has been associated with the formation of ovarian endometriomas. However, though hormonal stimulation during IVF treatment may play a role in the progression of the disease, little is known regarding this potential complication. To address this issue, Benaglia et al.[22] carried out a study including 64 women with surgical or echographic diagnosis of endometriosis and selected for IVF, being sonographically evaluated in the month preceding the IVF attempt and 3–6 months after the cycle. There was not either modification in size of ovarian endometriomas or development of new endometriomas or new deep nodules after the procedure. Therefore, IVF does not impair/enhance the progression of ovarian endometriosis.

Other Complications

The presence of ovarian endometriotic cysts may potentially lead to development of endometrioma rupture, potential contamination of follicular fluid and difficulty when retrieving oocytes during ovarian puncture. Furthermore, ovarian endometriosis has been associated with obstetric complications, such as preterm labor and intrauterine growth restriction. However, Benaglia et al.[23] recently demonstrated in a multicenter retrospective study that women with endometriomas achieving pregnancy through IVF do not seem to be exposed to a significant increased risk of obstetric complications.

Surgery

Ovarian responsiveness and the chance of conception during ART cycles are not the only factors that a physician has to consider prior to deciding whether or not the patient should undergo surgical treatment of an endometrioma. Surgery is costly and not free from complications. According to a meta-analysis published by Chapron et al.,[24] the incidence of major and minor complications associated with laparoscopy are 1.4% and 7.5% respectively. This aspect is of clinical relevance since patients diagnosed with endometriosis selected for endometriosis present and advanced stage of the disease and have generally been operated at least once before. Thus, these patients tend to develop thick adhesions and are at high risk of complications during the surgical procedure.

In addition, the incidence of severe ovarian damage, occurring in gonads operated for ovarian endometriomas, is not a rare event. Benaglia et al.[25] carried out a retrospective study to evaluate the rate of ovaries remaining silent when stimulated after surgery for endometriomas. In this study, the frequency of severe ovarian damage following surgery was 13%.[24] Thus, this point is of utmost relevance since the demonstration that surgery may be mainly responsible for the damage would strongly caution against systematic surgical removal of these lesions. Conversely, some authors consider that laparoscopy may still be useful for the treatment of endometriosis even after multiple IVF failures.[26] In this study, Littman et al. retrospectively evaluated 29 patients with prior IVF failures; 22 conceived after laparoscopic treatment of endometriosis, including 15 non-IVF pregnancies and 7 IVF pregnancies.

CONCLUSION

Laparoscopic management of endometrioma was the gold standard before IVF until recently. However, it has been shown that laparoscopic surgical removal of ovarian endometriotic cysts prior to IVF not only damages ovarian reserve, and impairs the responsiveness to hyperstimulation, but also does not offer any additional benefit in terms of fertility outcomes. This damage becomes of particular clinical relevance in women with previous interventions for endometriosis or bilateral disease, since the excision of ovarian endometriomas may result in a severe impairment of the ovarian reserve and even ovarian failure. In addition, it should be taken into account that laparoscopic cystectomy of an endometrioma increases the time to achieve a pregnancy, the treatment costs and exposes women to dangerous risks inevitably related to a demanding surgery, whereas risks associated with expectant management are mostly anecdotal or of doubtful clinical relevance.

The best treatment approach for ovarian endometrioma should be individualized, assessing both the advantages and complications of cyst removal prior to ART in each individual case. We recommend generally proceeding directly to IVF to reduce time to pregnancy in those patients with previous interventions for endometriosis, damaged ovarian reserved, absence of pain symptoms, bilateral disease and stable growth in order to avoid potential surgical complications and to limit patient costs. Conversely, surgery should be indicated in specific circumstances, such as to treat concomitant pain symptoms which are refractory to medical treatments, or when malignancy cannot be reliably ruled out, or in the presence of large cysts.

MESSAGE BOX

Laparoscopic management of endometrioma was the gold standard before IVF until recently. However, laparoscopic surgical removal of ovarian endometriotic cysts prior to IVF damages ovarian reserve, impairs the responsiveness to hyperstimulation, increases time to achieve pregnancy as well as treatment costs. Furthermore, it does not offer any additional benefit in terms of fertility outcomes.

We thus recommend generally proceeding directly to IVF to reduce time to pregnancy in those patients with previous interventions for endometriosis, damaged ovarian reserved, absence of pain symptoms, bilateral disease and stable growth in order to avoid potential surgical complications and to limit patient costs.

REFERENCES

1. Bulun SE. Endometriosis. N Engl J Med. 2009;360(3):268-79.
2. Vercellini P, Chapron C, De Giorgi O, et al. Coagulation or excision of ovarian endometriomas? Am J Obstet Gynecol. 2003;188(3):606-10.
3. Jenkins S, Olive DL, Haney AF. Endometriosis: pathogenetic implications of the anatomic distribution. Obstet Gynecol. 1986;67(3):335-8.
4. Sallam HN, Garcia-Velasco JA, Dias S, et al. Long-term pituitary down-regulation before in vitro fertilization (IVF) for women with endometriosis. Cochrane Database Syst Rev. 2006(1):CD004635.
5. Mesogitis S, Daskalakis G, Pilalis A, et al. Management of ovarian cysts with aspiration and methotrexate injection. Radiology. 2005;235(2):668-73.
6. Agostini A, De Lapparent T, Collette E, et al. In situ methotrexate injection for treatment of recurrent endometriotic cysts. Eur J Obstet Gynecol Reprod Biol. 2007;130(1):129-31.
7. Benaglia L, Somigliana E, Vercellini P, et al. Endometriotic ovarian cysts negatively affect the rate of spontaneous ovulation. Hum Reprod. 2009;24(9):2183-6.
8. García-Velasco JA, Motta L, Rodriguez S, et al. Decreased concentrations of AMH in follicular fluid of women with endometriosis: A hypothetical new marker of oocyte quality. J Endometriosis. 2009;1:1-5.
9. Gupta S, Agarwal A, Agarwal R, et al. Impact of ovarian endometrioma on assisted reproduction outcomes. Reprod Biomed Online. 2006;13(3):349-60.
10. Kumbak B, Kahraman S, Karlikaya G, et al. In vitro fertilization in normoresponder patients with endometriomas: comparison with basal simple ovarian cysts. Gynecol Obstet Invest. 2008;65(3):212-6.
11. Diaz I, Navarro J, Blasco L, et al. Impact of stage III-IV endometriosis on recipients of sibling oocytes: matched case-control study. Fertil Steril. 2000;74(1):31-4.
12. Muzii L, Bianchi A, Croce C, et al. Laparoscopic excision of ovarian cysts: is the stripping technique a tissue-sparing procedure? Fertil Steril. 2002;77(3):609-14.
13. Raffi F, Metwally M, Amer S. The impact of excision of ovarian endometrioma on ovarian reserve: a systematic review and meta-analysis. J Clin Endocrinol Metab. 2012;97(9):3146-54.
14. Horikawa T, Nakagawa K, Ohgi S, et al. The frequency of ovulation from the affected ovary decreases following laparoscopic cystectomy in infertile women with unilateral endometrioma during a natural cycle. J Assist Reprod Genet. 2008;25(6):239-44.
15. Nargund G, Cheng WC, Parsons J. The impact of ovarian cystectomy on ovarian response to stimulation during in-vitro fertilization cycles. Hum Reprod. 1996;11(1):81-3.
16. Demirol A, Guven S, Baykal C, et al. Effect of endometrioma cystectomy on IVF outcome: a prospective randomized study. Reprod Biomed Online. 2006;12(5):639-43.
17. Yu HT, Huang HY, Soong YK, et al. Laparoscopic ovarian cystectomy of endometriomas: surgeons' experience may affect ovarian reserve and live-born rate in infertile patients with in vitro fertilization-intracytoplasmic sperm injection. Eur J Obstet Gynecol. 2010;152(2):172-5.

18. Kuivasaari P, Hippelainen M, Anttila M, et al. Effect of endometriosis on IVF/ICSI outcome: stage III/IV endometriosis worsens cumulative pregnancy and live-born rates. Hum Reprod. 2005;20(11):3130-5.
19. Tsoumpou I, Kyrgiou M, Gelbaya TA, et al. The effect of surgical treatment for endometrioma on in vitro fertilization outcomes: a systematic review and meta-analysis. Fertil Steril. 2009;92(1):75-87.
20. Deligdisch L, Penault-Llorca F, Schlosshauer P, et al. Stage I ovarian carcinoma: different clinical pathologic patterns. Fertil Steril. 2007;88(4):906-10.
21. Benaglia L, Somigliana E, Iemmello R, et al. Endometrioma and oocyte retrieval-induced pelvic abscess: a clinical concern or an exceptional complication? Fertil Steril. 2008;89(5): 1263-6.
22. Benaglia L, Somigliana E, Santi G, et al. IVF and endometriosis-related symptom progression: insights from a prospective study. Hum Reprod. 2011;26(9):2368-72.
23. Benaglia L, Bermejo A, Somigliana E, et al. Pregnancy outcome in women with endometriomas achieving pregnancy through IVF. Hum Reprod. 2012;27(6):1663-7.
24. Chapron C, Fauconnier A, Goffinet F, et al. Laparoscopic surgery is not inherently dangerous for patients presenting with benign gynaecologic pathology: Results of a meta-analysis. Hum Reprod. 2002;17(5):1334-42.
25. Benaglia L, Somigliana E, Vighi V, et al. Rate of severe ovarian damage following surgery for endometriomas. Hum Reprod. 2010;25(3):678-82.
26. Littman E, Giudice L, Lathi R, et al. Role of laparoscopic treatment of endometriosis in patients with failed in vitro fertilization cycles. Fertil Steril. 2005;84(6):1574-8.

47

Myomas in Infertility

Sunita R Tandulwadkar, Devika Chopra

INTRODUCTION

Uterine myomas and their relationship to a woman's fertility has since long been a concern for infertility clinicians worldwide. This issue is gaining relevance in the developed world wherein there is a tendency to start a family at an age when natural female fertility is on a decline and the incidence of fibroids is increasing.[1] As a consequence, the proportion of infertile women diagnosed with fibroids is rising, and it may have important economic and clinical consequences associated with infertility treatment.[1]

Myomas are heterogeneous tumors that vary in composition, size, location and number, all of which may have an impact on a woman's fertility.[2] Myomas are the most common benign solid tumor of the genital system of females and are diagnosed in 25–30% of females during their lives.[3] Uterine myomas are speculated to be the sole cause of infertility in 1–3% of women and are proposed to be a contributing factor for infertility in 5–10% of women.[4] A number of studies have been performed to determine the influence of myomas on fertility all of which have widely varying findings.[2]

The causative role of fibroids in infertility remains controversial.[5] It has been proposed that fibroids alter the uterine contour, hamper the tubo-ovarian relationship, impinge on the tubal opening, interfere with sperm transport and compress cervical canal in some cases thereby hampering sperm capture. Additionally, fibroids compress the uterine cavity (some intramural and submucous type 1 and 2) cause venous ectasia over submucous (SM) components, release of vasoactive amines, hamper blood supply to the endometrium causing necrosis and inflammation and thus interfere with implantation.[6]

This chapter has focused on different types of myomas and their relationship to fertility. Additionally, this chapter has attempted to answer the following questions based on recent evidence: (1) Do uterine fibroids, of specific size or location, decrease fertility? (2) Does removal of the fibroid(s) enhances fertility as evidenced by clinical pregnancy and live birth rates?

RECENT EVIDENCE

Several studies have documented the effect of myomas on fertility and have documented the effect of myoma removal/no treatment on the results of infertility treatment. These studies study clinical characteristics such as patient age, abortion times before myomectomy, operation type, number, location and classification of myomas, uterine cavity penetration and uterine volume that could affect the pregnancy and live birth rate after myomectomy[2,7] **(Table 1)**.

EFFECT OF LOCATION OF MYOMA ON IVF OUTCOME

A study by Eldar-Geva et al. in 1998 found a lower implantation and clinical pregnancy rate in women with intramural (IM) and SM fibroids even when there was no compromise of the uterine cavity. They also concluded that subserosal (SS) fibroids had no effect on implantation and pregnancy rates. They proposed myomectomy prior to commencement of ART treatment.[8] Since then several studies have been published interpreting the relationship between the location of the myoma and IVF outcome. Similarly in 2009, Sunkara et al. also concluded that non-cavity distorting IM fibroids lowered IVF results when compared with patients with no fibroids.[9] A meta-analysis by Somigliana et al. also concluded that SM, IM and SS fibroids interfere with fertility in decreasing order of importance.[1]

The most recent update by the American Society of Reproductive Medicine (ASRM) stated that irrespective of the location, the clinical pregnancy, implantation and ongoing pregnancy rate were lower in women with fibroids compared to that of controls **(Table 2)**.

Table 1 Various studies documenting the effect of myomas on fertility[2]

Study	Design	Control	Infertility treatment	Age (years), control vs. study	Location and no. of patients	Size (mm)	No. of fibroids per patient	Myomec-tomy trial	Uterine cavity evaluation[b]	Uniform evaluation of subjects	Inclusion and exclusion criteria specified	Single subject per outcome specified	Outcome assessment methodology specified
Stovail	P	Infertile women without fibroids	IVF	35.9 vs. 35.8	SS 5, IM 86	Mean 24.2	1.8	No	HSG	No	Yes	No	No
Eldar-Geva	R	Infertile women without fibroids	IVF/ICSI	35.5 vs. 35.7	SS 41, IM 55, SM 10	Means SS 24, IM 23.7, IC 44.8	SS 1.3, IM 1.8, IC 2.7	No	Not stated	No	No	No	Yes
Farhi	R	Infertile women with tubal factor and without fibroids	IVF	33.5 vs. 34	SS/IM 28, SM 18	Not stated	Not stated	No	US	No	No	No	No
Narayan	P	Infertile women without fibroids	IVF/none	34.5 vs. 36.6	SM 28	Not stated	Not stated	Yes	US	No	No	No	No
Varasteh	R	Infertile women without fibroids	All treatments	37.2 vs. 35.2	SM 36	Not stated	Not stated	Yes	Hysteroscopy	No	Yes	Yes	No
Surrey 2001	R	Infertile women without fibroids	IVF/ICSI	36–42 vs. 37–43	IM 73 cycles	Mean 2.33	Not stated	No	Hysteroscopy	Yes	Yes	No	Yes
Seoud	R	Infertile women without fibroids and those with in situ fibroids	IVF	36.1 vs. 37.1	SS 10, IM 1	Myomec-tomy mean 89 myoma mean 31	Not stated	Yes	HSG	No	No	No	No
Ramzy	R	Infertile women without fibroids	IVF/ICSI	34.7 vs. 34.0	SS 32, IM 12	SS mean 38, IM mean 32	1.2	No	US	No	No	No	No
Bulletti 1999	R	Infertile women without fibroids and those with in situ fibroids	None	Not done	SS/IM/SM 106	Not stated	Not stated	Yes	US	No	No	Yes	Yes

Contd…

Contd...

Study	Design	Control	Infertility treatment	Age (years), control vs. study	Location and no. of patients	Size (mm)	No. of fibroids per patient	Myomectomy trial	Uterine cavity evaluation[b]	Uniform evaluation of subjects	Inclusion and exclusion criteria specified	Single subject per outcome specified	Outcome assessment methodology specified
Bernard	R	Infertile women without fibroids	None	35.7 vs. 34.5	IM 16	Range 10–50	1.4	No	Hysteroscopy	Yes	Yes	Yes	No
Dietterich	R	Oocyte and embryo donor recipients with fibroids	Oocyte and embryo done recipients	Recipient age 44.1 vs. 41.5	IM/SS 9	Rang 6–26	1–6	No	US	No	Yes	Yes	Yes
Wang 2001	P	Infertile women without fibroids	None	32.7 vs. 35.5[a]	SS 13, IM 13, SM 8	Not stated	Not stated	No	US	No	Yes	No	Yes
Wang 2004	P	Oocyte donation recipients without fibroids	Oocyte donor recipients	Recipient age 39.5 vs. 43[a]	SS/IM 49	30.3 or less	Not stated	No	US	No	Yes	Yes	Yes
Check	P	Infertile women without fibroids	IVF/ICSI	36.6 vs. 36.6	SS/IM 61	Range 6–51	1–7	No	HSG	No	Yes	Yes	Yes
Ng	P	Infertile women without fibroids	IVF/ICSI	35 vs. 37[a]	SS/IM 77	Range 10–60	1–6	No	US	No	Yes	Yes	Yes
Hart	P	Infertile women without fibroids	IVF/ICSI	34.6 vs. 36.4[a]	IM 112	Range 50 or less	1–4	No	US	No	Yes	Yes	No
Oliveira	R	Infertile women without fibroids	ICSI	35.1 vs. 35.1	SS 82, IM 130, SS/IM 33	Range 4–69	1–4	No	HSG	No	Yes	Yes	No
Yarali	R	Infertile women without fibroids	ICSI	35.6 vs. 36.0	SS 35, IM 73	Range 5–100	1–8	No	HSG	No	Yes	Yes	Yes
Bulletti 2004	P	In situ fibroids	IVF/ICSI	Not stated	SS/IM 84	At least one >50	1–5	Yes	US	Yes	Yes	Yes	No
Gianaroli	R	Infertile women without fibroids	IVF/ICSI	35.7 vs. 35.8	IM/SM 75	19–48	1–7	No	US	No	No	No	Yes

Contd...

Contd...

Study	Design	Control	Infertility treatment	Age (years), control vs. study	Location and no. of patients	Size (mm)	No. of fibroids per patient	Myomectomy trial	Uterine cavity evaluation[b]	Uniform evaluation of subjects	Inclusion and exclusion criteria specified	Single subject per outcome specified	Outcome assessment methodology specified
Surrey 2005	R	Infertile women without fibroids and oocyte donor recipients without fibroids	IVF/ICSI and oocyte donor recipients	37.8 vs. 38.0, 41.3 vs. 40.0	IM/SS 55, SM 46	14–68	1–4	Yes	Hysteroscopy	No	Yes	No	Yes
Klatsky	R	Infertile women without fibroids	Oocyte donor recipients	Donor age 26.2 vs. 24.7	IM/SS 94	Unknown range, mean 28 mm	Not stated	No	HSG	No	Yes	Yes	Yes
Casini	RCT	In situ fibroids	None	Not compared all less than 35	SM 94, IM 76	Unknown range	Not stated	Yes	HSG	Yes	Yes	Yes	Yes

Abbreviations: HSG, hysterosalpingography; ICSI, intracytoplasmic sperm injection; IM, intramural myoma; IVF, in vitro fertilization; P, prospective; R, retrospective; RCT, randomized control trial; SHG, sonohysterography; SM, submucous myoma; SS, subserosal myoma; US, ultrasound

[a]Statistically significantly older patients in the different groups

[b]Indicated the highest quality investigative tool used in all study subjects

Table 2 Effect of fibroids on fertility: all locations[2]

Outcome	Number of studies/substudies	Relative risk	95% confidence interval	Significance
Clinical pregnancy rate	18	0.849	0.734–0.983	P = 0.029
Implantation rate	14	0.821	0.722–0.932	P = 0.002
Ongoing pregnancy/live birth rate	17	0.697	0.589–0.826	P < 0.001
Spontaneous abortion rate	18	1.678	1.373–2.051	P < 0.001
Preterm delivery rate	3	1.357	0.607–3.036	Not significant

Table 3 Effects of fibroids on fertility: submucous fibroids

Outcome	Number of studies/substudies	Relative risk	95% confidence interval	Significance
Clinical pregnancy rate	4	0.363	0.179–0.737	P = 0.005
Implantation rate	2	0.283	0.123–0.649	P = 0.003
Ongoing pregnancy/live birth rate	2	0.318	0.119–0.850	P < 0.001
Spontaneous abortion rate	2	1.678	1.373–2.051	P = 0.022
Preterm delivery rate	0	–	–	–

In women with SM and IM fibroids all parameters, i.e. clinical pregnancy rate, implantation rate and ongoing pregnancy rate were significantly lower compared to controls **(Tables 3 and 4)**. Whereas SS fibroids had no effect on the aforementioned parameters between the two groups.[2]

Thus, the location of fibroids does impact clinical pregnancy and implantation rates in IVF.

EFFECT OF SIZE OF MYOMA ON IVF OUTCOME

While analyzing women with IM fibroids less than 5 cm, Hart et al. (2001) noted that implantation, pregnancy and ongoing pregnancy rate were significantly reduced compared to controls. They concluded that IM fibroids halve the chances of ongoing pregnancy after assisted conception cycles.[10] In 2004, Oliveira et al. found that patients having SS or IM leiomyomas of less than 4 cm not encroaching on the uterine cavity had IVF-ICSI outcomes comparable to those of patients without such leiomyomas. They therefore concluded that these patients did not require myomectomy before being scheduled for assisted reproduction cycles. However, they recommended caution for patients with IM fibroids greater than 4 cm, and such patients needed myomectomy before they were enrolled in IVF-ICSI cycles.[11]

Another study in 2007 noted that women with fibroids greater than 4 cm required higher number of cycles to achieve a pregnancy without myomectomy. They therefore recommended a myomectomy for IM fibroids greater than 4 cm. However, they did not recommend myomectomy prior to IVF cycles in small to moderate sized myomas irrespective of their location.[12] Their finding was further bolstered by a study in 2011 by Somigliana et al. wherein no difference was noted with respect to implantation and clinical pregnancy rates after IVF in women with small asymptomatic fibroids.[13]

Thus, IM myomas greater than 4 cm in size, even if they are non-cavity distorting may have an impact on IVF-ICSI success rates and warrant treatment before embryo transfer.

EFFECT OF MYOMECTOMY ON IVF OUTCOMES

In 2006, Casini et al. noted that among the patients who underwent myomectomy, the pregnancy rates obtained were 43.3% in cases of SM, 56.5% in cases of IM, 40% in cases of SM-IM and 35.5% in cases of IM-SS uterine fibroids, respectively. Among the patients who did not undergo surgical treatment, the pregnancy rates obtained were 27.2% in women with SM, 41% in women with IM, 15% in women with SM-IM and 21.43% in women with

Table 4 Effect of fibroid on fertility: intramural fibroids[2]

Outcome	Number of studies/substudies	Relative risk	95% confidence interval	Significance
A. All studies				
Clinical pregnancy rate	12	0.810	0.696–0.941	P = 0.006
Implantation rate	7	0.684	0.587–0.796	P < 0.001
Ongoing pregnancy/live birth rate	8	0.703	0.583–0.848	P < 0.001
Spontaneous abortion rate	8	1.747	1.226–2.489	P = 0.002
Preterm delivery rate	1	6.000	0.309–116.606	Not significant
B. Prospective studies				
Clinical pregnancy rate	3	0.708	0.437–1.146	Not significant
Implantation rate	2	0.552	0.391–0.781	P = 0.001
Ongoing pregnancy/live birth rate	2	0.465	0.291–0.744	P = 0.019
Spontaneous abortion rate	2	2.384	1.110–5.122	P = 0.002
Preterm delivery rate	0	–	–	–
C. Studies using hysteroscopy in all subjects				
Clinical pregnancy rate	2	0.845	0.666–1.071	Not significant
Implantation rate	1	0.714	0.547–0.931	P = 0.013
Ongoing pregnancy/live birth rate	2	0.733	0.383–1.405	Not significant
Spontaneous abortion rate	2	1.215	0.391–3.774	Not significant
Preterm delivery rate	1	6.000	0.309–116.606	Not significant

IM-SS uterine fibroids, respectively. Although the results were not statistically significant in the group of women with IM and IM-SS fibroids; this study confirmed the important role of the position of the uterine fibroid in infertility as well as the importance of myomectomy for SM fibroids in results of assisted conception.[14]

Somigliana et al. noted that surgical treatment appeared to increase the pregnancy rate greater than 50% for women who underwent myomectomy for infertility.[1] A comparative study has provided insight into the effectiveness of myomectomy prior to IVF (Bulletti et al.). Patients selected for the procedure, who were diagnosed with IM-SS fibroids, with at least one lesion with a mean diameter of 5 cm, were informed about the pros and cons of myomectomy. The cumulative delivery rate in women who did and did not undergo surgery was 25% and 12%, respectively.[15]

A systematic review by the ASRM in 2009 concluded that myomectomy caused a statistically significant increase in clinical pregnancy rate in women with SM fibroids. They did not find any difference in ongoing pregnancy and live birth rate in myomectomies performed for SM and IM fibroids[2] **(Tables 5 and 6)**.

Thus, evidence suggests that there is a definite improvement in clinical pregnancy rate after removal of SM myomas. There are however conflicting views regarding the removal of IM fibroids and their role in improving IVF outcomes.

■ CONCLUSION

Location of Myoma

The location of fibroids does affect the IVF outcome. SM fibroids negatively impact IVF results. IM fibroids, even if they are non-cavity distorting, reduce implantation and thereby hamper IVF results. SS fibroids do not have any effect on implantation in IVF cycles.

Size of Myoma

Myomas larger than 4 cm in size do have a negative impact on IVF results. Although the ASRM systematic review has failed to recognize any co-relation between the size of myomas and IVF outcomes; several studies use the cutoff as 4 cm to warrant removal of myomas prior to embryo transfer.

Table 5 Effect of myomectomy: submucous fibroids[2]

Outcome	Number of studies/substudies	Relative risk	95% confidence interval	Significance
A. Controls: fibroids in situ (no myomectomy)				
Clinical pregnancy rate	2	2.034	1.081–3.826	P = 0.028
Implantation rate	0	–	–	–
Ongoing pregnancy/live birth rate	1	2.654	0.920–7.658	Not significant
Spontaneous abortion rate	1	0.771	0.359–1.658	Not significant
Preterm delivery rate	0	–	–	–
B. Controls: infertile women with no fibroids				
Clinical pregnancy rate	2	1.545	0.998–2.391	Not significant
Implantation rate	2	1.116	0.906–1.373	Not significant
Ongoing pregnancy/live birth rate	3	1.128	0.959–1.326	Not significant
Spontaneous abortion rate	2	1.241	0.475–3.242	Not significant
Preterm delivery rate	0	–	–	–

Table 6 Effect of myomectomy: intramural fibroids[2]

Outcome	Number of studies/substudies	Relative risk	95% confidence interval	Significance
A. All studies				
Clinical pregnancy rate	12	0.810	0.696–0.941	P = 0.006
Implantation rate	7	0.684	0.587–0.796	P < 0.001
Ongoing pregnancy/live birth rate	8	0.703	0.583–0.848	P < 0.001
Spontaneous abortion rate	8	1.747	1.226–2.489	P = 0.002
Preterm delivery rate	1	6.000	0.309–116.606	Not significant
B. Prospective studies				
Clinical pregnancy rate	3	0.708	0.437–1.146	Not significant
Implantation rate	2	0.552	0.391–0.781	P = 0.001
Ongoing pregnancy/live birth rate	2	0.465	0.291–0.744	P = 0.019
Spontaneous abortion rate	2	2.384	1.110–5.122	P = 0.002
Preterm delivery rate	0	–	–	–
C. Studies using hysteroscopy in all subjects				
Clinical pregnancy rate	2	0.845	0.666–1.071	Not significant
Implantation rate	1	0.714	0.547–0.931	P = 0.013
Ongoing pregnancy/live birth rate	2	0.733	0.383–1.405	Not significant
Spontaneous abortion rate	2	1.215	0.391–3.774	Not significant
Preterm delivery rate	1	6.000	0.309–116.606	Not significant

Role of Myomectomy

Several studies have shown the benefit of removing SM fibroids and positive co-relation between IVF results and SM myoma excisions. Results are conflicting however, with respect to IM myomas.

Postoperative complications, like adhesions, infections, and intrapartum complications, like uterine rupture, need to be kept in mind prior to planning any myomectomy. An informed decision needs to be taken prior to myomectomy preceding an IVF cycle. Studies have shown that laparoscopic myomectomies have better postoperative results (less adhesion, less blood loss and less postoperative morbidity). However, the strength of the myomectomy scar in laparoscopic myoma excision is weaker than in open myomectomy and chances of antepartum/intrapartum uterine rupture is higher in laparoscopic myomectomies.

Thus, myomas have a definite impact on a woman's fertility and assessment of the myoma before undergoing an assisted conception cycle is of utmost importance. In conclusion, better studies and randomized trials are needed to reveal answers into the role of myomectomy for improving IVF results in IM fibroids.

■ REFERENCES

1. Somigliana E, Vercellini P, Daguati R, et al. Fibroids and female reproduction: a critical analysis of the evidence. Hum Reprod Update. 2007;13(5):465-76.
2. Pritts EA, Parker WH, Olive DL. Fibroids and infertility: an updated systematic review of the evidence. Fertil Steril. 2009;91(4):1215-23.
3. Mettler L, Schollmeyer T, Tinelli A, et al. Complications of uterine fibroids and their management, surgical management of fibroids, laparoscopy and hysteroscopy versus hysterectomy, haemorrhage, adhesions, and complications. Obstet Gynecol Int. 2012;2012:791248.
4. Kolankaya A, Arici A. Myomas and assisted reproductive technologies: when and how to act? Obstet Gynecol Clin North Am. 2006;33(1):145-52.
5. Kasum M. Fertility following myomectomy. Acta Clinica Croatica. 2009;48(2):137-43.
6. Practice Committee of the American Society for Reproductive Medicine. Myomas and reproductive function. Fertil Steril. 2004;82(Suppl 1):111-6.
7. Zhang Y, Hua KQ. Patients' age, myoma size, myoma location, and interval between myomectomy and pregnancy may influence the pregnancy rate and live birth rate after myomectomy. J Laparoendosc Adv Surg Tech A. 2014;24(2):95-9.
8. Eldar-Geva T, Meagher S, Healy DL, et al. Effect of intramural, subserosal, and submucosal uterine fibroids on the outcome of assisted reproductive technology treatment. Fertil Steril. 1998;70(4):687-91.
9. Sunkara SK, Khairy M, El-Toukhy T, et al. The effect of intramural fibroids without uterine cavity involvement on the outcome of IVF treatment: a systematic review and meta-analysis. Hum Reprod. 2010;25(2):418-29.
10. Hart R, Khalaf Y, Yeong CT, et al. A prospective controlled study of the effect of intramural uterine fibroids on the outcome of assisted conception. Hum Reprod. 2001;16(11):2411-7.
11. Oliveira FG, Abdelmassih VG, Diamond MP, et al. Impact of subserosal and intramural uterine fibroids that do not distort the endometrial cavity on the outcome of in vitro fertilization-intracytoplasmic sperm injection. Fertil Steril. 2004;81(3):582-7.
12. Vimercati A, Scioscia M, Lorusso F, et al. Do uterine fibroids affect IVF outcomes? Reprod BioMed Online. 2007;15(6):686-91.
13. Somigliana E, De Benedictis S, Vercellini P, et al. Fibroids not encroaching the endometrial cavity and IVF success rate: a prospective study. Hum Reprod. 2011;26(4):834-9.
14. Casini ML, Rossi F, Agostini R, et al. Effects of the position of fibroids on fertility. Gynecol Endocrinol. 2006;22(2):106-9.
15. Bulletti C, DE Ziegler D, Levi Setti P, et al. Myomas, pregnancy outcome, and in vitro fertilization. Ann N Y Acad Sci. 2004;1034:84-92.

48 Genital Tuberculosis and ART

Neena Malhotra

INTRODUCTION

Tuberculosis (TB) remains one of the major health problems primarily in the developing countries with high morbidity and mortality.[1] Genital tuberculosis (GTB) is one of the most common causes of female infertility among women particularly from Indian subcontinent with a variable reported incidence of 1–19%.[2,3] This stands as a stark contrast to the developed world where GTB is responsible for infertility in less than 1%.[4] While the exact burden of disease is unknown, it leaves behind sequelae with irreversible damage and infertility, mainly as a consequence of tubal, endometrial damage, requiring some form of assisted reproduction techniques (ART) for a successful pregnancy and live birth. ART in women with GTB is challenging not only because of the dismal outcome in terms of pregnancy or live births but also because it is difficult to identify women with the disease when it manifests in a subtle form that is not confirmed with the conventional tests available.

EPIDEMIOLOGY OF GENITAL TUBERCULOSIS

It is extremely difficult to ascertain the precise burden of disease as most cases are asymptomatic and remain undiagnosed. Even though GTB is an uncommon type of extra pulmonary tuberculosis (EPTB), it has a worldwide distribution with a high incidence in developing world, including India. Infertility is the most common presentation of female genital tuberculosis (FGTB) with a reported incidence of 40–80%.[5-7] GTB is one of the most common causes of female infertility varying worldwide from more than 1% in USA to 10–19% in some Indian studies.[2-4] The exact incidence of FGTB is not accurately known, perhaps because of under reporting and also due to lack of reliable confirmatory investigations.[8] Studies from other parts of the world including Iran were suggestive of a strong relationship between GTB and infertility.[9] In yet another prospective study from Ethiopia where clinically suspected cases of FGTB were subjected to investigations to confirm the diagnosis using histopathology, acid fast bacilli (AFB) smears, TB culture and polymerase chain reaction (PCR) for *Mycobacterium tuberculosis*, FGTB was confirmed in infertile women highlighting that FGTB is a significant clinical problem in Ethiopia.[10] In a recent prospective study from New Delhi, India, investigating infertile women, a suspicion of GTB was made on history and preliminary tests [Mantoux, erythrocyte sedimentation rate (ESR)] in 10–25%, and confirmation was made by a combination of tests including endometrial sampling, laparoscopy and peritoneal biopsy from suspicious lesions at laparoscopy and hysteroscopy in approximately 25% of women.[11] Even though these statistics do not reflect the true burden of disease in the community as they are common from tertiary hospital and are mostly retrospective data, nevertheless GTB is a major cause of infertility in the developing world.

ETIOPATHOGENESIS OF INFERTILITY IN GENITAL TUBERCULOSIS

Genital TB, an uncommon form of extrapulmonary TB is caused by *Mycobacterium tuberculosis* complex (*M. tuberculosis, M. bovis and M. africanum*) and is always secondary to pulmonary TB or extrapulmonary sites as gastrointestinal tract, renal, skeletal or military TB. The spread from lungs and other sites is via a hematogenous or lymphatic spread. The infection is variable in its extent and presentation, involving most pelvic organs but involvement of Fallopian tubes and endometrium notoriously causes harm sufficient to result in infertility. The pelvic organs involved include Fallopian tubes (90–100%), endometrium (50–80%), ovaries (20–30%), cervix (10–15%) and rarely vagina and vulva (<1%).[2,5,8,12]

Infertility in GTB is a consequence of involvement of tubes, endometrium peritoneum or ovary. Tubercular involvement of the Fallopian tubes may start from muscularis mucosa or the peritoneal surface depending on spread hematogenously or from intestines, and invariably involve the tubal mucosa. The disease involves ampulla, isthmus or interstitial part of tube in order of frequency, resulting in congestion, adhesive lesions (peritubal with surrounding pelvic organs) in initial stages. In chronic stage the disease is fibrotic resulting in thickened hard and beaded tubes with blockage and occasionally calcification. Microscopically tubal damage is due to endosalpingitis, exosalpingitis or interstitial salpingitis with granulomas containing Langhans giant cells in background of chronic inflammatory cells.

Involvement of the endometrium in initial stages may be unremarkable due to repeated shedding during menstruation but progresses to ulceration and caseation. The disease resolves with loss of glandular architecture resulting in atrophic endometrium or intrauterine adhesions and obliteration of cavity. In advanced stages with extensive damage, there may be total destruction of endometrium or Asherman's syndrome. Infertility results from failure to implant even in initial stages of disease due to immunologic factors. In advanced or extensive disease infertility is a consequence of mechanical factors with distorted cavity consequent to adhesions and obliteration of cavity or failure to implant on an atrophic endometrium. Peritoneal involvement with disease often presents with adhesions consequent to adhesive disease and is a mechanical cause of infertility. Rarely the disease manifests with miliary tubercles which in later stages forms thick plastic adhesions between pelvic organs resulting in infertility by distorting tubo-ovarian relationship. Less commonly ovarian involvement may be secondary to TB peritonitis, rarely due to tubercular oophoritis with tubercles, adhesions, caseation, and tubo-ovarian masses. Ovarian involvement albeit rare may deplete the ovarian reserves when the ovary is completely destroyed. However even with a subtle involvement ovarian reserves may be diminished as seen in our study comparing ovarian reserve in women with GTB with women of similar demographic profile without disease.[13] Attenuation of ovarian reserves is the mechanism contributing to infertility in these women.

■ DIAGNOSIS OF GENITAL TUBERCULOSIS

The diagnosis of GTB is a dilemma as there is yet no case definition of the disease. While most women may have no symptoms other than infertility, a battery of test may be required to reach to a diagnosis or prior to start of antitubercular therapy (ATT). The diagnosis of GTB is often difficult and elusive and a high index of suspicion is the first step in most asymptomatic women especially in our settings. Many more cases which may be labeled as unexplained infertility or present as repeated implantation failures after in vitro fertilization (IVF) and embryo transfer (ET) are subsequently detected to have FGTB.[14] The accepted diagnosis of GTB is identification of bacilli from endometrial samples sent for histology, culture and AFB staining, and is considered the "gold standard". But the paucibacillary nature of infection further adds to the diagnostic dilemma as the "gold standard" of AFB staining, culture of *Mycobacterium tuberculosis* and demonstration of tuberculous granulomas on histology on endometrial aspiration may detect up to 13–23% of cases.[8,15] Endometrium provides less diagnostic information because it is sloughed monthly and the time for granuloma formation is often inadequate. Thus there is a high chance of false negative, besides the low sensitivity even with the available gold standards. Endometrial involvement in the presence of typical granulomas may be detectable in up to 15–23% cases due to repeated shedding during menstruation.[7,15]

Preliminary investigations including complete blood tests, X-ray chest and tuberculin skin test as Mantoux are often done as part of the workup, but are less specific as they may be affected by systemic illnesses and immune-suppression. Chest X-ray may be less effective in FGTB and the Mantoux test may be positive in 40% of healthy Indian women consequent to prior vaccination and should not form basis to diagnose GTB.[16,17]

Molecular methods including PCR can be done on endometrial samples to improve detection as it may pick up the bacterial deoxyribonucleic acid (DNA) or ribonucleic acid (RNA) with as little as 10 bacilli. Considering the paucibacillary nature of infection PCR is more sensitive and specific.[18-20] The sensitivity of DNA PCR has been variably reported between 47% and 79% from studies on endometrial samples.[17,19,21] Therefore availability of PCR has improved diagnosis of GTB in absence of conventional tests on endometrial or other samples. But PCR has its inherent nuisances of false positive in up to 10% of cases and will even read a test positive in a treated case of GTB as the dead bacilli will be picked as positive on a DNA PCR.[21] Therefore it may be difficult to differentiate if the PCR on samples is indicative of previous old infection or latent and subclinical infection, which may be possible by mRNA-based reverse endometrial transcriptase (RT) PCR which detects only live bacilli.[20] Therefore, positive RT-PCR test on samples is indicative of active disease. But RT-PCR is labor intensive and may not be readily available in all microbiology laboratories.

Imaging modality of benefit in diagnosis of GTB is ultrasonography and hysterosalpingography (HSG); however, they have low sensitivity and specificity.[22,23]

While sonographic features as hydrosalpinx, encysted fluid collection, tubo-ovarian masses, are suggestive of tubal or peritoneal disease, persistent thin endometrium around day window of implantation (day 14 to 21 of periods), calcifications in endometrium, fluid collection in uterus suggest endometrial involvement[24] **(Figs 1 to 6)**. However these sonographic features, though suggested are not the sole criteria for diagnosis or treatment, but in presence of other tests such as molecular methods including a positive PCR on endometrial samples may be reason to treat. HSG findings as beaded tubes, blocks, hydrosalpinx, or peritubal adhesions may be useful in deciding for endoscopy or anti-tubercular treatment.

■ ENDOSCOPY PRIOR TO IN VITRO FERTILIZATION

Laparoscopy is not required prior to IVF per se if the decision for IVF is taken on account of blocked tubes or a case of confirmed GTB. Laparoscopy may be of value in defining disease in absence of positive conventional tests. Laparoscopy and dye hydrotubation is a reliable tool to identify tubal, peritoneal, and ovarian involvement. The findings on laparoscopy are classified into five categories and serve a useful guide in identifying patient when these are present despite a negative result on conventional tests. The classification by Rattan[25] et al. in a study conducted at All India Institute of Medical Sciences which was further confirmed by studies from the same institute has been useful in the diagnosis on laparoscopy.[20,22]

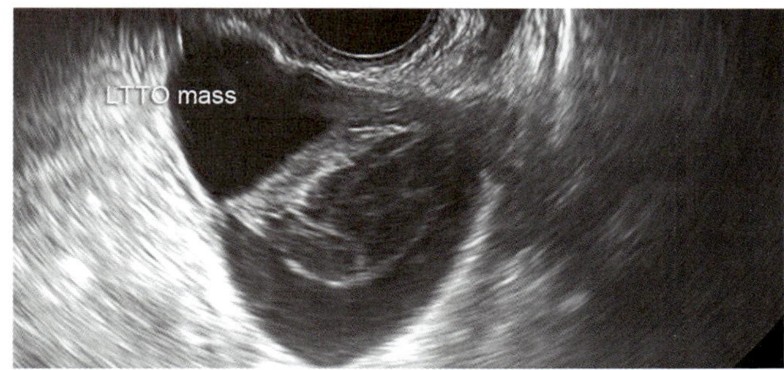

Fig. 3 Ultrasonography of tubercular tubo-ovarian (TO) masses with encysted fluid collection in pelvis

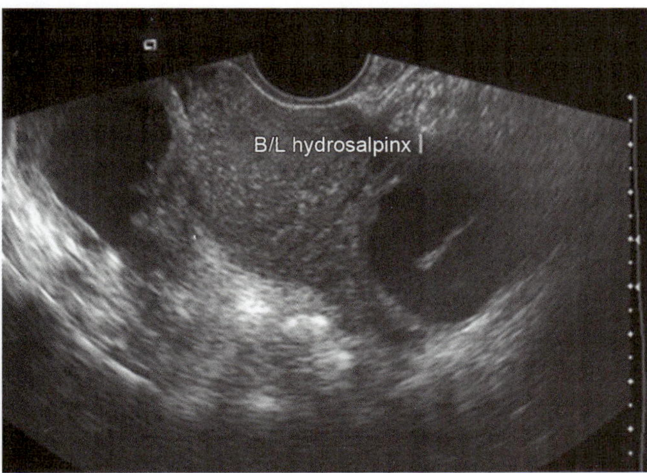

Fig. 1 Baseline ultrasonography scan showing bilateral hydrosalpinges in women with genital tuberculosis

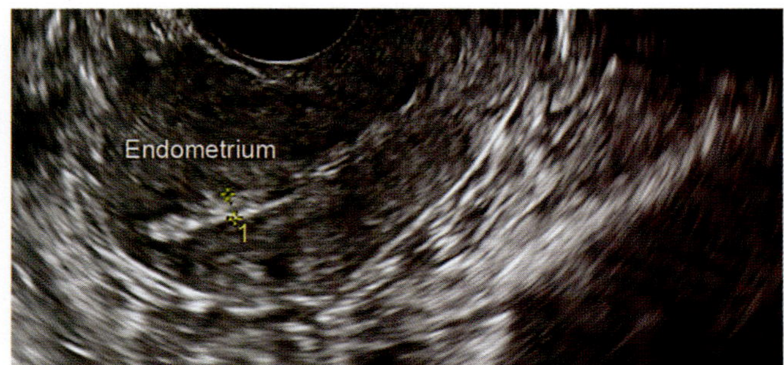

Fig. 4 Thin endometrium on ultrasonography around day 21

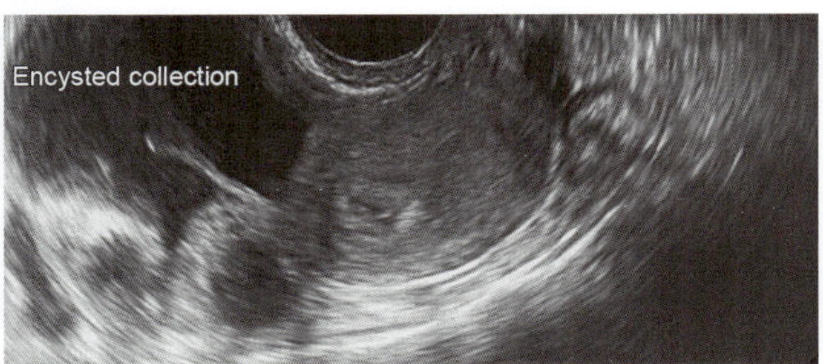

Fig. 2 Encysted collection in pelvis on baseline scan

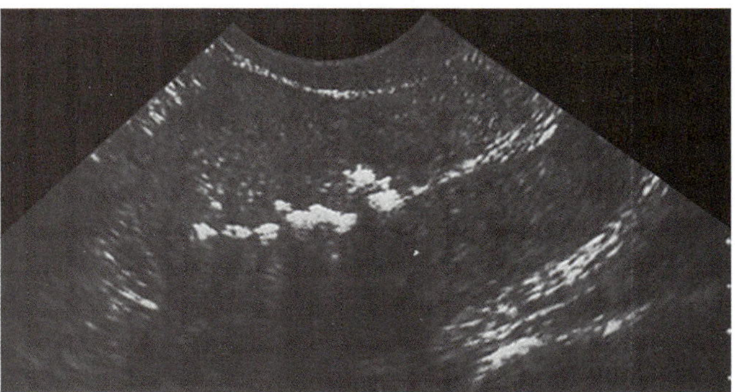

Fig. 5 Calcifications in endometrium seen on baseline ultrasonography

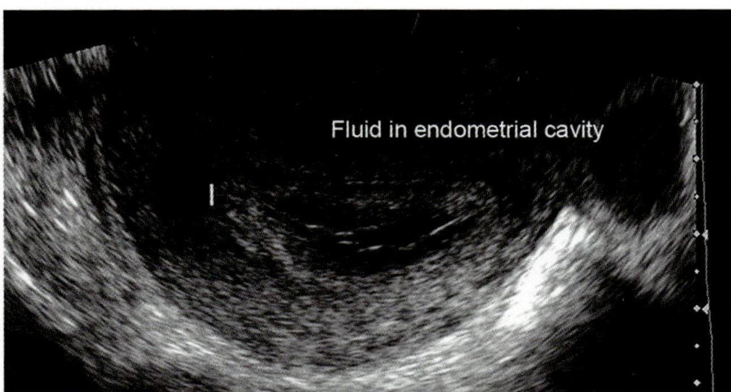

Fig. 6 Fluid collection on day 2–5 scan

A. *Definitive TB*: Presence of tubercles, caseation and beaded tubes.
B. *Probable TB*: Presence of straw-colored fluid in pouch of Douglas, extensive deep pelvic and/or peritubal/periovarian adhesions, hydrosalpinx, tubo-ovarian mass, thick fibrosed tubes, mid-tubal block, perihepatic adhesion and hyperemia of tubes/blue uterus on chromopertubation.
C. *Possible TB*: Mild/flimsy adhesions, dilated tortuous tubes, cornual/fimbrial block and fimbrial agglutination/phimosis.
D. *Incidental*: Fibroid, polycystic ovary, endometriosis with patent tubes and no suggestion of GTB.
E. Normal findings.

Findings on laparoscopy (level A and B) may be useful in the diagnosis in light of a positive PCR on endometrial or washings from pouch of Douglas.[20] Lesions identified can be biopsied and further fluid from encysted collections can be subjected for molecular methods including PCR or rapid culture to increase diagnostic yield.[20,21,23] The dilemma in diagnosis of GTB in women planned for ART arises when women on investigation are negative on conventional tests and have only positive PCR on endometrial samples. In such situations endoscopic evaluation of pelvis and or uterine cavity is useful. In a study by Jindal et al. laparoscopic findings for GTB correlated with PCR on endometrial samples in 84.6% of cases. Even in those with a negative PCR tests findings were detected in 18.2% of cases, thereby suggesting the role of endoscopy even in PCR negative cases with a strong clinical suspicion.[23]

Hysteroscopy has a definite role prior to IVF in appreciating the gland architecture and assessing capacity of uterine cavity as the diagnosis may be made only on a look inside the uterus.[26] These are more useful when the disease has not been identified on conventional tests of microscopy, histology and culture. In our published data, routine hysteroscopy improved the diagnosis of adhesions which would have been missed on routine baseline sonography in these women.[27] Hysteroscopy when combined with laparoscopy improves the diagnostic yield in women undergoing investigations. Lesions as tubercles or caseation seen on hysteroscopy signify active disease, and can be biopsied. Quiescent disease can be suspected in light of atrophic endometrium **(Fig. 5)** or loss of glandular architecture on hysteroscopy while extensive adhesions, obliterated cavity **(Fig. 6)** suggested end-stage disease with poor implantation and such patients can be counseled for surrogacy outright. Hysteroscopy may further be needed in those who have completed antitubercular drugs as improvements in endometrial adhesions, glandular structure and capacity may be identified on second look laparoscopy.[28] Minimal or mild adhesions may suggest better prognosis particularly after lysis of same when corroborated with endometrial blood flows as seen on Doppler studies combined with endometrial pattern from a cross-sectional study conducted at our center.[29]

■ INDICATIONS OF ASSISTED REPRODUCTION TECHNIQUES

Infertility resulting from GTB infection is multifactorial, but when the damage is irreversible and is beyond medical and surgical correction IVF remains the only choice. Frydman et al. suggest IVF as the most effective treatment option for tubercular infertility[30] and has been found in studies from Indian subcontinent as well.[3] Indications for IVF include:

- *Tubal disease*: When extensive, bipolar
- Diminishing ovarian reserve
- Endometrial damage justifying surrogacy.

In vitro fertilization remains as the only option with tubal disease; however, outcome in terms of pregnancy rate may not be as promising as for IVF indicated for tubal disease other than GTB.

Surrogacy is the only option when the endometrial damage is extensive or the uterine cavity is shrunken, distorted and may be unsuitable to house pregnancy.

■ PRE-IN VITRO FERTILIZATION EVALUATION

Evaluation in women with GTB is no different from women undergoing IVF for other indications. However special importance needs to be given to evaluating the ovarian reserves, as there is evidence that ovarian reserves are compromised in women with GTB when compared to women without the disease.[13] Further there is evidence these women require higher dosages of gonadotropins for stimulation when compared to those without TB undergoing stimulation during the IVF cycle.[14] This would entail a thorough evaluation with a battery of tests in the follicular phase[13] including hormone assays as serum follicle-stimulating hormone (FSH), anti-Müllerian hormone (AMH) and ultrasound markers including antral follicle counts and ovarian volume. Even in young women tests for ovarian reserve are of great value not just for counseling but also deciding protocols or doses of gonadotropins.

Further evaluation of the endometrium and uterine cavity is imperative as the disease involves the endometrium that affects receptivity and implantation. Exclusion of hydrosalpinges is mandatory as this is a sequel of irreversible tubal damage, and their presence adversely affects implantation. The fluid collection in the hydrosalpinges is embryotoxic, besides has a mechanical effects by lining the endometrium affecting receptivity.[31] Further this fluid contains cytokines and interleukins which are toxic to the transferred embryos.[32] In such a situation surgical removal or proximal occlusion of the tubes is bound to improve pregnancy rate and reduce miscarriage rate after IVF.[33,34]

Pre-IVF evaluation should therefore include:
- Baseline hormone assays including FSH, luteinizing hormone (LH) and AMH to evaluate ovarian reserve.
- Baseline transvaginal scan.
  - In follicular phase to evaluate ovaries including antral follicle count, ovarian volume, presence of ovarian calcifications, adherence to uterus, haziness of ovarian outline (suggestive of periovarian adhesions) and further useful in defining access to ovaries during oocyte recovery. This is the time to scan and define endometrium and adnexa. Findings as thin, irregular endometrium, calcification, and presence of fluid in cavity could suggest intrauterine adhesions or irreversibly scarred endometrium **(Figs 4 to 6)**. Adnexal evaluation excludes hydrosalpinx **(Fig. 1)**, or encysted pelvic collections **(Fig. 2)**.
  - Luteal phase scan for endometrial evaluation should be completed for endometrial thickness and pattern on 2D ultrasound **(Fig. 7)**. Endometrial and subendometrial blood flow with power Doppler and endometrial volume assessment with 3D/4D scan is useful at this time. Doppler flow indices are a good surrogate marker of receptivity particularly after ATT.[27] Assessment of the volume is particularly useful in suspected intrauterine adhesions as small volume cavity may define the women for a surrogacy program. 4D imaging may be useful as gives a vivid

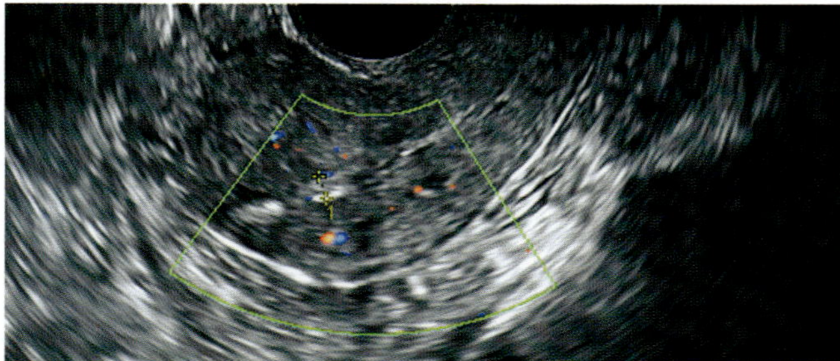

Fig. 7 Ultrasonography showing thin, irregular endometrial lining with poor flow on Doppler

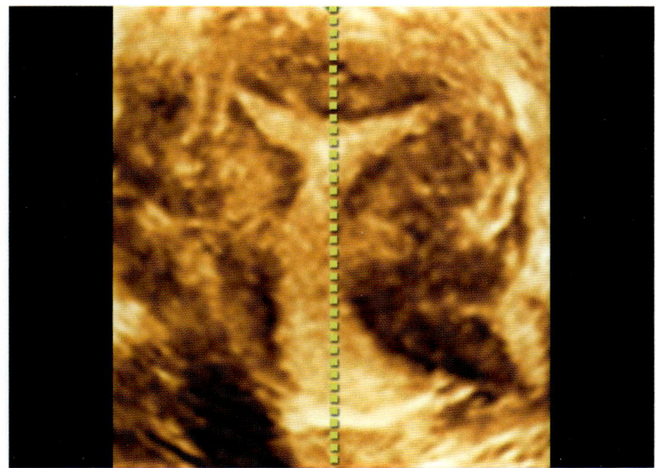

Fig. 8 Four-dimensional images of the uterine cavity showing mid-segment narrowing. This patient underwent lateral metroplasty prior to in vitro fertilization

picture of adhesions, segmental narrowing as an adjunct to hysteroscopy to roadmap operative correction prior to IVF **(Fig. 8)**.
  - During this scan, a repeat evaluation of adnexa for hydrosaplinx is helpful as many subtle ones may be better detected during the secretory phase once accumulated with secretions.
- Hysteroscopy to assess endometrial volume, glands and any sequel including intrauterine adhesions, fibrosis, and scarring. The gold standard to assess the endometrium and cavity is hysteroscopy. Hysteroscopy is thus imperative prior to IVF with findings on ultrasound or otherwise as it is useful in detection of mild adhesions, pale, atrophic endometrium, certainly not detectable with ultrasound alone **(Fig. 9)**. Hysteroscopy evaluation as in low resource settings it is still worthwhile and cost-effective as reported in a study by Bahadur et al. where workup with a routine

hysteroscopy prior to IVF detected abnormal findings in 14.2% cases including of intrauterine adhesions and pale endometrium which were not detected on ultrasound.[27] The decision for surrogacy is mostly dependent on hysteroscopy findings of obliterated cavity **(Fig. 10)** which is a manifestation of extensive damage and surgical corrections may not be of much benefit. Hysteroscopy evaluation is also useful after ATT in these women as many show improvement in endometrial findings after treatment.[28]

- A mock transfer can be often combined at the time of hysteroscopy as it is not uncommon to have a difficult transfer on account of adhesions in lower uterine cavity

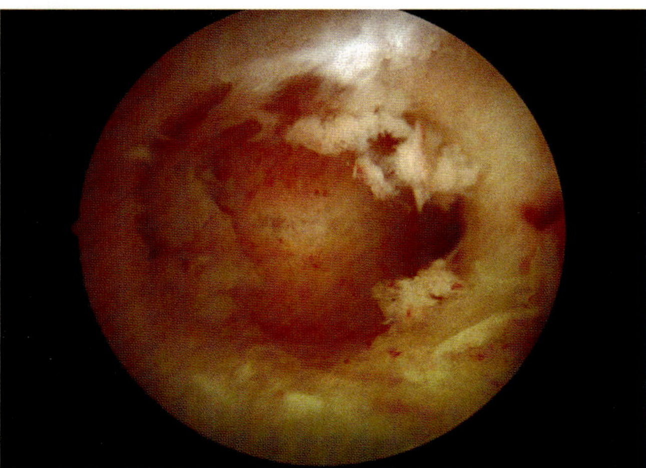

Fig. 9 Hysteroscopy images of pale looking endometrium depleted of glands

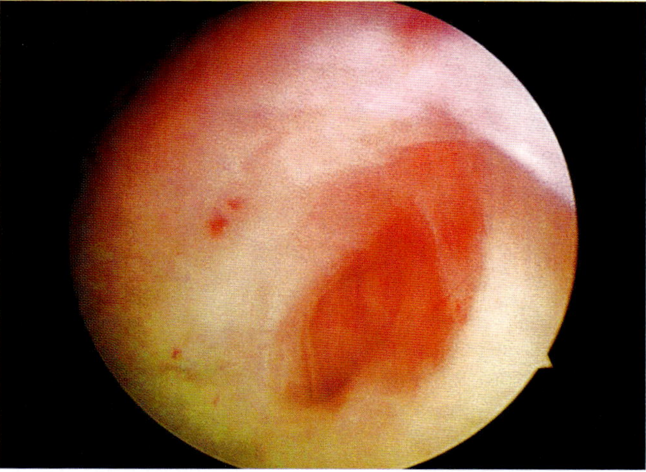

Fig. 10 Obliterated uterine cavity after endometrial tuberculosis

or cervical canal despite normal ultrasound findings. This could save a surprise difficult transfer as could arise in situations particularly with asymptomatic intrauterine adhesions mainly in the cervical canal or just above the internal orifice.

■ MEDICAL TREATMENT PRIOR TO IN VITRO FERTILIZATION

This involves ATT prior to IVF. When the endometrial samples test positive for the conventional tests including AFB staining, histopathology, or culture ATT is mandatory. The dilemma arises when only PCR tests positive on endometrial samples. The detection of PCR in absence of conventional tests may be indicative of either a latent or subclinical infection wherein the disease has not resulted in damage to be detectable on radiologic or endoscopic approach while evaluating the disease. In such cases early treatment in the course of disease may inhibit progression and prevent irreversible damage from fibrosis in tubes and endometrium. There is limited evidence on whether ATT is justified in women prior to IVF or in those with recurrent implantation failures on the basis of a positive PCR in endometrial samples alone. In a study by Dam et al. women with implantation failure at IVF, were given ATT and compared with their prior failed cycles to fresh and frozen ET after therapy. Those on ATT had required lower doses of gonadotropins with improved subendometrial blood flow and thickness when compared to previous failed cycles.[14] In a recent study, ATT was given for 6 months to infertile women solely on the basis of positive PCR on endometrial samples in absence of conventional tests. In this nonrandomized study those with a positive PCR receiving ATT were compared with women with negative PCR for pregnancy outcome either spontaneously or after ART. While overall pregnancy rate after ART were no different in both groups, those receiving ATT for a positive PCR had higher rate of spontaneous pregnancy, with the authors concluding that ATT early in the course of disease, without tubal or endometrial damage gives the best chance for spontaneous conception.[35] In absence of robust evidence without randomized trial there is yet no consensus to give ATT on the sole basis of PCR on endometrial samples in women prior to IVF cycles. However, PCR in light of early changes on laparoscopy or hysteroscopy justifies ATT. Yet it is to be observed that ATT may improve endometrial thickness and subendometrial flow in those with minimal damage, but is of limited value in those with dense adhesions as was seen in our observational study after hysteroscopic adhesiolysis.[29]

SURGICAL TREATMENT PRIOR TO IN VITRO FERTILIZATION

There is sufficient evidence that surgical treatment of hydrosalpinx prior to IVF improves pregnancy and live birth rates. Thus hydrosalpinx can undergo laparoscopic salpingectomy, tubal occlusion with Filshie clip or bipolar coagulation and even aspiration of hydrosalpinx fluid under ultrasound guidance. Which method is better than the other is still a matter of debate.[33] There is evidence sufficient to suggest that removal or delinking hydrosalpinges improves pregnancy.[34] The odds of clinical, ongoing pregnancy and live birth rate improved after surgical treatment of hydrosalpinx as well as a decrease in miscarriage rate in women undergoing IVF[33] as reported in a meta-analysis. Surgical options include salpingectomy or occlusion of the proximal ends of the Fallopian tubes; however no method is superior over the other with similar outcomes after IVF.[36,37] Proximal tubal occlusion may be an alternative when salpingectomy is technically not feasible as in dense pelvic adhesions.[37] Surgical treatment of hydrosalpinges therefore becomes an important intervention to improve the pregnancy rate after IVF-ET. Besides the surgical treatment of hydrosalpinx surgical treatment of intrauterine cavity for adhesions and lateral metroplasty is recommended in women planned for IVF. Intrauterine adhesiolysis improves intrauterine capacity but may be useful in improving implantation in some where the adhesions are mild or moderate. In severe adhesions while the cavity may be restored of its volume it may not translate of a receptive endometrium as those with sever and fibrotic adhesions are associated with depletion of subendometrial blood flow, a factor known to limit implantation.[29] Lateral metroplasty is particularly useful in cavity with tubercular narrowing along lateral walls of the lower half of uterus and is accomplished with incisions using monopolar cautery or mechanically with scissors **(Fig. 11)**. Likewise a mock trial ET is also important and should be added in the protocol of female evaluation prior to IVF.

PROBLEMS DURING IN VITRO FERTILIZATION

The procedure essentially is similar for any other indication including nontubercular tubal factor infertility. The choice of protocol and the type of gonadotropins are not dictated by the presence of the disease, and can be chosen as per unit policy. Both antagonist and agonist protocols are equally effective. However occasionally problem may arise including:

- *Poor response to gonadotropins*: Prolonged duration and increased dosages.

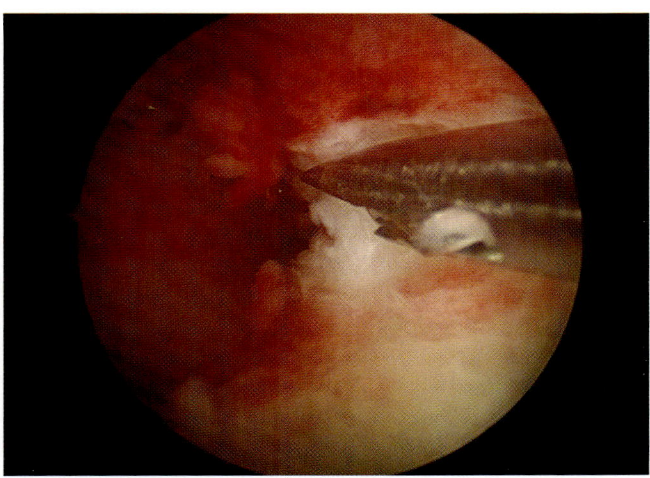

Fig. 11 Operative correction, lateral metroplasty with Bettochi scissors prior to in vitro fertilization in mid-segment narrowing of uterine cavity

- Appearance of hydrosalpinges during stimulation, which were undetectable during the baseline scan in follicular phase.
- Difficult ovum pick up especially if prior tubo-ovarian masses, adherent ovaries, encysted fluid collection or associated large hydrosalpinges making difficult access to ovaries.
- Appearance to fluid in endometrial cavity around time of ET.

This understanding is important as it helps patient's counseling prior to IVF and in preparedness during the cycle.

OUTCOME OF ASSISTED REPRODUCTION TECHNIQUES

Pregnancy rate after IVF-ET are dismal. Parikh et al. reported a pregnancy rate of 16.6% in 30 women who underwent IVF after ATT, while Gurgan et al. achieved a pregnancy rate of just 9.1% among women treated for GTB in contrast to 21.3% in women after IVF for tuboperitoneal infertility other than GTB. Even though results are low, IVF remains a reasonable option who would not achieve a pregnancy otherwise as was reported by Jindal et al. with conception rate of 17.3% with ART as compared to 4.3% with fertility enhancing surgery alone. One of the best results after IVF have been suggested by a study by Soussis et al. who reported a 28.6% intrauterine pregnancy (6 among 13 women undergoing 21 cycles) with histological proven GTB. The protocol included ATT and a thorough evaluation including hysteroscopy, laparoscopy and vaginal scan prior to IVF in each women in the unit. Even when pregnancy results after IVF there is a high chance of it being ectopic as the reported incidence of ectopic pregnancy varies between.

■ CONCLUSION

Genital tuberculosis is a major challenge when such women are to be undertaken for ART including IVF-ET. The diagnostic dilemma in absence of conventional tests and decision to start ATT prior to IVF need to be evaluated with large randomized trials as there is little evidence if such treatment solely on the basis of positive molecular methods as PCR alone would improve pregnancy rates. While IVF may be the only option of concluding a pregnancy in some of these women it may not be a feasible option considering the socio-economic background of such women in developing countries. Low cost IVF in GTB may be a viable and cost-effective option given the extensive damage this disease may cause to the genital organs.

■ KEY POINTS

- Genital tuberculosis is the most common cause of tubal factor infertility in developing countries including India.
- Assisted reproduction techniques including IVF remain the only hope when the tubal damage is irreversible.
- Prior assessment includes evaluation of ovarian reserves, endometrial and uterine cavity evaluation.
- A positive PCR on endometrial samples in absence of any other conventional tests needs confirmation with endoscopy including laparoscopy or hysteroscopy prior to start of antitubercular treatment.
- A pre-IVF hysteroscopy is mandatory and confirms status of uterine size, adhesions and health of the glands.
- Mock or trial ET should be done at the time of hysteroscopy for optimal outcome during IVF-ET.
- In vitro fertilization procedure is essentially similar in choice of protocol or gonadotropin as in any other tubal factor infertility other than GTB.
- Outcome in terms of pregnancy rate are lower than after other indications of IVF.

■ REFERENCES

1. WHO report on the TB epidemic (2007). TB, a global emergency. WHO/TB/94.177, World Health Organisation, Geneva.
2. Deshmukh KK, Lopez JA, Naidu TAK, et al. Place of laparoscopy in pelvic tuberculosis in infertile women. Arch Gynecol. 1985;237(Suppl):197-200.
3. Parikh FR, Nadkarni SG, Kamat SA, et al. Genital tuberculosis:a major pelvic factor causing infertility in Indian women. Fertil Steril. 1997;67:497-500.
4. Schaffer G. Female genital tuberculosis. Clin Obstet Gynecol. 1976;19:223-9.
5. Bazaz-Malik G, Maheshwari B, Lal N. Tubercular endometritis: a clinicopathological study of 1000 cases. Br J Obstet Gynaecol. 1983;138:974-7.
6. Bhide AG, Parulekar SV, Bhattacharya MS. Genital tuberculosis in females. J Obstet Gynaecol India. 1987;37:576-8.
7. Jindal UN. An algorithmic approach to female genital tuberculosis causing infertility. Int J Tuberc Lung Dis. 2006;10:1045-50.
8. Kumar S. Female genital tuberculosis In: Sharma SK, Mohan A (Eds). Tuberculosis, 1st edition. Delhi: Jaypee; 2001. pp. 311-24.
9. Jahromi NB, Parsanezhad ME, Shirazi RG. Female genital tuberculosis and infertility. Int J Gynaecol Obstet. 2001;75: 269-72.
10. Abede M, Lakew M, Kidane D, et al. Female genital tuberculosis in Ethiopia. Int J Gynaecol Obstet. 2004;84(3):241-6.
11. Gupta N, Sharma JB, Mittal S, et al. Genital tuberculosis in Indian infertility patients. Int J Gynecol Obstet. 2007;97(2): 135-8.
12. Sharma JB. Tuberculosis and obstetrics and gynecological practice. Progress in Obstetrics and gynecology. In: John Studd, Seang Lin Tan, Frank A. Chervenak (Eds). Churchill Livingstone; 2008. pp. 395-428.
13. Malhotra N, Sharma V, Bahadur A, et al. The effect of tuberculosis on ovarian reserve among women undergoing IVF in India. Int J Gynaecol Obstet. 2012;117(1):40-4.
14. Dam P, Shirazee HH, Goswami SK, et al. Role of latent genital tuberculosis in repeated IVF failure in the Indian clinical setting. Gynecol Obstet Invest. 2006;61:223-7.
15. Mani R, Nayak KS, Kagal A, et al. Tuberculous endometritis in infertility: a bacteriological and histopathological study. Indian J Tuberc. 2003;50:161.
16. Rozati R, Roopa S, Naga Rajeshwari C. Evaluation of women with infertility and genital tuberculosis. J Obstet Gynecol India. 2006;56:423-6.
17. Raut VS, Mahashir AA, Sheth SS. The Montoux test in the diagnosis of genital tuberculosis in women. Int J Gynaecol Obstet. 2001;72:165-9.
18. Baum SE, Dooley DP, Wright J, et al. Diagnosis of culture-negative female genital tract tuberculosis with involvement of polymerase chain reaction. J Reprod Med. 2001;46: 929-32.
19. Bhanu NV, Singh UB, Chakraborty M, et al. Improved diagnostic value of PCR in the diagnosis of female genital tuberculosis leading to infertility. J Med Microbiol. 2005;54:927-31.
20. Rana T, Singh UB, Kulshrestha V, et al. Utility of reverse transcriptase PCR and DNA-PCR in the diagnosis of female genital tuberculosis. J Med Microbiol. 2011;60:486-71.
21. Thangappah RBP, Paramasivan CN, Narayanan S. Evaluating PCR, culture and histology in the diagnosis of female genital tuberculosis. Ind J Med Res. 2011;134:40-6.
22. Kulshrestha V, Kriplani A, Agarwal N, et al. Genital tuberculosis among infertile women and fertility outcome

after antitubercular treatment. Int J Gynaecol Obstet. 2100;113: 229-34.

23. Jindal UN, Bala Y, Sodhi S, et al. Female genital tuberculosis: Early diagnosis by laparoscopy and polymerase chain reaction. Int J Tuberc Lung Dis. 2010;14(12):1629-34.

24. Fedele L, Binachi S, Dorta M, et al. Intrauterine adhesions, detection with transvaginal sonography. Radiology. 1996;199:757-9.

25. Rattan A, Gupta SK, Singh S, et al. Detection of antigens of *Mycobacterium tuberculosis* in patients of infertility by monoclonal antibody-based sandwich ELISA. Tuber Lung Dis. 1993;74:200-3.

26. Sharma JB, Roy KK, Pushparaj M, et al. Hysteroscopic findings in women with primary and secondary infertility due to genital tuberculosis. Int J Gynaecol Obstet. 2009;104(1):49-52.

27. Bahdur A, Malhotra N, Singh N, et al. Comparative study on the role of diagnostic hysteroscopy in the evaluation of the uterine cavity prior to in vitro fertilization in a developing country. Arch Gynecol Obstset. 2013;288(5):1137-43.

28. Bahadur A, Malhotra N, Mittal S, et al. Second look hysteroscopy after antitubercular treatment in infertile women with genital tuberculosis undergoing in vitro fertilization. Int J Gynecol Obstset. 2010;108:128-31.

29. Malhotra N, Bahadur A, Kalaivani M, et al. Changes in endometrial receptivity in women with Asherman's syndrome undergoing hysteroscopic adhesiolysis. Arch Gynecol Obstet. 2012;286(2):525-10.

30. Frydman R, Eibschitz I, Belaisch-Allart JC, et al. In-vitro fertilization in tuberculosis infertility. J In vitro Fert Embryo Transf. 1985;2(4):184-9.

31. Strandell A, Lindhard A. Why does hydrosalpinx reduce fertility? The importance of hydrosalpinx fluid. Hum Reprod. 2002;17(5):1141-5.

32. Mukherjee T, Copperman AB, McCaffrey C. Hydrosalpinx fluid has embryotoxic effects on murine embryogenesis: a case for prophylactic salpingectomy. Fertil Steril. 1996;66:851-3.

33. Johnson N, van Voorst S, Sowter MC, et al. Surgical treatment for tubal disease in women due to undergo in vitro fertilization. Cochrane Database of Systematic Reviews. 2010;(1):CD002125.

34. Strandell A, Lindhard A, Waldenstrom U, et al. Hydrosalpinx and IVF outcome: cumulative results after salpingectomy in a randomized controlled trial. Hum Reprod. 2001;16(11):2403-10.

35. Jindal UN, Verma S, Bala Y. Favorable infertility outcome following anti-tubercular treatment prescribed on the sole basis of positive polymerase chain reaction for endometrial tuberculosis. Hum Reprod. 2012;27(5):1368-74.

36. Ozmen B, Dierich K, Al-Hassani S. Hydrosalpinx and IVF: Assessment of treatments implemented prior to IVF. RBM Online. 2007;14(2):235-41.

37. Kontoravdis A, Makrakis E, Pantos K, et al. Proximal tubal occlusion and salpingectomy result in similar improvement in in-vitro fertilization outcome in patients with hydrosalpinx. Fertil Steril. 2006;86:1642-9.

49

Poor Ovarian Response

Sunita R Tandulwadkar, Parinaaz Parhar

INTRODUCTION

The past few years have seen the field of assisted reproductive technology (ART) grows by leaps and bounds, with introduction of new protocols and interventions making it possible to achieve success even in certain cases which were considered impossible until a decade ago. However, one group of patients whose management still continues to pose a difficult challenge to the ART practitioners is that of the poor ovarian responders.

The term poor ovarian response (POR) has been used to define a reduction in follicular response resulting in a reduced number of retrieved oocytes even after controlled ovarian hyperstimulation (COH) in In vitro fertilization (IVF) treatment. The goal of ovarian stimulation in IVF is the recruitment of multiple follicles in an effort to compensate for the inefficiencies of embryology culture, embryo selection for transfer and subsequent implantation.[1-3] Since this very goal seems to be defeated in patients with a POR to stimulation, their treatment is associated with disappointing results and hence is a cause of grave concern to ART specialists all over the world. These patients not only have impaired fertilization rates and lower embryo quality[4] but also the higher incidence of cycle cancelation and failure rates in them leads to an alarmingly reduced cost effectiveness of cycle.

In this chapter, we have discussed the various aspects of management of a poor ovarian responder in ART, right from their definition to their treatment.

DEFINITION

Considering the challenge posed by poor ovarian responders to ART specialists all around the globe, there has been a proportionate amount of research on the topic with various studies introducing various criteria and cutoff limits to define the group.

It was Garcia who in 1983 first described a poor responder as one who, on a standard stimulation regimen [150 IU human menopausal gonadotropin (hMG)], had a peak estradiol concentration of less than 300 pg/mL and poor follicle production leading to a smaller number of eggs retrieved and, therefore, a smaller number of embryos transferred.[5]

Ever since then, various studies have used numerous criteria like the number of dominant follicles developed (<3–<5) and oocytes retrieved (<3–<5),[6-11] peak estradiol levels at the time of trigger administration (<300–<500 pg/mL),[8,9] day 3 basal follicle-stimulating hormone (FSH) (>7–15 mIU/mL)[12-15] and estradiol levels (>60 pg/mL),[16] daily (>300 IU of FSH)[17] and total gonadotropin dosage required to produce an adequate response to define poor ovarian responders.

Table 1 from the Journal of Human Reproduction enumerates the various criteria used by different studies to define a POR in their study population.[18]

As is evident from the table, the heterogeneity of the criteria used and the lack of a uniform definition of a poor response makes it impossible to compare studies, and very difficult to develop or assess any protocol to improve the outcome of the patients. There was a globally felt need for an internationally acceptable and universally applicable definition for the condition which could be used in future studies to compare the results and interventions used in IVF in such patients.

In recognition of this need of the hour, a consensus was reached on the minimal criteria needed to define POR by the European Society of Human Reproduction and Embryology (ESHRE) in March 2010 at Bologna, Italy, which is now popularly known as the Bologna consensus. The Bologna consensus requires that to define a POR at least two of the following three features must be presented:

1. Advanced maternal age (≥40 years) or any other risk factor for POR;
2. A previous POR (≤3 oocytes with a conventional stimulation protocol) and
3. An abnormal ovarian reserve test (ORT) [i.e. antral follicle count (AFC) <5–7 follicles or anti-Müllerian hormone (AMH) <0.5–1.1 ng/mL].

Table 1 Criteria used to define poor ovarian response (POR)

Reference	Criteria
Garcia-Velasco et al. (2000)	At least one previous cycle canceled because of ≤3 follicles ≥18 mm
Ferraretti et al. (2000)	At least two previous cycles canceled or with ≤3 oocytes
Akman et al. (2001)	Two failed IVF attempts for one of the following reasons: Day 3 FSH >15 mIU/mL E2 <500 pg/mL at hCG <4 mature oocytes
Weissman et al. (2003)	One previous cycle with at least one of the following characteristics: <5 oocytes ≤3 follicles 16 mm or larger E2 <500 pg/mL at hCG
Marci et al. (2003)	One previous POR in a standard treatment
Goswami et al. (2004)	One to three failed IVF attempts due to POR to conventional long-agonist protocol
Kolibianakis et al. (2004)	One or more failed IVF cycles in which ≤5 oocytes were retrieved and day-3 FHS level >12 mIU/mL
Morgia et al. (2004)	One previous IVF cycle with ≤3 oocytes
Detti et al. (2005)	One or more of the following criteria present: age >38 years Previous canceled cycle Previous POR (≤3 oocytes or E2 <500 g/mL) Day-3 FSH >13 mIU/mL
Cheung et al. (2005)	One previous POR with ≤3 oocytes on a long-agonist protocol or repeated day-3 FSH >10 IU/L
Garcia-Velasco et al. (2005)	At least one previous canceled cycle doe to ≤4 follicles >16 mm and/or E2 level ≤500 pg/mL
Massin et al. (2006)	Two of the following criteria present: previous POR (E2 <1200 pg/mo at hCG and ≤5 oocytes) Day-3 FSH >12 Day-3 inhibin B <45 pg/mL
Aletebi (2007)	POR in previous cycle(s): ≤4 oocytes following stimulation for ≥15 days involving 300 IU of gonadotrpins daily
Schoolcraft et al. (2008)	At least one of the following criteria: Day-3 FSH >10 mIU/mL Age >41 years AFC <6 One previous cycle canceled One previous POR (E2 <500 pg/mL and/or <6 oocytes)
Franarelli et al. (2008a)	One or more of the following characteristics: Day-3 FSH >12 mIU/mL AFC ≤3 History of POR (≤5 oocytes. poor quality oocyte and/or poor quality embryos)
Frattarelli et al. (2008b)	Two previous POR (criteria not defined)
Barrenetxea et al. (2008)	Age ≥40 years and day-3 FSH ≥10 mIU/mL
Tazegul et al. (2008)	Previous POR: E2 <500 pg/mL or ≤3 mature follicles or <3 oocytes
Fabregues et al. (2009)	First IVF cycle canceled because of POR (criteria not defined)
Kahraman et al. (2009)	One or more of the following criteria present in at least one previous cycle: cycle canceled ≤3 oocytes E2 >500 pg/mL
Yarali et al. (2009)	Abnormal ORTs (FSH >10 mIU/mL or AFC <6) or previous POR (cycle canceled or E2 >500 pg/mL or ≤3 oocytes)
Weitzman et al. (2009)	One or more of the following criteria: age ≥40 years Day-3 FSH ≥10 mIU/mL Previous cycle canceled:previous cycle with ≤4 oocytes collected
Demirol and Gurgan (2009)	At least two previous POR (E2 <500 pg/mL or ≤3 oocytes) and day-3 FSH >15 IU/L
Tehraninejad et al. (2009)	At least one previous cycle canceled because of <3 mature follicles

Two episodes of POR after maximal stimulation are sufficient to define a patient as poor responder in the absence of advanced maternal age or abnormal ORT. By definition, the term POR refers to the ovarian response and, therefore, one stimulated cycle is considered essential for the diagnosis of POR. However, patients over 40 years of age with an abnormal ORT may be classified as poor responders since both advanced age and an abnormal ORT may indicate reduced ovarian reserve and act as a surrogate of ovarian stimulation cycle. In this case, the patients should be more properly defined as expected PORs.[18]

■ INCIDENCE

Based on the criteria utilized by various centers for its definition, the incidence of poor responders in literature varies from 9% to 24%.[19] Data from the ASRM/SART registry showed that out of 14.1% of initial cycles that were canceled; at least 50% were poor responders.[19,20]

■ ETIOLOGY

In spite of the wide research on the topic the cause of POR of a patient to a cycle of COH remains largely unknown. Though advanced maternal age is considered to be the main risk factor associated with the condition, its prevalence in younger age group refutes role of increased age as the sole cause responsible for the condition. It has largely been observed that the risk of POR in a cycle closely correlates with the resting residual pool of follicles or the ovarian reserve of a woman. Hence, even in the younger age group, women who have a low ovarian reserve due to various etiologies are the ones who respond inadequately to stimulation in an ART cycle.

Both genetic and acquired conditions which lead to a premature ovarian failure and poor ovarian reserve have been associated with a POR. Numerical and structural chromosomal aberrations like Turner syndrome, as well as mutations or variability in specific genes in reproductive aging, like FMR1 premutations,[21,22] are examples of genetic disorders leading to a poor ovarian reserve.

Molloy et al. in 1987 and Keay et al. in 1998 showed that pelvic infection, as evidenced by tubal damage and positivity to *Chlamydia* antibody testing and pelvic adhesions, is associated with poor response.[23,24] Similarly, patients with ovarian endometriomas and especially those who had undergone ovarian surgery for ovarian cysts were shown to be potential poor responders by Nargund et al. in 1996 and Garcia-Velasco and Somigliana in 2009.[25,26] Oktem and Oktay in 2007 studied how chemotherapy, especially when it includes an alkylating agent, has been reported to seriously reduce the pool of resting follicles and is associated with an increased risk for primary ovarian insufficiency.[27] Brodin et al. in 2008 further correlated how shortening of the menstrual cycle can represent another condition associated with increased risk for POR.[28]

Studies have shown how POR is the first sign of ovarian aging (early ovarian failure or early menopause) which is clinically displayed by a shortened follicular phase which limits the time available to recruit an adequate number of follicles.[29-31] Probable mechanisms for this POR include: decreased number of FSH receptors in granulosa cells, defective signal transduction after FSH receptor binding, an inappropriate local vascular network for the distribution of gonadotropins, the presence of autoantibodies against granulosa cells, an excess of vascular growth factor receptor (VEGFR-1), abnormality in IGF-I and IGF-II levels, and diminished circulating gonadotropin surge-attenuating factor (GnSAF) bioactivity.[32-38]

Ovarian response to FSH differs considerably among women leading to a growing interest in the probable hand of genetic makeup in the etiology of the condition. Recently, new insights have been gained in the investigation of variability in the gene that encodes FSH receptor (FSHR) or genes of the estrogen pathway. Efforts are being made to apply genetic markers as routine diagnostic tests before ovarian stimulation to predict ovarian response, determine the required FSH dose, and to avoid the possible complications related to FSH stimulation. As a result, several polymorphisms of the FSHR gene have been discovered, but Ser680Asn and Thr307Ala are the two most studied. While the Ser680Asn polymorphism of the FSHR gene has been found to influence the ovarian response to FSH stimulation in women undergoing IVF, in women with the genotype Ser/Ser, the FSHR appears to be more resistant to FSH action.[39,40]

■ PREDICTORS OF POOR OVARIAN RESPONSE

Prediction of POR is extremely difficult but yet necessary before the start of an IVF cycle to enable the treating ART specialist to individualize the treatment protocol accordingly. Accuracy of testing for the occurrence of POR to hyperstimulation appears to be modest. Whether the prior identification of actual poor responders in the first IVF cycle is of any prognostic value for their chances of conception in the course of a series of IVF cycles remains yet to be established. Most of these tests determine the resting follicular pool, i.e. the ovarian reserve since it has been observed to most closely correlate with the ovarian response in an IVF cycle. Thus, these tests help to identify women of relatively young age with clearly diminished reserve, as well as women around the mean age at which natural fertility on average is lost (41 years) but still with adequate OR.

The various tests employed to aid in predicting the response to stimulation can be divided into the static and dynamic test groups. The static tests can again be subdivided into the biochemical and the sonographic tests.

Static Tests[40]

Biochemical Tests

These test the ovarian reserve based on a single measurement in the early follicular phase (cycle days 2–4).
- High levels of serum FSH (>12 or >15 mIU/mL) on cycle days 2 or 3. In regularly cycling females, only high levels of basal FSH is an accurate prediction of poor response. This test is suitable only as a screening test for counseling purposes in the first IVF attempt.[41]
- Elevated FSH/luteinizing hormone (LH) on day 3 blood tests to more than 3.6. The FSH:LH ratio may increase before a dramatic increase in serum FSH is observed and appears to be a useful marker of ovarian reserve.[42]
- Elevated levels of serum estradiol (>30 or 75 pg/mL) on cycle days 2 or 3. The clinical applicability for basal estradiol as a test before starting IVF is limited by its very low predictive accuracy for poor response.[43] Combining day 3 FSH and E2 improved the prognostic ability of either of these hormones used alone.
- Decreased levels of serum inhibin B (45 pg/mL) on cycle days 2 or 3 are considered to be more predictive. In regularly cycling women, basal inhibin B is accurate only at a very low threshold level.[41]
- Reduced production and bioactivity of Gonadotropin Surge Attenuating Factor.[41]
- Low insulin-like growth factor (IGF-I) in the follicular fluid.[44,45]
- Decreased serum concentrations of AMH. AMH is a glycoprotein produced by the granulosa cells within preantral and early antral follicles and hence closely reflects the size of the growing cohort of small follicles which are sensitive to gonadotropin stimulation. AMH can be measured at any time of the menstrual cycle reducing the intercycle variability in test results.[46,47]

In 2002, de Vet et al. published a landmark paper that reported a 38% decline in AMH levels over a mean period of only 2.6 years in a group of young ovulatory women without any significant changes in AFC, serum FSH or inhibin B levels, suggesting that AMH was the most sensitive maker of ovarian reserve.[44]

Sonographic Tests[40]

Different sonographic tests have also been proposed as predictors of ovarian response. These include:
- *Decreased ovarian volume (OVVOL):* It is barely useful as a routine test for ovarian reserve assessment. A meta-analysis showed that ovarian volume measurement with a cutoff value of 3 cm^3, had the specificity for the prediction of cycle cancelation and non-pregnancy of 92% and 93%, respectively.[48]
- *Decreased AFC:* The accuracy of the AFC for predicting poor response in regularly cycling women is sufficient at low threshold levels.[49,50] Though unsuitable as a diagnostic test, but it may be used as a screening one directing further diagnostic steps in the first IVF attempt. A meta-analysis showed that women having AFCs less than four were more likely to have canceled cycles and less likely to get pregnant than women having AFCs of four or more.[48]
- *Decreased ovarian stromal blood flow:* The clinical value of Doppler studies for ovarian stromal blood flow has been unclear.[48]

Dynamic Tests

- *The clomiphene challenge test (CCT):* Baseline (day 2–3 of the menstrual cycle) and response levels (day 9–11) of FSH and 17-beta estradiol are measured before and after administration of 100 mg clomiphene on days 5–9 of the menstrual cycle. The test is abnormal if either the day 3 or day 10 FSH values are elevated or if the day 3 estradiol is more than 80 pg/mL. It performs no better than other tests like the AFC or basal FSH, especially because of a loss in specificity.
- *The exogenous FSH ovarian reserve test (EFORT):* EFORT is a simple and effective method for screening "good" and "poor" responders in IVF. In the study women received 300 IU of purified FSH IM on cycle day 3. Blood samples were taken just before the injection to measure plasma FSH and estradiol; 24 hours later, plasma estradiol concentration was determined. Around 90% of the women whose EFORT parameters were considered to be normal (bFSH ≤11 mIU/mL) had adequate responses to ovarian stimulation, and 81% of women in whom both parameters were considered to be altered (bFSH ≥11 mIU/mL and Δ<E2 <30 pg/mL) had poor responses to ovarian stimulation.
- *The GnRH agonist stimulation test (GAST):* When used in regularly cycling women, GAST showed a high degree of accuracy in the prediction of poor response that could match that of AFC. However, it can be a candidate for more extensive confirmation research.[41]

However, given the present level of evidence, dynamic ovarian tests should be completely abandoned.

In a systematic review and meta-analysis it has been conclusively proved that ORTs, such as basal FSH, AMH, inhibin B, basal estradiol, AFC, ovarian volume, ovarian vascular flow, ovarian biopsy, CCCT, EFORT, GAST and multivariate prediction models, have only little clinical value in the prediction of poor response.[41] However, recent evidence points that AMH and AFC may be superior to other tests, although other tests continue to be used and form the basis for the exclusion of women from fertility treatment.

■ TREATMENT

It is a well-researched fact that follicles require a period of approximately 70 days to mature into the preovulatory stage. However, in this period, the follicles are responsive to gonadotropins only for the final 20 days during the phase of recruitment and final follicular maturation. Hence, the treatment of poor ovarian responders can be discussed under two types of interventions: one as precycle adjuvants and the other as adjuvants at the initiation of a cycle aimed at the gonadotropin independent and the gonadotropin sensitive stages of the follicles respectively.

Precycle Adjuvants

Dehydroepiandrosterone

Dehydroepiandrosterone (DHEA) is an endogenous steroid that originates from the zona reticularis of the adrenal cortex and from ovarian theca cells. It is an essential prohormone in ovarian follicular steroidogenesis whose use as a supplementation in assisted reproduction was first described in a case series by Casson et al.[51,52] and a case report by Barad and Gleicher.[53] Studies have shown that circulating DHEA levels decrease with age. A daily dose of 80 mg for 2 months resulted in improved peak E2 levels and number of follicles in the subsequent COH cycles.

Since 2005, several studies have evaluated the role of DHEA supplementation in assisted reproduction. While certain studies have reported DHEA supplementation to improve the number of fertilized embryos and their quality others have documented a decrease in the cycle cancelation rate and an improved clinical pregnancy rate.[54] A retrospective study by Gleicher et al. showed decreased miscarriage rates with DHEA supplementation in a population undergoing IVF, while another showed an increase in serum AMH following DHEA supplementation.[55-57] Yet, DHEA supplementation for poor responders remains controversial as the majority of available data are derived from retrospective studies with limitations such as selection bias.

There is still considerable speculation regarding the mechanism of action of DHEA on the ovary. Possible mechanisms which have been described include:[58]

- Dehydroepiandrosterone can improve steroidogenesis, since it is a precursor of estradiol and testosterone[59] and during ovarian induction with exogenous gonadotropins, it is the prohormone of the follicular fluid testosterone.[60]
- Androgens may influence ovarian follicular growth, not only by acting as a metabolic precursor for steroid production, but also by serving as ligands for androgen receptors.[59,61]
- According to Casson et al. 1998, 2002,[62,63] there is a transient increase in insulin-like growth factor 1 (IGF-1) in patients undergoing exogenous gonadotropin ovulation induction after pretreatment with DHEA. This increase in IGF-1 may have been due to an increase in androgen production and may be responsible for the mechanism of action of DHEA supplements.
- Barad and Gleicher (2006)[64] postulated that the effect of DHEA was due to the creation of polycystic ovarian syndrome (PCOS)-like characteristics in the aging ovary. Long-term androgen exposure can induce histological and sonographic changes in normal ovaries similar to PCOS. The effect of DHEA is cumulative as more of the antral follicles become exposed to treatment. The theory of PCOS-like environment can explain the increase in response from cycle to cycle under DHEA exposure.
- It has also been postulated that DHEA supplementation reduces follicular apoptosis, thereby increasing the pool of primordial follicles.

Simple Cyst Drainage Prior to Stimulation Protocols

One of the most significant side effects of pituitary downregulation with gonadotropin-releasing hormone (GnRH) agonists in COH protocols is ovarian cyst formation with an incidence of 8% to 53%.[65] Formation of follicular cysts may be related to the endogenous gonadotropin flare in response to mid-luteal GnRH agonists. The impact of these ovarian cysts on IVF outcomes remains controversial with there being evidence of poor IVF performance in patients forming ovarian cysts in response to GnRH agonists in both poor responders and normal responders. While a study showed the worst outcomes with hormonally inactive cysts greater than

15 mm,[66] other studies however have failed to confirm the negative prognosis of follicular cyst formation on IVF outcome.[67]

Several studies have evaluated the effect of ovarian cyst aspiration on IVF outcomes. Most of them failed to show improved outcomes with precycle aspiration even though its one of the most commonly resorted to procedures on discovery of a cyst prestimulation.[68,69] While follicular cyst formation prior to IVF is probably a poor prognosticator, further studies are required to determine whether to proceed, wait or drain the cyst prior to the cycle.

The Benefits and Risk of Precycle Oral Contraceptive Pill or Antagonist Suppression Combined with Estrogen Priming

Oral contraceptive pills (OCPs) are commonly used in various IVF protocols. Patients with prior poor responses to ovarian stimulation may benefit from their use on multiple levels.

- OCP pretreatment in IVF protocols establishes an estrogenic environment and increases sex hormone-binding globulin levels while decreasing follicular androgen levels thus, delaying apoptosis.
- The progestin component of the OCP suppresses LH and may synchronize follicular development, leading to a more evenly sized follicular response.
- OCP pretreatment can prevent an early rise in progesterone by eliminating the corpus luteum in GnRH agonist flare cycles.
- OCPs also cause less pituitary downregulation when compared with GnRH agonists used in a long protocol.

Despite all these theoretical advantages of OCP use in IVF protocols for poor responders, numerous studies have failed to show any difference in IVF outcomes between patients pretreated with OCPs and those in whom OCPs were not used. Studies by Duvan et al.[70] and Kovacs et al.[71] failed to reveal any benefit of OCP pretreatment on IVF outcomes in patients with POR. In contrast to these studies, a study by Lindheim et al.[72] reported that short-term pituitary suppression with OCPs in poor responders may be beneficial; however, OCPs were shown to significantly prolong stimulation and increase the dose of gonadotropins. Pituitary suppression with OCPs may also blunt a GnRH agonist or letrozole flare response in follicular phase. However, it was demonstrated that, while the peak FSH level following a GnRH agonist flare is lower following OCPs, the percent and total rise in FSH is not different with or without OCP pretreatment.

A more recent precycle adjuvant studied for poor responders are GnRH antagonists used in the late luteal phase prior to a stimulation cycle. Fanchin et al.[73] showed that GnRH antagonists administered on day 25 of the menstrual cycle reduce size disparities among follicles. Recent studies have resulted in similar IVF outcomes when luteal E2/GnRH antagonists in GnRH antagonist protocols were compared with microdose GnRH agonist flare protocols. Several studies have found that luteal GnRH antagonists similar to OCPs increase the dose of gonadotropins required in subsequent COH cycles. Given the mixed results with GnRH antagonists in the luteal phase and their significantly higher cost, they are unlikely to replace precycle treatment with OCPs or E2.

Treatment with estrogen in the luteal phase prior to COH may promote granulosa cell FSH receptor induction and suppress premature follicular development. The increased number of FSH receptors and improved response to FSH stimulation may promote oocyte maturation. Several studies have demonstrated decreased cancelation rates, and improved number of oocytes and embryos following a luteal phase E2 patch; however, improved pregnancy rates have not been confirmed. Concern with suppression from the precycle use of oral contraceptives along with the need to prevent an early dominant follicle in poor responder cycles has generated interest in the use of E2 in the luteal phase prior to COH cycles in IVF. Its exact role, mechanism and potential benefit still require further study.

Adjuvants at the Initiation of a Cycle

GnRH Agonists

Most IVF programs use long GnRH agonist protocols for ovarian stimulation which work by inducing hypophyseal desensitization. GnRH agonists by suppressing endogenous LH surges and subsequent premature luteinization of oocytes, result in increased clinical pregnancy rates both per cycle and per embryo transfer. However, as a result of the extreme pituitary suppression caused by these agents and their direct inhibitory effect on the ovaries, their use results in a higher overall dose of gonadotropins and a longer duration of stimulation being required to achieve an adequate ovarian response. The reduced sensitivity to gonadotropins associated with the use of long GnRH agonist protocol has led to the introduction of various modified protocols which employ a reduced dose and duration of agonist in poor ovarian responders (**Table 2**).

Table 2 GnRH agonist stimulation protocols in poor responders

Sr. No	Protocol	Administration	Advantages (studies supporting use)	Disadvantages (studies opposing use)
1.	Mini dose protocol	Starts on cycle day 21 and dose of GnRH agonist reduces to half with onset of menses	Reduced gonadotropin requirement and shorter duration of stimulation Maximizes ovarian response, i.e. higher peak E2 levels, more oocytes recovered and embryos transferred[73,74]	Not helpful in true poor ovarian responders[75]
2.	Stop protocol	GnRH agonist from mid-luteal phase of previous cycle to onset of menstruation followed by high dose of gonadotropins	Retrieval of significantly higher number of oocytes[76]	Does not influence reproductive outcome[76]
3.	Flare protocol	Early follicular phase initiation of GnRH-a with minimal delay before commencing COH	Uses initial agonistic stimulatory effect of GnRH-a on endogenous FSH and LH secretion Eliminates excessive ovarian suppression due to prolonged agonist use Decreased gonadotropin requirement, higher pregnancy rates and decreased miscarriage rates[77-79]	Initial flare effect increases LH levels leading to raised intrafollicular androgen levels which lead to impaired folliculogenesis and significant reduction in fertilization and implantation capacity[77-79]
4.	Microdose flare protocol	Minimal doses of GnRH agonists such as 20–50 µg twice daily (bid) in the early follicular phase are usually combined with OCP pretreatment in the cycle prior to COH to prevent corpus luteum rescue	Increased ovarian response in the form of a more rapid and higher peak in E2 levels, recovery of larger number of mature oocytes Absence of enhanced LH, progesterone and androgen secretion seen with standard flare regimens[80,81]	

GnRH Antagonists

GnRH antagonists competitively block pituitary GnRH receptors, inducing a rapid, reversible suppression of gonadotropin secretion. Due to their distinct pharmacological mode of action, GnRH antagonists can be administered at mid-cycle to prevent a premature LH surge while not causing any suppression in the early follicular phase, which is a crucial time for follicular recruitment. This is particularly important in poor ovarian responders, allowing the ovaries to respond maximally to the administrated gonadotropins. Use of GnRH antagonists in poor responders was associated with a lower consumption of gonadotropins, a shorter duration of stimulation, a greater number of oocytes retrieved and a lower cycle cancelation rate besides the reduced risk of ovarian hyperstimulation syndrome (OHSS) and menopausal side effects.[82,83] However, no significant difference was found in clinical pregnancy rates, cycle cancelation rate, number of oocytes retrieved or number of mature oocytes retrieved.[84-86]

Clomiphene Flare Protocols

A flare of endogenous gonadotropins can also be achieved with early follicular phase clomiphene citrate (CC) administration. In these cycles, endogenous LH surge can be blocked with GnRH antagonists. CC flare was shown to reduce cancelation rates, increase the number of oocytes retrieved, and result higher implantation and pregnancy rates in poor responders.[87] However, its use does raise concerns about endometrial suppression especially in day 2–3 embryo transfer cycles. This concern is usually addressed by overlapping the CC flare with gonadotropins stimulation which not only reduces the dose and cost of the gonadotropins required but also improves the endometrial thickness. CC is commonly and successfully used both in minimal stimulation protocols and for its flare effect in high-dose protocols in poor responders who are undergoing freeze-all cycles.

Gonadotropins and their Stimulation Doses

Dose

A high starting gonadotropin dose in poor responders is widely practiced following a low response to a more standard dosing range of 150–300 IU of FSH. According to most authors, the starting dose for poor responders has been at least 300 IU/day, with a number of studies evaluating a daily dose of 450 IU of FSH.[88,89] No additional benefits in oocyte yield or pregnancy rates were found when the daily dose of FSH was greater than 450 IU by several studies carried out in this respect.[90] In fact, some studies have even supported the use of a step-down protocol in poor ovarian responders, starting with an initial dose of 450 IU, stepping the dose down to 300 IU and eventually down to 150 IU and shown it to be as effective as maintaining the standard maximum dose of 450 IU of FSH.[91] Since follicular recruitment occurs in the late luteal phase prior to menses and the early follicular phase, the maximal dosing, currently set at 450 IU of FSH, should be started as early in the stimulation cycle as possible. It may then be reduced once adequate response has been established.

hMG Versus Recombinant FSH

Although recombinant FSH (rFSH) introduced in the mid-1990s, was initially thought to improve stimulation and pregnancy rates when compared with the available equivalent dose of hMG. Recently, nearly all randomized prospective trials have documented equivalence without superiority of the various gonadotropins available on the market.

Role of LH in Stimulation Protocols for Poor Responders

Luteinizing hormone stimulation within a certain range, known as the LH window, is required to enable adequate folliculogenesis and steroidogenesis in a stimulation cycle to allow successful implantation and fertilization. It is seen that follicular maturation requires LH action to stimulate androstenedione biosynthesis to act as a substrate for aromatase activity. Apparently LH helps in improving the oocyte cytoplasmic maturation, through increased mitochondrial function and upregulated DNA repair enzymes, by indirectly increasing intraovarian E2 levels.

Luteinizing hormone supplementation is available as both a recombinant LH (rLH; MD Serono, MA, USA) and in the standard urinary hMG, which contains a 1:1 ratio of FSH and LH activity. Additional LH activity during stimulation for IVF can be obtained with low doses of urinary or recombinant hCG.

Patients with WHO type I anovulation, advanced maternal age, poor ovarian responders and those having been treated with GnRH agonist depot have been seen to benefit most from addition of LH preparations to their stimulation protocol. In women with advanced age, they help by overcoming the decreased biological activity of the circulating endogenous LH and the decreased number of functional LH receptors. LH supplementation as late as day 6–8 of cycle has been shown to improve the implantation and pregnancy rates in women aged more than 35 years according to various studies. In women with poor ovarian reserve and WHO type I anovulation, it helps by increased production of E2 precursor, androstenedione.

Minimal Stimulation

The role of minimal stimulation protocols to produce only a few oocytes per retrieval has been suggested for both normal and poor responders. Since in poor responders, a high dose of gonadotropins often produces no greater oocyte yield than a far less expensive cycle with oral medication or low-dose gonadotropins, minimal stimulation protocols are being particularly considered in them. In studies including poor responders, similar pregnancy rates were found following minimal stimulation IVF when compared with full-dose gonadotropins with IVF.[92,93]

■ NATURAL CYCLE IVF AND MODIFIED NATURAL CYCLE IVF

On lines with the reasoning for consideration of minimal stimulation protocol in poor responders, natural cycle and modified natural cycle IVF are good alternatives to conventional stimulation protocols in poor responders, being much cheaper and less invasive yet comparable in results.

Natural cycle IVF describes IVF carried out with oocytes collected from a woman's ovaries in a spontaneous menstrual cycle without administration of any medications during the cycle with the aim of collecting a naturally selected oocyte at the lowest possible cost.

Modified natural cycle is a terminology used to describe a natural, spontaneous cycle where exogenous hormones and drugs are used for reducing the risk of cycle cancelation while still aiming for collection of a naturally selected single oocyte. This is usually achieved by:

- Using hCG for final oocyte maturation and ovulation with or without luteal phase support administration.
- GnRH antagonist use to block spontaneous LH surge with/without usage of FSH or hMG as add-back therapy.

There are a limited number of studies comparing natural cycle IVF with full-dose gonadotropins in poor responders. A meta-analysis of 1,800 cycles of natural IVF in all types of infertility patients resulted in a 7.2% ongoing pregnancy rate per cycle and a 15.8% ongoing pregnancy rate per transfer. For normal responders, these ongoing pregnancy rates are unacceptably low. One randomized trial has shown that poor responders treated with natural cycles and intracytoplasmic sperm injection (ICSI) had higher implantation rates but similar clinical pregnancy rates per cycle and per transfer as patients treated with full-dose gonadotropins.[94] The improved implantation rate with natural cycles may be attributed to more physiologic follicular development and recruitment improving both the quality of the oocyte and endometrium.

OTHER ADJUVANTS

hGH

Human growth hormone is being widely researched for its potential use and benefits in infertile patients. Its potential to stimulate increase E2 production by follicular cells and enhance nuclear and cytoplasmic maturation of oocytes has been attributed to lead to improved fertilization rates, embryo development and pregnancy rates. These observations have called for increased research on their probable use in improving the cycle outcomes in poor responders.

Low Dose Aspirin

Low dose aspirin is known to improve organ perfusion by preferential inhibition of the vasoconstricting prostaglandins over the vasodilating ones. Earlier studies showed dramatic improvement in implantation and pregnancy rates following treatment with low dose aspirin. However, recent research has failed to show any improved ovarian or uterine blood flow or ovarian responsiveness in poor ovarian responder cycles supplemented with low dose aspirin, highlighting the need for further research on the topic.

LABORATORY OPTIONS IN POOR RESPONSE CYCLES

Intracytoplasmic Sperm Injection for Low Oocyte Yield

The low number of oocytes retrieved in poor responders, have been shown by some researchers to increase the likelihood of fertilization failure. This shortcoming has been shown to be overcome in some studies by utilizing ICSI even in non-male factor infertility patients to provide higher fertilization rates than standard IVF. In a larger prospective study, it was observed that, despite no clinical advantage of ICSI in terms of implantation or pregnancy rates, its use was associated with a higher fertilization rate per oocyte inseminated. Therefore, in couples with POR and fertilization failure, ICSI could have a potential advantage over IVF.[95] However, in the limited number of prospective studies in low responder couples without a male factor ICSI,[96,97] provided similar fertilization, pregnancy and implantation rates as conventional IVF as most oocyte defects in poor responders will not be overcome by ICSI.[97] Despite the lack of benefit of ICSI in limited prospective studies for poor responders, it is a common practice to perform ICSI on mature-appearing oocytes when fewer than five oocytes are retrieved. If either the oocytes appear immature, or the mature-appearing oocyte is immature after stripping, most employ standard IVF for the remaining oocytes.

Preimplantation Genetic Screening for Poor Responders

Couples with unexplained repeated IVF failures or advanced maternal age are at an increased risk of having chromosomally abnormal embryos.[98] Therefore, preimplantation genetic screening (PGS) utilizing fluorescent in situ hybridization (FISH), to select euploid embryos for implantation, has been studied for such patients with advanced maternal age, repeated miscarriage, repeated implantation failure and severe male factor infertility. However, either due to damage to the embryos or inaccuracy of the testing, clinical trials utilizing FISH technology decreased the LBRs in women of advanced reproductive age and poor responders. Hence, there has been a growing interest in other noninvasive methods of embryo chromosomal analysis like gene expression profiling of cumulus cells surrounding oocytes, metabolomics and proteomics. Newer methods such as comparative genomic hybridization (CGH) have been introduced with the ability to analyze the entire genome.

Studies using trophectoderm biopsies utilizing CGH for chromosomal analysis with the plan to transfer only euploid embryos after vitrification have shown an increased implantation rate without any improvement in the delivery rates.[99] Future randomized controlled trials are necessary to determine whether CGH can be utilized to increase delivery rates in poor responders. In addition there is a need to compare cleavage-stage biopsy with fresh transfer with trophectoderm biopsy of blastocysts with future frozen embryo transfer (FET). It is likely that poor responders with their low embryo number and poor blastulation rate will only be able to access cleavage-stage biopsy which too is likely be limited to younger patients seeking single-embryo transfer.

Assisted Hatching

Assisted hatching involves the artificial thinning or breaching of the zona pellucida of the developing embryo by use of acidified Tyrode's solution, laser photoablation, piezo micromanipulation or proteolytic enzymes, in an attempt to try and improve implantation and pregnancy rates following IVF. The procedure has been shown to benefit especially patients with poor prognostic factors for success, like those with previous multiple IVF failures and others with age above 38 years. Assisted hatching's selective application to embryos with poor prognosis based on their zona thickness, blastomere number, fragmentation rates and maternal age has also been shown to improve the implantation and pregnancy rates.[100] Considering its success in improving implantation and pregnancy rates in patients with poor prognostic factors, its use in women with poor ovarian reserve looks promising and needs further research.

Ideal Day of Transfer

The preferred day for embryo transfer has undergone a review in IVF over the past two decades, initially moving from day 2 to day 3 in the mid-1990s and now gradually to day 5, blastocyst transfer. Though, randomized trials have confirmed that despite transferring fewer embryos, day 5 transfer yields similar pregnancy rates in good responders,[101] the role of day 5 embryo transfer for poor responders is less clear. In fact, studies on poor responders have shown results ranging from some improvement in IVF clinical outcome[102,103] to no difference[104,105] in moving embryo transfer back to day 2 versus day 3 postretrieval. Although, extending in vitro culture allows the selection of embryos with higher implantation potential, embryos from poor responders are prone to cleavage arrest and their prolonged exposure to the deleterious effects of in vitro conditions may induce damage.[106] Hence, in poor responders where fewer oocytes and embryos are available for transfers, transferring embryos at an earlier cleavage stage appears to be safer and once the number of viable embryos is equal to the number planned to be transferred, further delay of transfer is likely to be more harmful than beneficial.

Number of Embryos for Transfer

There are limited prospective studies available to evaluate the optimal number of embryos to transfer in poor responders. In addition to advanced reproductive age, poor ovarian reserve and poor response may be an indication for increasing the number of embryos to transfer. The guidelines provided by American Society for Reproductive Medicine in 2009 for the number of embryos to transfer are age based and suggest up to two embryos in women aged below 35 years, up to three embryos in women aged below 38 years, and up to four embryos in women aged below 41 years.[107] These guidelines are generally adhered to for poor responders as well.

Donor Oocytes

The mainstay of management for poor responders with repeated IVF failure and very poor prognosis otherwise is oocyte donation. In 2009 reported data, the success rate of fresh oocyte donation (live births) was more than 50%, including all programs in the USA. Our very poor prognosis group includes nearly all patients over 43 years of age, or any patient with an FSH over 15 mIU/mL, or an undetectable AMH.

■ CONCLUSION

Poor ovarian responders, in spite of their wide prevalence, continue to pose a challenge to ART specialists even today. Even after numerous studies on the topic and a host of new adjuvants being introduced to improve PORs response to stimulation, there is still much to be done in terms of research in the field to help conclusively define helpful protocols. With carefully individualized management protocols, poor responders have been known to achieve reasonable pregnancy rates of up to 30%. However, until a scientific breakthrough achieves the ability to replenish the ever decreasing ovarian reserve with age, the management of poor ovarian responders will continue to daunt reproductive endocrinologists world over.

■ REFERENCES

1. Keay SD, Liversedge NH, Mathur RS, et al. Assisted conception following poor ovarian response to gonadotrophin stimulation. Br J Obstet Gynaecol. 1997;104:521-7.

2. Turhan NO. Poor response—the devil is in the definition. Fertil Steril. 2006;86:777.

3. Macklon NS, Stouffer RL, Giuduce LC, et al. The science behind 25 years of ovarian stimulation for in vitro fertilization. Endocr Rev. 2006;27:170-207.

4. Mahutte NG, Arici A. Poor responders: does the protocol make a difference? Curr Opin Obstet Gynecol. 2002;14:275-81.

5. Garcia JE, Jones GS, Acosta AA, et al. Human menopausal gonadotropin/human chorionic gonadotropin follicular maturation for oocyte aspiration: phase II, 1981. Fertil Steril. 1983;39:174-9.

6. Land JA, Yarmolinskaya MI, Dumoulin JC, et al. High-dose human menopausal gonadotropin stimulation in poor responders does not improve in vitro fertilization outcome. Fertil Steril. 1996;65(5):961-5.

7. Fridström M, Akerlöf E, Sjöblom P, et al. Serum levels of luteinizing and follicle-stimulating hormones in normal and poor-responding patients undergoing ovarian stimulation with urofollitropin after pituitary downregulation. Gynecol Endocrinol. 1997;11(1):25-8.

8. Raga F, Bonilla-Musoles F, Casañ EM, et al. Recombinant follicle stimulating hormone stimulation in poor responders with normal basal concentrations of follicle stimulating hormone and oestradiol: improved reproductive outcome. Hum Reprod. 1999;14(6):1431-4.

9. Loutradis D, Drakakis P, Milingos S, et al. Alternative approaches in the management of poor response in controlled ovarian hyper-stimulation (COH) Ann N Y Acad Sci. 2003;997:112-9.

10. Rombauts L, Suikkari AM, MacLachlan V, et al. Recruitment of follicles by recombinant human follicle-stimulating hormone commencing in the luteal phase of the ovarian cycle. Fertil Steril. 1998;69(4):665-9.

11. Surrey ES, Bower J, Hill DM, et al. Clinical and endocrine effects of a microdose GnRH agonist flare regimen administered to poor responders who are undergoing in vitro fertilization. Fertil Steril. 1998;69(3):419-24.

12. Droesch K, Muasher SJ, Brzyski RG, et al. Value of suppression with a gonadotropin-releasing hormone agonist prior to gonadotropin stimulation for in vitro fertilization. Fertil Steril. 1989;51(2):292-7.

13. Feldberg D, Farhi J, Ashkenazi J, et al. Minidose gonadotropin-releasing hormone agonist is the treatment of choice in poor responders with high follicle-stimulating hormone levels. Fertil Steril. 1994;62(2):343-6.

14. Olivennes F, Righini C, Fanchin R, et al. A protocol using a low dose of gonadotrophin-releasing hormone agonist might be the best protocol for patients with high follicle-stimulating hormone concentrations on day 3. Hum Reprod. 1996;11(6):1169-72.

15. Karande V, Morris R, Rinehart J, et al. Limited success using the "flare" protocol in poor responders in cycles with low basal follicle-stimulating hormone levels during in vitro fertilization. Fertil Steril. 1997;67(5):900-3.

16. Yarali H, Esinler I, Polat M, et al. Antagonist/letrozole protocol in poor ovarian responders for intracytoplasmic sperm injection: a comparative study with the microdose flare-up protocol. Fertil Steril. 2009;92(1):231-5.

17. Toth TL, Awwad JT, Veeck LL, et al. Suppression and flare regimens of gonadotropin-releasing hormone agonist. Use in women with different basal gonadotropin values in an in vitro fertilization program. J Reprod Med. 1996;41(5):321-6.

18. Ferraretti AP, La Marca A, Fauser BC, et al. ESHRE consensus on the definition of 'poor response' to ovarian stimulation for in vitro fertilization: the Bologna criteria. Hum Reprod. 2011;26(7):1616-24.

19. Venetis CA, Kolibianakis EM, Tarlatzi TB, et al. Evidence-based management of poor ovarian response. Ann N Y Acad Sci. 2010;1205:199-206.

20. Shanbhag S, Aucott L, Bhattacharya S, et al. Interventions for 'poor responders' to controlled ovarian hyperstimulation (COH) in in-vitro fertilisation (IVF). Cochrane Database Syst Rev. 2007;1:CD004379.

21. Gleicher N, Weghofer A, Oktay K, et al. Relevance of triple CGG repeats in the FMR1 gene to ovarian reserve. Reprod Biomed Online. 2009;19:385-90.

22. De Vos M, Devroey P, Fauser BC. Primary ovarian insufficiency. Lancet. 2010;11:911-21.

23. Molloy D, Martin M, Speirs A, et al. Performance of patients with a 'frozen pelvis' in an in vitro fertilization program. Fertil Steril. 1987;47:450-5.

24. Keay SD, Barlow R, Eley A, et al. The relation between immunoglobulin G antibodies to *Chlamydia trachomatis* and poor ovarian response to gonadotropin stimulation before in vitro fertilization. Fertil Steril. 1998;70:214-8.

25. Nargund G, Fauser BC, Macklon NS, et al. The ISMAAR proposal on terminology for ovarian stimulation for IVF. Hum Reprod. 2007;22:2801-4.

26. Garcia-Velasco JA, Somigliana E. Management of endometriomas in women requiring IVF: to touch or not to touch. Hum Reprod. 2009;24:496-501.

27. Oktem O, Oktay K. Quantitative assessment of the impact of chemotherapy on ovarian follicle reserve and stromal function. Cancer. 2007;15:2222-9.

28. Brodin T, Bergh T, Berglund L, et al. Menstrual cycle length is an age-independent marker of female fertility: results from 6271 treatment cycles of in vitro fertilization. Fertil Steril. 2008;90:1656-61.

29. Nikolaou D, Templeton A. Early ovarian ageing: a hypothesis, detection and clinical relevance. Hum Reprod. 2003;18(6):1137-9.

30. Beckers NG, Macklon NS, Eijkemans MJ, et al. Women with regular menstrual cycles and a poor response to ovarian hyperstimulation for in vitro fertilization exhibit follicular phase characteristics suggestive of ovarian aging. Fertil Steril. 2002;78(2):291-7.

31. de Boer EJ, den Tonkelaar I, te Velde ER, et al. A low number of retrieved oocytes at in vitro fertilization treatment is predictive of early menopause. Fertil Steril. 2002;77(5):978-85.

32. Martinez F, Barri PN, Coroleu B, et al. Women with poor response to IVF have lowered circulating gonadotrophin surge-attenuating factor (GnSAF) bioactivity during spontaneous and stimulated cycles. Hum Reprod. 2002;17(3):634-40.

33. Ulug U, Turan E, Tosun SB, et al. Comparison of preovulatory follicular concentrations of epidermal growth factor, insulin-like growth factor-I, and inhibins A and B in women undergoing assisted conception treatment with gonadotropin-releasing hormone (GnRH) agonists and GnRH antagonists. Fertil Steril. 2007;87(4):995-8.

34. Neulen J, Wenzel D, Hornig C, et al. Poor responder-high responder: the importance of soluble vascular endothelial growth factor receptor 1 in ovarian stimulation protocols. Hum Reprod. 2001;16(4):621-6.

35. Pellicer A, Ballester MJ, Serrano MD, et al. Aetiological factors involved in the low response to gonadotrophins in infertile women with normal basal serum follicle stimulating hormone levels. Hum Reprod. 1994;9(5):806-11.

36. Hernandez ER. Embryo implantation and GnRH antagonists: embryo implantation: the Rubicon for GnRH antagonists. Hum Reprod. 2000;15(6):1211-6.

37. Lee DW, Grasso P, Dattatreyamurty B, et al. Purification of a high molecular weight follicle-stimulating hormone receptor-binding inhibitor from human follicular fluid. J Clin Endocrinol Metab. 1993;77(1):163-8.

38. Zeleznik AJ, Schuler HM, Reichert LE, et al. Gonadotropin-binding sites in the rhesus monkey ovary: role of the vasculature in the selective distribution of human chorionic gonadotropin to the pre-ovulatory follicle. Endocrinology. 1981;109(2):356-62.

39. Loutradis D, Drakakis P, Vomvolaki E, et al. Different ovarian stimulation protocols for women with diminished ovarian reserve. J Assist Reprod Genet. 2007;24(12):597-611.

40. Ahmed B, Wageah A, El Gharib M, et al. Prediction and diagnosis of poor ovarian response: the dilemma. J Reprod Infertil. 2011;12(4):241-8.

41. Broekmans FJ, Kwee J, Hendriks DJ, et al. A systematic review of tests predicting ovarian reserve and IVF outcome. Hum Reprod Update. 2006;12(6):685-718.

42. Mukherjee T, Copperman AB, Lapinski R, et al. An elevated day three follicle-stimulating hormone:luteinizing hormone ratio (FSH:LH) in the presence of a normal day 3 FSH predicts a poor response to controlled ovarian hyperstimulation. Fertil Steril. 1996;65(3):588-93.

43. Licciardi FL, Liu HC, Rosenwaks Z. Day 3 estradiol serum concentrations as prognosticators of ovarian stimulation response and pregnancy out-come in patients undergoing in vitro fertilization. Fertil Steril. 1995;64(5):991-4.

44. Seifer DB, Maclaughlin DT. Müllerian inhibiting substance is an ovarian growth factor of emerging clinical significance. Fertil Steril. 2007;88(3):539-46.

45. Oosterhuis GJ, Vermes I, Lambalk CB, et al. Insulin-like growth factor (IGF)-I and IGF binding protein-3 concentrations in fluid from human stimulated follicles. Hum Reprod. 1998;13(2):285-9.

46. Seifer DB, Lambert-Messerlian G, Hogan JW, et al. Day 3 serum inhibin-B is predictive of assisted reproductive technologies outcome. Fertil Steril. 1997;67(1):110-4.

47. Van Rooij IA, Broekmans FJ, te Velde ER, et al. Serum anti-Müllerian hormone levels: a novel measure of ovarian reserve. Hum Reprod. 2002;17(12):3065-71.

48. Gibreel A, Maheshwari A, Bhattacharya S, et al. Ultrasound tests of ovarian reserve: a systematic review of accuracy in predicting fertility outcomes. Hum Fertil (Camb). 2009;12(2):95-106.

49. Chang MY, Chiang CH, Hsieh TT, et al. Use of the antral follicle count to predict the outcome of assisted reproductive technologies. Fertil Steril. 1998;69(3):505-10.

50. Bancsi LF, Broekmans FJ, Eijkemans MJ, et al. Predictors of poor ovarian response in in vitro fertilization: a prospective study comparing basal markers of ovarian reserve. Fertil Steril. 2002;77(2):328-36.

51. Fanchin R, de Ziegler D, Olivennes F, et al. Exogenous follicle stimulating hormone ovarian reserve test (EFORT): a simple and reliable screening test for detecting 'poor responders' in in-vitro fertilization. Hum Reprod. 1994;9(9):1607-11.

52. Casson PR, Lindsay MS, Pisarska MD, et al. Dehydroepiandrosterone supplementation augments ovarian stimulation in poor responders: a case series. Hum Reprod. 2000;15(10):2129-32.

53. Barad DH, Gleicher N. Increased oocyte production after treatment with dehydroepiandrosterone. Fertil Steril. 2005;84(3):756.

54. Barad D, Gleicher N. Effect of dehydroepiandrosterone on oocyte and embryo yields, embryo grade and cell number in IVF. Hum Reprod. 2006;21(11):2845-9.

55. Barad D, Brill H, Gleicher N. Update on the use of dehydroepiandrosterone supplementation among women with diminished ovarian function. J Assist Reprod Genet. 2007;24(12):629-34.

56. Gleicher N, Ryan E, Weghofer A, et al. Miscarriage rates after dehydroepiandrosterone (DHEA) supplementation in women with diminished ovarian reserve: a case-control study. Reprod Biol Endocrinol. 2009;7:108.

57. Gleicher N, Weghofer A, Barad DH. Improvement in diminished ovarian reserve after dehydroepiandrosterone supplementation. Reprod Biomed Online. 2010;21(3): 360-5.

58. Wiser A, Gonen O, Ghetler Y, et al. Addition of dehydroepiandrosterone (DHEA) for poor-responder patients before and during IVF treatment improves the pregnancy rate: a randomized prospective study. Hum Reprod. 2010;25(10):2496-500.

59. Hillier SG, Whitelaw PF, Smyth CD. Follicular estrogen synthesis: the '2-cell, two-gonadotrophin' model revisited. Mol Cell Endocrinol. 1994;100:51-4.

60. Haning RV Jr., Hackett RJ, Flood CA, et al. Plasma dehydroepiandrosterone sulfate serves as a prehormone for 48% of follicular fluid testosterone during treatment with menotropins. J Clin Endocrinol Metab. 1993;76:1301-7.

61. Dorrington JH, Moon YS, Armstrong DT. Estradiol-17beta biosynthesis in cultured granulosa cells from hypophysectomized immature rats; stimulation by follicle-stimulating hormone. Endocrinology. 1975;97:1328-31.

62. Casson PR, Santoro N, Elkind-Hirsch K, et al. Postmenopausal dehydroepiandrosterone administration increases free insulin-like growth factor-I and decreases high-density lipoprotein: a six-month trial. Fertil Steril. 1998;70:107-10.

63. Casson PR, Lindsay MS, Pisarska MD, et al. Dehydroepiandrosterone supplementation augments ovarian stimulation in poor responders: a case series. Hum Reprod. 2002;15:2129-32.
64. Barad D, Gleicher N. Effect of dehydroepiandrosterone on oocyte and embryo yields, embryo grade and cell number in IVF. Hum Reprod. 2006;21:2845-9.
65. Liu HC, Lai YM, Davis O, et al. Improved pregnancy outcome with gonadotropin releasing hormone agonist (GnRH-a) stimulation is due to the improvement in oocyte quantity rather than quality. J Assist Reprod Genet. 1992;9(4):338-44.
66. Keltz MD, Jones EE, Duleba AJ, et al. Baseline cyst formation after luteal phase gonadotropin-releasing hormone agonist administration is linked to poor in vitro fertilization outcome. Fertil Steril. 1995;64(3):568-72.
67. Herman A, Ron-El R, Golan A, et al. Follicle cysts after menstrual versus midluteal administration of gonadotropin-releasing hormone analog in in vitro fertilization. Fertil Steril. 1990;53(5):854-8.
68. Owj M, Ashrafi M, Baghestani AR. Ovarian cyst formation and in vitro fertilization outcome. Int J Gynaecol Obstet. 2004;87(3):258-9.
69. Rizk B, Tan SL, Kingsland C, et al. Ovarian cyst aspiration and the outcome of in vitro fertilization. Fertil Steril. 1990;54(4):661-4.
70. Duvan CI, Berker B, Turhan NO, et al. Oral contraceptive pretreatment does not improve outcome in microdose gonadotrophin-releasing hormone agonist protocol among poor responder intracytoplasmic sperm injection patients. J Assist Reprod Genet. 2008;25(2-3):89-93.
71. Kovacs P, Barg PE, Witt BR. Hypothalamic-pituitary suppression with oral contraceptive pills does not improve outcome in poor responder patients undergoing in vitro fertilization-embryo transfer cycles. J Assist Reprod Genet. 2001;18(7):391-4.
72. Lindheim SR, Barad DH, Witt B, et al. Short-term gonadotropin suppression with oral contraceptives benefits poor responders prior to controlled ovarian hyperstimulation. J Assist Reprod Genet. 1996;13(9):745-7.
73. Feldberg D, Farhi J, Ashkenazi J, et al. Minidose gonadotropin releasing hormone agonists is the treatment of choice in poor responders with high follicle stimulating hormone levels. Fertil Steril. 1994;62:343-6.
74. Olivennes F, Righini C, Fanchin R, et al. A protocol using a low dose of gonadotrophin releasing hormone agonist might be the best protocol for patients with high follicle stimulating hormone concentrations on day 3. Hum Reprod. 1996;11:1169-73.
75. Kowalik A, Barmat L, Damario M, et al. Ovarian estradiol production in vivo (inhibitory effect of leuprolide acetate. J Reprod Med. 1998;43:413-7.
76. Garcia-Velasco JA, Isaza V, Requena A, et al. High doses of gonadotrophins combined with stop vs non stop protocol of GnRH analogue administration in low responder IVF patients: a prospective, randomized, controlled trial. Hum Reprod. 2000;15:2292-6.
77. Garcia J, Padilla S, Bargati J, et al. Follicular phase gonadotropin-releasing hormone agonist and human gonadotropins (a better alternative for in vitro fertilization). Fertil Steril. 1990;53:302-5.
78. Katayama K, Roesler M, Gunnarson G, et al. Short-term use of gonadotropin-releasing hormone agonist (leuprolide) for in vitro fertilization. J In Vitro Fert Embryo Transfer. 1988; 5:332-7.
79. Padilla S, Dugan K, Shalika S, et al. Use of the flare-up protocol with high dose follicle stimulating hormone and human menopausal gonadotropins for in vitro fertilization in poor responders. Fertil Steril. 1996;65:796-9.
80. Kahraman K, Berker B, Atabekoglu CS, et al. Microdose gonadotropin-releasing hormone agonist flare-up protocol versus multiple dose gonadotropin-releasing hormone antagonist protocol in poor responders undergoing intracytoplasmic sperm injection-embryo transfer cycle. Fertil Steril. 2009;91(6):2437-44.
81. Scott RT, Navot D. Enhancement of ovarian responsiveness with microdoses of gonadotropin-releasing hormone agonist during ovulation induction for in vitro fertilization. Fertil Steril. 1994;61(5):880-5.
82. Nikolettos N, Al-Hasani S, Felberbaum R, et al. Gonadotrophin-releasing hormone antagonist protocol: a novel method of ovarian stimulation in poor responders. Eur J Obstet Gynecol Reprod Biol. 2001;97:202-7.
83. Craft I, Gorgy A, Hill J, et al. Will GnRH antagonists provide new hope for patients considered 'difficult responders' to GnRH agonist protocols? Hum Reprod. 1999;14:2959-62.
84. Akman MA, Erden HF, Tosun SB, et al. Comparison of agonistic flare-up-protocol and antagonistic multiple dose protocol in ovarian stimulation of poor responders: results of a prospective randomized trial. Hum Reprod. 2001;16(5):868-70.
85. Fasouliotis SJ, Laufer N, Sabbagh-Ehrlich S, et al. Gonadotropin-releasing hormone (GnRH)-antagonist versus GnRH-agonist in ovarian stimulation of poor responders undergoing IVF. J Assist Reprod Genet. 2003;20(11):455-60.
86. Berin I, Stein DE, Keltz MD. A comparison of gonadotropin-releasing hormone (GnRH) antagonist and GnRH agonist flare protocols for poor responders undergoing in vitro fertilization. Fertil Steril. 2010;93(2):360-3.
87. D'Amato G, Caroppo E, Pasquadibisceglie A, et al. A novel protocol of ovulation induction with delayed gonadotropin-releasing hormone antagonist administration combined with high-dose recombinant follicle-stimulating hormone and clomiphene citrate for poor responders and women over 35 years. Fertil Steril. 2004;81(6):1572-7.
88. Siristatidis CS, Hamilton MP. What should be the maximum FSH dose in IVF/ICSI in poor responders? J Obstet Gynaecol. 2007;27(4):401-5.
89. Tarlatzis BC, Zepiridis L, Grimbizis G, et al. Clinical management of low ovarian response to stimulation for IVF: a systematic review. Hum Reprod Update. 2003; 9(1):61-76.
90. Hofmann GE, Toner JP, Muasher SJ, et al. High-dose follicle-stimulating hormone (FSH) ovarian stimulation in low-responder patients for in vitro fertilization. J In Vitro Fert Embryo Transf. 1989;6(5):285-9.
91. Cedrin-Durnerin I, Bständig B, Hervé F, et al. A comparative study of high fixed-dose and decremental-dose regimens

of gonadotropins in a minidose gonadotropin-releasing hormone agonist flare protocol for poor responders. Fertil Steril. 2000;73(5):1055-6.

92. Weghofer A, Margreiter M, Bassim S, et al. Minimal stimulation using recombinant follicle-stimulating hormone and a gonadotropin-releasing hormone antagonist in women of advanced age. Fertil Steril. 2004;81(4):1002-6.

93. Elizur SE, Aslan D, Shulman A, et al. Modified natural cycle using GnRH antagonist can be an optional treatment in poor responders undergoing IVF. J Assist Reprod Genet. 2005;22(2):75-9.

94. Morgia F, Sbracia M, Schimberni M, et al. A controlled trial of natural cycle versus microdose gonadotropin-releasing hormone analog flare cycles in poor responders undergoing in vitro fertilization. Fertil Steril. 2004;81(6):1542-7.

95. Bhattacharya S, Hamilton MP, Shaaban M, et al. Conventional in-vitro fertilisation versus intracytoplasmic sperm injection for the treatment of non-male-factor infertility: a randomised controlled trial. Lancet. 2001;357(9274):2075-9.

96. Moreno C, Ruiz A, Simón C, et al. Intracytoplasmic sperm injection as a routine indication in low responder patients. Hum Reprod. 1998;13(8):2126-9.

97. Gabrielen A, Petersen K, Mikkelsen AL, et al. Intracytoplasmic sperm injection does not overcome an oocyte defect in previous fertilization failure with conventional in-vitro fertilization and normal spermatozoa. Hum Reprod. 1996;11(9):1963-5.

98. Gianaroli L, Magli MC, Ferraretti AP, et al. Preimplantation diagnosis for aneuploidies in patients undergoing in vitro fertilization with a poor prognosis: identification of the categories for which it should be proposed. Fertil Steril. 1999;72(5):837-44.

99. Schoolcraft WB, Katz-Jaffe MG, Stevens J, et al. Preimplantation aneuploidy testing for infertile patients of advanced maternal age: a randomized prospective trial. Fertil Steril. 2009;92(1):157-62.

100. Cohen J, Alikani M, Trowbridge J, et al. Implantation enhancement by selective assisted hatching using zona drilling of human embryos with poor prognosis. Hum Reprod. 1992;7:685-91.

101. Blake DA, Farquhar CM, Johnson N, et al. Cleavage stage versus blastocyst stage embryo transfer in assisted conception. Cochrane Database Syst Rev. 2007;4:CD002118.

102. Shen S, Rosen MP, Dobson AT, et al. Day 2 transfer improves pregnancy outcome in in vitro fertilization cycles with few available embryos. Fertil Steril. 2006;86(1):44-50.

103. Bahceci M, Ulug U, Ciray HN, et al. Efficiency of changing the embryo transfer time from day 3 to day 2 among women with poor ovarian response: a prospective randomized trial. Fertil Steril. 2006;86(1):81-5.

104. Frankfurter D, Silva CP, Mota F, et al. The transfer point is a novel measure of embryo placement. Fertil Steril. 2003;79(6):1416-21.

105. Dayal MB, Frankfurter D, Athanasiadis I, et al. Day 2 embryo transfer (ET) and day 3 ET afford similar reproductive outcomes in the poor responder. Fertil Steril. 2011;95(3):1130-2.

106. Laverge H, De Sutter P, Van der Elst J, et al. A prospective, randomized study comparing day 2 and day 3 embryo transfer in human IVF. Hum Reprod. 2001;16(3):476-80.

107. Practice Committee of the American Society for Reproductive Medicine and Practice Committee of the Society for Assisted Reproductive Technology. Guidelines on number of embryos transferred. Fertil Steril. 2009;92(5):1518-9.

50

ART in
Polycystic Ovary Syndrome

Jaideep Malhotra, Parul Arora

■ INTRODUCTION

Polycystic ovary syndrome (PCOS) is a polygenic multifactorial condition affecting 5–10% of the women of reproductive age group.[1] It is in fact the most common endocrinological disorder among the women accounting for the majority of the cases of hirsutism, menstrual disturbances and anovulatory infertility. Anovulation is common among females with PCOS and accounts for 80–90% of WHO group II anovulatory subfertility. The diagnosis of PCOS implies not only anovulation and infertility but also a variety of metabolic and endocrinological disturbances like obesity, hypertension, hyperglycemia, hyperlipidemia, coronary heart disease, and even the risk of endometrial hyperplasia and cancer.

Despite many debates and conferences conducted on this subject, the syndrome is surrounded by controversies regarding both its diagnosis and treatment. Various diagnostic criteria have been laid down by different expert groups for establishing the diagnosis of PCOS. These are discussed below.

NICHD/NIH criteria (1990): The diagnostic criteria according to this group require the simultaneous presence of hyperandrogenism (clinical and/or biochemical) and menstrual dysfunction, with the exclusion of other androgen excess disorders, thyroid disorders, hyperprolactinemia. The ultrasound criteria of polycystic ovaries were not included in definition.[2]

Rotterdam criteria (2003):[3] This criteria require the presence of at least two of the following:
- Clinical and/or biochemical evidence of hyper-androgenism
- Oligo-ovulation or anovulation
- Ultrasound evidence of polycystic ovaries: One or both the ovaries with greater than or equal to 12 follicles of 2–9 mm size, ovarian volume more than 10 cc. The distribution of the follicles and the stromal volume and echogenecity are now no longer included in the definition.

This criteria also require the exclusion of other disorders like congenital adrenal hyperplasia, androgen secreting ovarian tumors, Cushing's syndrome, hypo- or hyperthyroidism and hyperprolactinemia.

Androgen excess–PCOS society criteria (2009):[4] It require the presence of both hyperandrogenism and ovarian dysfunction. The ovarian dysfunction may be in the form of oligo-ovulation or anovulation or polycystic morphology of ovaries on ultrasound. The society also mandated the exclusion of other etiologies of androgen excess or ovulatory dysfunction. The criteria for PCO morphology of the ovaries were same as that in the Rotterdam criteria.

Although significant progress has been made toward establishing the universally accepted diagnostic criteria for PCOS, the optimal treatment of patients with PCOS has not yet been defined. PCOS patients present as a unique challenge to the reproductive medicine specialists, not only for their infertility treatment but also for other health concerns like obesity, hypertension, diabetes mellitus, coronary heart disease, hyperlipidemia, etc. These metabolic and endocrinological abnormalities need to be diagnosed and treated for maintaining an overall good health and ensuring good reproductive outcomes in such patients.

■ CHALLENGES IN PCOS

In addition to anovulation, there may be other factors that contribute to subfertility in women with PCOS. These include obesity and a variety of metabolic, inflammatory and endocrinological abnormalities. These abnormalities are thought to affect the oocyte quality and may have detrimental effect on the pregnancy outcome. The oocytes from patients with PCOS have reduced developmental competence, leading to aberrations in fertilization and increased chances of fertilization failure.[5] The intraovarian milieu in PCOS patients is also disturbed due to paracrine dysregulation, further contributing to impaired nuclear and cytoplasmic maturation of oocytes in such patients.

It is well known that females with PCOS are more prone to develop pregnancy complications like miscarriages, pre-eclampsia, gestational diabetes, intrauterine growth restriction, preterm births and stillbirths. *The aim of any treatment desired to achieve pregnancy, should not direct only toward achieving ovulation induction, but should take into consideration the entire range of risk factors that are present in a particular patient. These abnormalities need to be corrected before we aim at achieving pregnancy.*

It is well known that around 50% of the females with PCOS are obese.[6] Central obesity is a major factor influencing the outcomes of both treatment of symptoms and infertility in women with PCOS. Obesity worsens both symptomatology and endocrine profile, so the obese women [body mass index (BMI) >30 kg/m²] should be encouraged to lose weight. Weight loss improves endocrine profile, the likelihood of ovulation and the chances to have a healthy pregnancy. Even a 5–10% loss of body weight can improve the hormonal milieu and increase the chances of pregnancy.[1]

Body weight is also a major determinant of insulin sensitivity and ovarian hyperandrogenemia, independent of PCOS. It is believed that insulin resistance and secondary hyperinsulinemia are the major culprits in the pathophysiology of PCOS. Various studies have shown that patients with PCOS with ovulatory phenotype have less insulin resistance than those with classical phenotype (with anovulation).[7] It has also been observed that those without hyperandrogenemia have no insulin resistance.[8] In these two subtypes, the involvement of insulin resistance in the pathogenesis of disease is less important.

The preconceptional counseling in women with PCOS should identify risk factors for reproductive failure and correct them prior to treatment initiation. In this respect, it is important to recognize the presence of obesity and its centripetal distribution as well as to recommend folate supplementation in all women trying for conception. It is well known that obesity is associated with anovulation. It is also linked to resistance/delayed response to various ovulogens that are used in these patients for fertility treatment. The treatment of obesity is multifaceted and involves behavioral therapy, lifestyle modification with exercise, diet control, pharmacological interventions and bariatric surgeries. The effect of calorie restriction, increased physical activity and pharmacological interventions in the periconceptional period are largely unknown and may be potentially harmful to the health of newborn. So, these interventions should be undertaken prior to pregnancy, not concurrently with infertility treatment, until the risk benefit ratios of these strategies on pregnancy are better understood.[1]

In the Thessaloniki ESHRE/ASRM sponsored PCOS Consensus workshop group, it was concluded that lifestyle modification and weight loss with diet and exercise remain the first line of treatment for any PCOS woman who is overweight.[1] This is then to be followed by the use of clomiphene citrate (CC) for ovulation induction. The proposed second line therapy for infertility treatment in PCOS patients is either gonadotropins therapy or the use of laparoscopic ovarian drilling. Ovarian drilling may be considered an alternative to gonadotropin therapy for CC resistant anovulatory PCOS. It can also achieve unifollicular ovulation with no risk of ovarian hyperstimulation syndrome (OHSS) or high-order multiples. Various concerns for ovarian drilling are the need for surgery, with the risk of adhesion formation and destruction of normal ovarian tissue. This is also not indicated for non-fertility indications.

Assisted reproductive technology (ART) is indicated as a third-line treatment for PCOS patients not responding to the conventional treatment protocols that have been highlighted previously. It is also indicated for those PCOS subjects who have underlying other infertility factors like severe tubal damage, male factor infertility, severe endometriosis and those who require preimplantation genetic diagnosis.

■ PATHOPHYSIOLOGY AND OOCYTE ABNORMALITIES IN PCOS

A number of endocrinological disturbances have been implicated in the pathophysiology of disease. These include hyperinsulinemia, luteinizing hormone (LH) hypersecretion, follicle-stimulating hormone (FSH) deficiency, hyperandrogenemia, and a variety of paracrine disturbances in the intraovarian environment. Out of all these hormonal imbalances, hyperinsulinemia has been found to be the major culprit.

Polycystic ovary syndrome patients are typically characterized by increased number of oocytes retrieved during in vitro fertilization (IVF), but it has been found that these oocytes are often of poor quality and exhibit lower fertilization, cleavage and implantation rates and are associated with increased miscarriage rates. Mechanisms responsible for these outcomes are unclear, but may involve metabolism-induced changes in the oocyte quality.

The effects of these various endocrinologic disturbances and paracrine factors are discussed further.

Extraovarian Factors

The oocyte developmental process can be impaired by a number of extraovarian endocrine factors such as FSH deficiency, LH hypersecretion, hyperandrogenemia and hyperinsulinemia.

Hyperinsulinemia and Premature Follicle Luteinization

Insulin resistance coupled with hyperandrogenemia is a key factor in the pathophysiology of PCOS. Insulin resistance is thought to arise from aberrant phosphorylation of tyrosine and serine residues on insulin receptor resulting in increasing insulin resistance and accompanying hyperinsulinemia. As the insulin binds the insulin-like growth factor-1 (IGF-1) receptors on the theca cells, it stimulates the theca cell androgen production by stimulating 17 alpha-hydroxylase activity. Hyperinsulinemia also results in reduced hepatic synthesis of SHBG and insulin-like growth factor-binding protein-1 (IGFBP-1), which in turn increases the bioavailability of both androgens and IGF-1 and IGF-2 which are important regulators of ovarian follicular maturation and steroidogenesis.[9] Insulin also enhances the FSH-induced upregulation of LH receptors on the granulosa cells and increases their ability to produce P4 in response to LH. Consequently, small antral PCOS follicles exhibit P4 hypersecretion and show exaggerated shift in steroidogenesis from E2 to progesterone production.[10] This induces premature granulosa cell luteinization, leading to arrest of cell proliferation and follicle growth.

Insulin resistant PCOS women have been shown to have lower fertilization and implantation rates after IVF. A study by Teissier et al. reported a lower proportion of meiotically-competent oocytes obtained from follicles with increased androgen and P4 concentrations, suggesting that these oocytes have been obtained from prematurely luteinized follicles.

The insulin concentration in the human follicles is determined by body weight and fasting serum insulin levels and is highest in women with impaired glucose tolerance.[11] Therefore, the use of metformin has been suggested as a strategy to improve follicular growth and oocyte quality in PCOS. However, the results of various studies in this regard have been controversial, some supporting the use of metformin to improve follicular development while others showing no effect of the drug on oocyte quality. This makes the current use of metformin to improve development competence of PCOS oocytes controversial.[12]

FSH Deficiency

Follicle-stimulating hormone is an important hormone for recruitment, selection and dominance of ovarian follicle in each menstrual cycle. PCOS patients have lower FSH levels as compared to normal controls. The follicles are stimulated by chronic low levels of FSH, but do not attain complete maturity. This results in accumulation of small follicles between 2 mm and 8 mm size. These small follicles, however when exposed to exogenous FSH, can grow and form the dominant follicle. Consequently, PCOS patients when subjected to ovarian stimulation for IVF, commonly demonstrate high levels of E2, combined with a significantly higher number of oocytes retrieved although of poor quality. These oocytes exhibit poor fertilization rates, higher fragmentation rates, lower rate of blastocyst formation, lower implantation rates and higher miscarriage rates. It has been postulated that higher serum E2 levels may be detrimental outcomes of assisted reproduction.[13]

Luteinizing Hormone Hypersecretion

Polycystic ovary syndrome patients have tonic hypersecretion of LH during follicular phase of their cycle. This LH hypersecretion suppresses FSH release, promotes premature granulosa cell luteinization and causes premature oocyte maturation via inhibition of oocyte maturation inhibitors (OMIs). It may also cause premature meiotic maturation via damaging the oocyte nucleus. The impaired meiotic maturation results in impaired extrusion of first polar body, thus contributing to oocyte aneuploidy in PCOS subjects. This may explain the higher incidence of miscarriage in such patients.[14]

Hyperandrogenism

Increased androgen levels are common in PCOS, with a major contribution from the ovary, a substantial contribution from adrenal glands and to a lesser extent from fat tissue. Studies have shown the presence of androgen receptors (ARs) in human ovarian follicles at all stages of development. Comparison of the early growing follicles in normal and polycystic ovaries suggests that the AR protein expression is enhanced in follicles from PCOS patients. Androgens acting through its own receptors increases the number of primary, preantral and early antral follicles. As a result, intrinsic ovarian hyperandrogenism in PCOS is accompanied by hyperandrogenism in small antral follicles and development of PCO morphology. The increased intraovarian androgen levels are associated with decreased developmental competence of maturing oocytes. The mechanisms of testosterone activity within the oocyte may be related to decreased calcium oscillations in the oocyte which in turn impairs its cytoplasmic maturation with effect on meiotic maturation. *The complex effects of androgen on the follicular growth begin during preantral stage and continue during later follicle development.*[15]

The small follicles from polycystic ovaries from PCOS subjects also demonstrate increased 5 alpha-reductase activity which increases 5 alpha-reduced androgens in the ovary.[16] These androgens inhibit the aromatase activity in the follicles, thus reducing the estradiol levels in the small follicles. This decreases the E2/androgen ratio in the follicles, which again affects the nuclear and cytoplasmic maturation of the accompanying oocytes in these small follicles. Consequently, the disturbed E2/androgen ratios to which the immature human oocytes are exposed in the follicular phase appears to affect the quality of mature human oocytes obtained through IVF. The lower E2 levels in the follicular fluid negatively correlate with oocyte fertilization, cleavage and implantation, and have positive association with aneuploidies and miscarriages.

Intraovarian Factors

Oocyte development is regulated by a fine balance between intraovarian and extraovarian factors. Any pertubance in the balance may lead to disordered follicular development. There are a number of intraovarian factors that have been implicated in the orderly growth and maturation of oocytes. These include members of epidermal growth factor (EGF) family, fibroblastic growth factor (FGF) family, IGF, transforming growth factor-beta (TGF-β)-related proteins, vascular endothelial growth factor (VEGF) family, neurotrophic growth factor family, various cytokines and others.

Transforming Growth Factor—Beta-related Proteins

Both the granulosa cells and the oocyte produce a number of proteins of the TGF-β family. These include inhibins, activins, AMH, GDF9 and BMP15. These factors interact with each other to coordinate granulosa cell-oocyte interaction. In the human follicles, GDF9 secreted by the oocyte induces the follicular growth in vitro. GDF9 messenger ribonucleic acid levels have been showed to be reduced in oocytes obtained from PCOS subjects. This in turn is accompanied by impaired follicular growth and subsequent follicular arrest.[17]

Another important member of TGF-β family of proteins is AMH, which is produced by the granulosa cells of growing follicles. AMH normally acts to inhibit the growth and recruitment of adjacent primordial follicles while its deficiency has the opposite effect. AMH levels are low in primordial and primary follicles and increase to maximal levels in large preantral and small antral follicles, and again decline to low levels during final follicular maturation. Studies have shown that AMH levels in primordial and transitional follicles of PCOS patients are lower, implicating relative AMH deficiency

as an additional factor involved in abnormal growth of the primordial follicle and its oocyte.[18] In addition, the intraovarian levels of inhibin, activin and follistatin, which are produced from the granulosa cells of the developing follicles have been found to be abnormal in PCOS subjects. However, the clinical implications of the role of these glycoproteins on the oocyte development are yet to be defined.

The results of various studies regarding the role of EGF, FGF, neurotrophin derived growth factor, VEGFs, and their altered levels in serum and follicular fluid in PCOS patients remain controversial, and the impact of these growth factors on the oocyte and embryonic development needs to be clarified further.

Other factors which have been proposed to be altered and affecting the oocyte quality in PCOS subjects include renin, resistin, leptin, homocysteine, reactive oxygen species, etc. However, their exact role in oocyte maturation abnormalities needs to be elucidated further.

To summarize, a number of extra- and intraovarian factors regulating folliculogenesis, follicular growth and oocyte development have been identified. Whether these act directly through granulosa cell-oocyte interactions or act via paracrine/endocrine signaling is yet not clear. It remains a challenge for the clinical and the academic scientists alike to clearly define and elucidate the molecular mechanisms involved in the disease, especially the factors affecting the oocyte's developmental competence and meiotic maturation. Therefore, systematic screening for the key intraovarian factors which are related to PCOS (such as AMH, homocysteine, growth factors and cytokines) coupled with proper treatment for each PCOS phenotype are essential issues in achieving success for PCOS patients undergoing assisted reproduction, in an effort to effectively improve oocyte maturation and developmental competence.

■ OVARIAN STIMULATION PROTOCOLS FOR ART CYCLES IN PCOS

Ovarian stimulation for PCOS patients differs from the stimulation regimens used in patients with normal ovaries. One characteristic of ovulation induction in PCOS patients is the initial slow response which may then progressively changes into a picture of over-response, with a high risk of developing OHSS and cyst formation. When stimulated for IVF cycles, aiming for multifollicular recruitment, these women respond sensitively and are at a risk of developing OHSS.

The incidence of severe OHSS in PCOS patients undergoing IVF has been reported to be around 15% as compared to 2% in general IVF population. Different gonadotropin regimens have been used by various workers in an effort to reduce the OHSS incidence and severity in this group of patients.

Several stimulation protocols using different gonadotropin preparations have been used for the treatment of PCOS patients undergoing IVF. These include clomiphene citrate along with human menopausal gonadotropin (hMG), hMG alone, recombinant FSH (rFSH) alone, gonadotropin-releasing hormone (GnRH) agonist with rFSH/hMG and GnRH antagonist with rFSH/hMG. Finally, different formulations have been tried to trigger final maturation of oocytes in an attempt to reduce the risk and severity of OHSS.

Choice of Gonadotropin

Different gonadotropin preparations have been used for ovarian stimulation in PCOS patients. Since women with PCOS have elevated LH levels, theoretically it may be more prudent to use gonadotropin preparations devoid of LH activity. However, various studies done in this regard have shown little difference in outcomes with different gonadotropin preparations. The Cochrane systematic review comparing rFSH with urinary derived FSH gonadotropins in PCOS patients has shown that data are insufficient to determine which of the two preparations is preferable for ovarian stimulation in such subjects.[19] Also it has been shown that urinary FSH (uFSH) preparations do not improve pregnancy rates when compared with traditional and cheaper hMG preparations.

A study by Ayse et al. comparing hMG vs rFSH in PCOS women undergoing IVF, found the same clinical pregnancy and take home baby rates in the two groups.[20] In an another meta-analysis by Hesham Al-Inany et al. no statistically significant differences were found in the clinical pregnancy rate per cycle started between rFSH and urinary-derived FSH gonadotropins [odd ratio (OR) 1.07; 95% confidence interval (CI) 0.94–1.22].[21] At present, the evidence is insufficient to conclude that rFSH is more effective than uFSH/hMG in women with PCOS.

The newer preparations provide a greater flexibility with doses such that low doses with small incremental increases may be used, thus minimizing the risk of OHSS and at the same time maintaining the satisfactory pregnancy rates.

Which Protocol to be Used—GnRH Agonist vs GnRH Antagonist?

Use of GnRH agonists in long protocol for pituitary desensitization has been the gold standard protocol for controlled ovarian stimulation in IVF cycles for the last 20 years. The proponents in favor of using this protocol in PCOS patients, claim that suppression of endogenous LH by GnRH agonists may be advantageous for the sensitive polycystic ovary, allowing follicular recruitment to occur without exposure to high levels of LH. High LH levels have been reported to be associated with poor follicular development and hence lower oocyte quality. Studies have shown that the oocytes obtained from IVF cycles using GnRH analogs in long protocol fertilize better than those obtained in cycles without pituitary desensitization.

The more recent introduction of regimens using GnRH antagonist for pituitary suppression holds promise for PCOS patients. Antagonists suppress the gonadotropin release from pituitary within a few hours and do not produce any flare effect. Moreover, because of their short half-life, gonadal functions resume without a delay following their discontinuation.

A Cochrane meta-analysis 2011 [review of 45 randomized controlled trials (RCTs)] comparing GnRH antagonist regimen to long protocol GnRH agonist regimen has shown a statistically significant reduction in the incidence of OHSS using GnRH antagonist.[22] There was no evidence of a difference in live birth rates between the two protocols. When specifically the women with PCOS were compared, there was no significant difference in the ongoing pregnancy rates. Also it was noted that with the use of GnRH antagonist, the chance of cancelation or coasting due to high risk of developing OHSS was only 53% of that with GnRH agonist use.

Gonadotropin-releasing hormone agonist protocols allow more time for gonadotropin independent phase of follicular growth and hence synchronize a large cohort of follicles that have the capacity to respond to exogenous gonadotropins. This causes an increase in the number of developing follicles and hence higher levels of E2 in long protocol regimens. This in turn is associated with increased risk of OHSS with these regimens.

A number of studies have shown that a greater number of embryos are available and cryopreservation rates are higher in agonist group, there are no significant differences in the cumulative clinical pregnancy rates and live birth rates.[23]

In a meta-analysis by Griesinger et al. comparing GnRH agonist and antagonist protocol in a total of 305 PCOS subjects, the pregnancy rates were not statistically different between the two groups.[24] However, the incidence of severe OHSS was significantly lower in antagonist protocol. Another study by Ragini et al. also show similar results.[25]

However, Bahceci et al. demonstrated that there was no difference in terms of risk of OHSS in GnRH agonist and GnRH antagonist cycles in women with PCOS.[26]

Patient-friendly IVF is a repeated theme in the field of assisted reproductive technology and is a driving force for the formulation of new stimulation protocols. The GnRH antagonist protocols are considered more patient friendly than agonist protocols. The duration of treatment in the antagonist protocol is short by at least 14 days, and the dose and duration of gonadotropins required may also be low. Although this might not lead to a direct reduction in the cost of treatment, but if the cost considerations of hospitalization due to OHSS, number of working hours lost due to prolonged treatment and the inconvenience from multiple injections are taken into account, the final cost may be much less in antagonist protocol.

Unlike long protocol, where GnRH agonist is started from the midluteal phase of the previous menstrual cycle, GnRH antagonist is started after the commencement of ovarian stimulation, in either a fixed (day 6/7) or a flexible protocol. So, there is no risk that the antagonist is given inadvertently during early pregnancy as is the case may be with GnRH agonist long protocol.

Also there are no estrogen withdrawal symptoms like hot flushes, vaginal dryness, etc. and no risk of cyst formation with the antagonist protocol.

To summarize, although there is still no optimal ovarian hyperstimulation protocol for women with PCOS, various meta-analyses are in agreement about certain advantages of GnRH antagonist over agonist, in terms of duration of controlled ovarian hyperstimulation (COH), dose of gonadotropin required and the most important being a significantly lower risk of OHSS. Any protocol that virtually eliminates the risk of OHSS (which is purely an iatrogenic condition), while maintaining the satisfactory pregnancy rates, is welcomed. More multicenter RCTs are needed before a firm conclusion can be made.

Which Trigger for Final Oocyte Maturation?

Human chorionic gonadotropin (hCG) is usually used as a trigger for final oocyte maturation in IVF cycles (both agonist and antagonist cycles). However, because of the long half-life of hCG, the risk of OHSS is significantly high in PCOS patients.

Use of GnRH antagonist protocols in such high responders allows GnRH agonists to be used as final trigger for oocyte maturation. Native GnRH or GnRH agonist can displace the antagonist from pituitary GnRH receptors. This trigger is more physiological because of a shorter half life of endogenous LH (60 minutes) as compared to that of hCG (6–8 days).

The GnRH agonist-induced surge consists of two phases: a short ascending limb (>4 hours) and a long des-cending limb (>20 hours), in total around 24–36 hours. In contrast, the mid cycle LH surge of natural cycle is characterized by three phases: a rapidly ascending phase lasting for 14 hours, a plateau phase of 14 hours and a descending phase of 20 hours. This makes a total duration of 48 hours in a natural cycle. Thus, the total amount of gonadotropins released after GnRH agonist trigger is much less when compared to natural cycle and cycles where hCG is used as a trigger.[27] This is in turn is associated with a total elimination/much lesser incidence of OHSS after agonist trigger.

Another possible advantage of using GnRH agonist as a trigger for final oocyte maturation over hCG may be that there is simultaneous surge of FSH comparable to the natural cycle. Midcycle FSH surge has been found to induce the LH receptor formation on granulosa cells, thus optimizing the function of corpus luteum. The oocyte quality after using GnRH agonist (GnRHa) as a trigger is comparable or may be even better than that obtained after hCG trigger.

Thus, while the use of GnRH agonist as a trigger for final oocyte maturation is more physiological and associated with a significant decrease in the incidence of OHSS, it is associated with high pregnancy loss rates when not supplemented with intense luteal phase support. This can be explained by the massive premature luteolysis that occurs after using a single shot of GnRH agonist as a trigger. The luteolysis is due to the significantly shorter duration of LH surge after mid-cycle injection of GnRHa in combination with supraphysiological steroid levels during luteal phase and possibly the down regulation of pituitary GnRH receptors collectively resulting in a reduced LH support for the developing corpora lutea.

Various authors have used the modified luteal phase support for IVF cycles where GnRH agonist has been used as a trigger for final oocyte maturation. This *modified luteal phase* support consists of either intensive luteal supplementation with estradiol and progesterone or luteal LH activity supplementation with single/repeated boluses of hCG or recombinant LH.

The results of various meta-analyses, evaluating the effectiveness of adding estrogen to progesterone for luteal phase support in IVF cycles where hCG has been used as a trigger, have been controversial. These studies have been heterogeneous, precluding the extraction of clear and definitive conclusions. So, more studies need to be designed before final conclusions can be made.

However, it has been shown that when GnRH agonist triggering is used, estradiol levels are reduced by more than 50% compared with hCG triggering.[27] Hence, a beneficial effect of estradiol supplementation in addition to progesterone administration after GnRH agonist triggering cannot be excluded at present. Thus, it is recommended that all IVF/intracytoplasmic sperm injection (ICSI) patients having final oocyte maturation with GnRHa should continue luteal phase support with estradiol and progesterone until seventh gestational week when the luteo-placental shift normally occurs.

Some studies have shown that even intense luteal phase support with estradiol and progesterone in these patients may be inadequate, as suggested by high rates of early pregnancy loss. Therefore, it was speculated that not only the luteal endocrine environment, but possibly also the luteal endometrial milieu after GnRHa triggering might differ from what had previously been observed after hCG triggering. For that reason, the conventional luteal progesterone support, although supplemented with estradiol seemed to be insufficient, indicating a need for a more intense luteal steroid treatment or supplementation with LH activity.

Luteal Phase Rescue after GnRH Agonist Triggering—Modified Luteal Phase Support

Supplementation with hCG[27]

Various workers have used either a single bolus/repeated boluses of low doses of hCG to supplement luteal phase after GnRH agonist triggering. The doses used in different studies have been either 1500 IU as a single dose after oocyte retrieval or three doses of 500 IU each in luteal phase. These doses have been found to be safe and effective even in high responder patients, and allow fresh embryo transfers with no added risk of OHSS.

Supplementation with Recombinant LH

Some authors have advocated the use of recombinant LH instead of low doses of hCG. This is because of short half-life of LH, which could further reduce the risk of OHSS.[27]

A meta-analysis (published in 2010) of six RCTs revealed that with the use of modified luteal phase support (LPS), the delivery rates are similar to that reported with the use of hCG. However, a 6% difference in delivery rates still exists in favor of hCG use as a trigger. This is in contrast to when comparing the OHSS rates, which were 7% in hCG group and none in GnRHa group. These results indicate that modified luteal phase support has a significant positive effect on reproductive outcome in GnRHa triggering without an increase in OHSS rates. However, the best modified luteal phase support still needs to be explored.

■ INSULIN SENSITIZERS IN PCOS

Presence of insulin resistance and compensatory hyperinsulinemia are responsible for many of the clinical manifestations of the disease. In fact, numerous in vivo and in vitro data supports the central role of insulin resistance in the pathogenesis of PCOS. Hyperinsulinemia stimulates ovarian androgen production and increases the likelihood of developing diabetes, hypertension and cardiovascular disease. Hyperinsulinemia, together with increased LH levels also causes premature luteinization of granulosa cells in ovarian follicles and may be a cause of follicular arrest and hence anovulatory cycles in PCOS women. This has found a broad clinical application in the management of the syndrome, where the regulation of cycle abnormalities and the facilitation of pregnancy in PCOS patients, in addition to control of metabolic manifestations, is assisted by co-administration of agents such as the well-known insulin sensitizers.

Insulin sensitizers in addition to weight loss and lifestyle modification can improve both the reproductive and metabolic features of the disease which can have long-term health implications. Various studies have shown that insulin resistance is common in both obese and lean patients with PCOS.[28] The prevalence of insulin resistance has been found to be around 70% in all PCOS women.[29] Hence, the use of insulin sensitizers could therefore be suggested in most patients with PCOS.

The reduced fertility observed in PCOS patients cannot be attributed to anovulation alone. Other factors, including reduced oocyte and/or embryo quality, defects in endometrial development, and implantation abnormalities are also important. In addition, pregnant women with PCOS seem to have a significantly higher risk for miscarriage, gestational diabetes mellitus (GDM), gestational hypertension, pre-eclampsia (PE), and poor infant outcome. Finally, even if no well-controlled prospective data have demonstrated a higher mortality for cardiovascular disease in PCOS patients, an increased prevalence of several surrogate end-points, mainly type 2 DM and metabolic syndrome, have been demonstrated in PCOS. Use of insulin sensitizers in these patients has been found to reduce the derangements in the metabolic profile and improve the overall pregnancy outcomes.

Among all the available insulin sensitizers, metformin is the most comprehensively studied agent in this context and hence the most widely used agent. Among thiazolidinedione group of insulin sensitizers, troglitazone was withdrawn from market in the year 2000, due to reports of liver toxicity. Rosiglitazone and pioglitazone are FDA class C drugs and hence not recommended for treatment of infertile patients. Rosiglitazone has also been associated with cardiovascular toxicity. Among the newer insulin sensitizers, there is an another drug "D-chiro-inositol" and its derivative "myo-inositol" which have also been found to be beneficial in patients with PCOS and will be discussed later on in this chapter.

Metformin

It is a water soluble, second generation oral biguanide insulin sensitizer. It is an FDA category B drug. It inhibits hepatic gluconeogenesis and glycogenolysis, increases peripheral uptake of glucose and reduces intestinal absorption of glucose. Unlike sulfonylureas and insulin, metformin use does not result in increased insulin levels. There is also evidence that use of metformin in PCOS patients improves the follicular environment by reducing the ovarian androgens and improving hyperinsulinemia.

In March, 2007, in Thessaloniki, Greece, a second international ESHRE/ASRM-sponsored PCOS Consensus Workshop Group concluded that insulin sensitizers should not be used as first-choice agents in ovulation induction of women with PCOS, and their use should be restricted to patients with evidence of impaired glucose tolerance. This is probably due to the fact that knowledge regarding its effects and regimens of administration in PCOS patients is still incomplete.[1] However, this statement was based on the evaluation of results of two RCTs.[12,30]

However, studies conducted later on criticized these conclusions by ASRM/ESHRE group, maintaining an open debate on this issue. A number of studies have shown that metformin may significantly improve menstrual cycles (50–60%) and ovulation rates, both spontaneous and clomiphene-induced. A meta-analysis by Creanga et al. a result of 17 rigorously conducted studies showed a significant improvement in ovulation and pregnancy rates in women taking both clomiphene and metformin and also showed a better effect of combination therapy for live birth rate over clomiphene alone. However, the improvement in live birth rates was not statistically significant.[31]

The inconsistent results of the various studies could be explained by the design of the trial. For example, using live birth rate instead of pregnancy as the end-point may have biased some trials against metformin, which works slower than clomiphene. Another explanation may be different efficacy of metformin in different populations.[32] The trials which reported negative results with metformin contained a large percentage of obese and previously untreated people whose response to metformin may be weaker. More well-designed trials with homogenous study population and precisely defined end-points of the study are required to get the final answers.

Role of Metformin for COH Cycles for IVF-ICSI

Co-treatment with metformin has been shown to improve ovarian response to gonadotropins in women with PCOS. Its use has also been found to be associated with lower incidence of OHSS. Also an orderly pattern of ovarian stimulation has been found with the use of metformin in PCOS patients undergoing IVF cycle.[33] According to a Cochrane review 2009, no benefits in terms of clinical pregnancy rates/live birth rates were found with the use of metformin before or during ART cycle. However, the risk of developing OHSS in women with PCOS was reduced with the use of metformin.[34] In conclusion, metformin administration in infertile PCOS patients scheduled for IVF cycles is useful to reduce the OHSS risk.

As of now, there is a paucity of data regarding the use of metformin in hyperinsulinemic versus normoinsulinemic subjects with PCOS, and it remains unclear whether metformin use should be restricted to PCOS (both obese and lean) with biochemical or phenotypic (i.e. acanthosis nigricans) evidence of hyperinsulinemia.

Effect of Metformin on Pregnancy Outcomes

Effect on miscarriages: PCOS patients have a 30–50% risk of miscarriage after spontaneous or assisted conception. Although the exact reasons for miscarriages in these patients remain unclear, various mechanisms have been postulated. These include high LH levels, hyperinsulinemia, hyperandrogenism and hypofibrinolysis mediated by plasminogen activator inhibitor (PAI) activity. Studies have shown that PCOS patients have significantly lower serum glycodelin and IGFBP-1 concentrations during the first trimester of pregnancy, suggesting a deficient endometrial environment for implantation and pregnancy continuation.[35] Glycodelin is secreted by endometrial glands and acts by reducing the endometrial immune response against embryo development. IGFBP-1 modulates adhesion processes at the feto/maternal interface and hence may be important in the peri-implantation period. Besides being synthesized by the endometrium, IGFBP-1 is primarily synthesized in the liver, and insulin is known to inhibit hepatic IGFBP-1 production. Metformin exerts systemic actions by reducing body weight, insulin levels, PAI-1 levels, endothelin-1 levels, androgen and LH concentrations, and by increasing serum IGFBP-1 levels and glycodelin concentration.

It has been found that metformin use improves uterine artery blood flow indices and there is also an improvement in perifollicular blood flow.[36] This correlates with better oocyte quality due to better oxygenation of the developing follicles. This in turn also decreases the chromosomal and the cytoplasmic disorders related to poor vascularization.

Notwithstanding these hypothetical mechanisms by which metformin could reduce the abortion risk in PCOS women, the findings from RCTs do not seem to support the use of metformin in the preconceptional period concerning abortion risk reduction.

In another meta-analysis of 17 RCTs, designed to clarify the role of preconceptional metformin administration in PCOS patients, no significant overall benefit of metformin administration on abortion rate in the entire PCOS population was found.[37] On the other hand, encouraging data derived from retrospective or prospective nonrandomized studies were observed. A pilot study done by Glueck et al. demonstrated that PCOS women treated with metformin during pregnancy had a drastic reduction of spontaneous abortion when compared with historical outcome recorded in the same group of women not receiving treatment in previous pregnancies (73% vs 10%).[38] They also demonstrated that PAI-1 activity was directly related to the risk of having an abortion. It was speculated that the ability of metformin in reducing PAI-1 activity was related to an improvement in the insulin resistant state and, thus, in abortion rate. This hypothesis was subsequently confirmed in an another trial by Palomba et al.[39]

A further retrospective study by Jakubowicz et al. showed a significantly lower rate of early pregnancy loss in PCOS women who received metformin during pregnancy in comparison with women who did not receive metformin (8.8% vs 41.9%). The reduction in the abortion rate was remarkable if considering the historical miscarriage rate in the same population not treated with metformin in previous pregnancies (8.8% vs 70.6%).[40] The authors also proposed that the beneficial effect of metformin on the abortion rates was due to a reduction in androgen levels and increase in insulin sensitivity.

Another prospective cohort study by Khattab et al. clearly demonstrated the beneficial effects of metformin use during pregnancy in patients previously diagnosed with PCOS. The risk of an early pregnancy loss was 11.6% in women receiving metformin throughout pregnancy as compared to 36.3% in women who discontinued metformin at the time of conception or during pregnancy (OR, 0.23; 95% CI, 0.11 to 0.42; P = 0.0001).[41]

To summarize, regarding abortion prevention, no definitive conclusion on the efficacy of metformin administration during pregnancy may be reached because well-powered double blind RCTs having abortion rate as their aim are lacking. More well-powered and adequately designed study protocols are needed before drawing definitive conclusion on the beneficial effect of metformin on the abortion risk in PCOS patients.

Metformin and Gestational Diabetes Mellitus

Gestational diabetes mellitus (GDM) is more prevalent in PCOS women than controls, and it appears that PCOS is a significant risk factor for GDM. Studies have shown that around 20–40% women with PCOS develop GDM during pregnancy.[42] A number of studies have found the beneficial effects of metformin in reducing the risk of developing GDM during pregnancy. The proposed mechanisms by which metformin acts to reduce the likelihood of developing GDM are: the reduction of preconceptional weight, insulin levels, insulin resistance, insulin secretion and testosterone levels, and the persistence of these effects during pregnancy.

Glueck and colleagues (2002) have shown that metformin treatment throughout pregnancy in subjects with PCOS could reduce the prevalence of GDM from 31%, in women who did not take metformin in previous pregnancies, to 3% in current pregnancies. This implied a 10-fold reduction in the risk of developing GDM with the use of metformin.[43] In a subsequent study by the same authors (2008), metformin plus diet regimen during pregnancy was demonstrated to be effective for primary and secondary prevention of GDM. GDM developed in 12% of metformin-treated PCOS patients, in comparison with 30% of previous pregnancies without metformin.[44]

Although, metformin seems to prevent the development of GDM in PCOS patients, it should not be routinely used for this purpose as there is limited evidence of safety of this drug during pregnancy. In the Metformin in Gestational Diabetes (MiG) trial,[45] the largest study so far reported of metformin use in women with GDM, 751 women were randomized to receive either metformin or insulin. There was no significant difference in the composite fetal outcome between the two groups although preterm birth was found to be increased in the metformin group. Women in the metformin group had less weight gain compared with women in the insulin group. The infants born to women enrolled in this study were examined at 2 years of age. The children exposed to metformin in utero had increased subscapular and biceps skinfolds when compared with the unexposed infants, while total body fat was similar. It was hypothesized that this represents a possible benefit as this may signal a healthier fat distribution. However, it is well known that the earliest effect of the diabetes in pregnancy on long-term childhood obesity is not evident until 6–9 years of age. Hence, long-term studies are required to examine whether these infants of exposed women will subsequently be more insulin sensitive and healthier than their counterparts who were not exposed to the drug in utero.

So, the current clinical experience and the evidence published thus far support the safety and efficacy of metformin use in pregnancy with respect to the immediate pregnancy outcomes. However, more studies are needed to answer the long-term safety benefits of the drug on the offspring. In accordance with these outcomes, the drug may be stopped as soon as the pregnancy is confirmed.[46]

Metformin and Pre-eclampsia

Polycystic ovary syndrome increases the risk of developing hypertension during pregnancy. This could be explained by increased uterine artery resistance during first 12 weeks of pregnancy in subjects with PCOS.[47] Metformin administration to these patients in first trimester of pregnancy has been shown to reduce uterine artery resistance index (RI), with subsequent better trophoblastic invasion of spiral arterioles and better implantation with lesser risk of developing hypertension during pregnancy. In a small RCT by Salvesen et al. it was shown that metformin administration in PCOS patients during pregnancy reduced uterine artery impedance between 12 weeks and 19 weeks gestation, and this was associated with reduced complication rate.[48] The results of various other studies regarding the potential benefits of metformin in reducing the incidence and severity of preeclampsia in PCOS women have been controversial. Further studies are required to draw definitive conclusions in this regard.

Apart from decreasing the rates of pregnancy complications, metformin use has been found to be associated with the decreased levels of markers of metabolic inflammation such as endothelin-1, PAI-1, lipoprotein a, interleukin (IL)-1, tumor necrosis factor alpha (TNF-α), C-reactive protein (CRP). These inflammatory chemicals contribute to decreased insulin sensitivity, increased abdominal fat, endothelial dysfunction. The contribution of decreased insulin sensitivity to increased cardiovascular risk makes a strong case for the use of insulin sensitizers in PCOS in adults for benefits beyond those associated with reproductive integrity.

Side Effects of Metformin

Metformin use is associated with gastrointestinal side effects, like nausea, vomiting, diarrhea, bloating, etc. These can be minimized by slow titration of the medication to the desired dose over a 1-month period. A supervised incremental dosage protocol is usually used. During the first week, the patient takes 500 mg metformin with meals. This phase can be extended to 14 days in those who tolerate the drug poorly. The dose is then subsequently increased to 500 mg twice daily with meals for another 1 week. Finally, the dose may be increased to 500 mg thrice daily or 850 mg twice daily with meals. Other rare side effects that have been reported with metformin use are lactic acidosis which is mainly related to the underlying comorbid condition (liver, kidney or heart disease); pernicious anemia, vitamin B_{12} malabsorption, hyperhomocysteinemia.

Myo-inositol

Myo-inositol is a vitamin factor belonging to B-complex group of vitamins which is now being increasingly used as an insulin sensitizer in PCOS patients. It is also an important constituent of follicular microenvironment, playing an important role in cytoplasmic and nuclear maturation of oocyte. The higher levels of myo-inositol in the follicular fluid provide a marker of good quality oocytes.[49] It also decreases androgen concentration in the body and has been found to increase sex hormone binding globulin (SHBG) levels in the blood.

Use of myo-inositol in PCOS patients prior to and along with ovulation induction has been shown to be positively associated with increased number of mature oocytes retrieved and decrease in the number of atretic and degenerated oocytes.[50] Scientific evidence has also shown that supplementation with inositol decreases FSH requirement to induce ovulation and also improves the oocyte quality.

As the supplementation with myo-inositol decreases basal testosterone levels, its use has been found to be associated with lower estradiol levels on the day of hCG.[51] As a consequence, it can be supposed to be beneficial in reducing the incidence and severity of OHSS in PCOS patients.

In a study by Gerli et al. (2007), use of myo-inositol in dosages of 2 g twice daily for 16 weeks was associated with a significant decrease in BMI. There was also a significant increase in high density lipoprotein (HDL) concentration as compared to the placebo group. The low density lipoprotein (LDL) levels showed a downward trend with a significant improvement in HDL/LDL ratios. Also, there was a significant improvement in the ovulation rates as judged by increasing E2 levels in the early part of treatment (8d) and also increased P4 levels in the luteal phase of their cycle, suggesting that these cycles were ovulatory.[52]

These beneficial effects of myo-inositol support a future therapeutic role in women with PCOS.

■ COMPLICATIONS OF OVARIAN STIMULATION IN PCOS

The main dreaded complication of ovarian stimulation in PCOS is OHSS. In fact, it is the most serious iatrogenic complication of IVF treatment. Since PCOS patients have a large number of small antral follicles which are responsive to gonadotropin treatment, they are more prone to develop this complication.

The hallmark of OHSS is the increased capillary permeability, resulting in a loss of protein rich fluid from the intravascular compartment into the third space compartment. Loss of fluid into the third space causes a profound fall in intravascular volume, hemoconcentration, thrombosis, oliguria and a fall in plasma oncotic pressure which results in further loss of intravascular fluid. In addition, secondary hyperaldosteronism develops, which further aggravates the condition.

A number of chemical mediators and inflammatory cytokines have been implicated in the pathogenesis of this syndrome. These include VEGF, EGF, fibroblast growth factor, platelet derived growth factor, prostaglandins, renin-angiotensin-aldosterone system, ILs, TNF-α, endothelin-1 and histamine. While there is no doubt that VEGF is the most investigated cytokine in OHSS, it is still unclear whether this cytokine has a causative role, or is just an epiphenomenon. A study by Friedman et al. supports the notion that the increase in ovarian VEGF is an epiphenomenon rather than the cause of OHSS. In this study, they observed that follicular fluid from women of advanced reproductive age (not at risk to develop OHSS) showed increased VEGF concentrations compared with younger women, an increase that could be consistent with a hypoxic environment within follicles of older women.[53]

VEGF, also known as vascular permeability factor, is a potent angiogenic cytokine that stimulates growth of vascular endothelium. It also plays a role in follicular growth, corpus luteal function and ovarian angiogenesis. Studies have shown that hCG raises VEGF expression in ovarian granulosa cells and also raises serum VEGF concentration.

The clinical manifestations of OHSS reflect the extent to which the intravascular fluid shifts out into the third space. Symptoms range from mild abdominal distension due to enlarged ovaries alone or along with intra-abdominal ascitic fluid, to renal shut down and death as a result of hemoconcentration, disseminated intravascular coagulation (DIC) and reduced perfusion of kidneys, brain and heart.

Classification of Ovarian Hyperstimulation Syndrome

Based on the source of hCG, OHSS can be early or late. Early OHSS occurs 3–7 days after hCG administration for final oocyte maturation. While late OHSS occurs in conception cycles where there is increase in endogenous hCG secreted from implanting embryo. In general, late OHSS tends to be more serious and longer lasting than early OHSS, which is usually a self limited process in case no pregnancy occurs. In contrast to early OHSS, late OHSS is poorly correlated to ovarian response after stimulation. Multiple gestation and use of hCG in luteal phase are another risk factor for late OHSS.

Based on the severity of symptoms, OHSS can be classified as mild, moderate, severe and critical. However, the symptoms and signs exhibit a continuum of scope and severity that defies attempts at staging and classification. Mild manifestations of OHSS are relatively common and include:

- Mild lower abdominal pain/discomfort
- Nausea
- Vomiting
- Diarrhea.

In these cases, ovaries usually measure less than 8 cm. Mild OHSS is usually observed in 33% of superovulation cycles.

Progression of illness is recognized when the symptoms persist, worsen or include ascites that may become apparent by clinical examination, increased abdominal girth or by ultrasound examination. Serious illness exists when pain is accompanied by one or more of the following:

- Tense ascites
- Rapid weight gain
- Hemoconcentration
- Orthostatic hypotension, tachycardia
- Dyspnea, pleural effusion
- Progressive oliguria
- Laboratory abnormalities like hypoalbuminemia, hemoconcentration and deranged coagulation profile.

Hemoconcentration results from extravasation of protein rich exudates from intravascular compartment to the third space compartment. As a result, intravascular compartment shrinks, and the resulting hypotension causes a diminished blood flow to various organs and tissues of body. There is increased risk of thromboembolism due to hemoconcentration, diminished peripheral blood flow and decreased activity due to pain and ascites. In severe cases, renal failure, ARDS, thromboembolism, ovarian torsion and intra-abdominal hemorrhage may occur and may ultimately prove to be fatal. The incidence of clinically significant OHSS is 2–3%.

Strategies for Prevention of OHSS

Various methods for preventing or decreasing the severity of OHSS have been proposed. The criteria for placing the patient into a high-risk category to develop OHSS vary between different centers and include, the number of oocytes retrieved, size of ovaries at the time of retrieval, ascitic fluid, age of the patient and previous history of OHSS.

The oldest approach to prevent the development of OHSS has been to abandon the cycle. Although canceling the cycle and withholding hCG is the only method which totally avoids the risk of OHSS in ovarian induction cycles or in IVF, this approach may be frustrating for both the patient and the treating clinician as the IVF treatment implies a great commitment on the part of patient in terms of time, money and procedures. The treating doctor is also under pressure to give positive results from the planned cycle.

A number of other techniques and approaches have been used by various workers which usually succeed in decreasing the risk or severity of OHSS rather than totally eliminating it. These different strategies are discussed below:

Ovarian stimulation protocol: The protocol of choice for the potential hyperresponder patients prone to develop OHSS is GnRH antagonist protocol. This protocol has been shown to be associated with significantly lower incidence of OHSS as compared to the conventional long protocol of downregulation with the use of GnRH agonists. Furthermore, with antagonist protocol, GnRH agonist can be used as a trigger for final oocyte maturation, which is associated with a much lower risk of OHSS as compared to when hCG is used as a trigger. Furthermore, use of GnRH agonist allows embryo transfer to be done in hyper-responders with pregnancy outcomes comparable to those that with hCG trigger, provided an intense luteal phase support is used. Regardless of whether hCG or GnRH agonist is used as a ovulation trigger, use of exogenous progesterone for luteal phase support rather than hCG may further reduce the risk of OHSS.

Another important strategy in PCOS patients to decrease the incidence of OHSS is to start with a low dose of gonadotropins and increasing it gradually in a chronic low-dose step-up pattern, after serial ultrasound monitoring and close watch on estradiol levels.

The dose of gonadotropins should be reduced once the leading follicles reach the size of greater than or equal to 13 mm. This will allow the smaller and the intermediate size follicles to regress while allowing the growth of larger follicles. The net impact would be the lesser number of smaller follicles on the day of hCG trigger and hence lower estradiol levels, thereby lowering the occurrence of OHSS.

Coasting: It involves stoppage of gonadotropins and postponing the hCG trigger until the estradiol levels drop down to safer predefined levels (< 3,000 pg/mL). Coasting withdraws the gonadotropin support from smaller and intermediate size follicles, while allowing the growth of larger dominant follicles. The larger follicles are more resistant to atresia and apoptosis, and hence continue to grow even with declining FSH levels. Coasting reduces the functioning granulosa cell mass (from small and intermediate size follicles) available for luteinization, thereby resulting in a decline in vasoactive substances involved in the pathogenesis of OHSS. However, it has been shown that coasting when practiced for more than 3–4 days may result in a lower oocyte quality and lower implantation and pregnancy rates. Cancelation of oocyte retrieval should be considered if estradiol levels increase over 7,000 pg/mL or drop by more than 20% after hCG administration in coasted cycles, as implantation rates are generally poor when such a pattern is observed.[54] There is a lack of RCTs comparing coasting with no coasting or other interventions such as embryo freezing or intravenous (IV) albumin infusion for prevention of OHSS.

At present, the evidence is also insufficient to determine whether coasting is an effective strategy for preventing OHSS.[55]

Prophylactic intravenous administration of albumin or macromolecules such as hydroxyethyl starch (HES): Prophylactic administration of 20% albumin at the time of oocyte retrieval, in high-risk patients, has been suggested as a means to reduce the incidence and severity of OHSS in various studies. Albumin or HES administered at time of ovum pick up, may act by diminishing the severity of OHSS by increasing the intravascular volume and decreasing the third space fluid loss. Also, it has been proposed that albumin binds to OHSS mediators of ovarian origin, thus decreasing their concentration in serum.

The patients deemed to be at high risk include those with more than 20 follicles retrieved at the time oocyte pick up or those with high estradiol levels (>3000 pg/mL) at time of hCG trigger and patients with a previous history of OHSS.

An early Cochrane review (2002) of five RCTs clearly showed that prophylactic IV albumin administration at the time of oocyte retrieval in high-risk patients significantly reduces the risk of developing OHSS, with no effect on pregnancy rates.[56] It was seen that 18 women at high risk of developing OHSS would need albumin administration to avoid one severe case of OHSS.

In contrast, a further systematic review and meta-analysis of nine RCTs found that while there was no statistical benefit regarding the rate of OHSS compared with saline/no fluids, IV albumin significantly reduced pregnancy rates. This was supposed to be due the fact that albumin may bind to some of the mediators necessary for implantation.[57] In addition, the potential adverse effects of albumin administration should not be underestimated. There may be nausea, vomiting, febrile reactions, allergic reactions associated with the use of albumin. Since, albumin is a human product, there is a potential risk of transmission of viral/prion disease associated with its use.

To conclude, the prophylactic use of albumin as a plasma expander in hyperresponder patients at the time of oocyte retrieval remains controversial. Further studies which are more patient and population specific are required to be conducted to know the results.

Cryopreservation of embryos: Embryo cryopreservation is an another strategy for patients showing early signs of hyperstimulation and is a safety guard for the prevention of development of late OHSS, which can be even life threatening to the patient. This strategy also avoids the frustration of cycle cancelation and preserves the chance of live birth.

This strategy however has no effect on the risk of developing early OHSS and patients may still develop early, moderate to severe OHSS and require hospitalization for alleviation of their symptoms. The symptoms of early OHSS wane off gradually as the exogenous hCG given for final oocyte maturation is slowly eliminated from the body. This is in contrast to late OHSS which tends to be more severe, because of a continuous secretion of hCG from the developing placenta. Apart from reducing the incidence of OHSS in high responders, cryopreservation of embryos avoids the poor implantation rates that are associated with high estradiol levels in fresh embryo transfer cycles. Very high estradiol levels (>3500 pg/mL) have been found to be associated with endometrial glandular-stromal asynchrony, which results in low pregnancy rates in such cycles.

Variations in policies exist regarding the stage (pronuclear stage, 4-cell stage, blastocyst stage) and the protocol to be used for cryopreservation. The decision whether to cryopreserve all embryos or proceed with fresh embryo transfer of 1 or 2 embryos is largely determined by patient's symptoms. Late day 5 fresh embryo transfer with single blastocyst may be undertaken if no overt symptoms of moderate to severe OHSS are observed. It has been proposed that cryopreservation should be performed when prolonged coasting (≥ 3 days) has been performed.

Various studies evaluating the efficacy of elective embryo cryopreservation for reducing the risk of OHSS have been controversial. Cochrane review (2002) has questioned the efficacy of elective embryo cryopreservation as a preventive measure of OHSS. The authors of this review group concluded that there is a need for a large RCT, which clearly defines the women at risk of OHSS based on endocrinological, ultrasonographic and clinical criteria.[58] Hence, more uniform criteria need to be applied and uniform classification of OHSS needs to be used before any definitive opinion about the usefulness of this strategy can be laid down.

Use of dopamine agonists: There is evidence that administration of a dopamine agonist, such as cabergoline or quinagolide from the day of hCG trigger, can reduce the incidence of OHSS by inhibiting the phosphorylation of VEGF receptor-2, and thus reducing the release of vasoactive angiogenic agents. The two RCTs comparing the use of cabergoline with IV albumin have shown that cabergoline (0.5 mg/day) was more effective than albumin in preventing OHSS.[59,60]

Several other studies and meta-analyses have also demonstrated the efficacy of cabergoline as well as other dopamine agonists, quinagolide and bromocriptine in reducing the incidence of moderate OHSS, when given from the day of hCG administration through 6 days post-oocyte retrieval.[61-63]

A study by Gomez et al. (2011) showed that women with PCOS are less responsive to cabergoline compared with those without PCOS. This was probably due to a decreased production of dopamine and a reduced dopamine receptor expression in women with PCOS.[64]

Use of metformin with gonadotropins: Cochrane review 2009 showed that the use of metformin in patients scheduled for IVF has been associated with decrease incidence of OHSS.[34] A number of other studies have shown a more orderly growth of follicles and a reduction in multifollicular development with the use of metformin. It has been found that use of metformin in PCOS patients is associated with a shift in size of follicles, with a reduction in the number of smaller follicles in the recruited cohort. Clearly, though, more data are needed to fully elucidate the effects of metformin on OHSS in women with PCOS.

Ovarian suppression: Suppression of ovarian steroidal secretion through continued administration of GnRH agonists following oocyte retrieval, coupled with cryopreservation of all the embryos has been suggested to minimize the risk of developing OHSS. However, more studies need to be done in this regard, and this approach currently remains experimental.

Corticosteroids: It has been hypothesized that corticosteroids through their anti-inflammatory action may be helpful in preventing OHSS. However, outcomes of various studies in this regard have been contradictory, and currently the data is insufficient to recommend the use of these drugs.[65]

Role of calcium: The studies reporting the beneficial effects of calcium supplementation on the risk of developing moderate to severe OHSS have been limited. In two of the studies by Yakovenko et al. (2009) and Gurgan et al. (2011) respectively, IVF patients at risk of OHSS received IV infusion of calcium gluconate (10 mL of 10% solution) diluted in 200 mL of normal saline, on the day of ovum pick up and for 3 days thereafter. Patients receiving this infusion had a lower incidence of both mild and severe OHSS.[66,67] This prevention modality carries little risk and has a potential benefit, but because of insufficient evidence cannot be routinely recommended.

The mechanisms by which IV calcium reduces the incidence of OHSS is through alterations in renin-angiotensin system. Calcium infusion reduces the synthesis of cyclic adenosine monophosphate (cAMP), which in turn reduces the cAMP dependent renin synthesis by juxtaglomerular cells in kidneys. The decreased rennin secretion results in reduced angiotensin II synthesis, with a consequent decrease in angiotensin II mediated stimulation of VEGF synthesis. Yakovenko et al. also proposed that OHSS resulted from membrane depolarization and calcium acts by inducing membrane stabilization.[66]

Other strategies, like meticulous follicular aspiration, have been proposed as a means to reduce OHSS; this cannot be completely relied upon in the clinical settings to reduce the risk of development of OHSS.

To summarize, the keys to prevention of OHSS are experience with ovarian stimulation regimens and identification of the risk factors associated with this syndrome. Ovarian stimulation regimens should be highly individualized, monitored and based upon lowest possible dosages of gonadotropins for the minimum possible duration to achieve the desired therapeutic goal.

Caution is indicated when one or more of the following risk factors are identified:

- Rapidly rising serum estradiol levels
- Serum estradiol levels more than 4,000 pg/mL
- Multiple stimulated follicles (>20 in ART, >6 for ovulation induction)
- Young age (<35 years)
- Low body weight
- Polycystic appearing ovaries
- High serum anti-Müllerian hormone
- GnRH agonist down-regulated cycles.

IN VITRO MATURATION

In vitro maturation (IVM) and fertilization is an emerging technique in ART that is of great value in hyperresponder patients like PCOS. It is a technique that can totally prevent OHSS. It is indicated not only for patients with PCOS, but also for the patients who have polycystic ovarian morphology on ultrasound. Poor quality embryos or repeated IVF failures by conventional method is also another indication of IVM. This technique involves the aspiration of immature oocytes from the antral follicles of either unstimulated or minimally stimulated ovary. The oocytes are then cultured in a specially formulated medium for 24–48 hours. They are then fertilized, usually with ICSI, and the embryo transfer is done 2 or 3 days later.

Since the technique of IVM involves only few doses of gonadotropins and few days of ovarian stimulation, less monitoring is required, and more importantly, it avoids the risk of developing OHSS.

The maturation rates of the oocytes used in IVM procedure vary in different studies. While Gomez et al.[68] reported that approximately 16% of the immature oocytes retrieved from unstimulated patients reached MII stage after 48 hours of culture, the reported rates by Trouson et al.[69] were 60% and by Cha et al.[70] were 56%. A study by Child et al. (2002) showed that the maturation rates of oocytes retrieved from patients with PCOS were lower than those with normal ovaries.[71] Another study by Nicole et al. (1999) reported a maturation rate of 56% and a fertilization rate of only 10% in PCOS patients. However, no embryonic development occurred further, and hence no embryos were transferred.[72]

Various modifications in culture media are being tried and priming with hCG has been suggested by various authors to improve the maturation rates of oocytes obtained from unstimulated polycystic ovaries.

Also important to be considered is the effect of culture conditions on epigenetic profile of oocytes which are matured in vitro. The epigenetic changes brought about by these culture conditions largely remain unknown at present. Research continues into identifying prognostic indicators of the developmental potential of embryos, including metabolomics, secretomics and proteomics. Evaluation of cumulus layer is a potentially useful and simple procedure that may provide a scoring system in this evolving technique.

The implantation rates and pregnancy rates achieved with IVM technique are lower as compared to conventional IVF. The lower implantation rates could be due to a reduced oocyte developmental potential or due to the reduced/altered endometrial receptivity and also possibly due to asynchrony between endometrial and embryonic growth. Long-term studies are needed to confirm the safety of this new evolving technology on the health of children born through this technique.

In a Cochrane systematic review, it was concluded that no RCTs exist till date to recommend inclusion of IVM technique into routine practice.[73] More studies are needed before it can be routinely recommended and implemented for PCOS patients. With advancing technology, as the culture techniques and the fertilization rates may improve for in vitro matured oocytes, this may become the protocol of choice for PCOS patients.

■ CONCLUSION

Women with PCOS require different approach of ovarian stimulation as compared to patients with normal ovaries. Lifestyle modification and weight loss are the recommended first-line therapy in obese PCOS patients. This strategy has been found to increase the success rates and decrease the complication rates associated with ovulation induction. The GnRH antagonist protocol has now become the protocol of choice for PCOS patients, giving the same pregnancy rates and live birth rates as the long protocol, while being associated with low OHSS rates. Insulin sensitizers remain useful as adjunctive treatment especially in women with impaired glucose tolerance. IVM, though presently in its infancy, may hopefully eliminate all the complications associated with ovarian stimulation in future.

■ REFERENCES

1. The Thessaloniki ESHRE/ASRM sponsored PCOS Consensus Workshop Group. Consensus on infertility treatment related to polycystic ovary syndrome. Hum Reprod. 2008;23:462-77.
2. Ricardo A. Diagnosis of polycystic ovarian syndrome: the Rotterdam criteria are premature. J Clin Endocrinol Metab. 2006;91(3):3781-85.
3. The Rotterdam ESHRE/ASRM–sponsored PCOS consensus workshop group. Revised 2003 consensus on diagnostic criteria and long term health risks related to polycystic ovary syndrome (PCOS). Hum Reprod. 2004;19:41-7.
4. Azziz R, Carmina E, Dewailly D, et al. The Androgen Excess and PCOS Society criteria for polycystic ovary syndrome: the complete task force report. Fertil Steril. 2009;91:456-88.
5. Cano F, Garcia Velasco JA, Millet A. Oocyte quality in polycystic ovaries revisited: identification of a particular subgroup of women. J Assist Reprod Genet. 1997;14:254-60.
6. Rogers J, Mitchell GW. The relation of obesity to menstrual disturbances. N Engl J Med. 1952;247:53-6.
7. Adams JM, Taylor AE, Crowley WF Jr, et al. Polycystic ovarian morphology with regular ovulatory cycles: insights into the pathophysiology of polycystic ovarian syndrome. J Clin Endocrinol Metab. 2004;89(9):4343-50.
8. Barber TM, Wass JA, McCarthy MI, et al. Metabolic characteristics of women with polycystic ovaries and oligo-amenorrhoea but normal androgen levels: implications for the management of polycystic ovary syndrome. Clin Endocrinol (Oxf). 2007;66(4):513-7.
9. In: Balen AH, Conway GS, Homburg R, Legro RS (Eds). Polycystic Ovary syndrome: A Guide to Clinical Management. London: Taylor & Francis; 2005. pp. 47-67.
10. Franks S, Mason H, Willis D. Follicular dynamics in the polycystic ovary syndrome. Mol Cell Endocrinol. 2000;163:49-52.
11. Phy JL, Conover CA, Abbott DH, et al. Insulin and messenger ribonucleic acid expression of insulin receptor isoforms in ovarian follicles from nonhirsute ovulatory women and polycystic ovary syndrome patients. J Clin Endocrinol Metab. 2004;89(7):3561-6.
12. Legro RS, Barnhart HX, Schlaff WD, et al. Cooperative Multicenter Reproductive Medicine Network. Clomiphene, metformin or both for infertility in polycystic ovary syndrome. N Engl J Med. 2007;356:551-66.
13. Simon S, Cano F, Valbuena D, et al. Clinical evidence for a detrimental effect on uterine receptivity of high serum estradiol concentration in high and normal responder patients. Hum Reprod. 1995;10:2432-7.
14. Mann RJ, Keri RA, Nilson JH. Consequences of elevated luteinizing hormone on diverse physiological systems: use of the LH beta CTP transgenic mouse as a model of ovarian hyperstimulation-induced pathophysiology. Recent Prog Horm Res. 2003;58:343-75.
15. Daniel A, Dumesic MD, David H. Implications of polycystic ovary syndrome (PCOS) on oocyte development. Semin Reprod Med. 2008;26(1):53-61.
16. Jakimiuk AJ, Weitsman SR, Magoffin DA. 5a-reductase activity in women with polycystic ovary syndrome. J Clin Endocrinol Metab. 1999;84:2414-8.
17. Maciel GA, Baracat EC, Benda JA, et al. Stockpiling of transitional and classic primary follicles in ovaries of women with polycystic ovary syndrome. J Clin Endocrinol Metab. 2004;89:5321-7.
18. Stubbs SA, Hardy K, Da Silva-Buttkus P, et al. Anti-Müllerian hormone protein expression is reduced during the initial stages of follicle development in human polycystic ovaries. J Clin Endocrinol Metab. 2005;90(10):5536-43.
19. Bayram N, Van Waley M, Van Der Veen F. Recombinant FSH versus urinary gonadotrophins or recombinant FSH for ovulation induction in subfertility associated with polycystic ovary syndrome. Cochrane Database Syst Rev. 2001;(2):CD002121.
20. Ayse F, Berna S. Human Menopausal Gonadotropin versus recombinant FSH in polycystic ovary syndrome patients undergoing in vitro fertilization. Int J Fertil Steril. 2013;6(4):238-43.
21. Al-Inany H, Youssef M, Aboulghar M, et al. Gonadotrophin releasing hormone antagonists in subfertile couples undergoing ovulation induction as a part of an assisted conception program. Cochrane Database Syst Rev. 2011;(5):CD001750.
22. Kolibianakis EM, Collins J, Tarlatzis BC, et al. Among patients treated for IVF with gonadotrophins and GnRH analogues, is the probability of live birth dependent on the type of analogue

used? A systematic review and meta-analysis. Hum Reprod Update. 2006;12(6):651-71.

23. Lainas TG, Ioannis S, Zorzovillis IZ, et al. Flexible GnRH antagonist protocol versus GnRH agonist long protocol in patients with polycystic ovary syndrome treated for IVF: A prospective randomized controlled trial. Hum Reprod. 2011;25:683-9.

24. Griesinger G, Diedrich K, Tarlatzis BC, et al. GnRH-antagonists in ovarian stimulation for IVF in patients with poor response to gonadotropins, polycystic ovary syndrome, and risk of ovarian hyperstimulation: a meta-analysis. Reprod Biomed Online. 2006;13(5):628-38.

25. Ragni G, Vegetti W, Riccaboni A, et al. Comparison of GnRH agonists and antagonists in assisted reproduction cycles of patients at high risk of ovarian hyperstimulation syndrome. Hum Reprod. 2005;20:2421-5.

26. Bahceci M, Ulug U, Ben-Shlomo I, et al. Use of a GnRH antagonist in controlled ovarian hyperstimulation for assisted conception in women with polycystic ovary disease: a randomized, prospective, pilot study. J Reprod Med. 2005;50:84-90.

27. Humaidan P, Kol S, Papanilolaou EG. GnRH agonist for triggering of final oocyte maturation : time for a change of practice? Hum Reprod Update. 2011;17(4):510-24.

28. Sharma ST, Nestler JE. Prevention of diabetes and cardiovascular disease in women with PCOS: Treatment with insulin sensitizers. Best Pract Res Clin Endocrinol Metab. 2006;20:245-60.

29. Goodarzi MO, Korenman SG. The importance of insulin resistance in polycystic ovary syndrome. Fertil Steril. 2002;77:255-8.

30. Moll E, Bossuyt PM, Korevaar JC, et al. Effect of clomifene citrate plus metformin and clomifene citrate plus placebo on induction of ovulation in women with newly diagnosed polycystic ovary syndrome: randomised double blind clinical trial. BMJ. 2006;332(7556):1485-90.

31. Creanga AA, Bradley HM, McCormick, et al. Use of metformin in polycystic ovary syndrome: A meta-analysis. Obstet Gynecol. 2008;111(4):959-68.

32. De Leo V, Marca A, Ditto a, et al. Effects of metformin on gonadotropin–induced ovulation in women with polycystic ovary syndrome. Fertil Steril. 1999;72:282-5.

33. Stadtmauer LA, Toma SK, Riehl RM, et al. Metformin treatment of patients with polycystic ovary syndrome undergoing in vitro fertilization improves outcomes and is associated with modulation of the insulin like growth factors. Fertil Steril. 2001;75:505-9.

34. Tso Lo, Costello MF, Albuquerque LE, et al. Metformin treatment before and during IVF or ICSI in women with polycystic ovary syndrome. Cochrane Database Syst Rev. 2009;(2):CD006105.

35. Jakibowicz DJ, Paulina AE, Markku S, et al. Reduced serum glycodelin and insulin like growth factor binding protein-1 in women with polycystic ovary syndrome during first trimester of pregnancy. J Clin Endocrinol Metab. 2004;89(2):833.

36. Jakubowics D, Seppala M, Jakubowics S, et al. Insulin reduction with metformin increase luteal phase serum glycodelin and insulin- like growth factor-binding protein 1

concentration and enhances uterine vascularity and blood flow in the polycystic ovary syndrome. J Clin Endoc Metab. 2001;86:1126-33.

37. Palomba S, Falbo A, Orio F Jr, et al. Effect of preconceptional metformin on abortion risk in polycystic ovary syndrome: A systematic review and meta-analysis of randomized controlled trials. Fertil Steril. 2009;92:1646-58.

38. Glueck CJ, Phillips H, Cameron D, et al. Continuing metformin throughout pregnancy in women with polycystic ovary syndrome appears to safely reduce first trimester spontaneous abortion: a pilot study. Fertil Steril. 2001;75:46-52.

39. Palomba S, Orio F Jr, Falbo A, et al. Prospective parallel randomized, double blind, double-dummy controlled clinical trial comparing clomiphene citrate and metformin as the first line treatment for ovulation induction in nonobese anovulatory women with polycystic ovary syndrome. J Clin Endocrinol Metab. 2005;90:4068-74.

40. Jakubowicz DJ, Iuorno MJ, Jakubowicz S, et al. Effects of metformin on early pregnancy loss in the polycystic ovary syndrome. J Clin Endocrinol Metab. 2002;87:524-9.

41. Khattab S, Mohsen IA, Foutouh IA, et al. Metformin reduces abortion in pregnant women with polycystic ovary syndrome. Gynecol Endocrinol. 2006;22:680-4.

42. Radon PA, McMahon MJ, Meyer WR. Impaired glucose tolerance in pregnant women with polycystic ovary syndrome. Obstet Gynecol. 1999;94:194-7.

43. Glueck CJ, Wang P, Kobayashi S, et al. Metformin therapy throughout pregnancy reduces the development of gestational diabetes in women with polycystic ovary syndrome. Fertil Steril. 2002;77:520-5.

44. Glueck CJ, Pranikoff J, Aregawi D, et al. Prevention of gestational diabetes by metformin plus diet in patients with polycystic ovary syndrome. Fertil Steril. 2008;89:625-34.

45. Rowan JA, Hague WM, Gao W, et al and MiG Trial Investigators 2008. Metformin versus insulin for the treatment of gestational diabetes. N Engl J Med. 2008;358(19):2003-15.

46. Palomba S, Angela F, Fulvio Z, et al. Evidence–based and potential benefits of metformin in the polycystic ovary syndrome: a comprehensive review. 2009;30(1):1-50.

47. Palomba S, Russo T, Orio Jr F, et al. Uterine effects of metformin administration in anovulatory women with polycystic ovary syndrome. Hum Reprod. 2006;21:457-65.

48. Salvesen KA, Vanky E, Carlsen SM. Metformin treatment in pregnant women with polycystic ovary syndrome-is reduced complication rate mediated by changes in the uteroplacental circulation? Ultrasound Obstet Gynecol. 2007;29:433-7.

49. Chiu TT, Rogers MS, Law EL, et al. Follicular fluid and serum concentrations of myoinositol in patients undergoing IVF: relationship with oocyte quality. Hum Reprod. 2002;17: 1591-6.

50. Goud PT, Goud AP, Van OP, et al. Presence and dynamic redistribution of type I inositol 1,4,5–triphosphate receptors in human oocytes and embryos during in-vitro maturation, fertilization and early cleavage divisions. Mol Hum Reprod. 1999;5:441-51.

51. Iuorno MJ, Jakubowicz DJ, Baillargeon JP, et al. Effects of D-chiroinositol in lean women with polycystic ovary syndrome. Endocr Pract. 2002;8:417-23.

52. Gerli S, Papaleo E, Ferrari A, et al. Randomized, double blind placebo–controlled trial: effects of myoinositol on ovarian function and metabolic and metabolic factors in women with PCOS. Eur Rev Med Pharmacol Sci. 2007;11(5):347-54.

53. Friedman CI, Danforth DR, Herbosa-Encarnacion C, et al. Follicular fluid vascular endothelial growth factor concentrations are elevated in women of advanced reproductive age undergoing ovulation induction. Fertil Steril. 1997;68:607-12.

54. Benadiva C, Davis O, Kligman I, et al. Withholding gonadotropin administration is an effective alternative for the prevention of ovarian hyperstimulation syndrome. Fertil Steril. 1997;67(4):724-7.

55. D'Angelo, Amso N. "Coasting" (withholding gonadotropins) for preventing ovarian hyperstimulation syndrome. Cochrane Database Syst Rev. 2002;(3):CD002811.

56. Aboulghar M, Evers JH, Al-Inany H. Intravenous albumin for preventing severe ovarian hyperstimulation syndrome: a Cochrane review. Hum Reprod. 2002;17:3027-32.

57. Jee BC, Suh CS, Kim YB, et al. Administration of intravenous albumin around the time of oocyte retrieval reduces pregnancy rate without preventing ovarian hyperstimulation syndrome: a systematic review and meta-analysis. Gynecol Obstet Invest. 2010;70(1):47-54.

58. D'Angelo A, Amso NN. Embryo freezing for preventing ovarian hyperstimulation syndrome: a Cochrane review. Hum Reprod. 2002;17(11):2787-94.

59. Tehraninejad ES, Hafezi M, Arabipoor A, et al. Comparison of cabergoline and intravenous albumin in the prevention of ovarian hyperstimulation syndrome: a randomized clinical trial. J Assist Reprod Genet. 2012;29(3):259-64.

60. Carizza c, Abdelmassih V, Abdelmassih S, et al. Cabergoline reduces the early onset of ovarian hyperstimulation syndrome: a prospective randomized study. Reprod Biomed Online. 2008;17(6):751-5.

61. Spitzer D, Wogatzky J, Murtinger M, et al. Dopamine agonist bromocriptine for the prevention of ovarian hyperstimulation syndrome. Fertil Steril. 2011;95:2742-4.

62. Soares S, Gomez R, Simon C. Targeting the endothelial growth factor system to prevent ovarian hyperstimulation syndrome. Hum Reprod Update. 2008;14:321-33.

63. Humaidan P, Quartarolo J, Papanikolaou G. Preventing ovarian hyperstimulation syndrome: guidance for the clinician. Fertil Steril. 2010;94:389-400.

64. Gomez R, Soares SR, Busso C, et al. Physiology and pathology of ovarian hyperstimulation syndrome. Semin Reprod Med. 2010;28:448-57.

65. Lainas T, Petsas G. Administration of methylprednisolone to prevent severe ovarian hyperstimulation syndrome in patients undergoing in vitro fertilization. Fertil Steril. 2002;78:529-33.

66. Yakovenko SA, Sivozhelezov VS, Zorina IV, et al. Prevention of OHSS by intravenous calcium. Hum Reprod. 2009;24 (Suppl 1):i61.

67. Gurgan T, Demirol A, Guven S, et al. Intravenous calcium infusion as a novel preventive therapy of ovarian hyperstimulation syndrome for patients with polycystic ovarian syndrome. Fertil Steril. 2011;96:53-7.

68. Gomez E, Tarin JJ, Pellicer A. Oocyte maturation in humans: The role of gonadotropins and growth factors. Fertil Steril. 1993;60:40-6.

69. Trounson AO, Wood C, Kausche A. In vitro maturation and fertilization and developmental competence of oocytes recovered from untreated polycystic ovarian patients. Fertil Steril. 1994;62:353-62.

70. Cha KY, Koo JJ, Ko JJ, et al. Pregnancy after in vitro fertilization of human follicular oocytes collected from unstimulated cycles, their culture in vitro and their transfer in a donor oocyte program. Fertil Steril. 1991;55:109-13.

71. Child TJ, Philips SJ, Abdul-Jalil AK, et al. A comparison of in vitro maturation and in vitro fertilization for women with polycystic ovaries. Obstet Gynaecol. 2002;100:665-70.

72. Nicole GMB, Math HEC, Liliana R, et al. Retrieval, maturation and fertilization of immature oocytes obtained from unstimulated patients with polycystic ovary syndrome. J Assist Reprod Genet. 1999;16(2):81-6.

73. Siristatidis CS, Maheshwari A, Bhattacharya S. In vitro maturation in sub fertile women with polycystic ovarian syndrome undergoing assisted reproduction. Cochrane Database Syst Rev. 2009;(1):CD 006606.

51 — Gamete Donation

Abha Majumdar, Chauhan Kumudini

INTRODUCTION

Gamete donation is the use of third party for sperm or oocyte donation for fulfilling the desire of parenting a child by a couple who lacks either of these. In other words gamete donation is a process in which a man or woman donate sperms or oocytes respectively to help infertile couples.

Types of donor: A donor can be (1) anonymous and (2) non-anonymous. Anonymous donor is a person whose identity remains unknown to recipient and offspring. Non-anonymous donor means known or directed donor, who could be the couple's friend or a relative.

Family donor: Gamete donation within a family is an altruistic approach, which can overcome the problem of donor shortage and can avoid recipient couple being in long queue. If the family is involved in gamete donation, we should avoid using sperm and egg donation between close relatives to prevent consanguinity.

SPERM DONATION

This involves use of donor sperm to inseminate a woman for conception and the process is known as "artificial insemination by donor" (AID) or "therapeutic donor insemination" (TDI). Sperm donation is required in cases of noncorrectable male infertility when a couple is unable to have a child due to lack of adequate sperms to impregnate the woman. Men who need to resort to sperm donation for having a child in order to complete their family can be categorized as following:

- Azoospermic men
- Postvasectomy with no reversal or unsuccessful reversal
- Male partner carrier of a known hereditary disease
- Female Rh-isoimmunized and husband Rh-positive
- Severe Oligoasthenoteratozoospermia (OATs) but couple unable to afford in vitro fertilization–intracytoplasmic sperm injection (IVF–ICSI)
- Discordant couple for HIV with affected husband
- Single woman and lesbian couple.

Requirements of Recipient Female

- Recipient female has to sign a consent form (ICMR Form F)[1] **(Appendix 1)** along with her partner if applicable.
- Detailed medical and reproductive history needs to be taken.
- General and pelvic examination of the recipient female is mandatory along with necessary investigations relating to her health status to ensure healthy motherhood such as complete blood count, blood sugar levels and her thyroid status.
- She should be ovulating spontaneously or with help of ovulation inducing drugs and insemination need to be planned periovulatory.
- Tubal patency should be checked either by hysterosalpingography or laparoscopic chromopertubation test depending upon history and examination.

Preparation of Sperm Recipient

Therapeutic donor insemination can be done either in a natural ovulatory or in a stimulated cycle. Determination of ovulation is done prior to TDI either by ultrasonographic follicle monitoring or urine luteinizing hormone surge testing kits.

Requirements for a Sperm Donor (ICMR Guidelines)[2]

- The age of the donor must not be below 21 years or above 45 years.
- The individual must be free of HIV and hepatitis B and C infections, hypertension, diabetes, sexually transmitted diseases and identifiable and common genetic disorders such as thalassemia.

- Semen analysis must be carried out on the semen of the individual, preferably using a semen analyzer, and it must be found to be normal according to the World Health Organization 2010 manual for semen analysis, if intended to be used for assisted reproductive technology (ART).
- The blood group and the Rh status of the individual must be determined and placed on record.
- Other relevant information in respect of the donor such as height, weight, age, educational qualifications, profession, color of the skin and the eyes, record of major diseases including any psychiatric disorder, and the family background in respect of history of any familial disorder, must be recorded in an appropriate performa.

Semen Banks

Semen bank is a place where semen from sperm donors is collected, processed and preserved for future use for the purpose of intrauterine insemination (IUI), IVF and ICSI. In India, various semen banks have been established over a period of time but only in the last 10 years; they have had guidelines, laid down by the Indian Council of Medical Research (ICMR) to follow, which possibly guides them to some extent to follow practices used internationally.

Collection of Semen

Semen is collected by masturbation in a room known as donor cabin or "masturbatorium". This room may provide facilities like magazine and photographs to assist donor in sexual arousal.

Contract

Donor has to sign a contract, under which he has to provide semen sample for 6–24 months depending upon the number of intended pregnancies with that donor. Donor is also bound not to have had intercourse or masturbation for 2–3 days prior to collection.

Consent and Counseling of Donor

An informed consent should be taken after proper counseling of donor. According to ICMR consent form (Form L), **(Appendix 2)** donor should be fully informed that there will be no direct or indirect contact between donor and the recipient, and personal identity will not be disclosed to the recipient or to the child born through the use of his gamete. He shall have no rights whatsoever on the resulting offspring and vice versa.

Cryopreservation

This technique helps in preservation and stabilization of human cells at a very low temperature for future use. Cryopreservation of human spermatozoa was first introduced in the 1960s,[3] since then various methods of cryopreservation have been developed.

- *Slow freezing technique:* This method was proposed by Behrman and Sawada[4] where sperms are set to cooling over a period of 2–4 hours in two or three steps. This is done either manually or automatically using a semi-programmable freezer; hence the technique used is also known as semi-programmable freezing technique. This method is rarely used these days.
- *Rapid freezing technique:* This method of sperm freezing was first proposed by Sherman.[5] In this technique, the sperm straws are taken into direct contact with nitrogen vapors for 8–10 minutes before immersing them in liquid nitrogen at –196°C. This is done by holding the sperm straw 8 inches above the level of liquid nitrogen into vapors of liquid nitrogen for 10 minutes.
- *Vitrification*: Greg Fahy and William F Rall introduced vitrification to reproductive cryopreservation in the mid-1980s.[6] In this method, freezing is done by rapid cooling of sperm to a glassy state through extreme elevation of viscosity without intracellular ice crystallization.

Types of Frozen Preserved Semen Sample

- *Prewashed samples:* Semen sample is processed after collection by density gradient centrifugation for seminal fluid removal prior to freezing. This type of sample can directly be used for IUI.
- *Unwashed samples or conventional sample:* Semen sample is directly cryopreserved without washing. These samples need to be washed with density gradient method to remove contaminants and cryoprotectant agent after thawing the specimen prior to IUI or IVF.

Drawbacks and Benefit of Various Freezing Methods

Rapid freezing method gives superior post-thaw motility and cryosurvival as compared to the slow method of semi-programmable freezing and has almost replaced the slow freezing method of cryopreservation.[7] However, vitrification is now the most commonly used method due to better post-thaw motility of sperms.

Prewashed samples, which are IUI-ready preparation, have motile sperm recovery comparable to that of unwashed semen cryopreservation but have significantly better sperms morphologically.[8]

Screening of Semen Donor

The Indian Council of Medical Research recommends Form M **(Appendix 3)**[1] to be filled for semen donor; this form includes basic information of donor, medical history, general characteristic of donor, investigations and detailed physical examinations of all vital systems.

Information to be Given by Semen Donor in "ICMR Form M"

Basic information includes the identification number of the donor (donor ID), age, marital status, education and occupation of the donor and spouse as well as their monthly income and religion.

History includes the obstetric history of wife, number of deliveries, abortions and use of contraceptives. Along with the above, medical and family history as well as history of any abnormality in children of the donor is obtained. Information regarding previous or present blood transfusion or substance abuse is also to be taken.

The investigations recommended for all donors are blood group and Rh status, complete blood count, random blood sugar, blood urea/serum creatinine, SGPT, routine urine examination, status of HBsAg, hepatitis C and HIV with date of the tests done as well as thalassemia status and any other specific test if recommended.

Body features such as height, weight, color of skin, color of hair, color of eyes are noted. General physical examination includes pulse, blood pressure, temperature, respiratory system, cardiovascular system and abdominal examination. Other systems only if needed are examined.

Differences in Guidelines from Various Countries Regarding Gamete Donation

- *American Society for Reproductive Medicine (ASRM)* and *Society of Assisted Reproductive Technology (SART)* have recently published committee opinion regarding guidelines for gamete donation.[9] They have also incorporated the information from *Center of Disease Control, Food and Drug Administration* and *American Association of Tissue Bank.*
- The ASRM and SART committee have recommended some more investigations other than what we are doing in India. These investigations are hepatitis B core antibody, HTLV-I and -II (Human T cell lymphotropic virus), cytomegalovirus IgG and IgM), nucleic acid amplification test for *Chlamydia* and gonorrhea.
- *United Kingdom guidelines* published in 2008 also recommend the same infection profile to be done as laid down by ASRM. Regarding genetic screening the Royal College of Obstetricians and Gynaecologists

guideline recommends autosomal recessive gene screening specifically for cystic fibrosis, sickle cell disease, Tay-Sachs disease other than beta-thalassemia, which is the only genetic screening, offered to our donors in India.[10]

- Some *banks in Europe and America* screen for some more genetic diseases depending upon ethnicity of donor. However, chromosomal analysis, thalassemia screening and sickle cell disease screening is done for all donors irrespective of their ethnicity.
- *Selective screenings offered as per ethnicity by European banks.*[11]
- Cystic fibrosis screening for 33–86 mutations for all Caucasian donors.
- Tay-Sachs disease for donors with Ashkenazi Jewish or French Canadian ancestry.
- Canavan disease, familial Dysautonomia, Fanconi anemia type-C, Gaucher disease, Niemann-Pick type-A disease for donors with Ashkenazi Jewish ancestry.

ICMR Criteria for Running of a Semen Bank[2]

- Either an ART clinic, a law firm or any other suitable independent organization may set-up a semen bank. If bank is set-up by an ART clinic then it must operate as a separate identity.
- The bank will ensure that all criteria mentioned above for a sperm donor are met with (ART Draft Bill 2010, Section 3.6) and a suitable record of all donors is kept for 10 years after which, or if the bank closes during this period, the records shall be transferred to an ICMR repository.
- A bank may advertise suitably for semen donors who may be appropriately compensated financially.
- On request for semen by an ART clinic, the bank will provide the clinic with a list of donors (without the name or the address but with a code number) giving all relevant details such as those mentioned in Section 3.6. The semen bank shall not supply semen of one donor for more than ten successful pregnancies. It will be the responsibility of the ART clinic or the patient, as appropriate, to inform the bank about a successful pregnancy. The bank shall keep a record of all semen received, stored and supplied, and details of the use of the semen of each donor. This record will be liable to be reviewed by the accreditation authority.
- The bank must be run by professionally competent staff/scientist and must have facilities for cryopreservation of semen, following internationally accepted protocols. Each bank will prepare its own standard operating procedures (SOPs) for cryopreservation.
- Semen samples must be cryopreserved for at least 6 months (quarantine period) before first use.

At 6 months, the semen donor must be re-tested for HIV and hepatitis B and C infections, to allow the window period after sperm collection, to ensure freedom from the above-mentioned infections, before it is supplied for use.

- The bank must ensure confidentiality in regard to the identity of the semen donor.
- A semen bank may store a semen sample for exclusive use on the donor's wife or on any other woman designated by the donor. An appropriate charge may be levied by the bank for the storage. In the case of non-payment of the charges when the donor is alive, the bank would have the right to destroy the semen sample or give it to a bona fide organization to be used only for research purposes. In case of death of the donor, the semen would become the property of the legal heir or the nominee of the donor, nominated at the time of semen sample storage to the bank. All other conditions that apply to the donor would now apply to the legal heir, excepting that he cannot use it for having a woman of his choice inseminated by it. If after the death of the donor, there are no claimants, the bank would have the right to destroy the semen or give it to a bona fide research organization to be used only for research purposes.
- All semen banks will require accreditation.

■ OOCYTE DONATION

Use of donor oocyte to impregnate a recipient woman is known as oocyte donation.

Indications of Oocyte Donation

- Premature ovarian failure
- Gonadal dysgenesis
- Menopausal woman
- Repeated IVF failure due to poor quality of oocyte or poor oocyte recovery
- Female a carrier of a known genetic disease
- Recurrent miscarriage due to translocation defect in females karyotyping
- Single fathers or gay couples.

Requirements for an Oocyte Donor (ICMR Guidelines)

- Counseling and informed consent (Form K) **(Appendix 4)**.
- The individual must be free of HIV and hepatitis B and C infections, hypertension, diabetes, sexually transmitted diseases and identifiable and common genetic disorders such as thalassemia.

- The blood group and the Rh status of the individual must be determined and placed on record.
- Other relevant information in respect of the donor, such as height, weight, age, educational qualifications, profession, color of the skin and the eyes, and the family background in respect of history of any familial disorder, must be recorded in an appropriate performa.
- The age of the donor must not be less than 21 years or more than 35 years.
- Law firms and semen banks should be encouraged to obtain and maintain information on possible oocyte donors though appropriate advertisement. These organizations may appropriately charge the couple for providing an oocyte donor.
- The oocyte donor may be compensated suitably financially by the law firm or semen bank when the oocyte is donated. After many years of debate regarding donor compensation, it has been established that donor should be paid. There are various reasons to compensate the donor with monitory payment.

Requirements of Oocyte Recipient

- Consent for oocyte retrieval/embryo transfer (Form I) **(Appendix 5)** is to be signed by recipient female along with her partner.
- Detailed medical and reproductive history of recipient should be taken regarding mental and physical fitness for motherhood.
- General and pelvic examination should ascertain physical health.
- In case recipient is more than 40 years old, possibility of high-risk pregnancy should be informed and she should be counseled accordingly.
- Evaluation of uterine cavity by ultrasonography should be undertaken to ensure that uterus and its endometrial lining is normal.
- Preconception testing for blood grouping, HIV, syphilis, hepatitis B and C infections should be done before taking a female for embryo transfer. ASRM ethics committee also recommends for *Neisseria gonorrhoeae* and *Chlamydia trachomatis* testing. They also do varicella and rubella titer in recipient female and offer vaccination in unimmunized female.
- ICMR does not recommend routine genetic screening for recipient whereas ASRM ethics committee recommends genetic screening as per ethnicity of recipient, also.

Preparation of Oocyte Recipient

Endometrium should be well prepared before embryo transfer to uterus of the recipient female.

Methods of Endometrial Preparation

Natural cycle: In case of young ovulating females embryo transfer can be done in natural cycles on the endometrium which develops as a result of spontaneous ovulation with success rate equivalent to that of exogenous hormone treated endometrium.[12] Embryo transfer in natural cycle is not advisable in aged females due to their poor and inconsistent ovulatory performance thus the risk of high cycle cancelation rate.

Exogenous hormone replacement cycle: Exogenous hormones are used in women with non-ovulatory or irregular cycles to prepare endometrium appropriate for implantation. Various hormonal regimens have been tried for good endometrial preparation before embryo transfer.

- GnRH agonist downregulation of pituitary gonadotropins followed by estradiol valerate from day 2 of menstruation either given as constant dose of 2 mg 3 times a day or increasing dose regimen starting from day 2 or 3 of menstruation. The dose is started from 2 mg/day to 4 mg/day and is raised by 2–4 mg every 4–5 days till a maximum of 6–8 mg/day is given in divided doses, till appropriate endometrium develops.
- Estradiol valerate started from day 2 of periods in relatively higher dose (6–8 mg/day in divided doses) to suppress pituitary gonadotropins by negative feedback without GnRH agonist downregulation.
- Stimulated cycles by using low dose gonadotropin and human chorionic gonadotropin.

Artificial and stimulated cycles produce comparable pregnancy rates, implantation rates, cancelation rates and endometrial thickness, although stimulated cycles have a higher incidence of thin endometrium.[13]

Requirements for Partner of Oocyte Recipient

1. Consent for oocyte retrieval/embryo transfer (Form I) is to be signed
2. Detailed medical and reproductive history
3. Semen analysis
4. Infection profile including HIV, syphilis, hepatitis B and C should be evaluated.

Rights and Duties of Donor[14]

- Subject to the other provisions of this Act, all information about the donors shall be kept confidential and information about gamete donation shall not be disclosed to anyone other than the central database of the "Department of Health Research", except with the consent of the person or persons to whom the information relates, or by an order of a court of competent jurisdiction.
- Subject to the other provisions of this Act, the donor shall have the right to decide what information may be passed on and to whom, except in the case of an order of a court of competent jurisdiction.
- A donor shall relinquish all parental rights over the child which may be conceived from her gamete.
- No ART procedure shall be conducted on or in relation to any gamete of a donor under this Act unless such donor has obtained the consent in writing of her spouse, if there, to such procedure.
- The identity of the recipient shall not be disclosed to the donor.

Duties of ART Clinic in Reference Oocyte Donation

- No woman shall donate oocytes more than six times in her life, with not less than a 3-month interval between the oocyte pickups.
- Eggs from one donor can be shared between two recipients only, provided that at least seven oocytes are available for each recipient.
- No donor gamete shall be stored for a period of more than 5 years.

Problem of Donor Shortage

Couples are facing more problems in getting oocyte donors than sperm donor, because there is still no oocyte banking policy as in case of sperm donation. The reasons are manifold; on one side donation of oocyte is more complex as well as physically traumatic for the donor compared to sperm donation and also the technology for oocyte cryopreservation is not perfected yet. Though better than oocyte donation, need of sperm donation is also not met in many developed countries.

- *Oocyte sharing scheme:* The system of oocyte sharing involves two infertile couples; one of them need to raise resources for ART hence agrees to donate oocytes to an affluent infertile couple wherein the wife can carry a pregnancy through, but cannot produce her own oocyte for IVF. The affluent couple, for a monetary compensation would take care of the expenses of the ART procedure for the indigent couple. Concerns have been raised that egg sharing may cause psychological harm to the donor if she is unsuccessful with her treatment, but the recipient conceives.
- *Sperm sharing scheme:* In this, couples can get a reduction in treatment costs, or are moved up in waiting list, in return for the male partner (or another person they provide as a donor) donating their sperm.
- *Freeze sharing schemes:* This facility has become available at a small number of clinics more recently,

allowing women to store their eggs for future treatment (free for about 5 years) in exchange for donating some of these eggs.

■ CHANGING PRACTICE OF ANONYMITY

There have been a lot of concerns regarding the disclosure of information of the genetic parent to the desiring parents or to the offspring. ASRM ethics committee has raised the issue of disclosing the fact of gamete donation to offspring and information of donor to recipient parent and offspring both.

Some experts feel that gamete donation is just not a mechanical process of transferring gametes from one person to other but may also involve psychological and emotional turmoil in donor. These emotional changes if do not happen immediately, then may occur later on when the donor starts realizing the fact, that there are possibilities of existence of their genetic offspring whom they are unable to contact.

Traditionally, sperm banks tend to maintain anonymity of their sperm donors. However, in recent years, there has been a push toward the use of open-identity or ID-release donors. These donors generally agree to at least one contact by the child when the child reaches a certain age, usually at 18 years.[11] One recent study indicates that about 1/3rd of children conceived from open-identity sperm seek contact with their sperm donor, and several European countries no longer permit anonymous sperm donation. European Sperm Bank and USA only accept open-identity sperm donors into its sperm donation program.[11] One sperm bank in California has created a registry to aid children who want to meet siblings genetically related to them through gamete donation.[15]

■ LEVELS OF INFORMATION SHARING

The ASRM ethics committee outlined four levels of information sharing between donor, recipient and offspring.[16]

Level 1—Non-identifying information: Donor provides non-identifying medical or biographical information.

Level 2—Non-identifying contact for medical updates: Donor agrees to be contacted with anonymity intact by the program for medical updates and further information if requested.

Level 3—Non-identifying personal contact: Donor agrees to have non-identifying contact when the child reaches a certain age and both agree to the disclosure.

Level 4—Identifying personal contact: Donor agrees to have identifying information shared with the offspring when the child reaches the age of maturity and both agree to the disclosure.

Ethical principles related to gamete donation laid down by "Human Fertilization Embryology Authority"[17] take into consideration many facets of gamete donation; such as welfare of the future child, safety of donors and patients, respect for family life, altruism and fairness but with pragmatism, informed consent with free choice hence the importance of counseling and transparency.

■ CONCLUSION

We need to address the concerns of a couple's intrinsic need of forming a family. For some, donated sperm, eggs or embryos represents the only chance, other than adoption to fulfil this need. For such people, there needs to be adequate supply of donated gametes; therefore posing unjustifiable barriers to donation may be seen to impinge on one's ability to do so. Any change in policy by governing authorities should be easy for clinics to implement and also pose minimum burden on donors, patients and clinics. In other words, it is desirable to strike a balance between principle and practicality. The ultimate aim of the technology of gamete donation should be to fulfil the desire of a couple to form a family yet ensure no harm to the child born or intended mother, as a result of assisted reproduction with donor eggs or sperm.

■ MESSAGE BOX

- In family donation, we should avoid using sperm and egg donation between close relatives to avoid consanguinity.

- In India, ICMR has laid guidelines for gamete donation, and the ART bill has been drafted in 2010.

- Therapeutic donor insemination should only be offered for oligospermic men if the couple is unable to afford IVF–ICSI.

- Thalassemia screening is the only genetic test, which we offer in India in contrast to various genetic diseases testing which includes cystic fibrosis, sickle cell disease, Tay–Sachs disease, etc. in western world.

- Vitrification is the most common and recent method of sperm cryopreservation.

- Quarantine period of 6 months is necessary before release of semen for use.

- Method of oocyte cryopreservation has not been perfected to a stage to allow oocyte banking.

- Practice of anonymity in gamete donation has been changing and now more people are moving toward open identity (non-anonymous) donor for the sake of medical and psychological reasons.

APPENDIX 1: FORM F
Consent for Artificial Insemination or Intrauterine Insemination with Donor Semen

We, ________________________________ and ____________________________, being husband and wife and both of legal age, authorize Dr.____________________ to inseminate the wife artificially or intrauterine with semen/sperm of a donor (ART bank's no.____________________; obtained from ____________________ ART bank with valid registration no...................) for achieving conception.

We understand that even though the insemination may be repeated as often as recommended by the doctor, there is no guarantee or assurance that pregnancy or a live birth will result.

We have also been told that the outcome of pregnancy may not be the same as those of the general pregnant population, for example in respect of abortion, multiple pregnancies, anomalies or complications of pregnancy or delivery.

We declare that we shall not attempt to find out the identity of the donor.

I, the husband, also declare that should my wife bear any child or children as a result of such insemination(s), such child or children shall be as my own and shall be my legal heir(s).

The procedure carried out does not ensure a positive result, nor does it guarantee a mentally and physically normal body. This consent holds good for all the cycles performed at the clinic.

Endorsement by the ART Clinic

I/we have personally explained to ____________________ and ______________ the details and implications of his/her/their signing this consent/approval form, and made sure to the extent humanly possible that he/she/they understand these details and implications.

Name, address and signature of the Witness from the clinic

Signed:____________________________(Husband)
____________________________(Wife)

Name and signature of the Doctor
Name and address of the ART clinic
Dated:
____

Note: An appropriate modification of this form may be used for Artificial Insemination or Intrauterine Insemination of a single woman with donor semen

APPENDIX 2: FORM L
Consent Form for the Donor of Sperm

I, Mr ___________________________ consent to donate my sperm to couples/individuals who are unable to have a child by other means.

I have had a full discussion with Dr _________________ (name and address of the clinician) on ___________________,

I have been counseled by _____________________ (name and address of independent counselor) on___________

I understand that there will be no direct or indirect contact between the recipient, and me, and my personal identity will not be disclosed to the recipient or to the child born through the use of my gamete.

I understand that I shall have no rights whatsoever on the resulting offspring and vice versa.

(If applicable) My wife has agreed to the donation of my sperm. (Strike off if not applicable.)

Endorsement by the ART bank

I/we have personally explained to _____________________ the details and implications of his signing this consent/ approval form, and made sure to the extent humanly possible that he understands these details and implications.

Signed: _______________Name and address of the donor ____

Name and signature of the Doctor
Name, address and signature of the Witness from the ART bank
Name and address of the ART bank
Dated:

APPENDIX 3: FORM M
Information on Semen Donor

Date of filling the form:

Basic Information

1. Identification number (Donor ID)
2. Age/Date of birth
3. Marital status
4. Education:
   a. Donor
   b. Spouse
5. Occupation:
   a. Donor
   b. Spouse
6. Monthly income
7. Religion

History

8. Obstetric history of wife:
   a. Number of deliveries
   b. Number of abortions
   c. Other points of note
9. History of use of contraceptives
10. Medical history
11. Family history from the medical point of view
12. History of any abnormality in a child of the donor
13. History of blood transfusion
14. History of substance abuse

Investigations

15. Blood group and Rh status
16. Complete blood picture:
    a. Hb
    b. Total RBC count
    c. Total WBC count
    d. Differential WBC count
    e. Platelet count
    f. Peripheral smear
17. Random blood sugar

18. Blood urea/Serum creatinine
19. SGPT
20. Routine urine examination
21. HBsAg status
22. Hepatitis C status
23. HIV[1] status with date of the tests done
24. Hemoglobin A_2 (for thalassemia) status
25. HIV PCR[2] (positive or negative)
26. Any other specific test[3]

Features

27. Height
28. Weight
29. Color of skin
30. Color of hair
31. Color of eyes

Detailed Physical Examination

32. Pulse
33. Blood pressure
34. Temperature
35. Respiratory system
36. Cardiovascular system
37. Per abdominal examination
38. Other systems

Footnotes:
[1] To be carried out every 6 months
[2] To be carried out if donor leaves within 6 months of the previous HIV test
[3] Any additional test carried out on the basis of the history and examination of donor

All the tests should have been done within 15 days prior to the date of filling the form.

Name and signature with date, of the person filling the form

APPENDIX 4: FORM K
Consent Form for the Donor of Oocytes

I, Ms.___________________________ consent to donate my eggs to couples/individuals who are unable to have a child by other means.

I have had a full discussion with Dr_________________________(name and address of the clinician) on ____________________

I have been counseled by _______________________________ (name and address of independent counselor) on _________

I understand that there will be no direct or indirect contact between me and the recipient, and my personal identity will not be disclosed to the recipient or to the child born through the use of my gamete.

I understand that I shall have no rights whatsoever on the resulting offspring and vice versa.

I understand that the method of treatment may include:
- Stimulating my ovaries for multifollicular development.
- The recovery of one or more of my eggs under ultrasound-guidance or by laparoscopy under sedation or general anesthesia.
- The fertilization of my oocytes with recipients husbands or donor sperm and transferring the resulting embryo into the recipient.

(If applicable) My husband has agreed to the donation of my oocyte. (Strike off if not applicable.)

I understand and accept that the drugs that are used to stimulate the ovaries to raise oocytes have temporary side-effects like nausea, headaches and abdominal bloating. Only in a small proportion of cases, a condition called ovarian hyperstimulation occurs where there is an exaggerated ovarian response. Such cases can be identified ahead of time but only to a limited extent. Further, at times the ovarian response is poor or absent in spite of using a high dose of drugs. Under these circumstances, the treatment cycle will be canceled.

Endorsement by the ART Clinic

I/we have personally explained to ___________________ the details and implications of her signing this consent/ approval form, and made sure to the extent humanly possible that she understands these details and implications.

Signed: _________________ Name and address of the donor ____

Name, address and signature of the Witness from the clinic
Name and signature of the Doctor
Name and address of the ART clinic
Dated:

APPENDIX 5: FORM I
Consent for Oocyte Retrieval/Embryo Transfer

Name(s) and address(es) of commissioning person(s):

Name and address of the Clinic:

I have asked the Clinic named above to provide me with treatment services to help me bear a child. I consent to:

a. Being prepared for oocyte retrieval by the administration of hormones and other drugs

b. The removal of oocytes from my ovaries under ultrasound guidance/laparoscopy

c. The mixing of the following (using technologies such as IVF or ICSI):

    a. My oocytes b. the sperm of my husband

    c. Anonymous donor oocyte d. anonymous donor sperm

    d. The transfer in my _______________________ of

        1. __________ (no) of the oocytes mixed with the sperm

        2. ____________ (no) of the resulting embryos

        3. ____________ (no) of our cryopreserved embryos

        4. __________ (no) of embryo(s) obtained anonymously

    e. the transfer of resulting embryos (number________) into _______________who will act as my surrogate

(Tick the appropriate and strike off the others)

I/We had a full discussion with _______________ about the above procedures and I have been given oral and written information about them.

I/We consent that I/we shall be the legal parent(s) of the child and the child will have all the legal rights on me, in case of anonymous gamete/embryo donation.

I/We have been given a suitable opportunity to take part in counseling about the implications of the proposed treatment.

The type of anesthetic proposed (general/regional/ sedation) has been discussed in terms which I have understood.

Endorsement by the ART Clinic

I/we have personally explained to _______________ and _____________the details and implications of her signing this consent/approval form, and made sure to the extent humanly possible that she understands these details and implications.

Signature of Commissioning Person

Name, address and signature of the Witness from the clinic

Name and signature of the Doctor

Consent of Husband/Partner (As and if Applicable)

As the husband/partner, I consent to the course of the treatment outlined above. I understand that I will become the legal parent of any resulting child, and that the child will have all the normal legal rights on me.

Name, address and signature: ____________________

(Husband)

Name, address and signature of the Witness from the clinic:___________________________________

Name and signature of the Doctor: ____________________

Dated:

■ REFERENCES

1. Indian council of medical research. Information on semen donor. The Assisted Reproductive Technologies (Regulations) Rules. 2010.pp.56-8.
2. Radhey S Sharma, Pushpa M Bhargava, Nomita Chandhiok, Nirakar C Saxena (Eds). National Guidelines for Accreditation, Supervision and Regulation of ART Clinics in India. New Delhi: Narayan & Sons; 2005.
3. Sherman JK. Synopsis of the use of frozen human semen since 1964: state of the art of human semen banking. Fertil Steril. 1973;24(5):397-412.
4. Behrman J, Sawada Y. Heterologous and homologous inseminations with human semen frozen and stored in a liquid-nitrogen refrigerator. Fertil Steril. 1966;17(4):457-66.
5. Sherman J. Cryopreservation of human semen. In: Keel B, Webster BW, (Eds). Handbook of the Laboratory Diagnosis and Treatment of Infertility. Boca Raton, USA: CRC Press; 1990.
6. Rall WF, Fahy GM. Ice-free cryopreservation of mouse embryos at -196 degrees C by vitrification. Nature. 1985;313(6003): 573-5.
7. Vutyavanich T, Piromlertamorn W, Nunta S. Rapid freezing versus slow programmable freezing of human spermatozoa. Fertil Steril. 2010;93(6):1921-8.
8. Larson JM, McKinney KA, Mixon BA, et al. An intrauterine insemination-ready cryopreservation method compared with sperm recovery after conventional freezing and post-thaw processing. Fertil Steril. 1997;68(1):143-8.
9. The practice committee of American Society for Reproductive Medicine (ASRM) and the practice committee of Society of Assisted Reproductive Technology (SART). Recommendation for gamete and embryo donation: committee opinion. Fertil Steril. 2013;90:47-62.
10. Association of Biomedical Andrologists, Association of Clinical Embryologists, British Andrology Society, British Fertility Society, Royal College of Obstetricians and Gynaecologists. UK guidelines for the medical and laboratory screening of sperm, egg and embryo donors. Hum Fertil. 2008;11(4):201-10.
11. European sperm bank USA. 4915 25th Avenue NE, Suite 204, Seattle WA 98105. info@europeanspermbankusa.com.
12. Byrd W. Cryopreservation, thawing, and transfer of human embryos. Semin Reprod Med. 2002;20(1):37-43.
13. Wright KP, Guibert J, Weitzen S, et al. Artificial versus stimulated cycles for endometrial preparation prior to frozen-thawed embryo transfer. Reprod Biomed Online. 2006;13(3):321-5.
14. Indian council of medical research. Rights and duties of donors. The Assisted Reproductive Technologies (Regulations) Bill. 2010.pp.25.
15. The Sperm Bank of California. Available at: http://www.thespermbankofca.org. [Accessed on February, 2015].
16. Ethics committee of the American Society for Reproductive Medicine. Interests, obligations, and rights of the donor in gamete donation: Fertil Steril. 2009;91(1):22-7.
17. A review of the HFEA's sperm and egg donation policies-2011. Donating sperms and eggs. Have your say. Available from www.hfea.gov.uk/donationreview [Accessed on February, 2015].

52

Embryo Donation

Devika Gunasheela, Ashwini S, Jyothi Patil, Prathiba G

DEFINITION

Embryo donation is a form of third party reproduction. It is defined as the giving—generally without compensation—of embryos remaining after one couple's in vitro fertilization (IVF) treatments, to another person or couple, followed by the placement of those embryos into the recipient woman's uterus to facilitate pregnancy and childbirth in the recipient. The resulting child is considered the child of the woman who carries it and gives birth, and not the child of the donor.

Embryo donation could be the answer for couples who are unable to conceive and for those who have been successful in bearing a child, but are now struggling with the decision of what to do with their remaining embryos.

The child born after embryo donation has no genetic connection with his/her rearing parents, and the relationship between parents and child differs from that in conventional adoption in that the couples have the opportunity to experience pregnancy and childbirth. The question has been raised as to whether or not this treatment should be called embryo adoption or embryo donation.

One must be careful, however, in distinguishing the concept of *embryo donation* from *embryo adoption*. Adoption implies a legal process through which a child born to other parents is taken as one's own child.[1] While embryos certainly represent potential lives, regarding them as true persons is considered a fallacy. American Society for Reproductive Medicine (ASRM) explicitly rejects embryo *adoption* because it believes that the practice is deceptive and results in unethical administrative and legal procedures, as well as unnecessary costs for infertile recipient(s), who need donor embryos to become pregnant.[2] The legal term *adoption* does not apply to embryos, which hold the potential for life but are not persons. Within the published literature, it is mostly regarded as donation, as embryos are not considered to be persons and, as such, cannot be adopted.[3]

Cryopreservation of excess embryos for future use is a widely practiced component of assisted reproductive technologies (ARTs), and it is estimated that over 400,000 frozen embryos remain in storage in the USA.[4]

HISTORY

A careful reading of the 1983 clinical report often cited as the first instance of embryo donation reveals that the donated embryo was actually created for the recipient at the same time that four embryos were made for the donor couple's own use. The menstrual cycles of the donor and recipient women were synchronized using medications, and the transfers occurred on the same day. None of these embryos had been cryopreserved.[5]

Soon thereafter, reports were published documenting successful pregnancies and births from cryopreserved donor embryos. Again, however, these were embryos made from donor's gametes specifically for the recipients.[6,7] The use of donated embryos can provide patients a way to conceive that may be less complex and less expensive than gamete donation. It can also provide the donating patients with a sense of fulfillment as their donation helps other patients build a family. The ethical appropriateness of patients donating embryos to other patients for family building or for research, including stem cell research, is well established and has been affirmed by ASRM body and many others.[8-11]

TYPES

Embryo donation can be handled on an *anonymous basis* (donor and recipient parties are not known to each other) or on an *open basis* (parties' identities are shared and the families agree to a relationship). Occasionally, a *semi-open* arrangement is used in which the parties know family and other information about each other, but their real names and locating information are withheld in order to provide a layer of privacy protection.

■ SOURCE

The decision to donate the embryos is complex. Several factors contribute. First, egg retrieval is expensive, somewhat painful, and carries some degree of clinical risk to the woman both from the effects of the medications used and from the insertion of the needle into the ovary. Therefore, the incentive of freezing excess embryos is to avoid having to go back a second time to retrieve more eggs. At the same time, freezing and thawing of unfertilized eggs is not a favorable option compared to freezing and thawing of embryos. The cleavage stage embryo, on the other hand, is much more robust than an unfertilized egg and survives freezing and thawing much more reliably. Hence, couples undergoing ART end up freezing surplus embryos for future use.

Couples have four realistic choices for the disposition of their excess frozen embryos:
1. They can keep them in frozen storage in case they want to try for another child at a later time. Most of today's frozen embryos are, in fact, still designated in this way by the creating couples.
2. A couple can have them thawed and destroyed. This option is acceptable to relatively few couples; moreover, it is not acceptable to those who see the embryo as a life already.
3. A couple could also choose to donate them for research.
4. The fourth option is to donate the embryos to another couple to help them achieve pregnancy.

According to a survey by the ASRM, 54% of fertility patients want to preserve their remaining embryos for future use. Another 21% want to donate leftover embryos for research. The remaining 7% of those surveyed are willing to donate leftover embryos to another couple.[12]

■ INDICATIONS FOR EMBRYO DONATION

Ideal candidates for embryo donation include:
- Couples who are unable to conceive a genetically related child and therefore face the possibility of having to use both donor oocytes and donor sperm to conceive.
- Women who have poor quality embryos or decreased ovarian reserve are candidates for embryo donation.
- Couples with significant male factor infertility also may benefit from embryo donation.

Chemotherapy with alkylating agents specifically may predispose males to gonadal failure.[13] Males with certain genetic conditions, such as cystic fibrosis, may also suffer from significantly abnormal sperm counts or even azoospermia.[14] Such couples may first consider therapeutic donor insemination, but they may opt for embryo donation if costs of other infertility treatments with donor sperm become unacceptable.[15]
- Couples with repeated IVF or implantation failures may also consider the option of embryo donation.
- Finally, patients with genetic conditions or chromosomal abnormalities may also desire embryo donation to reduce transmission to offspring. Although, preimplantation genetic diagnosis for couples undergoing IVF is a viable option, there are significant costs associated with this technology; therefore, it may not be affordable to some couples.[15]

■ GUIDELINES

Guidelines for ART practices that offer embryo donation:[16]
I. *Guidelines for ART Practices that Offer Embryo Donation*
   - The practice may charge a professional fee to the potential recipients for embryo thawing, the embryo transfer procedure, cycle coordination, documentation and infectious disease screening and testing of both recipients and donors. However, the selling of embryos per se is ethically unacceptable.
   - Embryos should be quarantined for a minimum of 6 months before the potential donors are screened and tested or retested, with documentation of negative results.
   - Physicians and employees of an infertility practice should be excluded from participating in embryo donation as either donors or recipients within that practice.
II. *Embryo Donation:* The following guidelines apply to sexually intimate couples who decide to donate unused embryos that are the product of their own biological gametes:
   - The embryo donors must sign an informed consent document indicating their permission to use their embryos for embryo donation. Issues to be addressed in the consent form include:
     - Inadvertent loss or damage to the embryo(s)
     - Relinquishing all rights of the donor(s) to the embryo(s) and any child or children that may result from the transfer of such embryo(s)

- The right of the practice to refuse transfer to an inappropriate recipient.
 – The length of time that donated embryos will be maintained in cryostorage and the alternatives for their disposition thereafter.
 – Donors should receive no compensation for the embryos.
 – While there are no specifics on paternal age, some authorities advocate that female donors should be between the ages of 18 and 36.[17]

III. *Guidelines for Potential Recipients*
 – The recipient(s) must take full responsibility for the embryo(s) and any child or children that may result from the transfer.
 – The recipient(s) must release the gamete donors from any and all liability from any potential complications of the pregnancies, congenital abnormalities, heritable diseases or other complications of the embryo donation.
 – The ART program should also be absolved of liability from potential complications of pregnancy, congenital abnormalities and heritable diseases.
 – The ASRM recommends that the recipient(s) submit to the same blood tests for infectious disease testing as the donors.

■ RECORD KEEPING

- The US Food and Drug Administration (FDA) requires that records pertaining to each donor (screening and test results) be maintained for at least 10 years. However, in the opinion of the ASRM, a permanent record of each donor's screening and test results should be maintained. To the extent possible, the clinical outcome should be recorded for each donation cycle.
- *Indian Council of Medical Research (ICMR) guidelines—preservation, utilization and destruction of embryos:*
 – Couples must give specific consent to storage and use of their embryos. The Human Fertilization and Embryology Act, UK (1990), allows a 5-year storage period which India would also follow.
 – Consent shall need to be taken from the couple for the use of their stored embryos by other couples or for research, in the event of their embryos not being used by themselves. This consent will not be required if the couple defaults in payment of maintenance charges after two reminders sent by registered post.
 – No commercial transaction will be allowed for the use of embryos for research.

Protection of Confidentiality

Individuals participating in donor programs should be assured that their confidentiality will be protected.

Screening: Donors or Recipients

In the United States, embryo donation must meet established FDA guidelines for screening of the donors. Embryos lacking all the required screening, or having screened positive for an infectious condition, can still be transferred, but only if the donor and recipient couples are acquainted and only if full disclosure of the embryo's condition is made.

- Embryo donors must provide a medical and genetic history.
- The gamete donors used to create the embryos should be screened for relevant risk factors for HIV, other transmissible infections.
- There is no method to ensure completely that infectious agents will not be transmitted, but the following guidelines, combined with an adequate medical history and specific exclusion of individuals at high risk for HIV and other transmissible infections, should dramatically reduce these risks. The practice should determine if the cost of such tests will be borne by the donor couple, by the practice mediating the embryo donation or by the potential recipients. The following recommended tests should be performed using methods approved by the FDA for use in determining donor eligibility, on both partners, before gamete collection and more than 180 days after cryopreservation of the embryos to be donated:
 – HIV-1 antibody and nucleic acid testing (NAT)
 – HIV-2 antibody
 – Hepatitis B surface antigen
 – Hepatitis B core antibody (IgG and IgM)
 – Hepatitis C antibody and NAT
 – Serologic test for syphilis
 – *Neisseria gonorrhoeae* and *Chlamydia trachomatis* NAT
 – Although not required by the FDA, recommended tests also include:
 - Blood type and Rh factor
 In addition, the male gamete donor should be tested for:
 - Human T-cell leukemia virus type 1 (HTLV-1) and human T-cell leukemia virus type 2 (HTLV-2)
 - Cytomegalovirus (CMV) (IgG and IgM) antibody.
- If not already performed, appropriate genetic evaluation and testing should be conducted.

PROTOCOL

At Gunasheela IVF Center, the following protocol for frozen embryo transfer (FET) is followed:

The uterine cavity of the recipient is evaluated by transvaginal ultrasound (TVS) and hysteroscopy in the previous menstrual cycle. On the second or third day of spontaneous or induced menstrual cycle, TVS is done to look for ovarian cysts and the endometrial thickness. If the endometrial thickness is less than 5 mm and in the absence of ovarian cysts, incremental doses of estradiol valerate 2 mg for 3 days followed by 4 mg for 3 days and 6 mg for the next 3 days is given. TVS is done on the 10th day of hormone therapy to look for endometrial thickness. If the endometrial thickness is 7 mm or more, vaginal progesterone 600 mg is started and embryo transfer scheduled according to the day of freezing.

SUCCESS

According to Centers for Disease Control and Prevention (CDC) data (unpublished data), the pregnancy rate per donated embryo transfer cycle is 44% and the live birth delivery rate is 36%. The live birth rate for embryo donation is 36% compared to about 30% for autologous (a couple's own) frozen cycle IVF. This is because of the *selection factor*. Usually, though not always, embryos employed in a couple's own frozen cycle IVF come from a cohort where the first embryos have failed to achieve pregnancy. Conversely, embryos employed in an embryo donation cycle most often come from a cohort where the first embryos have been successful. (In this case, the donating couple had as many children as they wanted, and that is why they donated the embryos).

In a study by Keenan et al. the live birth rate for frozen embryo transfer cycles is 29% for non-donated embryos and 35.5% for donated embryos.[18] The higher rate for donated embryos appears to be due to better quality of the donated embryos because:
- Embryos are donated by couples who previously have had successful IVF cycles
- The embryos come from younger women.

However, there are contradictory results as well. In a study by Viveca Söderström-Anttila et al, the clinical pregnancy rate per donated embryo transfer was 27.8%.[19] There was no difference in pregnancy rate between embryos originating from treatment cycles, which resulted in pregnancy in the donor woman and those originating from non-pregnancy cycles.

LEGAL ISSUES

Fourteen nations forbid the practice altogether. In Italy, cryopreservation of embryos is also forbidden. In other nations, embryo donation is either governed by specific laws or carried on without any specific legal framework. In New Zealand, a couple must apply through a national committee in order to become parents by embryo adoption.

Embryo donation is not permitted in the following countries:
- Austria
- China
- Denmark
- Germany
- Israel
- Italy
- Latvia
- Norway
- Slovenia
- Sweden
- Switzerland
- Taiwan
- Tunisia
- Turkey.

In India, embryo donation is permitted by law. Offspring and social parents have right to non-identifying information on donors. Since April 2005, in UK identifying information about donors is held on the Human Fertilization and Embryology Authority (HFEA) Register and may be given to any child born from a donation once he/she is 18 years old.

ETHICAL ISSUES

The practice of embryo donation raises many ethical issues, since it involves several parties with separate interests: the donor couple, the recipient couple and the offspring.

However, there are those in the traditional adoption community who feel strongly that it is unethical to promote embryo donation when there are already born children living in foster care needing permanent homes. Others counter that the candidates for embryo adoption are looking for an infant to join their family, and are usually not the same people as those interested in undertaking parenting starting from the toddler, school age or adolescent stage. If anything, embryo donation might compete with adoption of already born newborn infants, but few of these are available for domestic adoption, and the cost of international adoptions was already prohibitively expensive for many even before the doors began to close on adoption from many countries in the past few years.

A second challenge comes from those in the pro-choice community who see embryo adoption as a competition to the donation of embryos for stem cell research. These individuals see the potential cure for chronic diseases as the priority, and the saving of the life of the embryo a much lower priority since, to them, it is not yet a human person.

Yet another challenge comes from those, particularly in the Roman Catholic community, who assert that the adoption of an embryo creates a new life outside the bonds of marriage. Those in favor advocated that from their perspective, the creation of embryos outside the body had not been legitimate, but once created, the saving of their lives was a positive act in keeping with the Catholic imperative of sanctity of human life.

The primary rate-limiting factors to the growth of the embryo adoption movement, however, are not the ideological oppositions from the outside, so much:

- As the reluctance of individual couples with remaining embryos to consider donating them.
- The hesitation of couples who are interested in adopting embryos to follow through with the process, at least in part because of costs.

For others, the issue is that they do not like the thought of their children meeting their own genetic siblings unexpectedly.

Some prospective donor parents have expressed the concern that they might feel guilty if they *brought a child into the world* to be raised by parents who then divorced or in some way were not satisfactory parents to the child.

DONOR ISSUES, OBSTACLES AND DILEMMAS

- *Time factor:* How long should they wait before making a final decision?
- *Profiling and preferences:* To what extent do they want to dictate their desires to the recipient couple? Should the recipient couple be allowed to have preferences?
- *Levels of openness:* Is remaining anonymous in the best interest of the offspring?
- *Relationship to recipients and to offspring:* Do they want to have access and visiting rights with the recipient family and potential offspring?
- *FDA regulations:* Do they want to have all the tests and screens to make sure they are not transmitting any infectious diseases? Who is going to pay for the tests and screens if a recipient couple is not identified right away for the stored donated embryos?
- *Psychological assessment:* Should a psychological assessment and background check be routine for both parties?
- *Ethical, legal and risk management issues:* They must be aware of these issues and seek council for advice.
- *Effectiveness of embryo transfer:* Is the quantity and quality of their embryos sufficient to warrant going through the donation process?
- *Cost:* Who is going to pay the medical, laboratory, consultation and legal fees?

CONCLUSION

With the controversy surrounding surplus embryo disposition being brought to the forefront, the choice of embryo donation has been deemed a *life-affirming parenthood choice*. As the number of excess embryos as a by-product of IVF increases, more couples may consider donating their embryos to other couples. This may serve as an ideal solution for couples who find embryo disposal unacceptable and wish to consider helping others who wish to become parents.

It would also be ideal if all couples who have cryopreserved embryos stored for 3 years or more would automatically receive an invitation to meet with a counselor or agency to discuss donation of their embryos to other couples with unmet family needs. We must encourage cooperation and teamwork between the ART clinics and social agencies.

Embryo donation, hence, provides another, less costly means of establishing a family. Perinatal outcomes in children born from either approach have been favorable and reassuring; however, obstetrical risks and complications in older recipients are significantly increased. Practice guidelines for the sage and ethical use of donated eggs and embryos have been published by both ASRM and European Society of Human Reproduction and Embryology (ESHRE) and should be adhered to in order to optimize outcomes of recipients while minimizing the risks to donors.

REFERENCES

1. Definition of adopted. [online] Available from www.merriam-webster.com [Accessed February 2015] 2012.
2. The Ethics Committee of the American Society for Reproductive Medicine. American Society for Reproductive Medicine: defining embryo donation. Fertil Steril. 2009;92:1818.
3. Robertson JA. Ethical and legal issues in human embryo donation. Fertil Steril. 1995;64:885-94.

4. Hoffman DI, Zellman GL, Fair CC, et al. Cryopreserved embryos in the United States and their availability for research. Fertil Steril. 2003;79(5):1063-9.

5. Trounson A, Leeton J, Besanko M, et al. Pregnancy established in an infertile patient after transfer of a donated embryo fertilized in vitro. British Medical J. 1983;286(6368):835-8.

6. Sauer MV, Paulson RJ. Human oocyte and pre-embryo donation: an evolving method for the treatment of infertility. Am J Obstet Gynecol. 1990;163(5 Pt 1):1421-4.

7. Van Steirteghem AC, Van den Abbeel E, Braeckmans P, et al. Pregnancy with a frozen-thawed embryo in a woman with primary ovarian failure. NEJM. 1987;317:113.

8. National Institutes of Health. Report of the human embryo research panel: final draft, September 27, 1994. Bethesda, MD: National Institutes of Health; 1994.

9. National Institutes of Health. Guidelines on human stem cell research. [online] Available from http://stemcells.nih.gov/policy/pages/2009guidelines.aspx [Accessed February 2015] 2009.

10. New York State Task Force on Life and the Law. Executive summary of assisted reproductive technologies, analysis and recommendations for public policy. [online] Available from http://www.health.ny.gov/regulations/task_force/reports_publications/execsum.htm [Accessed February 2015] 1998.

11. Human Fertilisation and Embryology Authority. Code of practice. [online] Available from www.hfea.gov.uk/code.html [Accessed February 2015].

12. Brown P. Controversial embryo adoptions on the rise. [online] Available from WJLA.COM [Accessed February 2015] 2012.

13. Howell SJ, Shalet SM. Fertility preservation and management of gonadal failure associated with lymphoma therapy. Curr Oncol Rep. 2002;4(5):443-52.

14. Stahl PJ, Schlegel PN. Genetic evaluation of the azoospermic or severely oligozoospermic male. Curr Opin Obstet Gynecol. 2012;24(4):221-8.

15. Lee J, Yap C. Embryo donation: a review. Acta Obstet Gynecol Scand. 2003;82(11):991-6.

16. The Practice Committee of the American Society for Reproductive Medicine and the Practice Committee of the Society for Assisted Reproductive Technology. Recommendations for gamete and embryo donation: a committee opinion. Fertil Steril. 2013;99(1):47-62.

17. Van Voorhis BJ, Grinstead DM, Sparks AE, et al. Establishment of a successful donor embryo program: medical, ethical, and policy issues. Fertil Steril. 1999;71(4):604-820.

18. Keenan J, Finger R, Check JH, et al. Favorable pregnancy, delivery, and implantation rates experienced in embryo donation programs in the United States. Fertil Steril. 2008;90:1077-80.

19. Söderström-Anttila V, Foudila T, Ripatti UR, et al. Embryo donation: outcome and attitudes among embryo donors and recipients. Hum Reprod. 2001;16(6):1120-8.

53 Surrogacy

Nayana Patel, Pankaj Kaingade

INTRODUCTION

Surrogacy, means an arrangement in which a woman agrees to a pregnancy achieved through assisted reproductive technology (ART), in which neither of the gametes belongs to her or her husband, with the intention to carry it to term and handover the child to the person or persons for whom she is acting as a surrogate.

INDIAN MYTHOLOGY

Krishna was the eighth child of Devaki and Vasudev. His maternal uncle (*Mama*), Kansa heard a prophecy that he would be killed by his sister Devaki's eighth child, and went on a mad spree killing all her first six children. Lord *Vishnu*, realizing the situation, arranged for the seventh child (*Balaram*) to be transferred into the womb of *Rohini* (*Nanda's* first wife), and requested Goddess *Maya* to be substituted for him in Devaki's womb.

BIBLE MYTHOLOGY

Surrogacy is not new. It has a history that dates back to Biblical times. The book of Genesis tells the story of *Sarah*, Abraham's wife, who said to her husband: "Behold now the Lord hath restrained me from bearing. I pray thee go to my maid, it may be that I may obtain children by her" (Genesis 16).

DEFINITIONS

Genetic couple, commissioning couple, intended parent—the couple who provide both sets of gametes.

Surrogate host or *host*—the woman receiving the embryos created from the gametes of the genetic couple.

Natural surrogacy, traditional surrogacy or *partial surrogacy*—where the egg belongs to the female carrying the pregnancy, the intended host is inseminated with the semen of the husband of the genetic couple.

Gestational surrogacy in vitro fertilization (IVF) surrogacy or *full surrogacy*—a treatment by which the gametes of the genetic couple or intended parents in a surrogacy arrangement are used to produce embryos and these embryos are subsequently transferred to a woman who agrees to act as a host for these embryos.

Commercial surrogacy arrangements—this is when the surrogate is paid over and above the necessary medical expenses.

Altruistic surrogacy arrangements—this is when the surrogate is paid only the necessary pregnancy-related expenses and at times nothing at all.

INDICATIONS FOR GESTATIONAL SURROGACY (FIG. 1)

- Absent uterus—either congenital absence of uterus (Mayer-Rokitansky-Küster-Hauser syndrome and other Müllerian anomalies) or post-hysterectomy
- Malformed uterus
- Severe intrauterine adhesions refractory to surgical lysis
- Recurrent pregnancy loss
- Repeated IVF implantation failures (> 6).

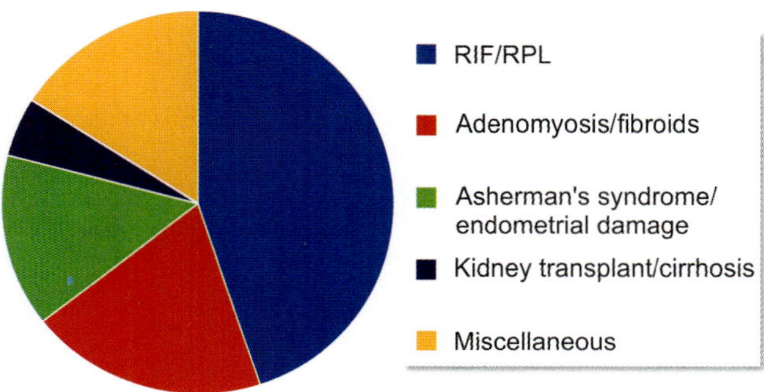

Fig. 1 Indications at Akanksha in vitro fertilization clinic

- Repeated ectopic pregnancies
- Medical reasons prohibiting continuation of pregnancy in the commissioning mother
- Posthumous conception using frozen embryos of a deceased woman, requested by the surviving partner or her parents.

■ STEPS IN SURROGACY

- Proper patient selection
- Source of surrogate (ART bank)
- Proper selection and screening of the surrogate
- Intensive counseling—the key factor
- Proper controlled ovarian stimulation and IVF technique
- Preparing the surrogate
- Synchronizing the cycles of the surrogate and the genetic mother
- Window period for embryo transfer
- Taking care of the legalities and financial contracts
- Transparency of the whole arrangement.

Patient Selection

The genetic couples are usually first seen alone and in-depth consultation and counseling of all the medical aspects of the treatment is conducted. If medically suitable for treatment, they are given some guidance on finding a host for themselves or take the help of a professional surrogate.

The genetic couple is screened for:
- Heritable diseases
- Family history of genetic diseases, chromosomal analysis
- Transmissible disease like sexually transmitted disease (STD), hepatitis B, human immunodeficiency virus and hepatitis C
- Hemoglobinopathies
- Pre-IVF investigations.

Counseling for the Intended Parents

- The medical and psychological risks of surrogacy
- Potential psychological risk to the child
- The chances of having a multiple pregnancy
- The possibility that the host may wish to retain the child after birth
- The importance of obtaining legal advice.

Selection of the Surrogate

The best surrogate is the genetic parent's mother or sister, or a best friend or cousin. There are no specific data on intrafamilial surrogacy. Surrogacy arrangements in general are less common than gamete donation.

The difficult aspect of the treatment is the extreme care with which the surrogate hosts must be selected by/for the genetic couple to ensure complete compatibility and also in-depth counseling is required for the short term and the long term in all aspects of the treatment.

Counseling of the Surrogate

- The full implications of undergoing treatment by IVF surrogacy
- The possibility of multiple pregnancy
- The possibility of her family and friends being against her having treatment
- The medical risks associated with pregnancy and delivery
- The implications of guilt on both sides, if the host spontaneously aborts a pregnancy
- The possible effect on her own children of acting as a surrogate
- The possibility that the host may feel a sense of bereavement when she gives the baby to the commissioning couple.

Screening of the Surrogate

- Age less than 35 years (preferably)
- No severe medical disorders or personal habit such as smoking, alcohol and drug abuse
- The woman satisfies all the testable criteria to go through a successful full-term pregnancy
- Screen for hereditary disorders, infectious diseases, hemoglobinopathies and STD
- Psychological assessment
- A physical examination and pap smear
- Infective disease testing
- Hysteroscopy
- A mock cycle.

Overview of Surrogacy Process

After completion of the orientation process and the selection of a surrogate, a comprehensive screening of all parties is undertaken. A physician needs to evaluate the intended parents for suitability for controlled ovarian hyperstimulation and egg retrieval. Several patients who have undergone a hysterectomy for malignancy have also had their ovaries moved high out of the pelvis to avoid harmful effects of radiation (in such cases, transabdominal ultrasound-guided egg harvesting is the preferred method).

Preparing the Surrogate for Embryo Transfer

Once the surrogate is selected, screened and counseled, endometrial lining preparation is done using oral estrogen preparations. If synchronization of cycles of genetic mother and surrogate host is considered, then the surrogate host is started on oral estradiol valerate at 6 mg/day, 2–3 days prior to ovulation induction of the commissioning mother. Regular ultrasound scanning for endometrial thickness is begun a week later and used to determine the need for modifying the estrogen replacement strategy.

With advancements in cryopreservation techniques, it is not necessary to synchronize the cycle of genetic mother with that of a surrogate host. Embryos of genetic parents are cryopreserved and used later once the surrogate host is ready.

Oral contraceptives/GnRH analogs are used for pituitary desensitization. The surrogate host is started on estradiol valerate 6 mg/day, increased as required, depending on ultrasound endometrial thickness is good enough, hCG trigger is given and progesterone supplementation started. Embryos are later transferred depending on the stage at which they are frozen. The number of embryos to be transferred depends on each institutes policies.

Luteal Phase Support

Intramuscular progesterone in oil, at a dose of 100 mg/day, or vaginal administration of natural progesterone suppositories or gel, is added to the drug regimen of the host mother, starting on the day after hCG administration.

Detection of Pregnancy

A quantitative serum beta-hCG is usually done 14 days post-egg retrieval. The surrogate will have a second quantitative hCG test 2 days later to verify that the levels are rising (they should double about every 2 days).

If a pregnancy has occurred, then an ultrasound is usually done about 2 weeks later for the detection of fetal sacs, and subsequently, a week later, to check for cardiac activity and confirm zygosity. Once the placenta starts taking over the hormone production, the surrogate is weaned off the hormone replacements. The rest of the pregnancy would follow the same course as any other pregnancy.

If the quantitative hCG is negative, then all external hormones are discontinued and a menstrual cycle will usually start within 5 days.

What are the Success Rates for Gestational Surrogacy?

The success rates of surrogacy procedures are entirely dependent upon the overall success rates for the given ART facility **(Fig. 2)**.

Surrogacy and Law

The Baby M in New Jersy. Here the surrogate mother Mary Beth Whitehead was reluctant to relinquish the child to Stern couple.

The recent case of baby Gammy where the Australian couple did not accept their surrogate baby who had Down's syndrome.

Indian Scenario and Legal Issues

The first Asian surrogate Grandmother case in January 2004, Akanksha IVF Clinic, Anand, Gujarat, India, where the grandmother carried the twins of her daughter (as she had Mayer-Rokitansky-Küster-Hauser syndrome). The genetic couple, i.e. the daughter and her husband, was UK citizen and the grandmother, an Indian national.

Baby Manji case in 2008, Akanksha IVF Clinic, Anand, Gujarat, India, where the couple got divorced during the pregnancy, but the contract was well in place, where in case of divorce, father was to take the custody of the baby.

A legal agreement between a gestational carrier, her husband, if married, and the intended parents, negotiated by an independent, separate legal counsel, is highly recommended. A gestational carrier contract should be as comprehensive as possible, setting forth for example, the parties intentions with respect to the parentage of the

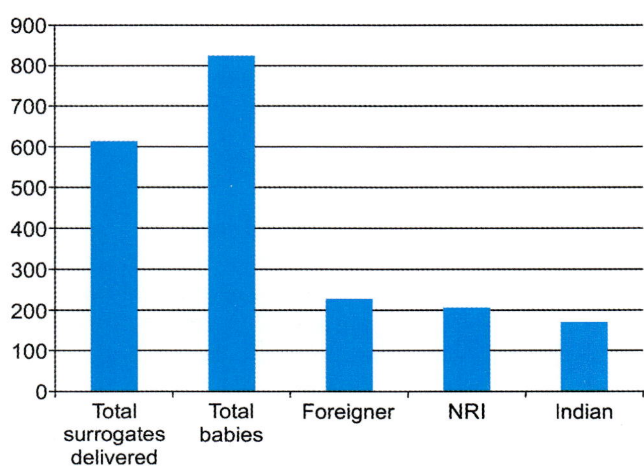

Fig. 2 Akanksha IVF clinic results

child, their financial arrangements, prenatal care, delivery plans, selective reduction, abortion, future contact among the parties, and cooperation on legal steps to establish parentage.

National Guidelines

Surrogacy being a grey area most doctors prefer to sign a consent form with the patients, to keep themselves out of legal and medical indemnity, although it can still be challenged.

Surrogacy has spawned a host of legal and emotional issues to which there are no "right" answers. For example:

- What will you do, if the surrogate insists on keeping the child?
- How much should you pay the surrogate?
- If she gets ill as a result of the pregnancy who will pay the medical costs?
- Is it possible to put the receiving mother's name as mother on the birth certificate?
- Will you tell the child about surrogacy?
- Will surrogates undertake pregnancy for profit?
- What happens, if the child is handicapped and is unwanted by the couple and the surrogate mother?
- What happens, if the surrogate dies during childbirth?

Highlights of Indian Council of Medical Research Guidelines

- The surrogates can be financially compensated by ART Bank.
- No ART clinic shall consider conception by surrogate for couple whom it would be normally be possible.
- Birth certificates will have the names of genetic parents.
- Surrogacy cannot be done with donor eggs and donor sperm both. At least either egg or sperm must be from intended parents.
- Surrogate has no right over the baby and duty toward the baby.

Ethical Issues

Unexpectedly, with the oncoming of surrogacy arrangements, concept of fatherhood and motherhood became subject to, too much controversy. Motherhood was never under such scrutiny. Paternity was a more controversial concept. But, little did one envisage, that a century later medical sciences would compartmentalize motherhood onto genetic, gestational and the social mother leading to a clash of interests, coincident in three women.

The Ethics Committee of the American Society for Reproductive Medicine has strongly recommended that surrogacy should not be widely practiced, but in spite of serious ethical reservations, they saw no reason to recommend legal prohibitions.

Ethical Consideration

In vitro fertilization surrogacy offers several advantages, but the role and outcome for all concerned remains subject to considerable uncertainty, particularly in some legislative jurisdictions.

There have been few instances where an IVF surrogacy has been considered for social reasons; that is, the parents have wished to have a child borne by a surrogate for other than medical reasons. This has generally been considered in appropriate.

■ OUR EXPERIENCE

See **Figure 3**.

Justification for Surrogate

- Becoming a surrogate empowers women with a sense of worth and authority.
- Surrogates could actually help liberate women.
- The domestic labor should be paid, so when reproduction and pregnancy becomes a job, we will look at the value of female labor in a new light. This would elevate the women's status in a patriarchal capitalist society.
- She has the right to fulfill her dreams—by not doing anything wrong or immoral—but by giving the greatest gift, that is creating a family.

Suggestions

While providing for rules and regulations, care must be taken to ensure that they are not so stringent, so as to indirectly encourage underground surrogacy arrangements. Harsh rules can have an adverse effect on

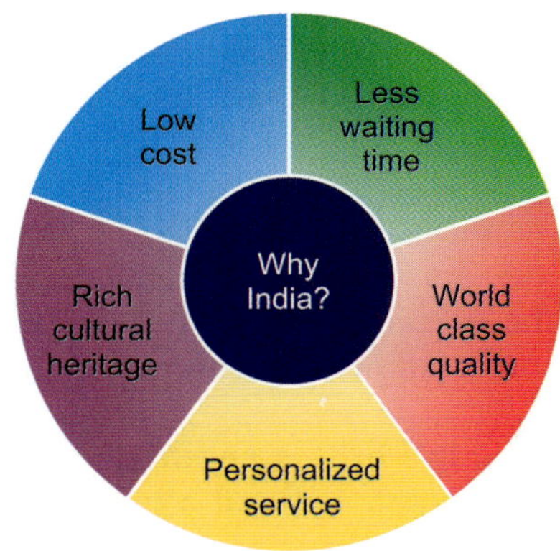

Fig. 3 Experiences for surrogacy in India

the parties to the arrangement. They shall then be forced to enter into private surrogacy arrangements thereby depriving themselves of the assistance of voluntary agencies working in this field. Therefore, the rules and regulations must be accommodative enough to take into account the interest of the parties.

- Rules must not be so strict whereby it leads to underground surrogacy arrangements
- To encourage altruistic surrogacy by allowing close members of the infertile couple to act as surrogate
- The vulnerability of the commissioning parents should be taken care of
- The welfare of the child should be given paramount importance in the surrogacy arrangements
- Assisted reproductive technology bank will recruit a surrogate. This means involvement of one more agency in the link—surrogate—ART clinic—couple. The problem will be—who would the surrogate trust? Who would the ART clinic put the confidence on? Where does the infertile couple stand?

Cost for Surrogacy

The costs of the basic procedures are quite complex and must be discussed with the patient in detail.

Below is a list of some potential unexpected costs of the surrogacy process:

- Pregnancy complications costs
- Maternal complications
- Fetal complications such as multiple pregnancy complications
- Costs for uterine evacuation procedures for spontaneous pregnancy losses
- Costs for selective reduction in multifetal pregnancies
- Costs for genetic amniocentesis
- Costs for termination of a genetically abnormal pregnancy (rare)
- Ongoing psychologic counseling costs
- Medical complications costs (rare).

Socioeconomic Upliftment of the Surrogates (Akanksha IVF Clinic)

Bought houses	163
Renovated houses and fixed deposit	74
Who invested in small business	45
Education of children	40
Saving account	89
Fixed deposit	138
Surgery—husband/children	25
For daughter's marriage/payment of debt	32

Surrogate House

There are so many problems that can come up during this entire procedure of surrogacy. The ultimate aim of surrogacy is to have a healthy baby and healthy surrogate, who willingly handover the baby to infertile couple. All throughout the pregnancy the well-being of the surrogate and the baby is of prime concern and this aspect will make the infertile couple extremely anxious. A *surrogate house* can be an answer to all these problems.

■ CONCLUSION

Gestational surrogacy is worth considering in women who have lost their uterus, were born without a uterus, have had repeated failures at implantation from a variety of sources, or have an underlying medical condition that prevents them from being pregnant. At experienced centers, the process of IVF surrogate pregnancy has thus far been uncomplicated and gratifying. This procedure offers hope for couples to produce their own genetic family. Perinatal and obstetric outcomes in patients undergoing surrogacy are also reassuring. This form of infertility treatment is now well established with a proven track record, and we endorse its continuation.

In India, surrogacy still needs public awareness and propaganda, as many childless couple who could benefit from this treatment modality, may be unaware of this option and lack of knowledge about the details of treatment.

In vitro fertilization surrogate gestation is an established, yet still controversial, approach to the care of infertile couples. The high success achieved with the current technology, and the possibility of having a genetically related offspring, continues to encourage the use of IVF surrogacy.

■ MESSAGE BOX

- Since most couples want their own genetic children, *IVF surrogacy* has become an accepted treatment option for women in certain countries with indications for surrogacy.
- Framing international guidelines on the practice of surrogacy is the challenge of the day. Hence, until such regulation is available, as others, we think that legal advice and formal and honest counseling to all the parties engaged in the surrogacy contract with a clear agreement on the terms of payment would be highly beneficial in protecting surrogacy from exploitation, avoiding legal, social and psychological complications, and further promoting the practice.
- Proper screening of surrogates is very important.
- In-depth counseling of the intended parents and surrogates is the key factor.
- Legal, ethical and moral issues along with medical issues should be assessed continuously in the surrogacy procedure, though the procedure itself is straight forward.

■ BIBLIOGRAPHY

1. British Medical Association Report. Changing Conceptions of Motherhood: The Practice of Surrogacy in Britain. London: BMA Publications; 1996.
2. Chang CL. Surrogate motherhood. Formos J Med Humanit. 2004;5(12):48-62.
3. Chen KC, Ng HT. Legal and ethical considerations of assisted reproductive technology and surrogate motherhood in AOFOG countries. J Obstet Gynaecol Res. 2001;27(2):89-95.
4. Cohen J, Jones H. Assisted reproduction. Rules and laws: International comparisons. Contracept Fertil Sex. 1999;27(4): I-VII.
5. Corson SL, Kelly M, Braverman AM, et al. Gestational carrier pregnancy. Fertil Steril. 1998;69(4):670-4.
6. Fasouliotis SJ, Schenker JG. Social aspects in assisted reproduction. Hum Reprod Update. 1999;5(1):26-39.
7. Goldfarb JM, Austin C, Peskin B, et al. Fifteen years experience with an in-vitro fertilization surrogate gestational pregnancy programme. Hum Reprod. 2000;15(5):1075-8.
8. Golombok S, Murray C, Jadva V, et al. Families created through surrogacy arrangements: parent-child relationships in the 1st year of life. Dev Psychol. 2004;40(3):400-11.
9. Goold I. Surrogacy: is there a case for legal prohibition? J Law Med. 2004;12(2):205-16.
10. Lalwani S, Berger M, Klipstein S, et al. Gestational surrogacy: A model to study the maximum success rates offered by an IVF program. Fertil Steril. 2002;78:143-4.
11. Rothenberg KH. Baby M. The surrogacy contract, and the health care professional: unanswered questions. Law Med Health Care. 1988;16(1-2):113-20.
12. Snowdon C. What makes a mother? Interviews with women involved in egg donation and surrogacy. Birth. 1994;21(2):77-84.
13. Utian WH, Goldfarb JM, Kiwi R, et al. Preliminary experience with in vitro fertilization-surrogate gestational pregnancy. Fertil Steril. 1989;52(4):633-8.
14. Van den Akker OB. Psychological trait and state characteristics, social support and attitudes to the surrogate pregnancy and baby. Hum Reprod. 2007;22(8):2287-95.
15. Van den Akker OB. Psychosocial aspects of surrogate motherhood. Hum Reprod Update. 2007;13(1):53-62.

Pregnancy and ART

54 First Trimester Screening in Pregnancies Conceived with ART

Pooja Lodha

INTRODUCTION

Pregnancy screening for Down syndrome and other chromosome abnormalities has become part of routine antenatal care over the last 20 years. The combined first trimester screening (FTS) consists of a detailed fetal ultrasound and maternal biochemistry (double marker) and is the most sensitive noninvasive clinical method of identifying a fetus as high risk for chromosomal abnormality.[1] FTS is not only limited to the diagnosis of chromosomal abnormalities, but also aids accurate dating of pregnancy, early diagnosis of fetal anomalies, screening for pre-eclampsia and preterm labor and determination of chorionicity in multiple gestation. There is no Indian law which makes it compulsory for a pregnant woman to undergo FTS, but fortunately the awareness of its importance is growing and increasingly higher numbers of women are now willingly opting for it.

FIRST TRIMESTER SCREENING

Effective screening for major aneuploidies can be provided in the first trimester of pregnancy. In the 1970s, the main method of screening for aneuploidies was by maternal age, and in the 1980s by maternal serum biochemistry and detailed ultrasonographic examination in the second trimester. In the 1990s, the emphasis shifted to the first trimester when it was realized that the great majority of fetuses with major aneuploidies can be identified by a combination of maternal age, fetal nuchal translucency (NT) thickness and maternal serum free β-human chorionic gonadotropin (β-hCG) and pregnancy-associated plasma protein-A (PAPP-A). In the last 10 years, several additional first trimester sonographic markers have been described which improve the detection rate of aneuploidies and reduce the false-positive rate.

The performance of the different methods of screening for trisomy 21 is summarized in **Table 1**.[1]

Twenty percent of pregnant women are 35 years or older, and this group constitutes 50% of trisomy 21 fetuses. Hence, half of the Down syndromes still occur in the younger age group women. Therefore, the standard of care is to perform detailed combined FTS for all pregnant women irrespective of the maternal age, and achieve a detection rate of 95% with a false-positive rate of less than 3%.[1,2]

How is FTS different in ART Pregnancies than Spontaneous Conceptions?

Although all pregnancies are *precious*, pregnancies conceived via assisted reproductive technologies (ART) are specifically considered *precious* because of related difficulty in conception and increased pregnancy complications.[3] The implications of FTS are different in ART pregnancies as compared to the spontaneous conceptions. Following may be few influencing factors:

- It can be hypothesized that women carrying pregnancies conceived via ART would be less likely to proceed to a diagnostic test because of the *precious* nature of these pregnancies and the risk of miscarriage associated with an invasive procedure. Therefore, it is of utmost importance that women conceived with ART undergo an effective noninvasive FTS with a very low false-positive rate, as the false-positive rate translates into invasive testing [chorionic villus sampling (CVS)/amniocentesis].

Table 1 Performance of methods of screening for trisomy 21[1]

Method	Detection rate (%)	False-positive rate (%)
Maternal age	30	5
First trimester		
Maternal age + nuchal translucency	75–80	5
Maternal age + double marker (PAPP-A + free β-hCG)	60–70	5
Maternal age + nuchal translucency + double marker (combined test)	85–95	5
Combined test + nasal bone/ductus venosus flow/tricuspid regurgitation (Figs 1 to 3)	93–96	2.5
Second trimester		
Maternal age + triple test (serum AFP, free β-hCG, uE3)	65–70	5
Maternal age + quadruple test (serum AFP, free β-hCG, uE3, inhibin A)	70–75	5
Integrated first and second trimester		
Maternal age + (nuchal translucency + double marker) + (quadruple marker)	90–94	5

Abbreviations: β-hCG, β-human chorionic gonadotropin; PAPP-A, pregnancy-associated plasma protein-A; AFP, alpha fetoprotein; uE3, unconjugated estriol

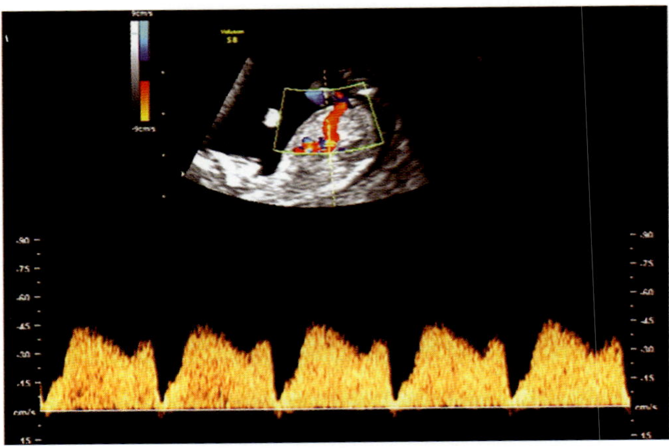

Fig. 2 Ductus venosus

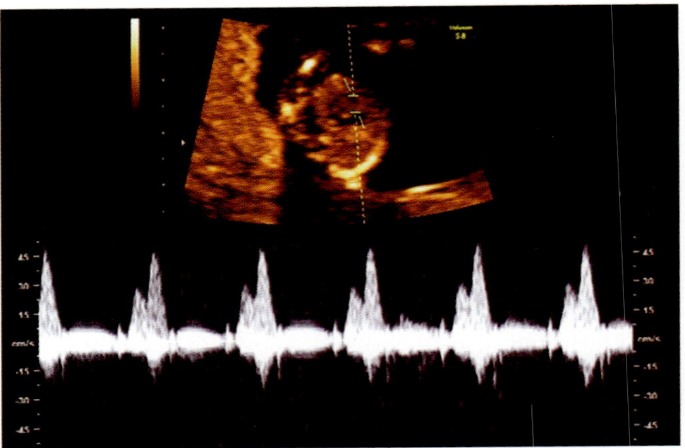

Fig. 3 Tricuspid valve flow

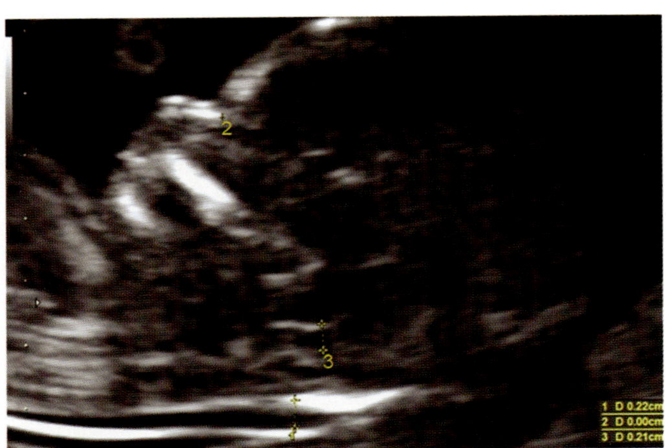

Fig. 1 Nuchal translucency and nasal bone

- The median age in women with ART conceptions is higher than that in a population of spontaneously conceived women. This also increases the anxiety among women and obstetricians, of being at an increased risk for chromosomal abnormalities due to a higher maternal age. But, it is important to note that advanced maternal age per se is not an indication for CVS or amniocentesis. In fact, the combined FTS (NT scan + double marker) performs better in the advanced maternal age group as compared to the younger women.
- Determination of a correct gestational age is an important pre-requisite for interpretation of FTS. The exact day of conception is known in pregnancies conceived after in vitro fertilization (IVF), but whether the early growth and development of the fetus

and/or placenta in these pregnancies differ from those in spontaneously conceived pregnancies is unknown.

- ART pregnancies being *precious*, there is a tendency of early withdrawal of blood sample for double marker. This remains a bias and may result in differences between the median values of double marker between ART and spontaneously conceived pregnancies.
- The higher incidence of twin/higher order pregnancies further complicates the interpretation of prenatal testing in women with ART pregnancies. ART increases the chances of dichorionic diamniotic pregnancies, due to the possibility of more than one embryo being implanted after embryo transfer. Because the overall incidence of twinning increased after ART, monochorionic twin pregnancies are also more commonly found in women conceived with ART.
- Rarely, the sample for double marker may be withdrawn immediately after the woman receives hCG injection (as a part of luteal support in some ART units). This can give a high value of free β-hCG and a false-positive double marker for Down syndrome, and trigger off an unnecessary panic.
- Vanishing twin, co-twin miscarriage, selective reduction of embryos (in higher order multifetal gestation) prior to double marker may cause confusion in interpretation of the combined FTS.
- Although, it is technically more difficult to perform selective embryo reduction at 12 weeks than at 7–9 weeks, it has an advantage of being able to differentiate the chromosomally normal fetus from the abnormal one before reduction. Also, when the FTS ultrasound is performed before reduction, the fetus is big enough to diagnose major structural abnormalities, which may be missed, if reduced at an earlier gestation (7–9 weeks). Hence, to optimize the results of *selective* embryo reduction, it is very important to carefully select a structurally and chromosomally normal embryo before the reduction.

Of the various components of FTS, the most profound effect is on PAPP-A levels, and it is found to be significantly different in ART pregnancies as compared to spontaneous ones. NT is affected to a lesser extent, and β-hCG is not significantly different among the two groups.

EFFECT OF ART ON FIRST TRIMESTER SCREENING

Cause of Infertility

It has been suggested that lower PAPP-A levels in ART pregnancies might be the result of metabolic impairments related to infertility of the mother.[4,5] However, few studies[6]

have found that PAPP-A levels were reduced, both in male-factor infertility, female-factor infertility, and the combination of female and male cause. Another group[7] found that PAPP-A values did not differ between male and female infertility. The same study group found higher median free β-hCG level values in non-male infertility compared with male infertility and spontaneous pregnancies. Various studies have found no correlation between the cause of infertility and the NT.

As of now, it is unlikely that the type of infertility affects the FTS.

Stimulation Protocol

Exogenous hormone treatment is the main reason for reduced PAPP-A levels in ART pregnancies.[7-9] When ART pregnancies conceived by exogenous hormonal stimulation are compared to those ART pregnancies without hormonal stimulation, the PAPP-A levels are significantly lower in the hormonally stimulated group. Also, the PAPP-A is reduced in hormonally-stimulated pregnancies irrespective of the type of ovarian stimulation.

A smaller NT thickness is noted in pregnancies treated with a long protocol hormone treatment compared with those with the short protocol hormone treatment. There is not any obvious biological explanation for these findings, and larger studies are needed in future to ascertain whether the difference is statistically significant so as to influence the screening risks.

Type of ART

The mode of the conception has an effect on NT: the NT thickness is thinner in IVF cases when compared with intracytoplasmic sperm injection (ICSI) cases. This is unlikely to have an effect on aneuploidy screening but warrants a thorough check of the other markers in fetuses of mother conceived by IVF, as the NT may apparently become less reliable.

Pregnancy-associated plasma protein-A concentration levels in fresh embryo transfers and frozen embryo transfers have also been studied. PAPP-A levels are reduced in both subgroups when compared with spontaneous pregnancies. However, fresh embryo transfers are associated with significantly lower PAPP-A levels as compared with FET pregnancies.[7] The additional ICSI procedure seems to produce the largest reduction in the PAPP-A level, especially after freezing and thawing of embryos. Embryos produced from ICSI are different as they have a tiny hole in the zona pellucida. The effect of ICSI, freezing and thawing might produce different effects on the placental development.[8]

Number of Oocytes Retrieved

It has been well established through large studies that there is a **greater reduction in PAPP-A following fresh embryo transfers in stimulation cycles in which a greater number of oocytes were retrieved,**[9] **further suggesting that hormone stimulation and the woman's response to hormone treatment is linked to the reduced PAPP-A.** The number of oocytes retrieved is directly proportional to the fall in PAPP-A levels, as shown in **Figure 4**.

■ EFFECT OF FTS ON ART PREGNANCY

Maternal Serum Biochemistry (PAPP-A, β-hCG)

In pregnancies affected by Down syndrome, the maternal serum level of PAPP-A is reduced to about half[10] and the level of free β-hCG is about twice as high when compared with values in chromosomally normal pregnancies.[11] Maternal serum PAPP-A and free β-hCG values are affected by the mode of conception, with values for PAPP-A being statistically significant in all studies till date. On an average, the PAPP-A in ART pregnancies is 10–18% less than the median PAPP-A in spontaneously conceived pregnancies. This is the most important factor which contributes to a high false-positive rate in ART pregnancies.

Free β-hCG values are not significantly different in ART pregnancies. But, in women with ovarian hyperstimulation, free β-hCG values are significantly higher than in women with spontaneous conception, as more number of oocytes secretes more β-hCG.

This typical trend of low PAPP-A and high free β-hCG increases chances of false-positive rates, and this may translate into unnecessary invasive testing for prenatal diagnosis of chromosomal abnormality.

Nuchal Translucency

As mentioned above, NT is lower in IVF pregnancies as compared to ICSI. Whether lower NT and lower PAPP-A is a cause or effect of the low birth weight in ART pregnancies, remains unknown.

False-positive Rates and Invasive Testing

Long-standing infertility or difficulty conceiving can evoke intense emotional responses and so consequently experiencing pregnancy loss could potentially lead to severe psychological issues. Hence, they may not be willing to take any additional risks, such as invasive testing during the pregnancy.[7,9,12-14] Therefore, it is important that the clinicians and the patients be aware that ART pregnancies may give a false-positive screening result and the pre- and post-test counseling should include this fact. This can help the couple take decisions against invasive testing based on the fact that false-positive rates are higher in these pregnancies, and they may not necessarily translate into invasive testing.

■ OTHER IMPLICATIONS OF FTS RESULTS FOR ART

The reduction in PAPP-A levels in ART pregnancies provides further evidence that ART pregnancies are different from non-ART pregnancies, an observation that may have implications beyond the combined screen. Low PAPP-A is known to be associated with severe fetal growth restriction, fetus small for gestational age and pre-eclampsia. These obstetric complications are more commonly seen in ART pregnancies as compared to spontaneous ones.[15-19] Whether low PAPP-A is a cause or result of impaired placental function and adverse pregnancy events, is unknown **(Fig. 5)**.

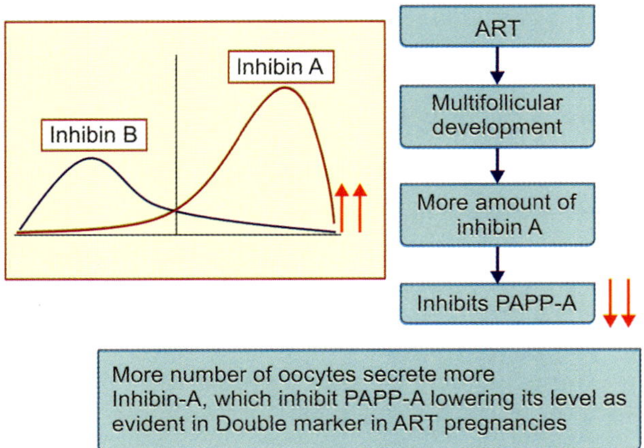

Fig. 4 Effect of response to stimulation on serum markers

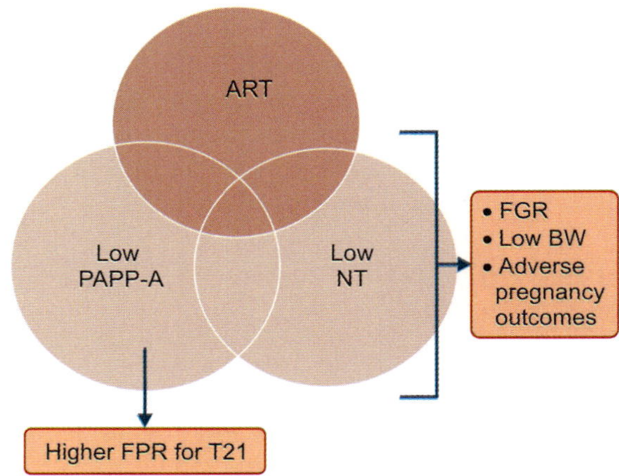

Fig. 5 Confounding factor for abnormal FTS in ART pregnancies
Abbreviations: FGR, fetal growth restriction; FPR, formyl peptide receptor

POSSIBLE EXPLANATIONS FOR DIFFERENCES IN FTS IN ART PREGNANCIES

The most marked effect of ART on FTS is reduction in PAPP-A levels. This has well been understood. Oocyte secretes inhibin which has an inhibitory effect on PAPP-A. Therefore, as the number of oocytes retrieved increased, the total Inhibin production increases and this reduces the PAPP-A. Low PAPP-A in turn gives a false-positive result for Down syndrome, increasing chances of invasive testing.

The endocrine changes that occur during early pregnancy, including the production of PAPP-A by the endometrium and placenta, are the result of a complex and poorly understood set of interactions between the corpus luteum, endometrium, placenta and embryo. Administration of exogenous hormones, occurring in fresh and artificial frozen-thawed ART cycles, interferes with the normal endocrine changes of early pregnancy, resulting in reduced PAPP-A levels. An explanation may be a delay in placental maturation because an ART pregnancy differs from spontaneously conceived pregnancies also in terms of growth and development of fetus and placenta. Moreover, a relationship with multiple corpora lutea, multiple implantation sites or drugs used in the ART treatment leading to an altered metabolism in both the fetus and the placenta has been suggested.[4,5,9]

Pregnancy-associated plasma protein-A is a growth factor that promotes growth by cleaving insulin-like growth factor binding proteins thereby increasing the bioavailability of insulin-like growth factors. When the PAPP-A is reduced, lesser insulin-like growth factors are available and this results in a low birth weight baby. The hormone treatment accompanying embryo transfers results in abnormal levels of ovarian steroid hormones and other factors yet to be identified, which in turn cause a reduction in PAPP-A production. Although PAPP-A is produced by the placenta, the reduction in PAPP-A is likely to be mediated via an effect of hormones on the endometrium because the effect is seen for hormone treatment administered prior to implantation and establishment of a placenta, possibly reflecting impairment of early implantation with some forms of ART.[15,18,19]

KEY POINTS

- Mode of conception is an important factor affecting FTS variables.
- The primary effect of ART treatment is a significant reduction in the serum PAPP-A level compared with spontaneous conceptions, whereas free β-hCG is not significantly altered.
- ART pregnancies have a lower NT than spontaneous pregnancies, and IVF conceptions have a significantly lower NT than ICSI.
- As the number of oocytes retrieved increases, the PAPP-A reduces. The amount of reduction in PAPP-A is directly proportional to the number of oocytes retrieved.
- The cause of infertility does not affect the FTS.
- Fresh embryo transfers are associated with significantly lower PAPP-A levels as compared with FET pregnancies.
- The reduction of PAPP-A is much more than the reduction in NT. Hence, there is a tendency for increase in false-positive rates for Down syndrome screening.
- Pregnancies conceived using ART are significantly less likely to be subjected to invasive testing than pregnancies conceived spontaneously in women of the same age and combined first trimester screen risk.

REFERENCES

1. Nicolaides KH. Screening for fetal aneuploidies at 11 to 13 weeks. Prenat Diagn. 2011;31:7-15.
2. Nicolaides K, Spencer K, Avgidou K, et al. Multicenter study of first trimester screening for trisomy 21 in 75 821 pregnancies: results and estimation of the potential impact of individual risk-orientated two stage first-trimester screening. Ultrasound Obstet Gynecol. 2005;25(3):221-6.
3. Harris J. Precious fertility and third-trimester tests. Prenat Diagn. 1999;19(8):753-4.
4. Maymon R, Shulman A. Serial first- and second-trimester Down's syndrome screening tests among IVF-versus naturally—conceived singletons. Hum Reprod. 2002;17(4):1081-5.
5. Maymon R, Shulman A. Integrated first- and second-trimester Down syndrome screening test among unaffected IVF pregnancies. Prenat Diagn. 2004;24(2):125-9.
6. Anckaert E, Schiettecatte J, Sleurs E, et al. First trimester screening for Down's syndrome after assisted reproductive technology: non-male factor infertility is associated with elevated free beta-human chorionic gonadotropin levels at 10–14 weeks of gestation. Fertil Steril. 2008;90(4):1206-10.
7. Amor DJ, Xu JX, Halliday JL, et al. Pregnancies conceived using assisted reproductive technologies (ART) have low levels of pregnancy-associated plasma protein-A (PAPP-A) leading to a high rate of false-positive results in first trimester screening for Down syndrome. Hum Reprod. 2009;24(6):1330-8.
8. Hui PW, Lam YH, Tang MH, et al. Maternal serum pregnancy-associated plasma protein-A and free beta-human chorionic gonadotrophin in pregnancies conceived with fresh and frozen thawed embryos from in vitro fertilization and intracytoplasmic sperm injection. Prenat Diagn. 2005;25(5):390-3.
9. Tul N, Novak-Antolic Z. Serum PAPP-A levels at 10–14 weeks of gestation are altered in women after assisted conception. Prenat Diagn. 2006;26(13):1206-11.

10. Brambati B, Macintosh MC, Teisner B, et al. Low maternal serum levels of pregnancy associated plasma protein A (PAPP-A) in the first trimester in association with abnormal fetal karyotype. Br J Obstet Gynaecol. 1993;100(4):324-6.
11. Spencer K, Macri JN, Aitken DA, et al. Free beta-hCG as first-trimester marker for fetal trisomy. Lancet. 1992;339(8807):1480.
12. Gjerris AC, Loft A, Pinborg A, et al. Prenatal testing among women pregnant after assisted reproductive techniques in Denmark 1995–2000: a national cohort study. Hum Reprod. 2008;23(7):1545-52.
13. Gjerris AC, Loft A, Pinborg A, et al. First trimester screening markers are altered in pregnancies conceived after IVF/ICSI. Ultrasound Obstet Gynecol. 2009;33(1):8-17.
14. Orlandi F, Rossi C, Allegra A, et al. First trimester screening with free beta-hCG, PAPP-A and nuchal translucency in pregnancies conceived with assisted reproduction. Prenat Diagn. 2002;22(8):718-21.
15. Giudice LC, Conover CA, Bale L, et al. Identification and regulation of the IGFBP-4 protease and its physiological inhibitor in human trophoblasts and endometrial stroma: evidence for paracrine regulation of IGF-II bioavailability in the placental bed during human implantation. J Clin Endocrinol Metab. 2002;87:2359-66.
16. Halliday J. Outcomes of IVF conceptions: are they different? Best Pract Res Clin Obstet Gynaecol. 2007;21:67-81.
17. Schieve LA, Meikle SF, Ferre C, et al. Low and very low birth weight in infants conceived with use of assisted reproductive technology. N Engl J Med. 2002;346:731-7.
18. Smith GC, Stenhouse EJ, Crossley JA, et al. Early-pregnancy origins of low birth weight. Nature. 2002;417:916.
19. Smith GCS, Shah I, Crossley JA, et al. Pregnancy-associated plasma protein A and alpha-fetoprotein and prediction of adverse perinatal outcome. Obstet Gynecol. 2006;107: 161-6.

55 Obstetric Outcome Following ART

Sunita R Tandulwadkar, Bhavana Mittal, Nirzari Mangeshikar

INTRODUCTION

The role of assisted reproductive technology (ART) increased from the 1990s. At present, nearly one child in every school class has been born after ART treatment in urban areas. Infertility has a major impact on the quality of life and the health experienced by affected couples. Psychological stress during treatment may also worsen the results of infertility treatment.[1] It has been proposed that the risks of ART may be due to underlying maternal factors associated with infertility, rather than the infertility treatment or technology.[2] It is well-documented that ART pregnancies, not only higher order births but also singletons, are at an increased risk of low birth weight, fetal growth restriction and preterm birth.[3]

The stressed infertile couple heaves a sigh of relief when they known that the pregnancy test is positive. But the next concern for the patient, family members and the treating doctor is a healthy outcome, i.e. a healthy mother and a healthy baby. The information provided to the patients on the risks of pregnancy outcomes and children's health should be accurate, to avoid adding unnecessary concerns to already stressed individuals.

The outcome of ART has been assessed by several studies over the last three decades.

To understand the obstetric outcomes following ART, we need to analyze data in four sections:

1. Comparison of pregnancy outcome in fertile vs subfertile women
2. Comparison of pregnancy outcome in subfertile women with naturally conceived pregnancies and after infertility treatment
3. Comparison of pregnancy outcome in fertile women vs ART pregnancies in subfertile women
4. Comparison of pregnancy outcome in natural conception in subfertile women/use of ovulation induction. (with or without intrauterine insemination), and use of in vitro fertilization (IVF).

COMPARISON OF PREGNANCY OUTCOME IN FERTILE VERSUS SUBFERTILE WOMEN

In a study[4] on 4,363 women, after adjusting for confounders, compared with controls, subfertile women had increased odds of:

Preeclampsia
- Antepartum hemorrhage
- Perinatal death
- Low birth weight
- Preterm birth less than 37 weeks or less than 31 weeks
- Cesarean delivery.

There was weak evidence for:
- Increased birth defects
- Gestational diabetes.

No increased risk was found for:
- Prelabor rupture of membranes
- Small for gestational age
- Postpartum hemorrhage.

Subfertile women with singleton births are at increased risk of several adverse outcomes. These risks should be considered during their antenatal care and when analyzing adverse effects of ART.

COMPARISON OF THE PREGNANCY OUTCOMES OF SUBFERTILE WOMEN AFTER INFERTILITY TREATMENT AND IN NATURALLY CONCEIVED PREGNANCIES

Altogether 428 ART pregnancies were compared with 928 spontaneously conceived pregnancies with time to pregnancy (TTP) of 2 years or more, during the period 1989–2007.

The main finding of the study was that the incidence of morbid pregnancy outcomes was similar in pregnancies conceived by ART-treated and those conceived naturally after a TTP of 2 years or more.

Outcomes of ART pregnancies have been previously compared with naturally conceived pregnancies of infertility clinic patients who had a TTP over 1 year[5] and in population-based cohorts.[6]

No difference between treated and untreated subfertile women has been reported for pregnancy duration and birth weight of primiparous women for estimates of small for gestational age.

Furthermore, a 1.1-fold risk of congenital malformations has been published.[6]

In the study of Kapiteijn et al., the rates of low and very low-birth weights, and preterm and very preterm infants born after natural pregnancies to subfertile women, were compared with the corresponding rates among women conceived after ovarian induction, IVF and controlled ovarian hyperstimulation or frozen embryo transfer in a natural cycle, which concluded that both the method and subfertility partly explained the observed impaired pregnancy outcomes, not solely subfertility.[7]

During childhood, also, psychomotor development and behavioral problems of these children has been compared, being very similar for both groups regardless of treatment.[6]

Association between a long TTP and adverse pregnancy outcomes is available in the literature. Specifically,
- 1.5–1.6-fold risk of poor neonatal health
- 1.2–2.7-fold risk of preterm birth
- 1.2-fold risk of fetal growth restriction
- 1.4–2.3-fold risk of low-birth weight
- 1.3–5-fold risk of preeclampsia
- 1.2-fold risk of congenital malformations, and
- 1.5-fold risk of cesarean section and induction of labor have been reported.[4]

Furthermore, after birth, it has also been reported associations with a 2.8-fold risk of neonatal mortality, an increased risk of a modest psychomotor developmental delay and even 1.9-fold risk of schizophrenia in the offspring. However, conflicting results showing no association between TTP and pregnancy outcome have also been published,[8] but different study design, incompletely reported TTPs and differences in populations planning pregnancies may have had a role herein.

Although the underlying mechanisms for adverse obstetric outcomes in pregnancies of subfertile women have not been resolved, possible explanations are the medical conditions that ultimately caused the subfertility, sperm factors, and in ART pregnancies, the ovarian stimulation, embryo culture and freezing (Romundstad et al. 2008).

The hypothesis of causality could be tested by, for example comparing patients treated by ART with patients treated by ovulation induction or insemination (Sutcliffe and Ludwig, 2007). One such study reported similarly reduced birth weights for both insemination pregnancies and IVF pregnancies, compared with those for fertile controls.[9] Another study comparing insemination and IVF pregnancies showed similar pregnancy duration, birth weight, cesarean section rate and need for neonatal intensive care in these groups.[10]

Recently, the question of causality has been studied by comparing subsequent pregnancies for the same woman, one after assisted-fertilization and another after spontaneous pregnancy. Interestingly, no differences were reported between these siblings. This result indicates that the adverse obstetric outcomes of ART pregnancies associate also with the underlying factors of subfertility, not only by the ART technique.[11]

In earlier studies of pregnancy outcome after ART, the comparative groups were a general obstetric population (Sutcliffe and Ludwig, 2007). Based on the present study, subfertile women who conceive without ART appear to represent a more informative reference population when the effect of the ART treatments on pregnancy outcome is the focus.

Another important finding in the current study was that women who had ART pregnancies had substantially better health behavior than women who conceived spontaneously after a long delay. Smoking, being overweight and drinking alcohol are all well-documented risk factors of subfertility.[12] Possibly, our data based on subfertile women in the general obstetric population is different from that for patients of infertility clinics:[5] these women with a long TTP may have had less knowledge of these effects and might benefit from preventive measures. On the other hand, better health-related behavior might lead to less need for using ART, and infertile couples might even be required to make lifestyle changes before active medical treatment.

Pregnancies of women with a long TTP were somewhat similar to IVF pregnancies. These results strongly support the hypothesis that the increased risks of impaired pregnancy outcomes of ART pregnancies are partly related to infertility itself, not only to the treatment.[13]

■ COMPARISON OF PREGNANCY OUTCOME IN FERTILE WOMEN VERSUS ART PREGNANCIES IN SUBFERTILE WOMEN

In accordance with the previously reported increased pregnancy risks of ART pregnancies over pregnancies in fertile women[5] Kaisa Raatikainen et al. in 2011 observed:
- 1.6–fold risk of cesarean section as the mode of delivery
- 1.5–fold risk of preterm birth

- 1.9–fold risk of low-birth weight
- 1.6–fold risk of need for neonatal intensive care.

Their results together with previously published results indicate that the adverse obstetric outcomes of ART pregnancies may be related partly to infertility itself, not to the treatment only.[11,13]

COMPARISON OF PREGNANCY OUTCOME IN NATURAL CONCEPTION IN SUBFERTILE WOMEN OR USE OF OVULATION INDUCTION (WITH OR WITHOUT INTRAUTERINE INSEMINATION) AND USE OF IN VITRO FERTILIZATION

A prospective database from a large multicenter investigation of singleton pregnancies, the first- and second-trimester evaluation of risk trial, was examined. Subjects were divided into three groups: (1) No ART use, (2) Use of ovulation induction (with or without intrauterine insemination) and (3) Use of IVF.

A total of 36,062 pregnancies were analyzed: 34,286 (95.1%) were spontaneously conceived; 1,222 (3.4%) used ovulation induction; and 554 (1.5%) used IVF.

- There was no association between ART and fetal growth restriction, aneuploidy, or fetal anomalies after adjustment for age, race, marital status, years of education, prior preterm delivery, prior fetal anomaly, body mass index, smoking history and bleeding in the current pregnancy.
- Ovulation induction was associated with a statistically significant increase in placental abruption, fetal loss after 24 weeks and gestational diabetes after adjustment.
- Use of IVF was associated with a statistically significant increase in preeclampsia, gestational hypertension, placental abruption, placenta previa and risk of cesarean delivery.

They concluded that patients who undergo IVF are at increased risk for several adverse pregnancy outcomes. Although many of these risks are not seen in patients undergoing ovulation induction, several adverse pregnancy outcomes are still increased in this group. But there was no increased incidence of fetal chromosomal or structural abnormalities in the women who used any type of ART compared with the women who conceived spontaneously (Level of evidence: II-2).[14]

CONCLUSION

The National Institute of Child Health and Human Development held a workshop on September 12–13, 2005, to summarize the risks for adverse pregnancy outcomes after ART; to develop an approach to counseling couples regarding these risks; and to establish a research agenda.

- Although the majority of ART children are normal, there are concerns about the increased risk for adverse pregnancy outcomes.
- More than 30% of ART pregnancies are twins or higher-order multiple gestations (triplets or greater) and more than half of all ART neonates are the products of multifetal gestations, with an attendant increase in prematurity complications.
- Assisted reproductive technology singleton pregnancies also demonstrate increased rates of perinatal complications—small for gestational age infants, preterm delivery and perinatal mortality—as well as maternal complications, such as preeclampsia, gestational diabetes, placenta previa, placental abruption and cesarean delivery.
- Although it is not possible to separate ART-related risks from those secondary to the underlying reproductive pathology, the overall increased frequency of obstetric complications, including preterm birth and small for gestational age neonates, should be discussed with the couple.
- Significant gaps in knowledge were identified, and the basic science and clinical and epidemiologic research required to address these gaps, is outlined.

REFERENCES

1. Ebbesen SM, Zachariae R, Mehlsen MY, et al. Stressful life events are associated with a poor in vitro fertilization (IVF) outcome: a prospective study. Hum Reprod. 2009;24(9): 2173-82.
2. Sutcliffe AG, Ludwig M. Outcome of assisted reproduction. Lancet. 2007;370(9584):351-9.
3. Reddy UM, Wapner RJ, Rebar RW, et al. Infertility, assisted reproductive technology, and adverse pregnancy outcomes: executive summary of a National Institute of Child Health and Human Development Workshop. Obstet Gynecol. 2007;109 (4):967-77.
4. Jaques AM, Amor DJ, Baker HW, et al. Adverse obstetric and perinatal outcomes in subfertile women conceiving without assisted reproductive technologies. Fertil Steril. 2010;94(7):2674-9.
5. De Geyter C, De Geyter M, Steimann S, et al. Comparative birth weights of singletons born after assisted reproduction and natural conception in previously infertile women. Hum Reprod. 2006;21(3):705-12.
6. Zhu JL, Basso O, Obel C, et al. Infertility, infertility treatment, and congenital malformations. Danish National Birth Cohort. BMJ. 2006;333(7570):679.
7. Kapiteijn K, de Bruijn CS, de Boer E, et al. Does subfertility explain the risk of poor perinatal outcome after IVF and ovarian hyperstimulation? Hum Reprod. 2006;21(12):3228-34.

8. Joffe M, Li Z. Association of time to pregnancy and the outcome of pregnancy. Fertil Steril. 1994;62(1):71-5.

9. Nuojua-Huttunen S, Gissler M Martikainen H, et al. Obstetric and perinatal outcome of pregnancies after intrauterine insemination. Hum Reprod. 1999;14(8):2110-5.

10. De Sutter P, Veldeman L, Kok P, et al. Comparison of outcome of pregnancy after intrauterine insemination (IUI) and IVF. Hum Reprod. 2005;20(6):1642-6.

11. Romundstad LB, Romundstad PR, Sunde A, et al. Effects of technology or maternal factors on perinatal outcome after assisted fertilisation: a population-based cohort study. Lancet. 2008;372(9640):737-43.

12. Homan G, Davies M, Norman R. The impact of lifestyle factors on reproductive performance in the general population and those undergoing infertility treatment: a review. Hum Reprod Update. 2007;13(3):209-23.

13. Raatikainen K, Kuivasaari-Pirinen P, Hippeläinen M, et al. Comparison of the pregnancy outcomes of subfertile women after infertility treatment and in naturally conceived pregnancies. Hum Reprod Update. 2011;27(4):1162-9.

14. Shevell T, Malone FD, Vidaver J, et al. Assisted reproductive technology and pregnancy outcome. Obstet Gynecol. 2005;106(5 Pt 1):1039-45.

56 ART to Antenatal Care

Sunita R Tandulwadkar, Parinaaz Parhar

INTRODUCTION

The absolute number of infertile couples in India is estimated to be around 17.9 million.[1] With the boom in the Indian economy and the sprouting of assisted reproductive technology (ART) centers in almost every town and city across the country, an increasing number of these infertile couples are now getting the chance to seek treatment for their condition.

Although helping a couple deemed infertile conceive is no mean feat by itself, continuation of such high-risk pregnancies to term is a challenge for most obstetricians owing to the unique nature of their conception. The adequate endocrinological support for the sustenance of such pregnancies is still a matter of much debate and research. Occurrence of certain antenatal complications, like pre-eclampsia gestational diabetes mellitus, intra-uterine growth restriction (IUGR), is increased in this population. Potential explanations for adverse obstetrical outcomes following ART are multiple gestations, increased maternal age, underlying infertility due to comorbidities like polycystic ovarian syndrome (PCOS) and obesity; increased immunological challenge in the case of donor gametes and iatrogenic reasons related to embryo culture conditions. Other conditions like ectopic gestation, multiple pregnancy and embryo reduction too are quite commonly encountered in these patients, depending on the prevailing institutional policies regarding the number of embryos transferred at a time. Besides, the increasing number of operative interventions that an infertility patient undergoes during the course of her treatment, like hysteroscopy and myomectomy, make these patients more prone to complications like incompetent os, preterm premature rupture of fetal membranes (PPROM), preterm labor, placenta previa and uterine rupture during the course of pregnancy.

Thus, it is indeed a daunting task for the obstetrician to simulate such a pregnancy as close to a spontaneous normal conception as possible and yet continue it till term.

The very "precious" nature of such pregnancies due to the whole ordeal endured for their conception leads to most consultants being overcautious in their management. A number of investigations, empirical procedures and medications are resorted to for their continuation, despite various randomized control trials proving no obvious benefit of the same. This, in turn, unnecessarily increases both the financial and the psychosocial burden associated with the continuation of such pregnancies on the couple seeking treatment.

In this chapter, we shall be discussing trimester wise, the challenges faced and their management at various stages of a pregnancy conceived with the aid of ART.

FIRST TRIMESTER

This is probably, the most tricky phase of the forthcoming 9 months. On one hand, the consultant has to try to establish and sustain this artificial conception by tapering the hormonal support to the individual's requirement, based on the number and stage of gestation and the underlying medical condition. On the other hand, conditions like ectopic gestation, anomalous baby, triplets and higher order gestation, which are detected at this stage, necessitate termination of pregnancy despite its precious nature. This leaves the obstetricians literally walking over eggshells as they try to reason against the patient's emotions, which are usually running high at this stage.

First Trimester Bleeding

First trimester bleeding might as well be called the curse of an ART conception. As opposed to spontaneous conceptions, these pregnancies seem to be at an increased risk for first trimester bleeding, probably due to the difference in implantation process following the procedure. Also, early vanishing twins (many being unrecognized) following multiple embryo transfer might be an explanation for the increased incidence of first trimester bleeding in ART pregnancies as it is seen that the incidence of this complaint is directly proportional to the number of embryos transferred. Inadequate luteal phase support for the artificially aided conception is another probable explanation for some of the cases of first trimester bleeding.

While in spontaneous pregnancies, first trimester bleeding incidence is about 20% of pregnancies,[2] after ART, the incidence is increased to 29–36%.[3-6] Such first trimester bleeding has been correlated with an increased risk for miscarriage both in spontaneous and in in vitro fertilization (IVF) pregnancies.

However, it may seem worthwhile to advise the patient to take bed rest, but in fact, there is no evidence that any precaution or treatment is beneficial. Neither progesterone[7] nor human chorionic gonadotropin (hCG) injections[8] have been demonstrated to be beneficial in improving pregnancy outcome in these cases.

Abortions

Compared to around 10–15% of all natural pregnancies ending in recognized spontaneous abortions,[9-11] a much higher incidence of spontaneous abortions is seen among ART pregnancies, in the range of 18–30%.[12-15] However, this comparison can be misleading as ART pregnancies are commonly under intense monitoring. Therefore, losses from a very early stage of such pregnancies are often carefully documented and reported, while in contrast, spontaneous abortion rates among natural conceptions can be easily underestimated.

The main reason for a higher incidence is the age of the patients, which on an average is 3–5 years higher than that of a fertile population at the time of a first pregnancy. In patients treated with ART, genetic defects, possibly due to the lack of gamete selection,[16] endometriosis,[17] obesity and high serum insulin concentration[18-20] and possibly hypersecretion of luteinizing hormone (LH)[21] all can be held responsible for the higher risk of spontaneous abortion. It is shown that the incidence of abortion in singleton IVF pregnancies drops from an overall high of 21.1 ± 12.2% at 6 weeks of gestation, when fetal heart activity is recorded to a residual risk of fetal demise at 13 weeks of gestation of 2.2%.

The only probable safeguard against abortion due to avoidable factors is to maintain adequate luteal phase support, primarily with progesterone preparations until 8–10 weeks of gestation when luteal placental transition takes place and then tapering off the hormonal support once placental function is established toward the end of first trimester.

Ectopic Gestation

The incidence of ectopic gestation in ART conceptions ranges from 2.1% to 4.8%. The incidence may vary depending on the type of ART procedure adopted with zygote intrafallopian transfer (ZIFT) associated with a higher incidence of ectopic gestations, the presence of history of pelvic inflammatory disease and tubal factor in the female partner and on the implantation potential of the embryos transferred, with embryos of high implantation potential associated with a lower risk.[22] Some studies have also found a higher risk of ectopic gestation associated with a higher volume of culture medium used at time of transfer and a higher progesterone to estradiol ratio on the day of embryo transfer. The higher incidence of ectopic gestation in ART conceptions due to the widely prevalent trend of multiple embryo transfer in several centers requires one to be ectopic minded and highly vigilant regarding the site of gestation on conception, especially in cases with disparity in the number of embryos transferred and the number of intrauterine gestational sacs visualized on first USG.

Congenital Malformations

In 1987, Lancaster first reported a greater than expected number of children with neural tube defects and transposition of the great arteries born to mothers after ART.[23] Recent meta-analyses suggest that the overall risk of major congenital malformation in children born after ART is around 30% higher than that in children conceived spontaneously.[24,25] In a study of a large cohort of children born after standard IVF and intracytoplasmic sperm injection (ICSI), the rate of major congenital malformations was around 4%, and another large prospective study comparing children born after ICSI with controls conceived spontaneously reported a relative risk of 1.24.[26,27] While there is an approximate fourfold increase in the frequency of cardiac defects and fivefold increased risk of spina bifida in children born after ART, there is also a notable increase in frequency of hypospadias in male ICSI-conceived infants.[28-30] Recently, there has reportedly been an unexpectedly high proportion of children born after assisted conception with imprinting disorders such as Beckwith-Wiedemann, Prader-Willi and Angelman syndromes **(Table 1)**.[31-36] It is unclear whether these associations are related to the underlying genetic predisposition of subfertile couples and/or to the interference of specific aspects of ART with epigenetic reprogramming during gametogenesis and early embryonic development as seen in the case of ovarian hyperstimulation with gonadotropins, the transfer

Table 1 Congenital malformations which occur with increased frequency in ART conceptions compared with spontaneous conceptions[37]

Types of malformation	Approximate OR of increased risk with ART vs spontaneous conception	Comments
All malformations	1.3–1.5	ICSI and IVF rates similar*
Cardiovascular defects	2–4	Especially cardiac septal defects
Neural tube defects	5	
Facial clefts	2	
Urogenital defects	2–5	Especially hypospadias with ICSI*
Imprinting defects	3–9	Especially Beckwith-Wiedemann syndrome

*While the rates of congenital malformations overall are similar following ICSI and IVF, there is a market association of urogenital defects, specifically hypospadias, with ICSI
Abbreviations: OR, odds ratio; ICSI, intracytoplasmic sperm injection; IVF, in vitro fertilization; ART, assisted reproductive technology

of embryos to the uterus and exposure to light, which may all be associated with epigenetic disturbance.[37]

In view of the increased risk and the precious nature of the pregnancy, it is important to screen such pregnancies for congenital anomalies at the earliest when termination is still an option and acceptable to the couple. First trimester screening tests like nuchal translucency and double marker tests and second trimester tests like triple test, quad test and detailed late second trimester anomaly scan are noninvasive, hence indispensable. Only patients considered to be at high risk for anomaly by these tests are subjected to the confirmatory invasive tests like amniocentesis and chorionic villus biopsy.

The clinical application of preimplantation genetic diagnosis must balance the benefits of avoiding disease transmission with the medical risks and financial burden of in vitro fertilization. In addition, men with severe oligozoospermia or azoospermia should be offered genetic or clinical counseling and offered karyotyping for chromosomal abnormalities before attempting IVF-ICSI allowing those affected to consider the option of donor insemination.

Multiple Gestations

At the European Society of Human Reproduction and Embryology (ESHRE) consensus meeting on risks and complications in ART in Maastricht on May 2002, it was agreed that the essential aim of IVF/ICSI is the birth of one single healthy child, with a twin pregnancy being regarded as a complication due to the associated high risk of maternal and perinatal complications.[38] Inspite of this, many physicians and patient couples continue to underestimate the risks associated with twin pregnancies and even today globally 25% of all pregnancies after IVF/

ICSI are twin pregnancies, 40% of all babies born after ART are born as part of a twin pair. Multiple gestations are the prime reason why ART-aided conceptions are so prone to obstetric complications despite being under constant surveillance. Although dichorionic twins are most common, the incidence of monochorionic twins is also increased. IVF pregnancies that occur after transferring blastocyst (5 days after fertilization) embryos are more often associated with monozygotic twinning (6%) than pregnancies that occur after transferring cleavage-stage (2–3 days after fertilization) embryos (2%).[39-41] Risks of multiple pregnancies include higher rates of perinatal mortality, preterm birth, low birth weight, gestational hypertension, placental abruption, placenta previa, and postpartum hemorrhage. Besides, parents of multiple births have more stress, and siblings of multiples are more likely to have behavior problems.[42,43]

In order to reduce the number of twin pregnancies after ART, elective single embryo transfer (eSET) has been introduced[44] with the primary aim of reducing the multiple pregnancy rate while maintaining an acceptable overall pregnancy rate. Patients with good prognosis for eSET are those who are less than 36 years of age, in their first or second ART cycle, and who have at least one good quality embryo. Hence, ESHRE 2002 consensus recommendations are:[38]

- eSET should be performed if a twin pregnancy is contraindicated and/or if a couple wishes to avoid a twin pregnancy at any cost.
- eSET should be proposed in a first or second IVF/ICSI cycle in women less than 36 years of age if at least one good quality embryo is available.
- Counseling for eSET should be done well in advance of embryo transfer, and in the ART center, the whole staff

should be convinced of the importance of avoiding twin pregnancies.

- Spare good quality embryos should be cryopreserved.

There is an urgent need for national guidelines to be developed to regulate the number of embryos transferred according to characteristics such as patient's age and grade of embryos.

Fetal reduction for high-order multiple pregnancies is a very difficult decision for couples who have gone through fertility treatment, particularly when the procedure may result in loss of the entire pregnancy. Even when successful, fetal reduction may have long-term adverse emotional consequences for the couple. Compared with spontaneously conceived twin pregnancies, twin pregnancies remaining after fetal reduction have a threefold to fourfold increase in low birth weight, very low birth weight and fetal growth restriction.

Fetal reduction is, however, still necessary, in spite of the associated risks, in order to improve the perinatal outcome of the surviving fetuses besides decreasing the maternal risks associated with higher order gestation. It involves an ultrasound-guided termination of the most accessible fetus using pharmacological agents like potassium chloride. These agents are instilled into the targeted fetal heart via a needle stab through transabdominal or transvaginal route until complete cessation of targeted fetal cardiac activity is obtained. At our center, we prefer to aspirate the intracardiac fetal blood until cessation of cardiac activity to eliminate the risk associated with accidental injection of toxic substances like potassium chloride into maternal circulation. The procedure is usually scheduled around 11–12 weeks of gestation. The dual purpose achieved by this is that firstly, by this age spontaneous fetal abortions which were to occur would have occurred and secondly by now the first trimester nuchal translucency scan is performed enabling selective fetal reduction of any anomalous fetus if present.

■ SECOND AND THIRD TRIMESTER

Preterm Labor and PPROM

Compared to spontaneous conception, ART pregnancies are at an increased risk of preterm delivery. The higher rate is mostly due to the higher incidence of multiple gestations, but it may also be attributed to various infertility cofactors such as uterine malformations, previous operative procedures that involved cervical dilatation and a history of pelvic infection. Especially, forceful cervical dilatation for operative hysteroscopy may lead to iatrogenic cervical incompetence. This observation is probably what prompts a number of obstetricians to prophylactically perform a cervical cerclage in ART conceptions despite no supportive evidence regarding its effectiveness.

The high stakes associated with such conceptions and the acknowledged higher risk of prematurity and preterm premature rupture of membranes (PPROM) lead to an increased number of practitioners administering steroids prophylactically for fetal lung maturity once conception has crossed the period of viability. Complications, such as premature rupture of membranes, are also more conservatively managed under higher antibiotic cover for as long as maternal and fetal condition permits.

Pre-eclampsia and IUGR

There is almost twofold to threefold increased risk of pre-eclampsia in IVF conceptions.[45-48] This increased risk may be due to the increased age of the IVF conceived patients, associated comorbidities like obesity and PCOS, and the higher incidence of multiple gestations which are seen in these pregnancies. The high incidence of pre-eclampsia in these patients in turn increases the incidence of intrauterine growth restriction (IUGR) in them.

However, the increased scrutiny and surveillance of these patients are subjected to due to the precious nature of the pregnancy, permits early diagnosis and a closer and better monitoring of maternal and fetal condition. Fetal growth restriction consequent to fetal reduction might represent placental insufficiency or be the result of abnormal implantation of the higher number of embryos. In addition, residual placental tissue from the reduced fetuses may promote a subclinical inflammatory response leading to preterm birth.

Diabetes Mellitus

Gestational diabetes mellitus is a relatively frequent complication in ART conceptions due to the demographic profile of the affected population, which is elderly, obese and may have underlying insulin resistance associated with PCOS. Many of these patients may have diabetes mellitus as the underlying cause of infertility that required treatment. Due to the high perinatal mortality associated with this condition if uncontrolled, it is extremely important to closely monitor the blood sugar levels while avoiding hypoglycemia which can be equally threatening. However, while diabetologists usually term A HbA_{1c} levels of 6.5–7% satisfactory control, obstetricians treating such patients usually aim for a better control with values below 6.2%. Many of them prefer using an insulin pump to help achieve a better control over blood sugar levels.

Antepartum Hemorrhage

A higher incidence of placenta previa and abruption placentae is associated with IVF conceptions. When pregnancy and the formation of the chorion are initiated in vitro, an inherent difference in the nature of the placenta itself may predispose the patient to develop these complications during gestation. Besides, according to some studies, since in ART embryos are placed in the uterine cavity by a catheter via the transcervical route, this procedure may induce uterine contraction, possibly due to the release of prostaglandins after mechanical stimulation of the internal cervical os.[49-51] Probably, these mechanically induced uterine contractions lead to higher frequencies of implantation in the lower uterine segment and thereby increase the risk of placenta previa. In addition, it may be a result of the large surface area of the placenta in multiple gestations encroaching on the lower uterine segment.

Cesarean Sections

Cesarean section is usually the preferred mode of delivery in IVF conceptions. Compared with spontaneous conception, singleton and twin pregnancies following IVF and IVF-ICSI have a twofold increased rate of induction of labor and cesarean delivery.[27,52,53] IVF-ICSI twin pregnancies are more likely to have cesarean delivery than IVF-ICSI singleton pregnancies, a trend also seen in spontaneously conceived pregnancies. This is attributable more to the obstetrician and patient preference than being a necessity due to the associated obstetric indications like placenta previa, malpresentation, fetal distress. Patient anxiety and the overcautious approach of the treating obstetrician are responsible for the increasing trend of elective cesarean sections in ART conceptions. However, patients with history of myomectomy leading to cavity entry during the course of infertility treatment make elective section at term essential.

■ CONCLUSION

Pregnancy post-ART conceptions might seem like the realization of a lifetime dream for an infertile couple. It is up to the treating obstetricians to realize and emphasize that it is just a part of their battle against infertility being won. The definite goal of delivering a healthy, term baby is still closely monitored three trimesters away, during which both the patient and the treating doctor will have to closely supervise the progress.

This does not mean that the couple should be burdened with the stress of the anxiety related to a healthy outcome. The couple needs to be well educated regarding the need to be cautious and to come for frequent and regular follow-up to rule out any impending complication while still in the initial treatable stages.

Most couples would be ready to go to great extents to follow the treating obstetricians' advice to ensure a healthy baby, especially if it is the same infertility specialist who made the miracle of pregnancy possible. This makes the doctor even more morally responsible to not subject the couple to any unnecessarily painful and traumatic treatments and investigations which might snatch away the very joy of experiencing what would probably be a once in a lifetime experience for these couples, while still maintaining a close vigil.

As we have already seen, the high risk nature of the pregnancy due to the age distribution of the patients and their coexisting comorbidities poses them at great risk for complications, and in need of close surveillance throughout pregnancy. An extremely meticulous yet caring and empathic approach by the entire treating team is what can make this apparently tedious routine a pleasant path and route to the couples' goal of a healthy bundle of joy.

■ REFERENCES

1. Shivaraya M, Halemani M. Infertility: psychosocial consequences of infertility on women in India. Indian Journal of Social Development. 2007;7(2);309-16.
2. Everett C. Incidence and outcome of bleeding before the 20th week of pregnancy: prospective study from general practice. BMJ. 1997;315:32-4.
3. Goldman JA, Ashkenazi J, Ben-David M, et al. First trimester bleeding in clinical IVF pregnancies. Hum Reprod. 1988;3(6):807-9.
4. Dantas ZN, Singh AP, Karachalios P, et al. Vaginal bleeding and early pregnancy outcome in an infertile population. J Assist Reprod Genet. 1996;13(3):212-5.
5. Hofmann GE, Gundrun C, Drake L, et al. Frequency and effect of vaginal bleeding on pregnancy outcome during the first 3 weeks after positive beta-hCG test results following IVF-ET. Fertil Steril. 2000;74(3):609-13.
6. Pezeshki K, Feldman J, Stein DE, et al. Bleeding and spontaneous abortion after therapy for infertility. Fertil Steril. 2000;74(3):504-8.
7. Oates-Whitehead RM, Haas DM, Carrier JAK. Progestogen for preventing miscarriage [Cochrane review]. The Cochrane Library. Chichester, UK: John Wiley & Sons, Ltd.; 2003.
8. Qureshi NS, Edi-Osagie EC, Ogbo V, et al. First trimester threatened miscarriage treatment with human chorionic gonadotrophins: a randomised controlled trial. BJOG. 2005;112(11):1536-41.
9. Wilcox AJ, Treloar AE, Sandler DP. Spontaneous abortion over time: comparing occurrence in two cohorts of women a generation apart. Am J Epidemiol. 1981;14(4):548-53.

10. Risch HA, Weiss NS, Clarke EA, et al. Risk factors for spontaneous abortion and its recurrence. Am J Epidemiol. 1988;128(2):420-30.

11. Nybo Andersen AM, Wohlfahrt J, Christens P, et al. Maternal age and fetal loss: population based register linkage study. Br Med J. 2000;320(7251):1708-12.

12. Seppälä M. The world collaborative report on in vitro fertilization and embryo replacement: current state of the art in January 1984. Ann N Y Acad Sci. 1985;442:558-63.

13. Saunders DM, Lancaster P. The wider perinatal significance of the Australian in vitro fertilization data collection program. Am J Perinatol. 1989;6(2):252-7.

14. Liu HC, Jones GS, Jones HW Jr, et al. Mechanisms and factors of early pregnancy wastage in in vitro fertilization-embryo transfer patients. Fertil Steril. 1988;50(1):95-101.

15. Breart G, de Mouzon J. Assisted reproduction vigilance. Bull Acad Natl Med. 1995;179(8):1759-64.

16. Koulischer L, Verloes A, Lesenfants S, et al. Genetic risk in natural and medically assisted procreation. Early Pregnancy. 1997;3(3):164-71.

17. Dicker D, Goldman JA, Levy T, et al. The impact of long-term gonadotropin-releasing hormone analogue treatment on preclinical abortions in patients with severe endometriosis undergoing in vitro fertilization-embryo transfer. Fertil Steril. 1992;57(3):597-600.

18. Craig LB, Ke R, Kutteh W. Increased prevalence of insulin resistance in women with a history of recurrent pregnancy loss. Fertil Steril. 2002;78(3):487-90.

19. Hamilton-Fairley D, Kiddy D, Watson H, et al. Association of moderate obesity with a poor pregnancy outcome in women with polycystic ovary syndrome treated with low dose gonadotrophin. Br J Obstet Gynecol. 1992;99(2):128-31.

20. Wang JX, Davies MJ, Norman RJ. Obesity increases the risk of spontaneous abortion during infertility treatment. Obes Res. 2002;10(6):551-4.

21. van Hooff M, Schoute E, Schoemaker J, et al. Hypersecretion of luteinizing hormone (LH) and ovarian steroids in women with recurrent abortion. Hum Reprod. 1994;9(1):179-80.

22. Clayton H, Schieve L, Peterson H, et al. Ectopic pregnancy risk with assisted reproductive technology. Obstetrics & Gynecology. 2006;107(3):595-604.

23. Lancaster PAL. Congenital malformations after in-vitro fertilization. Lancet. 1987;2:1392-3.

24. Rimm AA, Katayama AC, Diaz M, et al. A meta-analysis of controlled studies comparing major malformation rates in IVF and ICSI infants with naturally conceived children. J Assist Reprod Genet. 2004;21(12):437-43.

25. Hansen M, Bower C, Milne E, et al. Assisted reproductive technologies and the risk of birth defects—a systematic review. Hum Reprod. 2005;20(2):328-38.

26. Bonduelle M, Liebaers I, Deketelaere V, et al. Neonatal data on a cohort of 2889 infants born after ICSI (1991–1999) and of 2995 infants born after IVF (1983–1999). Hum Reprod. 2002;17(3):671-94.

27. Katalinic A, Rosch C, Ludwig M. Pregnancy course and outcome after intracytoplasmic sperm injection: a controlled, prospective cohort study. Fertil Steril. 2004;81:1604-16.

28. Kallen B, Finnstrom O, Nygren KG, et al. In vitro fertilization (IVF) in Sweden: risk for congenital malformation after different IVF methods. Birth Defects Res A Clin Mol Teratol. 2005;73(3):162-9.

29. Kurinczuk JJ, Bower C. Birth defects in infants conceived by intracytoplasmic sperm injection: an alternative interpretation. BMJ. 1997;315:1260-5.

30. Koivurova S, Hartikainen AL, Gissler M, et al. Neonatal outcome and congenital malformations in children born after in-vitro fertilization. Hum Reprod. 2002;17(5):1391-8.

31. Sutcliffe AG, Peters CJ, Bowdin S, et al. Assisted reproductive therapies and imprinting disorders—a preliminary British survey. Hum Reprod. 2006;21(4):1009-11.

32. Ludwig M, Katalinic A, Gross S, et al. Increased prevalence of imprinting defects in patients with Angelman syndrome born to subfertile couples. J Med Genet. 2005;42(4):289-91.

33. Lim D, Bowdin SC, Tee L, et al. Clinical and molecular genetic features of Beckwith-Wiedemann syndrome associated with assisted reproductive technologies. Hum Reprod. 2009;24(3):741-7.

34. Maher ER. Imprinting and assisted reproductive technology. Hum Mol Genet. 2005;14 Spec No 1:R133-8.

35. DeBaun MR, Niemitz EL, Feinberg AP. Association of in vitro fertilization with Beckwith-Wiedemann syndrome and epigenetic alterations of *LIT1* and *H19*. Am J Hum Genet. 2003;72(1):156-60.

36. Halliday J, Oke K, Breheny S, et al. Beckwith-Wiedemann syndrome and IVF: a case-control study. Am J Hum Genet. 2004;75(3):526-8.

37. Williams C, Sutcliffe A, Sebire NJ. Congenital malformations after assisted reproduction: risks and implications for prenatal diagnosis and fetal medicine. Ultrasound Obstet Gynecol. 2010;35:255-9.

38. Land JA, Evers JL. Risks and complications in assisted reproduction techniques: report of an ESHRE consensus meeting. Human Reprod. 2003;18(2):455-7.

39. Blickstein I. Estimation of iatrogenic monozygotic twinning rate following assisted reproduction: pitfalls and caveats. Am J Obstet Gynecol. 2005;192(2):365-8.

40. Schachter M, Raziel A, Friedler S, et al. Monozygotic twinning after assisted reproductive techniques: a phenomenon independent of micromanipulation. Hum Reprod. 2001;16(6):1264-9.

41. Milki AA, Jun SH, Hinckley MD, et al. Incidence of monozygotic twinning with blastocyst compared to cleavage-stage transfer. Fertil Steril. 2003;79(3):503-6.

42. Cook R, Bradley S, Golombok, S. A preliminary study of parental stress and child behaviour in families with twins conceived by in-vitro fertilization. Hum Reprod. 1998;13(11):3244-6.

43. Hay DA, McIndoe R, O'Brien PJ. The older sibling of twins. Aust J Early Child. 1988;13:25-8.

44. Vilska S, Tiitinen A, HydeÂn-Granskog C, et al. Elective transfer of one embryo results in acceptable pregnancy rate and eliminates the risk of multiple birth. Hum Reprod. 1999;14(9):2392-5.

45. Jackson RA, Gibson KA, Wu YW, et al. Perinatal outcomes in singletons following in vitro fertilization: a meta-analysis. Obstet Gynecol. 2004;103(3):551-63.

46. Schieve LA, Rasmussen SA, Buck GM, et al. Are children born after assisted reproductive technology at increased risk for adverse health outcomes? Obstet Gynecol. 2004;103(6):1154-63.

47. Wang JX, Knottnerus AM, Schuit G, et al. Surgically obtained sperm, and risk of gestational hypertension and pre-eclampsia. Lancet. 2002;359(9307):673-4.

48. Maman E, Lunenfeld E, Levy A, et al. Obstetric outcome of singleton pregnancies conceived by in vitro fertilization and ovulation induction compared with those conceived spontaneously. Fertil Steril. 1998;70(2):240-5.

49. Fraser IS. Prostaglandins, prostaglandin inhibitors and their roles in gynecological disorders. Baillieres Clin Obstet Gynaecol. 1992;6:829-57.

50. Fanchin R, Righini C, Olivennes F, et al. Uterine contractions at the time of embryo transfer alter pregnancy rates after in-vitro fertilization. Hum Reprod. 1998;13(7):1968-74.

51. Mansour R. Minimizing embryo expulsion after embryo transfer: a randomized controlled study. Hum Reprod. 2005;20(1):170-4.

52. Helmerhorst FM, Perquin DA, Donker D, et al. Perinatal outcome of singletons and twins after assisted conception: a systematic review of controlled studies. BMJ. 2004;328:261.

53. Smithers PR, Halliday J, Hale L, et al. High frequency of cesarean section, antepartum hemorrhage, placenta previa, and preterm delivery in in-vitro fertilization twin pregnancies. Fertil Steril. 2003;80(3):666-8.

57 Ovarian Hyperstimulation Syndrome

Nalini Mahajan

Ovarian hyperstimulation syndrome (OHSS) is a dreaded, potentially fatal[1] and in most parts an iatrogenic complication of ovarian stimulation. The incidence has been estimated at 3–6% for moderate, and 0.1–2% for severe OHSS.[2] It is mainly associated with the multifollicular response encountered in gonadotropin stimulations but can occur with use of clomiphene citrate and gonadotropin-releasing hormone (GnRH). Spontaneous OHSS[3] occurring in natural conception is rare, but cases have been reported.

Ovarian hyperstimulation syndrome is characterized by cystic enlargement of the ovaries, and transudation of fluid and proteins from the intravascular compartment into the third space due to increased capillary permeability. The trigger for initiation of this reaction appears to be human chorionic gonadotropin (hCG). OHSS is a self-limiting disorder and usually resolves spontaneously within 7–10 days. In conception cycles, symptoms may persist longer due to endogenous hCG stimulus. The clinical presentation can vary from mild to severe life threatening symptoms requiring hospital admission in 1.9% of cases.[4]

■ PATHOPHYSIOLOGY

The pathophysiology of this condition is still not completely elucidated, but it is believed to be mediated by an excessive secretion of vasoactive peptides and steroids from the hyperstimulated corpora lutea. Some of the factors that contribute to this condition are:[5]

- An increased secretion or exudation of protein-rich fluid from enlarged ovaries or peritoneal surfaces.
- Increased follicular fluid levels of prorenin and renin.
- Angiotensin-mediated changes in capillary permeability.

Vascular endothelial growth factor (VEGF), a member of the transforming growth factor β (TGF-β) superfamily, also known as vascular permeability factor, has emerged as one of the factors most likely involved in the pathophysiology of OHSS.[6] An angiogenic cytokine, it is known to stimulate the vascular endothelium and plays an integral role in follicular growth and ovarian angiogenesis.

It has been well established that the trigger for OHSS is hCG which appears to acts via VEGF. VEGF increases vascular permeability by interacting with its VEGF receptor 2 (VEGFR-2) allowing egress of protein rich fluid **(Fig. 1)**. It has been observed that hCG stimulates VEGF expression in granulosa cells, there is an increase in VEGF mRNA levels.[7] Blood levels of VEGF also correlate with the severity of OHSS.

Other factors like angiotensin II, insulin-like growth factor 1 (IGF-1), epidermal growth factor (EGF), TGFs α and β, basic fibroblast growth factor (BFGF), platelet-derived growth factor (PDGF), interleukin-1b (IL-1b), and interleukin-6 (IL-6) may also play a part in the pathogenesis either directly or via VEGF.[5]

Spontaneous OHSS has been reported to develop between 8 weeks and 14 weeks of amenorrhea in multiple pregnancies, molar pregnancies, pregnant women affected by hypothyroidism, polycystic ovary syndrome, gonadotropin-producing pituitary adenoma and also in normal pregnancies. Mutations of FSH receptors have been implicated as a cause for spontaneous OHSS.[8] Di Carlo et al. 2012 reported[9] a case of spontaneous, familial, recurrent OHSS in a 26-year-old primipara whose first-degree cousin, paternal grandmother and a number of other members of her father's family had suffered from a similar condition which points to a genetic predisposition.

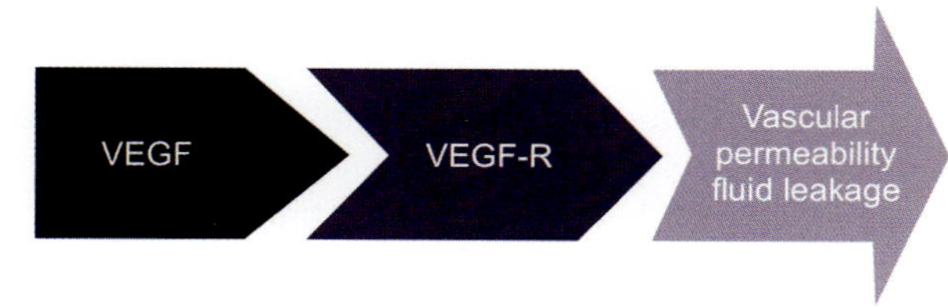

Fig. 1 VEGF in the pathogenesis of OHSS

CLINICAL PRESENTATION AND CLASSIFICATION OF OVARIAN HYPERSTIMULATION SYNDROME

Two forms of OHSS are described based on the onset of symptoms. Early OHSS occurs 2–3 days after oocyte retrieval (OR) as a result of the initial hCG trigger. Late OHSS occurs after 10 days of OR/7 days after embryo transfer (ET) in response to endogenous hCG secretion subsequent to successful implantation.[10] It can also be the result of hCG used for luteal support.

Patient can present with lower abdominal pain, mild distension, nausea, vomiting, or diarrhea in mild cases. With progression of disease accumulation of fluid in the abdomen leads to further distension, and eventually tense ascites. Nausea and vomiting increase, there is increasing tachypnea and decreased urinary output. Weight gain can be rapid, more than 1 kg/day. Ultrasound examination shows enlarged ovaries, and presence of ascites. Blood tests show hemoconcentration, elevated leukocytes, altered liver enzymes, electrolyte imbalance (hyperkalemia and hyponatremia), and in extreme cases increased creatinine levels. In severe OHSS, fluid can be seen in the pleural and pericardial cavities, leading to intense respiratory discomfort and hypovolemia. Life-threatening complications include hepatorenal failure, acute respiratory distress syndrome, hemorrhage from ovarian rupture and thromboembolism.[11]

Extravasation of protein-rich fluid and contraction of the vascular volume leads to hypotension, which in turn leads to reduced renal perfusion resulting in oliguria and anuria. Tense ascites elevates the diaphragm causing pulmonary compromise which is further aggravated by hydrothorax. Hemoconcentration and decreased peripheral blood flow increases the risk of thromboembolism.

Traditionally two classification have been used, Golan's classification in 1989 and that proposed by Rizk and Aboulghar in 1999. A recent classification more objectively related to symptoms than previous classifications **(Table 1)** incorporates vaginal ultrasound and laboratory parameters.[12] Mild, moderate and severe forms are distinguished by the extent of fluid shift into body cavities. Moderate OHSS involves fluid shifts of less than 500 mL. Severe OHSS involves presence of hemoconcentration and hypovolemia, and an alteration in the laboratory parameters. Since subjective signs and symptoms such as discomfort, pain, nausea, and vomiting, vary in individual cases, they have not been assigned to a particular grade of OHSS.

Golan Classification

- *Mild OHSS*
  - Grade 1, abdominal distension and discomfort
  - Grade 2, features of grade 1 plus nausea, vomiting and/or diarrhea; ovaries are enlarged from 5 cm to 12 cm
- *Moderate OHSS*
  - Grade 3, features of mild OHSS plus ultrasonic evidence of ascites
- *Severe OHSS*
  - Grade 4, features of moderate OHSS plus evidence of ascites and/or hydrothorax and breathing difficulties
  - Grade 5, all of the above, plus change in the blood volume, increased blood viscosity due to hemoconcentration, coagulation abnormality and diminished renal perfusion and function.

Rizk and Aboulghar Classification

- *Moderate OHSS*
  - Discomfort, pain, nausea, abdominal distension
  - No clinical evidence of ascites, but ultrasonic evidence of ascites and enlarged ovaries
  - Normal hematological and biological profiles
- *Severe OHSS*
  Grade A
  - Dyspnea, oliguria, nausea, vomiting, diarrhea, abdominal pain
  - Clinical evidence of ascites plus marked distension of abdomen or hydrothorax
  - Ultrasound scan showing large ovaries and marked ascites
  - Normal biochemical profiles
  Grade B
  - All symptoms of grade A, plus
  - Massive tension ascites, markedly enlarged ovaries, severe dyspnea and marked oliguria
  - Biochemical changes—increased hematocrit, increased creatinine and liver dysfunction
  Grade C
  - OHSS complicated by RDS, renal shutdown or venous thrombosis.

Categorization for Treatment

- Moderate OHSS—could be treated on outpatient basis with extreme vigilance
- Severe OHSS Grade A—inpatient or outpatient setting, depending on the physician's comfort, the patient's compliance and the medical facility

Table 1 Proposed new clinical grading system for OHSS

	Mild	Moderate	Severe
Objective criteria			
Fluid in Douglas pouch	✓	✓	✓
Fluid around uterus (major pelvis)		✓	✓
Fluid around intestinal loops			✓
Hematocrit >45%		✓a	✓
White blood cells >15,000/mm³		±a	✓
Low urine output <600 mL/24 h		±a	✓
Creatinine >1.5 mg/dL		±a	±
Elevated transaminases		±a	±
Clotting disorder			±c
Pleural effusion			±c
Subjective criteria			
Abdominal distention	✓	✓	✓
Pelvic discomfort	✓	✓	✓
Breathing disorder	±b	±b	✓
Acute pain	±b	±b	±b
Nausea/vomiting	±	±	±
Ovarian enlargement	✓	✓	✓
Pregnancy occurrence	±	±	✓

Note: The ± sign means may or may not be present.
Source: Humaidan P, Quartarolo J, Papanikolaou EG. Preventing ovarian hyperstimulation syndrome: guidance for the clinician. Fertil Steril. 2010;94:389-400.
a.   If two of these are present, consider hospitalization.
b.   If present, consider hospitalization.
c.   If present, consider intensive care.

- Severe OHSS Grade B—would be treated in an inpatient hospital setting with expert supervision
- Severe OHSS Grade C—which is critical, would be treated in an intensive care setting.

Identifying the Patient at Risk

Identification of risk factors is critical for prevention of OHSS as corrective measures can be taken before the onset of full blown disease. Predictive factors for OHSS can be divided into:
- *Primary risk factors:* Inherently present or identifiable before stimulation.
- *Secondary risk factors:* It become obvious during ovarian stimulation when patients with no known predisposing factors experience an excessive response to treatment.

Primary Risk Factors

- Young age
- Low body weight

- Polycystic ovary syndrome (PCOS), or isolated PCOS characteristics because of increased number of recruitable follicles
- History of previous OHSS, or increased response to gonadotropin therapy.

Unfortunately, there are no tests that can accurately predict OHSS but hormonal and ultrasound markers have been examined as predictors of ovarian response. Anti-Müllerian hormone (AMH) and antral follicle count (AFC) are two such markers that have shown great promise. AMH is expressed in the granulosa cells of preantral and small antral follicles and is a measure of ovarian reserve and a reliable predictor of ovarian response.[13] Lee et al. 2008 in a study[14] of 262 in vitro fertilization (IVF) cycles with 21 cases (8%) of moderate or severe OHSS found that baseline serum AMH levels were significantly correlated with development of OHSS [odds ratio (OR) 1.7856; p = 0.0004). An AMH cutoff value of 3.36 ng/mL gave a sensitivity of 90.5% and a specificity of 81.3% for prediction of OHSS.

Antral follicle count of greater than or equal to 12 antral follicles 2–8 mm in diameter is a diagnostic criteria of PCOS and an AFC of more than 14 may predict hyper-response to IVF treatment with a sensitivity of 0.82 and a specificity of 0.89.[15]

Secondary Risk Factors

Factors which become apparent during stimulation include:

- Absolute levels of estradiol (E2) greater than or equal to 3000 pg/mL or rate of increase of serum E2
- Follicular size and number (greater than or equal to 20) on both ovaries
- Number of oocytes collected.

It has been suggested that a combination of the above parameters may better predict OHSS. However, independently or together their accuracy is limited. Other factors being studied for their predictive ability are VEGF, inhibin B (increased inhibin B production may prime the follicle to over respond to hCG) and interleukins.

■ OVARIAN HYPERSTIMULATION SYNDROME PREVENTION

Any physician who has had to deal with severe OHSS would whole heartedly endorse the old adage that "Prevention is better than cure". Unfortunately, the measures for prevention available so far have not been very effective unless the cycle itself was canceled. Two seminal events changed this: introduction of GnRH antagonist which allowed use of GnRH agonist as ovulation trigger and the discovery that the dopamine agonist cabergoline (Cb2) could counter the increased vascular permeability by dephosphorylation of the VEGF2 receptor thus reducing the fluid shift[16] **(Fig. 2)**. Introduction and effectiveness of vitrification as a cryopreservation technique proved to be an additional boon. Use of antagonist cycle with an agonist trigger and elective vitrification of all embryos allows us to aim for an "OHSS Free" clinic today.

Prevention strategies can be divided into two types—primary and secondary.[12]

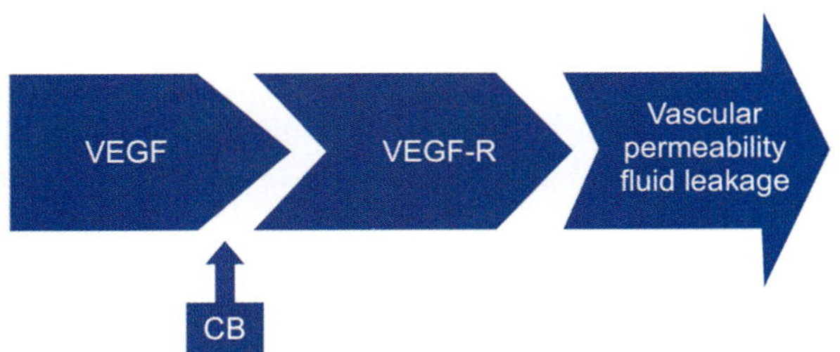

Fig. 2 Level of action of cabergoline in the prevention of OHSS

Primary prevention, involves using individualized ovarian stimulation protocols based on assessment of ovarian response using AMH, AFC, body mass index (BMI) and age as markers.

Secondary prevention methods are used to avoid progression to OHSS during stimulation.

Primary Prevention

Reducing Dose of Gonadotropin

Use of individualized stimulation protocols based on assessment of OR and response in assisted reproductive technology (ART) cycles, administration of chronic low dose protocol to promote monofollicular growth in ovulation induction cycles and soft stimulation to get 2–3 follicles in intrauterine insemination (IUI) cycles, aids in OHSS prevention.

Use of Gonadotropin-releasing Hormone Antagonist Protocols

Use of GnRH agonists in ART protocols lead to higher E2 levels and an increased incidence of OHSS [4.5% compared with 0.6% for non-GnRH agonists/human menopausal gonadotropin (hMG) cycles].[17] This was largely due to the increased dose of gonadotropins required for stimulation and in some part due to prevention of atresia of smaller antral follicles due to pituitary downregulation.[18]

The GnRH antagonist protocol has two advantages over agonist, one pituitary suppression is started after stimulation thus lower doses of gonadotropins can be used and two GnRH agonist trigger can be used for final oocyte maturation. Cochrane review 2011[19] demonstrated the lower incidence of OHSS with GnRH antagonist (29 trials: OR 0.43; 95% CI 0.33–0.57; p <0.00001). There was no evidence of a statistically significant difference in rates of live-births (OR 0.86; 95% CI 0.69–1.08) or ongoing pregnancy (OR 0.87; 95% CI 0.7–1.00). Severity of OHSS is also reduced with hospital admissions being significantly lower (OR, 0.46; 95% CI, 0.26–0.82; p = 0.01).

Avoid Human Chorionic Gonadotropin for Luteal Phase Support

Luteal phase support is essential in ART as the supra-physiological steroid levels (E2 and progesterone) lead to a negative feedback on the pituitary resulting in early luteolysis with reduced implantation rate, pregnancy rates, and an increased early pregnancy loss. Luteal support is given with progesterone and frequently hCG. Addition of hCG increases the risk of developing OHSS. Progesterone alone can be used without compromising results.[20]

In Vitro Maturation

In vitro maturation (IVM) has been promoted for patients with PCOS; however, the technical skill required coupled with lower pregnancy rates (10%) in most hands has limited its use. Some centers have reported pregnancy rates of between 20% and 54%.

Insulin-sensitizing Agents

Insulin resistance with compensatory hyperinsulinemia is thought to play a role in the ovarian dysfunction and hyperandrogenism associated with PCOS. In 1997 Velazquez et al.[21] reported that the insulin sensitizing agent metformin improved menstrual cyclicity and ovulation by reducing hyperandrogenism. An improvement in local and systemic hormonal and metabolic parameters, ovulation rates, clinical pregnancies and reduction in pregnancy complications were reported thereafter. Most of these claims were refuted by other authors; however, it was established that OHSS rate was significantly reduced in PCOS women undergoing ART (pooled OR 0.27; 95% CI 0.16–0.47) with use of metformin.[22]

Secondary Prevention Strategies

Coasting

Coasting involves withholding gonadotropins for a minimum of 48–72 hours with continued administration of GnRH agonist till the E2 levels decrease, and then giving the hCG trigger. Coasting has been employed since the 1980s and is popular with most physicians since it allows continuation of the cycle without compromising pregnancy, implantation or live-birth rates. The optimum time to start coasting is when the lead follicle reaches 16 mm in diameter and hCG should be given when E2 level drops below 3,000 pg/mL. It is recommended not to coast for more than 3 days as that leads to a significant drop in implantation and pregnancy rates.[23]

Coasting may act by diminishing the functioning granulosa cell cohort—stopping gonadotropin leads to atresia of smaller follicles, and reduces VEGF protein secretion (1,413 versus 3,538 pg/mL, p < 0.001) and gene expression (twofold decrease) in granulosa cells.[24]

Though coasting may decrease the severity and incidence, it does not eliminate the risk of OHSS. Contrary views were presented by the Cochrane database review 2011.[25] Significantly fewer oocytes were retrieved in coasting groups compared with GnRH agonists (OR –2.44; 95% CI –4.30 to –0.58; p = 0.01) or no coasting (OR –3.92; 95% CI –4.47 to –3.37; p < 0.0001). There was no evidence of a difference in the incidence of moderate and severe OHSS (OR 0.53; 95% CI 0.23–1.23) between groups, and the authors felt they could not recommend coasting above other methods of OHSS prevention. However this review has come under criticism because of the number and heterogeneity of the studies.

Coasting with GnRH Antagonist: Patients at high risk of OHSS (greater than or equal to 20) follicles/ovary and E2 levels greater than or equal to 3,000 pg/mL on long agonist protocol have been switched from agonist to daily administration of 0.25 mg antagonist for coasting. Seventy-five international units of hMG is continued with the antagonist till E2 levels fall to less than 3,000 pg/mL at which time an hCG trigger is administered. A significantly faster reduction in E2 (36% in 24 hours), more OR, more grade A embryos and shorter time to trigger were found with antagonist coasting. Clinical pregnancy rate and miscarriage rates were similar.[17]

Reduced Dose of Human Chorionic Gonadotropin Trigger

Long half-life of hCG results in a prolonged luteotropic effect which increases the risk of OHSS. This risk is similar for both urinary-derived and recombinant product.

Lowering the dose of hCG trigger has been promoted as a method of OHSS prevention. A dose of 5,000 IU instead of 10,000 IU does not compromise oocyte maturity or pregnancy rates. Doses as low as 3,300 IU and even 2,000 IU have been used successfully to trigger ovulation. Kashyap et al. 2010[26] reported success in OHSS prevention with a gentle stimulation and a sliding scale hCG trigger based on E2 levels. With E2 levels of 2,000–3,000 pg/mL between 5,000 IU and 3,300 IU of hCG is given. With E2 levels more than 3,000 pg/mL coasting is done until E2 falls below 3,000 pg/mL. A significant reductions in early OHSS (early; p < 0.001) and severe OHSS (late OHSS, p < 0.05) was reported in 792 cycles compared with 1,789 cycles given conventional hCG dose.

Unfortunately lowering the dose does not eliminate OHSS Schmidt et al. 2004[27] used doses of 5,000 IU and 3,300 IU based on E2 levels, and reported rates of mild OHSS of 8.5% and 6.3%, moderate OHSS of 2.1% and 10.6%, and severe OHSS of 0% and 4.2% respectively.

With better strategies available for OHSS prevention increasing the risk even if minimally is not justified.

Gonadotropin-releasing Hormone Agonist Trigger

Administration of a bolus of GnRH agonists results in a surge of luteinizing hormone (LH) and follicle-stimulating hormone (FSH) from the pituitary which mimics the natural mid-cycle gonadotropin surge resulting in final oocyte maturation and ovulation. Though this phenomenon has been known for some time, agonist trigger could not be used in ART cycles because of the prevalence of GnRH agonist downregulated cycles. Use of agonist trigger in antagonist protocols in women at risk revealed that OHSS was reduced or totally eliminated with this regime. Human chorionic gonadotropin triggering increased the risk of developing any form of OHSS by 3.79 times, and moderate to severe OHSS by 1.35 times compared with agonist trigger.[28] Unfortunately agonist trigger compromises the luteal phase reducing pregnancy rates and increasing miscarriage rates. Live birth rates too are significantly lower. The oocyte quality however is not compromised as is evident from donor cycles, where PR's and (Live viable births) LVB's in recipients do not show any reduction.[29]

Attempts to improve pregnancy rate and miscarriage rate by supplementing the luteal phase with high doses of estrogen and progesterone did not help. Supplementing the luteal phase additionally with small doses of hCG 500, 1,000, 1,500 given on the day of OR, or in luteal phase improved pregnancy rate but brought back the risk of OHSS. At present there is no consensus on the ideal luteal phase support in agonist triggered cycles.

Triggering with Recombinant Luteinizing Hormone

Triggering ovulation with recombinant LH has also been considered as a method of OHSS prevention. Recombinant LH trigger closely mimics the natural LH surge. The cost of the drug and the low pregnancy rates achieved do not support use of this agent.

Cryopreservation of All Embryos

Elective cryopreservation of all the embryos prevents the onset of late OHSS and has been used in high-risk patients. Embryos are replaced later in a natural or hormone replacement therapy cycle. Initially there were concerns of embryo loss because of freeze-thaw cycle and lower pregnancy rates;[12] however, elective embryo cryopreservation and deferred transfer in patients at risk of OHSS does not compromise the cumulative pregnancy rate per patient and also results in a low overall incidence of severe OHSS.[30] With the advent of vitrification, there has been a major improvement in the embryo survival and subsequent pregnancy rate. Cryopreservation alone cannot eliminate OHSS if hCG trigger is given, as the risk of early OHSS remains. A combination of the antagonist protocol with the agonist trigger and elective cryo-preservation can effectively eliminate both early and late OHSS.

Dopamine Agonists

Dopamine agonist Cb2 acts by dephosphorylation of the VEGF 2 receptor **(Fig. 2)**, thus reducing vascular permeability. In 2007 Alvarez[16] presented a proof of concept study for the use of Cb2 in OHSS prevention. Using oocyte donors in his study, he compared effect of Cb2 to placebo in women at high risk of OHSS. 0.5 mg of Cb2 was given from the day of hCG for 8 days, and this lead to a significant reduction in hematocrit, ascites and a 50% reduction in moderate OHSS. The anti-angiogenic effect did not compromise pregnancy rate. Though Cb2 is effective in reducing the severity, it does not eliminate OHSS. Further studies need to be done to compare Cb2 with established treatments such as intravenous albumin and coasting The non-ergot derived Dopamine agonist quinagolide is being promoted currently because of reports of valvular disorder with chronic use of Cb2 in Parkinson's disease.

Plasma Expanders: Intravenous Albumin and Hydroxyethyl Starch

Albumin administration corrects the osmotic pressure thus improving intravascular volume, and reducing effects related to hemoconcentration. It may also bind to the vasoactive agents responsible for development of OHSS, and facilitate their removal from the circulation. Though it is an effective agent in management of established OHSS, its role in prevention has been questioned.

Most studies do not support the use of intravenous albumin on the day of oocyte pickup as an effective measure of OHSS prevention though a reduction in severity has been suggested.[31] In a meta-analysis by Jee et al. 2010 lower pregnancy rates have been reported with its use.[32] There are potential side effects and risk of pulmonary edema in patients with diminished cardiac reserve. Hydroxyethyl starch (HES) solution has been suggested as an alternative to albumin as it is equally effective, cheaper and safer.

Cycle Cancelation

Cycle cancelation and withholding of hCG is one sure method to prevent OHSS; however, it is distressing to the patient and the physician and involves a huge financial loss. With better techniques available today this seems to be a bit extreme. It can only be considered in a setting where a long agonist cycle has been used, E2 levels are extremely high and cryopreservation is not available. In which case of course the physician should not be doing IVF at all. A word of caution in OI cycles without downregulation a natural LH surge may still result in ovulation and natural conception, hence contraception should be advised.

Other Strategies

Methylprednisolone has been used in OHSS prevention, the rationale being that glucocorticoids have an inhibitory effect on VEGF gene expression.[33]

Follicular aspiration: Follicles from one ovary are aspirated before hCG trigger. This reduces the functional granulosa cells and thereby the VEGF.

These methods cannot be promoted as much better options are available now.

■ MANAGEMENT OF OVARIAN HYPERSTIMULATION SYNDROME

Management depends on the symptoms and severity of disease. Tense ascites, significant hemoconcentration and oliguria require immediate hospitalization. The American Society for Reproductive Medicine (ASRM) practice committee 2008 guidelines[5] for management are given below.

Outpatient Management

Treatment usually requires only oral analgesics and antiemetics. Intercourse should be avoided as it may be painful and may increase the risk of ovarian rupture. Education of the patient regarding symptoms and close monitoring for disease progression is very important. Patient should be in touch with the doctor on a daily basis to give information regarding her symptoms.

Monitoring involves ultrasound examination for assessment of ascites and ovarian size, measurement of weight and abdominal girth, assessment of urinary output. Estimation of hematocrit, liver enzymes, creatinine and electrolytes whenever the clinical situations warrant it.

Recommendations for the Outpatient Management of Persistent and Worsening OHSS Include

- Oral fluid intake should be maintained at no less than 1 L per day; preferably electrolyte supplemented drinks
- Strenuous physical activity should be avoided to reduce risk of ovarian torsion. Light physical activity should be maintained. Strict bed rest is unwarranted and may increase risk of thromboembolism
- Weight and frequency and/or volume of urine output to be recorded daily. Weight gain of more than 2 pounds per day or decreasing urinary frequency should prompt repeated evaluation both ultrasound and laboratory tests

- Pregnant patients with OHSS must be monitored very closely because risk of progressing to severe disease.

Hospitalization

Hospitalization may be required based on severity of symptoms, analgesic requirements and social considerations. No one symptom or sign is an absolute indication, but hospitalization should be considered when one or more of the following are present:

- Severe abdominal pain or peritoneal signs
- Intractable nausea and vomiting that prevents ingestion of food and adequate fluids
- Severe oliguria or anuria
- Tense ascites
- Dyspnea or tachypnea
- Hypotension (relative to baseline), dizziness, or syncope
- Severe electrolyte imbalance (hyponatremia, hyperkalemia), Hemoconcentration, Abnormal liver function tests

Laboratory Findings in Severe OHSS

- Hemoconcentration (hematocrit >45%)
- Leukocytosis (white blood cell count >15,000)
- Electrolyte imbalances (hyponatremia: sodium <135 mEq/L; hyperkalemia: potassium >5.0 mEq/L)
- Elevated liver enzymes
- Decreased creatinine clearance (serum creatinine >1.2; creatinine clearance <50 mL/min)

Recommendations for Monitoring of Hospitalized Patients with OHSS include:

- Vital signs (every 2–8 hours, according to clinical status)
- Weight (recorded daily)
- Complete physical examination (daily, avoiding bimanual examination of the ovaries due to risk of ovarian rupture)
- Abdominal circumference (at the navel, recorded daily)
- Monitoring of fluid intake and output (daily, or more often as needed)
- Ultrasound examination (ascites, ovarian size), repeated as necessary to guide management or paracentesis
- Chest X-ray and echocardiogram (when pleural or pericardial effusion is suspected), repeated as necessary
- Pulse oximetry (for patients with symptoms of pulmonary compromise)
- *Laboratory investigations*
  - Complete blood count (daily, or more often as needed to guide fluid management)
  - Electrolytes (daily)

   – Serum creatinine or creatinine clearance, urine specific gravity, repeated as necessary
   – Liver enzymes, repeated as necessary

If a patients complaints of increasing abdominal pain and distension do not forget to look for evidence of ovarian rupture or acute intra-abdominal hemorrhage.

Fluid Management

Guidelines for Fluid Management of Hospitalized Patients

- Strict intake and output charting. Limit oral fluids
- Rapid initial hydration may be accomplished with a bolus of intravenous fluid (500–1,000 mL). Thereafter, fluids should be administered judiciously, in the volumes necessary to maintain adequate urine output (>20–30 mL/h) and reverse hemoconcentration. Five percent dextrose in normal saline (DNS) is preferable to lactated Ringer's solution, given the tendency to hyponatremia. Correction of hypovolemia, hypotension and oliguria has highest priority
- Albumin (25%) in doses of 50–100 g, infused over 4 hours and repeated at 4- to 12-hour intervals as necessary, is an effective plasma expander, and helps to maintain adequate urine output. Albumin is the preferred plasma expander, although others like HES, mannitol, fresh frozen plasma) may be used. Dextran has been associated with development of adult respiratory distress syndrome (ARDS) and is best avoided
- Treatment with diuretics (e.g., furosemide, 20 mg intravenous) may be considered after an adequate intravascular volume has been restored (hematocrit <38%). Premature or overzealous use of diuretics will increase risk of thromboembolism
- Onset of diuresis heralds resolution, and intravenous fluids should be strictly curtailed at this point
- Hyperkalemia is associated with risk of cardiac dysrhythmias, hence electrocardiography should be done, and appropriate treatment given. Electrocardiographic manifestations of hyperkalemia (prolonged PR and QRS intervals, ST segment depression, tall peaked T waves) indicate the need for immediate treatment with calcium gluconate.

Paracentesis

Ultrasound-guided paracentesis is indicated for patients with ascites that causes pain, compromised pulmonary function (e.g., tachypnea, hypoxia, hydrothorax),[32] or oliguria/anuria that does not improve with appropriate fluid management. A transvaginal or transabdominal approach may be used, under gentle ultrasound guidance. The volume of fluid that should be removed in one sitting is not defined, but generally the maximum possible is removed at a gradual pace. Pleural tap may be required if hydrothorax is causing dyspnea.

Where risk of thromboembolism is perceived prophylactic treatment with heparin (5,000 U subcutaneous, every 12 hours) should be considered. Low molecular weight heparin can also be given for prophylaxis. Full-length venous support stockings can be advised.

■ CONCLUSION

Ovarian hyperstimulation syndrome is a potentially life threatening complication of gonadotropin stimulation. Over time there has been an improvement in understanding the pathogenesis of the syndrome. An increased vascular permeability related to increased VEGF secretion is mainly responsible for the signs, and symptoms associated with the disease. It is important to look out for the risk factors and adopt preventive measures both prior to and during stimulation. Introduction of antagonist protocols in IVF and use of GnRH agonist trigger for final oocyte maturation have helped tremendously in reducing the incidence of OHSS. Elective vitrification when added to the above protocol, effectively eliminates OHSS.

GnRH agonist trigger is associated with a decreased pregnancy rate and an increased miscarriage rate due to luteal insufficiency. Strategies to supplement the luteal phase in agonist trigger cycles include use of high doses of estrogen and progesterone and small doses of hCG either at the time of OR, or in luteal phase. Adding hCG, however promotes the risk of OHSS. Dopamine agonist Cb2 has shown a lot of promise in reducing the vascular permeability thereby reducing severity of the disease without compromising pregnancy and implantation. It can be used in downregulated cycles where hCG trigger has been given. Intravenous albumin or HES given additionally can further reduce the symptoms. Coasting with agonist is still popular but coasting with antagonist recently reported, appears to be more effective.

We have come a long way in improving the safety of ART, and it is incumbent on the IVF specialist to be well versed with the latest developments to avoid the morbidity and mortality associated with this dreaded complication. An algorithm for OHSS **(Fig. 3)** prevention has been proposed by Papnikolaou et al.[34]

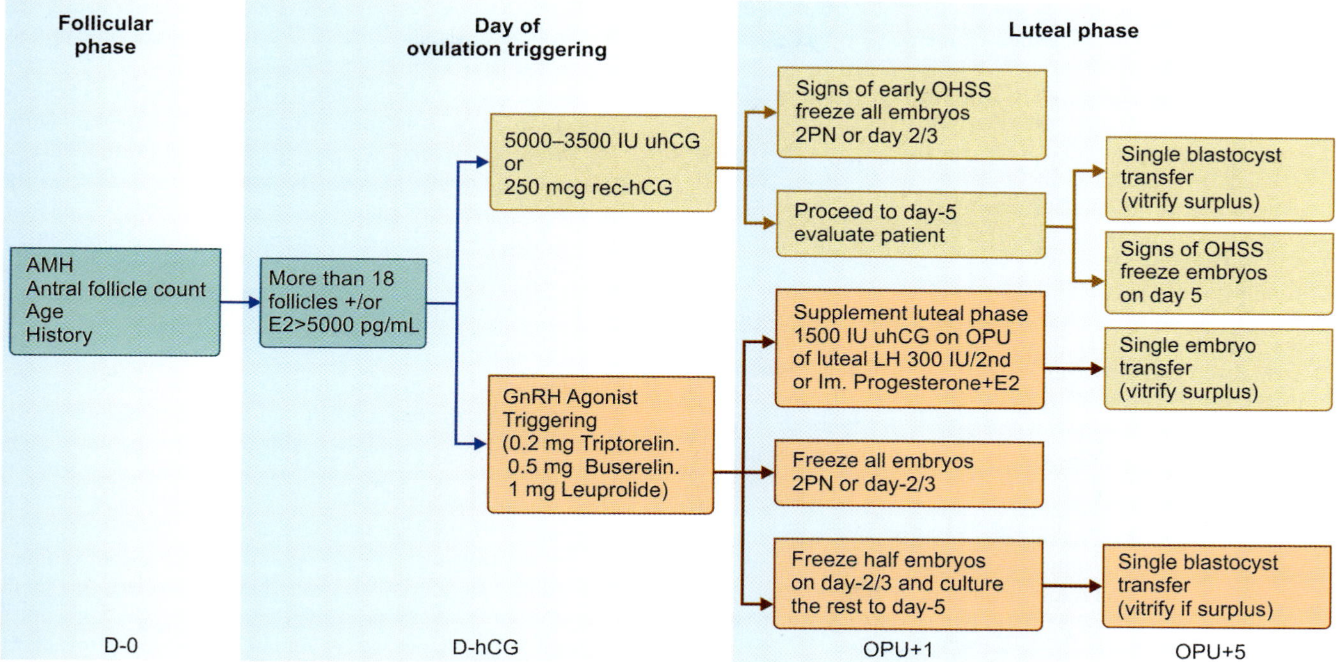

Fig. 3 Algorithm proposed by Papanikolaou

TAKE HOME MESSAGE

- Ovarian hyperstimulation syndrome is a life-threatening complication of ovarian stimulation
- It is mainly associated with gonadotropin stimulation
- Risk factors include young, lean PCOS women. High dose of gonadotropins and a previous history of OHSS
- The hallmark of the syndrome is an increased vascular permeability which allows shift of protein rich fluid into the third space. Increased VEGF is responsible for the increased vascular permeability
- Clinical symptoms are related to the fluid shift and consequent hemoconcentration
- Management includes giving albumin and or HES to improve hypovolemia and renal perfusion. Tapping of ascites/hydrothorax, antiemetics to give symptomatic relief
- Strategies to reduce risk include using chronic low dose protocol for OI, soft stimulation for IUI and individualized OS protocols based on estimation of ovarian response in ART
- AMH and AFC are good markers of ovarian reserve and response.
- Use of antagonist protocols in ART in all PCOS women.
- Use of GnRH agonist trigger instead of hCG in high risk cases.
- Use of Cabergoline for 8 days from the day of hCG trigger significantly reduces vascular permeability
- Antagonist protocol with GnRH agonist trigger, and elective cryopreservation of all embryos can completely eliminate the risk of OHSS

REFERENCES

1. Cluroe AD, Synek BJ. A fatal case of ovarian hyperstimulation syndrome with cerebral infarction. Pathology. 1995;27:344-6.
2. Aboulghar MA, Mansour RT. Ovarian hyperstimulation syndrome: classifications and critical analysis of preventive measures. Hum Reprod Update. 2003;9:275-89.
3. Francisco C, Júlio C, Pinto G, et al. Ovarian hyperstimulation syndrome in a spontaneous pregnancy. Acta Med Port. 2011;24(Suppl 3):635-8.
4. Mocanu E, Redmond ML, Hennelly B, et al. Odds of ovarian hyperstimulation syndrome (OHSS)—time for reassessment. Hum Fertil (Camb). 2007;10(3):175-81.
5. Ovarian hyperstimulation syndrome. The Practice Committee of the American Society for Reproductive Medicine. Fertil Steril. 2008;90:S188-93.
6. Koninckx PR, Renaer M, Brosens IA. Origin of peritoneal fluid in women: an ovarian exudation product. Br J Obstet Gynaecol. 1980;87:177-83.
7. Pellicer A, Albert C, Mercader A, et al. The pathogenesis of ovarian hyperstimulation syndrome: in vivo studies investigating the role of interleukin-1b, interleukin-6, and vascular endothelial growth factor. Fertil Steril. 1999;71:482-9.
8. Montanelli L, Delbaere A, Di Carlo C, et al. A mutation in the follicle-stimulating hormone receptor as a cause of familial spontaneous ovarian hyperstimulation syndrome. J Clin Endocrinol Metab. 2004;89(4):1255-8.
9. Di Carlo C, Savoia F, Ferrara C, et al. Case report: a most peculiar family with spontaneous, recurrent ovarian hyperstimulation syndrome. Gynecol Endocrinol. 2012;28(8):649-51.

10. Mathur RS, Akande VA, Keay SD, et al. Distinction between early and late ovarian hyper-stimulation syndrome. Fertil Steril. 2000;73:901-7.
11. Whelan JG 3rd, Vlahos NF. The ovarian hyperstimulation syndrome. Fertil Steril. 2000;73:883-96.
12. Humaidan P, Quartarolo J, Papanikolaou EG. Preventing ovarian hyperstimulation syndrome: guidance for the clinician. Fertil Steril. 2010;94:389-400.
13. Gnoth C, Schuring AN, Friol K, et al. Relevance of anti-Müllerian hormone measurement in a routine IVF program. Hum Reprod. 2008;23:1359-65.
14. Lee TH, Liu CH, Huang CC, et al. Serum anti-Müllerian hormone and estradiol levels as predictors of ovarian hyper-stimulation syndrome in assisted reproduction technology cycles. Hum Reprod. 2008;23:160-7.
15. Kwee J, Elting ME, Schats R, et al. Ovarian volume and antral follicle count for the prediction of low and hyper responders with in vitro fertilization. Reprod Biomed Online. 2007;5:9.
16. Alvarez C, Martí-Bonmatí L, Novella-Maestre E, et al. Dopamine agonist cabergoline reduces hemoconcentration and ascites in hyperstimulated women undergoing assisted reproduction. J Clin Endocrinol Metab. 2007;92(8):2931-7.
17. Aboulghar M. Antagonist and agonist coasting. Fertil Steril. 2012;97:523-6.
18. Jayaprakasan K, Hopkisson JF, Campbell BK, et al. Quantification of the effect of pituitary down-regulation on 3D ultrasound predictors of ovarian response. Hum Reprod. 2008; 23:1538-44.
19. Al-Inany HG, Youssef MA, Aboulghar M, et al. Gonadotrophin-releasing hormone antagonists for assisted reproductive technology. Cochrane Database Syst Rev. 2011;11(5): CD001750.
20. van der Linden M, Buckingham K, Farquhar C, et al. Luteal phase support for assisted reproduction cycles. Cochrane Database Syst Rev. 2011;(10):CD009154.
21. Velázquez E, Acosta A, Mendoza SG. Menstrual cyclicity after metformin therapy in polycystic ovary syndrome. Obstet Gynecol. 1997;90(3):392-5.
22. Tso LO, Costello MF, Albuquerque LE, et al. Metformin treatment before and during IVF or ICSI in women with polycystic ovary syndrome. Cochrane Database Syst Rev. 2009;(2):CD006105.
23. Mansour R, Aboulghar M, Serour G, et al. Criteria of a successful coasting protocol for the prevention of severe ovarian hyperstimulation syndrome. Hum Reprod. 2005;20:3167-72.
24. Garcia-Velasco JA, Zúñiga A, Pacheco A, et al. Coasting acts through downregulation of VEGF gene expression and protein secretion. Hum Reprod. 2004;19:1530-8.
25. D'Angelo A, Brown J, Amso NN. Coasting (withholding gonadotrophins) for preventing ovarian hyperstimulation syndrome. Cochrane Database Syst Rev. 2011;(6):CD002811.
26. Kashyap S, Leveille M, Wells G. Low dose hCG reduces the incidence of early and severe ovarian hyperstimulation syndrome. Fertil Steril. 2006;86(Suppl 2):S182–S183(P-138).
27. Schmidt DW, Maier DB, Nulsen JC, et al. Reducing the dose of human chorionic gonadotropin in high responders does not affect the outcomes of in vitro fertilization. Fertil Steril. 2004;82:841-6.
28. Engmann L, DiLuigi A, Schmidt D, et al. The use of gonado-tropin-releasing hormone (GnRH) agonist to induce oocyte maturation after cotreatment with GnRH antagonist in high-risk patients undergoing in vitro fertilization prevents the risk of ovarian hyperstimulation syndrome: a prospective randomized controlled study. Fertil Steril. 2008;89:84-91.
29. Bodri D, Guillén JJ, Galindo A, et al. Triggering with human chorionic gonadotropin or a gonadotropin-releasing hormone agonist in gonadotropin-releasing hormone antagonist-treated oocyte donor cycles: findings of a large retrospective cohort study. Fertil Steril. 2009;91:365-71.
30. Vyjayanthi S, Tang T, Fattah A, et al. Elective cryopreservation of embryos at the pronucleate stage in women at risk of ovarian hyperstimulation syndrome may affect the overall pregnancy rate. Fertil Steril. 2006;86(6):1773-5.
31. Aboulghar M, Evers JH, Al-Inany H. Intravenous albumin for preventing severe ovarian hyperstimulation syndrome: a Cochrane review. Hum Reprod. 2002;17(12):3027-32.
32. Jee BC, Suh CS, Kim YB, et al. Administration of intravenous albumin around the time of oocyte retrieval reduces pregnancy rate without preventing ovarian hyperstimulation syndrome: a systematic review and meta-analysis. Gynecol Obstet Invest. 2010;70(1):47-54.
33. Nauck M, Karakiulakis G, Perruchoud AP, et al. Corticosteroids inhibit the expression of the vascular endothelial growth factor gene in human vascular smooth muscle cells. Eur J Pharmacol. 1998;341:309-15.
34. Papanikolaou EG, Humaidan P, Polyzos N, et al. New algorithm for OHSS prevention. Reprod Biol Endocrinol. 2011;9:147.

Ovarian Cancer and ART

Priya Bhave Chittawar

INTRODUCTION

Ovarian cancer is the fifth most common cancer in women in the western world. It accounts for 4% of all malignancies in women. The lifetime risk of ovarian cancer in women is 1.75%. The peak incidence of ovarian cancer is at 62 years and most cancers are diagnosed in stage 3 or 4 (almost 70%). Women with ovarian cancer present with nonspecific symptoms including abdominal pain and bloating, changes in bowel habit, urinary and/or pelvic symptoms. Prognosis remains fairly poor with a 5-year relative survival of 30%. Epithelial ovarian cancers are the most common and account for 90% of ovarian cancers. Serous tumors are the most common epithelial ovarian tumors (75%) followed by mucinous (20%), endometrioid (2%) and clear cell (<1%). Several theories have been postulated regarding the pathogenesis of ovarian cancer **(Table 1)**. The high-risk factors for ovarian cancer are summarized in **Table 2**.

INFERTILITY AND OVARIAN CANCER RISK

Infertility is definitely associated with increased risk of ovarian cancer.[5] Whether this is an association or causation is unclear. The first study that pointed to a risk of ovarian cancer being caused by fertility treatments (and not infertility alone) was published in 1992. Data from 12 case control studies showed higher risk of epithelial cancer among women had used fertility drugs and those with long total duration of premenopausal sexual activity without birth control compared to normal population.[6] This study had several drawbacks including lack of information on type of infertility therapy, choice of controls, no adjustment for confounders like smoking status, etc.

To prove causation, randomized controlled trials are considered gold standard. However, when the result of an intervention [fertility medicines and in vitro fertilization (IVF)] is potentially harmful (ovarian cancer in this case), randomization is unethical. Hence, we have to rely on other study designs to prove causation.

To establish causation, following criteria must be fulfilled by the study of:[7]

- Assessment of strength of association
- Biological credibility
- Consistency with other investigations
- Time sequence
- Dose response relationship.

Many studies have shown a strong association between infertility and ovarian cancer risk. However, whether infertility per se that causes cancer or the treatments like ovulation induction and ovarian stimulation that contribute to cancer risk is still unproven. Various mechanisms are proposed by which fertility medications and IVF can contribute to cancer risk. They are summarized in **Table 3**.

Multiple studies have consistently shown that ovarian cancer risk is higher in women who are infertile. Cohort

Table 1 Hypothesis for origin of ovarian cancer

Incessant ovulation theory:[1] This theory suggests that ovarian cancer originated in the ovarian surface epithelium through repeated ovulation and the associated repair of the ovulatory wound

Gonadotropin theory:[2] High levels of FSH and LH result in high local estradiol levels which induce tumor genesis by molecular pathways

Extraovarian origin of epithelial ovarian cancers:[3] Ovarian epithelial tumors supposedly arise from the Fallopian tube epithelium. Animal studies in mice corroborate this theory. In addition, a large majority of serous epithelial cancers of ovaries are associated with endosalpinx involvement and tubal intraepithelial carcinoma and harbor the same p53 mutation[4]

studies and case control studies are the two available study designs to prove that ovarian cancer is caused by fertility treatments, specifically associated with fertility treatments **(Fig. 1)**.

Case control studies are useful in rare diseases. The "cases" of ovarian cancer are identified and comparable group without the disease are taken as control. The two groups are then investigated for exposure to putative causative agent (fertility therapy in this care). Cohort studies, on the other hand, start with exposure to fertility therapy and follow-up till development of the outcome of interest (ovarian cancer). Ovarian cancer has a low prevalence and peak incidence is in the sixth decade. Hence, cohort studies require a very large sample size and sufficiently long follow-up period to be adequately powered and meaningful. Cohort studies are free from recall bias (the affected women are more likely to remember exposure) and to a large extent selection bias. Case control studies are also not able to adjust for confounders like oral contraceptive pill use, smoking, etc.

Hence, for this chapter, we have analyzed cohort studies that follow-up infertile women who have undergone assisted reproductive therapy and compare them with fertile cohort and/or a cohort of infertile women who did not undergo assisted reproductive techniques. A total of nine such studies have been summarized in **Table 4**.

The outcomes (ovarian cancers) are compared as risk ratios (RRs), standardized incidence ratios (SIRs). RR is the ratio of the probability of an event occurring (ovarian cancer) in an exposed group (infertile women undergoing IVF) to the probability of the event occurring in a comparison, nonexposed group (normal population or women with infertility not undergoing IVF). SIR refers to the quotient of the observed and the expected number of ovarian cancer cases, the expected number of cases are derived from the local registry data for that age group. These nine cohort studies were combined in a meta-analysis which had a total of 109,969 women exposed to IVF with 76 cases of ovarian cancer.[9] When infertile women undergoing IVF were compared with general population, they found a statistically significant association between the use of IVF and an increased risk for ovarian cancer (RR 1.50; 95% CI: 1.17–1.92) **(Fig. 2)**. However, infertility is an independent risk factor for ovarian cancer as discussed before. When infertile women who underwent IVF were compared with infertile women who did not, there was no significant difference in ovarian cancer risk (RR 1.26; 95% CI: 0.62–2.55) **(Fig. 3)**.[9] This meta-analysis supports that

Table 2 Factors associate with ovarian cancer incidence

High-risk factors for ovarian cancer:
Ovulatory years (late menopause, low parity)
Nulliparous status
Smoking
Perineal talc exposure
Genetic predisposition
Protective factors:
Tubal ligation
Prophylactic salpingectomy, oophorectomy
Oral contraceptive use
Breastfeeding

Table 3 Biological mechanisms of cancer incidence associated with fertility treatments

Incessant ovulation resulting from induction and superovulation regimes[8]
Puncture trauma to ovarian surface during oocyte retrieval[9]
Depletion of ovarian follicles[10]
Stromal entrapment of surface epithelium[11]
Hormonal effect: High estradiol levels resulting in activation of c-myc proto-oncogene,[12] high FSH levels resulting in activation of protein kinase C and phosphatidylinositol-3-kinase[13,14]

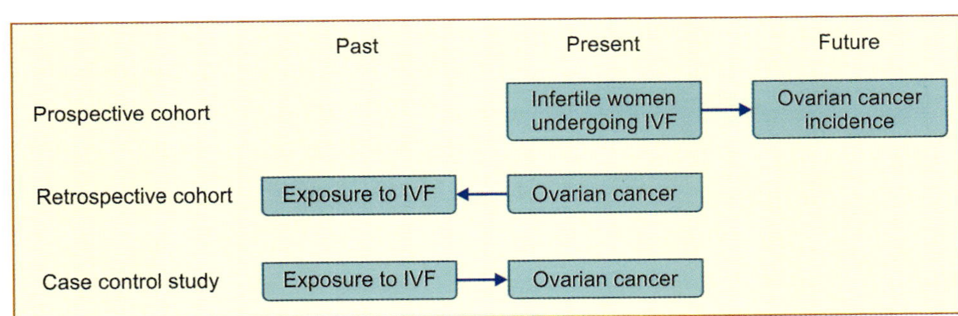

Fig. 1 Cohort studies and case control studies in studying ovarian cancer incidence and assisted reproductive techniques

Table 4 Cohort studies examining the effect of assisted reproductive techniques on ovarian cancer incidence

		Study population	Results
1.	Venn et al. (1995) Australia[15]	29,666 women, 3 cancers in exposed (evaluated for subfertility and exposed to IVF) 3 cancers in unexposed (referred for IVF but untreated or had "natural cycle" treatment without stimulation)	SIR in exposed = 1.7 (CI 95%: 0.55–5.27) SIR in unexposed = 1.62 (95% CI: 0.52–5.02) RR exposed vs unexposed = 1,45 (95% CI: 0.28–7.55)
2.	Venn et al. (1999)[16]	29,700 women, 7 ovarian cancers in exposed (evaluated for subfertility and had at least one IVF treatment cycle with ovarian stimulation) 6 in unexposed (referred for IVF but untreated or had "natural cycle" treatment without ovarian stimulation)	SIR in exposed = 0.88 (95% CI: 0,42–1.84) SIR in unexposed = 1.16 (95% CI: 0.52–2.59)
3.	Dor et al. (2002)[17]	Retrospective cohort of 5,026 women (treated for subfertility and had at least 1 cycle of IVF) 1 ovarian cancer case	SIR in exposed = 0.57 (95% CI: 0.01–3.20)
4.	Klip et al. (2002)[18]	23,592 women (diagnosed with subfertility problems and had at least 1 cycle of IVF, 17 ovarian cancers) vs subfertile women	No differences in risk exposed vs unexposed
5.	Lerner-Geva et al.[19]	1,082 women (diagnosed with subfertility problems and had at least 1 cycle of IVF), 3 ovarian cancers	SIR in exposed = 5.0 (95% CI: 1.02–14.6) SIR = 1.67 (0.02–9.27) when cancers developing within 1 year were excluded. No untreated group
6.	Van Leeuwen et al. (2011)[20]	19,146 IVF women, 6,006 subfertile women not treated with IVF	Risk of borderline ovarian tumors increased in the IVF group compared with the general population. SIR = 1.76 (95% CI: 1.16–2.56). The overall SIR for invasive ovarian cancer was not significantly elevated with longer follow-up after first IVF. SIR = 3.54 (95% CI: 1.62–6.72) after 15 years
7.	Källén et al. (2011)[21]	24,058 women (women who delivered an infant following IVF treatment), 26 ovarian cancers	RR exposed vs unexposed = 2.09 (95% CI: 1,39–3.12)
8.	Yli-Kuha et al. (2012)[22]	9,175 women, 9 invasive ovarian cancers, 4 borderline ovarian tumors	OR for invasive cancers = 2.57 (95% CI: 0.69–9.23) OR for borderline tumors = 1.68 (95% CI: 0.31–9.27)
9.	Brinton et al. (2013)[23]	87,403 women (infertile women undergoing IVF), 45 ovarian cancers	Global HR = 1.58 (95% CI: 0.75–3.29), HR among women receiving ≥ 4 IVF cycles = 1.78 95% CI: 0.76–4.13)

it is infertility per se which increases the risk of ovarian cancer and probably not the treatment for the same.

DRAWBACKS OF THE STUDIES EVALUATING IVF AND OVARIAN CANCER RISK

The follow-up period in most studies is less than 10 years, which is insufficient considering that most cases of ovarian cancer occur in fifth or sixth decade. Also it is known that more cases of ovarian cancer are diagnosed within the year that assisted reproduction is undertaken, due to better surveillance. Most studies did not exclude cancers diagnosed within 1 year of IVF and this could overestimate cancer risk in the IVF cohort. There is evidence that parity has a significant protective effect on the ovarian cancer risk.[24] Achieving live birth after IVF might thus actually protect infertile women from ovarian cancer later in life. Also, only one study evaluated the dose-result relationship, i.e. number of IVF cycles and the ovarian cancer risk.[23] Most patients with infertility already have predisposing factors like endometriosis, polycystic ovarian syndrome (PCOS), etc. which are high-risk factors for particular types of ovarian cancer and in the absence of adequate numbers of cases, subgroup analysis for type of ovarian cancer was not carried out in most of these

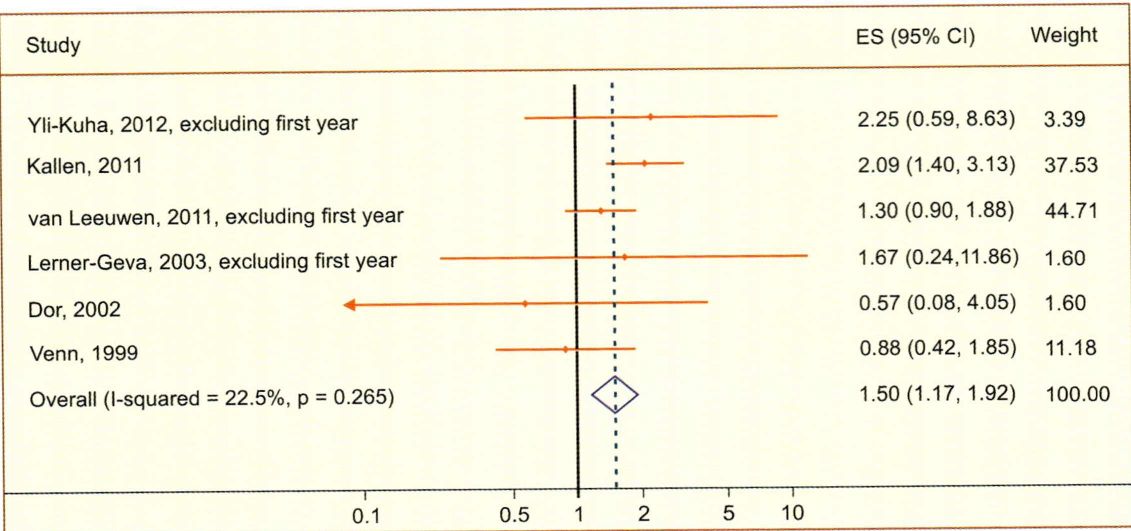

Fig. 2 Forest plot of studies for ovarian cancer in women exposed to IVF versus normal population: when compared to normal population, infertile women who underwent IVF had a significantly higher chance of ovarian cancer[9]

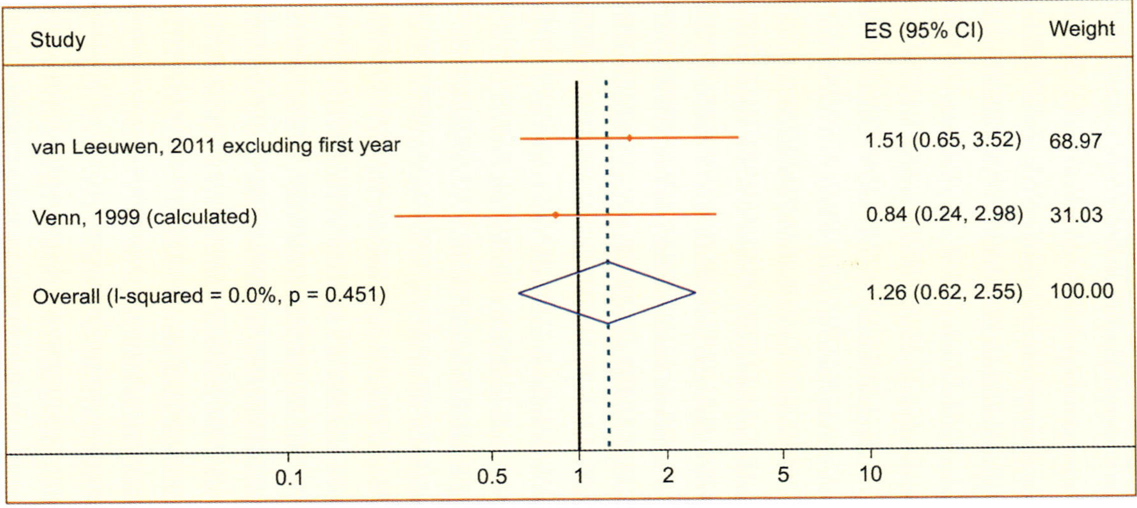

Fig. 3 Incidence rate ratios (IRRs) for ovarian cancer in women exposed to IVF versus infertile women showed no significant difference in ovarian cancer incidence[9]

studies.[25] Many patients of infertility undergo multiple cycles of ovulation induction with clomiphene and gonadotropins prior to enrolling for IVF. This data is not available in any of the nine studies. This could potentially be a confounder in the studies.

Future studies evaluating the role of IVF in causation of ovarian cancer must have a longer follow-up period and adjust for confounders like number of IVF cycles, treatment for infertility prior to undertaking IVF, smoking status, oral contraceptive pill use, etc. Women who do not achieve a live birth following IVF must be evaluated as a separate subgroup from those who succeed in IVF.

■ CONCLUSION

Data so far suggests that IVF does not add to the ovarian cancer risk over and above that conferred by infertility itself. More well designed large cohort studies with longer follow-up periods and information regarding exact infertility therapy and type of ovarian cancer are needed.

◼ REFERENCES

1. Fathalla MF. Incessant ovulation and ovarian cancer—a hypothesis re-visited. Facts Views Vis ObGyn. 2013;5(4):292-7.
2. Hilliard TS, Modi DA, Burdette JE. Gonadotropins activate oncogenic pathways to enhance proliferation in normal mouse ovarian surface epithelium. Int J Mol Sci. 2013;14(3):4762-82.
3. Hillier SG. Nonovarian origins of ovarian cancer. Proc Natl Acad Sci. 2012;109(10):3608-9.
4. Kindelberger DW, Lee Y, Miron A, et al. Intraepithelial carcinoma of the fimbria and pelvic serous carcinoma: evidence for a causal relationship. Am J Surg Pathol. 2007;31(2):161-9.
5. Gates MA, Rosner BA, Hecht JL, et al. Risk factors for epithelial ovarian cancer by histologic subtype. Am J Epidemiol. 2010;171(1):45-53.
6. Whittmore AS, Harris R, Itnyre J. Characteristics relating to ovarian cancer risk: collaborative analysis of 12 US Case-Control Studies II. Invasive epithelial ovarian cancers in white women. Am J Epidemiol. 1992;136(10):1184-203.
7. Kashyap S, Davis OK. Ovarian cancer and fertility medications: a critical appraisal. Semin Reprod Med. 2003;21(1):65-71.
8. Chene G, Penault-Llorca F, Bouëdec GL, et al. Ovarian epithelial dysplasia after ovulation induction: time and dose effects. Hum Reprod. 2009;24(1):132-8.
9. Siristatidis C, Sergentanis TN, Kanavidis P, et al. Controlled ovarian hyperstimulation for IVF: impact on ovarian, endometrial and cervical cancer—a systematic review and meta-analysis. Hum Reprod Update. 2013;19(2):105-23.
10. Smith ER, Xu X-X. Ovarian ageing, follicle depletion, and cancer: a hypothesis for the aetiology of epithelial ovarian cancer involving follicle depletion. Lancet Oncol. 2008;9(11):1108-11.
11. Cramer DW, Welch WR. Determinants of ovarian cancer risk. II. Inferences Regarding Pathogenesis. J Natl Cancer Inst. 1983;71(4):717-21.
12. Chien CH, Wang FF, Hamilton TC. Transcriptional activation of c-myc proto-oncogene by estrogen in human ovarian cancer cells. Mol Cell Endocrinol. 1994;99(1):11-9.
13. Choi K-C, Kang SK, Tai C-J, et al. Follicle-stimulating hormone activates mitogen-activated protein kinase in preneoplastic and neoplastic ovarian surface epithelial cells. J Clin Endocrinol Metab. 2002;87(5):2245-53.
14. Choi J-H, Choi K-C, Auersperg N, et al. Gonadotropins upregulate the epidermal growth factor receptor through activation of mitogen-activated protein kinases and phosphatidyl-inositol-3-kinase in human ovarian surface epithelial cells. Endocr Relat Cancer. 2005;12(2):407-21.
15. Venn A, Watson L, Lumley J, et al. Breast and ovarian cancer incidence after infertility and in vitro fertilisation. Lancet. 1995;346(8981):995-1000.
16. Venn A, Watson L, Bruinsma F, et al. Risk of cancer after use of fertility drugs with in-vitro fertilisation. Lancet. 1999;354(9190):1586-90.
17. Dor J, Lerner-Geva L, Rabinovici J, et al. Cancer incidence in a cohort of infertile women who underwent in vitro fertilization. Fertil Steril. 2002;77(2):324-7.
18. Klip H, Burger CW, Kenemans P, et al. Cancer risk associated with subfertility and ovulation induction: a review. Cancer Causes Control CCC. 2000;11(4):319-44.
19. Lerner-Geva L, Liat L-G, Rabinovici J, et al. Are infertility treatments a potential risk factor for cancer development? Perspective of 30 years of follow-up. Gynecol Endocrinol Off J Int Soc Gynecol Endocrinol. 2012;28(10):809-14.
20. Leeuwen FE van, Klip H, Mooij TM, et al. Risk of borderline and invasive ovarian tumours after ovarian stimulation for in vitro fertilization in a large Dutch cohort. Hum Reprod. 2011;26(12):3456-65.
21. Källén B, Finnström O, Lindam A, et al. Malignancies among women who gave birth after in vitro fertilization. Hum Reprod. 2011;26(1):253-8.
22. Yli-Kuha A-N, Gissler M, Klemetti R, et al. Cancer morbidity in a cohort of 9175 Finnish women treated for infertility. Hum Reprod. 2012;27(4):1149-55.
23. Brinton LA, Trabert B, Shalev V, et al. In vitro fertilization and risk of breast and gynecologic cancers: a retrospective cohort study within the Israeli Maccabi Healthcare Services. Fertil Steril. 2013;99(5):1189-96.
24. Merritt MA, Pari MD, Vitonis AF, et al. Reproductive characteristics in relation to ovarian cancer risk by histologic pathways. Hum Reprod. 2013;28(5):1406-17.
25. Daniilidis A, Karagiannis V. Epithelial ovarian cancer. Risk factors, screening and the role of prophylactic oophorectomy. Hippokratia. 2007;11(2):63-6.

59 Ethical and Stress Issues in ART

Ian Cook

ETHICAL ISSUES

General

Medical ethics underpin all actions in medicine and the basic elements of beneficence (doing good), non-maleficence (not doing harm), autonomy (exercising one's free will) and justice (fairness) have long been recognized. To these have recently been added dignity and honesty, covering informed consent and confidentiality. They have all evolved from the moral theories of consequentialism or utilitarianism (the greatest good for the greatest number), deontology (rights and duties), virtue ethics (focusing on the inherent character of an individual) and communitarianism (rights must be balanced by concern for others in a community.[1] Common elements in all these approaches are impartiality, rationality, consistency and reversibility. Impartiality is avoiding bias, rationality is using the scientific evidence derived from clinical data analysis.

Although, these moral values are applicable to all fields of medicine, reproductive medicine has been a focus since in vitro fertilization (IVF) was achieved in 1978. Debate started early in the United Kingdom (UK). It was appreciated that society's views needed to be taken into account so that this new activity could be appropriately regulated for the protection of those in society who could potentially benefit and of those involved in providing the services. The legal and moral framework was created by the Warnock Report (1988) on which the Human Fertilization and Embryology Act (1990) was based, which in turn created the Human Fertilization and Embryology Authority (HFEA) to oversee its implementation. It is important to emphasize that the Act provided a framework for regulation and subsequently detailed technical aspects were described in successive codes of practice,[2] which could be readily updated without changing the law. Changing the law would only be slow and difficult and the 1990 Act was not amended until 2008. The Indian Council for Medical Research (ICMR) has produced guidelines on assisted reproductive technologies (ART[3]); a draft ART (Regulation) Bill was promulgated in 2010[4] and remains before parliament.

Professional societies have played an important role in defining consensual standards of practice and these are based on the above principles. They have also defined the ethical aspects of many areas of practice and these sources of information can be readily accessed on the websites of the European Society of Human Reproduction and Embryology (ESHRE,[5] **Box 1**) and of the American Society of Reproductive Medicine (ASRM)[6] **(Box 2)**. Many countries have also issued guidelines for practice, which

Box 1 ESHRE documents of the task force on ethics and law

1. The moral status of the preimplantation embryo
2. The cryopreservation of human embryos
3. Gamete and embryo donation
4. Stem cells
5. Preimplantation genetic diagnosis
6. Multiple pregnancies
7. Cryopreservation
8. HIV
9. The application of preimplantation genetic diagnosis for human leukocyte antigen typing of embryos
10. Surrogacy
11. Posthumous assisted reproduction
12. Oocyte donation for nonreproductive purposes
13. The welfare of the child in medically assisted reproduction
14. Equity of access to assisted reproductive technology
15. Cross-border reproductive care
16. Providing infertility treatment in resource-poor countries
17. Life style factors and access to assisted reproduction
18. Oocyte cryopreservation for age-related fertility loss
19. Medically assisted reproduction within families

Abbreviations: ESHRE, European Society of Human Reproduction and Embryology; HIV, human immunodeficiency virus

Box 2 ASRM ethics committee documents

1. Sex selection and preimplantation genetic diagnosis (1999)
2. Preconception gender selection for non-medical reasons (2001)
3. Disposition of abandoned embryos (2004)
4. Informed consent and the use of gametes and embryos for research (2004)
5. Informing offspring of their conception by gamete donation (2004)
6. Oocyte donation to postmenopausal women (2004)
7. Posthumous reproduction (2004)
8. Fertility preservation and reproduction in cancer patients (2005)
9. Risk-sharing or refund programs in assisted reproduction (2006)
10. Financial compensation of oocyte donors (2007)
11. Access to fertility treatment by gays, lesbians and unmarried persons (2009)
12. Defining embryo donation (2009)
13. Child-rearing ability and the provision of fertility services (2009)
14. Donating spare embryos for stem cell research (2009)
15. Interests, obligations and rights of the donor in gamete donation (2009)
16. Human immunodeficiency virus and infertility treatment (2010)
17. Disclosure of medical errors involving gametes and embryos (2011)
18. Fertility treatment when the prognosis is very poor or futile (2012)
19. Human somatic cell nuclear transfer (cloning) (2012)
20. Using family members as gamete donors and surrogates (2012)

Abbreviation: ASRM, American Society of Reproductive Medicine

have been influenced by their religious and cultural morals, as reported in surveillance 2010.[7]

Although, the above principles arose from Greek culture with mediaeval Islamic and later Judeo-Christian influences and are now well established in western medicine, there are other systems which have a different historical tradition.[1] Buddhism has influenced Chinese and Japanese cultures and ethics and ayurvedic medicine has been a traditional practice in India. However literature has few references to ART in these disciplines. Ayurveda has emphasized whole body therapy with an emphasis on chronic disease, but there appears to be little specific to ART. Islamic tradition is a dominant feature of many countries, the principal objection being to third party gametes, although recently, differences have opened between Sunni and Shia traditions. This review will concentrate on western ethics, which appear to have been the principal system of reasoning in relation to ART practices, at least as reported in the literature in the past 5 years.

Current Ethical Issues

Definition of When Life (or "Personhood") Begins

This varies markedly in different countries. In Latin America, it is from the "moment" of conception. In Bangladesh, it is from 40 days of gestation, in Malaysia from 120, whereas in Greece it is from birth. In India and the UK, the embryo has protection from 14 days. Costa Rica, with its strong Catholic tradition, legislated against all IVF on the ground that it impacted on the right to life of the conceptus, as many failed to progress or were discarded. However, that law has recently been challenged by the Inter-American Court of Human Rights, which disputed the concept of the dignity of the embryo as espoused by the Catholic Church. The Court stated that concern should not be about the status of the embryo, but its interests and that the embryo could not be regarded as viable until after implantation. The Costa Rican government was instructed to repeal its law and provide access to ART for all its citizens.[8] A restrictive law in Italy had the same ethical basis—it stated that up to 3 oocytes could be fertilized and all had to be transferred; preimplantation genetic diagnosis (PGD) or embryo experimentation were not permitted. It was struck down by the Italian Supreme Court as it was shown that the outcome of such restrictions was a poorer delivery rate and encouraged multiple pregnancy with its higher risks of handicap, results disadvantageous to the child and to the parents. The Greek Orthodox view remains opposed to ART.

Stem Cells

Adult cells, such as skin cells, can be driven back to become induced pluripotent stem cells and subsequently be directed to transform into other cell types such as neurons, but still have the potential to induce tumors. However, only stem cells taken from the embryo's inner cell mass can so far be directed to any cell type and not induce tumors. The potential to grow mature cells for tissue or organ regeneration and replacement is a strong driver for research, and the benefits to the whole of society could be enormous, a utilitarian approach.[9] However, it is important that the couple with spare embryos gives informed consent (this is patient autonomy) and agrees to relinquish any future legal action in which a patient attempts to share profits from commercial development of those cells such as those that yield skin used for grafting. It could be argued that all "spare" embryos should be so utilized and that couples should routinely be asked for their consent to derive stem cells for research. Some stem cell research centers are building partnerships with large numbers of clinics as they seek such a source. Sperm have been derived from mouse stem cells and, were this to become a widely available technique in the human, it would transform the prospects for currently untreatable patients, who would be able to source gametes from their own mature cells.

Donor Gametes

Donation of spermatozoa has become a significant activity in those cultures where it is acceptable. Although its use has declined considerably since intracytoplasmic sperm injection (ICSI) was first reported in 1992, it is an option if no gametes are available. The area of conflicts have been whether students should be sought as donors, whether they should be paid and how much. They were the main source of donors when donations were anonymous to the recipient couple, but greater emphasis is now placed on donors being identified, so that their genetic provenance can be known to the offsprings, at least when they reach maturity, say at the age of 18. This has become all the more important when donation is used for single women and same sex partners. In the past, physical and some other characteristics were matched, but the identity was suppressed, making only some non-identifying information available. Recently, it has become more clearly, appreciated that one's sense of identity is connected to recognition of one's biological parents.

In preparation for treatment, the sociological impact of donation on a husband's self-esteem needs to be acknowledged and careful counseling of a recipient couple is required. Later, when the child is mature enough to understand, information about donation and the donor should be given to the offspring, using advice on how to do that. Keeping these details secret and later revealing them can have a disastrous impact on relations with the child leading to adverse psychological outcome. These consequences have led to the repeal of laws on anonymity in a number of countries. At the time of donation, the details are entered into a register and can be made available to the offspring at the age of 18. A society needs to decide how it wishes to deal with these problems and whether it puts greater emphasis on the child's right to know[10] or allows the parents to protect their secret to

the potential detriment of the child. It could be agued that the donor should be protected, but the child should know its origins.

Donor eggs are a later technical development and only became available once IVF was established. They resulted from superovulation yielding eggs that were surplus to an individual's requirements. These could be cryopreserved for a patient's own future use, donated to other infertile women or used for research. To take advantage of oocytes becoming available at a specific time, potential recipients had their cycles programmed to coincide. Various arrangements were made whereby a patient could donate half of her eggs to a recipient (egg sharer), provided she had six or more eggs, and in return reductions in fees were negotiated. These arrangements were agreed because of the shortage of eggs. Recipients were those that had failed IVF cycles, particularly for premature menopause or poor response to stimulation. The donor was beneficent and could make an autonomous decision to donate if sharing. Then the question arose as to the upper age limit for recipients; could they be postmenopausal patients when the menopause occurred at the usual age? Were they sufficiently fit and what would be the impact on the child to have elderly parents? Would this be to the child's disadvantage?

Later, with cryopreservation of oocytes, it became feasible to have elective transfer of embryos unrelated to the donor's cycle of treatment. With increasing demand for eggs, young women (often students not requiring IVF themselves) were invited to donate their eggs and were paid to do so. The sums offered could be quite large and be considered excessive inducements. Psychological evaluations would be carried out and some potential donors would be rejected, causing a considerable blow to their self-esteem. There were also the risks of the invasive procedure, of hyperstimulation, a potentially lethal condition, and the longer-term potential of the donor being unable subsequently to have her own children. For such donors, non-maleficence, honesty and truly informed consent are important.

Vitrification also allowed preservation of oocytes for patients about to be treated for a malignancy, such as cancer of the breast, although very few of those have subsequently been used. There needs to be an agreement about disposal of the oocytes in the case of death of the subject or, depending on the probability of recurrence, the time to elapse before the oocytes can be fertilized or embryos implanted. These technical developments also allow the possibility of preserving oocytes from single women, as a safeguard against their future reduced fertility. If a woman does not have a partner, at what age can she preserve her oocytes? If she does not find a partner, should she be able to use donor sperm as a single woman?

Given the increasing interest in identifying donors, the use of donors from abroad creates significant problems. Although frozen sperm can readily be transported, the provenance of those sperm needs to comply with the regulatory framework of the recipient's country, as applies to Danish sperm imported into the UK under the aegis of the HFEA. On the other hand, donor egg recipients travel to the country of the donor and are the major group involved in cross-border reproductive care. The quality of care received by the donor, the cost and the care provided to the recipient, compared to that available in their own country are valid issues. The provision of sufficient identifying information about the donor, which should match that available in the recipient's country, may be important for the child many years later when contact is not possible and the data have not been initially recorded.

Nonmedical Sex Selection

It is hard to justify nonmedical sex selection given the distortion of the sex ratio seen in both India and China. Its social impact later in life is being felt in China as too many young men seek too few young women, defying the concept of the greatest good for the greatest number. Yet the religious and cultural imperatives to have a son have outweighed the societal impact, in spite of legal prohibition and restricted access to sex selection in all countries. An induced abortion is likely to be preferred for a fetus of unwanted sex identified on ultrasound as it is less expensive than IVF and PGD to identify the sex of an embryo before implantation and avoids an abortion. The moral repugnance of abortion is unlikely be considered because of cost. PGD will continue to be used legitimately to avoid implanting an embryo with a specific disease or to replace a carrier of a dominant disease in preference to an affected embryo. If sperm sorting becomes widely available so that the selection of Y-bearing sperm pre-fertilization avoids resort to abortion, the argument for reproductive autonomy in family balancing, at present less powerful because of the consequences, will become much stronger. On the other hand, if it becomes possible to diagnose fetal sex very early in pregnancy using only a blood test for circulating fetal DNA, access to selective abortion, although morally problematic, may be very difficult to control.[11]

Surrogacy

In the UK, surrogacy attained such notoriety that a *review team* was set up by the Department of Health to review the social, legal and ethical issues involved. In 1988, they recommended that legislation should ban payments other than genuine expenses, require the registration of surrogacy agencies and give statutory force to a code of practice with legal sanctions for contravention. The Surrogacy Arrangements Act (1984) and Parental Orders (HFEA) Regulations (1994) regarding adoption were subsequently passed. The draft ICMR national guidelines, Chapter 3, consider a code of practice, ethical considerations and legal issues. However, the surrogacy arrangements have been heavily criticized for encouraging commercial surrogacy, failing to protect the gestational mother and giving greater prominence to protection of the commissioning parents than the child.[12] Further, it is alleged that the Bill disregards a number of important state policies, such as those against gender exploitation and the endorsement of the UN Rights of the Child. Surrogacy has resulted in increased cross-border reproductive care, where couples seek to take advantage of a less strictly regulated jurisdiction. They may have difficulty in arranging entry of their new offspring into their own country; it is important that appropriate legal advice be taken in advance, so that the laws of the country of the gestational mother and those of the commissioning parents are known to be compatible. Again, non-maleficence means that honesty and fully informed consent should lead to optimum care and no increased risk for the gestational mother.

Postmortem use of Gametes

Posthumous reproduction can take a number of forms: fertilization and pregnancy could take place before the death of a partner and birth of the child after death, fertilization and cryopreservation of embryos could both take place before death of the partner or fertilization and pregnancy could take place after the death of the partner. The last is possibly the most common. Retrieval of gametes, by electroejaculation or by testicular biopsy postmortem for posthumous insemination is permitted by statute in some countries and regulated by guidelines in others. Each requires written informed consent prior to death[7] and there may be a time limit by which the insemination must be carried out. It seems that few requests for use are subsequently pursued. Although, cryopreservation of sperm is relatively straightforward, posthumous retrieval of eggs or ovarian tissue is technically more difficult.

An explicit informed consent document is the best method for minimizing controversy, as many parties are involved: the deceased, the child to be born, the partner requesting the procedure, other living children and even society at large. There may be legal issues of inheritance or even of registration as the child of the deceased father.

With informed consent, the deceased's autonomy is respected. In Israel, practice does not always conform to guidelines promulgated by the attorney general, as judges grant permission for retrieval, even for unmarried males in response to family pressure, a much less persuasive claim. Although, it has been rarely practiced in Japan, there is considerable societal support, as there is a traditional religious belief that deceased family members watch the living ones. A US survey showed that almost half of the population supported posthumous reproduction from both men and women, but many were not aware of the possibilities, so there are opportunities for public education. A hospice and palliative care community survey provided a review of medical, legal and ethical issues and a list of resources for staff and patients as that community was likely to have to deal with these requests.[13]

Access and Cost in Low Resource Environments

A key element of a health system is prevention of infertility, but that does not preclude the provision of treatment services. In the presence of overpopulation, contraception and abortion services should be the preferred approach and ART does not contribute significantly to the numbers. Infertility services should be incorporated into family planning, maternity and reproductive health facilities and, as the provision of treatment respects reproductive autonomy, infertile couples should have the chance to attempt conception (ESHRE Task Force on Law and Ethics).[14] Restricting access to infertility management infringes the principle of justice, although the future child should be expected to have a fair chance of a reasonable quality of life.

As ART services are generally of high cost, and so not accessible to a majority of the population, there is a case for the provision of low cost services to a larger proportion. This should avoid multiple pregnancy and ovarian hyperstimulation as complications, so should aim for mild stimulation and single embryo transfer (SET). It is unlikely that the whole population can be offered even that but, as state expenditure on health varies from country to country, there is always an argument for increasing spending and for creating a more equitable service. In low resource countries, a woman's status is often dependent on her ability to have children and there may be severe consequences for the infertile. This reflects a poor public understanding of infertility and inadequate social support mechanisms, problems to be addressed by education and the development of suitable economic and social infrastructure.

Local Ethics Committees

The above comments may be appropriate for society as a whole or to guide individual decision making. However, large ethics committees are run in institutions to determine whether a research proposal is ethical. In that context, there is a need to see that the proposal is sound from the research perspective and whether appropriate patient safeguards for human rights, confidentiality and consent are in place. In a small clinic, the needs are different. They are to determine whether a couple should be treated if their characteristics or indications are borderline or if their chances of success are too limited. The local ethics committee's views provide reassurance for the clinician and maintain the reputation of the individual doctor and the clinic. They may provide strong support for not treating a couple. Such a committee should contain another clinician (not one working in the clinic), a scientist, someone versed in ethics, a religious person is often helpful and a member of the public should be included. A record of reasons should be kept for transparency and to provide confidence to all.

Conclusion

Ethical issues vary in different cultures at different times. These recent discussions from the literature reflect the concerns of infertile couples and of clinicians and embryologists and are influenced by their personal and societal histories. Although there may be particular circumstances where different conclusions are merited, the views presented reflect extensive debate. This is helped when professional organizations arrange discussions, consulting relevant disciplines as well as bioethicists and patients and publish their guidance. The UK Department of Health and the HFEA regularly publish reviews of specific issues in this field and invite comment from interested groups and members of society. Subsequently, the responses are assessed and used to influence their conclusions and recommendations; these may become the basis of draft laws. However, in many areas there will never be scientific data for a definitive view. It is important to recognize diversity of opinion and frame advice to take account of a plurality of views.

■ STRESS ISSUES

Principal Elements

Most couples find ART stressful.
- *Firstly, the condition:* Infertility is rarely expected; even when there is pre-existing recognized disease, fertility

aspects may never have been discussed with those providing care. An underlying anxiety of the patient may never have been expressed and this may be worse when cultural expectations are that all couples will soon conceive. If the consequences of infertility are that a wife will be rejected or another wife taken, these fears may be substantial and real. In many countries, investigation and treatment are not provided by the state and are only available in the private sector. The early referrals may be to doctors who are ill versed in the modern approach to management; the couple may have investigations delayed, inappropriate or unnecessary ones ordered or needless surgery performed. These may exhaust the financial resources of the family or through catastrophic expenditure (more than 30% of annual income) drive them into poverty. Even at that stage, they may not have been referred for definitive treatment such as IVF or they may be faced with another cycle they can ill afford, perhaps with poor advice about their chances of a successful delivery.

- *Secondly, the patients themselves:* They may have little knowledge of reproductive biology, they may not understand the problem that they have nor why that contributes to or causes their infertility. The personalities of each partner determine how each will deal with these stresses and influence the nature of their relationship. Are they supportive of one another? Does the underlying cause lie with the female, as society may expect? Does it lie with the male, more difficult to accept and to acknowledge? Is it unexplained infertility, where the lack of an explanation may be particularly hard to understand? Are they coping with these stresses? Has the process of investigation been efficient? Do they have a rational recommendation for definitive treatment? What has the outcome been: do they have a healthy baby to take home, do they have a multiple pregnancy with or without its complications? Does their attempt at treatment fail and are they left childless with no future prospects? How will they modify their lifestyle or indeed will they stay together?

- *Thirdly, the process of IVF itself:* It is mentally and physically demanding, it invades the couple's privacy; there are moments of high drama: do they respond to stimulation, is a sufficient number of eggs recovered, how many fertilize and develop, how many are available to transfer, how many are transferred, what happens to the remainder, is the pregnancy test positive, does the ultrasound show a fetal heart beat, do they have a multiple pregnancy? The timetable is demanding, are they away from home, what is happening there and can they continue to earn money when they are

away? Have all the expenses been clearly specified or are additional costs added?

These elements demand attention of those who provide treatment. How does one identify those couples or persons who are at risk by not coping with these stresses and what can be offered to minimize them? How should a clinic be organized to identify and reduce the problems as much as possible? What can be provided to help support couples during their journey?

Patient Screening

A number of Dutch clinics attempted to predict those women who may be at higher risk of emotional problems as they entered an IVF program.[15] The questionnaire (SCREENIVF) used a number of conventional psychological tools. Pretreatment distress was described in terms of anxiety and depression, a strong focus on the wish to have a child and difficulty in accepting that they had a fertility problem, a sense of helplessness and a lack of perceived social support. These elements identified those women at risk of emotional maladjustment before the start of their IVF treatment. The women were reassessed after the pregnancy test at the conclusion of their treatment cycle to see how well the preliminary assessment had identified those who did have problems. At the start of the program, 34% of women were found to have underlying problems and to be at risk of post-treatment psychological difficulty. Almost half of them did have problems identified at the conclusion of that cycle's treatment and of those, 80% had a negative pregnancy test.

The evaluation had more correctly identified those that would not have problems, but the early recognition of the patients at risk allowed the staff to pay more attention to them when giving instructions about treatment. They could be offered more help from a counselor with psychosocial support appropriate for their particular needs. The questionnaire could help predict those with emotional strain, an important reason for dropout.

A more general assessment of "quality of life" specifically directed to infertility is FertiQol, a downloadable questionnaire developed for international use and available in 20 languages including Hindi.[16] It was compiled with the help of and tested by men and women experiencing fertility problems as well as international ART experts. There are 26 items, the domains covered being emotional, mind or body, relationships and social with an option of a further 10 directed at treatment. Boivin et al. have validated it extensively so it can be used to identify people at risk of impaired quality of life.[17] It can also be used to monitor the quality of services and to optimize patient experiences. The standard of treatment and how it is tolerated are predictive of patient satisfaction and willingness to persist with treatment.

Patient Centered Care

As the objective in a clinic must always be to minimize the stress experienced by patients, it is helpful to consider the *patients' perspective* on fertility care. A systematic review of 51 studies has been carried out by Dancet et al.[18] and it is instructive to look at the criteria used for evaluation **(Table 1)**. The study attempted to assess the *patient centeredness* of fertility care reported in Europe, yet centers need to develop their own culture specific criteria. Patients with children or those who conceived had a more positive perspective on care. Those with higher educational levels or a longer duration of infertility had a more negative view. Personal control, feeling closer to their partner as a result of the infertility, satisfaction with their social network and marital satisfaction related well to how they viewed their care. A number of aspects were identified as needing attention, the quality of accommodation in the clinic, waiting times in the waiting room and during treatment, the frequency of appointments, organization in the clinic, quality information on alternatives and on emotional aspects and providing a clear plan for the future. Dealing with these issues contributed to the reduction of stress.

There has been criticism of the medical approach to ART in that clinics focus too much on effectiveness and success rates. Additional criteria have been proposed by Pennings and Ombelet[19] from Belgium, a country which provides state support for agreed treatments (reimbursement). The criteria are: cost-effectiveness, equity of access, minimal risk for mother and child and minimal burden for patients, all of which are derived from ethics base. Cost-effectiveness should be aimed at optimal use of community or family resources to maximize well-being. Equity of access embodies justice, minimal risk represents non-maleficence, and minimizing the burden of treatment is largely based on the principle of autonomy, where the patient's views are always respected. SET represents a big step toward minimizing risk for mother and child. The psychological distress that arises from treatment can be reduced by discussing all options, providing information and dealing with the patients' fear of the unknown, worry about injections and possible side effects of the drugs. Indeed, a Dutch study described how patients preferred three natural cycle treatments with a hypothetical 17% live birth rate rather than a single stimulated cycle with the same success rate. Anxiety about hormone injections was the only significant predictor of patient preferences.

Two additional points have been emphasized by Van Empel et al.[20] timeliness and patient centeredness (although, they recognize that these additional criteria are difficult to achieve where there are no reimbursement systems and where the female is older). Timeliness refers to reducing the waiting time for those who receive care and for those who provide care. Inaccurate scheduling of appointments or repeating tests unnecessarily cause delays, emotional distress and cost money. Patient

Table 1 Criteria used to evaluate studies on the patients' perspectives on fertility care

Principle	Examples
Access to care	Waiting times, geographical accessibility, availability of transport, ease of scheduling appointments
Respect for patient values, preferences and needs	Focus on the individual patient and their involvement in decision making
Coordination and integration of care	Coordination of clinical care, ancillary and support services and front-line patient care
Information, communication and education	Information on clinical aspects, prognosis, processes of care and education
Physical comfort	Pain management, assistance with daily activities and needs, hospital accommodation
Emotional support and alleviation of fear and anxiety	Clinical aspects, prognosis, impact of illness on themselves and their family, financial impact
Partner involvement	Support
Continuity and transition	Care after discharge: referral, treatment and support
Fertility clinic staff	Attitude and sensitivity of staff and their relationship with patients
Technical skills	Competence, comprehensiveness and quality of care

Source: Dancet EA, Nelen WL, Sermeus W, et al. The patients' perspective on fertility care: a systematic review. Hum Reprod Update. 2010;16(5):467-87

centeredness is being respectful of and responsive to individual patient preferences, needs and values and ensuring that the patients' values guide all clinical decisions. It also means that care is well coordinated, physical comfort is attended to and there is emotional support. Handover of care is seamless and there is continuity; family and friends are involved. There needs to be ready access to care and there is a need for good communication and appropriate education with supplementary written material. Patients want information about alternatives to treatment, such as adoption and lifestyle changes, although these will depend on culture and attitudes. This type of care can be delivered if patient organizations work with professionals, care providers and policymakers, an important liaison for professional societies to organize.

A major problem in all clinics is a significant discontinuation rate, which may reach very high levels. The couple may drop out before treatment starts or at the end of treatment, even those whom the medical staff thinks have a good prognosis. This problem has been analyzed by Boivin et al.[21] and it could be due to a conflict of values or the cost of treatment, but it could well be a direct result of the burden of treatment. The waiting time for the result of a pregnancy test after embryo transfer is probably the most stressful time for the patient and causes great strain, but disruption of the patient's daily routine or work by the treatment is also a factor. Poor organization of care can make the clinic look unstructured and seem like an assembly line, there may be excessive waiting times or patients may never see the same staff, making the patient feel depersonalized. Pregnancy test results can be received at work or when their partner is not present and so be stressful. The staff themselves can have time pressures or be overloaded, so that delivering the treatment can also be stressful for the staff. The interactions between patients and all staff, including embryologists, reception and administrative staff, may be problematic or unsympathetic. There may be poorly formulated explanations, the staff may have poor listening skills and may pay inadequate attention to the male partner. Patients may lose hope early. Some, as trade-off cost assessment has indicated, would accept a lower success rate for more reassuring communication.

Interventions

A variety of interventions to address the burden of ART is listed in **Table 2**. Structured checklists, such as the 34-item SCREENIVF or the 26-item FertiQol described

Table 2 Cause of the burden in ART and associated interventions

Factors	Cause	Interventions to address the burden
Patient	Fear and negative attitudes to treatment	Develop tailored patient information and educational materials using guidelines
		Use checklists and treatment questionnaires to ensure all treatment worries are addressed
	Psychological vulnerability and burden	Identify high-risk screening by questionnaire
		Implement general and/or tailored coping interventions for all patients
		Refer high-risk patients to appropriate mental health professionals for additional support
	Strain with partner	Ensure partner is fully involved in treatment
Clinic	Suboptimal care organization	Improve performance in areas known to be associated with discontinuation
		Monitor performance by questionnaires
		Involve patients in service evaluation and development
	Negative staff-patient interactions	Use communication strategies designed for brief patient staff interactions
		Address workload issues and teach staff stress management skills
Treatment	Physical burden	Simplify treatment protocols
	Poor prognosis	Incorporate persuasive communication in referrals for lifestyle change
		Accept that patients may want to end treatment

Abbreviation: ART, assisted reproductive technologies
Source: Boivin J, Domar AD, Shapiro DB, et al. Tackling the burden in ART: an integrated approach for medical staff. Hum Reprod. 2012;27(4): 941-50

above (in patient screening), can be very helpful. These would identify common misconceptions or worries about treatment that can be explored and cultural or religious perspectives can be appreciated during treatment discussions, although too much information at any one time can be unhelpful. It may need to be broken up or repeated appropriately.

Interventions, such as the self-administered Positive Reappraisal Coping Intervention,[22] **(Box 3)**, can be effective during the waiting period after embryo transfer, the patient repeating each sentence twice daily during the 14 days. Further education can also benefit the staff.

Substantial improvements have been made in clinic results, so it is now time to improve the clinic environment. Making time for more personalized care, such as introducing oneself, establishing the main reason for the visit, providing information about treatment procedures and asking whether the patient has other concerns, helps to make the patients more satisfied with their treatment. A named nurse program or improved leaflets may all help to make the program less stressful.

■ COUNSELING

Finally, the Special Interest Group of Psychology and Counseling of ESHRE[23] has published an introduction to infertility counseling as a guide for mental health and medical professionals. They detail the process for choosing the most appropriate type of infertility counseling and the use of assessment tools for understanding infertility related symptoms. These may relate to helping men prepare for semen analysis or deciding about fertility preservation and highlight the need for self-assessment

Box 3 Positive Reappraisal Coping Intervention (PRCI)

Source: Lancastle D, Boivin J. A feasibility study of a brief coping intervention (PRCI) for the waiting period before a pregnancy test during fertility treatment. Hum Reprod. 2008;23(10):2299-307

tools, as not all patients will require counseling (either as a group, a couple or individuals). Information gathering and analysis lead to implications and decision-making counseling; this is actually given by medical and nursing staff and is part of patient centered care. However, this may need to be supported by or extended to short-term crisis counseling, ideally done by mental health professionals. This may be needed for underlying anxiety, depression or marital or sexual problems, but also can be treatment related, such as after a failed cycle. More extensive therapeutic counseling includes psychotherapy but can also include long-term crisis counseling. These latter forms of counseling should be carried out by independent providers rather than by the medical team.

■ CONCLUSION

Men and women experience infertility differently: Women are more distressed, report more depression and anxiety and respond more poorly to treatment failure, but they are also more likely to seek help than men. Men appear to be less emotionally affected and are more willing to consider termination of treatment. Women seek more social support, but employ more avoidance strategies, which increases distress. Women want to share emotional experiences, but men prefer to keep their distance from other persons and these differences may impact on their partner and the relationship. The man tends to treat the process as a problem to be solved, but needs to allow his partner to experience her emotions and provide his support. Infertility can also have a powerful effect on a couple's sexual relationship. It may play a role in unexplained infertility and is an area that needs to be addressed by the counselor, as it is more likely to be a consequence of the infertility rather than its cause.

Donor conception and surrogacy are special situations that require extensive discussion and support with a great deal of information, including legal aspects, although these may require professional legal input, particularly with surrogacy. The discussion should relate not only to the treatment, but also to later disclosure to the child.

The literature that has been described relates almost entirely to European practice, so that its applicability may be questioned. However, the principles are sound, even although adaptation of the tools may require much effort.

Infertility is a life-changing event. With optimum practice and excellent communication in a patient-centered program, both patients and staff will feel fulfilled. Stress can be minimized while achieving the highest ideals of ethical practice.

■ MESSAGE BOX

Applying ethics in reproductive medicine means reviewing issues by criteria of beneficence, non-maleficence, autonomy, justice, dignity and honesty. Current issues considered are when does life begin, stem cells, donor gametes, nonmedical sex selection, surrogacy, postmortem use of gametes, access and cost in low-resource environments.

Stress is a major feature in ART and is due to the infertility, the patients' reaction and that caused by managing the treatment. High risk patients should be identified by screening; stress can be minimized by using a patient-centered approach. Interventions can be clinic based, but some counseling needs to be done by mental health professionals.

■ REFERENCES

1. MacDougall H, Ross Langley G. Medical ethics: past, present and future. [online] Available from http://www.royalcollege.ca/portal/page/portal/rc/resources/bioethics/primers/medical_ethics [Accessed February 2015].
2. Human Fertilisation and Embryology Authority (2009). Code of practice. [online] Available from http://www.hfea.gov.uk/code.html [Accessed February 2015].
3. Indian Council of Medical Research (2005). National guidelines for accreditation, supervision & regulation of ART clinics in India. [online] Available from http://icmr.nic.in/art/art_clinics.htm [Accessed February 2015].
4. MHFW, ICMR (2010). Draft ART (regulation) bill. [online] Available from http://www.icmr.nic.in/guide/ART%20REGULATION%20Draft%20Bill1.pdf [Accessed February 2015].
5. European Society of Human Reproduction and Embryology. Documents of the task force on ethics and law. [online] Available from http://www.eshre.eu/ESHRE/English/Specialty-Groups/SIG/Ethics-and-Law/Documents-of-the-Task-Force-Ethics-Law/page.aspx/136 [Accessed February 2015].
6. American Society of Reproductive Medicine. Ethics committee documents. Available from http://www.asrm.org/EthicsReports/ [Accessed February 2015].
7. International Federation of Fertility Societies (2010). Surveillance. [onine] Available from http://www.iffs-reproduction.org/documents/IFFS_Surveillance_2010.pdf [Accessed February 2015].
8. Inter-American Court of Human Rights, San Jose, Costa Rica Regula Realización de Técnicas de Reproducción Asistida. (2012). In Vitro o FIV (in Spanish), judgement delivered on 21 December, 2012. [online] Available from http://www.pgr.go.cr/scij/scripts/TextoCompleto.dll?Texto&nNorma=25469&nVersion=26946&nTamanoLetra=10&strWebNormativa=http://www.pgr.go.cr/scij/&strODBC=DSN=SCIJ_NRM;UID=sa;PWD=scij;DATABASE=SCIJ_NRM;&strServidor=%5C%5Cpgr04&strUnidad=D:&strJavaScript=NO [Accessed February 2015].
9. Ehrich K, Williams K, Farsides B, et al. Embryo futures and stem cell research: the management of informed uncertainty. Sociol Health Ill. 2012;34(1):114-29.
10. Mahlstedt PP, LaBounty K, Kennedy WT. The views of adult offspring of sperm donation: essential feedback for the development of ethical guidelines within the practice of assisted reproductive technology in the United States. Fertil Steril. 2010;93(7):2236-46.
11. Dondorp WJ, de Wert GMWR. The categorical ban on sex selection for non-medical reasons is in need of urgent reconsideration. Hum Reprod Suppl. 2011;1:263.
12. Qadeer I. The ART of marketing babies. Indian J Med Ethics. 2010;7(4):209-15.
13. Knapp C, Quinn G, Bower B, et al. Posthumous reproduction and palliative care. J Palliative Med. 2011;14(8):895-8.
14. ESHRE Task Force on Ethics and Law, Pennings G, de Wert, et al. Providing infertility treatment in resource-poor countries. Hum Reprod. 2009;24(5):1008-11.
15. Verhaak CM, Lintsen AM, Evers AW, et al. Who is at risk of emotional problems and how do you know? Screening of women going for IVF treatment. Hum Reprod. 2010;25(5):|1234-40.
16. Cardiff University. Fertility quality of life tool, FertiQol. [online] Available from http://psych.cf.ac.uk/fertiqol/download/index.html [Accesses February 2015].
17. Boivin J, Takefman J, Braverman A. The fertility quality of life (FertiQol) tool: development and general psychometric properties. Hum Reprod. 2011;26(8):2084-91.
18. Dancet EA, Nelen WL, Sermeus W, et al. The patients' perspective on fertility care: a systematic review. Hum Reprod Update. 2010;16(5):467-87.
19. Pennings G, Ombelet W. Coming soon to your clinic: patient-friendly ART. Hum Reprod. 2007;22(8):2075-9.
20. van Empel IW, Nelen WL, Hermens RP, et al. Coming soon to your clinic: high quality ART. Hum Reprod. 2008;23(6):1242-5.
21. Boivin J, Domar AD, Shapiro DB, et al. Tackling the burden in ART: an integrated approach for medical staff. Hum Reprod. 2012;27(4):941-50.
22. Lancastle D, Boivin J. A feasibility study of a brief coping intervention (PRCI) for the waiting period before a pregnancy test during fertility treatment. Hum Reprod. 2008;23(10):2299-307.
23. Peterson B, Boivin J, Norré J, et al. An introduction to infertility counseling: a guide for mental health and medical professionals. J Asst Reprod Genet. 2012;29(3):243-8.

Index

Page numbers followed by *f* refer to figure and *t* refer to table.